# Williams Hematology
# Hemostasis and Thrombosis

# Williams Hematology
# Hemostasis and Thrombosis

**Kenneth Kaushansky, MD, MACP**
Senior Vice President for Health Sciences
Dean, School of Medicine
SUNY Distinguished Professor
Stony Brook University
Stony Brook, New York

**Marcel Levi, MD, PhD**
Professor of Medicine and Chief Executive
University College London Hospitals
London, United Kingdom
University of Amsterdam
Amsterdam, the Netherlands

New York   Chicago   San Francisco   Athens   London   Madrid   Mexico City
Milan   New Delhi   Singapore   Sydney   Toronto

**Williams Hematology Hemostasis and Thrombosis**

1 2 3 4 5 6 7 8 9 0    LWI    22  21  20  19  18  17

ISBN 978-1-26-011708-0
MHID 1-26-011708-1

This book was set in Minion Pro by Cenveo® Publisher Services
The editors were Karen Edmonson and Harriet Lebowitz.
The production supervisor was Richard Ruzycka.
Project management was provided by Sonam Arora, Cenveo Publisher Services.
The cover designer was Randomatrix.
The designer was Eve Siegel.

This book is printed on acid-free paper.

**Library of Congress Cataloging-in-Publication Data**

Names: Kaushansky, Kenneth, editor. | Levi, Marcel, editor.
Title: Williams hematology hemostasis and thrombosis / [edited by] Kenneth
    Kaushansky, Marcel Levi.
Other titles: Hematology hemostasis and thrombosis | Separated from (work):
    Williams hematology. 2016. 9th ed.
Description: New York : McGraw-Hill Education, [2018] | This is an updated
    version of one section of Williams hematology / [editors] Kenneth
    Kaushansky, Marshall A. Lichtman, Josef T. Prchal, Marcel Levi, Oliver W.
    Press, Linda J. Burns, Michael A. Caligiuri. 9th edition. 2016. | Includes
    bibliographical references and index.
Identifiers: LCCN 2017042751| ISBN 9781260117080 (pbk. : alk. paper) | ISBN
    1260117081 (pbk. : alk. paper)
Subjects: | MESH: Hemostasis | Thrombosis | Blood Coagulation Disorders |
    Blood Platelet Disorders
Classification: LCC RC642 | NLM WH 310 | DDC 616.1/57—dc23 LC record available
    at https://lccn.loc.gov/2017042751

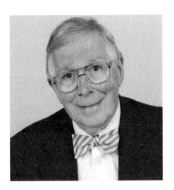

**William J. Williams, MD**
**1926 – 2016**

Medical educator, investigator, physician, mentor, academic leader,
colleague, and the founding editor of *Williams Hematology*

# CONTENTS

# CONTRIBUTORS

**Charles S. Abrams, MD**
Professor of Medicine, Pathology and Laboratory Medicine
Vice Chair for Research & Chief Scientific Officer
Department of Medicine
University of Pennsylvania School of Medicine
Philadelphia, Pennsylvania

**Doru T. Alexandrescu, MD**
Department of Medicine
Division of Dermatology
University of California, San Diego
VA San Diego Health Care System
San Diego, California
Instructor in Medicine
Dana-Farber Cancer Institute
Harvard Medical School
Boston, Massachusetts

**Joel S. Bennett, MD**
Professor of Medicine
Division of Hematology-Oncology
University of Pennsylvania School of Medicine
Philadelphia, Pennsylvania

**Mettine H. A. Bos, PhD**
Assistant Professor
Division of Thrombosis and Hemostasis
Leiden University Medical Center
Leiden, The Netherlands

**Paul Bray, MD**
Professor
Director, Division of Hematology
Jefferson University
Philadelphia, Pennsylvania

**Harry R. Buller, MD**
Professor of Medicine
Department of Vascular Medicine
Academic Medical Center
Amsterdam, The Netherlands

**Barry S. Coller, MD**
Head
Allen and Frances Adler Laboratory of Blood and Vascular Biology
Physician-in-Chief
Vice President for Medical Affairs
The Rockefeller University
New York, New York

**Michiel Coppens, MD, PhD**
Department of Vascular Medicine
Academic Medical Center
Amsterdam, The Netherlands

**Adam Cuker, MD, MS**
Assistant Professor of Medicine and of Pathology and Laboratory Medicine
Perelman School of Medicine at the University of Pennsylvania
Philadelphia, Pennsylvania

**Philippe de Moerloose, MD**
Professor
Division of Angiology and Hemostasis
University of Geneva Faculty of Medicine
Geneva, Switzerland

**Reyhan Diz-Küçükkaya, MD**
Associate Professor
Department of Internal Medicine
Division of Hematology
Istanbul University
Istanbul Faculty of Medicine
Istanbul, Turkey

**Miguel A. Escobar, MD**
Professor of Medicine and Pediatrics
Division of Hematology
University of Texas Health Science Center at Houston
Director, Gulf States Hemophilia and Thrombophilia Center
Houston, Texas

**David Ginsburg, MD**
Professor, Department of Internal Medicine, Human Genetics and Pediatrics
Investigator, Howard Hughes Medical Institute
Life Sciences Institute
University of Michigan
Ann Arbor, Michigan

**John H. Griffin, PhD**
Professor
Department of Molecular and Experimental Medicine
The Scripps Research Institute
La Jolla, California

**Katherine A. Hajjar, MD**
Professor of Pediatrics
Brine Family Professor, Department of Cell and Developmental Biology
Professor of Medicine
Well Cornell Medical College
Attending Pediatrician
New York Presbyterian Hospital
New York, New York

**Russell D. Hull, MD**
Professor
Department of Medicine
University of Calgary
Active Staff
Department of Internal Medicine
Foothills Hospital
Calgary, Alberta, Canada

**Joseph E. Italiano Jr., PhD**
Associate Professor of Medicine
Brigham and Women's Hospital
Harvard Medical School
Boston, Massachusetts

**Jill M. Johnsen, MD**
Assistant Member, Research Institute
Bloodworks Northwest
Puget Sound Blood Center
Assistant Professor, Division of Hematology
Department of Medicine
University of Washington
Seattle, Washington

**Kenneth Kaushansky, MD, MACP**
Senior Vice President, Health Sciences
Dean, School of Medicine
SUNY Distinguished Professor
Stony Brook Medicine
State University of New York
Stony Brook, New York

**Nigel S. Key, MB, ChB, FRCP**
Harold R. Roberts Distinguished Professor of Medicine
Director, University of North Carolina Hemophilia and Thrombosis
    Center
Chapel Hill, North Carolina

**Frank W. G. Leebeek, MD, PhD**
Professor of Hematology
Department of Hematology
Erasmus University Medical Center
Rotterdam, The Netherlands

**Marcel Levi, MD, PhD**
Professor of Medicine and Chief Executive
University College London Hospitals
London, United Kingdom
University of Amsterdam
Amsterdam, the Netherlands

**Ton Lisman, PhD**
Professor of Experimental Surgery
Surgical Research Laboratory and Section of Hepatobiliary Surgery
    and Liver Transplantation
Department of Surgery
University Medical Center, Groningen
Groningen, The Netherlands

**John S. (Pete) Lollar III, MD**
Aflac Cancer Center and Blood Disorders Services
Department of Pediatrics
Emory University
Atlanta, Georgia

**José A. López, MD**
Chief Scientific Officer
Bloodworks Northwest
Professor of Medicine and Biochemistry
University of Washington
Seattle, Washington

**Aaron J. Marcus, MD***
Professor of Medicine
Weill Cornell Medical College
Attending Physician
New York Harbor Healthcare System
New York, New York

**Shannon L. Meeks, MD**
Aflac Cancer Center and Blood Disorders Services
Department of Pediatrics
Emory University
Atlanta, Georgia

**Marzia Menegatti, MD**
Angelo Bianchi Bonomi Hemophilia and Thrombosis Center
Fondazione IRCCS Ca' Granda Ospedale Maggiore Policlinico
University of Milan
Milan, Italy

**Saskia Middeldorp, MD, PhD**
Department of Vascular Medicine
Academic Medical Center
Amsterdam, The Netherlands

**Emile R. Mohler III, MD**
Director, Vascular Medicine
Professor of Medicine
Division of Cardiovascular Medicine
Perelman School of Medicine at the University of Pennsylvania
Philadelphia, Pennsylvania

**Laurent O. Mosnier, PhD**
Associate Professor
Department of Molecular and Experimental Medicine
The Scripps Research Institute
La Jolla, California

**William A. Muller, MD, PhD**
Magerstadt Professor and Chair
Department of Pathology
Feinberg School of Medicine
Northwestern University
Chicago, Illinois

*Deceased

**Marguerite Neerman-Arbez, PhD**
Professor
Department of Genetic Medicine and Development
University of Geneva Faculty of Medicine
Geneva, Switzerland

**Flora Peyvandi, MD**
Angelo Bianchi Bonomi Hemophilia and Thrombosis Center
Fondazione IRCCS Ca' Granda Ospedale Maggiore Policlinico
University of Milan
Milan, Italy

**Mortimer Poncz, MD**
Jane Fishman Grinberg Professor of Pediatrics
Perelman School of Medicine at the University of Pennsylvania
Children's Hospital of Philadelphia
Philadelphia, Pennsylvania

**Jacob H. Rand, MD**
Professor of Pathology and Medicine
Director of Hematology Laboratory
Montefiore Medical Center
The University Hospital for the Albert Einstein College of Medicine
Bronx, New York

**A. Koneti Rao, MD**
Sol Sherry Professor of Medicine
Director of Benign Hematology, Hemostasis and Thrombosis
Co-Director, Sol Sherry Thrombosis Research Center
Temple University School of Medicine
Philadelphia, Pennsylvania

**Gary E. Raskob, PhD**
Dean, College of Public Health
Regents Professor, Epidemiology and Medicine
The University of Oklahoma Health Science Center
Oklahoma City, Oklahoma

**Pieter H. Reitsma, PhD**
Professor in Experimental Molecular Medicine
Division of Thrombosis and Hemostasis
Einthoven Laboratory for Experimental Vascular Medicine
Leiden University Medical Center
Leiden, The Netherlands

**Jia Ruan, MD, PhD**
Associate Professor
Department of Medicine
Weill Cornell Medical College
Associate Attending Physician
New York Presbyterian Hospital
New York, New York

**J. Evan Sadler, MD, PhD**
Ira M. Lang Professor of Medicine
Washington University School of Medicine
St. Louis, Missouri

**Andrew I. Schafer, MD**
Professor of Medicine,
Director, The Richard T. Silver Center for Myeloproliferative
    Neoplasms,
Weill Cornell Medical College
New York, New York

**Uri Seligsohn, MD**
Professor of Hematology and Director
Amalia Biron Research Institute of Thrombosis and Hemostasis
Sheba Medical Center
Tel-Hashomer and Sackler Faculty of Medicine
Tel Aviv University
Tel Aviv, Israel

**Sanford J. Shattil, MD**
Professor and Chief, Division of Hematology-Oncology
Department of Medicine
University of California, San Diego
Adjunct Professor of Molecular and Experimental Medicine
The Scripps Research Institute
La Jolla, California

**Susan S. Smyth, MD, PhD**
Jeff Gill Professor of Cardiology
Chief, Division of Cardiovascular Medicine
Medical Director, Gill Heart Institute
University of Kentucky
Lexington, Kentucky

**Sean R. Stowell, MD, PhD**
Department of Pathology and Laboratory Medicine
Emory University
Atlanta, Georgia

**Cornelis van't Veer, PhD**
Associate Professor
Center for Experimental and Molecular Medicine
Academic Medical Center
Amsterdam, The Netherlands

**Sidney Whiteheart, PhD**
Professor
Molecular and Cellular Biochemistry
University of Kentucky College of Medicine
Lexington, Kentucky

**Lucia Wolgast, MD**
Assistant Professor of Pathology (Clinical)
Director, Clinical Laboratories, Moses Division
Associate Director, Hematology Laboratories
Montefiore Medical Center/Albert Einstein College of Medicine
Department of Pathology
New York, New York

# PREFACE

Hemostasis and thrombosis are two sides of a finely balanced system of blood cells and proteins that protects the vasculature from injury-induced hemorrhage. Prior to the development of systematic farming and ranching, with its attendant dietary changes, and against a history of physical activity, hunting, and fighting, human evolution selected for a homeostatic system that favored blood clotting over hemorrhage. However, with current sedentary lifestyles and the "advent" of the "Western diet," hypertension, the ability to smoke two packs of cigarettes a day (something next to impossible when a smoker had to "roll their own"), and most recently, convenience foods that allow "super-sizing" dietary calories, sodium, and fats, atherosclerotic damage to the vasculature has, in many persons, turned physiologic hemostasis into pathologic thrombosis, responsible for more deaths in the Western world than any other category of disease. Based on careful descriptions of congenital bleeding and clotting disorders and biochemical fractionation of blood coagulation proteins and cells, our understanding of the molecular mechanisms of physiologic and pathologic blood coagulation is quite advanced. From such studies have come targets for new therapies that can intervene in pathologic thrombosis or help repair the blood coagulation system in states of pathologic hemorrhage.

Based on the extensive discussions of the pathophysiology of hemorrhage and thrombosis found in the 9th edition of *Williams Hematology* part XII, the thought leaders that contributed to this monograph have extensively updated the clinically relevant chapters to keep current with one of the fastest changing fields of medicine. The book is designed for the advanced medical student, who wishes a more thorough treatment of the (typically) 3-week block of the second year of medical school devoted to hematology; for medicine and pediatric residents and hematology/oncology fellows faced with patients with bleeding and clotting disorders on a myriad of medications; and for physicians at all levels of lifelong learning, in order to remain current with anticoagulant and antiplatelet therapies.

Kenneth Kaushansky
Marcel Levi

# CHAPTER 1
# MEGAKARYOPOIESIS AND THROMBOPOIESIS

Kenneth Kaushansky

## SUMMARY

Each day the adult human produces approximately $1 \times 10^{11}$ platelets, a level of production that can increase 10- to 20-fold in times of increased demand and an additional five- to 10-fold under the stimulation of exogenous thrombopoietin mimetic drugs. Production of platelets depends on the proliferation and differentiation of hematopoietic stem and progenitor cells to cells committed to the megakaryocyte lineage, their maturation to large, polyploid megakaryocytes, and their final fragmentation into platelets. The external influences that impact megakaryopoiesis and thrombopoiesis are a supportive marrow stroma consisting of endothelial and other cells, matrix glycosaminoglycans, and a family of protein hormones and cytokines, including thrombopoietin, stem cell factor, and stromal cell-derived factor-1. The role of the cytokines essential for these processes has been defined, the transcription factors critical for megakaryocyte development have been identified, the molecular mechanisms that underlie the two most unusual aspects of thrombopoiesis—endomitosis and proplatelet formation—have been studied, and reagents to specifically modify platelet production have been generated. This chapter focuses on the development of megakaryocytes, their precursors and their progeny, and the hematopoietic growth factors and transcriptionally active molecules that control the survival, proliferation, and differentiation of these cells.

## ● KINETICS OF THROMBOPOIESIS

The circulatory life span of a platelet is approximately 10 days in humans with normal platelet counts, but somewhat shorter in patients with moderate (7 days) to severe (5 days) thrombocytopenia, as a higher proportion of the total-body platelet mass is consumed in the day-to-day function of maintaining vascular integrity.[1] Based on a "normal" level of 200,000 platelets/$\mu$L, a blood volume of 5 L, and a half-life of 10 days, $1 \times 10^{11}$ platelets per day are produced. If 1 megakaryocyte produces approximately 1000 platelets, approximately $1 \times 10^8$ megakaryocytes are generated in the marrow each day.

Several independent lines of evidence indicate the transit time from megakaryocyte progenitor cell to release of platelets into the circulation ranges from 4 to 7 days. For example, following platelet apheresis, the platelet count falls, recovers substantially by day 4, and completely recovers by day 7.[2] In most physiologic and pathologic states, the platelet

Acronyms and Abbreviations: CAMT, congenital amegakaryocytic thrombocytopenia; FGF, fibroblast growth factor; GP, glycoprotein; HPS, Hermansky-Pudlak syndrome; IFN, interferon; IL, interleukin; ITP, immune thrombocytopenic purpura; MAPK, mitogen-activated protein kinase; P4P, polyphosphate-4-phosphatase; PI3K, phosphoinositol 3'-kinase; SDF, stromal cell-derived factor; TGF, transforming growth factor.

count is inversely related to plasma thrombopoietin levels. For example, liver failure is associated with moderate thrombocytopenia as a result of splenomegaly and thrombopoietin deficiency. Within the first week following orthotopic liver transplantation, the platelet count rises substantially, with kinetics matching those of thrombopoietin infusion.[3,4] These findings indicate expansion of the megakaryocyte mass takes from 3 to 4 days following a thrombopoietin stimulus in humans and, coupled with the approximate 12 hours required for platelet release,[5] results in a relatively brisk response to thrombocytopenia.

## ● CELLULAR PHYSIOLOGY OF THROMBOPOIESIS

Platelets form by fragmentation of megakaryocyte membrane extensions termed *proplatelets*, in a process that consumes nearly the entire cytoplasmic complement of membranes, organelles, granules, and soluble macromolecules. Although at first controversial, as the process was initially observed only *in vitro*, *in situ* microscopic studies have identified proplatelet formation and fragmentation in living animals.[6] Each megakaryocyte is estimated to give rise to 1000 to 3000 platelets[7] before the residual nuclear material is engulfed and eliminated by marrow macrophages. This process has been extensively reviewed.[8] The continuum of megakaryocyte development is arbitrarily divided into four stages. The major criteria differentiating these stages are the quality of the cytoplasm and the size, lobulation, and chromatin pattern of the nucleus (Table 1–1).

## MEGAKARYOBLAST

Stage I megakaryocytes, also termed *megakaryoblasts*, account for approximately 20 percent of all cells destined to form platelets. These cells in human marrow are 8 to 24 $\mu$m in spherical diameter (i.e., the actual size *in vivo*, as opposed to the apparent size of a cell on a flattened marrow smear) and contain a relatively large, minimally indented nucleus with loosely organized chromatin and multiple nucleoli, and scant basophilic cytoplasm containing a small Golgi complex, a few mitochondria and $\alpha$ granules, and abundant free ribosomes (Fig. 1–1).

### Surface Adhesion Molecule Expression

Although elegant experiments clearly demonstrated that the gene for integrin $\alpha_{IIb}$ is expressed as early as the erythroid-megakaryocytic progenitor stage[9] and possibly in the common myeloid progenitor, the cell-surface protein becomes demonstrable and functionally important only at the early stages of megakaryocyte development. Integrin $\alpha_{IIb}\beta_3$ is an integral transmembrane protein of two subunits, but only the $\alpha$ subunit is megakaryocyte-lineage specific. Absence of integrin $\alpha_{IIb}\beta_3$ leads to Glanzmann thrombasthenia resulting from failure of the defective platelets to engage fibrinogen and other adhesive ligands during hemostasis (Chap. 10). Megakaryocytes and platelets contain in their cytoplasmic membranes approximately twice the amount of integrin $\alpha_{IIb}\beta_3$ as is present on the cell surface. The granule compartment serves as a mobilizable pool that is exteriorized upon platelet activation. During the early and mid stages of megakaryocyte development, the granule content of integrin rises. Moreover, because developing megakaryocytes do not synthesize but contain fibrinogen in their $\alpha$-granules and cells from patients with Glanzmann thrombasthenia do not, integrin $\alpha_{IIb}\beta_3$ clearly begins to function, at least at the level of fibrinogen binding and uptake, long before platelet formation.

The glycoprotein (GP) Ib-IX complex is expressed only slightly after the appearance of integrin $\alpha_{IIb}\beta_3$.[10] Although endothelial cells reportedly express GPIb,[11] its levels are very low; otherwise, GPIb is the

**TABLE 1–1.** Maturation Stages of Megakaryocytes

| Term | Size (μM) | Morphology |
|---|---|---|
| Megakaryoblast (stage I) | >10 | Lobed nucleus, basophilic cytoplasm |
| Basophilic megakaryocyte (stage II) | >20 | Horseshoe-shaped nucleus, basophilic cytoplasm, azurophilic granules around centrosome |
| Granular megakaryocyte (stage III) | >25–50 | Large multilobed nucleus, acidophilic cytoplasm, numerous azurophilic granules |
| Mature megakaryocyte (stage IV) | >25–50 | Pyknotic nucleus, groups of 10–12 azurophilic granules |

second most abundant megakaryocyte-specific protein. Glycoprotein V also is expressed in complex with GPIb and GPIX, in a ratio of 1:2:2.[12] However, the genetic elimination of GPV has little effect on platelet adhesion,[13] and unlike GPIb and GPIX, no mutations of GPV are associated with Bernard-Soulier disease (Chap. 10).[14] Therefore, GPV does not appear to be required for the GPIb-V-IX complex to function as a von Willebrand factor receptor. Rather, GPV is a target of thrombin, potentially playing a role in platelet activation.[15]

### Demarcation Membranes

Another feature of the megakaryoblast is the initial development of demarcation membranes, which begin as invaginations of the plasma membrane and ultimately develop into a highly branched interconnected system of channels that course through the cytoplasm. The demarcation membrane system is in open communication with the extracellular space, based on studies using electron dense tracers.[16] Biochemical analysis indicates the composition of these membranes is very similar to the plasma membrane at each stage of megakaryocyte development. Over the 72 hours required for stage III/IV cells to develop from megakaryoblasts, the demarcation membrane system grows substantially. The demarcation membrane system provides the material necessary for development of proplatelet processes, structures that form in stage IV megakaryocytes and give rise upon fragmentation to mature platelets.[8,17]

### Endomitosis

One of the most characteristic features of megakaryocyte development is endomitosis, a unique form of mitosis in which the DNA is repeatedly replicated in the absence of nuclear or cytoplasmic division. The resultant cells are highly polyploid. Endomitosis begins in megakaryoblasts (Fig. 1–2) following the many standard cell divisions required to expand

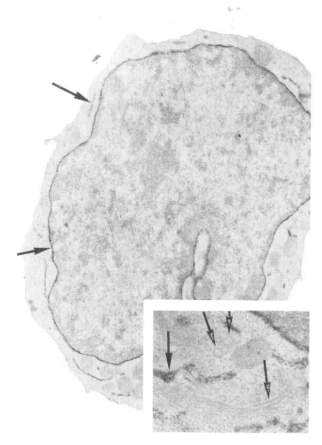

**Figure 1–1.** Electron micrograph of a normal human megakaryoblast stained for platelet peroxidase. The small cell (<9 μm) exhibits dense platelet peroxidase in the perinuclear space and endoplasmic reticulum (*arrows*) (magnification ×12,150). (*Inset*) Enlargement of the Golgi zone. The Golgi saccules and vesicles are devoid of platelet peroxidase (*open arrows*), whereas the endoplasmic reticulum contains platelet peroxidase activity (*closed arrow*) (magnification ×25,000). (*Used with permission of Dr. J. Breton-Gorius.*)

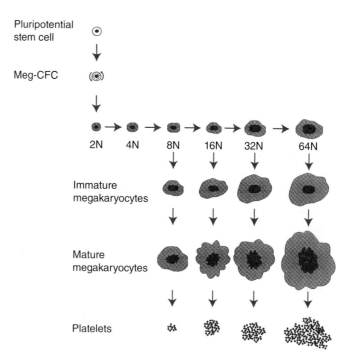

**Figure 1–2.** Origin and development of megakaryocytes. The pluripotential stem cell produces a progenitor committed to megakaryocyte differentiation (colony-forming unit–megakaryocyte [CFU-MK]), which can undergo mitosis. Eventually the CFU-MK stops mitosis and enters endomitosis. During endomitosis, neither cytoplasm nor nucleus divides, but DNA replication proceeds and gives rise to immature polyploid progenitors, which then enlarge and mature into morphologically identifiable, mature megakaryocytes that shed platelets. This figure does not necessarily imply that endomitosis and platelet formation are sequential but they can occur simultaneously. Meg-CFC, megakaryocyte colony-forming cells.

the number of megakaryocytic precursor cells and is completed by the end of stage II megakaryocyte development.[18] During the endomitotic phase, each cycle of DNA synthesis produces an exact doubling of all the chromosomes, resulting in cells containing DNA content from eight to 128 times the normal chromosomal complement in a single, highly lobated nucleus. Although poorly understood for many years, the ability to produce large numbers of normal megakaryocytes in culture has started to shed light on this enigmatic process. Endomitosis is not simply the absence of mitosis but rather consists of recurrent cycles of aborted mitoses.[19] Cell-cycle kinetics in endomitotic cells also are unusual, characterized by a short $G_1$ phase, a relatively normal DNA synthesis phase, a short $G_2$ phase, and a very short endomitosis phase.[20] During the endomitosis phase, megakaryocytic chromosomes condense, the nuclear membrane breaks down, and multiple (at advanced stages) mitotic spindles form upon which the replicated chromosomes assemble. However, following initial chromosomal separation, individual chromosomes fail to complete their normal migration to opposite poles of the cell, the spindle dissociates, the nuclear membrane reforms around the entire chromosomal complement, and the cell again enters $G_1$ phase.

### Regulation of Gene Expression

The promoters for integrin $\alpha_{IIb}$, GPIb, GPVI, GPIX, and platelet factor-4 genes have been the focus of several studies and are active at the megakaryoblast stage of development. Consensus sequences for both GATA-1 and members of the Ets family of transcription factors (e.g., Fli-1) are present in the 5′ flanking regions of these genes, deletion of which reduces or eliminates reporter gene expression,[21-24] at least in mature hematopoietic cells. MafB also enhances GATA-1 and Ets activity during megakaryoblast differentiation,[25] induced by activation of ERK1/2, one of the primary downstream events of thrombopoietin stimulation.[26]

Another target of GATA-1 in megakaryocytes is polyphosphate-4-phosphatase (P4P), which was first identified by subtraction cloning between normal and GATA-1 knockdown megakaryocytes.[27] One of the unexplained features of megakaryocytes in GATA-1 knockdown mice is that, rather than massive cell death as seen in GATA-1–deficient erythroid progenitors,[28] the aberrantly developing megakaryoblasts in GATA-1 knockdown marrow are highly abundant and proliferate *in vitro* far more than control cells.[29] P4P catalyzes hydrolysis of the D-4 position phosphate of $PI_{3,4}P$ and $PI_{3,4,5}P$. These membrane phospholipids are products of phosphoinositol 3′-kinase (PI3K) action on membrane phospholipids, and they play an important role in the proliferative and survival response to megakaryocyte growth factors. When reintroduced into the knockdown mice, P4P diminishes the exuberant growth characteristic of the knockdown cells.[27] These findings are similar to the phenotype of cells from PTEN or SHIP knockout mice, enzymes that hydrolyze the D-3 and D-5 positions of $PI_{3,4,5}P$.

Another transcription factor vital for megakaryoblast differentiation is RUNX1 (also termed CBFA2 and AML1), the gene responsible for thrombocytopenia seen in familial platelet disorder/predisposition to acute myelogenous leukemia (Chap. 9).[30] In this disorder, haploinsufficiency of RUNX1 is associated with thrombocytopenia. As its genetic elimination in mice leads to significant maturation defects in the megakaryocyte lineage,[31] the human disorder almost certainly results from this genetic alteration. During normal megakaryoblast differentiation, RUNX1 levels rise and, conversely, fall during erythroid differentiation. In response to phosphorylation by ERK1/2, RUNX1, in complex with CBFβ and together with GATA-1, induces integrin $\alpha_{IIb}$ and integrin $\alpha_2$ expression in megakaryoblast-like cells,[32] providing the beginnings of a molecular explanation for megakaryocyte development.

### Cytokine Dependency

The cytokines, hormones, and chemokines that affect the survival and proliferation of megakaryoblasts include thrombopoietin, interleukin (IL)-3, stem cell factor (also termed mast cell growth factor, steel factor, and c-kit ligand), and the chemokine CXCL12 (previously termed stromal cell-derived factor [SDF]-1). Thrombopoietin is the most critical (for additional details, see the more extensive discussion in "Hormones and Cytokines" below), as genetic elimination of the *TPO* gene in mice leads to circulating platelet levels approximately 10 percent of normal. Homozygous or complex heterozygous mutation of the gene encoding the thrombopoietin receptor cMPL leads to congenital amegakaryocytic thrombocytopenia, in which platelet levels are approximately 10 percent of normal because of a near absence of megakaryocytic progenitors and megakaryoblasts (Chap. 7). The importance of stem cell factor to megakaryoblast development is revealed by experimental findings both *in vitro* and *in vivo*. Genetic reduction in expression of stem cell factor or its receptor *c-kit* leads to a 50 percent reduction in circulating platelet levels.[33] The cytokine acts in synergy with thrombopoietin to enhance megakaryocyte production in semisolid and suspension culture systems.[34] Evidence that IL-3 contributes to normal or accelerated megakaryopoiesis *in vivo* is weak. Genetic elimination of the IL-3 gene fails to affect platelet counts, even when combined with thrombopoietin receptor deficiency,[35] but the cytokine can induce growth of marrow progenitors into colonies containing immature megakaryocytes *in vitro* in the absence of thrombopoietin.[36] The chemokine CXCL12 appears to play a role in megakaryocyte proliferation. *In vitro*, the chemokine acts in synergy with thrombopoietin to support the survival and proliferation of megakaryocyte progenitors.[37] The combination of fibroblast growth factor (FGF)-4 and CXCL12 restores megakaryopoiesis in *TPO* and *c-mpl* null mice.[38]

### Signal Transduction

The survival and proliferation of megakaryoblasts depend on at least two thrombopoietin-induced signaling pathways: PI3K and mitogen-activated protein kinase (MAPK). In the presence of chemical inhibitors of PI3K, the favorable effects of thrombopoietin on megakaryocyte progenitor survival and proliferation are eliminated,[39] although constitutively activating this pathway is not sufficient for thrombopoietin-induced growth. MAPK is another important signaling pathway stimulated by thrombopoietin. Using purified marrow megakaryocytic progenitors and model cell lines, several groups showed that inhibition of MAPK blocks megakaryoblast maturation[26,40-42] because of its effect of activating Ets transcription factors.

## STAGE II MEGAKARYOCYTES

Stage II megakaryocytes contain a lobulated nucleus and more abundant, but less intensely basophilic, cytoplasm. Ultrastructurally, the cytoplasm contains more abundant α granules and organelles. The demarcation membrane system begins to expand at this stage of development. Stage II megakaryocytes measure up to 30 $\mu$m in diameter, constitute approximately 25 percent of marrow megakaryocytes, and are the stage of development during which endomitosis is most prominent, generating cells displaying ploidy values of 8N to 64N.

### Endomitosis

Whereas megakaryoblasts are generally thought to be able to expand by cell division, at an early stage of their maturation, the cells begin to undergo endomitosis, in which cells diverge from the normal cell cycle during mid to late anaphase. Like normally mitotic cells, endomitotic megakaryocytes condense their chromatin into chromosomes, form a spindle, dissolve the nuclear membrane, and assemble the chromosomes on a metaphase plate, then the chromosomes begin to separate during early anaphase. However, rather than the dividing chromosomes migrating to opposite poles of the cell to allow the formation of a cleavage furrow, the chromosomes quickly decondense, the nuclear membrane reforms around the entire chromosomal complement, and the endomitotic cells reenter $G_1$ phase followed by S phase. A number of attempts to understand this process at the biochemical level have involved leukemic cell lines. Alterations in cyclin B, cdc2, cell-cycle kinase inhibitors, and aurora kinases have been claimed to be responsible for endomitosis.[43,44] Unfortunately, although these hypotheses possibly explain the polyploidy in various leukemic cell lines, the hypotheses have not been substantiated in studies of normal endomitotic megakaryocytes.[19,45] Endomitosis departs from a normal mitotic cell cycle at the late anaphase stage, when furrow invagination aborts short of cell abscission.[46] Additional studies indicate that disordered localization of the small G-protein RhoA may be responsible for this property.[46] Confirmation that a decrease in proper RhoA function is critical for endomitosis comes from the genetic elimination of RhoA from the megakaryocytic lineage; *RhoA* null megakaryocytes display enhanced polyploidy, although the released platelets are characterized by abnormal membrane rheology, resulting in their rapid clearance from the circulation.[47] Proper RhoA localization is controlled by its activation by the RhoA guanosine triphosphate (GTP) exchange factor (GEF) ECT2; ECT2 is down-modulated during the switch from mitosis to endomitosis in megakaryocytes, providing a mechanistic explanation for the onset of endomitosis.[48]

### Cytoplasmic Development

Early in megakaryocyte development, the cytoplasm acquires a rich network of microfilaments and microtubules. Toward stages III and IV, the proteins accumulate in the cell periphery, creating an organelle poor peripheral zone. Biochemically, the megakaryocyte cytoskeleton is composed of actin, $\alpha$-actinin, filamin, nonmuscle myosin (including the product of the *MYH9* gene, mutated in several giant platelet thrombocytopenic syndromes[49]; Chap. 7), $\beta_1$-tubulin, talin, and several other actin-binding proteins. Like platelets, megakaryocytes can respond to external stimuli by changing shape, transporting organelles around the cytoplasm, and secreting granules. These functions are dependent on the microfilament and microtubule systems of the cell. In addition, microtubules play a vital role during the later stages of platelet formation.[50]

### Regulation of Gene Expression

As discussed earlier, GATA-1 is vital for committing primitive multipotent progenitors to the erythroid–megakaryocyte pathway. However, the transcription factor also is critical later in megakaryopoiesis, for cytoplasmic development. The first convincing evidence that GATA proteins affect megakaryocyte development came from overexpression studies of *GATA-1* in a leukemic cell line, in which the transcription factor led to partial megakaryocytic differentiation.[51] Reduction in *GATA-1* expression also impairs cytoplasmic development in murine megakaryocytes, reducing demarcation membranes and platelet-specific granules.[29] Additional transcription factors expressed during stage II megakaryocyte development include RUNX-1, Tal1, and Fli1, but these transcription factors appear to play far greater a role in megakaryocyte maturation and platelet formation and are discussed in "Stage III/IV Megakaryocytes" below.

### Platelet Granule Formation

Although more prominent in later stages of differentiation (Fig. 1–3), platelet-specific $\alpha$ granules first begin to form adjacent to the Golgi apparatus as 300- to 500-nm round or oval organelles in stage II megakaryocytes. Three distinct compartments are recognized in $\alpha$ granules:

(1) a central, electron-dense nucleoid, containing fibrinogen, platelet factor-4, $\beta$-thromboglobulin, transforming growth factor (TGF)-$\beta_1$, vitronectin, and tissue plasminogen activator–like plasminogen activator; (2) a peripheral zone, containing tubules and von Willebrand factor (arranged much like that seen in endothelial cell Weibel-Palade bodies); and (3) the granule membrane, containing many of the critical platelet receptors for cell rolling (P-selectin), firm adhesion (GPIb-V-IX), and aggregation (integrin $\alpha_{IIb}\beta_3$). Proteins present in $\alpha$ granules arise from *de novo* megakaryocyte synthesis (e.g., GPIb-V-IX, GPIV, integrin $\alpha_{IIb}\beta_3$, von Willebrand factor, P-selectin, $\beta$-thromboglobulin, platelet-derived growth factor), nonspecific pinocytosis of environmental proteins (albumin and immunoglobulin G), or cell surface membrane receptor-mediated uptake from the environment (e.g., fibrinogen, fibronectin, factor V). Insights into platelet granule formation have come from a molecular understanding of Hermansky-Pudlak syndrome (HPS). In this disorder, characterized by oculocutaneous albinism and a qualitative platelet bleeding disorder, a complex of at least eight proteins form in various granule-associated complexes such as the biogenesis of lysosome-related organelles complexes, which affect $\delta$ granule formation.[52] These complexes are thought to be involved in cargo transport of a number of subcellular granules, such as lysosomes, melanosomes, and platelet $\delta$ granules.

## STAGE III/IV MEGAKARYOCYTES

Continued cytoplasmic maturation characterizes stage III/IV megakaryocyte development (Fig. 1–4). Cells are extremely large (40 to 60 $\mu$m in diameter) and display a low nuclear-to-cytoplasmic ratio. Cytoplasmic basophilia disappears as cells progress from stage III to stage IV. The demarcation membrane system gradually replaces the endoplasmic reticulum and Golgi apparatus during the final stages of maturation. The nucleus usually is eccentrically placed. Although the nucleus sometimes appears as several distinct nuclei in biopsy sections, it remains highly lobulated but single at all stages of megakaryocyte development. In occasional marrow sections (Fig. 1–4C), neutrophils or other marrow cells are seen transiting through the cytoplasm of the mature megakaryocyte, a process termed *emperipolesis*, and this is of no pathologic significance.

### Proplatelet Formation

Careful microscopic studies have localized marrow megakaryocytes to the abluminal surface of sinusoidal endothelial cells. In specially prepared specimens, the megakaryocytes can be seen issuing long, slender cytoplasmic processes between endothelial cells and into the sinusoidal lumen, structures termed *proplatelet processes* (Fig. 1–5).[53] The processes have been reproduced *in vitro* and *in vivo*.[6] The processes consist of a $\beta$-tubulin cytoskeleton and highway, transporting organelles and platelet constituents from the megakaryocyte to the terminal projection, the nascent platelet.[17]

### Membrane Composition

Most of the specific characteristics of platelet membranes are present at stages III and IV of megakaryocyte development. Megakaryocyte membrane lipid composition progressively changes through development, achieving approximately four times the content of phospholipids and cholesterol as found in immature cells. Megakaryocytes contain approximately the same amounts of membrane neutral lipid and phospholipid as platelets but contain relatively more phosphatidylinositol and less phosphatidylserine and arachidonic acid.

### Regulation of Gene Expression

One transcription factor that plays an important role in the final stages of megakaryocyte maturation is nuclear factor-E2 (NF-E2). Initially

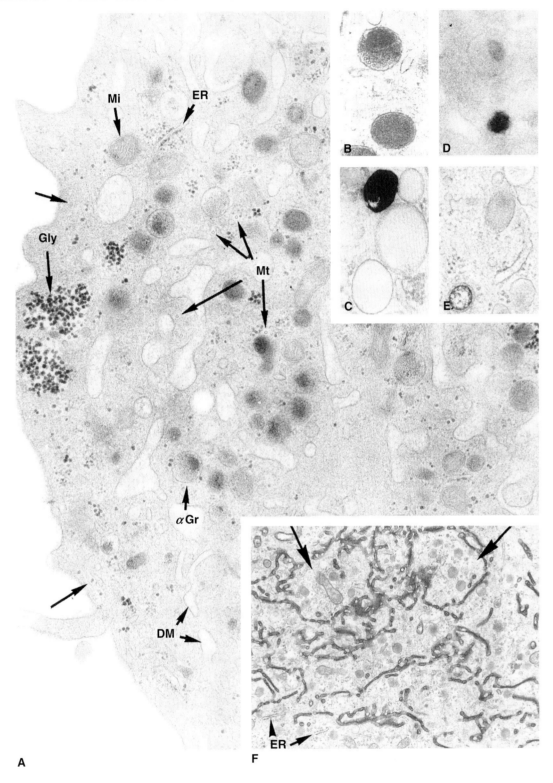

**Figure 1–3. A.** Ultrastructure of the cytoplasm of a mature megakaryocyte. The majority of the granules are *a* granules (*a*Gr) exhibiting dense nucleoid. Demarcation membranes (DM) are slightly dilated. Transverse sections of microtubules (Mt) are dispersed. At the periphery, a longitudinal microtubule runs under the cell membrane *(arrows)*. Dense aggregates of glycogen (Gly), small cisternae of endoplasmic reticulum (ER), and free ribosomes are seen (magnification ×30,320). **B.** Morphology of an *a* granule. Dense nucleoid is located at the *top*. In a clear zone at the opposite pole, four transverse sections of tubular structures are adjacent to the granule membrane (magnification ×37,200). **C.** Dense body can be distinguished from *a* granule by the black deposit when calcium is added to the fixative (magnification ×37,200). **D.** Cytochemical detection of acid phosphatase using β-glycophosphate as substrate and cerium as a trapping agent. Dense cerium–phosphate precipitates are present in lysosomal granules, whereas *a* granules are unreactive (magnification ×37,200). **E.** Microperoxisome visualized using alkaline diaminobenzidine. Note the small size of a reactive granule compared to the *a* granule. **F.** Distribution of a dense tracer filling the lumen of the demarcation membrane system in a maturing megakaryocyte *(arrows)*. In contrast to the demarcation membrane system, which is open to the extracellular space, the endoplasmic reticulum (ER) is not labeled (magnification ×9700). *(Used with permission of Dr. J. Breton-Gorius.)*

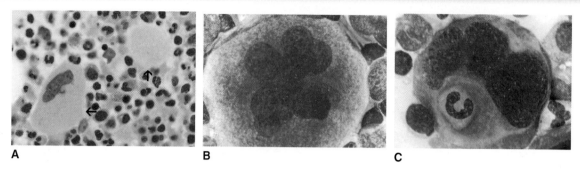

**Figure 1–4.** Megakaryocyte morphology. **A.** Normal human marrow biopsy. Two megakaryocytes are evident. In one case the section is through the cell at the level of the nuclei *(horizontal arrow)*, and in the other, it is through the cytoplasm above or below the nucleus *(vertical arrow)*. **B.** Normal human marrow aspirate. Mature (stage III) megakaryocyte with a multilobated nucleus and abundant cytoplasm. **C.** Normal human marrow aspirate. Mature megakaryocyte with a neutrophil embedded in the cytoplasm. Many ultrastructural studies have confirmed that this appearance represents marrow cells entering the canalicular system of megakaryocyte cytoplasm through its opening to the exterior of the cell (emperipolesis). *(Reproduced with permission from Lichtman's Atlas of Hematology, www.accessmedicine.com.)*

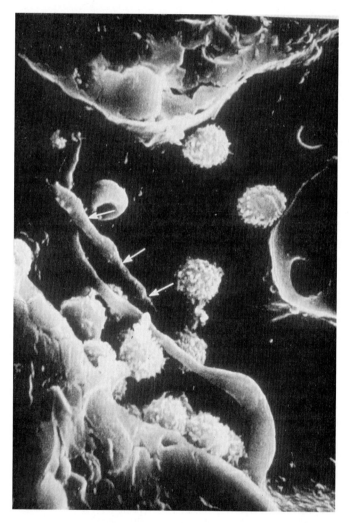

**Figure 1–5.** Megakaryocyte proplatelet processes in the marrow sinusoid. Scanning electron micrograph showing the luminal view of the confluence of two marrow sinusoids with two proplatelet processes protruding through the lining endothelial cells. One of the processes has intermittent constrictions *(arrows)*, indicating potential sites for platelet formation. Other cells depicted include lymphocytes and erythrocytes (magnification ×3000). *(Reproduced with permission from Becker RP, De Bruyn P: The transmural passage of blood cells into myeloid sinusoids and the entry of platelets into sinusoidal circulation; a scanning electron microscope investigation. Am J Anat 1976 Feb;145(2):183–205.)*

described as an erythroid-specific, heterodimeric protein belonging to the basic leucine zipper family of transcription factors, NF-E2 is composed of a ubiquitously expressed p18 subunit, and a 45-kDa protein (p45) expressed only in erythroid cells and megakaryocytes.[54] NF-E2 binds to tandem AP-1–like motifs, such as those seen in the second deoxyribonuclease (DNAse) hypersensitive site of the $\beta$-globin locus control region, and is required for $\beta$-globin expression.[55] However, genetic elimination of p45 failed to significantly affect erythropoiesis. Rather, p45-deficient mice display prominent alterations in megakaryocyte development and severe thrombocytopenia,[56] leading to death from widespread hemorrhage soon after birth. Examination of the animals reveals modest expansion of marrow megakaryocytes but failure of the cells to produce platelets because of defects in cytoplasmic maturation, including substantial reductions in platelet granules and demarcation membranes. Thus, the loss of either GATA-1 or NF-E2 results in failure of late aspects of cellular maturation. As p45 NF-E2 is induced by GATA-1/FOG,[57] the lack of cytoplasmic development in GATA-deficient mice likely is an indirect effect. The role of transcription factors in late megakaryopoiesis has been reviewed.[58]

Nearly all studies of megakaryopoiesis have focused on the marrow. The final stages of megakaryocyte fragmentation also are proposed to occur in the lung, at least for some cells, a theory based on the finding that platelet levels in pulmonary venous blood exceed those found in the pulmonary artery.[59] Whether this process represents the migration and fragmentation of intact megakaryocytes in the lung or merely the final size reduction of large fragments of megakaryocyte cytoplasm that also are released into the blood is not clear. Some data exist supporting the notion that lung megakaryocytes contribute to blood platelet production.[60] However, in mice administered high doses of thrombopoietin, with platelet counts as high as 4 million/$\mu m^3$, neither intact megakaryocytes nor denuded nuclei were found in the lungs of these animals.[61] One study found that canine lungs contain 2.5 megakaryocytes per $cm^3$.[62] Extrapolation of these data suggest human lungs contain approximately 6000 megakaryocytes, only enough to account for a small proportion (<0.1 percent) of daily platelet production.

## PLATELET FORMATION

Numerous studies have indicated thrombopoietin is the primary regulator of megakaryocyte maturation.[36,63] However, despite the importance of the hormone for generation of fully mature megakaryocytes from which platelets arise, elimination of the cytokine during the final stages of platelet formation is not detrimental.[64] Although proplatelet formation is possible under serum-free conditions,[65] most investigators have reported the presence of plasma and/or an integrin ligand-containing substratum (e.g., fibronectin or vitronectin) stimulates the process substantially.[64,66] These findings suggest external signals probably are required for normal platelet formation. One report suggests the thrombin–antithrombin complex with or without high-density lipoprotein particles mediates the favorable effect of plasma on proplatelet formation,[67] although other data suggest prothrombin and its conversion to thrombin by megakaryocytes inhibit the process.[68] Although the cytokine(s) required for this process is not known, activation of protein kinase C$\alpha$ clearly is necessary for the process to occur.[66]

Platelet formation involves massive reorganization of megakaryocyte cytoskeletal components, including actin and tubulin, during a highly active, motile process in which the termini of the process branch and issue platelets.[5] The size of the individual platelets formed is of interest. Unfortunately, little is known about this aspect of platelet formation except that tubulin is proposed to act as a measuring device for the proper site to pinch off platelets from proplatelet processes. The mechanism of platelet formation clearly must be affected in some way by the transcription factor GATA-1, the GPIb-IX complex, the Wiskott-Aldrich syndrome protein, and platelet myosin, as defects in each of these genes leads to unusually large or small platelets (Chap. 7).[69,70] Finally, localized cytoplasmic membrane proteolysis, a sublethal form of apoptosis, likely plays a role in initiating the final stages of platelet formation.[71]

# ● EXTRINSIC REGULATION OF MEGAKARYOCYTE PRODUCTION

## HORMONES AND CYTOKINES

Several cytokines, first identified using alternate hematopoietic activity assays, affect megakaryocyte development. IL-3, granulocyte-macrophage colony-stimulating factor, and stem cell factor support the proliferation of megakaryocytic progenitors in plasma-containing cultures.[72–74] In 1994, several groups reported the purification and/or cloning of thrombopoietin.[75] This cytokine clearly is the primary regulator of megakaryopoiesis but cannot explain thrombopoiesis in its entirety.

### Interleukin-3

IL-3 is a 25- to 30-kDa protein produced almost exclusively by T lymphocytes.[76] The mature human protein contains 133 amino acids, but N-linked carbohydrate modification accounts for the larger than expected Mr of the cytokine. Granulocyte-macrophage colony-stimulating factor is an 18- to 30-kDa protein also produced by T lymphocytes. However, endothelial cells, monocytes, and fibroblasts also produce the protein, and, like IL-3, granulocyte-macrophage colony-stimulating factor is highly modified with both N-linked and O-linked carbohydrate.[77] Although the two proteins display essentially no primary sequence homology, their tertiary structures are highly related,[78] and the receptors for the two cytokines share a common subunit.[79] However, the physiologic relevance of IL-3 and granulocyte-macrophage colony-stimulating factor for steady-state thrombopoiesis is uncertain. Administration of the cytokines to mice or humans has only minimal effects on thrombopoiesis, and genetic elimination of either has no impact on megakaryopoiesis, even when combined with elimination of other thrombopoietic cytokines.[80,81]

### Interleukin-6 and Related Cytokines

IL-6, cloned by several groups using multiple assays (hepatocyte growth, myeloma cell growth, immunoglobulin secretion, antiviral activity), enhances megakaryocyte maturation. IL-6 is a 26-kDa polypeptide produced by T lymphocytes, fibroblasts, macrophages, and stromal cells in response to inflammatory stimuli.[82] The mature protein is composed of 184 amino acids, contains two disulfide bonds, and displays both N-linked and O-linked carbohydrate modification. Although IL-6 alone fails to affect in vitro megakaryopoiesis, it augments the number of megakaryocyte colonies obtained in the presence of IL-3 or stem cell factor[83] and exerts primarily a differentiating effect.[84,85] Administration of IL-6 to mice or nonhuman primates or patients results in a modest thrombocytosis.[86–88] These findings suggest IL-6 contributes to megakaryopoiesis in vivo, a conclusion supported by its production by tumor cells in selected cases of paraneoplastic thrombocytosis.[89] However, genetic elimination of the cytokine fails to significantly affect basal platelet production.[90] Evidence suggests the cytokine affects platelet production indirectly[91] by stimulating thrombopoietin production.

IL-6 acts through a heterodimeric receptor, composed of a signaling subunit, termed GP130, and an affinity-converting subunit, termed IL-6R$\alpha$. GP130 also acts as the signaling subunit for several other cytokines, including IL-11 and leukemia inhibitory factor. Therefore, the finding that these cytokines also stimulate megakaryopoiesis in a manner similar to that of IL-6 is not surprising. IL-11 and leukemia inhibitory factor act in synergy with IL-3 or stem cell factor to augment megakaryocyte formation. IL-11 is a 23-kDa polypeptide, initially cloned from a gibbon marrow stromal cell line, whose activity can support the proliferation of an IL-6–responsive myeloma cell line.[92,93] Leukemia inhibitory factor displays a wide range of activities,[94] including (1) inducing the acute phase hepatic response, (2) inducing an adrenergic-to-cholinergic switch in neurons, (3) inhibiting lipoprotein lipase in adipocytes, and (4) maintaining pluripotentiality in embryonic cells.

Like IL-6, IL-11 and leukemia inhibitory factor enhance megakaryocytic maturation in vitro[95,96] and augment the effects of IL-3 and stem cell factor on primitive hematopoietic cells. Consistent with the in vitro findings, administration of either recombinant IL-11 or leukemia inhibitory factor to rodents, nonhuman primates, or humans produces modest thrombocytosis.[97–100] Despite the in vitro and in vivo findings, genetic elimination of either leukemia inhibitory factor or the IL-11 receptor has no effect on thrombopoiesis,[101] even when combined with elimination of the thrombopoietin receptor.[102]

### Stem Cell Factor

In contrast to the hematopoietic cytokine family, stem cell factor is more closely related to other hematopoietic proteins that utilize protein tyrosine kinase receptors, such as macrophage colony-stimulating factor and the flt-3 ligand.[103] Nevertheless, stem cell factor stimulates megakaryocyte colony growth when used in combination with other cytokines.[104] Moreover, genetic elimination of its receptor c-kit reduces megakaryocyte production[105] and the rebound thrombocytosis that occurs following immunosuppressive therapy.[106,107]

Stem cell factor was first identified using several different biologic assays (in addition to this term, the cytokine has been dubbed c-kit ligand, mast cell growth factor, and steel factor).[108] Later studies indicate the cytokine acts primarily on primitive cells of the hematopoietic, melanogenic, and germ cell lineages. Stem cell factor is a dimeric protein composed of two identical noncovalently linked polypeptides. The soluble form monomer contains 165 residues,[109] derived by proteolytic cleavage of a membrane-bound splice form of the molecule.[110] The membrane-bound form is more active than the soluble cytokine, as intracellular signaling in response to membrane-bound stem cell factor is prolonged in receptor-bearing cells.[111] Moreover, a naturally occurring mutant allele of the gene ($Sl^d$), which allows production of the soluble but not the membrane-bound form of the cytokine, results in a phenotype nearly identical to deletion of the entire locus,[112] again pointing to the importance of the membrane-bound form present on marrow stromal cells.

### Flt-3 Ligand

The flt-3 ligand initially was identified as a ligand for a novel member of the protein tyrosine kinase family of receptors.[103] This growth factor also affects megakaryocyte formation. Like stem cell factor, to which it is most closely related, flt-3 ligand is found in both soluble and membrane-bound forms, is a noncovalently linked dimer, and affects primarily primitive hematopoietic cells.[113] Although several studies have shown that flt-3 ligand used alone does not support megakaryocyte colony formation, some studies suggest it works in synergy with other megakaryocyte stimulatory agents to augment the proliferation of megakaryocytic progenitor cells in culture.[114,115] Administration of flt-3 ligand to mice expands the number of marrow and splenic progenitor cells that can give rise to megakaryocytes in vitro.[116] However, genetic elimination of either flt-3 ligand or its receptor does not produce a platelet phenotype.

### Thrombopoietin

The term thrombopoietin was first coined in 1958 to describe the primary regulator of platelet production.[117] A major impetus to the discovery of thrombopoietin in 1986 was the identification of the myeloproliferative leukemia virus (MPLV), which induces a vast expansion of hematopoietic cells.[118] The responsible viral oncogene was characterized in 1990,[119] and its cellular homologue c-Mpl was cloned in 1992.[120] Based on the presence of two copies of the hematopoietic cytokine receptor motif[121] and the ability of a fusion of c-Mpl and the IL-4 receptor to signal in factor-dependent cells,[122] c-Mpl clearly encoded a growth factor receptor, but its ligand was not known. Using three distinct strategies, four separate groups were able to clone complementary DNA for the corresponding hormone and report their results in 1994 (reviewed in Ref. 75). The gene for thrombopoietin encodes a 36-kDa polypeptide,[123] which also is predicted to be extensively posttranslationally modified, resulting in an approximately 50- to 70-kDa protein.

Thrombopoietin bears striking homology to erythropoietin, the primary regulator of erythropoiesis, within the amino-terminal half of the predicted polypeptide. The two proteins are more closely related than any other two cytokines within the hematopoietic cytokine family, sharing 20 percent identical amino acids, an additional 25 percent conservative substitutions, and identical positions of three of the four cysteine residues. Unlike any of the other cytokines in the family, thrombopoietin contains a 181-residue carboxyl-terminal extension, which bears homology to no known proteins. Two functions have been assigned to this region: it prolongs the circulatory half-life of the hormone,[3] and it aids in its secretion from the cells that normally synthesize the hormone.[124]

The biologic activities of thrombopoietin have been demonstrated in vitro and in vivo, in mice, rats, dogs, nonhuman primates, and humans. Incubation of marrow cells with thrombopoietin stimulates megakaryocyte survival and proliferation, alone and in combination with other cytokines.[34] In vivo, thrombopoietin stimulates platelet production in a log-linear manner to levels 10-fold higher than baseline[3,61,125] without affecting the blood red or white cell counts. In addition, because of its effect on hematopoietic stem cells, the numbers of erythroid and myeloid progenitors and mixed myeloid progenitors in marrow and spleen also are increased,[126,127] an effect that is particularly impressive when the hormone is administered following myelosuppressive therapy.[126,128,129] This effect likely results from the synergy between thrombopoietin and the other hematopoietic cytokines circulating at high levels in this condition.

Based on genetic studies, thrombopoietin clearly is the primary regulator of thrombopoiesis. Elimination of either the c-Mpl or Tpo gene leads to profound thrombocytopenia in mice as a result of a greatly reduced number of megakaryocyte progenitors, mature megakaryocytes,

and the reduced polyploidy of the remaining megakaryocytes.[130] A similar result occurs in humans. Patients with congenital amegakaryocytic thrombocytopenia (CAMT) display numerous homozygous or compound heterozygous nonsense or severe missense mutations of the thrombopoietin receptor c-Mpl (Chap. 7).[131,132] The effect of thrombopoietin on hematopoietic stem cells is particularly revealed by consideration of children with CAMT. Within 5 years of birth, nearly every patient with CAMT develops aplastic anemia as a result of stem cell exhaustion.

The thrombopoietin gene displays an unusual 5′ flanking structure. Unlike the majority of genes that initiate translation of the encoded polypeptide with the first ATG codon present in the mRNA, thrombopoietin translation initiates at the eighth ATG codon located within the third exon of a full-length transcript.[133] However, because the eighth ATG of thrombopoietin mRNA is embedded in the short, open reading frame of the seventh ATG, its translation is particularly inefficient because of the mechanism of ribosomal initiation.[134] As such, little thrombopoietin protein is produced for any given amount of mRNA. Although this molecular arrangement has no known physiologic consequences, it forms the basis for an unusual form of disease, a disorder of translation efficiency. Four cases of autosomal dominant familial thrombocytosis have been linked to mutations in the region surrounding the initiation codon. In two families, a single mutation in different nucleotides of the intron 3 splice donor sequence results in alternate splicing of the primary thrombopoietin transcript, eliminating the seventh and eighth ATG codons, creating a new aminoterminus by fusing of the fifth open reading frame with the thrombopoietin coding sequence. This novel thrombopoietin mRNA is efficiently translated, resulting in supraphysiologic levels of hormone production and nonclonal expansion of thrombopoiesis.[135,136] In another mutant thrombopoietin allele, deletion of a single nucleotide within the seventh open reading frame leads to its fusion with the thrombopoietin coding sequence and now enhanced translation of thrombopoietin from the seventh ATG codon.[137] A fourth mutation has been described within the seventh open reading frame, leading to premature termination of that short peptide, preventing its interference with translation initiation from the usual eighth initiation codon,[138] again enhancing thrombopoietin production (reviewed in Ref. 139). Of note, although reactive thrombocytosis is not thought to lead to hypercoagulability (Chap. 9), several patients in these pedigrees developed thromboses, raising the physiologic question of why chronic stimulation of platelets with enhanced levels of thrombopoietin should lead to hypercoagulability.

The physiologic regulation of thrombopoietin production has received much attention. Experimental induction of immune-mediated thrombocytopenia results in relatively rapid restoration of platelet levels, followed by a brief period of rebound thrombocytosis.[140] In these experimental cases and in most naturally occurring cases of thrombocytopenia, plasma hormone concentrations vary inversely with platelet counts, rising to maximal levels within 24 hours of onset of profound thrombocytopenia.[141] Two non–mutually exclusive models have been advanced to explain these findings. In the first model, thrombopoietin production is constitutive, but its consumption, and hence the level remaining in the blood to affect megakaryopoiesis, is determined by the mass of c-Mpl receptors present on platelets and megakaryocytes accessible to the plasma.[142] In this way, states of thrombocytosis result in increased thrombopoietin consumption (by the expanded platelet mass of c-Mpl receptors), reducing megakaryopoiesis. Conversely, thrombocytopenia reduces blood thrombopoietin destruction, resulting in elevated blood levels of the hormone that drives megakaryopoiesis and platelet recovery. This model is based on one of the mechanisms regulating macrophage colony-stimulating factor levels.[143] The invariable levels of thrombopoietin-specific mRNA present in the liver and kidney of experimental animals and patients with thrombocytopenia or thrombocytosis support this model.[144,145] Moreover, thrombopoietin knockout mice display a gene dosage effect.[146] Platelet levels in heterozygous mice are intermediate between those seen in wild-type and nullizygous animals, suggesting active regulation of the remaining thrombopoietin allele cannot compensate for the mild (60 percent of normal) thrombocytopenia induced by the loss of one allele.

A second model suggests thrombopoietin expression is a regulated event. Very low platelet levels can induce thrombopoietin-specific mRNA production. Several studies show that thrombopoietin mRNA levels are modulated in response to moderate to severe thrombocytopenia, at least in the marrow.[145,147] The signal(s) responsible for this form of thrombopoietin regulation is being uncovered but is, at least in part, mediated by transcriptional enhancement.[148] CD40 ligand, platelet-derived growth factor, FGF, TGF-$\beta$, platelet factor-4, and thrombospondin modulate thrombopoietin production from marrow stromal cells.[149,150]

The human thrombopoietin gene 5′ flanking region lacks a TATA box or CAAT motif and directs transcription initiation at multiple sites over a 50-nucleotide region.[151] Reporter gene analysis in a hepatocyte cell line identified an Ets2 transcription factor-binding motif responsible for high-level expression of the gene. The 5′ flanking region also includes SP-1, AP-2, and nuclear factor-$\kappa$B binding sites,[152] although the contribution of these transcription factors to thrombopoietin gene expression, either under steady-state or inflammatory conditions, has not been studied.

### CXCL12 (Stromal Cell-Derived Factor-1)

Chemokines are members of a rapidly growing class of molecules that play multiple roles in blood cell physiology.[153] Initially defined as substances that induce leukocyte chemotaxis, four classes of the 8- to 12-kDa polypeptides have been recognized, based on the spacing of cysteine residues close to the aminoterminus of the proteins. An equally rapidly growing family of chemokine receptors also has been discovered, classified by the subfamily of chemokines they serve. All chemokine receptors are members of the seven-transmembrane family of receptors that signal through heterotrimeric G proteins.

Most work has been conducted with the CC and CXC subfamilies of chemokines, molecules that display modest inhibitory effects on cell proliferation when used alone and potent effects when used in combination on hematopoietic progenitors at all levels of development.[154] On many levels, the CXC chemokine CXCL12 (previously termed SDF-1) and its receptor CXCR4 are notable exceptions to the many features shared by most members of the chemokine and chemokine receptor families. For example, although all the other genes for the known CXC chemokines reside on the long arm of human chromosome 14, CXCL12 localizes to the long arm of chromosome 10.[155] Moreover, most chemokine receptors can be activated by multiple ligands. For example, the chemokine CCL3 (macrophage inflammatory protein [MIP]-1$\alpha$) can bind and activate CCR1 and CCR5, and IL-8 can bind both CXCR1 and CXCR2.[156] In contrast, because the phenotypes of genetic elimination of both CXCR4 and CXCL12 are almost identical,[157,158] CXCR4 appears to be the only receptor for CXCL12, and CXCL12 is the only ligand for CXCR4.

The marrow stroma is the primary source of CXCL12, and most of the cell types known to express CXCR4 are hematopoietic in origin. One of the major phenotypes in CXCL12- or CXCR4-deficient neonatal mice is marrow aplasia, thought to be secondary to failure of perinatal hematopoietic stem cell homing.[159] In addition, megakaryocytes display CXCR4[160] and migrate in response to a CXCL12 concentration gradient.[161] Several groups have shown that CXCL12 augments thrombopoietin-induced megakaryocyte growth in suspension culture.[37,160] Later studies have shown the synergy between CXCL12 and other stimuli on megakaryocyte growth extends to cell surface adhesion.[38]

### Transforming Growth Factor-$\beta$

In addition to the many positive regulators of megakaryopoiesis, several substances down-modulate their development. Five isoforms of TGF-$\beta$ have been identified, all disulfide-linked homodimers each containing 112 residues.[162] TGF-$\beta_1$ is the predominant type of TGF found in hematopoietic tissues. Platelet $\alpha$ granules are a particularly rich source of the cytokine. In general, transforming growth factors are inhibitors of hematopoiesis,[163,164] particularly of megakaryocyte development.[165,166] The best understood TGF-$\beta$ growth inhibitory effects are exerted on cell-cycle progression. After binding to one of five receptors, two pathways that block cell-cycle progression are activated. pRb is hypophosphorylated,[167] antagonizing the effects of G$_1$-phase cyclin-dependent kinases, and cell-cycle inhibitors, including p27 and p15$^{INK}$, are upregulated, affecting cell-cycle progression.[168,169] In contrast to these negative effects of TGF-$\beta$ on cell proliferation, the cytokine enhances megakaryocyte differentiation.

### Interferon-$\alpha$

A second class of cytokines that negatively impact thrombopoiesis are the interferons (IFNs), proteins first defined by their ability to induce an antiviral state in mammalian cells.[170] Biochemical fractionation has revealed three classes of IFNs: IFN-$\alpha$, a family of 17 distinct but highly homologous molecules; IFN-$\beta$, a single molecule more distantly related to the various isoforms of IFN-$\alpha$; and IFN-$\gamma$, a unique molecule that shares functional properties but not structure with the others. IFNs exert profound inhibitory effects on hematopoiesis.[171]

The genes for the IFN-$\alpha/\beta$ subfamily cluster on the short arm of chromosome 9 and encode 165- to 172-residue polypeptides, of which 35 percent are invariant across the family of IFN-$\alpha$ molecules. IFNs of the $\alpha/\beta$ type are produced by transcriptional upregulation in fibroblasts and leukocytes in response to viruses and other infectious agents and to inflammatory cytokines. Once bound to the IFN receptors, a cascade of kinases and intracellular mediators are triggered, initiated by JAKs (Janus family kinases), STAT (signal transducer and activator of transcription) factors, and p38 MAPK, resulting in changes in gene transcription.

IFN-$\alpha$ inhibits megakaryopoiesis, the clinical use of which is responsible for modest to severe thrombocytopenia in a significant number of patients undergoing therapy for chronic viral hepatitis.[172,173] The mechanisms responsible for the inhibitory effect of IFN-$\alpha$ are multifactorial. Some studies suggest a direct inhibitory effect of IFN-$\alpha$ on growth factor–induced proliferation pathways. For example, the cytokine augments double-stranded RNA-activated protein kinase activity, inhibiting translation initiation factor-2, implicating reduction of the growth factor–induced protein synthesis necessary for growth factor response.[174] IFN-$\beta$ induces expression of the cell-cycle inhibitor p27$^{Kip1}$, arresting cells in G$_0$/G$_1$.[175] Other studies have demonstrated IFN-$\alpha$ induces a SOCS (suppressor of cytokine signaling)-1–based feedback mechanism that cross-reacts and depresses thrombopoietin signaling.[176] Thus, in addition to the multiple positive mediators of megakaryopoiesis, several cytokines block the process and can lead to thrombocytopenia.

## MEGAKARYOCYTE MICROENVIRONMENT

This chapter discusses aspects of the microenvironment particularly vital for megakaryocyte growth. The cellular concentration within the marrow is estimated to be 10$^9$/mL. Consequently, cell–cell and cell–matrix interactions will occur.[177] A particularly important interaction for thrombopoiesis is between the marrow sinusoidal endothelial cell and the mature megakaryocyte. Studies using *in situ* videomicroscopy indicate that proplatelet processes extend through the sinusoids into the vascular lumen, where the shear stress of flowing blood liberates single platelets.[6] Marrow stromal cells influence hematopoiesis in a number of other ways, perhaps the most prominent through production of several cytokines that positively or negatively affect megakaryocyte growth.[145,178–180] Stromal cells are the origin of a number of extracellular matrix proteins and glycomucins that either directly affect hematopoietic cells or indirectly affect hematopoietic cells by binding growth factors and presenting them in a functional context.[181,182] Stromal cells also bear ligands for Notch proteins, cell-surface receptors that are critical mediators of cell fate decisions.[183] Notch and its ligands Delta and Jagged play important roles as regulators of hematopoietic progenitor cell proliferation[184] and play a potential role in influencing the lineage fate choice between erythropoiesis and megakaryopoiesis.[185] Cell–cell interactions mediated by integrins present on hematopoietic cells and counterreceptors on stromal cells are very important for megakaryopoiesis,[186] both by bringing hematopoietic cells into close proximity to stromal cells producing soluble or cell-bound cytokines and more directly by triggering or augmenting intracellular signaling, promoting entry into the cell cycle, and preventing programmed cell death.

# ● THERAPEUTIC MANIPULATION OF THROMBOPOIESIS BY NATURALLY OCCURRING CYTOKINES

Thrombocytopenia is a major clinical problem with multiple origins (Chap. 7). Primary marrow diseases, certain infections, and solid tumors with a high propensity for marrow metastases directly affect platelet production. Nearly all leukemias, advanced lymphomas, and myelomas ultimately cause thrombocytopenia by this mechanism. Hypersplenism and thrombopoietin deficiency contribute to platelet sequestration and reduced platelet production in patients with hepatic failure. Consumptive coagulopathies, initiated by infection, tumors, or severe injury, can be responsible for severe thrombocytopenia. In other patients, autoimmune thrombocytopenia arises during the course of disease or is a primary disease. However, the most common cause of significant thrombocytopenia is iatrogenic: the use of potentially curative or palliative chemotherapy or radiation therapy in patients with malignancy. An estimated 300,000+ persons yearly worldwide undergo courses of chemotherapy adequate to produce clinically significant thrombocytopenia. Recovery from the marrow suppressive effects of most chemotherapeutic agents occurs within 1 to 3 weeks following discontinuation of therapy. However, some agents, including mitomycin C or nitrosoureas, can produce prolonged periods of marrow suppression. Moreover, the widespread use of IFN-$\alpha$ for chronic hepatitis C infection adds large numbers of patients who experience thrombocytopenia as a dose-limiting toxicity. Tumor- or treatment-related thrombocytopenia often delays much needed additional therapy, may necessitate potentially complicated platelet transfusions, and causes significant morbidity and occasional mortality. Given the increased understanding of the humoral basis for megakaryopoiesis and thrombopoiesis, numerous attempts have been made to manipulate these processes for therapeutic benefit.

## INTERLEUKIN-11

IL-11 augments the growth of megakaryocytic progenitors in the presence of IL-3[187,188] and acts to promote megakaryocyte maturation rather than proliferation.[189,190] The preclinical effects of IL-11 were evaluated in

mice, rats, and subhuman primates, and they revealed moderate activity in normal animals and following cytoreductive therapy.[98,191,192]

The first clinical trials of IL-11 were reported in abstract form in 1993 and 1994.[193,194] Randomized clinical trials were reported a few years later.[195–197] Most studies reported IL-11 ameliorated drug-induced thrombocytopenia. For example, IL-11 administered to patients with advanced stages of breast cancer undergoing multiple courses of anthracycline-based chemotherapy significantly reduced the need for platelet transfusions by 27 percent. However, use of the drug in patients undergoing autologous stem cell transplantation did not enhance platelet recovery or other indices of hematopoiesis. Although chemical evidence of an acute-phase response was noted in many of the patients treated in these studies, the drug was generally well tolerated, even though fluid retention has been a significant side effect, often necessitating concomitant use of diuretics. IL-11 (oprelvekin, Neumega) was approved by the FDA in 1998 for use in patients undergoing chemotherapy who have evidence of previous drug-induced thrombocytopenia (Chap. 9).

## INTERFERON-$\alpha$

As noted in "Hormones and Cytokines" above, IFN suppresses hematopoiesis and thrombopoiesis by multiple mechanisms. As a consequence, IFN-$\alpha$ has been used to reduce platelet counts in patients with many forms of myeloproliferative disease. The first reported clinical trial was performed in patients with a mixture of these disorders. The trial found the mean platelet count decreased significantly from $1050 \times 10^9$/L to $340 \times 10^9$/L.[198] Long-term therapy with IFN also was shown to be effective and safe.[199] From these and other studies, IFN (2 to 5 million units 3 times per week) clearly effectively reduces the platelet count toward normal in most patients with myeloproliferative disease. More aggressive regimens (2 to 6 million units daily) result in complete hematologic remissions but with no evidence that the clonal disorder responsible has been affected.[200] Not surprisingly, reduced energy level, weight loss, myalgia, and depression have been consistently reported, forcing discontinuation of the drug in approximately one-third of patients taking low to moderate doses of various forms of IFN-$\alpha$.[201] Of some concern and possibly related to its effects on the immune system, a significant number of patients treated with IFN for thrombocytosis have developed antibodies to the administered drug, with subsequent reduced efficacy.[202]

## THROMBOPOIETIN

Clinically, the most important activity of thrombopoietin likely is its effects on megakaryopoiesis, potentially ameliorating the thrombocytopenia that occurs in natural and iatrogenic states of marrow failure. In this regard, a number of promising results in preclinical trials of the cytokine were reported.[126,128,129,203] In general, in rodents, dogs, and nonhuman primates, almost every model of myelosuppression or immune-mediated platelet destruction has responded favorably to parenteral administration of thrombopoietin. In addition to the favorable effects on platelet recovery, many of these studies also reported enhanced recovery or hematopoietic progenitors of all lineages, accelerated recovery of erythrocytes or leukocytes, or both. The only exception to these generally favorable results has been reported in animal models of stem cell transplantation, where negligible to minimal acceleration of blood cell recovery was found, unless the stem cell donor was treated with the hormone.[204,205]

A number of clinical trials in patients with cancer undergoing cytotoxic therapy have been conducted. Results were varied, with the hormone helpful in many patients,[206–208] but not in all clinical situations.[209,210] In general, the hormone has been useful in patients who were administered moderately aggressive chemotherapeutic regimens that produce clinically important thrombocytopenia. However, the hormone has not been helpful in the setting of high-dose, prolonged cytotoxic therapy, as in the treatment of acute myelogenous leukemia, or in stem cell transplantation, unless, as in the animal studies, it is administered to the stem cell donor.[211] Thrombopoietin also increases platelet levels in patients with immune-mediated thrombocytopenia.[212] The timing of drug administration can significantly impact both the total amount of drug required and its efficacy.[213] For example, administration of one dose of drug before and once following myelosuppressive therapy was as effective as any other multidose regimen. This regimen resulted in significant reductions in nadir platelet counts and the need for platelet transfusion during chemotherapy cycles supplemented with thrombopoietin. Nevertheless, use of a modified form of recombinant thrombopoietin was associated with antibody formation to the drug, which cross-reacted with and neutralized the native hormone, resulting in thrombocytopenia.[214] Although this effect has not been reported with a nonmodified recombinant thrombopoietin, most efforts using thrombopoietin in patients with thrombocytopenia are focusing on small peptide or organic mimics that bind to and activate the thrombopoietin receptor[215-217] (reviewed in Ref. 218). Both types of thrombopoietin mimetic agents have been proven to be effective in clinical trials (Chap. 7). Two lead indications have been tested: primary immune thrombocytopenia (ITP) and IFN-induced thrombocytopenia in patients being treated for chronic hepatitis C infection. In a randomized controlled phase III clinical trial of a peptibody bearing four copies of a c-Mpl receptor-stimulating peptide on an immunoglobulin scaffold, 84 percent of heavily pretreated patients with ITP responded to treatment, with rates being slightly lower or higher depending on whether they had previously undergone splenectomy.[219] Likewise, the administration of a small, orally available organic thrombopoietin mimetic to patients with ITP resulted in 81 percent of patients achieving a platelet count above $50 \times 10^9/L$.[220] These studies have led to FDA approval of the two thrombopoietin agonists for use in patients with ITP. The same molecule was administered to patients with modest hepatic insufficiency undergoing IFN/ribavirin therapy for hepatitis C; 75 percent of such patients were able to complete 3 months of therapy without IFN dose reduction, compared to 6 percent of patients given placebo.[221]

Thrombopoietin mimics have also been tested in combination with other agents for the treatment of chronic ITP. For example, the combination of recombinant human thrombopoietin plus rituximab results in higher response rates and longer duration of response than rituximab alone.[222]

A number of studies have suggested that thrombopoietin mimics could lead to marrow fibrosis, particularly if used for long periods of time. However, thousands of patient-years of thrombopoietin receptor agonist therapy have been observed, and every potential complication, such as fibrosis or thrombosis, has been found no more frequently than expected.[223] Nevertheless, careful surveillance of these patients for complications of therapy should continue.

# REFERENCES

1. Hanson SR, Slichter SJ: Platelet kinetics in patients with bone marrow hypoplasia: Evidence for a fixed platelet requirement. *Blood* 66:1105, 1985.
2. Dettke M, Hlousek M, Kurz M, et al: Increase in endogenous thrombopoietin in healthy donors after automated plateletpheresis. *Transfusion* 38:449, 1998.
3. Harker LA, Marzec UM, Hunt P, et al: Dose-response effects of pegylated human megakaryocyte growth and development factor on platelet production and function in nonhuman primates. *Blood* 88:511, 1996.
4. O'Malley CJ, Rasko JE, Basser RL, et al: Administration of pegylated recombinant human megakaryocyte growth and development factor to humans stimulates the production of functional platelets that show no evidence of *in vivo* activation. *Blood* 88:3288, 1996.
5. Machlus KR, Italiano JE Jr: The incredible journey: From megakaryocyte development to platelet formation. *J Cell Biol* 201:785, 2013.
6. Junt T, Schulze H, Chen Z, et al: Dynamic visualization of thrombopoiesis within bone marrow. *Science* 317:1767, 2007.
7. Harker LA, Finch CA: Thrombokinetics in man. *J Clin Invest* 48:963, 1969.
8. Machlus KR, Italiano JE Jr: The incredible journey: From megakaryocyte development to platelet formation. *J Cell Biol* 201:785, 2013.
9. Tronik-Le Roux D, Roullot V, Schweitzer A, et al: Suppression of erythro-megakaryocytopoiesis and the induction of reversible thrombocytopenia in mice transgenic for the thymidine kinase gene targeted by the platelet glycoprotein alpha IIb promoter. *J Exp Med* 181:2141, 1995.
10. Debili N, Robin C, Schiavon V, et al: Different expression of CD41 on human lymphoid and myeloid progenitors from adults and neonates. *Blood* 97:2023, 2001.
11. Wu G, Essex DW, Meloni FJ, et al: Human endothelial cells in culture and *in vivo* express on their surface all four components of the glycoprotein Ib/IX/V complex. *Blood* 90:2660, 1997.
12. Hickey MJ, Hagen FS, Yagi M, Roth GJ: Human platelet glycoprotein V: Characterization of the polypeptide and the related Ib-V-IX receptor system of adhesive, leucine-rich glycoproteins. *Proc Natl Acad Sci U S A* 90:8327, 1993.
13. Kahn ML, Diacovo TG, Bainton DF, et al: Glycoprotein V-deficient platelets have undiminished thrombin responsiveness and do not exhibit a Bernard-Soulier phenotype. *Blood* 94:4112, 1999.
14. Lopez JA, Andrews RK, Afshar-Kharghan V, Berndt MC: Bernard-Soulier syndrome. *Blood* 91:4397, 1998.
15. Ramakrishnan V, DeGuzman F, Bao M, et al: A thrombin receptor function for platelet glycoprotein Ib-IX unmasked by cleavage of glycoprotein V. *Proc Natl Acad Sci U S A* 98:1823, 2001.
16. Breton-Gorius J, Reyes F: Ultrastructure of human bone marrow cell maturation. *Int Rev Cytol* 46:251, 1976.
17. Italiano JE Jr, Shivdasani RA: Megakaryocytes and beyond: The birth of platelets. *J Thromb Haemost* 1:1174, 2003.
18. Ebbe S, Stohlman F Jr: Megakaryocytopoiesis in the rat. *Blood* 26:20, 1965.
19. Vitrat N, Cohen-Solal K, Pique C, et al: Endomitosis of human megakaryocytes are due to abortive mitosis. *Blood* 91:3711, 1998.
20. Odell TT Jr, Reiter RS: Generation cycle of rat megakaryocytes. *Exp Cell Res* 53:321, 1968.
21. Tijssen MR, Ghevaert C: Transcription factors in late megakaryopoiesis and related platelet disorders. *J Thromb Haemost* 11:593, 2013.
22. Bastian LS, Kwiatkowski BA, Breininger J, et al: Regulation of the megakaryocytic glycoprotein IX promoter by the oncogenic Ets transcription factor Fli-1. *Blood* 93:2637, 1999.
23. Ramachandran B, Surrey S, Schwartz E: Megakaryocyte-specific positive regulatory sequence 5′ to the human PF4 gene. *Exp Hematol* 23:49, 1995.
24. Furihata K, Kunicki TJ: Characterization of human glycoprotein VI gene 5′ regulatory and promoter regions. *Arterioscler Thromb Vasc Biol* 22:1733, 2002.
25. Sevinsky JR, Whalen AM, Ahn NG: Extracellular signal-regulated kinase induces the megakaryocyte GPIIb/CD41 gene through MafB/Kreisler. *Mol Cell Biol* 24:4534, 2004.
26. Rojnuckarin P, Drachman JG, Kaushansky K: Thrombopoietin-induced activation of the mitogen-activated protein kinase (MAPK) pathway in normal megakaryocytes: Role in endomitosis. *Blood* 94:1273, 1999.
27. Vyas P, Norris FA, Joseph R, et al: Inositol polyphosphate 4-phosphatase type I regulates cell growth downstream of transcription factor GATA-1. *Proc Natl Acad Sci U S A* 97:13696, 2000.
28. Pevny L, Simon MC, Robertson E, et al: Erythroid differentiation in chimaeric mice blocked by a targeted mutation in the gene for transcription factor GATA-1. *Nature* 349:257, 1991.
29. Shivdasani RA, Fujiwara Y, McDevitt MA, Orkin SH: A lineage-selective knockout establishes the critical role of transcription factor GATA-1 in megakaryocyte growth and platelet development. *EMBO J* 16:3965, 1997.
30. Song WJ, Sullivan MG, Legare RD, et al: Haploinsufficiency of CBFA2 causes familial thrombocytopenia with propensity to develop acute myelogenous leukaemia. *Nat Genet* 23:166, 1999.
31. Ichikawa M, Asai T, Saito T, et al: AML-1 is required for megakaryocytic maturation and lymphocytic differentiation, but not for maintenance of hematopoietic stem cells in adult hematopoiesis. *Nat Med* 10:299, 2004.
32. Elagib KE, Racke FK, Mogass M, et al: RUNX1 and GATA-1 coexpression and cooperation in megakaryocytic differentiation. *Blood* 101:4333, 2003.
33. Ebbe S, Phalen E, Stohlman F Jr: Abnormalities of megakaryocytes in W-WV mice. *Blood* 42:857, 1973.
34. Broudy VC, Lin NL, Kaushansky K: Thrombopoietin (c-mpl ligand) acts synergistically with erythropoietin, stem cell factor, and interleukin-11 to enhance murine megakaryocyte colony growth and increases megakaryocyte ploidy *in vitro*. *Blood* 85:1719, 1995.
35. Gainsford T, Roberts AW, Kimura S, et al: Cytokine production and function in cmpl–deficient mice: No physiologic role for interleukin-3 in residual megakaryocyte and platelet production. *Blood* 91:2745, 1998.
36. Kaushansky K, Broudy VC, Lin N, et al: Thrombopoietin, the Mp1 ligand, is essential for full megakaryocyte development. *Proc Natl Acad Sci U S A* 92:3234, 1995.
37. Hodohara K, Fujii N, Yamamoto N, Kaushansky K: Stromal cell-derived factor-1 (SDF-1) acts together with thrombopoietin to enhance the development of megakaryocytic progenitor cells (CFU-MK). *Blood* 95:769, 2000.

38. Avecilla ST, Hattori K, Heissig B, et al: Chemokine-mediated interaction of hematopoietic progenitors with the bone marrow vascular niche is required for thrombopoiesis. *Nat Med* 10:64, 2004.

39. Geddis AE, Fox NE, Kaushansky K: Phosphatidylinositol 3-kinase is necessary but not sufficient for thrombopoietin-induced proliferation in engineered Mp1-bearing cell lines as well as in primary megakaryocytic progenitors. *J Biol Chem* 276:34473, 2001.

40. Miyazaki R, Ogata H, Kobayashi Y: Requirement of thrombopoietin-induced activation of ERK for megakaryocyte differentiation and of p38 for erythroid differentiation. *Ann Hematol* 80:284, 2001.

41. Pettiford SM, Herbst R: The protein tyrosine phosphatase HePTP regulates nuclear translocation of ERK2 and can modulate megakaryocytic differentiation of K562 cells. *Leukemia* 17:366, 2003.

42. Dorsey JF, Cunnick JM, Mane SM, Wu J: Regulation of the Erk2-Elk1 signaling pathway and megakaryocytic differentiation of Bcr-Abl(+) K562 leukemic cells by Gab2. *Blood* 99:1388, 2002.

43. Zhang Y, Nagata Y, Yu G, et al: Aberrant quantity and localization of Aurora-B/AIM-1 and survivin during megakaryocyte polyploidization and the consequences of Aurora-B/AIM-1-deregulated expression. *Blood* 103:3717, 2004.

44. Carow CE, Fox NE, Kaushansky K: Kinetics of endomitosis in primary murine megakaryocytes. *J Cell Physiol* 188:291, 2001.

45. Geddis AE, Kaushansky K: Megakaryocytes express functional aurora kinase B in endomitosis. *Blood* 104:1017, 2004.

46. Geddis AE, Fox NE, Tkachenko E, Kaushansky K: Endomitotic megakaryocytes that form a bipolar spindle exhibit cleavage furrow ingression followed by furrow regression. *Cell Cycle* 6:455, 2007.

47. Suzuki A, Shin JW, Wang Y, et al: RhoA is essential for maintaining normal megakaryocyte ploidy and platelet generation. *PLoS One* 8:e69315, 2013.

48. Gao Y, Smith E, Ker E, et al: Role of RhoA-specific guanine exchange factors in regulation of endomitosis in megakaryocytes. *Dev Cell* 22:573, 2012.

49. Seri M, Cusano R, Gangarossa S, et al: Mutations in MYH9 result in the May-Hegglin anomaly, and Fechtner and Sebastian syndromes. The May-Hegglin/Fechtner Syndrome Consortium. *Nat Genet* 26:103, 2000.

50. Hartwig J, Italiano J Jr: The birth of the platelet. *J Thromb Haemost* 1:1580, 2003.

51. Visvader JE, Elefanty AG, Strasser A, Adams JM: GATA-1 but not SCL induces megakaryocytic differentiation in an early myeloid line. *EMBO J* 11:4557, 1992.

52. Huizing M, Parkes JM, Helip-Wooley A, White JG, Gahl WA: Platelet alpha granules in BLOC-2 and BLOC-3 subtypes of Hermansky-Pudlak syndrome. *Platelets* 18:150, 2007.

53. Tavassoli M, Aoki M: Localization of megakaryocytes in the bone marrow. *Blood Cells* 15:3, 1989.

54. Andrews NC, Erdjument-Bromage H, Davidson MB, et al: Erythroid transcription factor NF-E2 is a haematopoietic-specific basic-leucine zipper protein. *Nature* 362:722, 1993.

55. Bean TL, Ney PA: Multiple regions of p45 NF-E2 are required for beta-globin gene expression in erythroid cells. *Nucleic Acids Res* 25:2509, 1997.

56. Shivdasani RA, Rosenblatt MF, Zucker-Franklin D, et al: Transcription factor NF-E2 is required for platelet formation independent of the actions of thrombopoietin/MGDF in megakaryocyte development. *Cell* 81:695, 1995.

57. Querfurth E, Schuster M, Kulessa H, et al: Antagonism between C/EBPbeta and FOG in eosinophil lineage commitment of multipotent hematopoietic progenitors. *Genes Dev* 14:2515, 2000.

58. Tijssen MR, Ghevaert C: Transcription factors in late megakaryopoiesis and related platelet disorders. *J Thromb Haemost* 11:593, 2013.

59. Howell WH, Donahue DD: The production of blood platelets in the lungs. *J Exp Med* 65:177, 1939.

60. Slater DN, Trowbridge EA, Martin JF: The megakaryocyte in thrombocytopenia: A microscopic study which supports the theory that platelets are produced in the pulmonary circulation. *Thromb Res* 31:163, 1983.

61. Kaushansky K, Lok S, Holly RD, et al: Promotion of megakaryocyte progenitor expansion and differentiation by the c-Mpl ligand thrombopoietin. *Nature* 369:568, 1994.

62. Kaufman RM, Airo R, Pollack S, et al: Origin of pulmonary megakaryocytes. *Blood* 25:767, 1965.

63. Harker LA, Marzec UM, Kelly AB: Effects of Mpl ligands on platelet production and function in nonhuman primates. *Stem Cells* 16(Suppl 2):107, 1998.

64. Choi ES, Nichol JL, Hokom MM, et al: Platelets generated *in vitro* from proplatelet-displaying human megakaryocytes are functional. *Blood* 85:402, 1995.

65. Norol F, Vitrat N, Cramer E, et al: Effects of cytokines on platelet production from blood and marrow CD34+ cells. *Blood* 91:830, 1998.

66. Rojnuckarin P, Kaushansky K: Actin reorganization and proplatelet formation in murine megakaryocytes: The role of protein kinase C alpha. *Blood* 97:154, 2001.

67. Ishida Y, Yano K, Ito T, et al: Purification of proplatelet formation (PPF) stimulating factor: Thrombin/antithrombin III complex stimulates PPF of megakaryocytes in vitro and platelet production *in vivo*. *Thromb Haemost* 85:349, 2001.

68. Hunt P, Hokom MM, Wiemann B, et al: Megakaryocyte proplatelet-like process formation *in vitro* is inhibited by serum prothrombin, a process which is blocked by matrix-bound glycosaminoglycans. *Exp Hematol* 21:372, 1993.

69. Geddis AE, Kaushansky K: Inherited thrombocytopenias: Toward a molecular understanding of disorders of platelet production. *Curr Opin Pediatr* 16:15, 2004.

70. Eckly A, Strassel C, Freund M, et al: Abnormal megakaryocyte morphology and proplatelet formation in mice with megakaryocyte-restricted MYH9 inactivation. *Blood* 113(14):3182, 2009.

71. De Botton S, Sabri S, Daugas E, et al: Platelet formation is the consequence of caspase activation within megakaryocytes. *Blood* 100:1310, 2002.

72. Quesenberry PJ, Ihle JN, McGrath E: The effect of interleukin 3 and GM-CSA-2 on megakaryocyte and myeloid clonal colony formation. *Blood* 65:214, 1985.

73. Kaushansky K, O'Hara PJ, Berkner K, et al: Genomic cloning, characterization, and multilineage growth-promoting activity of human granulocyte-macrophage colony-stimulating factor. *Proc Natl Acad Sci U S A* 83:3101, 1986.

74. Briddell RA, Bruno E, Cooper RJ, et al: Effect of c-kit ligand on *in vitro* human megakaryocytopoiesis. *Blood* 78:2854, 1991.

75. Kaushansky K: Thrombopoietin: The primary regulator of platelet production. *Blood* 86:419, 1995.

76. Yang YC, Ciarletta AB, Temple PA, et al: Human IL-3 (multi-CSF): Identification by expression cloning of a novel hematopoietic growth factor related to murine IL-3. *Cell* 47:3, 1986.

77. Wong GG, Witek JS, Temple PA, et al: Human GM-CSF: Molecular cloning of the complementary DNA and purification of the natural and recombinant proteins. *Science* 228:810, 1985.

78. Feng Y, Klein BK, Vu L, et al: 1H 13C, and 15N NMR resonance assignments, secondary structure, and backbone topology of a variant of human interleukin-3. *Biochemistry* 34:6540, 1995.

79. Lopez AF, Eglinton JM, Gillis D, et al: Reciprocal inhibition of binding between interleukin 3 and granulocyte-macrophage colony-stimulating factor to human eosinophils. *Proc Natl Acad Sci U S A* 86:7022, 1989.

80. Scott CL, Robb L, Mansfield R, et al: Granulocyte-macrophage colony-stimulating factor is not responsible for residual thrombopoiesis in Mpl null mice. *Exp Hematol* 28:1001, 2000.

81. Chen Q, Solar G, Eaton DL, de Sauvage FJ: IL-3 does not contribute to platelet production in c-Mpl–deficient mice. *Stem Cells* 16(Suppl 2):31, 1998.

82. Kishimoto T: The biology of interleukin-6. *Blood* 74:1, 1989.

83. Quesenberry PJ, McGrath HE, Williams ME, et al: Multifactor stimulation of megakaryocytopoiesis: Effects of interleukin 6. *Exp Hematol* 19:35, 1991.

84. Williams N, De Giorgio T, Banu N, et al: Recombinant interleukin 6 stimulates immature murine megakaryocytes. *Exp Hematol* 18:69, 1990.

85. Mei RL, Burstein SA: Megakaryocytic maturation in murine long-term bone marrow culture: Role of interleukin-6. *Blood* 78:1438, 1991.

86. Ishibashi T, Kimura H, Shikama Y, et al: Interleukin-6 is a potent thrombopoietic factor *in vivo* in mice. *Blood* 74:1241, 1989.

87. Asano S, Okano A, Ozawa K, et al: *In vivo* effects of recombinant human interleukin-6 in primates: Stimulated production of platelets. *Blood* 75:1602, 1990.

88. van Gameren MM, Willemse PH, Mulder NH, et al: Effects of recombinant human interleukin-6 in cancer patients: A phase I–II study. *Blood* 84:1434, 1994.

89. Blay JY, Favrot M, Rossi JF, Wijdenes J: Role of interleukin-6 in paraneoplastic thrombocytosis. *Blood* 82:2261, 1993.

90. Bernad A, Kopf M, Kulbacki R, et al: Interleukin-6 is required *in vivo* for the regulation of stem cells and committed progenitors of the hematopoietic system. *Immunity* 1:725, 1994.

91. Kaser A, Brandacher G, Steurer W, et al: Interleukin-6 stimulates thrombopoiesis through thrombopoietin: Role in inflammatory thrombocytosis. *Blood* 98:2720, 2001.

92. Du X, Williams DA: Interleukin-11: Review of molecular, cell biology, and clinical use. *Blood* 89:3897, 1997.

93. Gough NM: Molecular genetics of leukemia inhibitory factor (LIF) and its receptor. *Growth Factors* 7:175, 1992.

94. Hilton DJ: LIF: Lots of interesting functions. *Trends Biochem Sci* 17:72, 1992.

95. Debili N, Masse JM, Katz A, et al: Effects of the recombinant hematopoietic growth factors interleukin-3, interleukin-6, stem cell factor, and leukemia inhibitory factor on the megakaryocytic differentiation of CD34+ cells. *Blood* 82:84, 1993.

96. Teramura M, Kobayashi S, Hoshino S, et al: Interleukin-11 enhances human megakaryocytopoiesis *in vitro*. *Blood* 79:327, 1992.

97. Metcalf D, Nicola NA, Gearing DP: Effects of injected leukemia inhibitory factor on hematopoietic and other tissues in mice. *Blood* 76:50, 1990.

98. Neben TY, Loebelenz J, Hayes L, et al: Recombinant human interleukin-11 stimulates megakaryocytopoiesis and increases peripheral platelets in normal and splenectomized mice. *Blood* 81:901, 1993.

99. Farese AM, Myers LA, MacVittie TJ: Therapeutic efficacy of recombinant human leukemia inhibitory factor in a primate model of radiation-induced marrow aplasia. *Blood* 84:3675, 1994.

100. Gordon MS, McCaskill-Stevens WJ, Battiato LA, et al: A phase I trial of recombinant human interleukin-11 (Neumega rhIL-11 growth factor) in women with breast cancer receiving chemotherapy. *Blood* 87:3615, 1996.

101. Nandurkar HH, Robb L, Tarlinton D, et al: Adult mice with targeted mutation of the interleukin-11 receptor (IL11Ra) display normal hematopoiesis. *Blood* 90:2148, 1997.

102. Gainsford T, Nandurkar H, Metcalf D, et al: The residual megakaryocyte and platelet production in c-Mpl–deficient mice is not dependent on the actions of interleukin-6, interleukin-11, or leukemia inhibitory factor. *Blood* 95:528, 2000.

103. Lyman SD, James L, Vanden Bos T, et al: Molecular cloning of a ligand for the flt3/flk-2 tyrosine kinase receptor: A proliferative factor for primitive hematopoietic cells. *Cell* 75:1157, 1993.

104. Avraham H, Vannier E, Cowley S, et al: Effects of the stem cell factor, c-kit ligand, on human megakaryocytic cells. *Blood* 79:365, 1992.

105. Ebbe S, Phalen E, Stohlman F Jr: Abnormalities of megakaryocytes in S1-S1d mice. *Blood* 42:865, 1973.
106. Arnold J, Ellis S, Radley JM, Williams N: Compensatory mechanisms in platelet production: The response of Sl/Sld mice to 5-fluorouracil. *Exp Hematol* 19:24, 1991.
107. Hunt P, Zsebo KM, Hokom MM, et al: Evidence that stem cell factor is involved in the rebound thrombocytosis that follows 5-fluorouracil treatment. *Blood* 80:904, 1992.
108. Broudy VC: Stem cell factor and hematopoiesis. *Blood* 90:1345, 1997.
109. Langley KE, Bennett LG, Wypych J, et al: Soluble stem cell factor in human serum. *Blood* 81:656, 1993.
110. Cheng HJ, Flanagan JG: Transmembrane kit ligand cleavage does not require a signal in the cytoplasmic domain and occurs at a site dependent on spacing from the membrane. *Mol Biol Cell* 5:943, 1994.
111. Miyazawa K, Williams DA, Gotoh A, et al: Membrane-bound Steel factor induces more persistent tyrosine kinase activation and longer life span of c-kit gene-encoded protein than its soluble form. *Blood* 85:641, 1995.
112. Flanagan JG, Chan DC, Leder P: Transmembrane form of the kit ligand growth factor is determined by alternative splicing and is missing in the Sld mutant. *Cell* 64:1025, 1991.
113. Lyman SD, Jacobsen SE: C-kit ligand and Flt3 ligand: Stem/progenitor cell factors with overlapping yet distinct activities. *Blood* 91:1101, 1998.
114. Ramsfjell V, Borge OJ, Veiby OP, et al: Thrombopoietin, but not erythropoietin, directly stimulates multilineage growth of primitive murine bone marrow progenitor cells in synergy with early acting cytokines: Distinct interactions with the ligands for c-kit and FLT3. *Blood* 88:4481, 1996.
115. Piacibello W, Garetto L, Sanavio F, et al: The effects of human FLT3 ligand on *in vitro* human megakaryocytopoiesis. *Exp Hematol* 24:340, 1996.
116. Brasel K, McKenna HJ, Morrissey PJ, et al: Hematologic effects of flt3 ligand *in vivo* in mice. *Blood* 88:2004, 1996.
117. Kelemen E, Cserhati I, Tanos B: Demonstration and some properties of human thrombopoietin in thrombocythemic sera. *Acta Haematol* 20:350, 1958.
118. Wendling F, Varlet P, Charon M, Tambourin P: MPLV: A retrovirus complex inducing an acute myeloproliferative leukemic disorder in adult mice. *Virology* 149:242, 1986.
119. Souyri M, Vigon I, Penciolelli JF, et al: A putative truncated cytokine receptor gene transduced by the myeloproliferative leukemia virus immortalizes hematopoietic progenitors. *Cell* 63:1137, 1990.
120. Vigon I, Mornon JP, Cocault L, et al: Molecular cloning and characterization of MPL, the human homolog of the v-Mpl oncogene: Identification of a member of the hematopoietic growth factor receptor super-family. *Proc Natl Acad Sci U S A* 89:5640, 1992.
121. Cosman D: The hematopoietin receptor superfamily. *Cytokine* 5:95, 1993.
122. Skoda RC, Seldin DC, Chiang MK, et al: Murine c-Mpl: A member of the hematopoietic growth factor receptor superfamily that transduces a proliferative signal. *EMBO J* 12:2645, 1993.
123. Lok S, Kaushansky K, Holly RD, et al: Cloning and expression of murine thrombopoietin cDNA and stimulation of platelet production *in vivo*. *Nature* 369:565, 1994.
124. Linden HM, Kaushansky K: The glycan domain of thrombopoietin enhances its secretion. *Biochemistry* 39:3044, 2000.
125. Basser RL, Rasko JE, Clarke K, et al: Thrombopoietic effects of pegylated recombinant human megakaryocyte growth and development factor (PEG-rHuMGDF) in patients with advanced cancer. *Lancet* 348:1279, 1996.
126. Kaushansky K, Broudy VC, Grossmann A, et al: Thrombopoietin expands erythroid progenitors, increases red cell production, and enhances erythroid recovery after myelosuppressive therapy. *J Clin Invest* 96:1683, 1995.
127. Farese AM, Hunt P, Boone T, MacVittie TJ: Recombinant human megakaryocyte growth and development factor stimulates thrombocytopoiesis in normal nonhuman primates. *Blood* 86:54, 1995.
128. Akahori H, Shibuya K, Obuchi M, et al: Effect of recombinant human thrombopoietin in nonhuman primates with chemotherapy-induced thrombocytopenia. *Br J Haematol* 94:722, 1996.
129. Neelis KJ, Hartong SC, Egeland T, et al: The efficacy of single-dose administration of thrombopoietin with coadministration of either granulocyte/macrophage or granulocyte colony-stimulating factor in myelosuppressed rhesus monkeys. *Blood* 90:2565, 1997.
130. Gurney AL, Carver-Moore K, de Sauvage FJ, Moore MW: Thrombocytopenia in c-Mpl–deficient mice. *Science* 265:1445, 1994.
131. van den Oudenrijn S, Bruin M, Folman CC, et al: Mutations in the thrombopoietin receptor, Mpl, in children with congenital amegakaryocytic thrombocytopenia. *Br J Haematol* 110:441, 2000.
132. Ballmaier M, Germeshausen M, Schulze H, et al: C-mpl mutations are the cause of congenital amegakaryocytic thrombocytopenia. *Blood* 97:139, 2001.
133. Sohma Y, Akahori H, Seki N, et al: Molecular cloning and chromosomal localization of the human thrombopoietin gene. *FEBS Lett* 353:57, 1994.
134. Morris D: *Cis*-Acting mRNA structures in gene-specific translational control, in *Post-Transcriptional Gene Regulation*, edited by JB Harford, DR Morris, p 165. Wiley-Liss, New York, 1997.
135. Wiestner A, Schlemper RJ, Van der Maas AP, Skoda RC: An activating splice donor mutation in the thrombopoietin gene causes hereditary thrombocythaemia. *Nat Genet* 18:49, 1998.
136. Jorgensen MJ, Raskind WH, Wolff JF, et al: Familial thrombocytosis associated with overproduction of thrombopoietin due to a novel splice donor site mutation. *Blood* 92:205a, 1998.
137. Kondo T, Okabe M, Sanada M, et al: Familial essential thrombocythemia associated with one-base deletion in the 5′-untranslated region of the thrombopoietin gene. *Blood* 92:1091, 1998.
138. Ghilardi N, Wiestner A, Kikuchi M, et al: Hereditary thrombocythaemia in a Japanese family is caused by a novel point mutation in the thrombopoietin gene. *Br J Haematol* 107:310, 1999.
139. Cazzola M, Skoda RC: Translational pathophysiology: A novel molecular mechanism of human disease. *Blood* 95:3280, 2000.
140. Odell TT Jr, McDonald TP, Detwiler TC: Stimulation of platelet production by serum of platelet-depleted rats. *Proc Soc Exp Biol Med* 108:428, 1961.
141. Nichol JL, Hokom MM, Hornkohl A, et al: Megakaryocyte growth and development factor. Analyses of in vitro effects on human megakaryopoiesis and endogenous serum levels during chemotherapy-induced thrombocytopenia. *J Clin Invest* 95:2973, 1995.
142. Kuter DJ, Rosenberg RD: The reciprocal relationship of thrombopoietin (c-Mpl ligand) to changes in the platelet mass during busulfan-induced thrombocytopenia in the rabbit. *Blood* 85:2720, 1995.
143. Bartocci A, Mastrogiannis DS, Migliorati G, et al: Macrophages specifically regulate the concentration of their own growth factor in the circulation. *Proc Natl Acad Sci U S A* 84:6179, 1987.
144. Emmons RV, Reid DM, Cohen RL, et al: Human thrombopoietin levels are high when thrombocytopenia is due to megakaryocyte deficiency and low when due to increased platelet destruction. *Blood* 87:4068, 1996.
145. McCarty JM, Sprugel KH, Fox NE, et al: Murine thrombopoietin mRNA levels are modulated by platelet count. *Blood* 86:3668, 1995.
146. de Sauvage FJ, Carver-Moore K, Luoh SM, et al: Physiological regulation of early and late stages of megakaryocytopoiesis by thrombopoietin. *J Exp Med* 183:651, 1996.
147. Sungaran R, Markovic B, Chong BH: Localization and regulation of thrombopoietin mRNA expression in human kidney, liver, bone marrow, and spleen using in situ hybridization. *Blood* 89:101, 1997.
148. McIntosh B, Kaushansky K: Marrow stromal production of thrombopoietin is regulated by transcriptional mechanisms in response to platelet products. *Exp Hematol* 36:799, 2008.
149. Solanilla A, Dechanet J, El Andaloussi A, et al: CD40-ligand stimulates myelopoiesis by regulating flt3-ligand and thrombopoietin production in bone marrow stromal cells. *Blood* 95:3758, 2000.
150. Sungaran R, Chisholm OT, Markovic B, et al: The role of platelet alpha-granular proteins in the regulation of thrombopoietin messenger RNA expression in human bone marrow stromal cells. *Blood* 95:3094, 2000.
151. Kamura T, Handa H, Hamasaki N, Kitajima S: Characterization of the human thrombopoietin gene promoter. A possible role of an Ets transcription factor, E4TF1/GABP. *J Biol Chem* 272:11361, 1997.
152. Chang MS, McNinch J, Basu R, et al: Cloning and characterization of the human megakaryocyte growth and development factor (MGDF) gene. *J Biol Chem* 270:511, 1995.
153. Rollins BJ: Chemokines. *Blood* 90:909, 1997.
154. Broxmeyer HE, Mantel CR, Aronica SM: Biology and mechanisms of action of synergistically stimulated myeloid progenitor cell proliferation and suppression by chemokines. *Stem Cells* 15(Suppl 1):69, discussion 15(Suppl 1):78, 1997.
155. Shirozu M, Nakano T, Inazawa J, et al: Structure and chromosomal localization of the human stromal cell-derived factor 1 (SDF1) gene. *Genomics* 28:495, 1995.
156. Luster AD: Chemokines—Chemotactic cytokines that mediate inflammation. *N Engl J Med* 338:436, 1998.
157. Nagasawa T, Hirota S, Tachibana K, et al: Defects of B-cell lymphopoiesis and bone-marrow myelopoiesis in mice lacking the CXC chemokine PBSF/SDF-1. *Nature* 382:635, 1996.
158. Ma Q, Jones D, Borghesani PR, et al: Impaired B-lymphopoiesis, myelopoiesis, and derailed cerebellar neuron migration in CXCR4- and SDF-1-deficient mice. *Proc Natl Acad Sci U S A* 95:9448, 1998.
159. Aiuti A, Webb IJ, Bleul C, et al: The chemokine SDF-1 is a chemoattractant for human CD34+ hematopoietic progenitor cells and provides a new mechanism to explain the mobilization of CD34+ progenitors to peripheral blood. *J Exp Med* 185:111, 1997.
160. Wang JF, Liu ZY, Groopman JE: The alpha-chemokine receptor CXCR4 is expressed on the megakaryocytic lineage from progenitor to platelets and modulates migration and adhesion. *Blood* 92:756, 1998.
161. Hamada T, Mohle R, Hesselgesser J, et al: Transendothelial migration of megakaryocytes in response to stromal cell-derived factor 1 (SDF-1) enhances platelet formation. *J Exp Med* 188:539, 1998.
162. Daopin S, Piez KA, Ogawa Y, Davies DR: Crystal structure of transforming growth factor-beta 2: An unusual fold for the superfamily. *Science* 257:369, 1992.
163. Keller JR, Mantel C, Sing GK, et al: Transforming growth factor beta 1 selectively regulates early murine hematopoietic progenitors and inhibits the growth of IL-3-dependent myeloid leukemia cell lines. *J Exp Med* 168:737, 1988.
164. Dybedal I, Jacobsen SE: Transforming growth factor beta (TGF-beta), a potent inhibitor of erythropoiesis: Neutralizing TGF-beta antibodies show erythropoietin as a potent stimulator of murine burst-forming unit erythroid colony formation in the absence of a burst-promoting activity. *Blood* 86:949, 1995.
165. Ishibashi T, Miller SL, Burstein SA: Type beta transforming growth factor is a potent inhibitor of murine megakaryocytopoiesis *in vitro*. *Blood* 69:1737, 1987.
166. Kuter DJ, Gminski DM, Rosenberg RD: Transforming growth factor beta inhibits megakaryocyte growth and endomitosis. *Blood* 79:619, 1992.

167. Laiho M, DeCaprio JA, Ludlow JW, et al: Growth inhibition by TGF-beta linked to suppression of retinoblastoma protein phosphorylation. *Cell* 62:175, 1990.
168. Polyak K, Kato JY, Solomon MJ, et al: P27Kip1, a cyclin-Cdk inhibitor, links transforming growth factor-beta and contact inhibition to cell cycle arrest. *Genes Dev* 8:9, 1994.
169. Teofili L, Martini M, Di Mario A, et al: Expression of p15(ink4b) gene during megakaryocytic differentiation of normal and myelodysplastic hematopoietic progenitors. *Blood* 98:495, 2001.
170. Theofilopoulos AN, Baccala R, Beutler B, Kono DH: Type I interferons (alpha/beta) in immunity and autoimmunity. *Annu Rev Immunol* 23:307, 2005.
171. Broxmeyer HE, Cooper S, Rubin BY, Taylor MW: The synergistic influence of human interferon-gamma and interferon-alpha on suppression of hematopoietic progenitor cells is additive with the enhanced sensitivity of these cells to inhibition by interferons at low oxygen tension *in vitro*. *J Immunol* 135:2502, 1985.
172. Fattovich G, Giustina G, Favarato S, Ruol A: A survey of adverse events in 11,241 patients with chronic viral hepatitis treated with alfa interferon. *J Hepatol* 24:38, 1996.
173. Dusheiko G: Side effects of alpha interferon in chronic hepatitis C. *Hepatology* 26(Suppl 1):112S, 1997.
174. Jaster R, Tschirch E, Bittorf T, Brock J: Interferon-alpha inhibits proliferation of Ba/F3 cells by interfering with interleukin-3 action. *Cell Signal* 11:769, 1999.
175. Kuniyasu H, Yasui W, Kitahara K, et al: Growth inhibitory effect of interferon-beta is associated with the induction of cyclin-dependent kinase inhibitor p27Kip1 in a human gastric carcinoma cell line. *Cell Growth Differ* 8:47, 1997.
176. Wang Q, Miyakawa Y, Fox N, Kaushansky K: Interferon-alpha directly represses megakaryopoiesis by inhibiting thrombopoietin-induced signaling through induction of SOCS-1. *Blood* 96:2093, 2000.
177. Long MW: Blood cell cytoadhesion molecules. *Exp Hematol* 20:288, 1992.
178. Toksoz D, Zsebo KM, Smith KA, et al: Support of human hematopoiesis in long-term bone marrow cultures by murine stromal cells selectively expressing the membrane-bound and secreted forms of the human homolog of the steel gene product, stem cell factor. *Proc Natl Acad Sci U S A* 89:7350, 1992.
179. Yang L, Yang YC: Regulation of interleukin (IL)-11 gene expression in IL-1 induced primate bone marrow stromal cells. *J Biol Chem* 269:32732, 1994.
180. Linenberger ML, Jacobson FW, Bennett LG, et al: Stem cell factor production by human marrow stromal fibroblasts. *Exp Hematol* 23:1104, 1995.
181. Gordon MY, Riley GP, Watt SM, Greaves MF: Compartmentalization of a haematopoietic growth factor (GM-CSF) by glycosaminoglycans in the bone marrow microenvironment. *Nature* 326:403, 1987.
182. Roberts R, Gallagher J, Spooncer E, et al: Heparan sulphate bound growth factors: A mechanism for stromal cell mediated haemopoiesis. *Nature* 332:376, 1988.
183. Artavanis-Tsakonas S, Matsuno K, Fortini ME: Notch signaling. *Science* 268:225, 1995.
184. Karanu FN, Murdoch B, Miyabayashi T, et al: Human homologues of Delta-1 and Delta-4 function as mitogenic regulators of primitive human hematopoietic cells. *Blood* 97:1960, 2001.
185. Lam LT, Ronchini C, Norton J, et al: Suppression of erythroid but not megakaryocytic differentiation of human K562 erythroleukemic cells by notch-1. *J Biol Chem* 275:19676, 2000.
186. Fox NE, Kaushansky K: Engagement of integrin a4b1 enhances thrombopoietin-induced megakaryopoiesis. *Exp Hematol* 33:94, 2005.
187. Bruno E, Briddell RA, Cooper RJ, Hoffman R: Effects of recombinant interleukin 11 on human megakaryocyte progenitor cells. *Exp Hematol* 19:378, 1991.
188. Neben S, Turner K: The biology of interleukin 11. *Stem Cells* 11(Suppl 2):156, 1993.
189. Burstein SA, Mei RL, Henthorn J, et al: Leukemia inhibitory factor and interleukin-11 promote maturation of murine and human megakaryocytes *in vitro*. *J Cell Physiol* 153:305, 1992.
190. Yonemura Y, Kawakita M, Masuda T, et al: Synergistic effects of interleukin 3 and interleukin 11 on murine megakaryopoiesis in serum-free culture. *Exp Hematol* 20:1011, 1992.
191. Yonemura Y, Kawakita M, Masuda T, et al: Effect of recombinant human interleukin-11 on rat megakaryopoiesis and thrombopoiesis *in vivo*: Comparative study with interleukin-6. *Br J Haematol* 84:16, 1993.
192. Schlerman FJ, Bree AG, Kaviani MD, et al: Thrombopoietic activity of recombinant human interleukin 11 (rHuIL-11) in normal and myelosuppressed nonhuman primates. *Stem Cells* 14:517, 1996.
193. Gordon MS, McCaskill-Stevens W, Battiato L, et al: The *in vivo* effects of subcutaneously (SC) administered recombinant human interleukin-11 (neumega rhIL-11 growth factor; rhIL-11) in women with breast cancer (BC). *Blood* 82(Suppl 1):498a, 1993.
194. Champlin RE, Mehra R, Kaye JA: Recombinant human interleukin eleven (rhIL-11) following autologous BMT for breast cancer. *Blood* 84(suppl 1):395a, 1994.
195. Tepler I, Elias L, Smith JW 2nd, et al: A randomized placebo-controlled trial of recombinant human interleukin-11 in cancer patients with severe thrombocytopenia due to chemotherapy. *Blood* 87:3607, 1996.
196. Isaacs C, Robert NJ, Bailey FA, et al: Randomized placebo-controlled study of recombinant human interleukin-11 to prevent chemotherapy-induced thrombocytopenia in patients with breast cancer receiving dose-intensive cyclophosphamide and doxorubicin. *J Clin Oncol* 15:3368, 1997.
197. Vredenburgh JJ, Hussein A, Fisher D, et al: A randomized trial of recombinant human interleukin-11 following autologous bone marrow transplantation with peripheral blood progenitor cell support in patients with breast cancer. *Biol Blood Marrow Transplant* 4:134, 1998.
198. Tichelli A, Gratwohl A, Berger C, et al: Treatment of thrombocytosis in myeloproliferative disorders with interferon alpha-2a. *Blut* 58:15, 1989.
199. Gisslinger H, Ludwig H, Linkesch W, et al: Long-term interferon therapy for thrombocytosis in myeloproliferative diseases. *Lancet* 1:634, 1989.
200. Sacchi S, Gugliotta L, Papineschi F, et al: Alfa-interferon in the treatment of essential thrombocythemia: Clinical results and evaluation of its biological effects on the hematopoietic neoplastic clone. Italian Cooperative Group on ET. *Leukemia* 12:289, 1998.
201. Taylor PC, Dolan G, Ng JP, et al: Efficacy of recombinant interferon-alpha (rIFN-alpha) in polycythaemia vera: A study of 17 patients and an analysis of published data. *Br J Haematol* 92:55, 1996.
202. Tornebohm-Roche E, Merup M, Lockner D, Paul C: Alpha-2a interferon therapy and antibody formation in patients with essential thrombocythemia and polycythemia vera with thrombocytosis. *Am J Hematol* 48:163, 1995.
203. Hokom MM, Lacey D, Kinstler OB, et al: Pegylated megakaryocyte growth and development factor abrogates the lethal thrombocytopenia associated with carboplatin and irradiation in mice. *Blood* 86:4486, 1995.
204. Fibbe WE, Heemskerk DP, Laterveer L, et al: Accelerated reconstitution of platelets and erythrocytes after syngeneic transplantation of bone marrow cells derived from thrombopoietin pretreated donor mice. *Blood* 86:3308, 1995.
205. Molineux G, Hartley C, McElroy P, et al: Megakaryocyte growth and development factor accelerates platelet recovery in peripheral blood progenitor cell transplant recipients. *Blood* 88:366, 1996.
206. Fanucchi M, Glaspy J, Crawford J, et al: Effects of polyethylene glycol conjugated recombinant human megakaryocyte growth and development factor on platelet counts after chemotherapy for lung cancer. *N Engl J Med* 336:404, 1997.
207. Vadhan-Raj S, Murray LJ, Bueso-Ramos C, et al: Stimulation of megakaryocyte and platelet production by a single dose of recombinant human thrombopoietin in patients with cancer. *Ann Intern Med* 126:673, 1997.
208. Basser RL, Underhill C, Davis I, et al: Enhancement of platelet recovery after myelosuppressive chemotherapy by recombinant human megakaryocyte growth and development factor in patients with advanced cancer. *J Clin Oncol* 18:2852, 2000.
209. Archimbaud E, Ottmann OG, Yin JA, et al: A randomized, double-blind, placebo-controlled study with pegylated recombinant human megakaryocyte growth and development factor (PEG-rHuMGDF) as an adjunct to chemotherapy for adults with *de novo* acute myeloid leukemia. *Blood* 94:3694, 1999.
210. Bolwell B, Vredenburgh J, Overmoyer B, et al: Phase 1 study of pegylated recombinant human megakaryocyte growth and development factor (PEG-rHuMGDF) in breast cancer patients after autologous peripheral blood progenitor cell (PBPC) transplantation. *Bone Marrow Transplant* 26:141, 2000.
211. Somlo G, Sniecinski I, Ter Veer A, et al: Recombinant human thrombopoietin in combination with granulocyte colony-stimulating factor enhances mobilization of peripheral blood progenitor cells, increases peripheral blood platelet concentration, and accelerates hematopoietic recovery following high-dose chemotherapy. *Blood* 93:2798, 1999.
212. Nomura S, Dan K, Hotta T, et al: Effects of pegylated recombinant human megakaryocyte growth and development factor in patients with idiopathic thrombocytopenic purpura. *Blood* 100:728, 2002.
213. Vadhan-Raj S, Patel S, Bueso-Ramos C, et al: Importance of predosing of recombinant human thrombopoietin to reduce chemotherapy-induced early thrombocytopenia. *J Clin Oncol* 21:3158, 2003.
214. Li J, Yang C, Xia Y, et al: Thrombocytopenia caused by the development of antibodies to thrombopoietin. *Blood* 98:3241, 2001.
215. Kimura T, Kaburaki H, Tsujino T, et al: A non-peptide compound which can mimic the effect of thrombopoietin via c-Mpl. *FEBS Lett* 428:250, 1998.
216. de Serres M, Yeager RL, Dillberger JE, et al: Pharmacokinetics and hematological effects of the PEGylated thrombopoietin peptide mimetic GW395058 in rats and monkeys after intravenous or subcutaneous administration. *Stem Cells* 17:316, 1999.
217. Broudy VC, Lin NL: AMG531 stimulates megakaryopoiesis *in vitro* by binding to Mpl. *Cytokine* 25:52, 2004.
218. Kaushansky K: Hematopoietic growth factor mimetics. *Ann N Y Acad Sci* 938:131, 2001.
219. Kuter DJ, Bussel JB, Lyons RM, et al: Efficacy of romiplostim in patients with chronic immune thrombocytopenic purpura: A double-blind randomised controlled trial. *Lancet* 371:395, 2008.
220. Bussel JB, Cheng G, Saleh MN, et al: Eltrombopag for the treatment of chronic idiopathic thrombocytopenic purpura. *N Engl J Med* 357:2237, 2007.
221. McHutchison JG, Dusheiko G, Shiffman ML, et al: Eltrombopag for thrombocytopenia in patients with cirrhosis associated with hepatitis C. *N Engl J Med* 357:2227, 2007.
222. Qin P, Dong X, Li J, et al: Recombinant human thrombopoietin and rituximab vs. rituximab monotherapy in corticosteroid resistant primary immune thrombocytopenia: A multicenter randomized controlled study. *Blood* 122:329, 2013.
223. Nguyen TT, Palmaro A, Montastruc F, et al: Signal for thrombosis with eltrombopag and romiplostim: A disproportionality analysis of spontaneous reports within VigiBase®. *Drug Safety* 38:1179, 2015.

# CHAPTER 2
# PLATELET MORPHOLOGY, BIOCHEMISTRY, AND FUNCTION

Susan S. Smyth, Sidney Whiteheart, Joseph E. Italiano Jr., Paul Bray, and Barry S. Coller

## SUMMARY

The approximately 1 trillion platelets that circulate in an adult human are small anucleate cell fragments adapted to adhere to damaged blood vessels, to aggregate with one another, and to facilitate the generation of thrombin. These actions contribute to hemostasis by producing a platelet plug and then reinforcing plug strength by the action of thrombin converting fibrinogen to fibrin strands. To accomplish these tasks, platelets have surface receptors that can bind adhesive glycoproteins; these include the GPIb/IX/V complex, which supports platelet adhesion by binding von Willebrand factor, especially under conditions of high shear, and the $a_{IIb}\beta_3$ (GPIIb/IIIa) receptor, which is platelet-specific and mediates platelet aggregation by binding fibrinogen and/or von Willebrand factor. Other receptors for adhesive glycoproteins (integrin $a_2\beta_1$ [GPIa/IIa], GPVI, and perhaps others for collagen; integrin $a_5\beta_1$ [GPIc*/IIa] for fibronectin; integrin $a_6\beta_1$ [GPIc/IIa] for laminin; and CLEC-2 for podoplanin) also contribute to platelet adhesion, but their precise contributions are less well defined. Activated platelets express both surface P-selectin, which mediates interactions with leukocytes, and CD40 ligand, which activates a number of proinflammatory cells, and release chemokines and a soluble form of CD40 ligand, thus initiating an inflammatory reaction. Platelet coagulant activity results from the exposure of negatively charged phospholipids on the surface of platelets and the generation of platelet microparticles, along with release and activation of platelet factor V and perhaps exposure of specific receptors for activated coagulation factor. Platelets change shape with activation as a result of a complex reorganization of the platelet membrane skeleton and cytoskeleton. With activation, platelets undergo release of $a$ granules, dense bodies, and lysosomes, the contents of which work to restore vascular integrity. The activation process involves a number of receptors for agonists such as adenosine diphosphate, epinephrine, thrombin, collagen, thromboxane (TX) A$_2$, vasopressin, serotonin, platelet activating factor, lysophosphatidic acid, sphingosine-1-phosphate, and thrombospondin, as well as several signal transduction pathways, including phosphoinositide metabolism, arachidonic acid release and conversion into TXA$_2$, and phosphorylation of a number of different target proteins. Increases in intracellular calcium result from, and further contribute to, platelet activation. Platelet activation results in a change in the conformation of the integrin $a_{IIb}\beta_3$ receptor, leading to high-affinity ligand binding and platelet aggregation.

Platelets also act as storehouses for a variety of molecules that affect platelet function, inflammation, innate immunity, cell proliferation, vascular tone, fibrinolysis, and wound healing; these agents are actively released upon platelet activation. Other vasoactive and platelet-activating substances are newly synthesized when platelets are activated. Through cooperative biochemical interactions, platelets can communicate with, and are affected by, other blood cells and endothelial cells.

Quantitative and qualitative disorders of platelets produce hemorrhagic diatheses (Chaps. 9 to 12). In pathologic states, uncontrolled platelet thrombus formation can lead to vasoocclusion and ischemic tissue necrosis, as, for example, in myocardial infarction and stroke (Chap. 25). Platelets may also facilitate tumor cell growth and metastasis.

**Acronyms and Abbreviations:** AA, arachidonic acid; ADAM, a disintegrin and metalloprotease; ADMIDAS, adjacent to metal ion-dependent adhesion site; AngII, angiotensin II; APP, amyloid precursor protein; AP3, activator protein 3; BTK, Bruton tyrosine kinase; CIB, calcium and integrin binding protein; CLEC, C-type lectin-like receptor; COX, cyclooxygenase; DAG, diacylglycerol; DTS, dense tubular system; EDTA, ethylenediaminetetraacetic acid; EGF, epidermal growth factor; EMMPRIN, matrix metalloproteinase inducer; ERK, extracellular signal-regulated kinase; FAK, focal adhesion kinase; FOG, friend of GATA; FERM, four point one, ezrin, radixin, and moesin; GAS, growth arrest-specific gene; GP, glycoprotein; GPCR, G-protein–coupled receptor; GPI, glycosylphosphatidylinositol; GSK, glycogen synthase kinase; HDL, high-density lipoprotein; HPETE, hydroxyeicosatetraenoic acid; hTRPC, human canonical transient receptor potential; ICAM, intercellular adhesion molecule; IL, interleukin; IP$_3$, inositol-1,4,5-trisphosphate; ITAM, immunoreceptor tyrosine-based activation motif; ITIM, immunoreceptor tyrosine-based inhibitory motif; ITSM, immunoreceptor tyrosine-based switch motif; JAM, junctional adhesion molecule; LAMP, lysosome-associated membrane protein; LDL, low-density lipoprotein; LIBS, ligand-induced binding site; LIMBS, ligand-associated metal binding site; LOX, lipoxygenase; LPA, lysophosphatidic acid; LPC, lysophosphatidyl choline; LPS, lipopolysaccharide; LT, leukotriene; LX, lipoxin; MAPK, mitogen-activated protein kinase; MIDAS, metal ion-dependent adhesion site; miRNA, microRNA; MLC, myosin light chain; MMP, matrix metalloproteinase; MRP, myeloid-related protein; MVB, multivesicular body; NAP, neutrophil-activating peptide; NET, neutrophil extracellular trap; NMR, nuclear magnetic resonance; NO, nitric oxide; PAF, platelet-activating factor; PAR, protease-activated receptor; PDGF, platelet-derived growth factor; PDI, protein disulfide isomerase; PDZ, postsynaptic density protein (PSD95), *Drosophila* disk large tumor suppressor (Dlg1), and zonula occludens-1 protein (zo-1); PECAM, platelet-endothelial cell adhesion molecule; PG, prostaglandin; PH, pleckstrin homology; PI, phosphoinositol; PIP$_2$, phosphoinositol 4,5-bisphosphate; PIPK, phosphoinositol phosphate kinase; PKC, protein kinase C; PL, phospholipase; PNH, paroxysmal nocturnal hemoglobinuria; PPAR, peroxisome proliferator-activated receptors; PSGL, P-selectin glycoprotein ligand; PTB, phosphotyrosine binding; RIAM, Rap1GTP-interacting adapter molecule; SERT, serotonin transporter; SNP, single nucleotide polymorphism; S1P, sphingosine-1-phosphate; SR, scavenger receptor; STIM, stromal interaction molecule; SyMBS, synergy metal binding site; TFPI, tissue factor pathway inhibitor; TGF, transforming growth factor; TLR, toll-like receptor; TLT, TREM-like transcript; TNF, tumor necrosis factor; TP, thromboxane prostanoid receptor; TRAIL, TNF-related apoptosis-inducing ligand; TREM, triggering receptors expressed on myeloid cells; TSP, thrombospondin; TX, thromboxane; VASP, vasodilator-stimulated protein; VEGF, vascular endothelial growth factor; VWF, von Willebrand factor; WASP, Wiskott-Aldrich syndrome protein.

# OVERVIEW OF PLATELET ADHESION, AGGREGATION, AND PLATELET THROMBUS FORMATION

The hemostatic system is under elaborate control mechanisms lest the response be either inadequate to meet the hemorrhagic challenge or result in inappropriate thrombosis in response to trivial provocation. Evolutionary pressures have probably favored a more active hemostatic system as individuals with more active hemostatic systems were more likely to avoid death from hemorrhage prior to attaining sexual maturity or in association with childbirth. Our active hemostatic system may be less well adapted to our modern age, which is characterized by long life spans and progressive vascular disease, given that the deposition of a platelet-fibrin thrombus on a damaged atherosclerotic plaque is the cause of most myocardial infarctions and many strokes.

The platelet's major function is to seal openings in the vascular tree. It is appropriate, therefore, that the initiating signal for platelet deposition and activation is exposure of underlying portions of the blood vessel wall that are normally concealed from circulating platelets by an intact endothelial lining (Fig. 2–1).[1] Additional parameters that probably control the platelet response are: (1) the depth of injury, with deeper damage exposing more platelet-reactive materials and tissue factor (Chap. 5); (2) the vascular bed, with the blood vessels serving mucocutaneous tissues especially dependent on platelets for hemostasis, in contrast to the vascular beds in muscles and joints, which rely more on the coagulation mechanism; (3) the age of the individual, because the composition of the blood vessel wall probably changes with age; (4) the hematocrit, because increased numbers of erythrocytes enhance platelet interactions with the blood vessel wall by forcing platelets to the periphery of the bloodstream (as the erythrocytes disproportionately occupy the axial region), by imparting radially directed energy to platelets as the erythrocytes engage in flip-flop motions, and perhaps by releasing the platelet activator adenosine diphosphate (ADP) at sites of vascular injury[2–4]; and (5) the speed of blood flow and the size of the blood vessel, which will determine the number of platelets passing by a single point in a given time interval, the amount of time a platelet has to interact with the blood vessel wall or other platelets, the rate of dilution of platelet activating agents, and the forces tending to pull a platelet from the vessel wall or another platelet (shear rate).[2,4–6] The vasospastic response that accompanies vascular injury, to which platelets contribute by release of thromboxane (TX) $A_2$ and serotonin, probably plays a key role in decreasing hemorrhage and facilitating platelet and fibrin deposition via its effect on blood flow.

The initial adhesion of platelets occurs to the adhesive proteins within the subendothelial layer immediately subjacent to the endothelium[1,5] or to activated endothelium. The platelet expresses many receptors that participate in adhesive interactions (Table 2–1). Intravital microscopy and *ex vivo* flow chamber studies indicate that discoid platelets that show minimal or no evidence of activation can form the initial layers of platelet aggregates when laminar flow is disrupted by a stenotic lesion, but that stable thrombus development requires the generation and/or release of soluble activators.[6] Membrane tethers, which can undergo restructuring and stabilization, are important in achieving interactions with matrix proteins and other platelets.

The shear rate differentially affects platelet adhesion to surfaces.[3,4,7–12] Shear rates, which reflect the differences in flow velocity

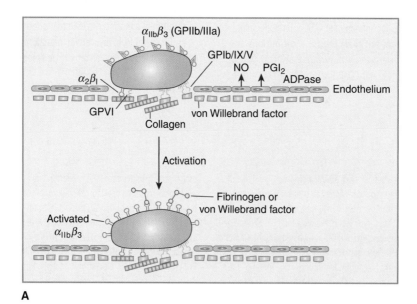

**A**

**Figure 2–1.** Platelet adhesion, activation, aggregation, and platelet–leukocyte interactions. **A.** Endothelial cells limit platelet deposition because they separate platelets from the adhesive proteins in the subendothelial area, produce two inhibitors of platelet function (nitric oxide [NO] and prostacyclin [PGI$_2$]), and contain a potent enzyme (CD39) that can digest adenosine diphosphate (ADP) released from platelets. Platelet adhesion is initiated by loss of endothelial cells (or, in the case of an atherosclerotic lesion, rupture or erosion of the plaque), which exposes adhesive glycoproteins such as collagen and von Willebrand factor (VWF) in the subendothelium. In addition, VWF and perhaps other adhesive glycoproteins in plasma deposit in the damaged area, in part by binding to collagen. Platelets adhere to the subendothelium via receptors that bind to the adhesive glycoproteins. Glycoprotein (GP) Ib binding to VWF plays a prominent role, but integrin $\alpha_2\beta_1$ (GPIa/IIa) and GPVI binding to collagen and other platelet receptors (see Table 2–4) probably also play a role. After platelets adhere, they undergo an activation process that leads to a conformational change in integrin $\alpha_{IIb}\beta_3$ receptors involving headpiece extension and leg separation (see Fig. 2–5), resulting in their ability to bind with high-affinity select multivalent adhesive proteins, most prominently fibrinogen and VWF, including the VWF that binds to collagen in the subendothelial area.

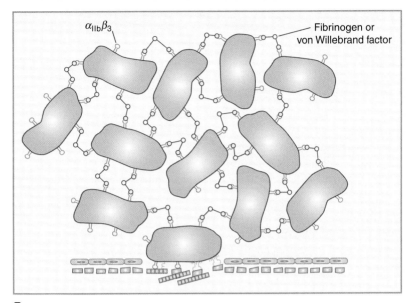

**B**

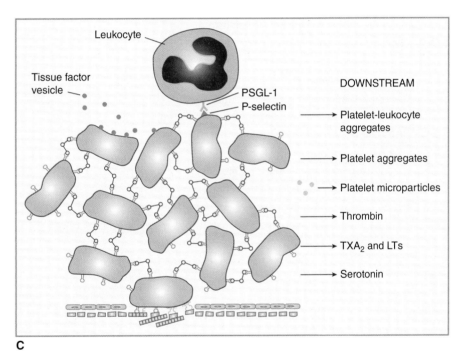

**C**

**Figure 2–1. B.** Platelet aggregation occurs when the multivalent adhesive glycoproteins bind simultaneously to integrin $\alpha_{IIb}\beta_3$ receptors on two different platelets, resulting in receptor crosslinking. Clustering of the receptors probably also contributes to the stability of the aggregates (not shown). **C.** After platelets adhere and aggregate, they help to initiate coagulation by binding tissue factor-containing vesicles circulating in the plasma, exposing negatively charged phospholipids on their surface (not shown), releasing platelet factor V (not shown), and releasing procoagulant microparticles. Activated platelets also express P-selectin on their surface, which leads to recruitment of leukocytes via interactions between platelet P-selectin and P-selectin glycoprotein ligand-1 (PSGL-1) expressed on the surface of leukocytes. Other interactions between platelets and leukocytes are detailed in Fig. 2–9. Thrombus formation is a dynamic cyclical process, with platelets repeatedly adhering, aggregating, and then breaking off and embolizing downstream. Platelet–leukocyte aggregates, platelet aggregates, platelet microparticles, thrombin, thromboxane $A_2$ (TXA$_2$), leukotrienes (LTs), and serotonin probably all go downstream and affect the microvasculature. Ultimately, the vessel either becomes fully occluded or loses its thrombogenic reactivity; that is, it becomes passivated.

as a function of distance from the blood vessel wall, vary considerably throughout the vasculature, being highest in small arterioles and lowest in large arteries and veins; very high rates are observed at the tips of severely stenotic atherosclerotic arteries.[6,11,12] Very high shear rates can cause platelets to aggregate via a mechanism that involves von

Willebrand factor (VWF) binding to glycoprotein (GP) Ib/IX followed by intracellular signaling, leading to activation of integrin $\alpha_{IIb}\beta_3$.[13–16] Platelets contribute more significantly to arterial thrombi than to venous thrombi, perhaps as a result of differences in the shear rates in the different beds.[5]

**TABLE 2–1.** Platelet Cytoskeletal Proteins*

| Protein | Properties |
|---|---|
| Actin[1805] | Mr = 42,000 |
| | 20–30% of total platelet protein (0.55 M; $2 \times 10^6$ per platelet) |
| | $\beta$ and $\gamma$ forms present at a ratio of 5:1 |
| | Monomeric actin (G-actin) bound to calcium-ATP (or adenosine diphosphate [ADP]) |
| | Polymerization requires energy (ATP→ADP) and produces F-actin |
| | F-actin filaments: two strands of intertwined helices with polarity based on ability to interact with myosin fragment ("pointed" and "barbed" ends) |
| | Steady-state polymerization: monomers lost from pointed end while others join barbed end ("treadmilling") |
| Profilin[1806] | Mr = 15,200 |
| | Forms 1:1 reversible complex with actin monomer |
| | Prevents actin polymerization |
| | May help "recharge" actin monomers with ATP |
| Gelsolin[1807] | Mr = 81,000 (5 $\mu$M; $2 \times 10^4$ per platelet) |
| | Binds to barbed end of F-actin filaments |
| | Severs actin filaments |
| | Facilitates nucleation |
| | Produces shorter filaments with gel→sol transformation |
| Thymosin $\beta_4$[267,268] | Mr = 5000 (0.55 M; $2 \times 10^6$ per platelet) |
| | Binds actin monomer |
| | Inhibits actin polymerization |
| Tropomyosin[1808] | Mr = 28,000; rod-shaped dimer of 35-nm length |
| | Binds to groove on actin filaments (6 actins:1 tropomyosin) |
| | Not all actin filaments have bound tropomyosin |
| Caldesmon[1809] | Mr = 80,000; asymmetric |
| | Binds to actin, tropomyosin, myosin, and calmodulin |
| | May control actin filament bundling and actomyosin adenosine triphosphatase (ATPase) |
| Filamin A (X) and B (3) (actin-binding protein)[133,154,216,249,1810,1811] | Filamin A-to-B = 10:1 |
| | Mr = 260,000 subunit; tail-to-tail dimer; elongated 162-nm flexible rod composed of 24 immunoglobulin-like domains; phosphorylated |
| | 2–3% of platelet protein |
| | Binds actin with 1 actin binding protein molecule per 14 actin molecules |
| | Binds glycoprotein (GP) Ib$\alpha$ and integrin $\beta$ subunit cytoplasmic domains and links GPIb/IX to actin |
| | Binds small guanosine triphosphatases (GTPases) ralA, ras, rho, Cdc-42, as well as kinases and phosphatases, and exchange factors |
| | Trio and Toll |
| | Crosslinks actin filaments to form a gel |
| | Dephosphorylation leads to loss of activity |
| Migfilin[142,1812] | Mr = 50,000; binds kindling-2 and vasodilator-stimulated protein (VASP) |
| | Can displace filamin from $\beta_3$ cytoplasmic domain, facilitating binding of talin |
| Talin[142,245,1812,1814] | Mr = 235,000 |
| | 3% of platelet protein |
| | Binds to $\beta_3$ integrin cytoplasmic tail to activate $\alpha_{IIb}\beta_3$; also binds vinculin and $\alpha$-actinin; cleaved and activated by calpain |
| $\alpha$-Actinin[1806] | Mr = 100,000 and 102,000; dimer |
| | Binds actin at 1:10 stoichiometry; binds $Ca^{2+}$ |
| | Forms gel with F-actin; cooperates with actin-binding protein; promotes actin polymerization |
| Vinculin[269,1815,1816] | Mr = 130,000 |
| | Binds to talin; may link actin to membrane proteins at adhesion sites |

*(Continued)*

**TABLE 2–1.** Platelet Cytoskeletal Proteins* (Continued)

| Protein | Properties |
|---|---|
| Myosin II[1817,1818] | Mr = 480,000 (2 × 200,000; 2 × 20,000; 2 × 16,000) |
| | 2–5% of platelet protein; 325 × 111-nm filaments |
| | Myosin light chain ($M_r$ = 20,000); phosphorylated; required for ATPase activity |
| Myosin light-chain kinase[1819] | Mr = 105,000 |
| | Phosphorylates myosin light chain and activates actomyosin ATPase leading to contraction |
| Calmodulin[1820] | Mr = 17,000 |
| | Binds four calciums and activates myosin light-chain kinase |
| CapZ[154,216] | Mr = 36,000 and 32,000 (5 $\mu$M; 2 × 10$^4$ per platelet) |
| | Heterodimer |
| | Binds barbed ends of actin filaments |
| Cofilin[154,216] | Mr = 20,000 |
| | Accelerates depolymerization of actin filaments |
| Fimbrin (L-plastin) | Mr = 68,000 |
| | Bundles actin filaments |
| | Found in microvilli |
| VASP[154,216] | Mr = 50,000 |
| | Tetrameric |
| | Binds profilin, vinculin, zyxin |
| GTPases[154,229,249] | Cdc42–filopodia |
| | Rho–stress fibers |
| | Rac–lamellipods and ruffles |
| | Rap1b–$\alpha_{IIb}\beta_3$ control |
| Tyrosine kinases | pp60$^{src}$ |
| | pp125$^{Fak}$–$\alpha_{IIb}\beta_3$ signaling |
| | pp72$^{syk}$–GPVI signaling |
| Adaptor proteins | 14–3–3$\zeta$–binds to GPIb$\alpha$ |
| | Pleckstrin–phosphorylated on activation |
| PI kinases | PI-3 kinase |
| | PI$_4$P-5 kinase |
| Spectrin | $\alpha,\beta$ heterodimers form head to head tetramers |
| | Bind to actin filaments |
| $\alpha,\gamma$ Adducins | Cap barbed ends of actin filaments and bind to spectrin |
| | Phosphorylated with platelet activation and cleaved by calpain |

*See Refs. 216,249,261,266, and 1821.

Platelets also interact directly with exposed collagen, including types I, III, and VI, via GPVI and integrin $\alpha_2\beta_1$ (GPIa/IIa), or perhaps one or more of the many other receptors implicated in platelet–collagen interactions (e.g., CD36 [GPIV], p65).[17-29] The interaction of platelets with collagen is most evident at relatively low shear rates. Depending on the vascular bed, available adhesive glycoproteins, and shear conditions, it is likely that various combinations of platelet receptors, including GPIb$\alpha$, integrin $\alpha_2\beta_1$ (GPIa/IIa), GPVI, and integrin $\alpha_{IIb}\beta_3$, act in concert to transform the tethering and slow translocation of platelets initiated by GPIb$\alpha$ interacting with VWF into stable platelet adhesion.[1,3,4,8,10,16,25,28]

For platelet plug formation to occur, platelets must undergo activation as well as adhesion. Adhesion of platelets to subendothelial structures, in particular VWF at high shear, may itself lead to platelet activation, including the generation of TXA$_2$, release of ADP and serotonin, and activation of the integrin $\alpha_{IIb}\beta_3$ receptors on the luminal side of the platelet so that they adopt their high-affinity ligand-binding conformation(s).[10] These positive feedback mechanisms ensure an adequate hemostatic response. Depending on the nature of the surface to which they adhere, platelets also undergo variable spreading reactions and become anchored by a process that at least partially involves integrin $\alpha_{IIb}\beta_3$ ligation and clustering, leading to "outside-in" signaling, cytoskeletal reorganization, and tyrosine phosphorylation; these reactions also contribute to initiating the release reaction.[30-36] In addition, platelet activators, such as ADP, are released or synthesized at the site of vascular injury, resulting in a local response. Cooperative biochemical interactions between erythrocytes and platelets may enhance platelet activation.[37]

Activated luminal integrin $\alpha_{IIb}\beta_3$ receptors on adherent platelets bind VWF, fibrinogen, and other adhesive glycoproteins, and await the interaction with another platelet, which itself may have undergone activation of its integrin $\alpha_{IIb}\beta_3$ receptors as a result of exposure to released ADP and $TXA_2$. Alternatively, a platelet may become activated and bind VWF or fibrinogen while still circulating, in which case the platelet-ligand complex may bind directly to an activated integrin $\alpha_{IIb}\beta_3$ receptor on the luminal surface. The binding of adhesive ligands to platelet receptors then repeats itself, resulting in the recruitment of additional layers of platelets, and ultimately the formation of a hemostatic plug. Intravital videomicroscopy of the mesenteric and cremasteric circulations of mice after endothelial cell damage demonstrates that, at least in these vascular beds, platelet thrombus formation is initially a very dynamic process, with many platelets depositing but then embolizing.[38] The thrombus grows relatively slowly compared to what its growth would be if all of the platelets that deposited remained attached to the surface.[39-41]

The integrin $\alpha_{IIb}\beta_3$ receptor occupies a central role in determining the extent of platelet aggregation, in part because it is present at an extraordinarily high density on the platelet surface (approximately 50,000 receptors per platelet, such that receptors are probably less than 20 nm apart).[30,42-45] This permits it to rapidly initiate platelet aggregation. On the other hand, the receptor is not in its high-affinity ligand-binding state on resting platelets but rather needs to be activated by agonists, including ADP, serotonin, thrombin, collagen, and $TXA_2$, that are localized to sites of vascular injury.[34,44,46] As a result, platelets can circulate in plasma containing high concentrations of the integrin $\alpha_{IIb}\beta_3$ ligands fibrinogen and VWF without ongoing platelet thrombus formation. The agonists that activate the integrin $\alpha_{IIb}\beta_3$ receptor are likely to work in combination *in vivo*. In fact, the mixture of agonists present is likely to change as the process unfolds, with collagen perhaps more important at the beginning, thrombin more important later on, and the other agonists in varying mixtures throughout. The platelet activation effects of multiple agonists may be additive or synergistic, depending on the mechanism(s) involved.[47,48]

A number of mechanisms stabilize platelet aggregates. These include absence of fibrinogen (presumably limiting fibrin formation),[41] leptin,[49-51] CD40 ligand,[52] growth arrest-specific gene 6 product (Gas6) and its receptors (Axl, Sky, and Mer),[53-57] Eph kinases and ephrins,[58] factor XII,[59] plasminogen activator inhibitor-1 and vitronectin,[50] or inhibition of select regions of fibrinogen.[60]

Activated platelets can facilitate thrombin generation by one or more different mechanisms, including recruitment of bloodborne tissue factor, synthesis or activation of tissue factor, formation of procoagulant microvesicles, exposure of activated factor V, exposure of negatively charged phospholipids, and perhaps activation of the contact system. The thrombin thus generated further activates platelets, leading to more extensive degranulation; it also further activates coagulation and initiates the deposition of fibrin strands that reinforce the platelet thrombus and serve as sites for additional VWF deposition.[61] Thrombin also helps to consolidate the plug by initiating platelet-mediated clot retraction (see section "Platelet Shape Change, Spreading, Contraction, and Clot Retraction" below). Finally, thrombin affects the surface membrane receptors, downregulating GPIb/IX and upregulating integrin $\alpha_{IIb}\beta_3$, perhaps facilitating the transition from platelet adhesion to platelet aggregation.[62-65]

Release of vasoactive and mitogenic agents, as well as chemokines, from platelets contributes to the inflammatory response, as does the appearance of P-selectin on the surface of activated platelets and endothelial cells, because P-selectin and other platelet receptors recruit leukocytes to the damaged region.[66-68] Finally, after contributing to hemostasis and initiating an inflammatory response, platelet-fibrin thrombi eventually resolve, most likely by a combination of embolization, fibrinolysis, and macrophage removal of debris.

Several inhibitory factors serve to balance platelet activation and thus prevent excessive platelet deposition. The dilutional effects of flowing blood are probably most important; thus, alterations in the surface of the blood vessel that produce local areas of stasis in which platelets

and coagulation factors may concentrate are prothrombogenic.[2,5] Endothelial cells can synthesize two potent inhibitors of platelet activation, prostacyclin and nitric oxide (Chap. 5).[69-72] Generation of prostacyclin at sites of vascular injury or inflammation may provide a mechanism to limit platelet accumulation. Nitric oxide, which is synthesized by endothelial cells, is a potent inhibitor of *ex vivo* platelet adhesion and aggregation. Endothelial cells and lymphocytes also have CD39, an ecto-ATP diphosphohydrolase (ecto-ADPase) that can digest ATP and ADP to adenosine monophosphate (AMP), and thus limit the effects of released ADP.[73,74] They also have CD73, which can convert AMP into the platelet inhibitor adenosine.

# ⬤ PLATELET MORPHOLOGY AND BIOCHEMISTRY

## MICROSCOPIC APPEARANCE

On films made from blood anticoagulated with the strong calcium chelating agent ethylenediaminetetraacetic acid (EDTA) and treated with Wright stain, platelets appear as small bluish-gray, oval-to-round–shaped cell fragments with several purple-red granules. The mean diameter of platelets varies in different individuals, ranging from approximately 1.5 to 3.0 $\mu m$, approximately one-third to one-fourth that of erythrocytes. There is also considerable variability in the size of platelets in a single individual, with occasional platelets in normal blood samples having diameters greater than half the diameter of erythrocytes. Overall, platelet size appears to follow a log normal distribution with an average volume of approximately 7 fL.[75] When unanticoagulated blood is used to prepare blood films, platelets undergo variable activation and spreading, and thus platelet aggregates are commonly seen; platelets from such specimens may demonstrate three or four very long fingerlike processes extending out from the body of the platelet (filopodia), and some platelets may be devoid of granules.

Electron microscopy reveals a fuzzy coat (glycocalix) extending 14 to 20 nm from the platelet surface, which is thought to be composed of membrane GPs, glycolipids, mucopolysaccharides, and adsorbed plasma proteins (Fig. 2–2).[76] Platelets move in an electric field as if they have a net negative surface charge; sialic acid residues attached to proteins and lipids are major contributors to this negative charge.[77] The electrostatic repulsion created by the negative surface charge may help prevent resting platelets from attaching to each other or to negatively charged endothelial cells.

Indentations on the platelet surface are thought to be the openings of the open canalicular system, which is an elaborate channel system composed of invaginations of the plasma membrane that extend throughout the platelet (see Fig. 2–2 and "Membrane Systems" below). The contents of platelet granules can gain access to the outside when the granules fuse with either the plasma membrane or any region of the open canalicular system. Similarly, glycoproteins contained within granule membranes can join the plasma membrane after granule fusion with either the plasma membrane or the open canalicular system.

## MEMBRANE SYSTEMS

### The Plasma Membrane

The plasma membrane is a trilaminar unit composed of a bilayer of phospholipids embedded with cholesterol, glycolipids, and glycoproteins.[76,78] Platelets prepared by the freeze–fracture technique demonstrate more intramembranous particles embedded in the outer platelet membrane leaflet than in the inner leaflet, which is the reverse of findings in erythrocytes; this observation presumably reflects the many external receptors that mediate platelet interactions. The plasma membrane is

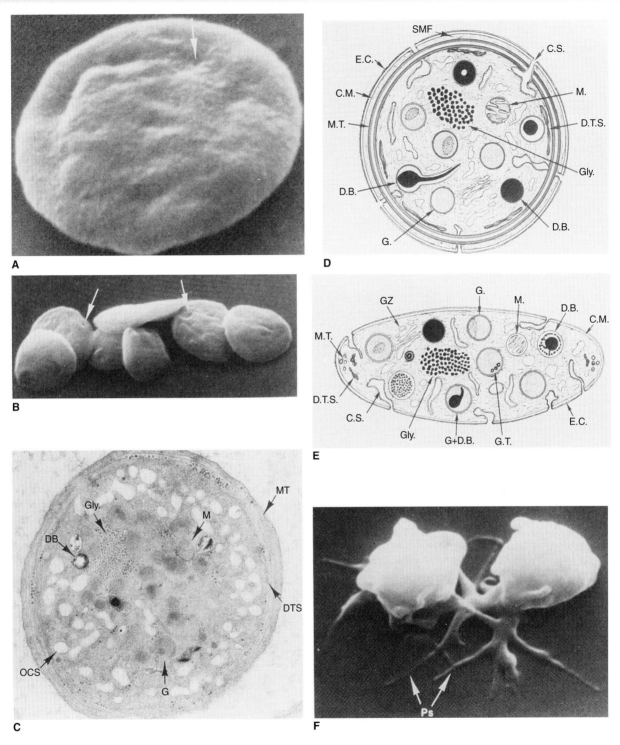

**Figure 2–2.** **A** and **B.** Discoid platelets. The lentiform shape of blood platelets is well preserved in samples fixed in glutaraldehyde and critical point dried for study in the scanning electron microscope. The indentations apparent on the otherwise smooth surfaces of the platelets *(arrows)* indicate sites where channels of the open canalicular system (OCS) communicate with the cell exterior. (Magnification: **A**, ×13,200; **B**, ×35,000.) **C, D,** and **E.** Ultrastructural features observed in thin sections of discoid platelets cut in the equatorial plane (**C** and **D**) or cross-section (**E**). Components include the exterior coat *(E.C.)*, trilaminar unit membrane *(C.M.)*, and submembrane area containing the specialized filaments of the membrane skeleton *(SMF)*. The plasma membrane indentations form the walls of the channels of the surface-connected open canalicular system (*C.S.* and *OCS*). The circumferential band of microtubules *(M.T.)* is seen as a continuous band beneath the plasma membrane on the equatorial section and as small open cylinders at the ends of the platelet on the cross-section. Glycogen granules *(Gly.)* are prominent punctate structures in the cytoplasm, and residual Golgi zones *(GZ)* can also be identified. Organelles include mitochondria *(M.)*, dense bodies *(D.B.)*, and α granules *(G.)*, many of which have regions of electron density (nucleoids). The dense tubular system *(D.T.S.)*, the platelet equivalent of the sarcoplasmic reticulum, sequesters calcium. (Magnification: **C**, ×30,000.) **F.** Platelet shape change. Platelets exposed to adenosine diphosphate and then fixed and examined by scanning electron microscopy. The platelets lose their discoid shape and become spiny spheres with long extensions, variably referred to as *filopodia* or *pseudopodia*. (Magnification: ×17,000.) *(Reproduced with permission from Bloom AL, et al: Hemostasis and Thrombosis. Edinburgh: Churchill Livingstone; 1994.)*

thought to contain the sodium- and calcium-adenosine triphosphatase (ATPase) pumps that control the intracellular ionic environment of the platelet. Approximately 60 percent of platelet phospholipids are contained in the plasma membrane. The phospholipids are asymmetrically organized in the plasma membrane; the negatively charged phospholipids are almost exclusively present in the inner leaflet, whereas the others are more evenly distributed.[79] The negatively charged phospholipids, especially phosphatidylserine, are able to accelerate several steps in the coagulation sequence, and so their presence in the inner leaflet of resting platelets, separated from the plasma coagulation factors, is thought to be a control mechanism for preventing inappropriate activation of the coagulation system.[80,81] During platelet activation induced by select agonists, the aminophospholipids may become exposed on the platelet surface or on the surface of microparticles (see "Platelet Coagulant Activity" below).[80-83]

The phospholipid asymmetry in resting platelets may be maintained by an ATP-dependent aminophospholipid translocase that actively moves phosphatidylserine and phosphatidylethanolamine from the outer to the inner leaflet.[80,84] Interactions of negatively charged phospholipids with cytoskeletal or other cytoplasmic elements may also contribute to the asymmetry.[80,81,85,86]

Lipid rafts are dynamic, cholesterol- and sphingolipid-rich membrane microdomains that are important in signaling and intracellular trafficking. In platelets, the cholesterol-to-phospholipid molar ratio is twofold higher in rafts than in bulk membranes, with sphingomyelin accounting for the majority of total raft lipids.[87] Platelet lipid rafts contain the marker proteins flotillin 1, flotillin 2, stomatin, and the ganglioside $GM_1$; the rafts are also notable for being devoid of caveolin. Other proteins, such as CD36, CD63, CD9, integrin $\alpha_{IIb}\beta_3$, and glucose transporter (GLUT)-3, are present in rafts prepared from resting platelets.[87] Upon activation of GPVI, Fc gamma chain, FcγRIIa, and GPIb/IX/V partition into the lipid rafts,[88,89] as do c-Src,[90] phosphatidic acid, and phosphoinositol (PI) 3'-kinase (PI3K) products.[87,91] Factor XI binds to extracellularly oriented lipid rafts and undergoes activation.[92] The calcium entry channel hTRPc1 is associated with lipid rafts in platelets and, upon platelet activation, contributes to calcium entry that is regulated by the state of intracellular calcium stores (store-mediated calcium entry).[93] The functionally detrimental effects of chilling platelets are thought to be mediated, at least in part, by the temperature-dependent coalescence of platelet lipid rafts.[94]

Open Canalicular System    The surface-connected open canalicular system is an elaborate series of conduits that begin as indentations of the plasma membrane and tunnel throughout the interior of the platelet.[76,95,96] Tracer studies demonstrate that the open canalicular system is contiguous with the exterior of the platelet, even though elements of the open canalicular system may appear as closed vesicles or vacuoles by electron microscopy of sectioned platelets.[76,95-97]

The open canalicular system may serve several functions. It provides a mechanism for entry of external elements into the interior of the platelet. It also provides a potential route for the release of granule contents to the outside, eliminating the need for granule fusion with the plasma membrane itself.[97,98] This latter function is especially important because, under most circumstances, platelet granules appear to move to the center of the platelet upon platelet activation rather than to the periphery.[76,95,99] Controversy remains, however, regarding the relative frequency with which secretion occurs via the open canalicular system versus direct fusion with the plasma membrane.[76,95,100]

The open canalicular system also represents an extensive internal store of membrane. Both filopodia formation and platelet spreading after adhesion require a dramatic increase in surface plasma membrane compared to the plasma membrane of resting platelets, and it is not possible for new membrane to be synthesized during the short time-course

of these phenomena. Thus, the membrane of the open canalicular system most likely contributes to the increase in plasma membrane under these conditions; the membranes of α granules, dense bodies, and, to a lesser extent, lysosomes may also contribute, but only if the stimulus is sufficient to induce the fusion of these organelles with the plasma membrane (release reaction). Finally, the membrane of the open canalicular system may serve as a storage site for plasma membrane glycoproteins. For example, under certain conditions, platelet activation by thrombin leads to a consistent, selective loss of GPIb/IX from the platelet surface, and data from electron microscopy indicate that the GPIb/IX becomes sequestered in the open canalicular system.[63,64,101] Plasmin may produce a similar phenomenon.[101,102] Platelet activation leads to an increase in surface integrin $\alpha_{IIb}\beta_3$, and although much of this receptor is thought to derive from α-granule membranes, at least some may come from integrin $\alpha_{IIb}\beta_3$ in the membranes of dense bodies and the open canalicular system.[101,103] Similarly, GPVI, the $P2Y_1$ ADP receptor, and the $TXA_2$ receptor, and perhaps other receptors, are present in the open canalicular system and can be recruited to the platelet surface with activation.[104,105]

Dense Tubular System/Sarcoplasmic Reticulum    The dense tubular system (DTS) is a closed-channel network of residual endoplasmic reticulum characterized histocytochemically by the presence of peroxidase activity.[76,106-108] The channels of the DTS are less extensive than those of the open canalicular system and tend to cluster in regions in close approximation to the open canalicular system.[76] The DTS is analogous to the sarcoplasmic reticulum of muscle because it can sequester $Ca^{2+}$ and release it when platelets are activated, leading to shape change, granule centralization, and secretion.[109,110] Calreticulin, a calcium binding protein found in the DTS/sarcoplasmic reticulum, probably helps to sequester ionized calcium.[111,112] Release of $Ca^{2+}$ from the DTS/sarcoplasmic reticulum involves the binding of inositol-1,4,5-trisphosphate ($IP_3$), a messenger molecule formed during signal transduction, to $IP_3$ type II receptors on the DTS/sarcoplasmic reticulum membrane (Fig. 2–3).[113,114] Cyclic AMP inhibits $Ca^{2+}$ release from the DTS/sarcoplasmic reticulum, either by enhancing the calcium pumping mechanism[115] or by inhibiting release induced by $IP_3$.[116] NO inhibits $Ca^{2+}$ uptake by the DTS/sarcoplasmic reticulum at high concentrations and stimulates uptake at low concentrations by effects on the calcium ATPase(s) SERCA26 and SERCA3.[117,118] Depletion of intracellular calcium stores activates store-operated calcium entry (SOCE) into platelets (reviewed in Ref. 119). The depletion of $Ca^{2+}$ from the DTS/sarcoplasmic reticulum is sensed by stromal interaction molecule 1 (STIM1), a transmembrane protein with a $Ca^{2+}$ binding motif (EF hand) in the DTS/sarcoplasmic reticulum.[120-122] Loss of $Ca^{2+}$ binding to STIM1 results in translocation and activation of Orai1, a calcium release activated calcium (CRAC) channel in the plasma membrane,[123,124] that allows $Ca^{2+}$ entry into the platelet. Although mice with defects in STIM1 and Orai1 have demonstrated abnormalities in platelet function,[120-122] humans with mutations in these proteins have had immune dysfunction, but no overt hemostatic or thrombotic abnormalities.[125-127] The human canonical transient receptor potential 1 (hTRPC1) has also been implicated in regulating platelet SOCE, but mice deficient in this protein do not have a defect in platelet $Ca^{2+}$ entry.[128-130]

The DTS membrane is also probably a major site of prostaglandin and TX synthesis[109,131]; in fact, the peroxidase activity used to identify the DTS is an enzymatic component of prostaglandin synthesis.[131,132]

## Cytoskeletal Elements

The discoid shape of the resting platelet is maintained by a well-defined and highly specialized cytoskeleton. This system of molecular struts and girders preserves the shape and integrity of the platelet as it encounters high shear forces in the circulation. The platelet cytoskeleton is operationally defined as proteins that are insoluble in the presence of the

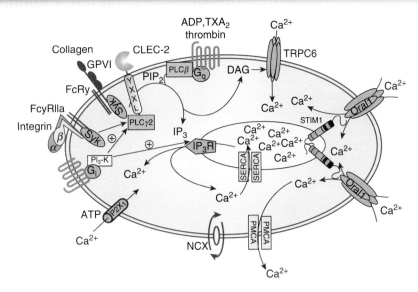

**Figure 2–3.** Platelet calcium homeostasis. Upon receptor activation, different phospholipase (PL) C isoforms hydrolyze phosphatidylinositol-4,5-bisphosphate (PIP$_2$) to inositol-1,4,5-trisphosphate (IP$_3$) and diacylglycerol (DAG). IP$_3$ releases Ca$^{2+}$ from the intracellular stores in the dense tubular system (DTS)/sarcoplasmic reticulum. The transmembrane protein stromal interaction molecule 1 (STIM1) senses the reduction in Ca$^{2+}$ through a decrease in Ca$^{2+}$ occupancy of its EF hand domain and then opens Orai1 Ca$^{2+}$ channels in the plasma membrane, a process called store-operated calcium entry, whereas DAG mediates calcium entry through canonical transient receptor potential channel 6 (TRPC6). Additionally, a direct receptor-operated calcium (ROC) channel, P2X$_1$, and an Na$^+$/Ca$^{2+}$ exchanger (NCX) contribute to the elevation in Ca$^{2+}$ in the platelet cytoplasm. The counteracting mechanisms to replenish DTS/sarcoplasmic reticulum Ca$^{2+}$ stores involve Ca$^{2+}$ adenosine triphosphatases (ATPases) (SERCAs). Plasma membrane Ca$^{2+}$ ATPases (PMCAs) pump Ca$^{2+}$ through the plasma membrane out of the cell. ADP, adenosine diphosphate; CLEC-2, C-type lectin-like receptor 2; FcR$\gamma$, Fc receptor $\gamma$ chain; FcγRIIa, Fc γ receptor IIa; GPVI, glycoprotein VI; IP$_3$R, IP$_3$ receptor; PI$_3$-K, phosphatidylinositol 3-kinase; Syk, spleen tyrosine kinase. Because of controversies about the localization and role of TRPC1 in the literature, this protein is not depicted in the figure. *(Adapted with permission from Varga-Szabo D, Braun A, Nieswandt B: Calcium signaling in platelets,* J Thromb Haemost. *2009 Jul;7(7):1057–1066.)*

nonionic detergent Triton X-100 under defined ionic conditions. The three major cytoskeletal elements are the spectrin membrane skeleton, the marginal microtubule coil, and the actin cytoskeleton.

**Membrane Skeleton** The plasma membrane and open canalicular system of the resting platelet are supported by a highly structured cytoskeletal system (see Figs. 2–2 and 2–4). This two-dimensional network, located just beneath the plasma membrane, has remarkable structural resemblance to its red blood cell counterpart. Thus, both involve the self-assembly of elongated spectrin strands that interconnect through their binding to actin filaments, generating triangular pores. Platelets contain approximately 2000 molecules of spectrin.[133–136] The spectrin network coats the cytoplasmic surfaces of both the plasma membrane and the open canalicular system. In contrast to the erythrocyte membrane skeleton, however, in which spectrin molecules connect on short actin filaments, in platelets, spectrin joins into a network by binding to the ends of actin filaments in close apposition to the plasma membrane. As a result, the spectrin lattice is assembled into a continuous network by its association with actin filaments. Moreover, tropomodulins, which are abundant in erythrocytes, are not expressed at significant levels in platelets and thus are unlikely to play a role in capping the pointed ends of actin filaments. Instead, these ends appear to be free in resting platelets. Finally, the protein adducin is abundantly expressed in platelets and appears to cap the majority of the barbed ends of the filaments making up the resting platelet cytoskeleton.[137] This serves to target them to the spectrin-based membrane skeleton, as the affinity of spectrin for adducin-actin complexes is greater than for either adducin or actin alone.[138–140]

The platelet spectrin-actin filament network is fortified by interactions with filamin A (actin binding protein), a noncovalent dimer of two identical Mr 280,000 protein subunits that fastens GPIb/IX/V complexes to the sides of actin filaments. By interacting with both the transmembrane glycoprotein GPIbα and the actin immediately below the membrane, filamin A connects these components to the spectrin network and the resulting membrane cytoskeleton, probably contributing to the platelet's discoid shape. In addition, the association of GPIbα with the membrane skeleton restricts the expansion of the spectrin network and probably helps to organize receptors into linear arrays on the platelet surface, thus enhancing receptor cooperation (see Fig. 2–4).[133] Filamin also binds to the cytoplasmic domains of the $\beta_3$ subunits of integrin receptors, and this keeps the receptor in a low-affinity state.[141–143] Other proteins that have been found in the membrane skeleton include talin, vinculin, dystrophin-related protein, molecules implicated in signal transduction, and several isoenzymes of protein kinase C.[133]

Talin has been implicated in controlling integrin $\alpha_{IIb}\beta_3$ activation, by binding to the cytoplasmic domain of integrin $\beta_3$ when phosphorylated and/or cleaved by calpain (see "Integrin $\alpha_{IIb}\beta_3$," below and Fig. 2–4).[144–148] Migfilin (filamin-binding LIM protein-1) is a 373-amino-acid protein of Mr 50,000 that can displace filamin from the integrin $\beta_3$ cytoplasmic domain, thus facilitating talin binding and activation. Moreover, joining integrin $\alpha_{IIb}\beta_3$ to the membrane skeleton via an integrin $\beta_3$ linkage creates the possibility for an actin–myosin contraction process to supply sufficient force to integrin $\alpha_{IIb}\beta_3$ to induce conformational changes in the receptor that result in high-affinity ligand binding.[149] The protein vimentin (Mr 58,000), which is an important component of intermediate filaments, is present in platelets and contributes to the membrane cytoskeleton. When platelets are activated, vitronectin–plasminogen activator inhibitor-1 (PAI-1) complexes bind to surface vimentin where they are strategically located to inhibit fibrinolysis.[150] With platelet activation, integrins $\alpha_{IIb}\beta_3$ and $\alpha_2\beta_1$ join the cytoskeleton. Thus, the cytoskeleton may affect whether receptors are free to move in the plane of the membrane; it may also have a role in moving certain receptors from the surface to the interior of platelets and vice versa via

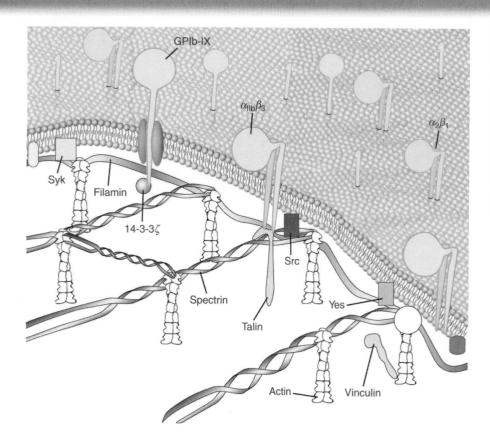

**Figure 2–4.** Diagrammatic depiction of established and hypothetical connections between select platelet transmembrane glycoproteins and the underlying membrane skeleton. Although evidence exists for direct interactions between IIb 3 with talin and Src and between GPIb with 14–3–3 and filamin, the remainder of the interactions are only hypothetical and are based on the recovery of proteins in the membrane skeleton fraction of solubilized platelets. *(Adapted with permission from Colman RW:* Hemostasis and Thrombosis: Basic Principles and Clinical Practice. *4th edition. Philadelphia, PA: Williams & Wilkins; 2001.)*

the open canalicular system.[101,133] The membrane skeleton may also be important in platelet spreading after adhesion.

**Microtubules** One of the most distinguishing features of the resting platelet is its marginal microtubule coil (see Fig. 2–2). Located below the plasma membrane, it plays an important role in platelet formation from megakaryocytes and maintaining the platelet's discoid shape.[76,151–153] Microtubules are the largest cytoskeletal filaments (25 nm) and are comprised of hollow polarized polymers composed of 13 protofilaments made up of $\alpha\beta$ tubulin dimers (each of Mr 110,000) that associate with several high-molecular-weight proteins (microtubule-associated proteins).[153–155] Motor proteins of the dynein and kinesin families are also associated with microtubules.[156–158] In cells, $\alpha\beta$ tubulin subunits are in dynamic equilibrium with assembled microtubules such that reversible cycles of assembly and disassembly of microtubules are frequently observed.[159] The critical concentration for tubulin polymerization is 5 $\mu$M, which is well below the tubulin concentration in platelets (70 $\mu$M), and thus, 60 percent of platelet tubulin is present as polymer.[154,160] On cross-section, approximately eight to 12 separate hollow structures are observed at the tapered ends of the platelet (see Fig. 2–2). Direct visualization of microtubule assembly in resting mouse platelets indicates that the circumferential coil in platelets is composed of at least eight actively polymerizing microtubules.[159] Microtubule dynamics allow for necessary changes in platelet shape that occur during the platelet life span and with activation. Tubulin is acetylated in resting platelets and undergoes deacetylation by histone deacetylase (HDAC) 6 with activation in association with the dissolution of the marginal band.[161,162]

Platelets contain four different tubulin isoforms ($\beta_1$, $\beta_2$, $\beta_4$, $\beta_5$), but $\beta_1$ is dominant and is specific for megakaryocytes and platelets. Targeted gene deletion of $\beta_1$-tubulin in mice results in thrombocytopenia and abnormal platelet and microtubule morphology.[153] $\beta_1$-Tubulin–deficient platelets are spherical in shape, probably as a result of having defective

marginal bands with fewer (approximately two to three) than normal (approximately eight) microtubule coils.[163] A heterozygous polymorphism of human $\beta_1$-tubulin (Q43P) has been described in association with macrothrombocytopenia,[164] but it is probably not causal,[165] and individuals homozygous for the Q43P variant have low platelet counts, abnormal platelet ultrastructure, and decreased tubulin, but normal platelet length, width, and area.[166] A heterozygous $\beta_1$-tubulin mutation (R207H) in a strategically located region of the molecule has been reported in association with macrothrombocytopenia, as has an F260S mutation[167] and an R318W mutation[165] (Chap. 10).[168]

**Actin Filaments** Actin is the most abundant of all platelet proteins, with 2 million molecules expressed per platelet (0.5 mM).[169] Like tubulin, actin is in dynamic monomer-polymer equilibrium, with 40 percent of the actin subunits polymerized to form 2000 to 5000 linear actin filaments in resting platelets (Fig. 2–5). The rest of the actin in the platelet cytoplasm is maintained in storage as a 1:1 complex with $\beta_4$-thymosin; this stored actin is converted to filaments during platelet activation to drive cell spreading.[170] Thus, actin filaments crisscross the interior of the cell, interconnected at various points into a rigid cytoplasmic network by abundantly expressed actin crosslinking proteins, including filamin and $\alpha$-actinin.[171–173] Filamin exists in solution as homodimers of subunits that themselves are elongated strands composed primarily of 24 repeats, each approximately 100 amino acids in length, that are folded into immunoglobulin (Ig) G-like $\beta$ barrels.[174,175] There are three filamin genes, and they are located on the X chromosome, chromosome 3, and chromosome 7.[176,177] Filamin A and filamin B are expressed in platelets, with filamin A accounting for approximately 90 percent of total filamin.

Filamin is a prototypical scaffolding protein that attracts binding partners, including the small guanosine triphosphatase (GTPase), RalA, Rac, Rho, and Cdc42,[178] and positions them adjacent to the plasma membrane.[179] Approximately 90 percent of the filamin in resting

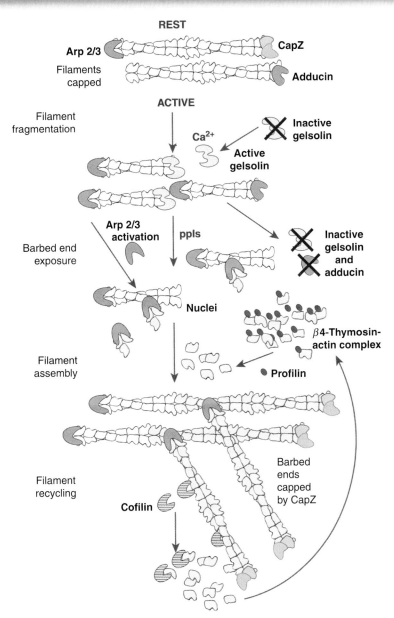

**Figure 2–5.** Control of platelet actin assembly. *(Rest)* Forty percent of the actin in the resting cell is filamentous. The rest of the actin is soluble (60 percent) and is in a 1:1 complex with $\beta_4$-thymosin. Filaments are stable because they are capped on their barbed ends by capZ. *(Active)* Shape change begins when calcium rises into the micromolar level and gelsolin becomes active. Gelsolin binds to actin filaments, interdigitates, and causes filaments to fragment. After fragmentation, gelsolin remains bound to the barbed filament end. Assembly of actin begins when capping proteins are dissociated from the barbed ends of the filament fragments formed in the rounding step by polyphosphoinositides (ppls) and when the actin-related protein (ARP2/3) complex in platelets is activated to nucleate de novo filaments. Actin monomers, stored in complex with $\beta_4$-thymosin, are the source of the actin for this polymerization event. Transfer of actin from $\beta_4$-thymosin to the barbed ends of actin filaments is facilitated by profilin. Once assembly is complete, CapZ recaps the barbed filament ends. *(Adapted with permission from Michelson A: Platelets. 2nd edition. Boston, MA: Academic Press/Elsevier; 2007.)*

platelets interacts with the cytoplasmic tail of the GPIbα subunit of the GPIb-IX-V complex via a binding site in filamin's second rod domain (repeats 17 to 20).[180,181] This interaction has three consequences. First, it positions filamin's self-association domain and associated partner proteins at the plasma membrane while presenting filamin's actin-binding sites into the cytoplasm. Second, because a large fraction of filamin is also bound to actin, it aligns the GPIb-IX-V complexes into rows on the plasma membrane surface of the platelet over the underlying actin filaments. Third, because the filamin linkages between actin filaments and the GPIb-IX-V complex pass through the pores of the spectrin lattice, it restrains the molecular movement of the spectrin strands in this lattice and holds the lattice in compression. The filamin–GPIbα connection is essential for the formation and release of discoid platelets by megakaryocytes, as platelets lacking this connection are produced in lower numbers and the ones that are produced are abnormally large and fragile. Platelets deficient in GPIb (Bernard-Soulier syndrome; Chap. 10) are very large, perhaps as a result of abnormalities in organizing the cytoskeleton.

## ● PLATELET ENERGY METABOLISM

Platelets have sizable stores of glycogen that can often be seen on electron microscopy (see Fig. 2–2). Glycogen can be broken down into glucose 1-phosphate, and platelets can also take up glucose from their surrounding medium. Platelet glycolysis rates significantly exceed those of erythrocytes and skeletal muscle.[182] Oxidative metabolism probably contributes to energy production in resting platelets, but it has been estimated that less than 1 percent of the pyruvate produced by glycolysis actually enters the citric acid cycle. The remainder is either converted to lactate or remains as pyruvate; both leave the platelet.[183] Platelet mitochondria are capable of oxidation of fatty acids, but its importance to energy production is unclear.[184–187] Platelets can actively metabolize acetate, which has been exploited to improve platelet storage conditions.[185,188] Amino acids may also serve as energy sources and feed into the citric acid cycle, but their contributions are uncertain.

As in all cells, ATP consumption by platelets is partially devoted to maintaining ionic and osmotic homeostasis.[189,190] In addition, the continuous polymerization and depolymerization of actin involves conversion of ATP to ADP, and this may account for as much as 40 percent of the ATP consumption in resting platelets.[191] The continuous polymerization and depolymerization of tubulin that occurs in the coil of resting platelet involves conversion of guanosine triphosphate (GTP) to guanosine diphosphate (GDP), and thus consumes energy.[159] Continuing dephosphorylation and rephosphorylation of phosphatidylinositols, which are important in signal transduction, has been estimated to consume as much as 7 percent of the total ATP produced.[192] Protein phosphorylation also occurs as an ongoing process, but its fractional use of ATP is not clear in resting cells. Platelet stimulation leads to a marked increase in both glycolytic activity and oxidative ATP production, perhaps as a result of the abrupt decrease in ATP that occurs with platelet activation or the increase in cytoplasmic pH.[187] The increased ATP appears to be used, at least in part, for phosphatidylinositide and protein phosphorylation.

Platelet stimulation is accompanied by a marked increase in both glycolytic activity and oxidative ATP production, perhaps through a feedback mechanism in response to the abrupt decrease in ATP that occurs with platelet activation or as a result of the increase in cytoplasmic pH.[193] The increased ATP appears to be utilized, at least in part, in phosphoinositide phosphorylation and protein phosphorylation.

### Organelles

**Peroxisomes** In platelets, some of the main metabolic functions of peroxisomes include fatty acid $\beta$-oxidation, plasmalogen (a phospholipid) synthesis, and synthesis of platelet-activating factor (PAF).[194] They contain acyl-CoA:dihydroxyacetone phosphate acyltransferase, which catalyzes the first step in the synthesis of ether-containing phospholipids. Deficiencies of this enzymatic activity have been identified in the cerebrorenal Zellweger syndrome, and the platelet activity can be used to diagnose the disorder.[195,196]

**Mitochondria** Platelets contain approximately four to seven mitochondria of relatively small size, often located near the plasma membrane; they are involved in oxidative energy metabolism.[197–199] Control of mitochondrial Bcl-2 family proteins, including Bcl-x1 and Bak, directly affects a platelet's life span, and alterations in these proteins can produce thrombocytopenia (Chaps. 1 and 7).[200] Release of mitochondria upon platelet activation, either in microparticles or free in the circulation, may contribute to inflammation and nonhemolytic transfusion reactions.[199] Abnormalities of mitochondrial enzymes, including the reduced form of nicotinamide adenine dinucleotide (NADH) coenzyme Q reductase (complex I), have been implicated in the pathophysiology of aging and several neurodegenerative disorders, including Alzheimer disease, schizophrenia, and some forms of Parkinson disease. Assays of platelet mitochondrial enzyme levels have been used in these studies.[201–206] In addition, hyperglycemia-induced mitochondrial superoxide generation may contribute to the enhanced platelet aggregation observed in diabetes.[207] Loss of the mitochondrial inner leaflet potential has been associated with surface expression of platelet procoagulant activity and coated platelet formation (see "Platelet Coagulant Activity" below).[208–211]

## ● PLATELET SHAPE CHANGE, SPREADING, CONTRACTION, AND CLOT RETRACTION

### OVERVIEW

The cytoskeleton establishes the platelet's native structure and its ability to respond to stimuli through changes in shape and force generation; as such, the cytoskeleton can be considered analogous to an animal's bones and muscles. Table 2–1 lists the major components of the platelet contractile system. These elements are thought to contribute to platelet shape change, secretion, and clot retraction after platelet activation.

When exposed to a variety of agonists, platelets undergo dramatic changes in shape within seconds. Shape change follows a reproducible sequence of events during which the resting platelet cytoskeleton is dismantled and reorganized. The first noticeable change following activation is the dismantling of the microtubule coil and conversion from discs to spheres. Filopodia and lamellipodia, generated by new actin filament assembly, then extend from the plasma membrane. At the same time, intracellular organelles and granules and the dismantled microtubule coil are compressed into the center of the platelet. Once shape change is finished, the actin cytoskeleton is used as a platform for contraction, and contractile tension is exerted between platelets and between platelets and the adjacent fibrin strands.

### PLATELET SHAPE CHANGE

Platelet shape change occurs in response to many different agonists. It involves loss of the platelet's normal discoid shape (approximately 1.5 to 2.5 $\mu$m diameter and approximately 0.5 to 0.9 $\mu$m width) and transformation to a spiny sphere with long, thin filopodia extending several micrometers out from the platelet and ending in points that are as small as 0.1 $\mu$m in diameter (see Fig. 2–2).[95,212] In the aggregometer, it has been generally assumed that the initial decrease in light transmission immediately after adding certain agonists is a reflection of platelets undergoing shape change,[213] but this interpretation has been challenged by the suggestion that microaggregation, rather than shape change, accounts for this phenomenon.[214] Although the reason platelets undergo shape change is unclear, one possibility is that it reduces electrostatic repulsion between two negatively charged platelets or between a platelet and a negatively charged surface or cell without the need to reduce surface charge density. Thus, after changing shape, the tip of a platelet filopodium can more easily approach and make contact with a surface or a cell because the great bulk of the repulsive surface charge is now at a distance from the tip.[215]

A change in platelet shape from disk to sphere is the first event that is observed as the platelet is activated. Agonist binding to select receptors activates phospholipase (PL) C$\beta$, which hydrolyzes membrane-bound PI-4,5-bisphosphate to inositol-1,4,5-triphosphate (IP$_3$) and diacylglycerol. IP$_3$ then binds to receptors on the DTS/sarcoplasmic reticulum, generating a rise in cytosolic calcium concentrations to 5 to 10 $\mu$M. While calcium can influence the activity of many actin-binding proteins, one of the major proteins that is activated is gelsolin, which is present in platelets at a concentration of approximately 5 $\mu$M. Actin filaments in resting platelets are relatively stable because their barbed ends (the end from which they can grow by adding additional actin monomers) are capped with the protein CapZ and $\alpha,\gamma$-adducins (see Fig. 2–5). Calcium-activated gelsolin both severs existing actin filaments and caps the newly created barbed ends. This increases the number of actin filaments by an estimated 10-fold and substitutes gelsolin for CapZ and $\alpha,\gamma$-adducins as the actin filament capping protein.[216] Severing of actin filaments that interact with the planar lattice composed of filamin A (actin binding protein), GPIb/IX, and spectrin in the membrane cytoskeleton releases the constraints on the spectrin network. This allows the membrane skeleton to swell (but not produce filopodia) (see Fig. 2–5) by incorporating into the plasma membrane the membranes from the open canalicular system and, later, the membranes from the granules that release their contents.

The protrusive force for lamellipodia and filopodia formation comes from new actin polymerization, such that there is a doubling of actin filament content. This burst of actin filament assembly is powered by the generation of barbed-end nucleation sites after receptor activation. These nucleation sites are generated *de novo* by the activation of the Arp2/3 complex or by the exposure of the barbed ends of preexisting filaments.[217] Because barbed ends have a higher affinity for actin molecules than do the actin sequestering proteins, they have the capacity to initiate actin filament polymerization.

Platelets contain two proteins whose main function is to bind and sequester actin monomers. The first is profilin, which is present at a concentration of 50 $\mu$M. Profilin can sequester actin monomers from the pointed ends of actin filaments, but not the barbed ends. Profilin also functions as a major transfer factor in actin filament polymerization. The second and more abundant protein involved in sequestration of actin monomers and stimulation of the polymerization of actin is thymosin-$\beta_4$. With a platelet concentration of 55 mM, it is equimolar to actin. Thymosin-$\beta_4$ binds actin molecules with an affinity that is greater than that of the pointed end of the actin filament, allowing it to compete effectively for molecules from the pointed end. Thymosin-$\beta_4$ has a lower affinity for actin monomer than actin has for the barbed end of the filament, resulting in filament assembly when barbed ends are free. Thymosin-$\beta_4$ maintains a large pool of unpolymerized actin, and 60 percent of the total actin in the platelet is bound to thymosin-$\beta_4$. The affinity of thymosin-$\beta_4$ for actin monomer is regulated by the nucleotide that is bound to actin.[218]

The platelet actin assembly reaction that follows the addition of agonists starts when free barbed ends are formed (see Fig. 2–5). Barbed ends are generated by the uncapping of filament ends and the *de novo* assembly of filaments by the Arp2/3 complex. Platelets contain high concentrations of barbed-end capping proteins that regulate the accessibility of these ends to regulate actin dynamics. Platelets contain 5 $\mu$M each of gelsolin[219] and capZ,[220] and 3 mM of adducin.[221] Uncapping of the actin filaments appears to be accomplished by the inactivation of capping proteins by phosphoinositides that are produced during platelet activation, including PI-3,4-bisphosphate (PI$_{3,4}$P$_2$), PI$_{4,5}$P$_2$, and PI$_{3,4,5}$P$_3$.[216] The uncapped actin filaments act as nuclei onto which actin monomers (which are maintained in an available pool by association with thymosin-$\beta_4$) can assemble on the barbed ends of the filaments. Profilin accelerates actin polymerization by facilitating the transfer of actin from the actin-thymosin-$\beta_4$ complex to the barbed ends of the actin filaments. In addition to exposing new filament ends as a source of nuclei, new nucleation sites are generated by activation by the Arp2/3 complex. The Arp2/3 complex mimics the pointed ends of actin filaments and stimulates barbed-end assembly of actin filaments. The Arp2/3 complex is made up of seven polypeptides, two of which have actin-related sequences, Arp2 and Arp3.[222,223] Platelets contain high concentrations of the Arp2/3 complex (2 to 10 $\mu$M). Approximately 30 percent of the Arp2/3 complex is bound to the resting platelet cytoskeleton. Once platelets are activated, the Arp2/3 complex redistributes to the cytoskeleton, increasing three-fold and concentrating in the lamellipodial zone of actin filament assembly. Several signaling pathways regulate the activity of the Arp2/3 complex, including Wiskott-Aldrich syndrome protein (WASP) family members. Mutations in the *WASP* gene result in Wiskott-Aldrich syndrome, an inherited X-linked recessive disorder characterized by thrombocytopenia and T-cell immunodeficiency (see Chap. 11).

Simultaneous with these changes, the peripheral microtubule coil becomes constricted and fragmented and is ultimately compressed into the center of the cell. As the filopodia form, the platelet's granules and organelles move to the center, surrounded by the microtubule coil, resulting in an increase in electron density. Activation of myosin II via phosphorylation of myosin light chain kinase contributes to the inward contractile force by its interaction with the actin fibers.

## PLATELET SPREADING AND SURFACE-INDUCED ACTIVATION

After platelets adhere to surfaces, they undergo variable degrees of spreading and activation. The patterns of spreading and activation depend primarily on the protein surface on which they spread, with collagen consistently inducing the most activation.[224,225] In addition to the nature of the surface, the protein density, especially in the case of fibrinogen, can dramatically affect the signaling systems that are activated in the adherent platelets.[226] Activation can result in release of granule contents and exposure of activated integrin $\alpha_{IIb}\beta_3$ receptors on the luminal surface of the platelets, where they are strategically located to bind adhesive glycoprotein ligands that can recruit additional platelets.[227] If the surface density of platelets is sufficient, the platelets can also enter into lateral associations, which appear to depend on integrin $\alpha_{IIb}\beta_3$.[228] In general, platelet spreading results in the development of broad lamellipodia rather than spike-like filopodia (see Fig. 2–2).[216,229] The different morphologies of platelet spreading reflect differences in the organization of the network of actin filaments. Ultrastructural examination of lamellipodia reveals them to be replete with actin filaments that are organized into orthogonal networks. This organization is established by the actin filament crosslinking protein filamin A. In contrast, filopodia contain long actin filaments that are organized as tight bundles. These structural differences reflect the different signals initiated by the adhesion process, and both PIs and the small GTPase molecules Rac and Cdc42 appear to be particularly important in this process.[154] In platelets, Rac is activated by thrombin receptor ligation, and it stimulates actin filament uncapping.[230] Proteins that have been implicated in organizing the tips of the filopodia where the actin bundles attach to the plasma membrane are the small GTPase Cdc42, the exchange protein WASP, vinculin, vasodilator-stimulated protein (VASP), zyxin, and profilin.[111] Pleckstrin, a platelet protein that is phosphorylated during platelet activation, appears to participate in this process by binding to PIs and affecting Rac via an exchange factor.[231,232] Platelets from mice deficient in pleckstrin have a defect in granule secretion, integrin $\alpha_{IIb}\beta_3$ activation, and aggregation mediated by protein kinase C. Thrombin can overcome this abnormality via a pathway involving PI3K.[233] Signaling after adhesion results from the assembly of protein complexes on the cytoplasmic surfaces of the receptor(s) involved in the adhesion process, including focal adhesion kinase (FAK), which is activated by integrin ligation and colocalizes with a number of cytoskeletal proteins. Deletion of FAK in megakaryocytes and platelets results in defects in platelet spreading.[234] These complexes then initiate local cytoskeletal rearrangements as well as the generation of signaling molecules that act throughout the platelet to produce a variety of effects, including the translation of new proteins.[235–238] The nature and extent of the signaling may determine whether the adherent platelets recruit additional platelets or white blood cells. In particular, the conversion of spread platelets to a microvesiculated procoagulant form has been associated with the recruitment of neutrophils.[239] Additionally, spread platelets can assemble fibronectin matrix on their surface, which may be important in stabilizing platelet–platelet interactions.[240]

Membrane glycoproteins are affected by cytoskeletal rearrangements associated with platelet shape change and spreading. Activation of platelets in suspension under certain conditions results in movement of GPIb/IX receptors from the surface of platelets to the open canalicular system.[241,242] With adherent platelets, the GPIb internalization is much slower.[111] The initial effect of activation on integrin $\alpha_{IIb}\beta_3$ is an approximate doubling of these receptors on the plasma membranes, as preassembled receptors in $\alpha$ granules, and perhaps dense bodies and the open canalicular system, join the plasma membrane. Inside-out activation of integrin $\alpha_{IIb}\beta_3$ has been associated with cytoskeletal changes, in particular, the binding of talin to the integrin $\beta_3$ cytoplasmic domain.[243-246] Tyrosine kinases, including FAK[33,247] and Src,[247] may play a role in this process, along with cortactin, a protein of Mr 85 kDa that is phosphorylated on tyrosine, and small GTP binding proteins such as Rho, Rac, and Cdc42.[216,229,248,249] When the attachment of integrin $\alpha_{IIb}\beta_3$ to the cytoskeleton includes actin and myosin, the force produced by the cytoskeleton on the integrin may supply the energy to produce the conformational changes that lead to higher ligand binding affinity.[250] After activation, more integrin $\alpha_{IIb}\beta_3$ molecules become associated with the cytoskeleton, and this presumably reflects the interaction with talin and other cytoskeletal proteins and ligand-induced integrin clustering, resulting in the development of protein complexes, including cytoskeletal proteins, on the cytoplasmic surface of the receptor.[237,245,251] When ligand-coated beads are added to adherent platelets and bind to integrin $\alpha_{IIb}\beta_3$ receptors, the beads are transported to the center of the platelets, indicating that the cytoskeleton can move integrin receptors that have bound ligand.[252,253]

Platelets contain calpains, which are calcium-dependent, sulfhydryl-containing, neutral proteases composed of two subunits that preferentially cleave cytoskeletal proteins, in particular filamins and talin,[229,254] but have also been reported to cleave the cytoplasmic domain of integrin $\beta_3$ and a number of molecules involved in signaling, including kinases and phosphatases (see "Calcium-Dependent Proteases [Calpains]" below). $\mu$-Calpain requires micromolar calcium, and m-calpain requires millimolar calcium for activation. It has been proposed that calpains are involved in cytoskeletal reorganization upon platelet activation, specifically via cleavage of the integrin $\beta_3$ cytoplasmic tail and talin upon ligand engagement.[245,255-257] Calpain cleavage of the integrin $\beta_3$ cytoplasmic tail may switch the function of the integrin from promoting platelet spreading to mediating clot retraction.[258] Calpains have also been implicated in platelet spreading, microparticle formation, and the generation of platelet coagulant activity.[229,256,259] Mice lacking $\mu$-calpain have reduced platelet aggregation and clot retraction, but normal bleeding time.[260]

## PLATELET CONTRACTION AND CLOT RETRACTION

The contractile mechanism involving actin and myosin is thought to facilitate granule secretion, but the details remain obscure.[261,262] In fact, mice with nearly complete disruption of the platelet heavy-chain myosin gene, Myh9, have a defect in secretion, but only in response to low concentrations of select agonists.[263] The cytoskeleton of resting platelets consists of the membrane skeleton described above, which lies just beneath the membrane, and a lacy cytoplasmic actin filament network composed of 2000 to 5000 linear actin polymers that also contains $\alpha$-actin, filamins (actin binding proteins) A and B, tropomyosin, vinculin, and caldesmon.[176,177,248,249,264-268] The contractile response is also thought to be initiated by an increase in cytosolic calcium, which results in the formation of a calcium-calmodulin complex that then activates myosin light-chain kinase; phosphatases and cyclic adenosine monophosphate (cAMP) kinase can modulate this response. After the initial platelet shape change, actin becomes organized centrally into thick filamentous masses, where it probably associates with phosphorylated myosin filaments.[269,270] The centralization of organelles within a contractile ring correlates with secretion.[95] There is controversy, however, as to whether platelets secrete their granular contents by fusion with the open canalicular system in the center of the platelet or by direct fusion with the plasma membrane, or both.[95,100]

When blood initially clots in vitro, the fibrin mesh extends throughout, trapping virtually all of the serum in a gel-like state. If platelets are present, within minutes to hours, the clot retracts,

extruding a very large fraction of the serum.[271] This process is thought to mimic in vivo phenomena that result in consolidation of thrombi and perhaps enhancement of wound healing. Clot retraction has also been implicated in decreasing porosity and solute transport so as to concentrate intrathrombus thrombin,[272] as well as decreasing the efficiency of thrombolysis, which may partially account for the resistance of platelet-rich thrombi to fibrinolytic agents.[273] The platelet requirement for clot retraction is indisputable, as is a requirement for integrin $\alpha_{IIb}\beta_3$ and a contractile mechanism involving actin and myosin.[274,275] In fact, nearly complete selective disruption of the myosin Myh9 gene in murine megakaryocytes gives rise to a phenotype characterized by macrothrombocytopenia; absence of clot retraction; reduced secretion in response to low concentrations of agonists, but not high concentrations; prolonged bleeding time; and protection from thrombus formation.[263] The mice do not, however, spontaneously bleed.[263] Myosin activation involves phosphorylation of the myosin light chain, a process that is governed by calcium-regulated myosin light-chain kinase activity and Rho kinase–regulated myosin phosphatase activity. Calpain cleavage of the cytoplasmic tail of integrin $\beta_3$ may promote RhoA activity and serve as a molecular switch to convert platelet spreading to clot retraction.[258] Other signaling molecules appear to contribute to clot retraction, including the Eph kinase EphB2,[276] protein phosphatase 2B,[277] and PI3K.[278] Despite these data, no model describing the details of the clot retraction process has gained acceptance.[279] Proposed mechanisms include movement of platelet filopodia along fibrin strands, tugging of fibrin strands by filopodia, and internalization of fibrin by the action of the membrane skeleton.[274,275,279-282]

Platelet integrin $\alpha_{IIb}\beta_3$ is required for clot retraction, as demonstrated by studies of patients with Glanzmann thrombasthenia (Chap. 11) and studies of normal platelets in the presence of agents that block either the integrin $\alpha_{IIb}\beta_3$ receptor[280,283-288] or the fibrinogen $\gamma$-chain C-terminal sequence that mediates interactions with the integrin.[289] It also requires disulfide bond exchange[290] and the tyrosine residues on the integrin $\beta_3$ subunit that are phosphorylated upon platelet activation and contribute to outside-in signaling.[291] Clot retraction correlates temporally with an integrin $\alpha_{IIb}\beta_3$-dependent decrease in protein tyrosine phosphorylation, presumably via activation of one or more phosphatases,[292] and may require both integrin-mediated mitogen-activated protein kinase (MAPK) activation[293] and translation of proteins such as Bcl-3, with the latter facilitated by ligand binding to integrin $\alpha_{IIb}\beta_3$.[294] However, results with integrin $\alpha_{IIb}\beta_3$ antagonists demonstrate differences in their ability to inhibit clot retraction that do not correlate with their ability to block fibrinogen binding to platelets,[280,287] and patients with Glanzmann thrombasthenia differ in the extent of their defect in clot retraction. Some integrin $\alpha_{IIb}\beta_3$ mutations, such as integrin $\beta_3$ L262P, interfere with interactions with fibrinogen but do not prevent interactions with fibrin and clot retraction.[295] Of particular note, fibrinogen lacking the $\gamma$-chain C-terminal sequence (amino acids 400 to 411) that mediates binding to platelet integrin $\alpha_{IIb}\beta_3$, as well as the two Arg-Gly-Asp (RGD)-containing regions in fibrinogen, is still capable of supporting clot retraction.[296,297] It is well established that when fibrinogen converts to fibrin, new sites become exposed on the surface of the molecule. Therefore, one possible explanation for this paradox is that additional or alternative integrin binding sequences in the fibrinogen $\gamma$-chain (e.g., 316 to 322, 370 to 383, or other regions) may be able to mediate clot retraction.[298,299] Potential binding sites for the $\gamma$370 to 381 sequence, which is better expressed on fibrin than fibrinogen, on the integrin $\alpha_{IIb}$ $\beta$-propeller region, were identified, and peptides from these regions inhibit clot retraction.[300] Factor XIII also plays an important role in clot retraction; it has been proposed to mediate the translocation of the fibrinogen/fibrin–integrin $\alpha_{IIb}\beta_3$ complex to sphingomyelin-rich lipid rafts in the platelet membrane as well as crosslink the complex to cytoskeletal and contractile elements.[301,302] It is also possible that GPIb/IX contributes to clot retraction by virtue of the binding of GPIbα to the thrombin and/or VWF bound to the fibrin.[303,304] Thus, although integrin $\alpha_{IIb}\beta_3$ is required for clot retraction, the process is not a simple reflection of fibrinogen binding to integrin $\alpha_{IIb}\beta_3$.

# ● PLATELET SECRETORY MACHINERY AND SECRETION

Platelets possess secretory granules and mechanisms for cargo release to amplify responses to stimuli and influence the surrounding environment. Platelet granule structures include α and dense granules, lysosomes, and peroxisomes.

## SECRETORY ORGANELLES

### Lysosomes

Lysosomes are produced from the endosomal membrane system through a complex mechanism involving membrane and protein sorting and trafficking.[305] Platelet lysosomes contain acid hydrolases typical of these organelles (e.g., β-glucuronidase, cathepsins, aryl sulfatase, β-hexosaminidase, β-galactosidase, endoglucosidase [heparitinase], β-glycerophosphatase, elastase, and collagenase).[197] With activation, platelets secrete some of these enzymes; however, lysosomal contents are more slowly and less completely released than are those from α granules and dense bodies.[306-308] Thus, stronger agonists are required to induce lysosomal enzyme release than release from the other granules, and their appearance on the platelet plasma membrane serves as a marker of high-level platelet activation.[309,310] The elastase and collagenase activities released from platelet lysosomes may contribute to vascular damage at sites of platelet thrombus formation.[311] The heparitinase may be able to cleave heparin-like molecules from the surface of endothelial cells, and the resulting soluble molecules appear to inhibit growth of smooth muscle cells.[312]

### Dense Bodies

Platelets contain approximately three to eight electron-dense organelles, 20 to 30 nm in diameter (see Fig. 2–2).[76,262] The intrinsic electron density of dense bodies when viewed as unstained whole mounts derives from their high content of calcium[76,197]; the granules are also dense when viewed by transmission electron microscopy because they are highly osmophilic.[262] Dense granules contain high concentrations of serotonin, which is taken up from plasma by a plasma membrane carrier and then trapped in the dense bodies.[262] Trapping of serotonin may occur as a result of the lower pH (approximately 6.1) maintained in dense granules as a result of the action of a proton pumping ATPase on the dense-body membrane.[262] ADP and ATP are also highly concentrated in dense bodies.[197] There is more ADP than ATP in the dense bodies (ATP to ADP ratio = 2:3), which is the reverse of their relative concentrations in the cytoplasm (ATP to ADP ratio = 8:1). As there is little connection between the pools of adenine nucleotides in the cytoplasm and the dense bodies, they have been respectively designated as the *metabolic* and *storage pools* of adenine nucleotides.[197] Storage of adenine nucleotides at such a high concentration in dense bodies appears to be achieved by stacking the ATP and ADP purine rings vertically in aggregates that are stabilized by the interactions of calcium ions with the polyphosphate groups.[313,314] The planar hydroxyindole rings of serotonin may also enter these stacks, providing a molecular basis for the trapping mechanism. Trapping of serotonin must differ from that of adenine nucleotides, however, because dense granule serotonin exchanges readily with external serotonin.[197] Transport and delivery of platelet-derived serotonin may play an important role in a variety of biologic phenomena including vasospasm, platelet coagulant activity, and liver regeneration.[315]

The membrane of dense granules contains glycoproteins that are also found on the plasma membrane and the membranes of α granules and lysosomes, including CD36, LAMP-2, CD63, P-selectin, $\alpha_{IIb}\beta_3$, and GPIb/IX. Abnormalities of eight different genes have been implicated in the Hermansky-Pudlak syndrome (HPS) (Chap. 11), an autosomal disorder characterized by a deficiency of dense bodies, and so these genes are presumed to participate in dense body formation. As with lysosomes, dense bodies are thought to derive from endosomes, via different types of multivesicular bodies (MVBs). The eight genes associated with HPS are thought to affect sorting and/or trafficking of membrane structures through participation in protein complexes that mediate these phenomena.[316,317] These complexes include three biogenesis of lysosome-related organelles complexes (BLOCs) and the activator protein 3 (AP3) complex.[305] Similarly, the product of the *LYST* gene, which is abnormal in some patients with Chédiak-Higashi syndrome (who also have abnormal dense bodies), has been proposed to associate with the dense granule membrane (Chap. 11).[318] The *LYST* gene product may associate with the AP3 complex.[305]

The abnormalities of *in vitro* platelet function in patients with HPS suggest that released dense granule contents contribute to platelet activation through a positive feedback mechanism. Release of ADP, which is a potent platelet activator, and serotonin, a weaker agonist (see section "Signaling Pathways in Platelets" below), probably accounts for most of the positive feedback effects on platelet aggregation. ATP is a partial antagonist of ADP-induced activation, but as ATP is rapidly catabolized to ADP in plasma ($T_{1/2}$ = 1.5 min), and ADP is rapidly catabolized to AMP ($T_{1/2}$ = 4 min) and then to adenosine,[197] a platelet inhibitor,[319] it is difficult to predict the overall effect of ATP release. Adding to the complexity *in vivo* is the presence of an ecto-ADPase (CD39; ecto-ADPase) present on endothelial and lymphoid cells, which can metabolize ATP and ADP to AMP and thus probably limits the amount of ADP present.[74] ATP released from platelets may also serve as a high-energy phosphate source for platelet ecto-protein kinases, which can phosphorylate several proteins, including CD36 (GPIV).[320-322]

### α Granules

An important platelet function is storage and release of a variety of bioactive substances packaged in α granules. α Granules are the most abundant granule type of platelets, numbering approximately 50 to 80 per platelet.[323,324] They are approximately 200 nm in diameter on cross-section and demonstrate internal variation in electron density, often with an eccentric area of accentuated electron density, termed a *nucleoid*, in which β-thromboglobulin, platelet factor 4 (PF4), and proteoglycans are concentrated (see Fig. 2–2).[325] The more electron-lucent areas contain tubular elements in which VWF, multimerin, and factor V are preferentially localized.[76] Proteomic analysis of the releasate of activated human platelets has identified more than 300 proteins, most of which are stored within α granules.[326-328] The list of α-granule proteins includes adhesive proteins, coagulation factors, protease inhibitors, chemokines, and angiogenesis regulatory proteins. Some of the most important proteins present in α granules are described in detail below. Platelets contain distinct subpopulations of α granules that undergo differential release of α-granule cargo during activation. For example, some α granules contain proangiogenic proteins, such as vascular endothelial growth factor (VEGF), whereas others contain antiangiogenic factors, such as endostatin (Fig. 2–6).[329] These two subclasses of α granules can be differentially induced to undergo degranulation by exposure of human platelets to agonists specific for either protease-activated receptor (PAR)-1 or PAR-4. Fibrinogen and VWF are localized

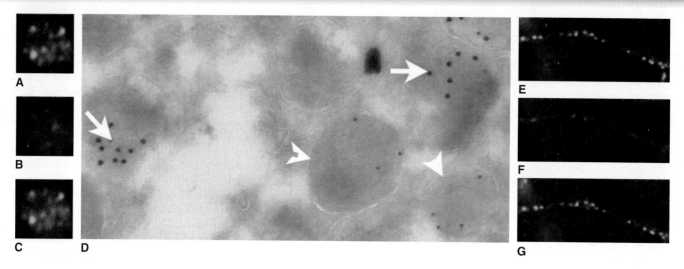

**Figure 2–6.** Platelets contain separate and distinct α-granule populations. **A, B,** and **C.** Specific pro- and antiangiogenic regulators organize into separate, distinct α granules in resting platelets. Double immunofluorescence microscopy of resting platelets using antibodies against vascular endothelial growth factor (VEGF) **(A)** and endostatin **(B)** and an overlay **(C). D.** Localization of proteins in resting, human platelets using immunoelectron microscopy of ultrathin cryosections. Double immunogold labeling on platelet sections was performed with the use of anti-VEGF antibody and antiendostatin antibodies. Large gold particles representing anti-VEGF staining (15 nm, *arrows*) are evident on one population of α granules, and small gold particles (5 nm) representing endostatin staining are abundantly present on a different population of α granules (*arrowheads*). **E, F,** and **G.** Pro- and antiangiogenic regulatory proteins are also segregated into separate, distinct α granules in megakaryocyte proplatelets. Megakaryocytes generate platelets by remodeling their cytoplasm into long proplatelet extensions, which serve as assembly lines for platelet production. Distinct α granules are visualized along proplatelets. Shown is a double immunofluorescence microscopy experiment of proplatelets using antibodies against VEGF **(E)** and endostatin **(F),** and an overlay **(G).** *(Reproduced with permission from Italiano JE, et al: Angiogenesis is regulated by a novel mechanism: pro- and antiangiogenic proteins are organized into separate platelet alpha granules and differentially released, Blood. 2008 Feb 1;111(3):1227–1233.)*

in separate α granules,[330] and glass activation of platelets results in the selective release of the fibrinogen-containing granules.

The α granule acquires its protein content by both biosynthesis (predominantly at the megakaryocyte level) and endocytosis (at both the megakaryocyte and circulating platelet levels). Small amounts of virtually all plasma proteins are nonspecifically taken up into α granules, and thus, the plasma levels of these proteins determine their platelet levels.[331,332] For example, the α-granule pool of immunoglobulins contains most of the platelet immunoglobulin; therefore, total platelet immunoglobulin is more affected by changes in plasma immunoglobulin levels than by changes in surface immunoglobulin.[331,332]

The cell biologic pathways that regulate α-granule assembly are not fully understood, but several studies suggest MVBs play a crucial intermediary role in α-granule biogenesis.[316,333] These membranous sacs, containing numerous small vesicles, develop from budding vesicles in the Golgi complex within megakaryocytes and can interact with endocytic vesicles. They are abundant in immature megakaryocytes and decrease in number with cellular maturation, suggesting that they are the precursors of α granules and/or dense bodies. MVBs may also function as a sorting hub to rout proteins into distinct classes of α granules.

The platelet-specific proteins (PF4 and the β-thromboglobulin family) are present in α granules at concentrations that are approximately 20,000 times higher than their plasma concentrations (when each is expressed as a fraction of total protein in platelets or plasma, respectively).[334,335] These Mr 7000 to 11,000 proteins all bind to heparin, but with varying affinities. They also share amino acid sequence homology with each other and with other members of the "intercrine-cytokine" family of molecules, such as interleukin (IL)-8 (neutrophil-activating peptide 1 [NAP1]), which are active in inflammation, cell growth, and malignant transformation.[336–338]

PF4 is a CXC chemokine (CXCL4) that does not contain the Glu-Leu-Arg (ELR) conserved sequence.[339,340] It binds to heparin with high affinity and can neutralize heparin's anticoagulant activity.[335,341–343]

PF4 tetramers complex with a proteoglycan carrier.[344,345] Specific PF4 lysine residues (amino acids 61, 62, 65, and 66) are implicated in its binding to heparin, and x-ray crystallography indicates that these lysines are on the surface of the PF4 tetramer and interact with negatively charged heparin molecules that wind around this core.[346–348]

After PF4 is released from platelets, it binds to heparin-like molecules on the surface of endothelial cells.[346] Heparin administration can mobilize this endothelial-bound pool of PF4 into the circulation.[346] PF4-heparin complexes and PF4-heparin-like molecule complexes on endothelial cells have been implicated as the target antigens in heparin-induced thrombocytopenia with thrombosis.[349,350] PF4 also binds to hepatocytes, which take it up and catabolize it.[351] PF4 is a weak neutrophil and fibroblast attractant.[340,352] It inhibits angiogenesis, perhaps through inhibition of endothelial cell proliferation.[353] A large number of other activities have been ascribed to PF4, including histamine release from basophils[354]; inhibition of both tumor growth[353] and megakaryocyte maturation[355–357]; reversal of immunosuppression[352,358]; enhancement of fibroblast attachment to substrata[359]; potentiation of platelet aggregation[360]; inhibition of contact activation[361]; and enhancement of both polymorphonuclear leukocyte responsiveness to the activating peptide f-Met-Leu-Phe and monocyte responsiveness to lipopolysaccharide.[362,363]

The β-thromboglobulin family of proteins are CXC chemokines that contain the conserved Glu-Leu-Arg (ELR) sequence.[340] They include platelet basic protein, low-affinity PF4 (connective tissue-activating peptide III [CTAP-III]), β-thromboglobulin, and β-thromboglobulin-F (NAP2, CXCL7).[334,364–366] All of these proteins share the same carboxy terminus but differ in the length of their amino termini, presumably as a result of proteolytic digestion of the parent molecule, platelet basic protein. These proteins bind to heparin but with lower affinity than PF4, and thus neutralize heparin less well. Unlike PF4, they are cleared from the circulation by the kidney rather than the liver.[367] CTAP-III is a weak fibroblast mitogen, and β-thromboglobulin is a chemoattractant for fibroblasts.[340] $\beta$-Thromboglobulin-F NAP2 (CXCL7) binds to CXCR2 and is chemotactic for granulocytes and activates them to undergo endocytosis.[339,340,366] Platelet $\alpha$ granules also contain additional chemokines that can variably activate leukocytes and platelets.[339]

The biochemistry of the adhesive glycoproteins contained in $\alpha$ granules and others variably present in plasma and extracellular matrix is described in Table 2–2 and in other chapters (e.g., Chaps. 3 and 15 for fibrinogen and Chap. 16 for VWF). Their relative concentrations in $\alpha$ granules varies significantly. Their localization in platelet $\alpha$ granules allows them to achieve high local concentrations when released from platelets at the site of vascular injury.

Multimerin comprises a family of disulfide-linked homomultimers, ranging in molecular weight from 450,000 to many millions.[368] The Mr 450,000 multimer is thought to be a trimer of a single subunit of either Mr 167,000[369] or Mr 155,000[368] that is synthesized in megakaryocytes and endothelial cells and stored in the electron-lucent region of $\alpha$ granules in platelets and dense-core granules in endothelial cells.[370] It colocalizes with VWF in platelets, but not endothelial cells. Although multimerin's multimeric structure is similar to that of VWF, the deduced amino acid sequence of its subunit is not homologous to that of VWF.[368] The pre-promultimerin subunit contains 1228 amino acids. It undergoes glycosylation and proteolysis during synthesis. It is composed of a number of domains, including an aminoterminal region that includes an RGD sequence, coiled coil sequences, epidermal growth factor (EGF)-like domains, and a carboxyterminal globular head similar to that found in the complement protein C1q. Multimerin binds both factor V and factor Va, and all of the biologically active factor V in platelets is bound to multimerin.[325] With thrombin activation of platelets, factor V separates from multimerin, and the higher molecular weight multimerin multimers bind to platelets. Multimerin does not circulate in plasma at an appreciable concentration, but it may act as an adhesive extracellular matrix protein.

Fibrinogen is concentrated in $\alpha$ granules as judged by the ratio of platelet-to-plasma fibrinogen. Megakaryocytes do not appear to synthesize fibrinogen; instead, it is taken up from plasma by a process that involves the $\alpha_{IIb}\beta_3$ receptor.[371] Because fibrinogen molecules that contain altered sequences in the $\gamma$ chain are not stored in $\alpha$ granules, even when the molecules are heterodimeric (i.e., contain one normal and one abnormal $\gamma$ chain), it is possible that uptake requires simultaneous binding of a single fibrinogen molecule to two different $\alpha_{IIb}\beta_3$ receptors via the $\gamma$-chain carboxyterminal sequence (see $\alpha_{IIb}\beta_3$ in the section "Platelet Membrane Glycoproteins" below and Chap. 11).[371,372]

The VWF stored in platelet $\alpha$ granules appears to contribute to hemostasis because in certain pathologic states it correlates better with bleeding symptoms than does plasma VWF concentration (Chap. 16). VWF is synthesized in megakaryocytes and endothelial cells. The multimeric structure of platelet VWF is thought to reflect endothelial VWF more nearly than plasma VWF, as higher Mr multimers are present.

Fibronectin is present in $\alpha$ granules, but no clear role in platelet function under normal conditions has been identified for this adhesive protein. Paradoxically, in murine models, fibronectin has been reported to both support platelet thrombus formation and inhibit platelet aggregation and thrombus formation[41,373]; the former effect may be mediated by insoluble fibronectin fibrils, whereas the latter may be mediated by soluble fibronectin.[374]

Vitronectin, which gets its name from its propensity to bind to glass, also binds to PAI-1, the urokinase receptor (uPAR), collagen, and heparin; it also forms ternary complexes with serine proteases and serpins in the coagulation and complement systems. It is present in platelets at levels that suggest it is concentrated,[375] but it does not appear to be synthesized in megakaryocytes. The binding of PAI-1 with vitronectin stabilizes PAI-1 in its active conformation, and it has been proposed that only the approximately 5 percent of PAI-1 complexed with vitronectin in platelet $\alpha$ granules is active.[150] Mice deficient in vitronectin have been reported to be protected from, or have a predisposition to develop, thrombosis, depending on the method of inducing thrombosis.[376–378]

Thrombospondin-1 is unique among the adhesive glycoproteins in blood in that it is present almost exclusively inside the platelet.[379–381] It constitutes approximately 20 percent of the released platelet proteins. Thrombospondin-1 is synthesized by megakaryocytes, cultured endothelial cells, and other cultured cells.[382,383] Although integrin $\alpha_{IIb}\beta_3$, GPIb/IX, integrin $\alpha_V\beta_3$, proteoglycans, integrin-associated protein (CD47 or IAP), and CD36 (GPIV) have all been implicated as receptors for thrombospondin,[384–390] CD47 appears to be most important in initiating platelet activation by thrombospondin (see "Signaling Pathways in Platelet Activation and Aggregation" below).[386,387,391] The phosphorylation state of CD36 (GPIV) may affect its ability to bind thrombospondin.[385] Thrombospondin contains an Arginine-Glycine-Aspartate (RGD) sequence, which may contribute to its binding to platelets, but other regions are probably also involved.[381,392] The conformation of thrombospondin varies with the calcium concentration of the surrounding environment. Thrombospondin can interact with many other adhesive glycoproteins, including fibronectin and fibrinogen,[210,393,394] and it is a component of the extracellular matrix.[395] Thrombospondin appears to stabilize platelet aggregates that are formed[396]; it may also act as a negative regulator of angiogenesis, modulate fibrinolysis, and contribute to activation of latent transforming growth factor (TGF)-$\beta_1$ released from platelets (see below in this section).[397,398]

Platelets contribute approximately 20 percent of the factor V present in whole blood, with nearly all of it in $\alpha$ granules.[399–401] Human platelet factor V appears to be taken up from plasma rather than being synthesized in megakaryocytes, which is in stark contrast to the situation in mice. When stored in $\alpha$ granules, factor V associates with multimerin.[402,403] Platelet-derived factor V appears to undergo unique posttranslational modifications and proteolytic activation, resulting in resistance to protein C-catalyzed inactivation.[404–406] Evidence from patients with inhibitors and deficiencies of plasma and platelet factor V indicate that platelet-derived factor V has an important role in hemostasis.[399,407,408] Platelets undergo microvesiculation when activated, and the microvesicles, which are rich in factor V, are potent promoters of coagulation.[409]

Protein S (Chap. 4), plasminogen activator-1 (Chap. 25), and $\alpha_2$-plasmin inhibitor (Chap. 25) are also contained in $\alpha$ granules and can be released from platelets. Similarly, tissue factor pathway inhibitor (TFPI; Chap. 4), $\alpha_1$-protease inhibitor, and C-1 inhibitor (Chap. 4) have also been identified in $\alpha$ granules.

Gas6 is a 75-kDa vitamin K-dependent protein that contains $\gamma$-carboxyglutamic acids and is similar in structure to protein S.[410,411] Gas6 was originally isolated as a growth arrest-specific gene from quiescent fibroblasts but subsequently was found to enhance platelet aggregation and secretion in response to several agonists.[412] Mice deficient in Gas6 have abnormalities in platelet aggregation and are protected from experimental thrombosis.[412] Gas6 is present in $\alpha$ granules and secreted with platelet activation. Platelets also express Mer, a tyrosine kinase receptor for Gas6, and mice deficient in Mer demonstrate both abnormalities in platelet aggregation and protection from thrombosis, but not to the same extent as mice deficient in Gas6.[413,414] Other Gas6 receptors in the same family as Mer also appear to contribute to platelet thrombus stability.[413–417]

Platelet-derived growth factor (PDGF) is a disulfide-linked dimeric molecule of approximately Mr 30,000 that is mitogenic for smooth muscle cells.[418] Platelet $\alpha$ granules contain a mixture of the homodimer PDGF-BB (30 percent) and the heterodimer PDGF-AB (70 percent); the different forms appear to have different functional activities.[419] PDGF may play a role in normal cell proliferation, as well

**TABLE 2–2.** Adhesive Glycoproteins

| Protein | Subunit, kDa | Unusual 1° Structural Features & Modifications | Domain Homologies & Binding Regions | Mature Protein Composition | Mature Protein Mr | Known Interactions |
|---|---|---|---|---|---|---|
| Collagens | 95–180 | Gly-Pro-X repeating sequence Hydroxylysine Hydroxyproline | RGD Right-handed triple helix | Tropocollagen = 3 chains | | Variable Thrombospondin |
| Type I | $\alpha_1(I)$ $\alpha_2(I)$ | | DGEA† VWFC | $[\alpha_1(I)]_2\alpha_2(I)$ (major component) $[\alpha_1(I)]_3$ | | Fibronectin von Willebrand factor |
| Type III | $\alpha_1(III)$ | | VWFC | $[\alpha_1(III)]_3$ | | |
| Type VI | $\alpha_1(VI)$ $\alpha_2(VI)$ $\alpha_3(VI)$ | | 3 VWFA 3 VWFA 12 VWFA | $\alpha_1(VI)\alpha_2(VI)\alpha_3(VI)$ | | |
| von Willebrand factor | 220 (2050 amino acids) | Large propeptide (741 amino acids); A, B, C, D, E repeats | $\alpha_{IIb}\beta_3$ – RGD 1789–1791 I Domains GPIb – 230–310 | Dimer = protomer Multimers of protomers from 2–~40 via disulfide bonds | 880,000– ~20,000,000 | Collagen Heparin Factor VIII Fibrin |
| Fibrinogen | A$\alpha$ = 63 (625 amino acids) B$\beta$ = 56 (461 amino acids) $\gamma$ = 47 (427 amino acids) | Alternately spliced $\gamma$ chains Phosphorylation of A$\alpha$ | 2 RGDs in A$\alpha$ (95–97 and 572–574) $\alpha_V\beta_3$ – RGD 572–574 $\alpha_{IIb}\beta_3$–C-terminal $\gamma$- chain dodecamer (400–411) | 2 A$\alpha$, 2 B$\beta$, 2 $\gamma$ via disulfide bonds | 340,000 | Thrombospondin ?Collagen Staphylococci Factor XIII Thrombin |
| Vitronectin | 1 chain = 75 (458 amino acids) 2 chain = 65 + 10 via disulfide bonds | Met → Thr polymorphism | RGD Somatomedin B 2 Hemopexin | Same as subunits | 75,000 and 65,000+10,000 | Glass Plastic Heparin Serine protease: serpin complexes PAI-1 uPAR Factor XIII |
| Fibronectin | 220 (2355 amino acids) | Types I, II, and III repeats Alternately spliced forms | RGD (1493–1495) | Heterodimer via disulfide bonds | 440,000 | Fibrin Heparin Collagen DNA Staphylococci |
| Thrombo-spondin 1 | 180 (1150 amino acids) | | RGD (?functional) VTCG† $\alpha_1(I)$ Collagen Epidermal growth factor Malaria antigen | Trimer via disulfide bonds | 450,000 | Calcium Plasminogen Collagen Fibrinogen Histidine-rich glycoprotein Fibronectin Laminin Heparin |
| Osteopontin | 32 (298 amino acids) | Phosphorylation Sulfation | RGD | | | Hydroxyapatite Plaque components |
| Laminin | A = 400 B$_1$ = 215 (1765 amino acids) B$_2$ = 205 (1576 amino acids) | | YIGSR† RGD (?functional) EGF | A, B$_1$, B$_2$, via disulfide bonds | 850,000 | Collagen type IV Nidogen/entactin Osteonectin Heparin sulfate C1q Plasminogen Plasmin |
| Multimerin | 155 or 167 kDa | Large prepro-peptide (1228 amino acids) | RGD in N-terminal region EGF | | 450,000– ~5,000,000 | Factor V |

EGF, epidermal growth factor; PAI-1, plasminogen activator-1; RGD, arginine-glycine-aspartic acid sequence; uPAR, urine-type plasminogen activator receptor; VWFA, VWFC, von Willebrand factor A and C repeats.

| Known Platelet Receptors | Electron Microscopy Structure | Plasma Concentration, mcg/mL | Platelet Concentration,* mcg/mL | Ratio Platelet/ Plasma | Sites of Synthesis |
|---|---|---|---|---|---|
| $\alpha_2\beta_1$ (GPIa/IIa; CD49b/CD29; VLA-2) GPVI<br>GPIV (CD36)? | Tropocollagen = rodlike coil, 15 × 3000; other forms have variable degrees of fibril formation | – | – | – | Fibroblasts |
| GPIb (CD42b, c)<br>$\alpha_{IIb}\beta_3$ (GPIIb/IIIa; CD41/CD61) | Elliptical, nodular coil, length 5000, but with some 11,000 Å | 10 | 34 | 3.4 | Endothelial cells<br>Megakaryocytes |
| $\alpha_{IIb}\beta_3$ (GPIIb/IIIa; CD41/CD61)<br>$\alpha_V\beta_3$ (CD51/CD61) | Trinodular, asymmetrical; 475 Å diameter | 3000 | 7300 | 2.4 | Hepatocytes |
| $\alpha_{IIb}\beta_3$ (GPIIb/IIIa; CD41/CD61)<br>$\alpha_V\beta_3$ (CD51/CD61) | | 350 | 800 | 2.3 | ?Hepatocytes |
| $\alpha_5\beta_1$ (GPIc*/IIa (CD49e/CD29; VLA-5)<br>$\alpha_{IIb}\beta_3$ (GPIIb/IIIa; CD41/CD61) | Extended antiparallel dimeric structure | 300 | 315 | 1.1 | Hepatocytes<br>Fibroblasts<br>?Endothelial cells<br>Megakaryocytes<br>Monocytes, etc. |
| GPIV (CD36)<br>$\alpha_{IIb}\beta_3$ (GPIIb/IIIa; CD41/CD61)?<br>Integrin associated protein (CD47) | 3 Asymmetrical dumbbells, joined near smaller globular domains | 0.16 | 4900 | 30,625 | Megakaryocytes<br>Many cultured cells |
| $\alpha_V\beta_3$ | | – | – | – | Bone<br>?Other cells |
| $\alpha_6\beta_1$ (GPIc/IIa; CD49/CD29; VLA-6) | Cross-like structure | – | – | – | Fibroblasts<br>Many other cell types |
| Unknown | Unknown | – | – | – | Megakaryocytes<br>Endothelial cells |

*Assumes $10^{11}$ platelets per mL of packed platelets.

†DGEA, VTCG, and YIGSR are other amino acid sequences involved in function.

as in the development of atherosclerosis, tumor growth, wound repair, and fibroproliferative responses.[420–422] After it was discovered in platelets and termed PDGF, other tissues were found to produce the same factor; thus, despite its name, PDGF is not exclusively derived from platelets. PDGF is structurally related to the transforming protein p28[sis] of simian sarcoma virus,[423,424] and its receptor is in the tyrosine kinase family.[425] Recombinant human PDGF-BB (becaplermin) is approved as adjunctive therapy to improve healing of foot ulcerations in diabetics.[426]

Platelets contain high concentrations of VEGF, an important stimulator of angiogenesis, and can release VEGF after stimulation *in vitro* and during the hemostatic response to a bleeding time wound.[427–429] Megakaryocytes express mRNA of the three VEGF isoforms (121, 165, and 189 amino acids),[430] and by immunoblot, VEGF protein bands of apparent molecular weights 34,000 and 44,000 are identifiable in platelets.[431] Platelets and megakaryocytes also express the gene transcript for the VEGF receptor termed KDR.[432] Another endothelial growth factor structurally related to VEGF, VEGF-C, has also been identified in platelets.[433] Platelet levels of VEGF have been reported to be increased in malignancies, and so elevated levels of platelet VEGF may be a cancer biomarker.[434,435] Platelet VEGF has also been postulated to play a role in tumor growth[436] and proliferative retinopathy in sickle cell disease.[437,438]

EGF has also been identified in platelets, but the kinetics of its release upon thrombin or collagen stimulation differs from that of other granule proteins.[439]

Platelets contain the highest levels of all peripheral tissues of amyloid precursor protein (APP), which contains the sequence for the self-aggregating 40- to 43-amino-acid-residue peptide, A$\beta$, that has been strongly implicated in the pathogenesis of Alzheimer disease.[440,441] The isoforms containing the Kunitz protease inhibitor domain (APP 770 and APP 751) predominate in platelets. Although synthesized as a membrane protein, platelet APP is cleaved by $\alpha$-, $\beta$-, and $\gamma$-secretase activities, producing all of the fragments produced by neurons, as well as the soluble sAPP$\alpha$, sAPP$\beta$, and A$\beta$ peptides, and the corresponding remaining C-terminal membrane-associated fragments.[440,442,443] Calpain, which is present in platelets, can also cleave platelet APP.[444] Approximately 90 percent of platelet APP is soluble and stored in $\alpha$ granules, but full-length APP surface expression is increased threefold by thrombin stimulation.[445] Platelets are the major source of plasma sAPPs and A$\beta$.[443,446] APPs released by platelets are potent inhibitors of factor XIa[447] and IXa,[448,449] and also can inhibit platelet aggregation induced by ADP or epinephrine. In contrast, A$\beta$ appears to enhance ADP-induced platelet aggregation and support platelet adhesion. It is possible, but not certain, that plasma A$\beta$ contributes to brain A$\beta$ in Alzheimer disease.[441] Patients with Alzheimer disease have been reported to display altered platelet APP metabolism.[450–455]

Factor XIII is present in the cytoplasm of platelets; it differs from plasma factor XIII in having only the "a" subunits (Chap. 3).[456–459] Platelet factor XIII accounts for approximately 50 percent of total blood factor XIII,[456,457] and platelet factor XIII may contribute to the plasma pool.[460] Upon platelet activation, factor XIII redistributes to the platelet periphery where it associates with the cytoskeleton and crosslinks filamin and vinculin.[461] It may also crosslink thymosin $\beta_4$ to fibrin after thrombin stimulation[462] and, in concert with calpain, decrease integrin $\alpha_{IIb}\beta_3$ adhesive function in thrombus formation on collagen.[463] Transglutaminase-mediated conjugation of serotonin to $\alpha$-granule proteins after platelet stimulation with collagen and thrombin results in the generation of a subpopulation of platelets that are coated with fibrinogen, thrombospondin, factor V, VWF, and fibronectin, either directly through ligand–receptor interactions or through interactions between the serotonin conjugates and platelet surface fibrinogen or thrombospondin (COAT platelets).[464,465]

Platelet $\alpha$ granules contain a high concentration of TGF-$\beta_1$, an Mr 25,000 homodimeric protein that promotes the growth of certain cells and inhibits the growth of others.[466–469] For example, TGF-$\beta$ can increase thrombopoietin production by marrow stromal cells. In turn, thrombopoietin induces both increased megakaryocyte production and megakaryocyte expression of TGF-$\beta$ receptors. The interaction of TGF-$\beta$ with these receptors then results in inhibition of megakaryocyte maturation.[470] TGF-$\beta_1$ also induces synthesis of extracellular matrix proteins, PAI-1, and metalloproteinases. It has been implicated in wound healing, malignancy, and tissue fibrosis.[471] In addition, TGF-$\beta_1$ has been reported to enhance platelet aggregation through a nontranscriptional effect.[472] Migration of endothelial cells is inhibited by TGF-$\beta_1$, but it acts as a chemoattractant for monocytes and fibroblasts. TGF-$\beta$ exists in three isoforms (TGF-$\beta_1$, TGF-$\beta_2$, and TGF-$\beta_3$), but platelets contain only TGF-$\beta_1$. TGF-$\beta_1$ released from platelets can stimulate smooth muscle cells to express and release VEGF, thus perhaps supporting reendothelialization after vascular injury.[473]

TGF-$\beta_1$ released from platelets is inactive (latent) because it is complexed with the remaining portion of its precursor protein (latency-associated peptide [LAP]).[474] LAP, in turn, is covalently coupled to another protein, the latent TGF-$\beta$–binding protein-1 (LTBP-1), which localizes the complex to the extracellular matrix.[475] Activation of latent TGF-$\beta_1$ is a complex process that is thought to involve a conformational change in LAP that results in altering its ability to shield the active site in TGF-$\beta_1$.[475] Activation of latent TGF-$\beta_1$ can be achieved by several different mechanisms, including acidification; proteolysis by plasmin, a furin-like enzyme, or other enzymes; traction produced by LTBP-1 binding to extracellular matrix and LAP interaction with integrin $\alpha_V\beta_6$ or $\alpha_V\beta_8$; interaction with thrombospondin-1 or a small peptide derived from thrombospondin-1; or exposure to stirring or shear.[475–479] The interaction of LAP with integrin receptors via its RGD sequence probably plays a dominant role as mice with a mutation in this sequence have a phenotype like that of TGF-$\beta_1$ null mice.[480] The ability of thrombospondin-1 to activate TGF-$\beta_1$ is of special interest because both TGF-$\beta_1$ and thrombospondin-1 are present in $\alpha$ granules. However, data from mice suggest a minor role for platelet thrombospondin in either TGF-$\beta_1$ packaging or activation.[481–483] Only a very small percentage of the TGF-$\beta_1$ released from platelets with thrombin stimulation becomes activated, but this amount is sufficient to activate synthesis of PAI-1.[479,481,482,484] Based on animals models, TGF-$\beta_1$ released from platelets has been implicated in promoting tumor metastases and cardiac fibrosis in response to constriction of the aorta or aortic valve stenosis.[485–487] Active TGF-$\beta$ can bind to three different cell surface proteins, a proteoglycan ($\beta$-glycan), and two serine/threonine kinases.[471,485–488]

Platelets may also release proteins that affect the uptake of oxidized low-density lipoproteins by macrophages, furnishing another potential link between platelet activation and atherosclerosis.[489]

## Exosomes

In addition to the contents of $\alpha$ granules, activated platelets release both microparticles (see "Platelet Coagulant Activity" below), which are derived from the plasma membrane, and exosomes, which are internal membrane MVBs.[490] Exosomes are smaller than microparticles (40 to 100 nm vs. 100 to 1000 nm), enriched in CD63 and tetraspanins (see section "Platelet Membrane Glycoproteins" below), and relatively deficient in membrane proteins such as GPIb/IX and platelet-endothelial cell adhesion molecule (PECAM)-1. Unlike microparticles, exosomes are not highly procoagulant as judged by their inability to bind prothrombin or factor X or to present negatively charged phospholipids on their surface. They may, however, contain NAD(P)H oxidase activity, which has the potential to generate reactive oxygen species that contribute to endothelial cell apoptosis in sepsis.[491]

# PLATELET SECRETION

An intricate pathway of protein–protein interactions has been proposed for platelet secretion in which granules tether and dock to the inner leaflet of the plasma membrane, after which fusion of the two opposing lipid bilayers mediates cargo release.[492] Docking and tethering are thought to be, in part, mediated by small GTP-binding proteins of the Rab family. Platelets have been reported to contain at least 11 Rabs, although only a few have been shown to be functionally relevant. Rab27s a and b are important for both granule biogenesis and secretion,[493] whereas Rab 4 appears to have a role in secretion.[494] The α-granule–associated Rab6 was shown to be phosphorylated upon thrombin stimulation in a protein kinase C (PKC)-dependent manner, and phosphorylation seems to increase its GTP loading.[495]

Platelet granule–plasma membrane fusion is analogous to exocytosis in neurons, where detailed studies have shown the importance of a core set of integral membrane proteins called soluble N-ethylmaleimide-sensitive factor (NSF) attachment protein receptors (SNAREs).[496] It is generally accepted that vesicle/granule-target membrane fusion is governed by the binding of a SNARE from the cargo-containing granule or vesicle (v-SNARE) with a heteromeric protein complex in the target membrane (t-SNAREs). The resulting, *trans*-bilayer complex is minimally sufficient for membrane fusion.[497] In human platelets, the v-SNAREs are vesicle-associated membrane protein (VAMP)-2/synaptobrevin, VAMP-3/cellubrevin, VAMP-7/TI-VAMP, and VAMP-8/endobrevin, with the latter being most abundant.[498–502] There are two classes of t-SNAREs: the synaptosome-associated protein (SNAP)-23/25/29 type and the syntaxin type. Human platelets contain syntaxins 2, 4, 7, and 11[498–502] as well as SNAP-23, -25, and -29.[503,504] Functional studies using *in vitro* assays and genetically engineered mice have established that VAMP-8 is the primary v-SNARE required for secretion from all three classes of platelet granules.[501,502] VAMP-2 or VAMP-3 can also play a role at higher levels of stimulation. As for t-SNAREs, SNAP-23 and syntaxin 2 are required for each secretion event. Syntaxin 4 appears to also play a role, but only in α-granule and lysosome release.[505–508]

Although the SNARE proteins are sufficient to mediate membrane fusion, they do so inefficiently and thus require accessory proteins to control where and when they interact. Many of these regulators may be sensitive to second messengers such as diacylglycerol (DAG) and Ca²⁺, whereas others are substrates for kinases, such as PKC. The Munc18 family (a, b, and c) controls syntaxins and is critical for platelet secretion.[509–511] Studies show that Munc18a and c are phosphorylated by PKC upon platelet activation and that this affects Munc18/syntaxin binding affinity.[510,511] At least two members of the Munc13 family are present in platelets (Munc13–1 and Munc13–4) (Schraw TD, Ren Q, and Whiteheart SW, unpublished data).[512] Munc13–4 appears to be important for dense granule release and functions through its interactions with Rab27.[513,514] Munc13s have Ca²⁺ and DAG binding sites and thus may be regulated by the secondary messengers generated during platelet activation.

Munc13–4 has drawn particular attention based on its involvement in familial hemophagocytic lymphohistiocytosis (FHL) and Griscelli syndrome. Munc13–4 is mutated in type 3 FHL[515] and interacts with the protein mutated in type 2 Griscelli syndrome, namely Rab27a.[516] One feature common to both diseases is the inability of T cells to properly organize the cytotoxic synapse required for toxin secretion and target cell killing.[515] For FHL patients, it is not clear whether they have bleeding-time defects because they generally receive marrow transplants very early in life.

# PLATELET EXOCYTOSIS

Platelet granule–plasma membrane fusion is mechanistically analogous to exocytosis in neurons and other secretory cell types, where detailed studies have demonstrated the importance of a core set of integral membrane

proteins called SNAREs.[517,518] It is generally accepted that vesicle/granule-target membrane fusion and, thus, granule content release require the binding of a SNARE from the cargo-containing granule or v-SNARE, with a heteromeric protein complex in the t-SNAREs. The resulting, *trans*-bilayer complex is minimally sufficient for membrane fusion.[519] In human platelets, the detectable v-SNAREs are VAMP-2/synaptobrevin, VAMP-3/cellubrevin, VAMP-4, VAMP-5, VAMP-7/TI-VAMP, and VAMP-8/endobrevin, with VAMP-8 being most abundant.[501,502,520–523] There are two classes of t-SNAREs: the SNAP-23/25/29 type and the syntaxin type. Human platelets contain syntaxins 2, 4, 6, 7, 8, 11, 12, 16, 17, and 18.[501,502,520–524] SNAP-23, -25, and -29 are all detectable, but SNAP-23 is the most abundant.[521,525,526] Functional studies, using *in vitro* assays and genetically altered mice, established that VAMP-8 is the primary v-SNARE required for secretion from all three classes of platelet granules; however, platelets lacking VAMP-8 do release their contents at attenuated rates, suggesting roles for other VAMPs.[502] Differential usage of the VAMPs may allow platelets to fine tune their release of cargo. For t-SNAREs, patients with FHL4, who are deficient in syntaxin 11, show robust platelet secretion defects from all three granule types.[527] Studies of mouse platelets suggest a minor role for syntaxin 8,[524] but loss of syntaxin 2 and/or syntaxin 4 had no effect.[527] Syntaxins form a heterodimeric complex with SNAP-23/25–like t-SNAREs. In platelets, SNAP-23 is the critical family member, based on its abundance and results from *in vitro* assays.[505,506,528] SNAP-23 phosphorylation, by IκB kinase (IKK), is important for SNARE complex assembly, membrane fusion, and secretion. Platelet-specific loss of IKK or its pharmacologic inhibition leads to bleeding.[529]

Although the SNARE proteins mediate membrane fusion, they do so inefficiently and thus require accessory proteins to control where, when, and how they interact. Many of these regulators are sensitive to second messengers (e.g., calcium). The Sec1/Munc18 (SM) proteins are syntaxin chaperones that control how the t-SNAREs interact with other SNAREs.[510,530–533] Although several isoforms are present, only Munc18b is important for platelet exocytosis.[530,532,534] It chaperones syntaxin 11 and is defective in FHL5 patients. Other SM proteins (e.g., Vps33a/b) are important for granule biogenesis.[535,536] Another syntaxin regulator, tomosyn-1/syntaxin binding protein 5 (STXBP5), binds to syntaxin/SNAP-23 heterodimers and affects access to v-SNAREs.[537] Genome-wide association studies (GWAS) suggest that alterations in STXBP5 are linked to venous thrombosis risk resulting from increased plasma VWF.[537–539] Surprisingly, mice lacking STXBP5 have a severe arterial bleeding diathesis as a result of their defective platelet secretion.[537,539]

Munc13 family members contain binding sites for calcium, phosphatidylserine, DAG, and calmodulin.[540] Two major family members, Munc13–2 and Munc13–4, are detectable in platelets, although only Munc13–4 is functionally relevant.[521,541] Munc13s are generally thought to be docking factors that localize granules for membrane fusion. Both FHL3 patients and the Unc13d^jinx mouse strain lack Munc13–4 and have robust granule-release defects and bleeding diatheses.[541,542] Munc13–4 binds to a small GTP-binding protein called Rab27, which is also important for platelet exocytosis and is defective in Griscelli syndrome.[543] Another Rab27-binding protein, called synaptotagmin-like protein 4/granuphilin, is also reported to be important for platelet exocytosis.[544]

Three types of FHL are caused by defects in genes encoding proteins that are important in platelet secretion: Munc13–4/FHL3, syntaxin 11/FHL4, and Munc18b/FHL5. Rab27a is defective in a related disease, Griscelli syndrome. One feature common to both diseases is the inability of T cells to properly organize the cytotoxic synapse required for toxin secretion and target cell killing. This suggests that these T-cell populations and platelets share common secretory machinery elements. For FHL patients, it is unclear whether bleeding or defective platelet function can be used as diagnostic criteria, but they have been reported as symptoms.[545]

# ● PLATELET GENOMICS, THE PLATELET TRANSCRIPTOME, AND PLATELET PROTEOMICS

## PLATELET GENOMICS

The *Homo sapiens* genome is comprised of approximately 3.2 billion base pairs and has approximately 3.5 million single nucleotide polymorphisms (SNPs) that occur at frequencies of 1 percent or greater, but continued sequencing of more genomes indicates there are at least an additional 43 million rare or "private" SNPs. dbSNP (www.ncbi.nlm.nih.gov/projects/SNP) maintains information about sequence variation, allele frequencies, differences in frequencies between populations of different ethnicity, and their functional consequences. New technologies, such as next-generation sequencing, and new analytic methodologies have driven and continue to drive expansion of genomics at a very rapid pace. Both epidemiologic and experimental approaches have been and are used to assess significance and functionality of platelet gene variants and gene expression, including genetic epidemiology, biochemistry, cell biology, physiology, and animal studies.

## GENE VARIANTS ASSOCIATED WITH DISEASE

### Candidate Genes

Because platelets play a central role in acute ischemic syndromes, antiplatelet therapy is a mainstay of therapy. Platelets may also contribute to the pathophysiology of the chronic process of atherosclerosis,[546] although the data are less consistent than with thrombosis. The earliest platelet genetic association studies considered associations between atherothrombotic disease outcomes and candidate platelet gene variants that altered amino acids in platelet membrane adhesion receptors. Numerous studies reported associations between myocardial infarction and stroke with SNPs in integrin $\beta_3$ (*ITGB3*), integrin $\alpha_2$ (*ITGA2*), and GPIb$\alpha$ (*GP1BA*), and GPVI (*GP6*).[547] In these relatively small studies, positive associations were more likely to be observed in patients with acute thrombosis and less likely in patients with stable atherosclerosis. However, there were inconsistent and conflicting results in these candidate studies.

### Genome-Wide Associations Studies

No unbiased GWAS has been performed using documented arterial thrombosis as the clinical phenotype, but many have been performed with coronary artery disease (CAD). Multiple studies have demonstrated that the Chr9p21.3 locus is associated with both myocardial infarction (MI) and CAD. A meta-analysis of all CAD GWAS studies that included 63,746 patients with acute and chronic CAD and 130,681 controls identified 46 loci meeting genome-wide significance.[548] These loci explain less than 11 percent of CAD heritability, and although a substantial proportion of the identified genes regulate lipid metabolism and inflammation, most loci are not located in previously well-known or well-characterized platelet genes. Few of these loci have been tested for functional effects in platelets. There are numerous possible explanations for the nonassociation with well-studied platelet candidate genes, including small platelet gene effect sizes in underpowered heterogeneous clinical phenotypes.[549]

### Whole-Exome Sequencing

Whole-exome sequencing is well suited to identify variants in protein-coding genes and was used to identify *NBEAL2* as the causative gene in the gray platelet syndrome.[550,551]

### Pharmacogenetics

The *CYP2C19*2* allele (681G>A; rs4244285) causes a loss of function of the CYP2C19 enzyme and reduced platelet inhibition by clopidogrel as a result of decreased conversion to the active metabolite.[552] It could account for approximately 12 percent of the variation in platelet inhibition in response to clopidogrel.[553] Several large meta-analyses have shown the loss-of-function *CYP2C19*2* allele is associated with both stent thrombosis and cardiovascular ischemic events or death in patients undergoing percutaneous coronary interventions.[554,555]

## GENE VARIANTS ASSOCIATED WITH PLATELET TRAITS

Many cellular pathways in multiple tissues contribute to the pathogenic processes resulting in an atherothrombotic event (Fig. 2–7), increasing the "noise" in genetic epidemiology studies testing for associations with

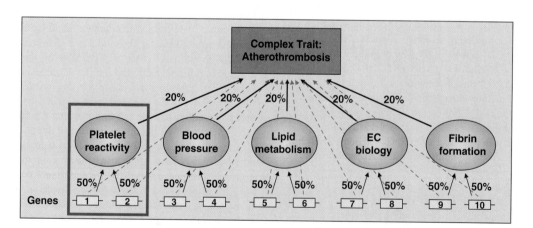

**Figure 2–7.** Intermediate phenotypes in association studies. Atherothrombosis is a complex phenotype that is regulated by many intermediate traits, of which platelet reactivity is only one. Because a large number of genes contribute to multiple traits, the effect of any one gene on atherothrombotic events, such as myocardial infarction, is small. This highly simplified diagram assumes five traits each contribute 20 percent to the complex trait (*heavy solid arrows*) and two different genes equally regulate each intermediate trait. Thus, each gene contributes 50 percent to the intermediate trait (*thin arrows*), but only 10 percent to the clinical end point (*faint dashed arrows*). Thus, for any given sample size, there is more power to detect genetic associations with intermediate phenotypes than with complex traits. (*Reproduced with permission from Bray PF: Platelet genomics beats the catch-22,* Blood. *2009 Aug 13;114(7):1286–1287.*)

complex phenotypes. The use of intermediate phenotypes as outcomes in genetic association studies has enhanced power to detect gene associations because the number of genes potentially responsible for the phenotype is reduced, thereby increasing the fraction of the variance explained by any single factor or gene. Despite large interindividual variability in platelet reactivity, light transmission aggregometry has been shown to be reproducible and heritable, with the reproducibility persisting for years.[556,557]

### Candidate Functional Platelet Genes

The Leu33Pro variant of integrin $\beta_3$ (rs5918 of *ITGB3*) is responsible for human platelet alloantigen 1a/b (Pl$^{A1}$/Pl$^{A2}$).[558] Fibrinogen and prothrombin binding is enhanced to the Pro$^{33}$ isoform of purified integrin $\alpha_{IIb}\beta_3$.[559] Compared to cell lines expressing Leu33 variant of integrin, Pro33 cells have increased adhesion, spreading, actin cytoskeletal reorganization, and migration under static[560,561] and shear conditions.[562] This prothrombotic phenotype of Pro33 is mediated by *enhanced outside-in platelet signaling* through integrin $\alpha_{IIb}\beta_3$.[563,564] Notably, this variant does *not* affect inside-out signaling, as assessed by standard platelet light transmission aggregometry of human platelets.[565] Additional support for the prothrombotic nature of the Pro33 variant of integrin $\beta_3$ comes from mice made homozygous for Pro33. These animals have reduced bleeding, increased *in vivo* thrombosis and enhanced outside-in integrin $\alpha_{IIb}\beta_3$ signaling, but normal inside-out signaling.[566]

Laboratory evidence for functional effects of genetic variants in the gene encoding GPIb$\beta$ has been inconsistent. Variants in the two platelet collagen receptors, GPVI and integrin $\alpha_2$ subunit (of integrin $\alpha_2\beta_1$) alter receptor expression and adhesion to collagen using *in vitro* perfusion assays.[567-569] Functional variants in the genes encoding Fc$\gamma$RIIA (*FCGR2A*), P2Y$_{12}$ (*P2RY12*), GPIV (*CD36*), and PAR-1 (*F2R*) have also been reported.

Associations between SNPs in 97 hematopoietic cell genes were tested, and 17 novel associations with platelet responses to crosslinked collagen-related peptide (CRP) and ADP were identified, including genes encoding cell surface receptors (*CD36*, *GP6*, *ITGA2*, *PEAR1*, and *P2Y12*), kinases (*JAK2*, *MAP2K2*, *MAP2K4*, and *MAPK14*), and other signaling molecules (*GNAZ*, *VAV3*, *ITPR1*, and *FCERG1*).[570] Variants at the Chr9p21.3 locus are associated with the platelet aggregation response to low (0.5 mcg/mL) but not higher concentrations of collagen in a large cohort with two replication studies.[571]

### Genome-Wide Association Studies

The first GWAS reported for platelet reactivity tested association of 2.5 million SNPs with platelet aggregation responses to ADP, collagen, and epinephrine.[565] The primary cohorts were generally healthy, European-ancestry populations from the Framingham Heart Study (FHS) (n = 2753) and the GeneSTAR cohorts (n = 1238). SNPs at seven loci (*PEAR1*, *MRVI1*, *SHH*, *ADRA2A*, *PIK3CG*, *JMJD1C*, and *GP6*) met genome-wide statistical significance and were replicated in an African-ancestry cohort (n = 840). A second platelet function GWAS identified SNPs in *SVIL* (encodes supervillin) as associated with closure time in the *in vitro* platelet function analyzer PFA-100.[572] Human platelet gene expression studies and data with *Svil* –/– mice demonstrated an inhibitory role for supervillin in platelet adhesion and thrombus formation under high-shear but not low-shear conditions. A meta-analysis by the HaemGen consortium of 66,867 individuals identified 43 and 25 loci associated with platelet number and mean platelet volume (MPV), respectively.[573] These loci accounted for 4.8 percent of the phenotypic variance in platelet number and 9.9 percent in MPV and included well-known platelet regulators (*ITGA2B*, *GP1BA*, and *F2R*). These investigators identified 11 of the genes as novel regulators of blood cell formation using gene silencing in *Danio rerio* and *Drosophila melanogaster*.

## PLATELET GENE EXPRESSION

### TRANSCRIPTOMICS

The *Homo sapiens* genome includes approximately 21,000 protein-coding genes (genome build GRCh38). To date, more than 10 times this number of protein-coding transcripts have been identified, primarily as a result of alternate exon splicing, and more are being continually discovered. Platelets from healthy subjects contain approximately 2.20 femtograms (fg) of total RNA per cell, which is approximately 1000-fold less than nucleated blood cells. Platelets can splice pre-mRNA into mature mRNA, which is translated into proteins.[574,575] Characterization of the transcriptome enables quantitative assessment of gene expression in the tissue of interest and identification of alternately spliced transcripts. Genome-wide transcriptome studies have enabled dissection of the molecular basis of inherited platelet disorders and a better understanding of the relationship between gene expression and megakaryocyte and platelet differentiation. In addition, platelet RNA profiles may have utility as biomarkers.[576]

Technologic advances have greatly facilitated understanding the platelet transcriptome. Early studies using serial analysis of gene expression and microarrays estimated approximately 6000 mRNAs in the human platelet.[577,578] Platelet RNA sequencing (RNA-seq) has demonstrated an unexpected complexity to the transcriptome and substantive differences between the human and mouse platelet transcriptome.[579] The exquisite sensitivity of RNA-seq provided estimates of approximately 9000 protein-coding genes in platelets (Fig. 2–8),[580,581] although only approximately 7800 are commonly expressed[582] in human platelets. Approximately half of the transcripts in platelets encode mitochondrial genes.[581] Platelet mitochondrial mRNAs are inversely correlated with subject age,[582] and mitochondrial function may regulate platelet apoptosis[583] and support optimal platelet function during storage,[584] but platelet mitochondria diseases have not been described. The S-shaped curves in Fig. 2–8 illustrate several features of the human platelet transcriptome: (1) estimates of expressed protein-coding genes are more similar among different subjects for high-abundance genes (leftward in Fig. 2–8), and (2) there is substantial interindividual variation in total transcript estimates when considering the less abundant genes (rightward in Fig. 2–9). Furthermore, it is not known what is the biologically relevant copy number of transcripts in any cell, and the arbitrary choice of "threshold" could dramatically affect the number of reported genes expressed in platelets. Transcriptomes of *primary* megakaryocytes have not been determined, but RNA profiling of megakaryocytes derived from cultured CD34+ hematopoietic stem cells has identified transcripts that are differentially expressed upon differentiation and between normal subjects and patients with essential thrombocytosis.[585,586]

### Platelet mRNAs Associated with Disease

Platelet mRNA profiling in patients with acute ST-segment elevation MI and stable CAD demonstrated that *S100A9* (myeloid-related protein-14 [MRP-14]) was expressed at higher levels in patients than controls.[587] This discovery was validated in the Women's Health Study and PROVE IT-TIMI 22 trials.[587,588] Platelet mRNA expression profiling can distinguish essential thrombocythemia (ET) patients from healthy subjects,[589] and levels of *HIST1H1A*, *SRP72*, *C20orf103*, and *CRYM* can predict JAK2 V617F–negative ET in 87 percent of patients.[590] mRNA expression profiling identified reduced *MYL9* transcripts in platelets of a patient with an inherited platelet defect.[591] Platelet RNA-seq was also used to identify *NBEAL2* as causing the gray platelet syndrome.[592]

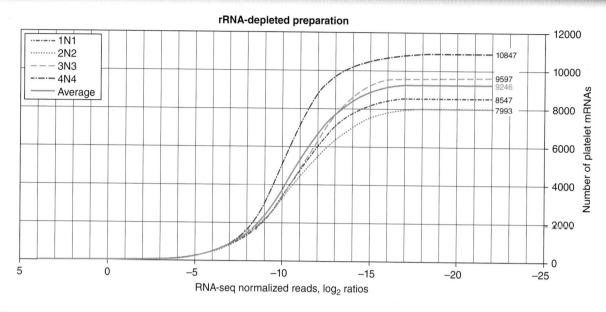

**Figure 2–8.** Estimates of platelet-expressed mRNAs. Platelet total RNA was extracted from four normal donors, depleted of ribosomal RNA (rRNA), and subjected to RNA sequencing (RNA-seq). The number of platelet-expressed mRNAs *(y axis)* was plotted against RNA-seq read number in log2 ratios normalized to β-actin. *(Reproduced with permission from Bray PF, et al: The complex transcriptional landscape of the anucleate human platelet, BMC Genomics 2013 Jan 16;14:1)*

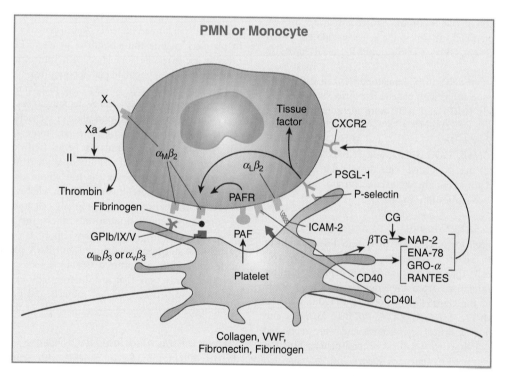

**Figure 2–9.** Platelet–leukocyte interactions. A number of interactions can occur between platelets and leukocytes, including neutrophils and monocytes. The interaction between platelet P-selectin and leukocyte P-selectin glycoprotein ligand-1 (PSGL-1) probably is the most important initial interaction (and can lead to tissue factor synthesis by monocytes), but fibrinogen binding simultaneously to activated $\alpha_M\beta_2$ on leukocytes and either $\alpha_{IIb}\beta_3$ or $\alpha_V\beta_3$ on platelets may play a role under certain circumstances. Platelets can release platelet-activating factor (PAF), which can interact with a PAF receptor (PAFR) on leukocytes, leading to $\alpha_M\beta_2$ activation and binding of fibrinogen and factor X. Leukocyte $\alpha_M\beta_2$ can also interact with platelet junctional adhesion molecule-3 (JAM-3) or GPIb. Platelets can release chemokines (e.g., ENA-78, GRO-α, and RANTES [regulated upon activation, normal T-cell expressed and secreted]), and β-thromboglobulin (βTG) released by platelets can be converted by leukocyte cathepsin G (CG) into the potent chemotactic CXC chemokine NAP-2. Some of the chemokines, in turn, activate leukocytes by binding to the chemokine receptor CXCR2. Platelets also contain the potent immune-stimulating molecule CD40 ligand (CD40L), and both express it on the platelet surface and release it into the circulation upon platelet activation. The interaction between thrombospondin and CD36 molecules on both platelets and some leukocytes and the presence of CD40 on platelets are not shown. VWF, von Willebrand factor.

### Platelet mRNAs Associated with Platelet Traits

An unbiased genome-wide platelet RNA expression study identified an association between expression of PEAR1 and platelet activation.[593] A similar approach identified 290 differentially expressed transcripts between hyperreactive versus hyporeactive platelets.[594] mRNA and protein levels of VAMP-8, a critical v-SNARE involved in platelet granule secretion, were significantly higher in hyperreactive platelets. Another study identified 63 genes differentially expressed according to platelet activation by ADP and/or CRP.[595] Two of these genes, COMMD7 and LRRFIP1, were associated with early-onset MI.[595] The Platelet RNA and Expression-1 (PRAX1) study phenotyped platelet function and performed genome-wide platelet RNA expression profiling on 70 black and 84 white subjects.[596] PAR4-mediated platelet aggregation and calcium mobilization were greater in black subjects than white subjects. A novel platelet gene encoding phosphatidylcholine transfer protein (PC-TP) showed a strong correlation with race and with PAR-4 reactivity, and a PC-TP–specific inhibitor blocked PAR-4– but not PAR-1–mediated platelet aggregation. This finding underscores the genetic basis for interindividual variation in platelet function and the potential need to consider race and genetic factors when treating patients with antiplatelet therapies.

### Platelet Noncoding RNAs

The best studied of the noncoding RNAs are microRNAs (miRNAs), which regulate expression of more than 60 percent of protein-coding genes.[597,598] Human platelets express approximately 200 annotated miRNAs, some of which are differentially expressed according to platelet reactivity and may predict platelet responsiveness to activation[599] and some of which are differentially expressed by age, gender, and race.[582,596] Indirect evidence indicates strong correlations between megakaryocyte and platelet miRNA levels.[600] miR-155 maintains megakaryocyte progenitors in an undifferentiated state,[601] whereas miR-150 and miR-125b-2 drive megakaryocyte differentiation.[602,603] Loss of expression of miR-145 in the 5q– syndrome leads to an increase in the megakaryocyte Fli-1 transcription factor, thus enhancing megakaryocyte production.[604]

Platelet miRNA profiles are more stable than mRNA profiles and are useful as biomarkers.[576] Levels of miR-26b and miR-28 are associated with myeloproliferative neoplasms,[605,606] whereas levels of miR-10a, miR-148a, and miR-490–5p discriminate ET from secondary thrombocytosis.[607] Specific sets of platelet miRNAs have been associated with MI.[608,609] Antiplatelet therapies alter platelet miRNA levels.[610,611] Relationships between platelet miRNAs, mRNAs, and physiology in the same subjects permit prediction of miRNA function and discovery of novel platelet genes.[599] This approach identified PRKAR2B as associated with platelet reactivity, and a functional effect was confirmed in murine platelets lacking Prkar2b.[599] A similar approach was used to demonstrate that platelet miR-376c levels were higher in white subjects compared to black subjects and that these levels correlated with PCTP mRNA, PC-TP protein, and platelet PAR-4 reactivity.[596] miR-376c directly targets the PCTP 3′UTR and represses its expression.[596]

## PROTEOMICS

Disease pathophysiology is dictated by the effects of proteins, including their levels, structures, and posttranslational modifications. Cataloging platelet proteomes in health and disease and under different activation states provides information not achievable from genomics or transcriptomics, including protein isoforms, localization, stoichiometry, and posttranslational modifications. Early proteome-wide studies of platelet lysates used two-dimensional gel electrophoresis (2D-GE).[612] However, technologic advances using nongel approaches

with proteolytic peptide analyses have largely replaced 2D-GE and include surface-enhanced laser desorption/ionization (SELDI), isotope-coded affinity tags (iCAT), and isotope tags for relative and absolute quantification (iTRAQ).[613,614] These improved technologies have provided an estimate of approximately 20 million protein molecules per platelet and have updated estimates of the number of detectable different proteins in the platelet proteome to nearly 5000.[615] Pathway and gene ontology analyses reveal most highly expressed platelet proteins localize to the cytoplasm, with substantial percentages in the membrane or secretome,[616] and fall into expected functional categories of cytoskeletal rearrangement, membrane trafficking, and intracellular signal transduction.[615]

Platelet protein levels are regulated by mRNA translation in megakaryocytes and platelets, uptake of plasma proteins, and protein degradation,[574,617] although the relative contribution of each mechanism to the platelet proteome in health and disease is unknown. The dynamic nature of the platelet proteome is illustrated by alterations with disease, aging, gender, and other environmental factors,[616] as well as differential sorting of proteins between megakaryocytes and platelets.[618] Infectious agents, such as dengue virus, stimulate blood platelet mRNA translation into protein.[619] Posttranslational modifications of platelet proteins, such as phosphorylation, have critical effects on platelet activation. Platelets from healthy individuals exhibit marked interindividual variation in function,[556] and unbiased genome-wide approaches have identified variation in proteins regulating the corresponding function.[594] Components of protein ubiquitination and degradation have been identified in platelets, but their function is poorly understood.

### Cataloging the Platelet Proteome

Most platelet proteomic analyses to date have studied platelets from small numbers of healthy donors. Analyses of resting whole platelets have provided global protein profiles.[612,620] Fractionation of platelet lysates has been used to assess the $\alpha$ granule,[621] dense granule,[622] and membrane proteomes.[623,624] Proteins with posttranslational modifications have been identified for phosphorylation,[625,626] palmitoylation,[627] and glycosylation.[628] After platelet activation, hundreds of proteins have been identified in releasates (secretomes)[629,630] and microparticles.[631,632]

### Platelet Proteome Association Studies

Platelet proteome-wide analyses were used to identify NBEAL2 as the gene responsible for the gray platelet syndrome[551] and to unravel the molecular basis of the Quebec platelet disorder.[633] Differentially expressed platelet proteins involved in integrin $\alpha_{IIb}\beta_3$ signaling were observed in the myelodysplastic syndrome.[634] Proteomic approaches have consistently identified platelet septin and actin as increasing over time in storage.[635-637] A small study suggested platelet protein posttranslational modifications may be associated with acute coronary syndromes.[638]

### Relationship Between Platelet Proteome and Transcriptome

Transcriptomic approaches have identified about twice as many genes expressed in platelets as have proteomic approaches, primarily because the former has greater sensitivity. Correlations between 10 platelet RNA-seqs and the most quantitatively robust proteomic analyses to date have been reported.[639] Most (87.8 percent) proteins had a detectable corresponding mRNA, and the relative abundances showed a significantly positive, albeit weak, correlation. Platelet proteins that lack a corresponding mRNA are likely to be taken up from plasma rather than being synthesized in megakaryocytes, and include fibrinogen, albumin, and immunoglobulins, all of which were suspected to fall into this category based on other studies.[640] Platelet mRNAs that lack a corresponding protein may be vestigial from the megakaryocyte. Some of these could be translated subsequently by the platelet under physiologic demands. Combining "multiomic" data with phenotyping can provide important insights as demonstrated by a study in which transcriptomic and proteomic analysis identified six platelet transcripts associated with aspirin resistance.[641] The expression of these genes was associated with death or MI. In addition, platelet phenotyping and genome-wide genotyping and platelet mRNA and miRNA profiling led to the identification of novel protein-coding and noncoding transcripts associated with platelet activation.[596]

# PLATELET COAGULANT ACTIVITY

In resting platelets, negatively charged phospholipids, including phosphatidyl serine (PS) and phosphatidylethanolamine (PE), are almost exclusively present in the inner leaflet of the cell membrane and phosphatidylcholine predominates in the outer leaflet. This asymmetry is maintained by ATP-dependent "flippase" transporters, which restrict PS to the inner membrane surface, and "floppases," which promote outward-directed lipid transport.[84,85,642,643] When platelets are activated by strong agonists, negatively charged phospholipids redistribute to the outer leaflet of the platelet plasma membrane. This involves a putative calcium-dependent "scramblase" that transports lipids bidirectionally and, when active, collapses membrane asymmetry and results in PS exposure on the outer leaflet. The eight-transmembrane domain containing protein TMEM16F serves as a $Ca^{2+}$-activated, nonselective cation channel that is crucial for $Ca^{2+}$-dependent phospholipid scrambling and PS exposure on activated platelets.[644]

Platelet activation with strong agonists also results in the formation of microparticles, which are particularly rich in surface-exposed negatively charged phospholipids. Microparticles also are rich in factor Va and thus actively support thrombin generation.[82,645,646] Microparticle formation can be induced in vitro by activation of platelets with ionophore A23187, complement C5b-9, or the combination of thrombin and collagen; by adding tissue factor to recalcified platelet-rich plasma; or by high shear stress.[645,647-652] Elevations of cytosolic $Ca^{2+}$, calpain activation, cytoskeletal reorganization, protein phosphorylation, and phospholipid translocation have all been implicated in microparticle formation.

The biologic relevance of platelet microparticles is supported by the finding of increased circulating levels of platelet microparticles in patients with activated coagulation and fibrinolysis, diabetes mellitus, sickle cell anemia, human immunodeficiency virus infection, unstable angina, heparin-induced thrombocytopenia with thrombosis, and respiratory distress syndrome.[645,653] Microparticles can bind to fibrin thrombi via one or more of the receptors present on their surface, including integrin $\alpha_{IIb}\beta_3$, GPIb/IX, P-selectin, and possibly P-selectin glycoprotein ligand (PSGL)-1.[654]

Microparticles bind factors VIII, Va, and Xa, allowing them to form both the factor Xase and prothrombinase complexes on their surface.[645] They can also bind protein S and facilitate inactivation of factors Va and VIIIa, which could serve an anticoagulant function.[655,656] In addition, microparticles can activate platelets by supplying arachidonic acid.

Evidence supporting the importance of platelet microparticle formation to platelet coagulant activity has been gathered from observations of patients who have significant bleeding diatheses in association with defects in platelet microparticle formation (Scott syndrome; Chap. 11).[657-659] Platelets from the most intensively studied patient had an impaired ability to accelerate the activation of both factor X and prothrombin. In addition, this patient's platelets exhibited both abnormal factor V binding and abnormal exposure of negatively charged phospholipids.

Activated platelets synthesize tissue factor by splicing pre-mRNA into mature mRNA and then translating the tissue factor protein.[660,661] Additionally, platelet thrombi can recruit tissue factor from blood by binding leukocyte-derived, tissue factor-containing microparticles or by binding an alternatively spliced, soluble form of tissue factor.[466,472,662-665] The interaction between PSGL-1 on the surface of leukocyte-derived microparticles and P-selectin on the surface of activated platelets appears to play an important role in the binding of microparticles to platelet thrombi.[664] Interactions between platelets and leukocytes, and perhaps leukocyte-derived microparticles, reportedly enhance ("de-encrypt" or decrypt) tissue factor activity, probably by supplying negatively charged phopholipids[666] and/or the oxidoreductase enzyme protein disulfide isomerase (PDI).[667]

Platelet-dense granules contain polyphosphate, a linear polymer of inorganic phosphate synthesized by inositol hexakisphosphate 6 kinase. Polyphosphates are released during platelet activation and promote clot formation. Polyphosphates affect many steps in coagulation. Polyphosphates accelerate factor V and factor XII[668] and alter the structure of fibrin clots. In the presence of polyphosphates, fibrin clots have thicker fibers and are more resistant to fibrinolysis.[669] In contrast to bacterial polyphosphates, which are long-chain structures, platelet polyphosphates have shorter chain length and are more effective in increasing factor V and TFPI activity.

Incontrovertible evidence exists that platelets accelerate thrombin formation.[658,659,670-672] Platelets accelerate the activation of factor X by factors IXa and VIIIa and the activation of prothrombin by factors Xa and Va.[659,670] However, only a subpopulation of platelets develops a procoagulant phenotype with activation, as only a fraction of activated platelets display high levels of factors Va and Xa, termed "coat" platelets.[464,465,670,673] The assembly of the factor IXa/factor VIIIa/platelet complex increases the catalytic efficiency of factor X activation ($k_{cat}/K_m$ [turnover number/Michaelis-Menten dissociation constant]) by a factor of $2.4 \times 10^6$.[670] Prothrombin binds to approximately 20,000 sites on activated platelets with a $K_D$ equal to its plasma concentration (approximately 0.15 $\mu$M).[674] Integrin $\alpha_{IIb}\beta_3$ binds prothrombin through its RGD domain and may contribute to the localization of prothrombin to the surface of unactivated and activated platelets.[675]

In addition to accelerating coagulation, the binding of activated coagulation factors to the surface of platelets appears to protect them from inactivation by inhibitors in plasma and platelets.[399] The bleeding diathesis in patients with Quebec platelet syndrome, who have proteolysis of their platelet $\alpha$-granule factor V, supports the potential importance of platelet factor V in normal hemostasis (Chap. 11), as do the studies of another patient with abnormal platelet factor V.[659]

Other connections between platelets and the coagulation system include: (1) the presence of fibrinogen in platelet $\alpha$ granules and perhaps on the surface of platelets, where it is strategically located for interactions with locally generated thrombin[371,399]; (2) the presence of intracellular VWF and the binding of extracellular VWF to platelets (via GPIb/X and integrin $\alpha_{IIb}\beta_3$), with the potential colocalization of factor VIII attached to the VWF (Chap. 16); (3) activation of factor XI by thrombin on the platelet surface,[676,677] with the dimeric structure of factor XI allowing it to interact both with the platelet and factor IX simultaneously[678]; (4) a factor XI-like protein associated with platelet membranes, which may be an alternatively spliced form of factor XI lacking exon V; the level of this factor appears to correlate better with hemorrhagic symptoms than does the level of plasma factor XI[399,679]; (5) the presence of cytoplasmic factor XIII (Chap. 3); (6) the presence of inhibitors of coagulation ($\alpha_1$-protease inhibitor, C-1 inhibitor, TFPI, the thrombin inhibitor protease nexin I, and the factors IXa and XIa inhibitor protease nexin II or $\beta$-APP)[399,448]; and (7) promotion of factor XII activation by ADP-treated platelets.[399]

# ● PLATELETS AND THROMBOLYSIS

The interactions between platelets and the fibrinolytic system are complex; Table 2–3 contains a partial listing of reported findings.[680–684] Both profibrinolytic[398,685–692] and antifibrinolytic[693–701] effects of platelets have been described, and so it is difficult to predict the net effect. Since platelet-rich thrombi are known to resist thrombolysis in animal models, the antifibrinolytic effects of platelets appear to predominate *in vivo*.[702]

---

**TABLE 2–3.** Platelets and Thrombolysis

*Profibrinolytic effects of platelets*

Tissue plasminogen activator (t-PA) and single-chain urokinase-type t-PA identified on or in platelets.

Unactivated platelets bind plasminogen, and binding is enhanced by thrombin.

Thrombospondin, a plasminogen-binding protein, is expressed on the surface of platelets after activation.

Activation of plasminogen by t-PA is enhanced by platelets.

Clot lysis is enhanced by platelets in some model systems.

*Antifibrinolytic effects of platelets*

Plasminogen activator inhibitor-1 and $a_2$-antiplasmin are present in platelet granules.

Platelets contain protease nexin-1, a serpin that inhibits plasminogen activators and plasmin.

Platelets contain factor XIII, which can crosslink fibrin, making it resist fibrinolysis, and can crosslink $a_2$-antiplasmin to fibrin, enhancing its antifibrinolytic effects.

Platelets contain tissue factor pathway inhibitor-2, which inhibits t-PA.

Platelet $a_{IIb}\beta_3$ can bind plasma factor XIIIa directly or indirectly, localizing it to the site of thrombus formation.

Platelets facilitate clot retraction, which diminishes the efficiency of fibrinolysis.

*Platelet-activating effects of thrombolytic agents*

Streptokinase and t-PA activate platelets *in vivo* and *in vitro*.

Plasmin, at high doses, can aggregate platelets.

Thrombolytic agents may paradoxically generate the potent platelet agonist thrombin or release it from thrombi.

Thrombolytic agents may blunt the prostacyclin increase that accompanies acute thrombosis.

*Platelet-inhibiting effects of thrombolytic agents*

Plasmin, at low doses, can inhibit platelet activation and aggregation.

Platelets can be disaggregated by t-PA by selective lysis of platelet-bound fibrinogen.

Plasmin can cause redistribution and/or cleavage of platelet glycoprotein Ib.

Inhibition of platelet aggregation by the depletion of plasma fibrinogen, if severe, and generation of fibrin (ogen) degradation products.

Proteolysis of plasma von Willebrand factor.

Prolongation of the bleeding time.

Adapted with permission from Fozzard HA, Haber E, Jennings RB: *The Heart and Cardiovascular System*, 2nd edition. New York: Raven Press; 1991.

---

The effects of fibrinolytic agents on platelets are similarly complex. For example, there is considerable evidence that fibrinolytic agents can activate platelets soon after administration,[703–709] via either a direct effect of plasmin,[710–713] perhaps acting on PAR-4,[714] or an indirect effect through the paradoxical generation of thrombin.[683,715–718] Interpretation of the latter studies is complicated by the ability of tissue plasminogen activator to release fibrinopeptides from fibrinogen, one of the biomarkers used to assess thrombin activation.[719]

Stimulation of platelets by thrombolytic agents may prolong the time required for reperfusion of thrombosed blood vessels and may contribute to reocclusion after successful reperfusion.[680,720] In animal models and in humans, potent antiplatelet agents can, in fact, speed reperfusion, abolish reocclusion, and diminish the size of myocardial infarcts.[721–723] In human studies, the benefits of combining integrin $\alpha_{IIb}\beta_3$ antagonists with fibrinolytic agents in enhancing coronary thrombolysis have been counterbalanced by an increase in major hemorrhage.[724] Combining a potent integrin $\alpha_{IIb}\beta_3$ antagonist with a reduced dose of a fibrinolytic agent in acute ST-segment elevation MI when patients are rapidly treated with percutaneous coronary intervention has demonstrated evidence for more rapid reperfusion, but clinical benefit has been variable and bleeding has been increased.[725,726] In experimental models of stroke, paradoxically, early treatment with integrin $\alpha_{IIb}\beta_3$ antagonists reduces the hemorrhage associated with thrombolytic therapy, perhaps by preventing platelet aggregation in the microcirculation and the release of agents that can damage the vasculature and diminish its integrity.[727–729] In human studies, however, a potent integrin $\alpha_{IIb}\beta_3$ antagonist given alone did not improve clinical outcomes.[730,731]

With prolonged use of thrombolytic agents, inhibition of platelet function can occur via a variety of mechanisms.[102,707,708,732–744] These effects may contribute to some of the hemorrhagic phenomena observed with this therapy. One proposed mechanism is that the thrombolytic agents make platelets refractory to further stimulation by agonists.

# ● PLATELETS IN INFLAMMATION AND INFECTION

Leukocytes can bind to activated platelets and in model systems transmigrate through a platelet monolayer (reviewed in Ref. 745; see Fig. 2–9). Animal models and studies of human tissue demonstrate that within hours after vascular injury, leukocytes become enmeshed in platelet thrombi and/or transiently form a monolayer on top of adherent or aggregated platelets.[746,747] These interactions may be important at sites of vascular injury or inflammation where leukocytes have been shown to deposit on adherent and aggregated platelets. Platelet recruitment of leukocytes has been associated with a number of systemic and inflammatory processes in animal models, including the development of intimal hyperplasia after vascular injury,[748] ischemia–reperfusion injury, alloimmunity-mediated transplant rejection,[749] obesity,[750] and acute lung injury.[751] By depositing chemokines such as CCL5 (also termed RANTES [regulated upon activation, normal T-cell expressed and secreted]) on activated endothelium[752,753] or by direct interactions with leukocytes,[754] platelets may also enhance leukocyte recruitment to inflamed or atherosclerotic endothelium and thereby promote the development and progression of atherosclerosis.

Many mechanisms of platelet–leukocyte interactions have been defined, but the initial interaction appears to be mediated primarily by the interaction between P-selectin (CD62P) expressed on the surface of activated platelets and PSGL-1 on the surface of neutrophils and monocytes.[755–761] P-selectin–PSGL-1 interactions are characterized by rapid on-and-off rates that promote tethering and rolling of leukocytes along adherent platelets. In addition to PSGL-1, leukocyte CD24 may also bind P-selectin. The transient P-selectin–mediated interactions are stabilized by subsequent contacts mediated, in large part, by activation of leukocyte $\beta_2$ integrins. Platelet surface-immobilized and released chemokines promote firm leukocyte adhesion and arrest by acting through G-protein–coupled receptors to activate leukocyte $\beta_2$ integrins. Platelets can synthesize and release PAF, which can activate leukocyte $\alpha_M\beta_2$. CCL5 and the CXC chemokines ENA-78 and GRO-$\alpha$, released by activated platelets, can also activate leukocytes. The chemokine neutrophil-activating peptide-2 (NAP-2) can be produced by the action of leukocyte cathepsin G on $\beta$-thromboglobulin secreted by platelets.[762,763] Activated $\alpha_M\beta_2$ on leukocytes can interact with platelet GPIb$\alpha$[764] as well as with platelet-bound fibrinogen via a region(s) on the $\gamma$ chain (amino acids 190 to 202[765] and 377 to 395). Thrombospondin may serve as a bridging molecule between CD36 (GPIV) receptors, which are expressed on both platelets and mononuclear cells.[766] Platelets also have intercellular adhesion molecule (ICAM)-2 on their surface, which is a ligand for the leukocyte integrin receptor $\alpha_L\beta_2$; although this ligand–receptor interaction appears to have only a minor role in platelet–leukocyte adhesion, it may be more important in leukocyte tethering.[763] Platelet junctional adhesion molecule (JAM) 3 has also been suggested as a counterreceptor for leukocyte $\alpha_M\beta_2$.[767] The immunoreceptor tyrosine-based activation motif (ITAM)-associated receptors GPVI and C-type lectin-like receptor-2 (CLEC-2) also promote platelet–leukocyte interactions during inflammation via their respective counterreceptors matrix metalloproteinase inducer (EMMPRIN) on neutrophils and macrophages and podoplanin on inflammatory macrophages.

Transcellular metabolism of eicosanoids can result in production of unique products (Fig. 2–10), and leukocytes can modify platelet activation.[768] In a complementary fashion, the intimate relationship between leukocytes and platelets allows the latter to contribute to the inflammatory response, including the release of chemokines that can activate leukocytes; PDGF can affect fibroblast and smooth muscle cells; TGF-$\beta_1$ both stimulates and inhibits cellular growth; and PF4 primes neutrophils and has antiangiogenic activity. Platelets synthesize the cytokine IL-1$\beta$, an important mediator of the inflammatory response.[769] Platelets contain Fc$\gamma$IIA receptors that can localize IgG and immune complexes, resulting in complement activation. Platelets express CD40L on their surface after activation, and this molecule can interact with CD40, a member of the tumor necrosis factor (TNF) receptor family, on leukocytes and endothelial cells, leading to their activation and their elaboration of a number of proinflammatory molecules[770-772] (see "CD40 Ligand [CD40L, CD154] and CD40"). Platelet CD40L also promotes procoagulant activity in endothelial cells.[773] Finally, platelet–leukocyte interactions can promote the generation of reactive oxygen species, but platelets can also generate signals to stop their production.[774]

Platelet–leukocyte interactions may be important in the initiation of coagulation and fibrin formation through a P-selectin–dependent pathway. In fact, platelet–leukocyte aggregates facilitate thrombin generation to a greater extent than either platelets or leukocytes alone.[775,776] Coincubation of platelets and leukocytes generates tissue factor activity, in part, through P-selectin–PSGL-1 interactions. The induction of tissue factor activity involves both de novo protein synthesis and exposure ("deencryption") of latent tissue factor. The latter may occur by P-selectin–mediated production of tissue factor containing microparticles from leukocytes. Real-time imaging of platelet thrombus formation in vivo indicates that tissue factor accumulates in growing thrombi before leukocytes become associated with the thrombus. The accumulation of tissue factor and fibrin formation in thrombi depend on both platelet P-selectin and PSGL-1. These observations, coupled with the finding of bloodborne tissue factor antigen in the circulation,[777]

have led to a model in which platelet P-selectin recruits tissue factor-containing leukocyte microparticles to platelet-rich thrombi.[778] Neutrophil-derived microparticles express active integrin $\alpha_M\beta_2$, which can interact with platelets by binding to GPIb$\alpha$. This, in turn, can initiate platelet P-selectin expression, which will enhance the interactions with neutrophil microparticles containing the counterreceptor PSGL-1.[779] In mice, increases in soluble P-selectin levels promote a procoagulant state associated with elevated levels of leukocyte-derived microparticles,[780] and a P-selectin–immunoglobulin chimeric molecule can increase levels of leukocyte-derived microparticles in vitro and normalize the bleeding time in hemophilia A mice.[781]

Several clinical observations support a potential role for platelet–leukocyte interactions in vascular disease, including the presence of circulating platelet–leukocyte aggregates in patients with unstable angina[792] and after coronary artery angioplasty[783]; in the latter situation, the presence of such aggregates appears to confer a worse prognosis for ischemic vascular complications.[783] Circulating platelet–leukocyte aggregates are perhaps the most sensitive indicator of systemic platelet activation, reflecting the expression of P-selectin on the surface of platelets.[784] Analysis of polymorphisms of PSGL-1 involving variable numbers of tandem repeats indicates that the longer PSGL-1 molecules are better able to form platelet–leukocyte aggregates; in some, but not all, studies, the longer molecules were associated with increased risk of some forms of thrombotic vascular disease.[785-790] The S100 calcium-modulated protein family member MRP-14 (also known as S100A9), which is abundant in neutrophils and released by activated platelets, promotes platelet thrombus, at least in part through CD36.[791]

Platelets can contribute to both innate and adaptive immunity in several ways. Bacterial endotoxin binding to toll-like receptors can activate platelets (see "Toll-Like Receptors 1, 2, 4, 6, 9"), enhance platelet–neutrophil interactions, and promote bacterial trapping by stimulating the production of neutrophil extracellular traps (NETs) composed of DNA, histones, and enzymes that degrade pathogens.[792-794] The production of NETs confers resistance to a variety of pathogens, including gram-positive (Staphylococcus aureus, Streptococcus pneumoniae, and group A streptococci) and gram-negative (Salmonella typhimurium, Shigella flexneri, and Escherichia coli) bacteria. A number of gram-positive bacteria can activate and aggregate platelets, and the platelet immune receptor Rc$\gamma$RIIA, integrin $\alpha_{IIb}\beta_3$, Src, and Syk, along with PF4, ADP, and TXA$_2$, all play a role in the process.[795] Platelets release mitochondria, which are related to bacteria in composition, when activated either in microparticles or free into plasma, where they associate with neutrophils and the platelet enzyme PLA2 IIA, which hydrolyzes mitochondrial and bacterial membranes, releasing a variety of proinflammatory molecules, including mitochondrial DNA, arachidonic acid, and lysophospholipids that are themselves capable of initiating NET formation.[796] Release of platelet mitochondria during storage for transfusion has been suggested as being a contributor to platelet-associated nonhemolytic transfusion reactions.[796]

Thrombocytopenia is often present in association with bloodborne bacterial infections (sepsis), and the severity of the thrombocytopenia mirrors the severity of the infection and prognosis. Platelet factor V contributes to resistance to group A streptococcal infection[797] by promoting thrombin generation and fibrin deposition, which may help to wall off the bacteria.[797] Platelets also influence the function of lymphocytes.[798] They enhance cytolytic T-cell proliferation and antibody production by B cells. Platelets can inhibit the responses of helper T cells and, via release of TGF-$\beta_1$, increase regulatory T (Treg) cells. Finally, platelets can bind to malarial-infected erythrocytes and both suppress the growth of the parasites and destroy the intraerythrocytic malarial parasites.[799]

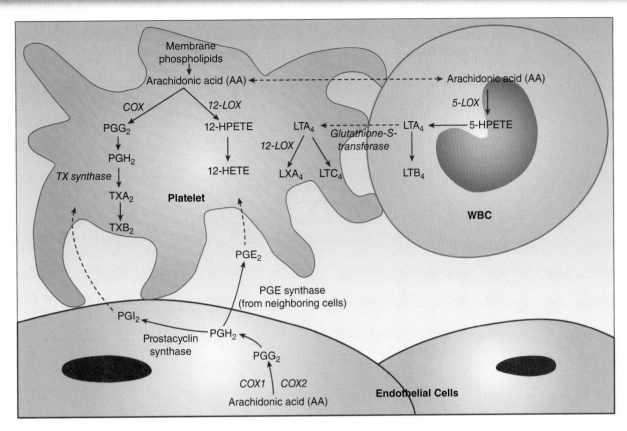

**Figure 2–10.** Select aspects of transcellular eicosanoid metabolism. At sites of platelet–white blood cell (WBC) interactions, free arachidonic acid (AA) can be generated by both activated platelets and leukocytes and exchanged between the cells. In the platelet, cyclooxygenase 1 (COX-1), the target for aspirin, generates the major AA metabolite prostaglandin (PG) G$_2$, the precursor for PGH$_2$ that, in turn, is converted by thromboxane (TX) synthase to TXA$_2$. TXA$_2$ and PGH$_2$ promote platelet activation and inflammation through binding to thromboprostanoid (TP) receptors. TXA$_2$ is rapidly converted to TXB$_2$. Platelets also express platelet-type 12-lipoxygenase (LOX), which converts AA to the relatively unstable intermediate 12-hydroperoxy-5,8,10,14-eicosatetraenoic acid (12-HPETE), which is subsequently converted to 12-hydroxyeicosatetraenoic acid (12-HETE). Platelets from most mammalian species do not possess 5-LOX and, therefore, cannot generate leukotriene A$_4$ (LTA$_4$) from AA. However, LTA$_4$ produced by leukocytes can be transferred to interacting platelets, where it can be metabolized by glutathione-*S*-transferase to LTC$_4$ or by platelet 12-LOX to the antiinflammatory mediator lipoxin (LXA$_4$). In endothelial cells, AA can also be released from membrane phospholipids, but unlike in the platelet, it is sequentially metabolized by COX-1 or COX-2 and prostacyclin synthase to PGI$_2$, which inhibits platelet activation by effects on the platelet inhibitory prostanoid (IP) receptor. Endothelial cells can also serve as a source of PGH$_2$ that is metabolized by PGE synthase to PGE$_2$. At high concentrations, PGE$_2$ inhibits platelet activation, and at lower concentrations (<10$^{-6}$ M), it activates platelets through the EP3 receptor. *(Used with permission of Matt Hazzard, Teaching and Academic Support Center, The University of Kentucky.)*

# ● PLATELETS IN VESSEL INTEGRITY AND DEVELOPMENT

Platelets are essential to maintain the integrity of the vasculature, especially in inflammatory sites, although the mechanisms are not fully understood. Platelets store a number of barrier-stabilizing cytokines and growth factors that may be released constitutively or in a stimulus-dependent manner, including sphingosine-1-phosphate (S1P), which is essential for barrier function, ADP, serotonin, VEGF, and thrombospondin. While platelet G-protein–coupled signaling is essential for hemostasis and thrombosis after vascular injury, these pathways do not appear to be required for hemostasis during inflammation. And functional platelet ITAM motif receptors, CLEC-2 and GPVI, are required to maintain vascular integrity during inflammation, likely by triggering a unique response in the setting of inflammation.[800]

The partitioning between lymphatic and blood vessels during development requires normal platelet function. Platelets regulate lymphangiogenesis, at least in part, through interactions between platelet CLEC-2 and podoplanin on lymphatic endothelial cells. In addition, downstream ITAM signaling, mediated by Syk, SLP-76, and PLCγ$_2$, is also required. Platelet activation along lymphatic endothelium may result in secretion of angiogenic factors. Importantly, platelet adhesion may result in intravascular hemostasis that promotes the lymphovenous junction, in that mouse embryos lacking CLEC-2, podoplanin, Syk, or SLP-76 display blood-filled lymphatic vessels. The requirement for platelets in maintaining blood–lymphatic separation extends beyond embryogenesis into adulthood. Importantly, the requirements for lymphovenous hemostasis are different from arterial and venous hemostasis, likely because of the low-flow, low-shear environment and intact lymphatic endothelium.

# ● PLATELET MEMBRANE GLYCOPROTEINS

Platelet membrane glycoproteins mediate most of the interactions between platelets and their external environment. Receptors can receive signals from outside the platelet and transmit signals inside. In addition, glycoprotein receptors receive signals from inside the platelet that affect their external domain functions. Platelet glycoprotein receptors are grouped into several different receptor families (integrins, leucine-rich glycoproteins, immunoglobulin cell adhesion molecules, selectins, tetraspanins, and seven-transmembrane domain receptors; see Table 2–4). One member

**TABLE 2–4.** Important Platelet Surface Proteins

| Gene Family | Common Name | Platelet Chain Designation | Integrin Designation | VLA† Designation | CD† Designation | | Mr Nonreduced | | Reduced |
|---|---|---|---|---|---|---|---|---|---|
| Integrin | Fibrinogen/receptor | | $\alpha_{IIb}\beta_3$ | | $\alpha_{IIb}\beta_3$-CD41a $\alpha_{IIb}$-CD41b $\beta_3$-CD61 | $\alpha_{IIb}$ $\beta_3$ | 145,000 90,000 | $\alpha_{IIb}\,\alpha$ $\alpha_{IIb}\,\beta$ | 125,000 23,000 114,000 |
| | Collagen receptor | GPIa/IIa | $\alpha_2\beta_1$ | VLA-2 | $\alpha_2$-CD49b $\beta_1$-CD29 | $\alpha_2$ $\beta_1$ | 150,000 138,000 | | 148,000 |
| | Fibronectin receptor | CPIc*/IIa | $\alpha_5\beta_1$ | VLA-5 | $\alpha_5$-CD49e $\beta_1$-CD29 | $\alpha_5$ $\beta_1$ | 140,000 138,000 | | 148,000 |
| | Laminin receptor | GPIc/IIa | $\alpha_6\beta_1$ | VLA-6 | $\alpha_6$-CD49f $\beta_1$-CD29 | $\alpha_6$ $\beta_1$ | 140,000 138,000 | | 148,000 |
| | Vitronectin receptor | $\alpha_\sqrt{}$/GPIIIa | $\alpha_v\beta_3$ | | $\alpha_v$-CD51 $\beta_3$-CD61 | $\alpha_v$ $\beta_3$ | 150,000 90,000 | $\alpha_v$ $\alpha_v$ | 125,000 25,000 114,000 |
| Leucine-rich repeat glycoproteins | von Willebrand factor receptor | GPIb/Ix | | | Ib/Ix-CD42 Ib/α-CD42b Ib/β-CD42c Ix-CD42a | GPIb GPIX | 170,000 17,000 | GPIbα GPIbβ | 145,000 22,000 17,000 |
| | | GPV | | | | GPV | 82,000 | | 82,000 |
| Immuno-globulin family cell adhesion modecules | PECAM-I | | | | CD31 | | 130,000 | | |
| | Fcγ-RII | | | | CD32 | | 40,000 | | |
| | HLA-Class 1 | | | | | | | | |
| | ICAM-2 | | | | CD102 | | | | 59,000 |
| | GPVI | | | | | | 62,000 | | 65,000 |
| | IAP | | | | CD47 | | 50,000 | | |
| Selectins | P-Selectin (GMP 140; PADGEM) | | | | CD62P | | 140,000 | | |
| Tetraspanins | p24 | | | | CD9 CD63 | | 24,000 | | |
| | PETA-3 | | | | CD151 | | 27,000 | | |
| | Lamp 3 (granulophysin) | | | | CD63 | | 53,000 | | |
| Miscellaneous | GPIV | | | | CD36 | | 88,000 | | |
| | CLEC-2 | | | | CD94 | | | | |
| | TLR(1-6) | | | | | | | | |
| | Lamp 1 | | | | CD107a | | 110,000 | | |
| | Lamp 2 | | | | CD107b | | 120,000 | | |
| | 67 kDa Laminin receptor | | | | | | 67,000 | | |
| | ADP P2X1 receptor | | | | | | 70,000 | | |
| | Leukosialin, sialophorin | | | | CD43 | | 90,000 | | |
| Seven-trans-membrane domain (G protein-linked) | PAR-1 | | | | | | 70,000 | | |
| | PAR-4 | | | | | | | | |
| | Thromboxane A$_2$ receptor | | | | | | | | 55,000 |
| | $\alpha_2$-Adrenergic receptor | | | | | | | | 64,000 |
| | Vasopressin receptor | | | | | | 125,000 | | |
| | ADP P2Y$_1$ receptor | | | | | | | | |
| | ADP P2Y$_{12}$ receptor | | | | | | | | |
| | Serotonin 5-HT2A | | | | | | 53,000 | | |

Fib, fibrinogen; Fn, fibronectin; GP, glycoprotein; HLA, human leukocyte antigen; IAP, integrin-associated protein; ICAM, intercellular adhesion molecule; lamp, lysosome-associated membrane protein; PAR, protease-activated receptor; PECAM, platelet-endothelial cell adhesion molecule; PSGL-1, P-selectin glycoprotein ligand-1; TSP, thrombospondin; TX, thromboxane; Vn, vironectin; VWF, von Willebrand factor.

| Amino Acids | Carbohydrate | Lipid | Phosphorylated | Chromosome | Ligands | Platelet Specific | Function | Molecules on Platelet Surface (S) or Internal (I) |
|---|---|---|---|---|---|---|---|---|
| $\alpha_{IIb}$ 1039 | + | – | – | 17 | Fib, VWF, Fn, Vn, ?TSP | + | Adhesion, aggregation, protein trafficking | (S) 80,000 |
| $\beta_3$ 762 | + | – | + | 17 | | + | | (I) 40,000 |
| $\alpha_2$ 1152 | | | | 5 | Collagen | – | Adhesion | (S) 1000 |
| $\beta_1$ 778 | | | | 10 | | – | | |
| $\alpha_5$ 1008 | | | | 12 | Fn | – | Adhesion | (S) 1000 |
| $\beta_1$ 778 | | | | 10 | | | | |
| $\alpha_6$ 1067 | | | | 2 | Laminin | – | Adhesion | (S) 1000 |
| $\beta_3$ 778 | | | | 10 | | | | |
| $\alpha_v$ 1048 | | | | 2 | Vn, Fib, VWF, Fn, ?TSP, Osp | – | ?Adhesion, ?Protein trafficking | (S) 100 |
| GPIIIa 762 | + | – | | 17 | | | | |
| GPIbα 610(8)* | + | – | – | 1 | VWF, thrombin | +? | Adhesion (high shear), ?thrombin activation | (S) 25,000 |
| GPIbβ 181(1)* | + | + | + | 22 | | +? | | (S) 25,000 |
| GPIX 160(1)* | + | + | | 3 | | +? | | (S) 25,000 |
| GPV 544(15)* | + | + | + | 3 | | +? | | (S) 12,500 |
| PECAM-1 738 | + | ? | + | 17 | Heparin | – | ?Adhesion | (S) 8000 |
| FcγRII 324 | + | | + | 1 | Immune complexes | – | Immune complex binding | (s) ~1000 |
| HLA | + | | | 6 | – | | Histocompatibility | (S) |
| ICAM-2 274 | | | | 17 | LFA-1 | – | Platelet-leukocyte adhesion | (S) 2600 |
| GPVI 316 | + | – | | ? | Collagen | + | Activation | (S) ~2000 |
| IAP 287 | + | | | 3 | TSP | – | Activation | |
| P-Selectin 830 | + | + | + | 1 | Sialyl-le$^x$ PSGL-1 | | Platelet-leukocyte adhesion | (I) 20,000 |
| CD9 228 | + | | | | ? | – | Activation | (S) 40,000 |
| CD151 253 | + | – | – | 11 | ? | – | Activation | (I) ~2000 |
| Lamp 3 238 | + | | | | | | | (I) 10,000 |
| GPIV 471 | + | | + | 7 | Collagen, TSP | – | Adhesion | (S) 20,000 |
| CLEC-2 229 | + | | + | 12 | Podoplanin | – | Adhesion/activation | |
| TLR | | | | | Pathogen-associated molecular patterns | – | Activation | |
| Lamp 1 389 | + | | | 13 | ? | – | ? | (I) 1200 |
| Lamp 2 381 | + | | | X | ? | | | |
| 67 kDa ?295 | | | | X | Laminin | – | Adhesion | |
| P2X$_1$ 399 | + | | | 17 | ATP, ADP | – | Activation | (S) 13–130 |
| CD43 400 | + | | + | 16 | ICAM-1 | – | Adhesion | |
| PAR-1 425 | | | | 5 | Thrombin | – | Activation | (S) ~1800 |
| PAR-4 385 | + | | + | 19 | Thrombin | – | Activation | |
| TXA$_2$ 343 | | | | 19 | PGH$_2$/thromboxane A$_2$ | – | Activation | ~200 |
| $\alpha_2$-Adrenergin 450 | | | | 10 | Epinephrine | – | Activation | ~250 |
| Vasopressin 418 | | | | ?x | Vasopressin | – | Activation | ~75 |
| P2Y$_1$ 373 | + | | | 3 | ADP | – | Activation | |
| P2Y$_{12}$ 342 | | | | 3 | ADP | + | Activation | |
| 5-HT2A | + | | + | 13 | Serotonin | – | Activation | |

*Number of leucine-rich repeats.

†CD, cluster of differentiation; VLA, very-late antigen.

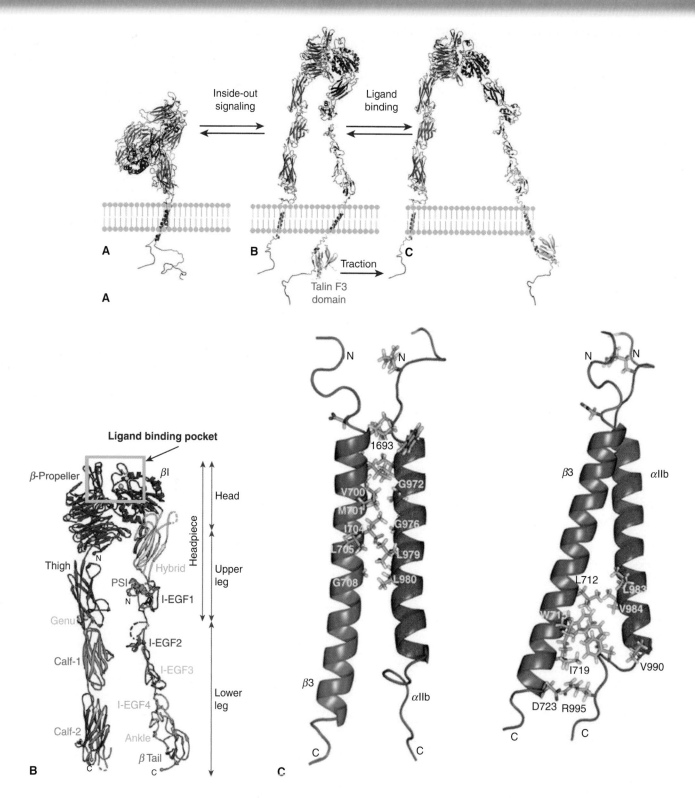

**Figure 2–11.** $\alpha_{IIb}\beta_3$ Integrin structure and activation. **A.** Model for $\alpha_{IIb}\beta_3$ integrin inside-out activation and outside-in signaling. The $\alpha$ subunit is in *blue*, and the $\beta$ subunit is in *red*. The bent, inactive receptor is depicted in *(A)*. Under resting condition, the integrin $\beta_3$ cytoplasmic domain appears to interact with filamin. Cellular stimulation induces migfilin to displace filamin from the integrin $\beta_3$ cytoplasmic domain as well as a conformational change in talin that alters the interactions between the talin head and rod domains and exposes the talin head domain. The FERM F3 domain in the head then binds to the integrin $\beta_3$ cytoplasmic domain, which unclasps the inter-subunit cytoplasmic and transmembrane domains from their complex with the integrin $\beta_3$ cytoplasmic and transmembrane domains. Kindlin-3 binding to the integrin $\beta_3$ cytoplasmic domain may facilitate talin binding and appears to be required for the conversion hos the high-affinity state. The binding of talin then leads to separation of the ectodomain sub-unit tails and may diminish the interaction of the integrin headpiece with the tails. Although small ligands can bind to the receptor without headpiece extension, the large glycoprotein ligands may require extension to facilitate access to the ligand binding site. Extension *(B)* may occur spontaneously after leg separation or may result from traction force exerted on the integrin $\beta_3$ cytoplasmic domain via talin's association with the cytoskeleton

of the integrin family, integrin $\alpha_{IIb}\beta_3$, is virtually unique to platelets (and their precursors, megakaryocytes), whereas the leucine-rich glycoproteins GPIb/IX and GPV appear to have highly restricted but not uniquely platelet expression patterns, including cytokine-activated endothelial cells.[801,802] All of the other receptors are expressed more widely on other cell types.

## INTEGRINS

Integrin receptors are heterodimeric complexes composed of an $\alpha$ subunit containing three or four divalent cation binding domains and a $\beta$ subunit rich in disulfide bonds. Both subunits are transmembrane glycoproteins and are coded by different genes. There are at least 18 $\alpha$ subunits and eight $\beta$ subunits.[43,803,804] Three major families of integrin receptors are recognized based on the $\beta$ subunit: $\beta_1$, $\beta_2$, and $\beta_3$. Integrins are widely distributed on different cell types, and each integrin demonstrates unique ligand-binding properties. Integrin receptors mediate interactions between cells and proteins or proteins on cells; they are also involved in protein trafficking in cells. Integrin receptors can also transduce messages from outside the cell to inside the cell and from inside the cell to outside the cell.

### Integrin $\alpha_{IIb}\beta_3$ (Also Termed GPIIb/IIIa, Fibrinogen Receptor, and CD41/CD61)

The integrin $\alpha_{IIb}\beta_3$ complex, a member of the $\beta_3$ integrin receptor family, is the dominant platelet receptor, with 80,000 to 100,000 receptors present on the surface of a resting platelet (Fig. 2–11).[805-812] Another 20,000 to 40,000 receptors are present inside platelets, primarily in $\alpha$-granule membranes, but also in dense bodies and membranes lining the open canalicular system; these receptors are able to join the plasma membrane when platelets are activated and undergo the release reaction.[813-815] On average, integrin $\alpha_{IIb}\beta_3$ receptors are less than 20 nm apart on the platelet surface and thus are among the most densely expressed adhesion/aggregation receptors present on any cell type.

On resting platelets, integrin $\alpha_{IIb}\beta_3$ has low affinity for fibrinogen in solution, but when platelets are activated with ADP, epinephrine, thrombin, or other agonists, integrin $\alpha_{IIb}\beta_3$ binds fibrinogen relatively strongly.[808,816] Activation induces changes in the integrin $\alpha_{IIb}\beta_3$ receptor itself that are responsible for the change in fibrinogen-binding affinity, but changes in the microenvironment surrounding integrin $\alpha_{IIb}\beta_3$ may also be involved. The integrin $\alpha_{IIb}\beta_3$ receptors in $\alpha$ granules appear to cycle to and from the plasma membrane.[817] This recycling helps to explain the ability of the integrin to take up fibrinogen from plasma and transport it to $\alpha$ granules, where it is concentrated.[375,818]

Data from other integrin receptors identified a cell recognition sequence composed of RGD in the ligand fibronectin,[819,820] and this same sequence is important in ligand binding to integrins $\alpha_v\beta_3$ and $\alpha_{IIb}\beta_3$. Fibrinogen contains one RGD sequence near the carboxy terminus of each of the two A$\alpha$ chains (amino acids 572 to 574) and another at amino acids 95 to 97.[821] In addition, the carboxyterminal 12 amino acid region of each of the two $\gamma$ chains (amino acids 400 to 411) contains a sequence that includes Lys-Gln-Ala-Gly-Asp-Val, which is the most important in the binding of fibrinogen to platelets.[822-826] VWF contains an RGD sequence in its carboxyterminal domain, and that region mediates the binding to integrin $\alpha_{IIb}\beta_3$.[809,810,812] Small, synthetic peptides containing the RGD or $\gamma$-chain sequence inhibit the binding of fibrinogen to platelets, and these observations have been exploited to produce therapeutic agents (tirofiban and eptifibatide) to inhibit platelet thrombus formation[827] (Chap. 24). Similarly, monoclonal antibodies that inhibit binding of ligands to integrin $\alpha_{IIb}\beta_3$ have been developed, and a mouse/human chimeric Fab fragment of one of them has been developed into a drug (abciximab) that is an effective antiplatelet agent.

The binding of fibrinogen to integrin $\alpha_{IIb}\beta_3$ appears to be a multistep process[808,828-833]: (1) the initial interaction is most likely via the $\gamma$-chain carboxyterminal region(s) and divalent cation-dependent[823-826]; (2) subsequent interactions enhance the binding and internalization of the fibrinogen[834] and render it irreversible, even when divalent cations are removed[835]; (3) binding of fibrinogen induces changes in the receptor that can be recognized by antibodies (ligand-induced binding sites [LIBSs])[442,826]; (4) binding of fibrinogen to integrin $\alpha_{IIb}\beta_3$ induces changes in fibrinogen (receptor-induced binding sites) that can be recognized by antibodies and may involve exposure of the A$\alpha$ chain Arg-Gly-Asp-Phe sequence at amino acids 95 to 98[836,837]; and (5) fibrinogen binding induces receptor clustering.[251,838]

By electron microscopy, the receptors have a globular head of $8 \times 12$ nm and two 18-nm long tails representing the carboxyterminal regions of each subunit, including their hydrophobic transmembrane domains.[839,840] Crystallographic, electron microscopic, electron and neutron scattering, and biochemical data from integrin $\alpha_{IIb}\beta_3$ and the related integrin $\alpha_v\beta_3$ receptor indicate that the unactivated receptors are in a bent conformation and that activation involves both extension of the receptor head and a swing out motion in the $\beta_3$ subunit.[149,827,841-853] A three-dimensional reconstruction of integrin $\alpha_{IIb}\beta_3$ in a lipid bilayer nano disc from negative-stain electron microscopy images supports a compact conformation of the inactive receptor, but unlike the crystal structure of the ectodomain, the legs are not parallel and straight.[848]

---

and actin-myosin contractile force. Ligand binding to the integrin is associated with a swing out motion of the integrin $\beta_3$ hybrid domain from the $\beta$A(I) domain *(C)*, which results in both increased ligand affinity via alterations in the ADMIDAS (adjacent to metal ion-dependent adhesion site) and MIDAS (metal ion-dependent adhesion site) regions of integrin $\beta_3$ and greater leg separation. This conformational change may initiate outside-in signaling. The ligated integrins may then cluster (not shown). The structure in panel *(A)* is based on the crystal structure of the ectodomain (PDB 3FCS)[250] and the nuclear magnetic resonance (NMR) structure of the transmembrane and cytoplasmic domains (PDB 2K9J).[894] The structure in *(B)* is based on the same ectodomain crystal structure, but with extension at the genus of the subunits (PDB 3FCS),[250] the NMR structures of the separated transmembrane and cytoplasmic domains,[894] and the structure of the complex between the $\beta_3$ cytoplasmic domain and the talin F3 domain (PDB 2H7E).[896] The structure in *(C)* is based on crystal structure of the liganded receptor (PDB 2VDN) headpiece,[827] the extended structure of ectodomain (PDB3FCS),[250] and the monomeric transmembrane structures connected to unstructured cytosolic tails. **B.** Domain structure of structure of integrin $\alpha_{IIb}\beta_3$. The individual domains and the ligand binding pocket are identified in the model of the extended integrin. I-EGF, integrin epidermal growth factor; PSI, plexins, semaphorins, integrins. **C.** The integrin transmembrane complex. Selected views of the NMR structure of the $\alpha_{IIb}$ *(red)* and $\beta_3$ *(blue)* transmembrane complex. The *left* panel depicts contacts involved in the outer membrane clasp, and the *right* panel depicts the contacts involved in the inner membrane clasp. Note that after the integrin $\alpha_{IIb}$ helical region ends at V990, the next 5 residues (GFFKR) reenter the membrane; the two aromatic F residues make hydrophobic contacts with $\beta_3$, and $\alpha_{IIb}$ R995 makes a salt bridge with integrin $\beta_3$ D723. *(A, reproduced with permission from Lau TL, Kim C, Ginsberg MH, et al: The structure of the integrin alphaIIbbeta3 transmembrane complex explains integrin transmembrane signalling, EMBO J 2009 May 6;28(9):1351–1361. B, reproduced with permission from Zhu, J., et al: Structure of a complete integrin ectodomain in a physiologic resting state and activation and deactivation by applied forces, Mol Cell 2008 Dec 26;32(6):849–861. C, Reproduced with permission from Lau TL, Kim C, Ginsberg MH, et al: The structure of the integrin alphaIIbbeta3 transmembrane complex explains integrin transmembrane signalling, EMBO J 2009 May 6;28(9):1351–1361.)*

Integrin $\alpha_{IIb}\beta_3$ shares the same basic structural features of all integrin receptors (see Table 2–4).[30,848] The $\alpha$ subunit, $\alpha_{IIb}$, is a transmembrane protein with four characteristic divalent cation-binding sites (see Fig. 2–11). The mature protein contains 1008 amino acids[43,854] with one transmembrane domain; during processing, it is cleaved into a heavy chain and a light chain connected by a disulfide bond. The $\beta$ subunit, $\beta_3$, contains 762 amino acids and is rich in cysteine residues, with a characteristic cysteine-rich region near its transmembrane domain.[43,855] The integrin $\alpha_{IIb}$ and $\beta_3$ cytoplasmic tails consist of 20 and 47 amino acids, respectively. The genes coding for $\alpha_{IIb}$ and $\beta_3$ are very close to each other on chromosome 17 at q21.32, but are not so close as to share common regulatory domains.[856,857] Both proteins are synthesized in megakaryocytes and join to form a calcium-dependent, noncovalent complex in the rough endoplasmic reticulum.[858] Calnexin probably serves as a chaperone for integrin $\alpha_{IIb}$,[859] but it is unclear which chaperone(s) are involved in integrin $\beta_3$ folding and/or integrin $\alpha_{IIb}\beta_3$ complex formation. The integrin $\alpha_{IIb}\beta_3$ complex subsequently undergoes further processing in the Golgi apparatus, where the carbohydrate structures undergo maturation and the pro-GPIIb molecule is cleaved into its heavy and light chains by furin or a similar enzyme.[860,861] Approximately 15 percent of the mass of both integrins $\alpha_{IIb}$ and $\beta_3$ are composed of carbohydrate.[862] The mature integrin $\alpha_{IIb}\beta_3$ complex is then transported to the plasma membrane or the membranes of $\alpha$ granules or dense bodies. If integrins $\alpha_{IIb}$ and $\beta_3$ do not form a proper complex, either because of a structural abnormality in either subunit or the failure to synthesize one of the subunits, the subunit(s) that are synthesized are rapidly degraded and so are not expressed on the membrane surface (Chap. 11). Degradation of integrin $\alpha_{IIb}$ appears to involve retro-translocation from the endoplasmic reticulum into the cytoplasm, ubiquitination, and proteolysis by the megakaryocyte proteasome.[859]

Both integrins $\alpha_{IIb}$ and $\beta_3$ are composed of a series of domains (see Fig. 2–11). The aminoterminal region of integrin $\alpha_{IIb}$ contains a seven-blade $\beta$-propeller domain, and each blade is composed of four $\beta$ strands connected by loops. The propeller interacts with the $\beta A$ (I-like) domain of integrin $\beta_3$, forming the globular head region observed in electron micrographs. The four calcium ions bound by the propeller domain interact with $\beta$ hairpin loops in blades four to seven that extend away from the interface with integrin $\beta_3$. In addition, there is a unique integrin $\alpha_{IIb}$ cap subdomain made up of four loops from blades one to three that are unique to $\alpha_{IIb}$ and contribute to its ligand binding specificity. The remainder of the extracellular components of integrin $\alpha_{IIb}$ are made up of a thigh, genu (knee-like), and two calf domains,[250] much like the structure of the related integrin $\alpha_V$ subunit.[841,844] The cytoplasmic domain of integrin $\alpha_{IIb}$ interacts with the cytoplasmic domain of integrin $\beta_3$ and the interaction is important in controlling activation of the holoreceptor.[863–866] The cytoplasmic domain of integrin $\alpha_{IIb}$ has a GFFKR sequence near the membrane that is thought to control inside-out activation of the integrin receptors because mutations or deletions in this region result in the receptor adopting a conformation with high affinity for fibrinogen.[867–871] A number of studies using mutagenesis and nuclear magnetic resonance (NMR) identified different structures for the transmembrane and cytoplasmic domains, and differences in the relative roles of heterodimeric and homodimeric associations.[864,872–875] Disrupting the conformation of this region also results in a constitutively high-affinity receptor,[876,877] which has led to the conclusion that inside-out activation of integrin $\alpha_{IIb}\beta_3$ requires separation of the transmembrane and cytoplasmic domains, but it remains possible that more subtle changes in the cytoplasmic and transmembrane domains may be sufficient.[848]

The integrin $\beta_3$ subunit domains are not linearly arranged because the first domain (PSI [plexins, semaphorins, and integrins]) was subjected to the insertion of a hybrid domain, which itself was subjected to the insertion of a $\beta A$ (I-like) domain; the latter domain is homologous to the VWF A domain and integrin I domains, both of which bind ligands

(see Fig. 2–11).[827,878] The double insertion in the PSI domain explains why there is a "long range" disulfide bond extending from C13 to C435; thus, even though the $\beta A$ domain makes contact with the integrin $\alpha_{IIb}$ propeller (via Arg261 and other residues that interact with two rings of hydrophobic residues in the integrin $\alpha_{IIb}$ "cage"), it is not the aminoterminus of the molecule. The PSI domain contains Leu33, which defines the Pl$^{A1}$ (HPA-1a) specificity, as opposed to the alloantigen Pl$^{A2}$ (HPA-1b), which is produced by a Pro33 polymorphism. The integrin $\beta_3$ leg is composed of four integrin EGF domains that are rich in disulfide bonds. In the crystal structure, this region interacts with the integrin $\alpha_{IIb}$ stalk region and the globular head in the bent, unactivated receptor, but these interactions are less prominent in the three-dimensional reconstruction of the inactive receptor not in the activated receptor.[250,827,848] Mutations in the integrin EGF domains, including cysteine residues, can activate the receptor as can the binding of monoclonal antibodies.[879–882] The importance of the normal disulfide bond pairings in integrin $\beta_3$ is further supported by data demonstrating that certain reducing agents can cause activation of integrin $\alpha_{IIb}\beta_3$, fibrinogen binding, and platelet aggregation,[883,884] and an enzyme capable of catalyzing the exchange of thiol groups and disulfide in proteins (PDI) has been identified on the surface of platelets and in platelet releasates.[883,885–887] Thiol-disulfide exchange in integrins $\alpha_{IIb}\beta_3$ and $\alpha_V\beta_3$ is implicated as a contributor to clot retraction.[888] Moreover, regions in integrin $\beta_3$ itself have the same consensus sequence (CGXC) present in PDI that is thought to mediate the catalysis.[889] One model suggests that integrin $\alpha_{IIb}\beta_3$ can achieve a low level of activation without alterations in disulfide bonds, but that maximal activation requires PDI or similar activity along with a source of thiols such as plasma glutathione or a membrane NAD(P)H oxidoreductase system.[883] Inhibition of PDI and other enzymes that mediate thiol-disulfide exchange (ERp57, ERp5) reduces platelet thrombus formation.[890,891] It is still unclear, however, whether disulfide bond alterations contribute to activation *in vivo* under physiologic or pathologic conditions.

Transmembrane domain structures of integrin $\alpha_{IIb}$ and integrin $\beta_3$ have been proposed based on NMR and structural modeling studies.[871,873,874,892–896] Because the integrin $\alpha_{IIb}$ transmembrane helix is shorter than the integrin $\beta_3$ helix, they traverse the membrane at an angle of approximately 25 degrees. The association of the integrin $\alpha_{IIb}$ and integrin $\beta_3$ ectodomains near the site of entry into the membrane results in the transmembrane helices being directly juxtaposed in the region of the membrane closest to the ectodomain (outer membrane clasp). Near the cytoplasmic end of the membrane, the helices are held together by an inner membrane clasp composed of the integrin $\alpha_{IIb}$ residues immediately after the end of the helix (GFFKR), with the membrane reimmersion of F992 and F993 filling the gap and interacting with integrin $\beta_3$ W715 and I719, with integrin $\alpha_{IIb}$ R995 creating a salt bridge with integrin $\beta_3$ 723 and perhaps residue 726.[897,898] Of note, these regions are conserved in many other integrins receptors, and so the basic mechanism may be common to many of the receptors.

Inside-out signaling is accomplished by the talin F3 domain binding to the integrin $\beta_3$ cytoplasmic domain, which is proposed to disrupt the inner membrane clasp.[34,244,245,863,865,866,869,870,872,876,892,899,900] This may be facilitated by migfilin displacing filamin from the integrin $\beta_3$ cytoplasmic domain as the latter interaction may prevent talin binding.[901] Talin binding results in dissociation of the transmembrane helices and reorganization of the cytoplasmic region of integrin $\beta_3$ into a more extended helix. Integrin $\alpha_{IIb}\beta_3$ ectodomain chain separation, headpiece extension, and integrin $\beta_3$ swing out then follow, either spontaneously or as a result of the traction force generated by the cytoskeleton on integrin $\beta_3$ through talin.[149] Outside-in signaling is presumed to be initiated by loss of ectodomain interactions between the membrane-proximal regions of integrins $\alpha_{IIb}$ and $\beta_3$, perhaps as a result of ligand binding producing even greater integrin $\beta_3$ swing out, resulting in disruption of the outer membrane clasp and subsequent dissociation of the transmembrane helices. This potentially may facilitate the interaction of the cytoplasmic domains with cytoskeletal elements and signaling molecules.

The integrin $\beta_3$ tail also contains two NXXY motifs, and Y747 and Y759 within one of these motifs are phosphorylated upon platelet aggregation, thus producing docking sites for signaling molecules.[235] Studies in mice and in recombinant systems demonstrate a role for the sites in clot retraction and platelet aggregate stability.[291,902]

A number of proteins have been shown to bind to the cytoplasmic domains of integrin $\alpha_{IIb}$ and/or $\beta_3$, either directly or through interactions with other proteins, including signaling molecules (Src, Shc, FAK, paxillin, and ILK, all of which bind to integrin $\beta_3$), cytoskeletal proteins (kindlin-3, skelemin, $\alpha$-actin, and myosin, which bind to integrin $\beta_3$, and filamin and talin, which bind to integrins $\alpha_{IIb}$ and/or $\beta_3$), and other proteins ($\beta_3$-endonexin and CD98, which bind to integrin $\beta_3$, and CIB and calreticulin, which bind to $\alpha_{IIb}$) (Fig. 2–12).[244,866,903-919] These interactions are important in mediating inside-out signaling and outside-in signaling.[235] JAM-A is a negative regulator of outside-in activation by integrin $\alpha_{IIb}\beta_3$ that acts by regulating activation of Src.[920] Similarly, PECAM-1 serves as an inhibitor of integrin $\alpha_{IIb}\beta_3$ activation through a sequential phosphorylation mechanism.[921,922] Force on the integrin $\beta_3$ cytoplasmic domain by actin–myosin action may supply the energy for the conformational change in integrin $\alpha_{IIb}\beta_3$ from bent to extended.[250]

The junction between the integrin $\alpha_{IIb}$ propeller and the $\beta_3$ $\beta A$ (I-like) domain is the site of ligand binding to integrin $\alpha_{IIb}\beta_3$ (see Fig. 2–11). This region of integrin $\beta_3$ contains three divalent cation binding sites: MIDAS (metal ion-dependent adhesion site), ADMIDAS (adjacent to MIDAS), and SyMBS (synergy metal binding site).[250] The latter was previously termed the ligand-associated metal binding site (LIMBS) based on the crystal structure of integrin $\alpha_V\beta_3$.[844,845]

The crystal structure of integrin $\alpha_V\beta_3$ demonstrated that an RGD peptide is bound primarily via interactions between the Arg in the peptide and two Asp residues (D150 and D218) in integrin $\alpha_V$ and between the Asp in the peptide and the MIDAS cation.[845] The binding pocket in integrin $\alpha_{IIb}\beta_3$ is similar but differs in that only one Asp in integrin $\alpha_{IIb}$ (D224) is available to interact with an Arg (or Lys as in the fibrinogen $\gamma$-chain peptide), the distance between D224 in integrin $\alpha_{IIb}$ and the MIDAS cation is longer, and a cap subdomain of the integrin $\alpha_{IIb}$ propeller contributes Phe160 to a hydrophobic exosite in combination with

Tyr190.[149,827] As a result, the pocket is able to accommodate the longer fibrinogen $\gamma$-chain C-terminal peptide better, with the peptide's Asp and C-terminal Val carboxyls interacting with the MIDAS and ADMIDAS cations, respectively.[826] It also explains why integrin $\alpha_{IIb}\beta_3$ can bind peptides containing the longer Lys residue (KGD peptides).[923] Crystal structures are also available for the integrin $\alpha_{IIb}\beta_3$ receptor with the drugs eptifibatide and tirofiban, which are effective antithrombotic agents because of their ability to block ligand binding to integrin $\alpha_{IIb}\beta_3$, and demonstrate specificity for integrin $\alpha_{IIb}\beta_3$ compared to integrin $\alpha_V\beta_3$.[827] The basis of the specificity of these agents involves in part their interaction with the integrin $\alpha_{IIb}$-specific exosite and the greater length between their positive and negative charges.[827] The third integrin $\alpha_{IIb}\beta_3$ antagonist drug, abciximab, is a chimeric murine monoclonal antibody Fab fragment. Its epitope has been localized to a region on integrin $\beta_3$ very close to the MIDAS, suggesting that it works by steric interference with ligand binding, disruption of the binding pocket, or both mechanisms.

Two major conformational changes in integrin $\alpha_{IIb}\beta_3$ have been described in association with activation: headpiece extension and integrin $\beta_3$ hybrid and PSI domain swing-out (see Fig. 2–11).[250,827,853] Headpiece extension can contribute to ligand binding by enhancing access to the binding site; it can also contribute to platelet aggregation by extending the receptor out further from the platelet surface,[924] thus facilitating the ability of fibrinogen to bridge between platelets.[846] The integrin $\beta_3$ hybrid and PSI domain swing-out motion appears to enhance ligand binding, but the precise mechanism is unclear.[826,847,850] Swing-out is associated with movement of the ADMIDAS metal ion and the $\alpha_1$-$\beta_1$ loop toward the MIDAS with the latter movement stabilized by the interaction of two backbone nitrogens in the $\alpha_1$-$\beta_1$ loop with the ligand carboxyl oxygen, thus reinforcing the binding to the MIDAS metal ion.[149,826] Mutations that produce swing-out of the hybrid and PSI domains result in constitutive ligand binding to integrin $\alpha_{IIb}\beta_3$.[925]

Binding of fibrinogen to platelet integrin $\alpha_{IIb}\beta_3$ leads to platelet aggregation, presumably via crosslinking of integrin molecules on two different platelets by fibrinogen.[840] The dimeric and relatively rigid structure of fibrinogen and the location of the binding sites at the ends of the $\gamma$ chains are all consistent with such a model as the two binding sites on a single fibrinogen molecule are probably more than 45 nm apart. Soon after fibrinogen binds, it can be dissociated from the platelet by chelating the divalent cations, but the binding becomes irreversible

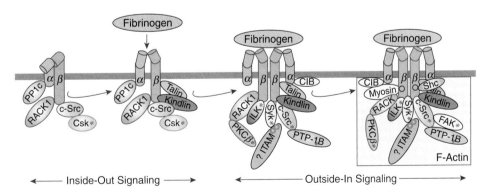

**Figure 2–12.** Protein interactions with the cytoplasmic domains of $\alpha_{IIb}\beta_3$ regulate inside-out and outside-in signaling. Shown are some, but not all, of the proteins reported to associate with the $\alpha_{IIb}\beta_3$ cytoplasmic domains, many in a dynamic fashion. Some are associated with resting platelets, while others are recruited to, or dissociate from, the integrin during inside-out or outside-in signaling, leading to F-actin assembly. In addition, several proteins with enzymatic function become activated *(asterisks)* after fibrinogen binding to $\alpha_{IIb}\beta_3$. Not shown are the many additional adapter molecules, enzymes, and substrates that may become recruited through more indirect interactions. CIB, calcium and integrin-binding 1; Csk, c-Src tyrosine kinase; ILK, integrin-linked kinase; ITAM, a yet-to-be identified protein with one or more immunoreceptor tyrosine activation motifs; PKC$\beta$, protein kinase C$\beta$; PP1c, protein phosphatase 1c; RACK1, receptor for activated C kinase 1; Syk, spleen tyrosine kinase. *(Reproduced with permission from Coller, B.S. and S.J. Shattil, The GPIIb/IIIa (integrin alphaIIbbeta3) odyssey: a technology-driven saga of a receptor with twists, turns, and even a bend, Blood 2008 Oct 15;112(8):3011–3025.)*

within an hour.[835] Fibrinogen binding alone is not sufficient for platelet aggregation, but the events necessary after fibrinogen binding, which probably include ligand- and/or cytoskeletal-mediated receptor clustering, are not well understood.[95,835,926,927] After ligands bind to integrin $\alpha_{IIb}\beta_3$, "outside-in" signaling through the integrin can occur, resulting in a number of phosphorylation events, changes in the platelet cytoskeleton, platelet spreading, and even initiation of protein translation.[236,237,928]

In addition to fibrinogen, several other proteins can bind to integrin $\alpha_{IIb}\beta_3$ on activated platelets, including VWF, fibronectin, vitronectin, thrombospondin, and prothrombin[390,675,929]; each of these contains an RGD sequence in the region implicated in the initial interaction with platelets. There are subtle differences in the binding of each of these ligands, however, with regard to divalent cation preference and competent activating agents. The binding of all of these other ligands can also be inhibited by RGD-containing peptides, indicating a common requirement for the interaction between the RGD sequence in the protein and the RGD-binding site in integrin $\alpha_{IIb}\beta_3$.[930,931]

Platelet aggregation measured in the aggregometer *ex vivo* depends upon fibrinogen binding to integrin $\alpha_{IIb}\beta_3$. It is less clear whether fibrinogen is the most important ligand supporting platelet aggregation *in vivo* since studies performed in model systems under flowing conditions indicate that VWF is the major ligand at higher shear rates.[932] Even in the aggregometer, VWF can partially substitute for fibrinogen if the fibrinogen concentration is very low.[933] *In vivo*, mice deficient in both VWF and fibrinogen still make platelet thrombi in response to vascular injury.[934–936] Although fibronectin was initially implicated in supporting the development of such thrombi, mice deficient in fibrinogen, VWF, and fibronectin have paradoxically increased platelet aggregation and thrombus formation, suggesting that fibronectin may play an inhibiting role in thrombus formation under certain circumstances.[373]

Although resting platelets do not bind soluble fibrinogen (or other adhesive glycoproteins) to an appreciable extent, they can adhere to fibrinogen immobilized on a surface.[825,937] This activation-independent adhesion may be from alterations in the structure of fibrinogen when it is immobilized on a surface.[836,938] Alternatively, there may always be a few integrin $\alpha_{IIb}\beta_3$ receptors that are transiently in the proper conformation to bind fibrinogen, and immobilization may result in high local density of fibrinogen and favorable kinetics for adhesion. Finally, it is possible that even low-affinity fibrinogen interactions with integrin $\alpha_{IIb}\beta_3$ are sufficient to initiate integrin interactions with the cytoskeleton such that actin-myosin–induced contraction provides the energy required for the conformational changes needed to achieve higher affinity binding.[250]

Fibrinogen and/or fibrin have been identified on the surface of damaged blood vessels; thus, it is possible that integrin $\alpha_{IIb}\beta_3$ mediates platelet adhesion under those circumstances.[939] In contrast, integrin $\alpha_{IIb}\beta_3$ on resting platelets does not appear to be able to mediate adhesion to VWF or fibronectin[940]; if platelets are activated, however, integrin $\alpha_{IIb}\beta_3$ can support adhesion to these glycoproteins.[930] In models of platelet accumulation under flowing conditions, $\alpha_{IIb}\beta_3$ acts in synergy with GPIb/IX, VWF, and fibrinogen at the apex of thrombi, where shear forces are greatest.[28,941,942] The integrin $\alpha_{IIb}\beta_3$ has also been implicated in platelet spreading after adhesion,[227,228,943] and it is necessary for clot retraction (see above) and the uptake of plasma fibrinogen into platelet $\alpha$ granules.[818,944]

Less well-defined roles for integrin $\alpha_{IIb}\beta_3$ have been suggested in the binding of plasminogen,[688] calcium transport across the platelet membrane,[945–947] IgE binding to platelets leading to parasite cytotoxicity,[948] and interactions with the *Borrelia* species spirochetes that cause Lyme disease[949] and hantavirus.[950] Integrin $\alpha_{IIb}\beta_3$ also mediates factor XIIIa binding to platelets, but this is primarily as a result of factor XIII's association with fibrinogen.[456] Factor XIIIa and calpain have also been

implicated in limiting platelet–platelet interactions after activation by adhesion to collagen.[951]

### Integrin $\alpha_2\beta_1$ (Also Termed GPIa/IIa, Collagen Receptor, VLA-2, and CD49b/CD29)

Integrin $\alpha_2\beta_1$ (GPIa/IIa) is widely distributed on different cell types and can mediate adhesion to collagen.[19,20,952–957] The integrin $\alpha_2$ subunit (GPIa) contains a region of 220 amino acids inserted in the aminoterminal $\beta$-propeller region (I domain) that is homologous to similar regions in other proteins that are known to interact with collagen, including VWF and cartilage matrix protein.[958] This region has a MIDAS, and crystallographic data of the $\alpha_2$ I domain in complex with a CRP containing the type I collagen sequence GFOGER (where O indicates hydroxyproline) demonstrated that the glutamic acid in the peptide coordinates $Mg^{2+}$ binding in the MIDAS.[959–961] The integrin $\alpha_2\beta_1$ I domain can assume a variety of conformations, going from inactive (closed), through intermediate or low affinity, to active high affinity.[952,962]

Both integrin $\alpha_2\beta_1$ and GPVI appear to participate in platelet interactions with collagen.[963–965] Bleeding defects have been described in patients with decreased levels of integrin $\alpha_2\beta_1$ and GPVI, but the precise contributions of the decreases in these receptors is uncertain (Chap. 11). Although integrin $\alpha_2\beta_1$ is capable of supporting adhesion to collagen without exogenous activators, like integrin $\alpha_{IIb}\beta_3$, it appears to be able to increase its affinity for ligand in response to inside-out activation.[966,967] Potential initiators of integrin $\alpha_2\beta_1$ activation include signaling after GPVI interaction with collagen and GPIb-mediated adhesion to VWF, perhaps acting via actin polymerization.[959,968–970] Thus, one possible scenario is that following GPIb-mediated adhesion to VWF and collagen adhesion and activation mediated by GPVI, integrin $\alpha_2\beta_1$ may promote firm adhesion to collagen, stabilize thrombus growth on collagen, and promote procoagulant activity.[971,972] In addition, the affinity of integrin $\alpha_2\beta_1$ may also be modulated by alterations in disulfide bonds since inhibition of platelet PDI and sulfhydryl blocking agents inhibit integrin $\alpha_2\beta_1$-mediated platelet adhesion to type I collagen and to the related peptide GFOGER.[883,973] The state of the collagen may also influence whether integrin $\alpha_2\beta_1$ or GPVI mediates the interaction with collagen, because GPVI appears to mediate adhesion to fibrillar collagen, whereas integrin $\alpha_2\beta_1$ preferentially adheres to collagen that has been treated with partial protease digestion.[28,974]

Ligand binding to integrin $\alpha_2\beta_1$ is enhanced in the presence of magnesium or manganese and is inhibited by calcium, and thus the conditions in human blood, where calcium concentrations are higher than those of magnesium, do not provide optimal cation concentrations for the receptor's function.[975] Integrin $\alpha_2\beta_1$ can, however, mediate platelet adhesion to collagen in heparinized blood,[956,975] and inhibitors of integrin $\alpha_2\beta_1$ inhibit thrombus formation in animal models.[976–978] Regions of collagen type I have been implicated as potential binding sites for integrin $\alpha_2\beta_1$[979]; the peptide sequence 502 to 516 of collagen type I $\alpha_1$ chain, which contains a Gly-Glu-Arg (GER) sequence, may be of particular importance,[980] but other regions of the collagen molecule may also be important.[981] In type III collagen, amino acids 522 to 528 of fragment $\alpha_1$ (III) CB4 contain a binding region for $\alpha_2\beta_1$.[982]

Three different alleles for the integrin $\alpha_2$ gene, which differ at nucleotides 807 (T or C) and 1648 (G or A), have been described.[983] The 807 substitution does not affect the amino acid sequence, but the 1648 substitution causes a change from Glu to Lys, resulting in the Br$^b$ and Br$^a$ alloantigens (HPA-5a and HPA-5b). Allele 1 (T-G) is present in 39 percent of individuals, allele 2 (C-G) in 53 percent, and allele 3 (C-A) in 7 percent.[984,985] Individuals with allele 1 have higher integrin $\alpha_2\beta_1$ platelet density than individuals with allele 2, and individuals with allele 3 have the lowest density; the density of integrin $\alpha_2\beta_1$ correlates with platelet deposition on collagen under flow. The association of these polymorphisms with cardiovascular disease morbidity and mortality, including the risk of developing MI[986,987] and stroke,[988] has been extensively study without firm conclusions, although there is some suggestion that they may be associated with cardiovascular risk.[983,989-992]

Integrin $\alpha_2\beta_1$ is probably linked to the membrane skeleton.[993] Its ligand specificity appears to be determined by the cell on which it is expressed, since on endothelial cells it functions as a laminin receptor as well as a collagen receptor.[994,995] Engagement of integrin $\alpha_2\beta_1$ is capable of initiating platelet protein synthesis.[236] Integrin $\alpha_2\beta_1$ has been implicated in megakaryocyte development and platelet formation. In particular, loss of activated integrin $\alpha_2\beta_1$ receptors on the surface of megakaryocytes, as a result of interacting with collagen, has been implicated in the transition from the marrow to the peripheral circulation,[967] and conditional targeting of megakaryocyte and platelet integrin $\alpha_2\beta_1$ in mice is associated with reduced MPV.[996]

### Integrin $\alpha_5\beta_1$ (Also Termed GPIc*/IIa, Fibronectin Receptor, VLA-5, and CD49e/CD29)

Integrin $\alpha_5\beta_1$ is a receptor that is expressed on a wide variety of different cells and mediates adhesion to fibronectin.[804,819,820] It is important for interactions with extracellular matrix, and data from cells other than platelets indicate a role for this receptor in developmental biology and metastasis formation. The RGD sequence in fibronectin is crucial for cell adhesion, but other regions in fibronectin probably also contribute. RGD-containing peptides can inhibit cell adhesion mediated by integrin $\alpha_5\beta_1$. As with other integrin receptors, adhesion depends on the presence of divalent cations. Integrin $\alpha_5\beta_1$ is competent to mediate adhesion of resting platelets to fibronectin,[997,998] but its affinity may be modulated by activation.[999] The biologic role of this receptor on platelets is not clear. Although it may be involved in hemostasis and/or thrombosis, it is also possible that its function is primarily related to megakaryocyte binding to marrow matrix and proplatelet formation.[1000] Integrin $\alpha_5\beta_1$ is not the only fibronectin receptor on platelets, since with appropriate activation, integrin $\alpha_{IIb}\beta_3$ can also bind fibronectin.[804,1001]

### Integrin $\alpha_6\beta_1$ (Also Termed GPIc/IIa, Laminin Receptor, VLA-6, and CD49f/CD29)

Platelet adhesion to select laminins, which are variably found in basement membranes and extracellular matrix, can be mediated by integrin $\alpha_6\beta_1$.[804,1002-1004] Because VWF can bind to some laminins, GPIb can also contribute to platelet adhesion to laminin.[1002] This adhesion is best demonstrated with magnesium and manganese; calcium does not support adhesion. This receptor is competent on resting platelets, but its role in platelet physiology is not clear. Mice deficient in integrin $\alpha_6\beta_1$ do not bleed pathologically but are protected against thrombosis.[1002] The integrin appears to be able to signal in platelets via PI3 kinase to induce morphologic changes.[1005] An approximate Mr 67,000 laminin receptor has also been identified on platelets; this receptor is present on other cells as well.[1006]

### Integrin $\alpha_v\beta_3$ (Also Termed Vitronectin Receptor and CD51/CD61)

Integrin $\alpha_v\beta_3$ receptor shares the same $\beta$ subunit as integrin $\alpha_{IIb}\beta3$ (GPIIb/IIIa) (see Fig. 2–11).[804,855,1007-1009] The integrin $\alpha_v$ and $\alpha_{IIb}$ subunits display 36 percent sequence identity.[1010] Integrin $\alpha_v\beta_3$ differs dramatically, however, from integrin $\alpha_{IIb}\beta_3$ in its platelet surface density, because there are only approximately 50 to 100 integrin $\alpha_v\beta_3$ receptors per platelet.[1011] The crystal structure of the external domains of integrin $\alpha_v\beta_3$ alone and in complex with a peptide containing the RGD cell recognition sequence found in a number of ligands has been solved at high resolution.[844,845] Such RGD peptides inhibit ligand binding to integrin $\alpha_v\beta_3$. The most important findings were: (1) the receptor adopts

a bent conformation in which the globular headpiece composed of the N-terminal $\beta$-propeller region of $\alpha_v$ and the $\beta$A (I-like) domain of integrin $\beta_3$ lies near the legs of the integrin $\alpha_v$ and $\beta_3$ subunits, and (2) the RGD peptide binds to the headpiece with the Arg (R) making contact with integrin $\alpha_v$ and the Asp (D) making contact with the MIDAS domain in $\beta_3$. Current evidence suggests that the bent conformation is the inactive one and that activation results in extension of the headpiece and pivoting between the integrin $\beta_3$ $\beta$A and hybrid domains in association with leg separation.[827,843,1007,1009] Integrin $\alpha_v\beta_3$ can mediate adhesion to vitronectin, but only in the presence of magnesium or manganese, not calcium.[1011] It can also mediate interactions with fibrinogen, VWF, prothrombin, and thrombospondin.[389,1012-1015] Platelet stimulation can activate integrin $\alpha_v\beta_3$, analogous to activation of integrins $\alpha_{IIb}\beta_3$ and $\alpha_2\beta_1$. Activated integrin $\alpha_v\beta_3$ may uniquely mediate adhesion to osteopontin, a protein found in high concentrations in atherosclerotic plaque.[1016] The receptor's role in platelet physiology is not defined, but it may contribute to the development of platelet coagulant activity.[1017]

The integrin $\alpha_v\beta_3$ receptor is also present on endothelial cells,[822,1013] osteoclasts,[1018] smooth muscle cells, and other cells; it has been implicated in bone resorption,[1019-1021] endothelial–matrix interactions,[822,1013] lymphoid cell apoptosis,[1022] neovascularization,[1023] tumor angiogenesis,[1023-1025] intimal hyperplasia after vascular injury,[1026-1028] sickle cell disease,[1029-1031] focal segmental glomerulosclerosis,[1032,1033] and scleroderma.[1034]

The presence or absence of integrin $\alpha_v\beta_3$ on the platelets of patients with Glanzmann thrombasthenia can help localize the abnormality to either integrin $\alpha_{IIb}$ (if integrin $\alpha_v\beta_3$ is present in normal or increased amounts) or integrin $\beta_3$ (if integrin $\alpha_v\beta_3$ is reduced or absent) (Chap. 11).

## LEUCINE-RICH REPEAT GLYCOPROTEIN RECEPTORS

### GPIb/GPIX/V (CD42)

GPIb is composed of GPIb$\alpha$ (CD42b) (610 amino acids) disulfide-bonded to two GPIb$\beta$ subunits (CD42c) (122 amino acids).[801,1035-1043] GPIb appears to exist on the surface of platelets in a 1:1 complex with GPIX (160 amino acids) and a 2:1 complex with GPV (Fig. 2–13). The GPIb$\alpha$ gene is on the short arm of chromosome 17, and the GPIb$\beta$ gene is on the long arm of chromosome 22. The GPIX gene is on the long arm of chromosome 3.[1044-1046] GPIX is required for efficient surface expression of GPIb,[1047] but beyond that, its function is unknown. GPIb/IX is expressed on megakaryocytes and platelets; there is controversy as to whether GPIb/IX is expressed on endothelial cells, either constitutively or after cytokine activation.[802] The promoters for GPIb/IX lack TATA or CAAT boxes, but contain binding sites for the GATA and ETS families of transcription factors, which, along with the expression of the cofactor FOG (friend of GATA-1), may account for the limited expression of GPIb/IX.[1048-1056]

A genetic polymorphism in GPIb$\alpha$ affects the number of repeating 13-amino-acid units (1, 2, 3, or 4) and produces changes in the molecular weight of GPIb$\alpha$.[1057] The 2 repeat variant is most common, but there is considerable ethnic variation in the frequency of the different numbers of repeats. This molecular weight polymorphism has been linked to the Sib and Ko alloantigens, which have been localized to a T→M variation at amino acid 145 of GPIb$\alpha$, with M associated with either 3 or 4 repeats and T associated with either 1 or 2 repeats.[984] Some, but not all, reports suggest an association between the alleles with the larger number of repeats and vascular disease.[983,991,1058,1059] Two other GPIb$\alpha$ polymorphisms have been described: (1) C or T at position –5 from the ATG start codon (RS system), and (2) a nucleotide dimorphism at the third bases of the codon for Arg 358.[1038,1060,1061] A C at position –5 is present in only 8 to 17 percent of individuals and more closely resembles

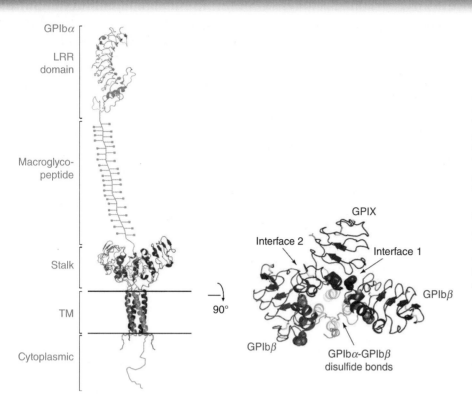

**Figure 2–13.** The organization of GPIb/IX complex. GPIbα *(green)*, GPIbβ *(blue)*, and GPIX *(purple)* subunits are colored differently. *Left:* A cartoon illustration of the GPIb/IX complex largely drawn in ribbon diagrams. Various parts of GPIbα are labeled on the left. *Right:* The top view of the membrane-proximal portion of GPIb/IX that contains the stalk region of GPIbα, the extracellular domains of GPIbβ and GPIX, and a portion of the transmembrane (TM) helical bundle. The disulfide bonds between GPIbα and GPIbβ are highlighted in *red*. Side chains of Tyr106 in GPIbβ are shown in *blue spheres*, one of which is located at the interface 1 between GPIbβ and GPIX. Residue Pro74 in GPIbβ is shown in *orange spheres*, one of which is located at or close to the interface 2. *(Reproduced with permission from Li R, Emsley J: The organizing principle of the platelet glycoprotein Ib-IX-V complex. J Thromb Haemost 2013 Apr; 11(4):605–614.)*

the sequence surrounding the ATG start codon (Kozak sequence) considered optimal for translation. In fact, this polymorphism is associated with higher levels of platelet surface GPIb and may be a risk factor for ischemic vascular disease.[1062–1070] GPIb has been implicated as a target antigen in autoimmune thrombocytopenia and in quinine and quinidine-induced thrombocytopenia (Chap. 7).

GPIbα has a large number of *O*-linked carbohydrate chains terminating in sialic acid residues,[1071] and the latter contribute significantly to the negative charge of the platelet membrane.[215] Electron micrographic analysis indicates that GPIb exists as a long flexible rod (approximately 60 nm) with two globular domains of approximately 9 and 16 nm.[1072] Thus, GPIb probably extends much further out from the platelet's surface than does integrin $\alpha_{IIb}\beta_3$, which may account for its primacy in platelet adhesion, as well as the increased risk of cardiovascular disease in individuals with longer GPIb molecules because of an increased number of 13-amino-acid repeats. The long extension may also make it susceptible to conformational changes induced by shear forces.[801] The extracellular region of GPIbα is readily cleaved by a variety of proteases, including platelet calpains,[1073] yielding a soluble fragment named *glycocalicin* that circulates in normal plasma at 1 to 3 mg/L.[1074] *In vivo*, platelet shedding of glycocalicin from GPIbα is mediated by a disintegrin and metalloprotease (ADAM)-17 (also termed TACE) cleaving a juxtamembrane sequence[1075,1076]; shedding is controlled by GPIbβ interactions with an unidentified protein, calpain, and reactive oxygen species.[1077–1079] Levels of plasma glycocalicin correlate with platelet production and thus can be used to differentiate thrombocytopenia based on decreased platelet production from thrombocytopenia as a result of increased platelet destruction.[1080–1085]

GPIbβ and GPIX have free sulfhydryl groups in their cytoplasmic domains that undergo palmitoylation, at least in part, further anchoring the protein to the membrane.[1086,1087] The penultimate serine residue at the C-terminus of GPIbα is phosphorylated, providing an attachment site for the signal-complex protein 14-3-3ζ.[1088] Similarly, GPIbβ can undergo phosphorylation of Ser 166 in its cytoplasmic domain as a result

of protein kinase A activation via cAMP, providing another binding site for 14-3-3ζ (see Fig. 2–13).[1089–1091] The cytoplasmic domain of GPIbα connects GPIb to filamin A (actin-binding protein), thus connecting GPIb to the platelet cytoskeleton.[993,1092,1093] Coordinated expression of GPIbα and filamin is required for efficient expression of both proteins, and imbalances result in abnormalities in platelet size.[1094,1095] Alterations in the cytoskeleton can affect GPIb functional activity.[1096–1098] 14-3-3ζ can bind PI3 kinase and has been implicated in GPIb-mediated intracellular signaling that results in integrin $\alpha_{IIb}\beta_3$ activation; Lyn, Vav, Rac1, Alet, and Lim kinase-1 also have been implicated in GPIb/IX–mediated signaling.[9,1099–1101] GPIb also appears to be in close proximity to FcγRIIA and the Fc receptor γ-chain, two receptors that can initiate signaling via tyrosine phosphorylation of their cytoplasmic ITAM sequences by Src family kinases and recruitment of the tyrosine kinase syk.[1102–1105] Engagement of GPIb by VWF may lead to clustering of GPIb-IX–V complexes in glycolipid-enriched microdomains or lipid rafts, which may serve to concentrate signaling molecules; clustering also increases ligand avidity.[1106]

GPIbα has eight leucine-rich repeats in the aminoterminal region of its extracellular domain, whereas GPIbβ and GPIX have one each.[1039,1042,1045] These repeats are consensus sequences of 24 amino acids with seven regularly spaced leucines; well-defined disulfide loop sequences flank the repeats.[801] Similar leucine-rich repeats are present in a variety of other proteins.

Crystal structures of the N-terminus of GPIbα (amino acid residue 1–305) alone and in complex with native and mutated A1 domains of VWF provide important information on the interactions between these proteins (Fig. 2–14).[1107,1108] This region of GPIbα adopts a curved shape made up of an N-terminal β-hairpin flanking sequence (finger) containing a C4-C17 disulfide loop (H1-D18), eight leucine-rich repeats (K19-W204), a β-switch region (V227-S241), and a C-terminal sulfated anionic region (D269-D287), with Y276, Y278, and Y279 undergoing posttranslation sulfation.[1108–1110] The VWF-A1 domain, which has alternating β strands and α helices organized into a central β-sheet

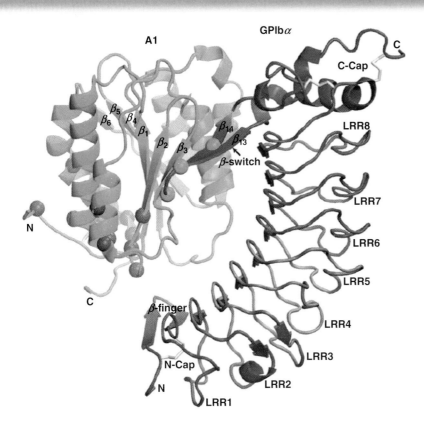

**Figure 2-14.** Structural, binding, and mutational features of the A1 domain (cyan) bound to GPIbα (magenta). Disulfides are in yellow stick. The A1-GPIbα complex forms a super β-sheet at the interface between the A1 β3 and GPIbα β14 strands. Platelet-type von Willebrand disease (VWD) mutations (green Cα atom spheres) stabilize the β-switch in its bound over its unbound conformation. VWD type 2B mutations (red Cα spheres) locate distal from the GPIbα interface, near to the A2 termini where elongational force is applied. VWD type 2B mutations are hypothesized to stabilize an alternative, high-affinity conformation. A region of GPIbα that is important for interaction with A1 in high shear (leucine-rich repeats [LRR] 3–5) and with ristocetin is shown in gray. *(Adapted with permission from Li R, Emsley J: The organizing principle of the platelet glycoprotein Ib-IX-V complex. J Thromb Haemost 2013 Apr; 11(4):605–614.)*

surrounded by amphiphatic α helices, interacts with the concave face of GPIbα with two areas of tight interactions, at the N-terminal β-hairpin + first leucine-rich repeat (with VWF A1 domain loops $α_1β_2$, $β_3α_2$, and $α_3β_4$), and a more extensive interaction at leucine-rich repeats 5 to 8 + the β switch region (with VWF A1 domain helix $α_3$, loop $α_3β_4$, and strand $β_3$). The structure of the VWF A1 domain when not bound to GPIbα differs from that of the bound VWF A1 in that the $α_1β_2$ loop protrudes in a way that would prevent interaction with GPIbα.[1108] This observation and others related to differences in the ability of different-sized fragments of VWF and GPIbα to interact indicate that other regions of both proteins probably contribute to both the binding and activation of the receptor. The crystal structure of GPIbα with the naturally occurring mutation M239V in the β-hairpin region that results in platelet-type (pseudo-) von Willebrand disease (Chap. 16) has also been obtained,[1109] and demonstrates a more stable β-hairpin conformation, which probably accounts for the approximately sixfold increase in binding affinity, primarily through an increase in the association rate. Leucine-rich repeats 3 to 5 do not demonstrate interaction with the normal VWF A domain in the crystal structure, but they are important in ristocetin-induced platelet agglutination and platelet adhesion at high shear; they do participate to some extent in crystal structures with gain-of-function mutations in VWF A1.[1107,1111,1112] It has been proposed that hydrodynamic forces produced at high shear alter the A1 domain and expose regions that interact with these repeats in GPIb.[1113] Other natural and site-directed mutations causing the platelet-type von Willebrand disease pattern of enhanced VWF binding (G233V, V234G, D235V, K237V) also affect the β-hairpin region. A number of Bernard-Soulier syndrome mutations that cause loss of VWF binding to GPIbα localize to the concave face of leucine-rich repeats 5, 6, and 7 (L129P, A156V, and L179del) and to the sides of leucine-rich repeat 2 (C65R and L57P).[1110]

The GPIb ectodomain crystal structure has been determined, confirming the four predicted conserved disulfide bonds (C1-C7, C5-C14, C68-C93, and C70-C116), along with the unpaired C122, which crosslinks to GPIbα.[1114] The two former disulfides are in the N-capping region, and the two latter are in the C-capping region flanking the single leucine-rich repeat.[1040] Using a chimeric GPIbβ/GPIX ectodomain protein, the likely contacts between GPIb and GPIX were identified. The structure proposed is a tetramer of one GPIbα, two GPIbβs, and one GPIX in which GPIX interacts with one of the GPIbβ molecules.[1037,1040,1043]

Plasma VWF will not bind to GPIb under static conditions unless the antibiotic ristocetin or the snake venom botrocetin is added. The mechanism by which ristocetin induces VWF binding to GPIb is unclear, but effects on VWF as well as on platelet surface charge have been described, and dimerization of ristocetin molecules and multimerization of VWF, as well as stabilization of an A1 domain conformation with high affinity for GPIb, have also been implicated.[801,1113,1115-1118] Botrocetin binds to VWF, exposing the site that binds to GPIb.[1119] Peptide studies implicate the anionic, sulfated tyrosine region of GPIb as the binding site for botrocetin-treated VWF.[801]

Unlike integrin $α_{IIb}β_3$, which requires intact, activated platelets to bind to VWF, GPIb-mediated VWF binding does not require platelet activation or even platelet metabolic integrity, because fixed platelets are readily agglutinated in the presence of VWF and either ristocetin or botrocetin.[1116] This observation forms the basis of the assay of plasma VWF activity.

Platelets will adhere to VWF when the latter is immobilized on a surface, even in the absence of ristocetin or botrocetin.[1116,1120-1122] Under these circumstances, the VWF is believed to undergo a conformational change that allows for direct interactions. It may not, however, be necessary to propose a change in VWF conformation as the interaction between VWF and GPIb appears to have both high association and dissociation rates, permitting tethering and translocation on a surface coated with a high density of VWF, but minimal interaction in fluid phase.[809] Similarly, VWF associated with fibrin can interact with platelet GPIb without ristocetin or botrocetin.[61,1123] The C1C2 domains of VWF appear to contain a fibrin binding site.[304]

Shear stress is an important factor in GPIb-mediated adhesion of platelets to immobilized VWF and subendothelial surfaces.[1042,1113,1120–1122,1124,1125] Platelets deficient in GPIb or platelets in which GPIb has been blocked with monoclonal antibodies[1122,1124] adhere poorly to subendothelial surfaces at all shear rates, but the defect in blood from patients with von Willebrand disease is manifest primarily at higher shear rates.[10,11,1122] In what may be a related phenomenon, subjecting platelets to high shear stresses can induce platelet aggregation, which is mediated by VWF binding to GPIb, followed by platelet activation and integrin $\alpha_{IIb}\beta_3$-dependent platelet aggregation.[13,15,1126] Whether the shear rates generated *in vivo* in stenotic blood vessels are of sufficient magnitude and duration to produce a similar degree of platelet activation is unknown. It is also uncertain as to whether the effect of shear is acting on GPIb, on VWF, or on both,[15,801,809,1042] but shear-induced changes in the structure of VWF, leading to a more extended conformation and conformational changes in the A1 domain, have been defined.[1113,1127] GPIb forms catch bonds with VWF, meaning that increasing force first prolongs and then shortens bond lifetimes.[1113,1128]

GPIb also functions as a platelet binding site for thrombin.[801,1129,1130] The regions between amino acids 216 and 240 and amino acids 269 and 287 were proposed as thrombin binding sites based on biochemical data, with the latter region demonstrating similarity to hirudin, a thrombin-binding protein.[801,1131] Sulfation of the three tyrosine residues in the latter region is particularly important for thrombin binding.[1093]

Two somewhat different crystal structures of the interactions between thrombin and the negatively charged tail region of GPIb have been reported, but in both cases two molecules of thrombin bind to each GPIb molecule using different regions on thrombin (exosites I and II). This raises the possibility that free thrombin or thrombin adherent to fibrin can cluster GPIb/IX/V complexes.[1132]

Binding of thrombin to platelet GPIb appears to contribute to thrombin-induced activation of platelets, even when PAR-1 and PAR-4 are desensitized, and platelets lacking GPIb (Bernard-Soulier syndrome) do, in fact, have blunted responses to thrombin. GPIb has been proposed as the high-affinity binding site for thrombin,[1129,1133] but there are only approximately 50 high-affinity thrombin-binding sites and approximately 25,000 GPIb molecules per platelet,[1129,1130] raising the possibility that only the subpopulation of GPIb molecules in lipid rafts are able to function in activating platelets.[1134] Binding of thrombin to GPIb may also facilitate its effect on one or more of the other thrombin receptors, and there is experimental support for this hypothesis.[1135,1136]

GPIb has also been demonstrated to interact with P-selectin in a cation-independent manner.[764,1035,1093] Although GPIb shares a number of features with the P-selectin ligand, PSGL-1 (both are sialomucins and have analogous anionic/sulfated tyrosine sequences), the interaction between GPIb and P-selectin appears to be more like the interaction between P-selectin and heparin.[1035,1093] In inflamed mesenteric venules in animals, platelets are observed to roll on the activated endothelium,[1137] and so it is possible that platelet GPIb interacts with endothelial P-selectin in this interaction.[1093] PSGL-1, a well-documented ligand for P-selectin on leukocytes, has also been identified on the surface of platelets,[1138] and so may also contribute to this interaction.

GPIbα also binds to high-molecular-weight kininogen and factor XII, and both of these interactions interfere with thrombin-induced platelet activation.[1139,1140] Factor XI also binds to GPIbα, where it undergoes activation by thrombin.[1141] Activated leukocyte integrin $\alpha_M\beta_2$ also can bind to GPIbα via the I-domain of the integrin,[1142] and this interaction has been proposed to play an important role in transmigration of leukocytes through platelet thrombi at sites of vascular injury. GPIb plays complex roles in inflammation and endotoxemia in murine models, demonstrating both proinflammatory and antiinflammatory effects.[1143,1144] GPIb has also been implicated in supporting metastases in murine models.[1145]

GPV, the third member of the GPIb/IX/V complex, has an Mr of 82,000 and is composed of 544 amino acids, including 15 leucine-rich repeats. GPV appears to form a noncovalent complex with GPIb, mediated through association of their transmembrane domains,[1146] but because the number of GPV molecules on the surface of platelets is approximately 50 percent of the number of GPIb and GPIX molecules,[1147] it has been suggested that the basic unit consists of two GPIb molecules, two GPIX molecules, and one GPV molecule.[801,1035,1038] GPV is deficient in platelets from patients with Bernard-Soulier syndrome (Chap. 11), but GPV is not required for surface expression of the GPIb/IX complex.[1148] A soluble fragment of Mr 69,000 is cleaved from GPV by thrombin, but cleavage does not correlate with thrombin-induced platelet activation.[1149] Platelets from mice lacking GPV appear to respond more actively to thrombin and ADP than wild-type mice, raising the possibility that GPV inhibits platelet activation.[1150] The platelets from these mice also adhere to immobilized VWF and can bind VWF in the presence of botrocetin, indicating that GPV is not required for the interaction between VWF and the GPIb/IX/V complex.[1150] It has been proposed that removing a portion of GPV by thrombin proteolysis allows thrombin access to GPIbα, thus facilitating its ability to activate platelets. In support of this model, thrombin's ability to activate platelets does not require proteolytic activity if GPV is absent, suggesting a direct nonproteolytic effect mediated via GPIbα.[1151]

# IMMUNOGLOBULIN FAMILY OF CELL-SURFACE ADHESION RECEPTORS AND THEIR ASSOCIATED MEMBRANE PROTEINS

## Platelet-Endothelial Cell Adhesion Molecule-1 (Also Termed CD31)

PECAM-1 is a transmembrane glycoprotein of the immunoglobulin gene family with six immunoglobulin-like domains of the C2 group and an Mr of 130,000.[1152–1155] In addition to platelets and endothelial cells, PECAM-1 is expressed on monocytes, myeloid cells, and some lymphocyte subsets. There are approximately 8000 PECAM-1 molecules on the surface of platelets.[1156] PECAM promotes homophilic interactions via a homophilic binding domain in the immunoglobin-like repeats. The cytoplasmic tail of PECAM is 118 amino acids in length and contains a palmitoylation site (C595), an immunoreceptor tyrosine-based inhibitory motif (ITIM) including Y663, an immunoreceptor tyrosine-based switch motif (ITSM) including Y686, and a lipid-interacting $\alpha$ helix that contains Y686 and S702, which undergoes inducible phosphorylation.[1152,1157] Upon phosphorylation, the ITIMs recruit and activate phosphatases, such as SHP-2 and to a lesser extent SHP-1, SHIP, and PP2A,[1158] via their SH2 domains.[1152] PECAM-1 undergoes homotypic interactions that lead to signaling and crosslinking.[1159] PECAM-1 activation overall thus induces inhibitory activity as the phosphatases counteract the effects of stimulating kinases but are complex and agonist specific. PECAM-1 activation decreases platelet responses to ADP and thrombin, and PECAM-1 platelet expression correlates inversely with platelet sensitivity to these agonists.[1160] PECAM-1 also negatively regulates collagen-induced platelet activation mediated by the ITAM-bearing GPVI/FcRγ-chain complex, GPIb/IX/V signaling, and laminin-induced activation.[1159] Platelets from mice lacking PECAM-1 are hyperresponsive to subthreshold doses of collagen and, when compared to those from wild-type mice, form larger platelet thrombi on VWF and in experimental settings *in vivo*.

Crosslinking PECAM-1 molecules on the platelet surface with antibodies enhances platelet adhesion and aggregate formation, suggesting that under certain circumstances PECAM-1 might be a costimulatory agonist, working in concert with platelet integrin $\alpha_{IIb}\beta_3$.[1161] Moreover, mice lacking PECAM-1 can undergo normal inside-out activation of integrin $\alpha_{IIb}\beta_3$ but have a partial defect in integrin $\alpha_{IIb}\beta_3$-mediated outside-in signaling.[1162] PECAM-1 crosslinking may also lead to GPIb internalization, resulting in decreased platelet adhesion.[1163]

In endothelial cells, PECAM-1 is localized to the contact areas between endothelial cells, in the lateral border recycling compartment, where it is involved in controlling stimulus-specific transmigration of leukocytes.[1155,1164] It appears to be capable of both homotypic and heterotypic interactions, with the latter mediated by CD177 on neutrophils (and perhaps glycosaminoglycans, integrin $\alpha_v\beta_3$, or CD38) interacting with the fifth or sixth PECAM-1 immunoglobulin domain.[1155,1165] PECAM-1 engagement triggers signaling and leukocyte integrin receptor activation that facilitates transmigration, with activation of the laminin receptor, integrin $\alpha_6\beta_1$, of particular importance. Endothelial PECAM-1 is also important in maintaining vascular integrity, and endothelial and leukocyte PECAM-1 mediate both proinflammatory and antiinflammatory phenomena in model systems.[1155]

### Triggering Receptors Expressed on Myeloid Cells–Like Transcript-1

Triggering receptors expressed on myeloid cells (TREM)–like transcript-1 (TLT-1) is a receptor whose external domain is homologous to those in the family termed TREM. Like those receptors, it contains a single V-set immunoglobulin domain, but its cytoplasmic domain is much longer, is palmitoylated, and carries a canonical ITIM capable of becoming phosphorylated and binding the Src homology-containing protein, tyrosine phosphate-1 (SHP-1).[627,1166] The phosphatase can then dephosphorylate signaling molecules, leading to inhibition of platelet activation. PECAM-1 has a similar ability to bind SHP-1. TLT appears to be restricted in expression to platelets and megakaryocytes. It is primarily in $\alpha$-granule membranes in resting platelets and joins the plasma membrane when platelets are activated.

### GPVI

GPVI is an Mr 62,000 transmembrane glycoprotein of 316 amino acids.[18,804,1167,1168] It belongs to the immunoglobulin superfamily and is the major platelet signaling receptor for collagen. It may also mediate platelet interactions with monocytes by binding the ligand EMMPRIN.[1169] GPVI on the platelet surface exists in a complex with Fc receptor (FcR) $\gamma$-chain. Because the latter is a dimer, two GPVI molecules associate with one FcR $\gamma$-chain, forming a high-affinity complex.[1168] The GPVI extracellular region contains two immunoglobulin C2-like domains, and its transmembrane domain contains an Arg residue that is essential for association with the FcR$\gamma$-chain. The 51-amino-acid cytoplasmic domain contains a proline-rich sequence that binds SH3 (Src homology 3) domains of Src family tyrosine kinases. GPVI signals through the FcR$\gamma$-chain, which contains an ITAM. An unpaired thiol in the cytoplasmic tail of GPVI can undergo oxidation, resulting in homodimer formation,[1170] required for high-affinity interactions with collagen peptides and GPVI-mediated signaling.[1171,1172] Resting platelets have approximately 29 percent of their GPVI molecules in dimers, and interactions with CRPs or thrombin activation increase the percentage of GPVI in dimers.[1171] When GPVI binds collagen, the ITAM domain of the FcR$\gamma$-chain becomes phosphorylated by the Src kinases Fyn and/or Lyn, resulting in the formation of large complex of signal-transducing proteins (for a discussion of the role of GPVI as a receptor for collagen, see "Signaling Pathways in Platelets" below).[1041,1104] GPVI is required for stable platelet thrombus formation on collagen surfaces *in vitro*.

Mice lacking GPVI have a relatively mild phenotype and are protected from thrombosis in some but not all experimental models. GPVI and FcR$\gamma$-chain appear to play important roles in ferric chloride-mediated arterial thrombosis in mice, but not in laser-induced thrombosis, perhaps because the former, but not the latter, injury elicits collagen exposure along the damaged vessel. Inherited and acquired defects in human platelet GPVI have been reported (Chap. 11), and the associated bleeding disorders have been variably described as mild to severe.[1172–1176] Two alternatively spliced forms and several polymorphisms have been identified for GPVI and variably linked to alterations in platelet function or risk of thrombotic disease.[1177,1178]

### Fc Receptor γ-Chain

The FcR$\gamma$-chain[1179] exists as a homodimer of Mr 20,000 that physically and functionally associates with GPVI[1180] and GPIb/IX.[1102] In mouse platelets, the absence of FcR$\gamma$-chain results in lack of surface expression of GPVI. The FcR$\gamma$-chain, along with Fc$\gamma$RIIA, are the only known platelet proteins with ITAMs.[1104] Phosphorylation of the ITAM domain serves to recruit proteins with Src homology 2 (SH2) domains, which are essential for collagen-mediated signaling through the GPVI/FcR$\gamma$-chain pathway.[1041,1104,1181] The FcR$\gamma$-chain may also contribute to GPIb/IX-mediated intracellular signaling after VWF binding.[1035,1102,1105]

### Fcγ Receptor IIA (FcγRIIA, Also Termed CD32)

The Fc$\gamma$RIIA is a low-affinity immunoglobulin receptor of Mr 40,000 that is widely distributed on hematopoietic cells.[804] Three different mRNA transcripts (A, B, and C) make similar Fc$\gamma$RIIA molecules,[1182] and these are preferentially expressed on different cells. Fc$\gamma$RIIA contains an ITAM domain and thus may be important for signaling by its associated proteins, including GPIb and select integrins, as well as through direct stimulation by immune complexes. Crosslinking of Fc$\gamma$RIIA initiates tyrosine phosphorylation, PI metabolism, activation of PLC$\gamma_2$, calcium signaling, and cytoskeletal rearrangements.[960,961] Fc$\gamma$RIIA appears to be in close proximity to the GPIb/IX/V complex in lipid rafts,[212] and signal transduction that accompanies VWF binding to GPIb may be mediated at least in part through Fc$\gamma$RIIA.[885,971] Fc$\gamma$RIIA is also important in mediating integrin $\alpha_{IIb}\beta_3$ outside-in signaling, including effects on platelet spreading, clot retraction, and thrombus formation.[1183,1184] Platelet 12(S)-lipoxygenase (LOX) is required for platelet activation mediated by Fc$\gamma$RIIA.[1185]

The Fc$\gamma$RIIA on platelets may bind immune complexes generated in certain diseases, and by engaging these complexes, the platelets may become sensitized to other stimuli.[1186–1188] It may also provide a second binding site for antibodies that bind to platelets via their antibody-binding site (see "CD9" below). This second interaction can potentially lead to bridging between platelets, with the antibody binding to an antigen on one platelet and an Fc$\gamma$RIIA receptor on another platelet.[1189] It is also possible that antibodies can bind to both an antigen and an Fc$\gamma$RIIA on a single platelet. These interactions can lead to platelet activation through engagement of Fc$\gamma$RIIA, followed by crosslinking of Fc$\gamma$RIIA receptors, which can lead to tyrosine phosphorylation, PI metabolism, activation of PLC$\gamma_2$, calcium signaling, and cytoskeletal rearrangements.[1190,1191] This type of interaction appears to play an important role in heparin-induced thrombocytopenia (Chap. 7). Fc$\gamma$RIIA undergoes proteolysis when platelets are activated, and Fc$\gamma$RIIA proteolysis has been proposed as an assay for heparin-induced thrombocytopenia.[1192,1193] Cooperation between Fc$\gamma$RIIA and C1q receptor has been reported.[1194] A variety of viruses and bacteria can interact with and activate platelets, and this is variably mediated by Fc$\gamma$RIIA, with or without immunoglobulin.[795,1195,1196] Fc$\gamma$RIIA may also contribute to cancer cell activation in platelets.[1197]

FcγRIIA expression on platelets shows considerable variation among individuals (approximately 600 to 1500 molecules per platelet), and this variation correlates with FcγRIIA-mediated function.[1188] This variation in receptor density may explain individual differences in immune-mediated disorders such as heparin-induced thrombocytopenia with thrombosis.[1198] An H131R polymorphism within FcγRIIA affects the binding of different IgG subclasses.[1199,1200] The H131R polymorphism may also have clinical significance because the R131 allele is associated with increased binding of activation-dependent antibodies to platelets.[1201] A variety of associations have been identified between the H131ER polymorphism and different aspects of heparin-induced thrombocytopenia and immune thrombocytopenia, but the data differ from study to study and no consensus has yet emerged.[1202–1207]

### Intercellular Adhesion Molecule-2 (CD102)

ICAM-2, a member of the immunoglobulin family of receptors, is an endothelial cell ligand for the $\beta_2$-integrin $\alpha_L\beta_2$ (LFA-1) on lymphocytes and myeloid cells.[1208] Approximately 2600 ICAM-2 molecules are present on platelets, distributed on the membrane surface and open canalicular system.[1208] Platelet ICAM-2 may contribute to platelet–leukocyte interactions (see "Platelet–Leukocyte Interactions" below).

### FcεRI

Platelets express the high-affinity IgE receptor FcεRI and appear to participate in both defense against parasitic diseases, including malaria, and allergic phenomena.[799,1209–1211]

### Junctional Adhesion Molecule-A (Also Termed F11)

JAM-A was identified on platelets by the ability of a monoclonal antibody directed against the receptor to initiate platelet activation via crosslinking to FcγRIIA.[1212–1216] It is phosphorylated during platelet activation, and loss of JAM-A in a mouse model results in a prothrombotic phenotype.[1217] JAM-A appears to inhibit outside-in signaling via integrin $\alpha_{IIb}\beta_3$ by recruiting Csk, which, in turn, phosphorylates Src at Y529.[1217,1218] It is also able to interact with the integrin $\alpha_L\beta_1$ receptor on leukocytes, and in endothelial cells, it participates in tight junction formation and leukocyte recruitment and transmigration.[920]

### Junctional Adhesion Molecule-C

The JAM-C transmembrane protein has an Mr of 43,000 and 279 amino acids. It contains two C2-type immunoglobulin domains in its extracellular domain and three potential tyrosine phosphorylation sites in its cytoplasmic domain.[767,920] JAM-C is expressed on platelets but not granulocytes, monocytes, lymphocytes, or erythrocytes. It shares 32 percent homology with JAM-A. Based on monoclonal antibody binding studies, platelets contain approximately 1600 copies of JAM-C. Platelet JAM-C acts as a counterreceptor for leukocyte integrins $\alpha_M\beta_2$ and $\alpha_X\beta_2$ and contributes to platelet–leukocyte interactions under some conditions.[767] Its precise role in platelet physiology is uncertain, but it has been implicated in binding CD34 stem cells.[1219]

## LECTIN-CONTAINING RECEPTORS

### P-Selectin (Also Termed GMP140, PADGEM, and CD62P)

P-selectin, which has an Mr of 140,000, is a glycoprotein present in α-granule membranes in resting platelets that joins the plasma membrane when platelets are activated.[759,1220–1222] Approximately 13,000 P-selectin molecules are detected by antibodies on the surface of activated platelets. The expression of P-selectin on circulating platelets has, therefore, been used as an indicator of their *in vivo* activation.[1223,1224] It is also present in the Weibel-Palade body membranes of endothelial cells; as in platelets, it joins the plasma membrane when endothelial cells are activated.[759,1222]

P-selectin has a modular structure in which the aminoterminal region has a calcium-dependent lectin domain that binds carbohydrates. Adjacent to the lectin domain is an EGF domain, followed by nine repeats that are homologous to complement regulatory proteins ("sushi" domains), a transmembrane domain, and a cytoplasmic domain.[759,1220] The cytoplasmic domain contains Ser, Thr, Tyr, and His residues that can be phosphorylated. In addition, a Cys residue becomes acylated with stearic or palmitic acid. Alternatively spliced forms of P-selectin may be produced in which sushi domains are omitted. The selectin family also includes E-selectin (ELAM-1; CD62E), which is expressed on the surface of activated endothelial cells, and L-selectin (LAM-1; CD62L), which is expressed on the surface of myeloid and lymphoid cells.[1225]

Soluble P-selectin is present in plasma from humans and mice. Alternative splicing generates a soluble form of human P-selectin that lacks the transmembrane domain.[1226] In mice, at least a portion of soluble P-selectin is derived from proteolytic cleavage of surface P-selectin by an unidentified protease.[1227]

Recognition of ligand by P-selectin requires specific carbohydrate and protein structures. Fucose and sialic acid are important carbohydrate components, with sialyl-3-fucosyl-N-acetyllactosamine (SLe$^x$; CD15S) a preferred ligand structure.[756,1228–1230] Myeloid and tumor cell sulfatides may also act as ligands for P-selectin.[1231,1232] PSGL-1, a mucin-like transmembrane glycoprotein homodimer (Mr 220,000) expressed on neutrophils, monocytes, lymphocytes, and to a small extent platelets, is an important ligand for P-selectin.[1138,1233–1235] Both sulfation of tyrosine residues contained in an anionic region and branched fucosylation of O-linked carbohydrates are required for optimal binding to P-selectin.

P-selectin can mediate the attachment of neutrophils and monocytes to platelets and endothelial cells. Thus, neutrophils and monocytes may be recruited to sites of vascular injury where platelets deposit and become activated (see "Platelet–Leukocyte Interactions" below). Platelet P-selectin can also recruit procoagulant monocyte-derived microparticles containing both PSGL-1 and tissue factor to growing thrombi *in vivo*.[1236] Binding of P-selectin to PSGL-1 on monocytes can trigger tissue factor synthesis,[1237] and infusing a P-selectin chimeric molecule into mice results in the generation of procoagulant microparticles.[781] In a reciprocal fashion, P-selectin engagement of PSGL-1 may lead to platelet activation.[1238] Soluble P-selectin may also promote a prothrombotic state in humans by increasing tissue factor–expressing microparticles in plasma. Indeed, the risk of future cardiovascular events is elevated in apparently healthy women with the highest levels of soluble P-selectin.[1239]

In intact blood vessels, the rapid on and off rates of the interactions between PSGL-1 on neutrophils and P-selectin on endothelial cells allow leukocytes to roll on the endothelium, the first step in leukocyte transmigration.[1240] The rapid upregulation of P-selectin after endothelial cell activation allows for a quick response. Platelets have been reported to roll on activated endothelium, and this appears to result from an interaction between endothelial P-selectin and perhaps either platelet GPIbα[1093,1137] or platelet PSGL-1.[1138,1241] Upon their corelease from endothelial Weibel-Palade bodies, P-selectin may tether ultralarge VWF to the surface of activated endothelium, and thereby promote platelet GPIbα-mediated platelet rolling.[1242]

Genetic and pharmacologic targeting of P-selectin or PSGL-1 in experimental animal models suggests that these receptors may modulate thrombolysis, sickle cell vasoocclusion, restenosis, deep venous thrombosis, cerebral ischemia and infarction, atherosclerosis, metastasis, and thrombotic glomerulonephritis (reviewed in Refs. 1243 to 1246).

### C-Type Lectin-Like Receptor-2

Podoplanin is a sialoglycoprotein present on a variety of tumor cells, lymphatic endothelial cells, kidney podocytes, lung epithelial cells, lymph node stromal cells, and the choroid plexus epithelium that can aggregate platelets.[1247–1250] Its receptor on platelets is CLEC-2, a C-type lectin-like receptor selectively expressed on megakaryocytes and platelets (approximately 2000 copies per platelet) that binds podoplanin and the snake venom platelet-activating protein rhodocytin.[1251–1253] The cytoplasmic tail of CLEC-2 contains an atypical ITAM (hemITAM) with a single YITL sequence that can be tyrosine phosphorylated by Src kinases when platelets are activated. Because CLEC-2 exists as a dimer, it can supply two ITAMs and lead to activation of Syk and, ultimately, $PLC\gamma_2$.[1254] This signaling system is similar to that of GPVI in combination with the $FcR\gamma$-chain. Activation of CLEC-2 leads to proteolytic cleavage of GPVI and $Fc\gamma$RIIa.[1255] In experimental tumor models, inhibiting the podoplanin/CLEC-2 system reduces metastases.[1256] CLEC-2 interaction with podoplanin on lymphatic endothelial cells, followed by platelet activation and CLEC-2-podoplanin clustering, is required for the separation of blood and lymph vessels during development.[1257–1259] CLEC-2 also plays a role in lymph node development and maintenance.[1260] HIV-1 can also bind to CLEC-2.

## TETRASPANINS

Tetraspanins are a family of four-transmembrane-domain-containing proteins that have conserved Cys residues that form crucial disulfide bonds. The extracellular and intracellular loops in these proteins contain many motifs that mediate interactions with other proteins.[1261] While the specific function(s) of tetraspanins is not yet clear, these proteins are able to associate with several membrane proteins and have been reported to modulate integrin function, perhaps in part by organizing membrane and intercellular signaling molecules in cholesterol-associated microdomains distinct from lipid rafts.[1262] CD9, CD63, and CD151 have juxtamembrane Cys residues that can be palmitoylated, and this modification may contribute to assembly of complexes with other proteins and localization to lipid microdomains.[1263] Studies in mice implicate CD151 and TSSC6 in outside-in signaling of integrin $\alpha_{IIb}\beta_3$.[1264] Oligomers of tetraspanins are known to facilitate the formation of larger complexes of membrane proteins that could serve as scaffolds for several platelet signaling events.[1265] CD9 is the most abundant platelet tetraspanin (approximately 40,000 molecules per platelet), followed by CD151, Tspan9, and CD63.[1266] The levels of TSSC6 are not known.

### CD9 (5H9; BA2; P24; GIG2; MIC3; MRP-1; BTCC-1; DRAP-27; TSPAN29)

CD9 is a 228-amino-acid tetraspanin that is present on platelets, endothelial cells, smooth muscle cells, cultured fibroblasts, some lymphoblasts, eosinophils, basophils, and other cells.[1267–1269] It colocalizes with integrin $\alpha_{IIb}\beta_3$ on the inner surface of $\alpha$ granules in resting platelets and on pseudopods of activated platelets.[1270] Binding of monoclonal antibodies specific for CD9 to platelets results in platelet aggregation by triggering phosphatidylinositol metabolism via a mechanism that also requires binding to the platelet $Fc\gamma$RIIA receptor.[1271–1273] The platelet activation induced by the binding of such antibodies requires external calcium and results in an association between CD9 and integrin $\alpha_{IIb}\beta_3$.[1274] CD9 has been proposed to play a role in microparticle release from platelets.[1275] Studies in mice lacking CD9 suggest that CD9 is a negative regulator of integrin $\alpha_{IIb}\beta_3$ signaling, as the mice have enhanced platelet aggregation, fibrinogen binding, and thrombus formation.[1276]

### CD63 (Also Termed Granulophysin and LAMP-3)

CD63 (Mr 53,000) appears to be present in both lysosomal and dense granule membranes in platelets.[310,1263,1277] CD63 is also present in Weibel-Palade bodies in endothelial cells, the lysosomal membranes of a variety of other cells, and the membranes of melanosomes. It appears on the surface membrane when platelets are activated, making it a useful marker for platelet activation.[310,1224] CD63 colocalizes with integrin $\alpha_{IIb}\beta_3$ and CD9 on the surface of activated platelets in a process that appears to require CD63 palmitoylation.[1263] CD63 is markedly reduced or absent from the dense bodies of patients with Hermansky-Pudlak syndrome,[1277] who have oculocutaneous albinism and a defect in platelet dense bodies (Chap. 11). The amino acid sequence of CD63 has been deduced from complementary DNA (cDNA) cloning.[1278]

### CD151 (Also Termed GP27, MER2, RAPH, SFA1, PETA-3, and TSPAN24)

CD151, a glycoprotein of Mr 27,000, is present on platelets, endothelial cells, and many other cells.[1279–1281] Antibodies to CD151, like those to CD9, can initiate platelet aggregation by binding to both CD151 and $Fc\gamma$RIIA.[1280] The role of CD151 in platelet physiology remains to be firmly established, but it may participate with $Fc\gamma$RIIA as a signal transduction complex.[1280] CD151 appears to functionally associate with integrin $\alpha_{IIb}\beta_3$, and in mice, loss of CD151 impairs platelet aggregation, clot retraction,[1282] and thrombus formation.[1283]

### TSSC6 (PHMX, PHEMX FLJ17158, FLJ97586, MGC22455, TSPAN32)

TSSC6 is a 340-amino-acid tetraspanin that is expressed in marrow, spleen, thymus, and several hematopoietic cell types.[898] It is present in platelets and has been reported to interact with integrin $\alpha_{IIb}\beta_3$. Mice deficient in TSSC6 display a slightly prolonged bleeding time and significantly increased rebleeding.[1265] Platelets lacking TSSC6 show impaired aggregation and clot retraction.

## GLYCOSYLPHOSPHATIDYLINOSITOL-ANCHORED PROTEINS (CD55, CD59, CD109, PRION PROTEIN)

At least five separate platelet proteins are attached to the membrane through a GPI link. These include proteins involved in complement regulation (CD55, decay accelerating factor, and CD59, membrane inhibitor of reactive lysis)[1284]; CD109, an Mr 170,000 protein present on platelets, endothelial cells, hematopoietic cells, and fibroblasts that carries both ABO oligosaccharides and an alloantigen (HPA-15, Gov) involved in neonatal isoimmune thrombocytopenia[1285,1286]; and an Mr 500,000 protein of unknown identity. Patients with paroxysmal nocturnal hemoglobinuria (PNH) have abnormalities in the GPI anchor and thus variably lack all of the GPI-linked proteins. The diagnosis of PNH can be established by assessing platelet expression of these proteins.[897,1287,1288] Patients with PNH have been reported to have platelet function abnormalities,[1287] raising the possibility that one or more of these proteins has a role in platelet function, but no specific platelet function roles have yet been assigned to the proteins. Of particular interest is the presence of the normal prion protein, which is an Mr 27,000 to 30,000 GPI-linked protein that is both upregulated and shed from the platelet surface with platelet activation.[1289–1292] In fact, platelets contain the majority of the prion protein present in normal blood.

## TYROSINE KINASE RECEPTORS

### Eph Kinases and Ephrin Ligands

Eph kinase receptors compose the largest family of cell-surface–associated tyrosine kinases with 14 members identified in mammals. Eph kinases have a conserved structure consisting of an N-terminal extracellular ephrin-binding domain, two fibronectin type II repeats, and intracellular kinase, sterile $\alpha$ motif (SAM), and PDZ binding domains [defined by the first three proteins to display this protein–protein domain, postsynaptic density protein (PSD95), *Drosophila* disk large tumor suppressor (Dlg1), and zonula occludens-1 protein (zo-1)]. A total of eight ephrins have been identified that serve as cell-surface ligands for the Eph kinases. In general, Eph A kinases recognize ephrins that contain a GPI anchor (ephrin A family), while Eph B kinases bind to ligands with a transmembrane domain (ephrin B family). The Eph receptors and the ephrins appear to signal bidirectionally at sites of cell-to-cell contact. Platelets contain Eph kinases EphA4 and EphB1, and their ligand ephrin B1, as well as EphB2.[276,1293] Messenger RNA for ephrinA3 has also been detected in platelets, but confirmation of the presence of ephrinA3 protein in platelets is lacking. Forced clustering of either Eph kinases or ephrins in platelets promotes cytoskeletal reorganization, adhesion, granule secretion, and Rap1b activation in concert with other platelet stimuli.[1293,1294] Eph kinase–ephrin interactions may stabilize platelet aggregates and thrombus formation after platelet–platelet contact has occurred.[276,1295]

### Thrombopoietin Receptor (c-mpl, CD110)

The thrombopoietin receptor (c-mpl; Mr 80,000 to 85,000) is expressed at low levels on platelets (approximately 25 to 224 per platelet) and binds thrombopoietin with high affinity ($K_D$ approximately 0.50 nM).[1296–1299] Steady-state plasma levels of thrombopoietin are maintained, in part, by platelets and megakaryocytes, which bind thrombopoietin via the thrombopoietin receptor and then internalize and degrade the growth factor. Additional mechanisms for regulation of thrombopoietin levels have been described (Chap. 1). Although its major function is to stimulate megakaryocyte growth and maturation (Chap. 1), thrombopoietin also is able to sensitize platelets to activation by agonists.[1300–1305] Mutations of the receptor have been associated with inherited thrombocytopenia (Chap. 7) and myeloproliferative neoplasms.[1306,1307] It can also contribute to hematopoiesis through effects on hematopoietic stem cells and other progenitors.

## SCAVENGER RECEPTORS

### CD36 (GPIV)

CD36 (GPIV) is an Mr 88,000 glycoprotein that is highly, but variably, expressed on platelets (approximately 20,000 copies per platelet).[1308–1313] The nucleotide sequence of CD36 (GPIV) cDNA encodes a protein of 471 residues with a predicted Mr of 53,000 and 10 potential N-linked glycosylation sites,[1314] accounting for the difference between predicted and experimentally determined Mr. It is unusual in having two putative transmembrane domains and two short cytoplasmic tails. The cytoplasmic regions may associate with intracellular tyrosine kinases of the Src family and undergo phosphorylation.[1315] Antibodies to CD36 (GPIV) have been reported to produce neonatal alloimmune thrombocytopenia (Chap. 7).[1316] Biochemical data suggest that it may form dimers and multimers.[1317] Increased platelet surface expression of CD36 (GPIV) has been described in patients with myeloproliferative neoplasms.[1318] CD36 (GPIV) is also expressed on phagocytic cells (with the exception of neutrophils), fat and muscle cells, cardiac myocytes, and microvascular endothelial cells. The phosphorylation status of the extracellular region of the protein may control its ligand-binding properties,[1319] offering a potential explanation for some of the variable results obtained under different conditions.[1308,1319,1320]

CD36 (GPIV) plays an important role in long-chain fatty acid transport in the heart, fat, and muscle, and may contribute to atherosclerosis and insulin sensitivity.[1321,1322] Oxidized low-density lipoproteins (LDL), which can be produced by the effects of endothelial cell or platelet nitric oxide (NO) on LDL, bind to CD36 and, perhaps in concert with scavenger receptor (SR)-A, can increase platelet reactivity to agonists via signal transduction mediated in part by Src kinases

and a MAPK.[1323–1325] The variability in platelet CD36 expression may account for the variability in platelet hyperreactivity in response to elevated levels of oxidized LDL.[1326] CD36 can also mediate microparticle binding to platelets, which augments platelet-mediated thrombosis in model systems.[1327] Thus, CD36 has been reported to contribute to atherogenesis, diabetes, the metabolic syndrome, angiogenesis, and inflammation.[1328–1331] CD36 also interacts with the S100 calcium-modulated protein family member myeloid-related protein (MRP)-14 (also known as S100A9), which can be released from activated neutrophils and platelets. It has been proposed as a platelet receptor for thrombospondin[1332] and collagen,[1333,1334] but the functional significance of these interactions remains unclear because individuals who lack CD36 on an inherited basis (Nak$^a$-negative) do not have a bleeding disorder[1335] (Chap. 11). CD36 may play a role in the thrombospondin-mediated interaction reported between platelets and sickle erythrocytes,[1336] apoptosis, innate immunity, and the binding of *Plasmodium falciparum*-infected erythrocytes to endothelial cells and monocytes.[1310,1314]

### Scavenger Receptor-BI (SCARB1; CLA-I)

The class B SR-BI (CLA-I) is related to CD36 and is expressed on platelets, endothelial cells, and hepatocytes.[1313] It transports the cholesteryl esters from high-density lipoprotein (HDL) cholesterol and facilitates bidirectional flux of free cholesterol between cells and lipoproteins. Oxidized, but not unoxidized, HDL can inhibit platelet aggregation via binding to SR-BI.[1337] SR-BI has many other lipid ligands, however, and it is uncertain how these interact under physiologic conditions. A number of mutations are associated with elevated HDL levels.[1338] A heterozygous missense mutation has been associated with increased platelet unesterified cholesterol and both increased and decreased platelet function.[1338] Mouse studies indicate that disrupting the SR in nonhematopoietic tissues can affect platelet function via alterations in plasma lipids and alterations in the platelet SR can protect against hyperactivity induced by increased platelet cholesterol content.[1326]

## MISCELLANEOUS

### CD40 Ligand (CD40L, CD154) and CD40

CD40 ligand (CD40L, CD154) is a trimeric transmembrane protein (Mr 33,000) of the tumor necrosis family that localizes to α granules in resting platelets and rapidly appears on the surface of platelets upon activation. Within minutes to hours of platelet activation, an Mr 18,000 fragment of CD40L is released from the platelet surface, perhaps mediated in part by matrix metalloproteinase (MMP-2) bound to integrin $\alpha_{IIb}\beta_3$.[1339] This soluble form of CD40L circulates as a trimer. The bulk of soluble CD40L in plasma is derived from activated platelets and, hence, can serve as a marker for platelet activation *in vivo*. Elevated levels of soluble CD40L are observed in acute coronary syndromes, after percutaneous coronary intervention, in the setting of coronary artery bypass surgery, and in peripheral vascular disease[1340] (reviewed in Refs. 1341 and 1342). Soluble CD40L activates neutrophil integrin $\alpha_M\beta_2$, enhances neutrophil adhesion, and induces the neutrophil oxidative burst.[1343] Moreover, elevated levels of soluble CD40L are associated with recurrent cardiovascular events in the setting of acute coronary syndromes[1340,1344] and restenosis following percutaneous coronary intervention.[1345] CD40L and, to a lesser extent, its counterreceptor CD40 have been implicated in the progression of atherosclerosis in animal models.[1346,1347]

The extracellular portion of CD40L binds to CD40, an Mr 48,000 transmembrane receptor. Approximately 600 to 1000 copies of CD40 are present on both resting and activated platelets,[1348] and although

CD40L has been reported to initiate platelet activation via binding to CD40,[1349] the functional significance of CD40–CD40L interactions in platelet physiology remains to be determined. CD40L also contains a KGD sequence (RGD in mice) that has been implicated in binding to integrin $\alpha_{IIb}\beta_3$. In mice, CD40L–$\alpha_{IIb}\beta_3$ interactions appear to stabilize thrombus growth,[1348] perhaps by activating receptor-mediated signaling.[1350] Additionally, integrin $\alpha_{IIb}\beta_3$ antagonists block the release of soluble CD40L from activated platelets. Both platelet-associated and soluble CD40L may stimulate leukocytes to release proinflammatory cytokines; CD40L may also inhibit endothelial cell migration after vascular injury.[1351] The inhibitory effects of CD40L on reendothelialization may partially explain why elevated levels of soluble CD40L are associated with higher rates of clinical restenosis.[1345] Finally, platelet CD40L may modulate adaptive immunity by serving as a costimulatory signal for antigen-presenting cells.[1352,1353]

### Fas Ligand, LIGHT, and TRAIL

Fas ligand (FasL), LIGHT (also termed TNF superfamily member 14), and TNF-related apoptosis-inducing ligand (TRAIL), along with CD40L, belong to the TNF family of cytokines.[1354] With activation, platelets express FasL, LIGHT, and TRAIL on their surface and release soluble forms of these receptors,[1354–1356] analogous to activation-dependent CD40L platelet expression and release. The receptor Fas (Apo-1, CD95) is expressed on a wide variety of normal and malignant cells. Engagement of Fas by FasL initiates signaling that results in apoptosis, and this process is important in embryonic development, cellular hemostasis, and immune regulation.[1354] The surface-expressed FasL on platelets is biologically active and can initiate apoptosis. The soluble form of FasL may act as an inhibitor of apoptosis induced by surface-expressed FasL.[1354] Similarly, platelet-derived LIGHT is biologically active and can initiate inflammatory responses in monocytes and endothelial cells.[1356]

### Lysosome-Associated Membrane Proteins 1 and 2 (CD107a, CD107b)

LAMP-1 and LAMP-2 are lysosome-associated membrane proteins that are approximately 30 percent homologous and constitute approximately 50 percent of lysosomal membrane proteins.[1357] They are integral membrane glycoproteins of Mr 110,000 and 120,000, respectively, that are contained within lysosomal membranes.[1358] When platelets undergo the release reaction, they join the plasma membrane. Each protein has two extracellular disulfide-bonded loops containing 36 to 38 amino acids. The loops are separated by a region rich in Pro and Ser that shares homology with the hinge region of IgA. There are multiple N-linked glycosylation sites on each glycoprotein, and they contain more than 60 percent carbohydrate. Among the carbohydrate residues are polylactosaminoglycans that may possess sialylated Lewis$^x$ structures, which are thought to interact with selectins. LAMP-1 and LAMP-2 play roles in control of lysosome fusion in autophagosomes and phagosomes.[1357]

### C1q Receptors

Platelets have several receptors for C1q, an Mr 460,000 glycoprotein composed of six globular domains attached to a short collagen-like triple helix.[1359–1361] One is for the collagen-like domain (cC1qR, Mr 60,000 to 67,000 nonreduced and 72,000 to 75,000 reduced), and another is for the globular domain (gC1qR, Mr 28,000 to 33,000).[1362,1363] A third receptor of Mr 126,000 enhances phagocytosis.[1364] C1q circulates with C1r and C1s as a calcium-dependent complex, but interaction with immune complexes leads ultimately to dissociation of the complex and release of free C1q, with its collagen-like domain exposed. cC1qR has sequence homology to calreticulin and can modulate platelet–collagen interactions at low collagen concentrations. It may also localize

immune complexes, and when crosslinked by aggregated C1q, it can initiate platelet activation, aggregation, secretion, and expression of platelet coagulant activity.[1365,1366] Thus, the binding of C1q monomers to platelets inhibits collagen-induced platelet aggregation but has little effect on platelet adhesion to collagen.[1367] C1q multimers support platelet adhesion and can induce aggregation via activation of integrin $\alpha_{IIb}\beta_3$.[1368] C1q can also augment platelet aggregation induced by aggregated IgG.[1194] The gC1qR may self-associate to form a doughnut-shaped ternary complex.[1369] In addition to binding C1q, this receptor can bind *S. aureus* protein A on endothelial cells, where it functions as a receptor for high-molecular-weight kininogen.[1363] It may, therefore, participate in contact activation.

### GMP-33 (Thrombospondin N-Terminal Fragment)

An Mr 33,000 $\alpha$-granule membrane protein was initially identified as an activation-dependent protein that joins the plasma membrane when platelets undergo the release reaction. Approximately 4000 antibody molecules directed against GMP-33 bind to resting platelets, and 19,000 bind to activated platelets.[1370] Subsequent studies identified this antigen as a membrane-associated fragment from the N-terminal of thrombospondin.[1371]

### Leukosialin, Sialophorin (CD43)

Leukosialin, a glycoprotein of Mr 90,000, may act as a ligand for ICAM-1.[1372] It is expressed on myeloid and some lymphoid cells. Abnormalities in leukosialin have been described in Wiskott-Aldrich syndrome (Chap. 11).

### Toll-Like Receptors 1, 2, 4, 6, 9

Toll-like receptors (TLRs) are involved in innate immunity by virtue of their ability to sense products of protozoa, fungi, viruses, and bacteria, including endotoxin (lipopolysaccharide [LPS]), and then activate intracellular signaling pathways to initiate the inflammatory response.[1373] TLRs 1, 2, 4, 6, and 9 have been identified in platelets.[1373,1374] Activation of TLR-1 and TLR-2 can lead to platelet activation via a GPVI-like mechanism with TLR-4 through the nuclear factor (NF)-$\kappa$B pathway.[1375] All of the components of the LPS signaling complex, including relatively high levels of TLR-4[1376] and CD14, MD2, and MyD88, have been identified in platelets. LPS binding to platelets stimulates secretion and potentiates agonist activation by signaling through the TLR-4 complex.[1377] LPS binding to platelet TLR-4 causes release of CD40L[1378] and modulates the release of cytokines by platelets.[1379,1380] In experimental animal models, TLR-4 may mediate LPS-induced microvascular thrombosis and thrombocytopenia.[1376,1381] TLR-4–null mice have prolonged times to vasoocclusion after vascular injury, but endothelial TLR-4 rather than platelet TLR-4 seems to be more important in supporting platelet thrombus formation.[1382] The interaction of LPS, produced by toxigenic *E. coli*, with platelet TLR-4 has been proposed to contribute to the pathophysiology of hemolytic uremic syndrome.[1378] Ligand binding to platelet TLR-4 also promotes platelet–neutrophil interactions, neutrophil activation, and along with TLR-2, the formation of NETs, which capture and sequester bacteria from the circulation.[792,1383] Activation of TLR-9 with protein adducts leads to Src-dependent platelet activation.[1374]

### Peroxisome Proliferator-Activated Receptors

Peroxisome proliferator-activated receptors (PPARs) belong to a nuclear hormone receptor family of ligand-activated transcription factors.[1384] PPAR$\gamma$ is one of the three PPAR family members and is widely expressed in white adipose tissue, macrophages, B and T lymphocytes, smooth muscle cells, fibroblasts, and endothelial cells. It has been implicated in metabolism, insulin responsiveness, adipocyte differentiation, immune function, and inflammation. The thiazolidinedione class of insulin-sensitizing drugs used to treat type 2 diabetic patients act by binding PPAR$\gamma$. Both PPAR$\beta$/$\delta$ and PPAR$\gamma$ are present in platelets. PPAR$\gamma$ agonists decrease thrombin-induced platelet aggregation and release of ATP, TX, and CD40L.[1384] Thus, PPAR$\gamma$ appears to downregulate platelet activation. Activated platelets release PPAR$\gamma$ complexed with the retinoid X receptor.[1385] Treatment with select thiazolidinediones has been associated with reductions in markers of platelet activation, including aggregation and P-selectin expression. PPAR$\beta$ ligands synergize with NO to inhibit platelet function.[1386,1387] The antiplatelet effects of the calcium channel blocker nifedipine may be mediated through PPAR receptors.[348]

### Matrix Metalloproteinases

Platelets contain a number of MMPs, as well as MMP activators and inhibitors.[1388,1389] MMP-1 can be activated by collagen and, in turn, cleave PAR-1 at a site two amino acids N-terminal to the site of thrombin cleavage.[1390] This cleavage, like thrombin's, activates PAR-1 by activating a tethered ligand. Thus, MMP-1 can augment collagen-induced platelet activation mediated by GPVI and integrin $\alpha_2\beta_1$. MMP-2 cleavage has been implicated in enhancing platelet aggregation via cleavage of talin and activation of integrin $\alpha_{IIb}\beta_3$.[1389] It exists in an inactive form in resting platelets and is cleaved into its active form when platelets are activated, probably by platelet-type von Willebrand disease (MT1-MMP).[1391] It then moves to the surface via binding to integrin $\alpha_{IIb}\beta_3$ and may then go on to cleave CD40 ligand.[1339] MMP-2 is released into the coronary circulation of patients with acute coronary syndromes.[1392] ADAM-17 (TACE) is important in the cleavage of GPIb and the release glycocalicin.[1076] MMP-9, which is increased in plasma in models of sepsis, can also cleave platelet CD40L.[1393] Other related proteins in platelets include MMP-9 and -14, ADAM-10, and tissue inhibitor of metalloproteinase (TIMP)-1, -2, and -3. Platelets also contain ADAMTS-13, which cleaves VWF, thus controlling hemostasis and thrombosis (Chap. 16).

## ⬤ SIGNALING PATHWAYS IN PLATELETS

### OVERVIEW

Platelets generally circulate in a quiescent state, but are poised to be activated in response to a variety of agonists that become available at sites of vascular injury or ruptured atherosclerotic plaques. Agonists differ in their intrinsic ability to produce these phenomena, and added complexity derives from differences in dose responses to each agonist and the synergistic effects of agonists used in combination. Agonists are diverse and include small and large soluble molecules, enzymes, and immobilized adhesive glycoproteins. They can be classified as either "strong" or "weak," depending on whether full activation, including the release reaction, can be initiated without the augmenting effect of platelet aggregation itself. Low doses of strong agonists behave like weak agonists. Most agonists are released, synthesized, or formed at the site of vascular injury, and this undoubtedly serves to localize the response.

Agonists bind to receptors of two general categories: seven-transmembrane G-protein–coupled receptors and receptors that can initiate phosphorylation of target proteins (Fig. 2–15). In both cases, a sequence of signaling events ultimately leads to platelet activation. Physiologic responses of platelets to agonists lead to the activation of the integrin $\alpha_{IIb}\beta_3$ receptor to a high-affinity ligand-binding state and subsequent platelet aggregation. Moreover, binding of ligands to platelets and platelet aggregation itself further propagate signals that are required for stabilization of the platelet aggregates and clot retraction. In this section, the major agonists, receptors, and signaling pathways involved in early stages of platelet activation that lead to shape change, granule secretion, and platelet aggregation, as well as postaggregation signaling events, are described.

## AGONIST-INDUCED PLATELET ACTIVATION

Many platelet agonists initiate platelet activation by binding to seven-transmembrane heterotrimeric G-protein–coupled receptors (see Fig. 2–15).[1394] When such receptors are activated, the G$\alpha$ subunit exchanges GDP for GTP and dissociates from the $\beta$/$\gamma$ complex. The free G$\alpha$ subunit and, in some cases, the $\beta$/$\gamma$ complex can activate some relatively common downstream pathways and initiate positive feedback loops. Activation of these pathways is usually intertwined. One common pathway involves the activation of one or more isozymes of PLC, leading to phosphoinositide hydrolysis. Three classes of PLC ($\beta$, $\gamma$, and $\delta$) have been described, and multiple isozymes exist within each class.[1395] The best-studied PLCs in platelets include PLC$\beta$ and PLC$\gamma_2$. PLC$\beta$ is often activated downstream of the seven-transmembrane, G-protein–coupled, receptor family, whereas PLC$\gamma_2$ can be activated by phosphorylation on tyrosine, which is a downstream signal from other types of agonist receptors. PLC of either type hydrolyzes phospholipids between the glycerol backbone and the phosphate moiety; the PLC$\beta$ class is relatively specific for phosphoinositides, whereas PLC$\gamma$ can cleave other types of phospholipids as well. The hydrolysis of one particular phosphoinositide, PI 4,5-bisphosphate (PIP$_2$), by either class of PLC is critical in platelet function, since it results in the formation of two important products, IP$_3$ and DAG. IP$_3$ binds to specific receptors on the DTS/sarcoplasmic reticulum, causing a release of intracellular Ca$^{2+}$. Increases in intracellular Ca$^{2+}$ are important for activation of a number of signaling enzymes and proteins involved in cytoskeletal reorganization. Increases in calcium are also important in granule fusion and the release reaction. DAG binds to PKC and participates in its conversion to an active enzyme. For many agonists, activation of one or more of the multiple isozymes of PKC is an obligatory step in the conversion of integrin $\alpha_{IIb}\beta_3$ to a high-affinity fibrinogen receptor and subsequent platelet aggregation.[918,1396,1397] One consequence of PKC activation is to cause the release of ADP from dense granules. Released ADP acts at its own seven-transmembrane G-protein–coupled receptor(s) to potentiate the action of numerous agonists. The precise mechanism(s) by which PKC causes integrin $\alpha_{IIb}\beta_3$ activation, however, remains unclear.

Activation of a number of receptors also leads to the activation of PLA$_2$, which releases arachidonic acid from membrane lipid stores. Arachidonic acid is rapidly converted to prostaglandin (PG) products, PGH$_2$ and TXA$_2$, which are themselves potent activators of platelet aggregation.

### Adenosine Diphosphate: P2Y$_1$, P2Y$_{12}$, P2X$_1$

Platelets express receptors for both ADP and ATP. Both nucleotides are present in platelet dense granules and are secreted when platelets are activated by adequate concentrations of most, if not all, agonists. Another source of these nucleotides is the red blood cell (RBC); damaged RBCs or those subjected to high shear stress may release ADP and ATP, increasing their local concentrations. ADP is an especially important physiologic agonist, not only because it can induce platelet aggregation independent of other agonists, but because secreted ADP contributes significantly to the full aggregation response induced by many other agonists. This has been convincingly demonstrated in experimental systems in which secreted ADP is rapidly degraded or inhibited. Moreover, submaximal concentrations of ADP synergize with other agonists, and this has been best studied with epinephrine. ADP induces or contributes to a variety of responses in platelets: shape change, granule release, TXA$_2$ production, activation of integrin $\alpha_{IIb}\beta_3$, and platelet aggregation.[1398,1399] Recent pharmacologic and cloning and sequencing studies suggest that ADP exerts its full effect on platelets through at least two different receptors. These receptors, P2Y$_1$ and P2Y$_{12}$, are G-protein–coupled and are responsible for most of the physiologic effects of ADP.[1400]

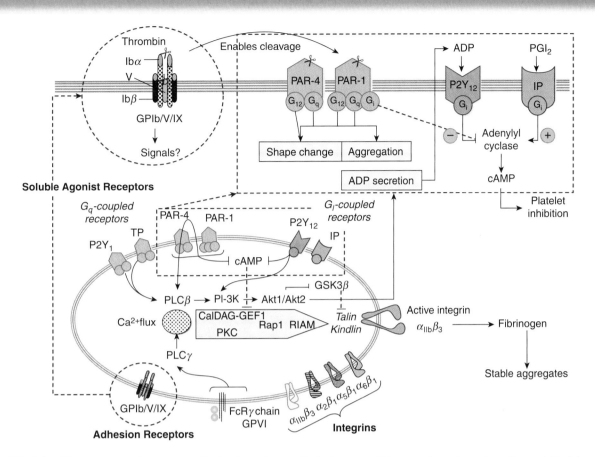

**Figure 2–15.** Role of G-protein–coupled receptors in platelet activation. Under basal conditions, prostacyclin produced by endothelial cells inhibits platelet activation by binding to its platelet receptor IP and increasing cyclic adenosine monophosphate (cAMP). When the endothelium is denuded, collagen interaction with GPVI can initiate signaling via the FcRγ-chain. In addition, the GPIb/V/IX complex can mediate adhesion of platelets to the newly exposed or deposited von Willebrand factor. This, in turn, can lead to platelet activation directly by a pathway not shown. GPIb/V/IX can also contribute to platelet activation by thrombin by facilitating the cleavage of protease-activated receptor (PAR)-1. Not shown is another pathway to PAR-1 cleavage and activation via collagen-induced release of matrix metalloproteinase (MMP)-1. In concert with PAR-4, cleaved PAR-1 initiates intracellular signaling pathways through molecular switches from the $G_q$, $G_{12}$, and $G_i$ protein families. This results in adenosine diphosphate (ADP) secretion and subsequent activation of both $P2Y_{12}$ and $P2Y_1$. A number of signals can also initiate the synthesis of thromboxane (TX) $A_2$, which can exit from the platelet and activate the same or other platelets by binding to its own receptor, TP. Ultimately, activation of phospholipase C (PLC) β and γ and released calcium ($Ca^{2+}$) initiate a series of steps that terminate in talin and kindlin binding to the cytoplasmic domain of $β_3$ and activation of the glycoprotein (GP) $α_{IIb}β_3$ receptor to its high-affinity ligand-binding state. CalDAG-GEF1, calcium and diacylglycerol-regulated guanine-nucleotide exchange factor 1; PKC, protein kinase C; RIAM, Rap1-guanosine triphosphate (GTP)-interacting adapter molecule. *(Reproduced with permission from Smyth SS, Woulfe DS, Weitz JI, et al: G-protein-coupled receptors as signaling targets for antiplatelet therapy,* Arterioscler Thromb Vasc Biol 2009 Apr; 29(4):449–457.)

The platelet $P2Y_{12}$ receptor, which is the target of the thienopyridine class of drugs (ticlopidine, clopidogrel, prasugrel, and ticagrelor) that are used in the treatment of acute coronary syndromes and peripheral vascular disease, as well as to prevent thrombosis following percutaneous vascular interventions, has been cloned and sequenced.[1401] It couples to Gαi[1402–1404] to inhibit adenylyl cyclases, a class of enzymes that produce cAMP, which, in turn, activates type A protein kinases that inhibit platelet activation by a variety of effects. VASP is phosphorylated in response to $P2Y_{12}$-mediated activation of protein kinase A, and so the extent of VASP phosphorylation in response to a combination of ADP and an agent that stimulates cAMP formation can be used as a marker for receptor blockade (see "Nitric Oxide" below). Decreases in cAMP level alone are likely insufficient to activate platelets,[1405,1406] and ADP activation of platelets requires synergistic effects between the signaling pathways of the $P2Y_1$ and $P2Y_{12}$ receptors (and perhaps the $P2X_1$ ATP receptor.) Regulation of $P2Y_{12}$ is complex and involves homologous desensitization, internalization, and recycling.[1407] Studies of $P2Y_{12}$ knockout mice demonstrate that $P2Y_{12}$ contributes to multiple steps during thrombosis, including platelet adhesion and activation, thrombus growth, and thrombus stability.[1408] Platelets obtained from $P2Y_{12}$-deficient mice respond only weakly to ADP and less vigorously than normal to other agonists such as collagen and thrombin.[1409] A minor $P2Y_{12}$ haplotype (H2) has been associated with enhanced ADP-induced platelet aggregation, as well as resistance to the antiplatelet effects of clopidogrel.[1410,1411]

The platelet $P2Y_1$ receptor, the other G-protein–coupled ADP receptor on platelets, has been cloned and sequenced, and a high-resolution crystal structure demonstrating two disparate ligand binding sites is available.[1412] Data from experiments with inhibitors of $P2Y_1$ and mice lacking $P2Y_1$ suggest that stimulation of this receptor is necessary, but not sufficient, to induce platelet aggregation. Thus, platelets from $P2Y_1$-null mice are unable to change shape or aggregate in response to ADP; however, ADP activation does cause a decrease in cAMP via its effects on $P2Y_{12}$.[1413,1414] $P2Y_1$ couples to heterotrimeric G-proteins containing Gαq. The importance of Gαq can be inferred from the observation that platelets from mice that do not express Gαq do not aggregate in response to ADP and that patients with abnormalities in Gαq have a bleeding disorder and abnormal platelet function (Chap. 11).[1415] Activation of PLCβ and subsequent phosphoinositide hydrolysis have been linked to both shape change and platelet activation.

P2X$_1$, the third purine nucleotide receptor on platelets, is a member of the P2X family of ligand-gated ion channels rather than a G-protein–coupled receptor.[1416] This receptor is predicted to span the plasma membrane twice and is largely extracellular.[1417] While P2X$_1$ has been described as both an ATP and an ADP receptor, the bulk of current evidence suggests that it is an ATP receptor that is antagonized by ADP.[1418,1419] Because ATP antagonizes the P2Y$_{12}$ receptor, the overall contribution of P2X$_1$, which is stimulated by ATP, to platelet activation, is not clear. Nonetheless, ATP is released from platelets upon stimulation with agonists such as collagen,[1420] and ATP binding to P2X$_1$ causes a rapid Ca$^{2+}$ influx.[1421] However, Ca$^{2+}$ influx induced by stimulation of this receptor alone appears to be insufficient to induce platelet shape change or aggregation.[1405] It does, however, synergize with the P2Y platelet ADP receptors.[1421] This synergy is likely caused by the specific downstream signaling events evoked by ATP stimulation of this receptor, which include Ca$^{2+}$ influx and MAPK activation.[1420] Support for a biologically important role for this receptor comes from data in both mice with targeted deletions of P2X$_1$, which have impaired *in vivo* thrombus formation,[1422] and mice that overexpress P2X$_1$, which have a prothrombotic phenotype.[1423] A variant of P2X$_1$, P(2X1del), which lacks 17 amino acids, has been described in megakaryocyte-like cell lines,[1424] but its functional role is uncertain.[1418,1419]

Several antiplatelet agents inhibit ADP-induced platelet activation. Thus, metabolites of ticlopidine, clopidogrel, and prasugrel inhibit the P2Y$_{12}$ receptor[1425] (Chap. 24), whereas soluble CD39 catabolizes ADP and ATP.[1426]

### Epinephrine: α2A Adrenergic Receptors

When added to platelet-rich plasma, epinephrine uniquely initiates a first phase of aggregation without first inducing shape change; after a plateau period, a second wave of aggregation occurs. The ability of epinephrine to synergize with other agonists, such as ADP, is well documented, but there is controversy as to whether epinephrine, in the absence of released ADP or TXA$_2$, is sufficient to initiate platelet aggregation.[1427-1429] Epinephrine can cause an elevation in intracellular Ca$^{2+}$, even in aspirin-treated platelets,[1427] possibly by opening an external channel or causing release of calcium from membrane sources[1428,1429]; it does not appear to mobilize intracellular Ca$^{2+}$ or generate measurable amounts of IP$_3$. Analysis of the purified epinephrine receptor and its nucleotide sequence identified it as a seven-transmembrane, G-protein–coupled, α2A adrenergic receptor of Mr 64,000.[1430,1431] It couples to Gαi family members, primarily Gαz, to inhibit adenylyl cyclase and thus prevent formation of cAMP.[1432] The reduction in cAMP caused by epinephrine is probably not sufficient, however, to initiate platelet aggregation, and it is likely that other effectors are required for platelet activation.[1433-1436] Platelets from a patient with a chronic bleeding disorder contained reduced amounts of Gαi1 and displayed impaired epinephrine-induced aggregation, suggesting that Gαi1 may also contribute to epinephrine-mediated responses.[1437] Polymorphisms of the α2A adrenergic receptor have been associated with enhanced platelet reactivity and signaling.[1438,1439]

The physiologic and pathologic significance of epinephrine-induced platelet activation remains unclear, but there is a possibility that sympathetic stimulation may contribute to enhanced platelet activation.[1440] In particular, in animal models, infusion of epinephrine can enhance platelet thrombus formation and can overcome the inhibition produced by aspirin.[1441,1442] Increased sympathetic tone may thus account for the resistance to antiplatelet agents during acute coronary syndromes.[1443]

### Thromboxane A$_2$ and Other Arachidonic Acid Metabolites: Thromboxane Prostanoid Receptor

The metabolism of arachidonic acid (AA) to TXA$_2$ is a fundamental pathway contributing to agonist-induced platelet activation and aggregation. Many agonists stimulate the release of AA from phosphatidylcholine (PC) and PE in the plasma membrane.[1444] Most AA is released by the action of PLA$_2$, but some is also released by the concerted actions of PLC and DAG kinase, followed by PLA$_2$, and perhaps by the action of PLC followed by the action of DAG lipase. PLA$_2$ is a cytosolic enzyme, with multiple isoforms in platelets.[1445] PLA$_2$ acts on the C2 position of triacylglycerols such as PC and PE to form free AA and the resulting lysophospholipid. PLA$_2$ also converts phosphatidic acid into lysophosphatidic acid, which is also a platelet agonist. Some PLA$_2$ isozymes are activated by the rise in intracellular platelet Ca$^{2+}$ that occurs during agonist-stimulated activation, whereas other isozymes are activated in a Ca$^{2+}$-independent manner. Studies in mice[1446] and in a patient with recurrent small intestinal ulcers and platelet dysfunction[1447] have identified cytosolic PLA$_2\alpha$ as the principal PL responsible for the liberation of the AA that is essential for eicosanoid biosynthesis in platelets. Ligand binding to integrin α$_{IIb}\beta_3$ activates cytosolic PLA$_2\alpha$, perhaps through one or more intermediary proteins.[1448]

AA is subsequently metabolized by cyclooxygenase (COX) to generate PGs and TX and by LOX to generate leukotrienes (LTs) and hydroxyeicosatetraenoic acids (HPETEs). The main COX in platelets, COX-1, metabolizes AA to PGG$_2$, which is subsequently converted to PGH$_2$.[1449,1450] TX synthase next converts PGH$_2$ to TXA$_2$, which is spontaneously and rapidly converted to the inactive metabolite, TXB$_2$.[1451] TXA$_2$ and its precursor, PGH$_2$, can both stimulate platelet TX receptors to induce platelet aggregation.[1451-1453] An inducible COX (COX-2) is present in many cells involved in mediating the inflammatory response and megakaryocytes, but only trace amounts are present in normal platelets.[1454,1455] COX inhibitors such as aspirin inhibit platelet function by inhibiting COX-1 and decreasing TXA$_2$ production.[1451] It has been hypothesized that some patients whose platelets are resistant to aspirin inhibition may have increased amounts of COX-2, which is not as readily inhibited by aspirin as COX-1.[1452] Selective COX-2 inhibitor drugs are associated with increased risk of thrombosis, and this is ascribed to their inhibition of endothelial cell prostacyclin production without the compensatory inhibition of TXA production via COX-1.[1456]

TXA$_2$ is a potent platelet agonist that exerts its effects via interaction with specific members of the thromboxane prostanoid receptor (TP) family of G-protein–coupled receptors. There are two TP isoforms in human platelets (TPα and TPβ), which arise from alternative splicing of exon 3 of the TP gene; TPβ, but not TPα, undergoes agonist-induced internalization.[1457] Although both TPα and TPβ mRNA can be detected in platelet lysates, it appears that TPα is the dominant form.[1458] The TXA$_2$ receptor has been localized to the platelet plasma membrane, and on sodium dodecylsulfate (SDS)-polyacrylamide gel electrophoresis, it migrates as a broad band of Mr 55,000 to 57,000,[1459,1460] the range a result of variability in glycosylation.[1458] Pharmacologic studies suggest the existence of two distinct TXA$_2$ receptor subtypes based on differing affinities for agonist ligands. The low-affinity binding sites may mediate platelet aggregation and granule secretion, whereas the high-affinity sites seem to be associated with platelet shape change.[1461] Studies of TP-deficient mice demonstrate that this gene locus is responsible for most, if not all, the biologic effects attributed to TXA$_2$.[1462] Bleeding times in these mice are prolonged, confirming the importance of this pathway in normal hemostasis. Platelet aggregation to collagen, but not ADP, is delayed, demonstrating the importance of TXA$_2$ production to the collagen response in platelets. TXA$_2$ pathways activate Gαq,[1415,1463] Gα12 and Gα13,[1464,1465] Gα11,[1466] and Gαi2.[1467,1468] Activation of Gαq is essential for aggregation and secretion, whereas the Gα12/13 pathways contribute to shape change and aggregation.[1469-1471] It is unclear whether TP directly couples to GαI[1472] or activates this pathway indirectly via released ADP.[1467,1470] A significant portion of PGH$_2$/TXA$_2$-induced platelet aggregation is actually mediated by secreted ADP, because ADP scavenger systems inhibit aggregation induced by a stable PGH$_2$/TXA$_2$ analogue either partially (30 percent)[1473] or totally.[1472]

AA can also be converted to LTs and lipoxins by the sequential actions of LOX and other enzymes. Platelets from most animal species lack 5-LOX, but possess 12-LOX. Consequently, AA liberated by cytosolic PLA$_2$α can be oxygenated by 12-LOX to generate 12-HPETE, an unstable intermediate that is reduced by glutathione peroxidase or other mechanisms to generate HETE. The generation of 12-HPETE in platelets is slower and more sustained than the generation of TXA.[1474] Platelets from mice deficient in the platelet-type 12-LOX are hypersensitive to stimulation by ADP, suggesting an inhibitory role for this pathway in platelet activation by ADP.[1475] 12-LOX activity in platelets can be regulated by signaling through the GPVI collagen receptor.[1476] Because they lack 5-LOX, platelets do not generate LTB$_4$, nor do they appear to possess LTB$_4$ receptors.[1477] However, they participate in LT and lipoxin (LX) generation through transcellular metabolism involving leukocytes. Leukocyte metabolism of AA, some of which may be derived from platelets, by 5-LOX generates LTA$_4$, which is then released and can be transformed by glutathione-S-transferase in platelets to LTC$_4$.[1478] The generation of LTC$_4$ by platelets requires P-selectin–mediated adhesion to leukocytes.[1479] Leukocyte-derived LTA$_4$ can also be converted by platelets to the antiinflammatory metabolite LXA$_4$ by the actions of 12-LOX in platelets.[1480]

### Thrombin

Thrombin is derived from the inactive zymogen, prothrombin, which circulates in plasma. When acted upon by the prothrombinase complex (FXa, FVa, Ca$^{2+}$) assembled on the membrane of activated platelets and other cells, prothrombin is cleaved into thrombin[1481] (Chap. 3), one of the most potent platelet agonists. The proteolytic activity of thrombin is required for its role as a platelet agonist.[1482] Thrombin activates PAR-1, a seven-transmembrane G-protein–coupled receptor on platelets and other cells,[514,1483,1484] by cleaving an extracellular 41-amino-acid peptide from the N-terminus of the receptor (Fig. 2–16). Removal of this peptide results in a new aminoterminus, which acts as a "tethered ligand," by binding to another region of PAR-1 to activate the receptor and initiate signal transduction. Short peptides modeled after the "tethered ligand" region (e.g., SFLLRN) also activate PAR-1 signaling. The 41-amino-acid cleavage product of PAR-1 can also induce platelet aggregation by a poorly defined mechanism.[1485] PAR-1 can also be cleaved to an active form by MMP-1 when platelets are stimulated with collagen, but the cleavage site is two amino acids N-terminal to the thrombin cleavage.[1390] A crystal structure of PAR-1 bound to vorapaxar, a small-molecule antagonist recently approved for secondary prophylaxis of cardiovascular disease,[1486] has been solved and provides insights into PAR-1 activation by the SFLLRN-tethered ligand.[1487]

Cloning of PAR-1 and gene deletion experiments in mice led to the discovery of additional members of the PAR family[1483,1488,1489]: PAR-1 and PAR-4 are the main thrombin signaling receptors on human platelets; PAR-3 and PAR-4 mediate thrombin activation on mouse platelets; and PAR-2 is a receptor for trypsin and other proteases. Short endogenous peptide sequences that function as selective agonists have been identified for PAR-1 (SFLLR), PAR-2 (SLIGK), and PAR-4 (GYPGQV). On human platelets, a full response to thrombin requires both PAR-1 and PAR-4.[1489,1490] The receptors display distinct kinetics of activation and desensitization; PAR-1 mediates a substantial portion of thrombin signaling, but PAR-4 contributes at high doses of thrombin.[1490-1493] PAR-3 and PAR-4 serve as thrombin receptors on murine platelets,[1488] where PAR-4 is the primary signaling molecule[1494] and PAR-3 functions as a

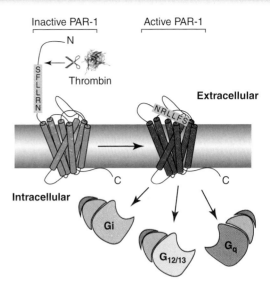

**Figure 2–16.** Protease-activated receptor (PAR)-1 activation by thrombin. Thrombin cleaves PAR-1 N-terminus and exposes a new N-terminal peptide SFLLRN, which can bind to and activate the transmembrane core of PAR-1. PAR-1 can activate several G proteins, including G$_i$, G$_{12/13}$, and G$_q$. *(Reproduced with permission from Zhang C, Srinivasan Y, Arlow DH, et al: High-resolution crystal structure of human protease-activated receptor 1, Nature 2012 Dec 20;492(7429):387–392.)*

cofactor for the cleavage and activation of PAR-4 by thrombin.[1495] Deficiency of either PAR-4 or PAR-3 results in a bleeding defect and protection from experimental thrombosis in mice.[1494,1496]

When platelets are exposed to a subaggregating concentration of thrombin, they become relatively insensitive to subsequent stimulation with an aggregating concentration of thrombin, a process termed homologous desensitization. This involves rapid receptor internalization and alterations in the thrombin receptor signaling systems.[1497] Trafficking of the thrombin receptor to lysosomes is dictated by the amino acid sequence in the cytoplasmic tail of PAR-1 and requires phosphorylation.[1498] In comparison with PAR-1, activation-dependent internalization of PAR-4 occurs to a lesser extent, and termination of PAR-4 signaling occurs more slowly,[1493] resulting in distinct patterns of signaling through each receptor.

PAR-1 activation can be either proinflammatory or antiinflammatory, depending on the dose of thrombin. PAR-1 activation in nonhematopoietic cells contributes to the innate immune response to viral infection with influenza A and coxsackievirus B3 in animal models,[1499] but in other models, PAR-1 activation enhances influenza A pathogenicity in response to severe infection and PAR-1 deficiency offers protection.[1500] Thus, the relative roles of platelet PAR-1 and tissue-specific PAR-1 in viral infections are complex.[1501]

Thrombin can bind to GPIbα, and platelets from patients lacking the GPIb/IX complex (Bernard-Soulier syndrome) have decreased thrombin-induced platelet aggregation (Chap. 11). A region on GPIbα with three sulfated tyrosines and a large number of anionic amino acids, with homology to the high-affinity thrombin inhibitor hirudin, contains the thrombin binding site.[1132,1502] Tertiary structures of the extracellular, aminoterminal domain of GPIbα bound to thrombin indicate that two thrombin molecules interact with each GPIbα.[1503,1504] This bivalent interaction may allow thrombin to serve as a bridge linking GPIbα receptors on the same or adjacent platelets.[1132,1502] Binding of thrombin to GPIb may also enhance activation via PAR-1. Thrombin can activate platelets via interaction with GPIb even when both PAR-1 and PAR-4 have been desensitized, and there may be a still unidentified mechanism by which thrombin activates platelets independent of PAR-1, PAR-4, and GPIb.[1505]

### Tachykinins: Substance P and Endokinins A and B

The tachykinin neurotransmitter substance P induces platelet aggregation and the release reaction at micromolar concentrations and enhances aggregation induced by other agonists at lower concentrations.[1506] Platelets express two seven-transmembrane G-coupled receptors for substance P ($NK_1$ and $NK_2$), and $NK_1$ has been implicated in mediating the response to substance P.[1507] In addition, an amidated peptide from the C-terminus of the related tachykinins, endokinins A and B (GKASQFFGLM-NH$_2$), initiates platelet aggregation. Substance P has also been identified in platelets, and platelets secrete substance P when activated.

### Chemokines: Chemokine Receptors CCR1, CCR3, CCR4, CXCR1, CXCR4

Based on monoclonal antibody binding and/or mRNA expression studies, platelets and/or megakaryocytes have been reported to express the seven-transmembrane G-protein–coupled chemokine receptors CCR1, CCR3, CCR4, CXCR1, and CXCR4 (reviewed in Refs. 762 and 1508). These receptors may play a role in megakaryopoiesis and platelet production. In addition, a number of chemokines, in particular PF4 (CXCL4), CXCL12, CCL13, and CCL22, have been variably found to be able to either augment platelet activation and aggregation induced by other agonists or actually fully initiate platelet adhesion, activation, and aggregation. Because high concentrations of the chemokines relative to plasma concentrations are required to demonstrate these effects, it is unclear what role these receptors play in platelet physiology, but it is possible that local chemokine levels are higher in areas of inflammation.

### Lipid Mediators (Platelet-Activating Factor, Lysophosphatidic Acid, and Sphingosine-1-Phosphate)

PAF (a mixture of 1-$O$-hexadecyl-2-acetyl-sn-glycero-3-phosphocholine and 1-$O$-octadecyl-2-acetyl-sn-glycero-3-phosphocholine[1509]) is a phospholipid ether produced by platelets, leukocytes, and other cells. PAF is a potent platelet agonist and mediator of inflammation. Cellular responses to PAF are mediated by a specific seven-transmembrane G-protein–coupled receptor.[1510,1511] PAF induces G-protein–dependent inhibition of adenylyl cyclase and activation of PLC,[1512] which cause phosphoinositide turnover, leading to the activation of PKC and an increase in intracellular $Ca^{2+}$.[1511] PAF also indirectly activates $PLA_2$, which causes release of AA from the platelet membrane.[1513] All of these effects contribute to the overall platelet response to PAF. PAF is catabolized by PAF acetylhydrolase, and this enzyme may play an important role in inflammation and atherosclerosis.[1514]

LDLs activate human platelets, and oxidized LDLs are more potent platelet activators. One active component in oxidized LDLs is oxidized phosphatidylcholine ($oxPC_{36}$), which increases with diet-induced hyperlipidemia. $oxPC_{36}$ signals through CD36[1325] via phosphorylation of the MAPKs p38 and c-Jun N-terminal kinase.[1323] Platelet activation by oxidized LDLs in the absence of hyperlipidemia may also require SR A.[1324] Increases in levels of $oxPC_{36}$ with hyperlipidemia may provide an explanation for observations that atherogenic mice have a prothrombotic phenotype as indicated *in vivo* by decreased tail-bleed time and propensity to thrombosis in response to either ferric chloride or photochemical injury, and *in vitro* by increased platelet aggregation.[1325,1515]

Activated platelets likely contribute to lysophosphatidic acid (LPA) generation in blood[1516] via lysophospholipase D (lysoPLD)-catalyzed hydrolysis of a lysophosphatidyl choline (LPC).[1517] Autotaxin, initially identified as a tumor-cell–derived motility factor, appears to be responsible for the majority of lysoPLD activity in serum; it is also responsible for the formation of LPA from LPC,[1518] and release of autotaxin from platelets may promote tumor cell metastasis through the generation of

LPA.[1519] Mild oxidation of LDL generates LPA, and the LPA component of oxidized LDL in the lipid-rich thrombogenic core of atherosclerotic lesions exposed during plaque rupture may be an important platelet activator.[1520]

In human platelets, LPA elicits shape change,[1521] platelet-monocyte aggregate formation,[1522] and fibronectin-matrix assembly[1523]; it also potentiates ADP-induced platelet aggregation. LPA signaling pathways couple by activation of the small G-protein Rho,[1521] Src kinase activity, and calcium entry,[1524] with little activation of Gq-dependent pathways.[1525] Some of the platelet responses to LPA in whole blood are attenuated by $P2Y_1$ and $P2Y_{12}$ receptor antagonists, suggesting that released ADP may play an important role in mediating aspects of the response to LPA.[1524] The platelet receptor(s) responsible for LPA signaling are not known.

S1P is a weaker activator of platelets than LPA and requires high concentrations (>10 $\mu$M) to induce platelet aggregation,[1526] raising the possibility that a contaminant or an S1P-derived metabolite may account for its biologic activity.[1527] S1P elicits platelet shape change,[1528] activates protein kinases, and stimulates fibronectin matrix assembly.[1523] Paradoxically, S1P has also been reported to inhibit thrombin- and epinephrine-induced platelet aggregation.[1529]

### Serotonin

Platelets serve as the major serotonin (5-hydroxytryptophan [5HT]) storage site in the circulation because they have the capacity to take it up actively and store it in dense granules. The release of serotonin from dense granules during platelet activation may amplify platelet aggregation and granule release. Serotonergic receptors, which are seven-transmembrane G-protein–coupled receptors, exist in seven main subfamilies termed $5HT_1$ to $5HT_7$.[1530] The receptor that mediates serotonin's effects on platelet function is of the $5HT_{2A}$ subtype and is identical to the $5HT_{2A}$ receptor present in the brain frontal cortex.[1531–1534] The $5HT_2$ receptor-blocking compound ketanserin antagonizes serotonin's stimulatory effects on platelets and neurons.[1535] Two naturally occurring amino acid substitutions have been identified in the receptor.[1536] Platelets from patients heterozygous for the H452Y polymorphism have a blunted calcium response when stimulated with serotonin compared to platelets from patients homozygous for H452.[1536] Silent polymorphisms in the $5HT_{2A}$ gene (T102C in exon 1 and –1438A/G in the promoter region) have been correlated with nonfatal acute MIs and enhanced $5HT_{2A}$ receptor-mediated small platelet aggregate formation.[1537] Many studies have been performed correlating platelet serotonin transporter activity and $5HT_{2A}$ receptors with a number of neuropsychiatric disorders.[1538–1542] There is some concern, however, about the correlation between $5HT_{2A}$ receptors on platelets and those in the brain.[1543] Hyperresponsive $5HT_{2A}$ receptors have been implicated in the association between depression and increased risk of cardiovascular events.[1544]

Addition of serotonin in micromolar concentrations to platelets *in vitro* causes elevation of intracellular calcium, PLC activation, protein phosphorylation, and mild aggregation.[1545,1546] In whole blood, serotonin does not itself cause platelet aggregation, but it does enhance aggregation induced by ADP and thrombin.[1547] Serotonin released from platelets can cause vasoconstriction of blood vessels that have suffered endothelial damage,[1548] further promoting thrombus formation. Inhibition of serotonin's action has a favorable effect in animal models of thrombosis and vascular damage, but it is not clear whether the benefit derives from effects on platelet aggregation or vasoconstriction.[1549] Mice deficient in serotonin have prolonged bleeding times, suggesting a physiologic role for serotonin in hemostasis.[1550]

A role for serotonin in linking procoagulant proteins to activated platelets has been described. Serotonin can attach via a transglutaminase-dependent reaction to multiple substrates, including fibrinogen, VWF, thrombospondin, fibronectin, and $\alpha_2$-antiplasmin. These serotonylated proteins then associate to a subpopulation of activated platelets termed "coated" platelets, perhaps via interactions with fibrinogen or thrombospondin.[1550,1551] Tissue transglutaminase in platelets can also catalyze the addition of serotonin to the small G-proteins Rab4 and RhoA in a reaction that renders them constitutively active and promotes $\alpha$-granule secretion.[1552]

The serotonin transporter (SERT), which takes up and releases serotonin, contributes to platelet stores of serotonin. Expression of SERT is required for normal ADP- and thrombin-mediated aggregation of mouse platelets.[1553] Furthermore, SERT activity is enhanced by ligand binding to integrin $\alpha_{IIb}\beta_3$. Case reports have suggested an association between the use of a serotonin reuptake inhibitor and bleeding abnormalities.[1554] Reports conflict as to whether these antidepressants may protect from MI or reduce the complications of acute thrombosis. In mice, platelet release of serotonin is essential for liver regeneration following partial hepatectomy.[1555]

### Vasopressin: V₁-Type Receptor

Vasopressin interacts with platelets to induce shape change, aggregation, and dense granule release.[1556] These events follow an induced rise in intracellular calcium and PLC activation.[1557] The platelet binding site is classified pharmacologically as a $V_1$-type receptor,[1558] and radiolabeled vasopressin binds with a $K_D$ of 1 to 10 n$M$.[1559] Unlike the case with $V_2$ receptors that activate adenylate cyclase, the $V_1$ receptors appear to activate PLC,[1560] perhaps via coupling through G$\alpha$q11.[1561] There are fewer than 100 binding sites for vasopressin per platelet,[1562] and there is controversy as to whether physiologic concentrations of vasopressin are sufficiently high to activate platelets directly[1563,1564]; even if vasopressin does not directly activate platelets, it may be able to enhance platelet activation induced by other agonists. Vasopressin $V_{1a}$ receptor antagonists inhibit vasopressin-induced platelet aggregation.[1565,1566]

### Angiotensin II: AT1-Type Receptor

Platelets express angiotensin II (AngII) AT1-type receptors.[1567] AngII treatment of platelet-rich plasma results in shape change but not platelet aggregation.[1568,1569] Infusion of AngII into normal volunteers results in platelet activation as assessed by plasma $\beta$-thromboglobulin levels and platelet surface expression of P-selectin and fibrinogen binding sites.[1570] Certain AT1 receptor antagonists, such as losartan and irbesartan, competitively inhibit TXA$_2$ receptors on platelets.[1569,1571,1572] AT1 receptor antagonists stimulate NO release from isolated platelets.[1573] In hypertensive rats treated with losartan, platelet function appears to be attenuated,[1574] but data in humans on the effects of administering AT1 receptor antagonists are inconsistent.[1575–1578]

### Thrombospondin: Integrin-Associated Protein (CD47)

Thrombospondin (TSP), a large disulfide-bonded trimer (subunit Mr 160,000), is both a platelet $\alpha$-granule protein and an extracellular matrix protein present in the subendothelium. TSP is rapidly released from platelets upon thrombin stimulation. In addition to its role as an adhesive protein, TSP also functions as an agonist to stimulate integrin $\alpha_{IIb}\beta_3$-mediated platelet aggregation.[386,1579] Multiple potential TSP receptors are present on platelets, including CD36, integrins $\alpha_{IIb}\beta_3$ and $\alpha_v\beta_3$, and integrin-associated protein (termed CD47). Of these receptors, CD47 is most strongly implicated as the major signaling receptor in response to TSP. CD47 was first discovered as a protein that copurifies with integrins, including integrins $\alpha_{IIb}\beta_3$,[386] $\alpha_v\beta_3$,[1580] and $\alpha_2\beta_1$.[1581] The sequence of CD47 indicates that it has a single immunoglobulin-like extracellular domain, five membrane-spanning regions, and a short cytoplasmic tail.[391,1579,1580] CD47 probably generates signals independent of integrins and affects integrin function via downstream effects. CD47 couples physically and functionally to the large G-protein, G$\alpha$I,[1582] which is of note because all known large G-proteins couple to receptors with seven rather than five transmembrane-spanning regions. Further downstream signaling probably involves the activation of tyrosine kinases, including Syk, Lyn, and Fak, as well as PLC$\gamma$2.[1583] Studies of mice with targeted deletions of CD47 indicate that it may block the inhibitory effects of NO on platelets,[1584] which may contribute to its role in stimulating platelet adhesion to activated endothelium under low shear rates.[1585]

How other TSP binding sites on platelets contribute to the overall response induced by TSP is not clear. CD36 copurifies with several tyrosine kinases, including Fyn, Lyn, and Yes.[1315] However, whether TSP binding to CD36 activates these kinases and whether they then contribute to the observed platelet response is unknown.

TSP also functions as a reductase for VWF; in $\alpha$ granules, it appears to reduce VWF multimer size.[1586,1587] In contrast, TSP also binds to the A3 domain of plasma VWF, where it competes for ADAMTS-13 binding, thus slowing the rate of VWF cleavage and favoring large multimers.[1587] TSP also makes a small, but significant, contribution to the conversion of latent TGF-$\beta_1$ released from platelets to active TGF-$\beta_1$.[478]

### Collagen: GPVI and Integrin α₂β₁

Upon vascular injury, collagens in the subendothelium become exposed to flowing blood and promote both platelet attachment and activation, thereby contributing to normal hemostasis. Collagen is also one of the most thrombogenic substances in atherosclerotic plaques, and upon plaque rupture, it is believed to contribute to platelet aggregation and thrombus formation, leading to ischemic damage (Fig. 2–17).[1588] The types of collagen present in the subendothelium include: I, III, IV, V, VI, VIII, and XIII,[1589] with the most abundant being types I and III (greater than 95 percent). Under conditions that mimic physiologic blood flow, platelets adhere tightly to collagen types I, III, and IV, weakly to types VI, VII, and VIII, and not at all to type V. However, under static conditions, platelets can adhere to types I to VIII.[1335] Collagens are normally acid insoluble fibers, but can form spiral microfibrils when subjected to proteolysis. Differences in the nature of the collagen surface influence its recognition by platelets.[1590]

Collagen-induced platelet activation probably involves multiple receptors, most notably GPVI and integrin $\alpha_2\beta_1$, with indirect activation of PAR-1 via activation of MMP-1.[1390] GPVI is an Mr 62,000 glycoprotein from the immunoglobulin superfamily[1591–1594] that functions in concert with the FcR$\gamma$-chain, with the latter initiating intracellular signaling.[804,1167,1168,1595–1598] Other collagen receptors on platelets include CD36[1309] and an Mr 65,000 protein termed GP65.[1599] The I (inserted) domain in the $\alpha_2$ subunit of integrin $\alpha_2\beta_1$ is homologous to a number of collagen-binding domains in other proteins and mediates adhesion of the receptor to collagen. Integrin $\alpha_2\beta_1$ recognizes spiral microfibrils, but not the acid-insoluble form of collagen in which the monomers assume a banded pattern.[1590] The potential interrelation of all of the collagen receptors is unknown, but GPVI appears to be responsible for platelet interactions with insoluble collagens, and GPVI and $\alpha_2\beta_1$ work in concert to recognize collagen spiral microfibrils, perhaps by assembling intracellular proteins into complexes.[964,1600,1601]

GPVI exists as both monomer and dimer in a stable physical complex with the dimeric FcR$\gamma$-chain; FcR$\gamma$-chain is absent from GPVI-deficient platelets.[1168,1171,1180] The tertiary structure of GPVI revealed a dimeric structure with parallel orientation of the collagen binding domains, separated by a distance (5.5 nm) that matches the orientation of the collagen triple helix.[1596] Molecular docking studies suggested that collagen interacts with a shallow groove on the surface. The addition of either collagen or an antibody that can crosslink GPVI induces tyrosine phosphorylation of the FcR$\gamma$-chain.[1180] The kinases contributing to this event are probably Fyn and/or Lyn.[1041,1104,1602]

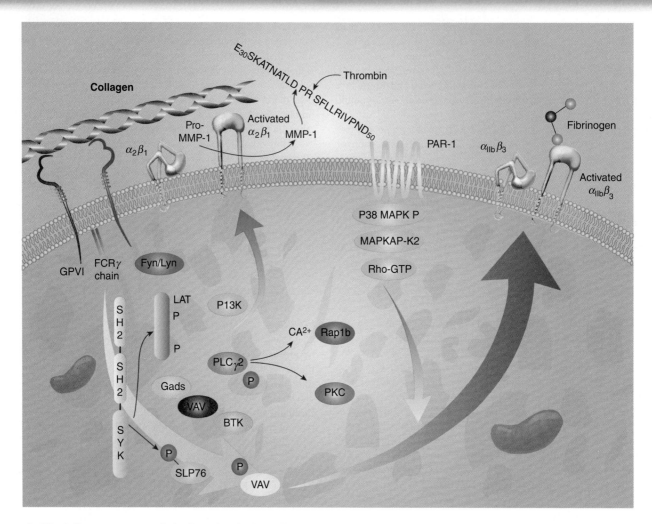

**Figure 2–17.** Collagen activation of platelets. The platelet collagen receptor GPVI is physically and functionally coupled to the immunoreceptor tyrosine-based activation motif (ITAM)-containing FcRγ chain. Upon collagen binding to GPVI, GPVI dimerizes as a result of oxidation of intracytoplasmic thiol groups (not shown) and then tyrosine motifs within the FcRγ chain are phosphorylated (P) by the Src family kinase Fyn. This action initiates a chain of events that includes recruitment of the tyrosine kinase Syk, which is phosphorylated and activated by Fyn and Lyn, and phosphorylation of adaptor proteins LAP and SLP76. A signaling cascade activates Bruton tyrosine kinase (BTK), phospholipase C (PLC)-2, protein kinase C (PKC), and phosphoinositol 3′-kinase (PI3K). Ultimately integrins $\alpha_2\beta_1$ and $\alpha_{IIb}\beta_3$ are converted to a high-affinity ("active") state. Activation of $\alpha_2\beta_1$ promotes firm adhesion to collagen and reinforces intracellular signaling pathways.

Tyrosine phosphorylation of the ITAM on the FcRγ-chain increases the motif's affinity for proteins containing SH2 domains, resulting in the recruitment of such proteins to the FcRγ-chain.[1041,1104] The non-receptor tyrosine kinase Syk contains two adjacent SH2 domains and a tyrosine kinase domain. In platelets from normal mice, Syk physically associates with the FcRγ-chain and becomes phosphorylated and activated after collagen stimulation,[1180] whereas in platelets from mice lacking FcRγ-chain, collagen is unable to induce Syk phosphorylation and activation.[1597] Similarly, in platelets lacking GPVI or in platelets in which integrin $\alpha_2\beta_1$ is blocked, collagen-induced Syk phosphorylation is also inhibited, demonstrating that GPVI, integrin $\alpha_2\beta_1$, and Syk all participate in the platelet response to collagen. The $\beta$ subunit of the integrin $\alpha_2\beta_1$ also displays Tyr residues spaced in a manner reminiscent of an ITAM motif, and thus it is possible that Syk might also associate with this collagen receptor. In addition to Syk,[1603] Src also becomes tyrosine phosphorylated in response to collagen. Although Src is an abundant kinase in platelets, its role in platelet signaling is unclear, as mice lacking Src do not suffer from any obvious bleeding disorder.[1605] Syk, on the other hand, appears to play a critical role in collagen activation of platelets as platelets from mice lacking Syk do not aggregate

or undergo secretion in response to collagen.[1597] Collagen stimulation of platelets also results in tyrosine phosphorylation and activation of PLCγ2,[1606] and activation of this enzyme causes PI hydrolysis, leading to integrin $\alpha_{IIb}\beta_3$ activation. PLCγ2 activation occurs downstream of Syk, as evidenced by the findings that collagen is unable to activate PLCγ2 in platelets pretreated with a Syk-selective inhibitor[1607] or in platelets from Syk knockout mice.[1597] It is unknown whether Syk activates PLCγ2 directly, but Bruton tyrosine kinase (BTK) might be positioned between Syk and PLCγ2 because patients lacking BTK not only exhibit the B-cell deficiency X-linked agammaglobulinemia, but also show reduced platelet responsiveness to collagen and diminished phosphorylation of PLCγ2.[1608] Signaling via GPVI also activates the other major collagen receptor integrin $\alpha_2\beta_1$,[1609,1610] perhaps via talin binding to the $\beta_1$ cytoplasmic domain,[245] elimination of an inhibitory influence of the $\alpha_2$ cytoplasmic domain,[245] and/or extracellular disulfide exchange.[973]

Intermediate events of GPVI signaling involve the activation of a small G-protein, Rap-1, which has been implicated in integrin activation in platelets and megakaryocytes.[1611] Full GPVI-induced Rap-1 activation appears to involve both release of ADP (acting on the P2Y12 ADP receptor) and ADP receptor-independent pathways.[1612] GPVI signaling also results in the activation of at least one negative regulator of platelet function, c-CBL, which is tyrosine phosphorylated and activated downstream of Src kinases. Platelets deficient in c-CBL show enhanced aggregation responses in response to GPVI engagement.[1613] While much of the GPVI-mediated signaling occurs via the associated FcRγ, the cytoplasmic domain of GPVI also contains a highly basic region that binds calmodulin and a Pro-rich region that binds Src kinases, which also appear to contribute to GPVI-mediated signaling.[1614] GPVI signaling also leads to the generation of reactive oxygen species.[1615]

Integrin $\alpha_2\beta_1$ can also signal in response to collagen, independent of GPVI and induce phosphorylation and activation of many of the same signaling components attributed to the GPVI-induced signaling cascade, such as Src, Syk, SLP-76, and PLC2. Other components include plasma membrane calcium ATPase and FAK.[1616] However, separate studies indicate that integrin $\alpha_2\beta_1$ must be in an active conformation in order to participate in this signaling.[967,1617] Thus it appears that collagen-induced signaling via GPVI activates integrin $\alpha_2\beta_1$, allowing both receptors to participate in the signaling necessary for a full response to collagen.[1617]

The inactive form of MMP-1 (proMMP-1) is associated with integrin $\alpha_2\beta_1$,[1390] as well as integrin $\alpha_{IIb}\beta_3$.[1618] With collagen activation, MMP-1 becomes activated and then can cleave the N-terminal region of PAR-1, resulting in the generation of a new N-terminal that can insert into the receptor and initiate downstream signaling through the p38 MAPK, Rho-GTP pathway. Of note, the cleavage of PAR-1 by MMP-1 is at a site two amino acids N-terminal to the cleavage site of thrombin. The combined activation of PAR-1, integrin $\alpha_2\beta_1$, and GPVI may account for the high thrombogenicity of collagen surfaces.

The levels of GPVI and integrin $\alpha_2\beta_1$ expressed on platelets vary among individuals, but it is unclear whether there is a correlation between the levels of expression of each of them.[983,1619-1621] The level of expression of these receptors correlates with the ability of platelets to be stimulated by collagen. GPVI is present on the membranes of the open canalicular system and α granules, but these pools are not detectable on the surface of resting platelets. These pools merge with the plasma membrane pool in stimulated platelets, increasing the apparent surface expression of GPVI by approximately 60 percent.[1622]

CD36 can also bind collagen, and antibodies to CD36 partially inhibit platelet adhesion to collagen.[1623,1624] Platelets from patients lacking CD36 responded normally to collagen in one study,[1625] but showed a minor defect in adhesion to collagen under flow conditions in another.[1626]

Platelets stimulated with collagen exhibit several distinct responses. Although elevated cAMP levels normally inhibit platelet aggregation, collagen-stimulated platelets are relatively resistant to inhibition by cAMP.[1627] This may be related to the fact that collagen stimulates the PLCγ isotype, which is insensitive to cAMP-mediated inhibition, whereas other agonists such as thrombin stimulate PLCβ, which is inhibited by cAMP. In addition, phosphatase inhibition decreases collagen- but not thrombin- or ADP-induced platelet aggregation,[1628] suggesting that one or more phosphatases are critical in collagen-induced platelet aggregation.

### GPIb/IX/V

The GPIb/IX/V complex promotes the initial interactions of platelets with VWF, particularly under conditions of high shear, resulting in platelet tethering. GPIb/IX/V can also initiate signals that activated the integrin $\alpha_{IIb}\beta_3$ receptor, resulting in firm platelet adhesion and aggregation.[1035] Some of the first evidence that the GPIb/IX/V complex could serve as a signaling receptor came from studies in which antibodies to integrin $\alpha_{IIb}\beta_3$ partially inhibited ristocetin-induced platelet

aggregation.[284] Subsequently, ristocetin-mediated interaction of VWF with platelets was observed to cause $PIP_2$ metabolism, activation of PKC, and an increase in intracellular $Ca^{2+}$. Likewise, shear forces initiate signaling through the binding of VWF to GPIb/IX/V.[1629] In heterologous systems such as Chinese hamster ovary (CHO) cells expressing both GPIb/IX and integrin $\alpha_{IIb}\beta_3$, occupancy of GPIb/IX by VWF can lead to activation of $\alpha_{IIb}\beta_3$.[1630,1631] In platelets, the GPIb/IX/V complex associates with signaling proteins with ITAM motifs, such the FcγRIIA receptor[1632] and FcRγ-chain[1105]; however, engagement of GPIb/IX/V alone is sufficient to activate integrin $\alpha_{IIb}\beta_3$.[1633] The signaling pathway triggered by engagement of GPIb/IX/V is incompletely understood but appears to involve activation of Src[1523,1633,1634] and PI3K, and recruitment of the adaptor proteins SLP-76 and ADAP (SLAP-130).[1633] The result is activation of $PLC\gamma_2$,[1635] PKC, and integrin $\alpha_{IIb}\beta_3$. Signaling through the GPIb/IX/V complex also causes release of AA and generation of $TXA_2$. A cyclic guanosine monophosphate (cGMP) and MAPK-dependent pathway for GPIb/IX-mediated activation of integrin $\alpha_{IIb}\beta_3$ has also been reported.[1636] The GPIb/IX/V complex binds several intracellular proteins, including filamin (actin binding protein),[1092] calmodulin,[1637] and 14-3-3ζ.[1090,1638,1639] Activation of c-RAF by 14-3-3ζ may link GPIb/IX/V signaling to the MAPK signaling pathway; moreover, protein 14-3-3ζ exists as a dimer, which may allow it to bridge and dimerize GPIb molecules.[1639] In CHO cells, clustering of GPIb/IX promotes stable adhesion via integrin $\alpha_{IIb}\beta_3$.[1640]

The GPIb/IX/V complex also appears to be involved in transmitting at least one cAMP-dependent inhibitory signal. Thus, elevated cAMP, which activates protein kinase A (PKA), induces phosphorylation of GPIbβ on Ser 166.[1091] Elevated cAMP also normally inhibits agonist-induced platelet actin polymerization. However, in platelets from patients with Bernard-Soulier syndrome, which lack GPIb/IX/V, actin polymerization proceeds normally after collagen stimulation, even when cAMP is elevated, suggesting that cAMP-mediated phosphorylation of GPIbβ may be required for the cAMP-mediated inhibition.[1641]

GPV, an Mr 82,000 membrane-spanning protein that is a member of the leucine-rich repeat family and complexes with GPIb/IX, is a substrate for thrombin.[1642] GPV-null platelets display enhanced responses to thrombin,[1150] and GPV-null mice have accelerated thrombus growth in response to vascular injury.[1643] Proteolytically inactive thrombin selectively activates mouse platelets lacking GPV and induces thrombosis in GPV-deficient but not wild-type mice.[1151] Together, these observations suggest that GPV may function as a negative regulator of thrombin signaling through GPIb/IX, and in its absence, thrombin may function as a ligand for GPIb/IX.

## ADDITIONAL INTERMEDIATE SIGNALING MOLECULES

### Calcium

Elevation of intracellular $Ca^{2+}$ has a multitude of effects on platelet physiology.[1435,1644] The concentration of $Ca^{2+}$ in resting platelets (100 to 500 nM) is very low compared to the plasma concentration of $Ca^{2+}$ (approximately 2 mM). Exposure of platelets to most agonists is accompanied by a rapid, transient rise in the intracellular free $Ca^{2+}$ concentration to micromolar levels, followed by a less-rapid return to normal resting levels. The cytoplasmic $Ca^{2+}$ concentration at any given time is a result of the rates of passive $Ca^{2+}$ influx, active $Ca^{2+}$ extrusion across the plasma membrane, and both active release and/or uptake of $Ca^{2+}$ by the DTS/sarcoplasmic reticulum (see "Dense Tubular System/Sarcoplasmic Reticulum" above), which is a $Ca^{2+}$ storage depot in platelets analogous to the sarcoplasmic reticulum in muscle. Active $Ca^{2+}$ extrusion and uptake of $Ca^{2+}$ are mediated by several pumps (see Fig. 2–3). The cytosolic pool of $Ca^{2+}$ turns over rapidly as a result of a plasma membrane

Na$^+$/Ca$^{2+}$ antiporter, whereas the DTS/sarcoplasmic reticulum contains a more slowly exchanging pool of Ca$^{2+}$ regulated by a Ca$^{2+}$/Mg$^{2+}$ ATPase (sarco-/endoplasmic reticulum Ca$^{2+}$-ATPase 3 [SERCA3]), a pump that also appears to be located in the plasma membrane.[1645] During agonist stimulation, most Ca$^{2+}$ enters the platelet cytosolic compartment through receptor-operated calcium channels (reviewed in Ref. 1646) in the plasma membrane. Collagen, for example, causes Na$^+$ entry into platelets, which reverses the Na$^+$/Ca$^{2+}$ antiporter to promote Ca$^{2+}$ entry, thus contributing to platelet aggregation.[1647] Release of intracellular Ca$^{2+}$ from the DTS/sarcoplasmic reticulum also occurs rapidly in response to agonist stimulation, in large a result of the IP$_3$ generated as part of the phosphoinositide cycle.[1646,1648] The release of internal stores of Ca$^{2+}$ results in translocation of STIM1 from the DTS/sarcoplasmic reticulum, followed by activation of the plasma membrane Ca$^{2+}$ channel Orai1, leading to store-operated Ca$^{2+}$ entry.[119] Calcium entry is also supported by TRPC6 mediating non–store-operated mechanisms, induced by DAG.[93,119,1646] The role of TRPC1 remains to be defined.[93,119,1646] Integrin $\alpha_{IIb}\beta_3$ may also participate in Ca$^{2+}$ entry.[1649]

An intracellular rise of Ca$^{2+}$ levels induces numerous downstream events, including activation of Ca$^{2+}$-sensitive forms of PLA$_2$[1650] and PKC[1651]; calmodulin-dependent enzymes such as myosin light-chain kinase, which phosphorylates myosin light chain[1652] and promotes cytoskeletal rearrangements required for platelet shape change; and gelsolin, which facilitates actin severing and rearrangement, secretion, and aggregation. In addition, Ca$^{2+}$ probably plays a direct role in controlling the secretory machinery, which mediates the membrane fusion events that result in degranulation and the release reaction. Calcium-dependent proteases or calpains also become activated and play an important role in postaggregation events. The Ca$^{2+}$ binding protein CIB (calcium and integrin binding protein)[1653] binds to the membrane proximal region of $\alpha_{IIb}$[1654] and contributes to platelet spreading.[31]

## Phosphoinositide 3'-Kinases

PI3Ks are a family of lipid kinases that phosphorylate the D-3 hydroxyl group of the myoinositol ring of phosphoinositides.[1655,1656] Class I PI3Ks are heterodimeric protein complexes containing both adaptor and catalytic subunits that use PI, PI(4)P, and PI(4,5)P$_2$ as substrates to form PI(3)P, PI(3,4)P$_2$, and PI(3,4,5)P$_3$, respectively. Class Ia (PI3K$\alpha$, PI3K$\beta$, and PI3K$\delta$) and class Ib (PI3K$\gamma$) have distinct subunits and regulatory features. The catalytic subunit of class Ia PI3K is an Mr 110,000 to 120,000 protein; the adaptor subunit, p85 (PI3K p85$\alpha$), has two SH2 domains, a breakpoint cluster region homology domain, a Pro-rich region, and a single SH3 domain. Members of this class of PI3K possess intrinsic serine-threonine protein kinase activity in addition to lipid kinase activity, and they appear to be regulated, at least in part, by binding of the p85 subunit to tyrosine-phosphorylated proteins. Although platelets possess PI3K$\alpha$ and PI3K$\delta$, the main class Ia member that is thought to contribute to platelet function is PI3K$\beta$. PI3K$\gamma$ has been isolated from platelets and neutrophils and contains both regulatory (p101) and catalytic (p110$\gamma$) subunits; the latter is activated by the $\beta/\gamma$ subunit of heterodimeric G proteins. Both isoforms of PI3K appear to associate with the platelet cytoskeleton after agonist activation.

In platelets, 3-phosphorylated phosphoinositides are produced in response to a variety of agonists, including thrombin, TXA$_2$, LPA, ADP, and collagen, and may mediate early signaling events that precede integrin $\alpha_{IIb}\beta_3$ activation, as well as late events involved in stabilizing fibrinogen binding and platelet aggregation.[1655–1657] Thrombin stimulates rapid accumulation of PI(3,4,5)P$_3$ and PI(3,4)P$_2$[1658] and late production of PtdIns(3,4)P$_2$; the latter requires fibrinogen binding to $\alpha_{IIb}\beta_3$ and calpain activity.[1659] Collagen promotes the association of class Ia PI3K via the SH2 domains with tyrosine-phosphorylated forms of FcR$\gamma$-chain and the regulatory protein, linker-for-activator T cells, to

modulate PI3K.[1660] Platelets from mice lacking PI3K p85$\alpha$ aggregate normally to ADP, thrombin, U46619, and phorbol esters, but display impaired responses to collagen and CRP and diminished tyrosine phosphorylation of the PI3K effectors Btk, Tec, Akt, and PLC$\gamma_2$.[1661] Fc$\gamma$RIIA-induced platelet aggregation requires PI3K activity, which is upstream of PLC$\gamma_2$ in the pathway.[1662] Genetic deletion of PI3K$\beta$ in mice results in embryonic lethality, but mice possessing a kinase dead form of the enzyme have been generated. Platelets from these mice have defects in G-protein–coupled receptor (GPCR)-, collagen-, and integrin-mediated signaling pathways.[1663] Platelets from mice lacking PI3K$\gamma$ isoform aggregate normally to thrombin and collagen but have impaired responses to ADP, and PI3K$\gamma$-deficient mice are protected from ADP-induced thromboembolism.[1664] Platelets from mice expressing a kinase dead form of PI3K$\gamma$ have defective GPCR-induced activation of Rap1 and aggregation, but normal responses through GPVI-activated pathways.[1663] A working model to explain the observations is that PI3K$\beta$ serves as a common intermediary of signals elicited by GPCR, collagen, and integrin ligation, whereas PI3K$\gamma$ primarily affects GPCR-initiated pathways. Many of the biologic actions of PI3K are mediated by their phospholipid products, which bind to specific sequences in proteins.[1665] The pleckstrin homology (PH) domains (approximately 100-amino-acids long) present in pleckstrin and other platelet proteins involved in signal transduction recognize either PI(3,4)P$_2$ or PI(3,4,5)P$_3$. Binding of PI(3,4,5)P$_3$ to the aminoterminal PH domain in PLC$\gamma$ enhances its activity.[1666] PI(3,4,5)P$_3$ binding to PH domains in BTK[1667] targets BTK to the plasma membrane, where it is further phosphorylated and activated.[1668] PI(3,4)P$_2$ or PI(3,4,5)P$_3$ binding to the PH domains in the serine/threonine kinase Akt (or protein kinase B) changes the conformation of Akt, permitting it to become activated by phosphorylation on Ser and Thr by Akt-kinase (PDK1).[1669,1670] Akt activation is biphasic, occurring before and after platelet aggregation.[1659] Two isoforms of Akt are present in human platelets (Akt1 and Akt2).[1671] The Akt isoforms have multiple substrates in platelets. One prominent substrate is glycogen synthase kinase (GSK)-3$\beta$, which is inactivated by Akt-mediated phosphorylation. GSK-3$\beta$ suppresses platelet function and thrombosis in mice.[1672] Akt activation also stimulates NO production and resultant protein kinase G (PKG)-dependent degranulation.[1673] Finally, Akt has been implicated in activation of a cAMP-dependent phosphodiesterase (PDE3A), which plays a role in reducing platelet cAMP levels after thrombin stimulation.[1674] Each of these Akt-mediated events is expected to contribute to platelet activation. Deficiency of Akt2 in mice impairs platelet aggregation, secretion, and fibrinogen binding in response to low doses of thrombin and U46619, but has minimal effects on collagen signaling.[1675] Akt2-null mice have normal bleeding times, but are protected from experimental thrombosis, as are mice with a deficiency of Akt1.[1675,1676] Interestingly, in platelets containing either kinase dead PI3K$\beta$ or PI3K$\gamma$, activation of Akt by ADP was abolished, and yet under the same condition, aggregation was only modestly affected,[1663] which raises questions about the role of Akt in these events.

## Small G Proteins

**Overview** The Ras superfamily of small GTPases are intracellular transducers that act as "on–off" switches to facilitate the response to extracellular stimuli. Platelets contain members of the Ras subfamily (Ras, Ral, and Rap), the Rho subfamily (Rho, Rac, and Cdc42), the Rab subfamily (Rab 1, 3, 4, 6, 8, 11, 27, 31, 32),[1677–1680] and the Arf subfamily (Arf1 or 3 and 6).[1681]

Rho family GTPases are regulators of cytoskeletal remodeling: Cdc42 for filopodia formation, Rac for lamellipodia and membrane ruffling, and Rho for focal adhesion and stress fiber formation.[1682,1683] Platelets have Cdc42,[1684] Rac1,[1685] and RhoA.[1679] Resting platelets have very low levels of the GTP-bound forms of these GTPases,[1686–1688] but all are converted to their GTP-bound states upon platelet activation.[1689,1690] Thus, receptor-mediated signaling activates Rho family GTPases. Cdc42 and Rac1 are activated at a very early phase of stimulation (approximately 10 seconds) and reach maximal activation 30 seconds after stimulation with collagen, thrombin, or ADP.[1687,1688,1690,1691] This temporal response is consistent with an early role for these GTPases in filopodia and lamellipodia formation. Integrin-dependent secondary signaling is required for full activation of RhoA,[1686] but not Cdc42 or Rac1,[1687,1690] suggesting a role for RhoA in both early (adhesion/aggregation) and late (clot retraction) stages of platelet activation. More detailed descriptions of each subfamily follows.

**Ras** Platelets contain at least one Ras isoform (H-Ras).[1692] Despite its intensively studied functions in proliferation, differentiation, and cell survival in nucleated cells,[1693,1694] the exact role of Ras and its signaling in platelets is unclear. Platelets do contain most of the downstream Ras effectors: Raf-1, MEK (MAPK/ERK kinase), and ERK (extracellular signal-regulated kinase).[1695] Ras and ERK are both known to be activated upon platelet stimulation.[1696]

**Rho** Inactivation of RhoA with C3 exoenzyme treatment inhibits agonist-induced shape change,[1697–1699] adhesion/aggregation,[1686,1698,1700,1701] and formation of focal adhesions.[1701] Platelets treated with the exoenzyme also show decreased stress fiber formation, a process mediated by Rho kinase-dependent phosphorylation of myosin light chain (MLC).[1686,1697,1700]

**Rac** In nucleated cells, Rac1 functions in actin remodeling via activation of three downstream effectors: phosphatidylinositol 4-phosphate 5-kinase type Iα, p21-Cdc42/Rac-activated kinase, and suppressor of cyclic AMP receptor/WASP-family verprolin-homologous protein.[1702] The roles of Rac1 in lamellipodia formation and aggregation have been examined using platelets from mice lacking Rac1. Rac1 deletion does not affect platelet production[1703–1705] or filopodia formation, but does affect lamellipodia formation upon stimulation with thrombin and collagen.[1704] Aggregation was diminished in Rac1$^{-/-}$ platelets when stimulated with low doses of thrombin or collagen or when subjected to shear stress under flow condition.[1704,1705]

**Cdc42** The assessment of Cdc42 function in platelets is less clear. Wiskott-Aldrich syndrome is caused by a defect in WASP, which is a downstream effector of Cdc42. However, the platelets from affected individuals have normal shape change, including filopodia formation and Arp2/3 activation (Chap. 11).[1706] One study suggested that Cdc42 might function in GPVI-mediated integrin $\alpha_2\beta_1$ activation and subsequent platelet adhesion on collagen-coated surfaces.[969]

**Rap** Rap GTPases participate in cell adhesion, cell–cell junction formation, and the development of cell polarity in nucleated cells.[1707] In platelets, Rap1a, Rap1b, and Rap2 are all activated upon platelet stimulation.[1708,1709] Platelets from Rap1b$^{-/-}$ mice have a defect in platelet aggregation and decreased integrin $\alpha_{IIb}\beta_3$ activation upon platelet stimulation with ADP or PAR-4 peptide.[1710] With the discovery of the important role of CalDAG-GEF1, an exchange factor for Rap1 in platelet function, Rap1's role in integrin signaling has been a major focus of research.[1711] Platelets lacking CalDAG-GEF1 have decreased Rap1B activation and integrin $\alpha_{IIb}\beta_3$ activation.[1712] Integrin $\alpha_{IIb}\beta_3$ activation could be completely blocked by treating CalDAG-GEF1$^{-/-}$ platelets with a PKC inhibitor, suggesting that CalDAG-GEF1 and PKC function independently to activate integrin $\alpha_{IIb}\beta_3$.[1713] Studies using CHO cells reconstituted with integrin $\alpha_{IIb}\beta_3$, talin, and Rap1GTP-interacting adapter molecule (RIAM) showed that Rap1GTP-dependent talin recruitment to integrin $\beta_3$ by RIAM is required for integrin $\alpha_{IIb}\beta_3$ activation.[1714] The function of Rap2 remains to be determined; CalDAG-GEF1 does not interact with it.[1715]

**Ral** In nucleated cells, Ral GTPases (RalA and RalB) are thought to function in regulated exocytosis by recruiting a multisubunit complex termed "exocyst" for targeting secretory vesicles to specific plasma membrane domains.[1716] Both RalA and RalB in platelets are associated with platelet dense granules[1717] and become rapidly activated in a Ca$^{2+}$-dependent manner upon platelet activation.[1718] A recombinant Ral-interacting domain of Sec5, a downstream effector of RalA in exocyst complex, inhibits serotonin release from platelet-dense bodies, suggesting a role for Ral exocyst in platelet granule release.[1719]

**Rab** Rab GTPases are the largest family of small GTPases; 63 members are detected in the human genome.[1720] They are highly compartmentalized to different organelle membranes and function by coordinating vesicle transport, including vesicle formation and tethering to their target compartments.[1720] Rab proteins have been shown to play roles in both granule biogenesis and secretion.

**Arf** Arf family GTPases, in nucleated cells, function in secretory and cytoskeletal processes. Platelets contain Arf1 or 3 and Arf6. Functional studies of Arf6 show that unlike other platelet GTPases, it is in the GTP-bound state in resting platelets and there is a conversion to the GDP-bound state upon platelet activation.[1681] Inhibitors of this transition disrupt aggregation, secretion, and clot retraction. Further analysis suggests that the Arf6-GTP to Arf6-GDP transition is required for activation of Rho family proteins in platelets.

### Calcium-Dependent Proteases (Calpains)

After ligand binding, integrin clustering, and platelet aggregation, neutral cysteine proteases termed *calpains* become activated by a rise in intracellular Ca$^{2+}$.[229] The most important and best-studied calpains in platelets are: μ-calpain (calpain-1), which is activated by micromolar concentrations of Ca$^{2+}$ and accounts for 80 percent of the Cys protease activity in platelets, and m-calpain (calpain-2), which requires millimolar levels of Ca$^{2+}$ for activation.[1721] Each calpain consists of a common Mr 30,000 regulatory subunit paired with a unique catalytic subunit of Mr 80,000. Activated μ-calpain cleaves numerous proteins,[229] including cytoskeletal proteins (e.g., filamin [actin binding protein], talin, WASP, and cortactin), tyrosine kinases (e.g., BTK, Src, Syk, and FAK), tyrosine phosphatases (e.g., protein tyrosine phosphatase 1B [PTP1B; also called PTPN1], SHP-1, and PTPMEG), other important platelet proteins (e.g., integrin $\beta_3$, SNAP-23, Vav, PLC-β), and certain isoforms of PKC.[1721] Cleavage of talin by calpain *in vitro* enables talin to activate integrin $\alpha_{IIb}\beta_3$,[148] but the role of calpain in activation of integrin $\alpha_{IIb}\beta_3$ by talin in intact platelets is uncertain. Calpain also appears to be upstream of, and able to affect, the activation of the small G proteins Rac and RhoA. Calpain's role in platelet secretion has not been defined, although it is clear that the t-SNARE SNAP-23 is inactivated by calpain-mediate cleavage.[1722] Thus calpains, through their effects on structural and signaling molecules, appear to affect multiple aspects of platelet function. Mice deficient in μ-calpain demonstrate abnormal platelet aggregation, decreased clot retraction, and reduced tyrosine phosphorylation of several platelet proteins, including the β subunit of integrin $\alpha_{IIb}\beta_3$. These abnormalities in platelet function can be reversed by inhibition of tyrosine phosphatases or by deletion of PTP1B, suggesting that μ-calpain's effects on platelet kinases and phosphatases may be central to its role in platelet function.[1723]

### Inside-Out Activation of Integrin $\alpha_{IIb}\beta_3$ and Outside-In Signaling by Activated Integrin $\alpha_{IIb}\beta_3$

The active state of integrin $\alpha_{IIb}\beta_3$ is defined as the conformation that is competent to bind large, soluble, adhesive proteins, such as fibrinogen and VWF, with relatively high affinity. Precise regulation of the activation state of integrin $\alpha_{IIb}\beta_3$ is essential for maintenance of normal hemostasis, such that integrin $\alpha_{IIb}\beta_3$ activation only occurs upon vascular injury. Crystallographic and electron microscope studies suggest that the extracellular portion of both integrin $\alpha_{IIb}\beta_3$ and the related integrin $\alpha_V\beta_3$ are in a bent conformation when inactive and in an extended conformation when activated.[149,843,844] The activation state of integrin $\alpha_{IIb}\beta_3$ is controlled by the cytoplasmic domains of this integrin in concert with specific intracellular binding proteins. Thus, under basal conditions, interactions between the cytoplasmic domains of integrins $\alpha_{IIb}$ and $\beta_3$ maintain the receptor in the resting state. Interrupting the interactions between the cytoplasmic domains results in long-range conformational changes that convert the extracellular portion of the integrin to an active state.[1724] Interactions between regions of the integrins $\alpha_{IIb}$ and $\beta_3$ transmembrane and cytoplasmic domains near the membrane involve upper and lower membrane clasps and a salt bridge between acidic and basic amino acid residues of each subunit (see "Integrin $\alpha_{IIb}\beta_3$" above).[871,894,1725,1726] Mutations that disrupt these interactions result in integrin $\alpha_{IIb}\beta_3$ activation.[871,894,1726] Cytoskeletal restraints appear to further maintain integrin $\alpha_{IIb}\beta_3$ in an inactive conformation, because treatment of platelets with low doses of the actin depolymerizing agents activate the integrin.[243] Upon agonist activation, the binding of the cytoskeletal linking proteins talin and kindlin to integrin $\beta_3$ may play a key role in the conversion of integrin $\alpha_{IIb}\beta_3$, as well as several other integrins, to an active conformation.[245] One model suggests that filamin binding to the $\beta$ subunit cytoplasmic tail maintains the receptor in an inactive state by presenting talin binding. The cytoskeletal adapter protein migfilin can displace filamin from the integrin $\beta_3$ subunit and facilitate the binding of talin.[901] Talin itself can exist in a conformation that is either less or more favorable for binding to integrin $\beta_3$ at multiple sites. The affinity of talin for $\beta$ integrins increases in response to $PI(4,5)P_2$ binding to talin.[1727] $PIP_2$ may be generated locally from PI via the enzyme phosphatidylinositol phosphate kinase type $1\gamma$, which can bind to talin.[1728,1729] Talin is composed of an Mr 47,000 head domain and an Mr 190,000 rod domain. The head contains a "FERM" domain, named for the proteins four point one (4.1), ezrin, radixin, and moesin, that promotes specific interactions with cytoplasmic regions of multiple proteins. The F3 region of the FERM domain, which resembles a phosphotyrosine binding (PTB) domain,[1730] binds sequentially to membrane distal and proximal regions of integrin $\beta_3$ in addition to establishing electrostatic interactions with the lipid head groups, disrupting its interaction with the membrane and integrin $\alpha_{IIb}$.[244,871,894,896,1730-1734] This binding site is not available when PI phosphate kinase (PIPK)I is bound to talin, so presumably any prebound PIPKI would be displaced from talin upon talin interaction with integrin $\beta_3$.[1735] After talin binding, the reorganization of the transmembrane and intracytoplasmic domains disrupts the interaction of integrins $\alpha_{IIb}$ and $\beta_3$, and this is transmitted to the ectodomain.[871,894,1724] The $\beta_3$ cytoplasmic domain can also bind proteins that connect it to the cytoskeleton such as $\alpha$-actinin, ICAP1, filamin, Src, and skelemin, and so it has been proposed that interactions of the integrin $\beta_3$ subunit with the actin–myosin contraction apparatus via the cytoskeleton may supply the energy needed to adopt the extended conformation of integrin $\alpha_{IIb}\beta_3$ with the swing out of the integrin $\beta_3$ hybrid domain away from the $\beta A$ (I-like) domain.[250] The rod-like region of talin has also been reported to interact with integrin $\beta_3$,[1736] and an unknown region of talin has been reported to interact with integrin $\alpha_{IIb}$.[1737] While these interactions may serve to stabilize or subsequently cluster the integrin, their exact roles are unknown.

Members of the kindlin family of focal adhesion proteins that contain PTB domains serve as integrin activators,[1738-1740] perhaps functioning to facilitate talin–integrin interactions. Kindlin-2 binds the C-terminus of integrin $\beta_3$ in a region containing the conserved TS(752) T sequence and NITY(759) motif and acts synergically with talin to promote integrin $\alpha_{IIb}\beta_3$ activation in a recombinant expression system.[1738] Whereas kindlin-2 is widely distributed, kindlin-3 expression is limited to hematopoietic cells, including platelets. Genetic deletion of kindlin-3 in mice results in a severe bleeding phenotype and defective

activation of integrin $\alpha_{IIb}\beta_3$ on platelets.[1741] Mutations in kindlin-3 have been described in patients with leukocyte adhesion deficiency III, which is characterized by abnormalities in leukocyte and platelet integrin activation and function (Chap. 11).[1742-1745] In fact, the bleeding symptoms are even more severe than those in Glanzmann thrombasthenia, and the platelet aggregation defects are similar. Mutational analysis also identified the NXXY motif (Tyr795) and preceding threonine-region in kindlin binding to integrin $\beta_1$.[1746] Finally, based on model systems, it has been proposed that $\alpha_{IIb}$ transmembrane and cytoplasmic domains from adjacent integrin $\alpha_{IIb}\beta_3$ receptors may form homodimers and integrin $\beta_3$ transmembrane and cytoplasmic domains may form homotrimers, resulting in stabilization of the activated state and clustering of integrin $\alpha_{IIb}\beta_3$ receptors,[251,1747] but it is not clear that these interactions are favored under biologic conditions.[871,894]

Platelet aggregation is commonly described as progressing through two phases: an initial reversible aggregation phase, which is often the response observed with low concentrations of agonists, followed by a stronger, irreversible phase. The irreversible phase of aggregation correlates with $TXA_2$ production and platelet secretion of ADP. Fibrinogen binding to integrin $\alpha_{IIb}\beta_3$ and the platelet–platelet contacts that occur during the initial phase of aggregation initiate specific signal transduction events, resulting in positive feedback loops that promote irreversible aggregation, maintain secretion, and initiate later events like clot retraction.[291]

Fibrinogen or VWF binding to the extracellular region of integrin $\alpha_{IIb}\beta_3$ transmits long-range conformational changes to the integrin cytoplasmic domains, perhaps via a pivot action between the integrin $\beta_3$ $\beta A$ (I-like) and hybrid domains[827] that induce signaling from outside the platelet to inside the platelet (outside-in signaling).[876,879] These conformational changes, along with integrin clustering,[838] are likely to be the basis for outside-in signal transduction through integrin $\alpha_{IIb}\beta_3$, perhaps by altering the association of the cytoplasmic domains with one another and initiating recruitment of proteins with enzymatic activity to the cytoplasmic tails, forming complexes capable of generating signaling molecules.

One important signaling molecule that is constitutively associated with the integrin $\beta_3$ cytoplasmic tail is the tyrosine kinase, Src.[1748-1750] Src binds to the C-terminus of the integrin in resting platelets via its SH3 domain independent of its catalytic activity.[1748] This pool of Src in unstimulated platelets appears to exist in a minimally active state with its activity suppressed in part by the Src regulator Csk, which phosphorylates Src at Tyr 529. Platelet adhesion to fibrinogen increases the Src activity associated with integrin $\alpha_{IIb}\beta_3$ in part because of the dissociation of Csk and subsequent dephosphorylation of Src 529.[1750] Full Src activation occurs upon integrin $\alpha_{IIb}\beta_3$ clustering and transphosphorylation of Src on Tyr 418. Src activation is required for several subsequent signaling events such as the activation of the tyrosine kinase Syk. Syk, along with Src, is required for platelet spreading on fibrinogen.[1748] Syk binds to unphosphorylated integrin $\beta_3$ via its N-terminus.[1751,1752] Some of these events have now been visualized in living platelets.[1753] Negative regulators of Src activation include PECAM-1, which can recruit the protein tyrosine phosphatases SHP-1 and SHP-2 via its ITIMs[1749,1754-1757]; carcinoembryonic antigen-related cell adhesion molecule-1, which also possess ITIMs[1758]; and perhaps G6b-B[1759-1761] and TLT-1.[1166]

When platelets are aggregated in response to one of multiple agonists, the integrin $\beta_3$ cytoplasmic domain becomes phosphorylated on Tyr.[902,910] Two sites of potential tyrosine phosphorylation exist on the $\beta_3$ cytoplasmic domain and both may be utilized. Several molecules have been identified that bind specifically to the tyrosine-phosphorylated cytoplasmic domain of integrin $\beta_3$. A synthetic integrin $\beta_3$ cytoplasmic domain peptide containing phosphate groups on the two candidate Tyr residues binds to the contractile protein myosin,[902] and this interaction may facilitate the transmission of cytoskeletal tension from inside the platelet to outside, and thus initiate clot retraction. Recombinant, mutated integrin $\beta_3$ that cannot be phosphorylated is unable to support extensive clot retraction when expressed in a cell line.[902] Other proteins that bind to the diphosphorylated integrin $\beta_3$ cytoplasmic domain include the SHC adapter proteins,[906] which also become tyrosine phosphorylated during platelet aggregation. Therefore, it is possible that the SHC adapter proteins may link diphosphorylated integrin $\beta_3$ to the MAPK pathway.[906,1762] Mice containing mutated integrin $\beta_3$ molecules that cannot be phosphorylated exhibit a mild bleeding disorder as evidenced by occasional rebleeding of tail cuts. Moreover platelets derived from these mice form abnormally loose thrombi when activated by shear forces.[1763] Other integrin $\beta_3$ cytoplasmic domain binding proteins have been described, including skelemin, a member of a family of proteins that regulate myosin,[914] and talin.

Some signaling events that occur downstream of integrin $\alpha_{IIb}\beta_3$ require only integrin clustering, whereas other events require clustering, ligand binding, and/or platelet aggregation. For example, the tyrosine kinase Syk becomes activated in response to integrin $\alpha_{IIb}\beta_3$ clustering, independent of cytoskeletal assembly, whereas activation of the tyrosine kinase FAK requires integrin clustering, ligand binding and cytoskeletal assembly.[1764] In studies conducted in cell lines, activation of Syk downstream of integrin $\alpha_{IIb}\beta_3$ leads to phosphorylation of Vav1, a guanine nucleotide exchange factor for Rac, and lamellipodia formation. Syk and Vav1 cooperate to activate Jun N-terminal kinase, ERK2, and Akt.[1764] These pathways are also likely to be involved in postaggregation events in the platelet.

Proteins other than the well-described integrin $\alpha_{IIb}\beta_3$ ligands fibrinogen and VWF also induce signaling events via binding to integrin $\alpha_{IIb}\beta_3$. One such protein is CD40L, a TNF family member that is expressed on a variety of cells including activated platelets. Platelets are also the major source of a soluble form of CD40L.[1765] In addition to binding to its classical receptor, CD40, CD40L also binds to integrin $\alpha_{IIb}\beta_3$ on platelets and induces signaling events[1350] that are required for normal arterial thrombus formation in mice.[1348] CD40L may also initiate platelet aggregation by binding to CD40 on platelets.[1349]

## INHIBITORY PATHWAYS IN PLATELETS

### Prostaglandins

Prostaglandins that inhibit platelet activation include $PGE_2$ (at high concentrations) and $PGI_2$ (at low concentrations) (also termed *prostacyclin*) (reviewed in Refs. 1766 and 1767). In the vasculature, the endothelium produces $PGI_2$ and $PGE_2$, which are important in maintaining vascular patency.[1768] Inhibition is initiated by the binding of these PGs to their own specific GPCR.[1769,1770] PG receptor occupancy converts the G$\alpha$ subunit to the GTP bound, active form, which then activates adenylyl cyclase. Adenylyl cyclase catalyzes the formation of cAMP. The exact amount of cAMP present in the cell is also determined by its rate of breakdown by phosphodiesterases (PDEs). Biochemical studies and studies from gene targeted mice support a primary role for PDE3A in platelets.[1771-1773] Therefore, agents that inhibit PDE, such as theophylline, caffeine, and the drug cilostazol, also elevate cAMP levels in platelets and other cells.[1774] cAMP then activates PKA, which phosphorylates specific target proteins. PKA inhibits platelet activation by several pathways. One mechanism involves PKA-dependent phosphorylation of VASP (discussed under "Nitric Oxide" below). A separate mechanism involves the phosphorylation and inhibition of G$\alpha$13, which couples to the $TXA_2$ receptor, thus impairing this activation pathway.[1775] Also, PKA phosphorylates GPIb$\beta$ on Ser 166 and negatively regulates the ability of GPIb to bind VWF.[1776] In addition, PKA may phosphorylate and inhibit the $IP_3$ receptor, which would repress agonist-induced intracellular $Ca^{2+}$

mobilization.[1777] PI metabolism is also affected, as the activities of both PLC and $PLA_2$ are suppressed.[1778] Moreover, PKA also phosphorylates Raf kinase on three sites, which inhibits Raf kinase function in part by inhibiting its binding to the activating protein RasGTP.[1779,1780] Finally, the small G protein, Rap1b, which contributes to integrin $\alpha_{IIb}\beta_3$ activation,[1611] is phosphorylated by PKA,[1781] although it appears that this phosphorylation event does not inhibit platelet function[1782] and may, in fact, contribute to Rap1b activation.[1783]

Paradoxically, in contrast to the inhibitory effects of high levels of $PGE_2$, low levels of $PGE_2$ ($<10^{-6}$ M) potentiate agonist-induced platelet aggregation by acting via the EP3 receptor to decrease intraplatelet cAMP levels.[1784,1785] Mice lacking the EP3 receptor are protected from AA-induced thrombosis[1786]; thus it is possible that $PGE_2$ present in atherosclerotic lesions contributes to atherothrombosis.

### Nitric Oxide

NO is synthesized from L-arginine by NO synthase in endothelial cells, platelets, and other cells. The formation of NO is enhanced at sites of shear stress and by platelet agonists (e.g., thrombin or ADP),[1787] and it readily diffuses into platelets.[1788,1789] Similar to $PGI_2$ or $PGE_2$, NO pretreatment of platelets inhibits platelet activation and can reverse platelet aggregation soon after initiation. However, NO works not by elevating cAMP, but instead by increasing cGMP.[1790] NO synthase activity in platelets increases during platelet activation, suggesting that NO production is a normal negative feedback mechanism that limits further platelet aggregation. NO and $PGI_2$ act together synergistically to inhibit platelet activation.[1791]

Elevation in intracellular cGMP levels activates cGMP-dependent PKG, whose downstream targets include ERK and the $TXA_2$ receptor.[1792] In mice, the absence of PKG results in enhanced platelet accumulation along damaged vessels after ischemic injury, supporting an important role for PKG in platelet deposition.[1793] VASP, a member of the Pro-rich, actin-regulatory Ena/VASP protein family, is phosphorylated in response to elevations in either cAMP or cGMP,[1794] and both PKA and PKG phosphorylate VASP *in vitro*.[1795] A role for VASP in inhibition of platelet function was established in studies of VASP-deficient mice: platelets obtained from the mice display increased P-selectin expression and integrin $\alpha_{IIb}\beta_3$ activation in response to agonists,[1796] and platelet adhesion at sites of vascular injury or atherosclerosis is enhanced in VASP-deficient mice.[1797] The enhanced platelet adhesion in VASP-null mice is not corrected by NO, suggesting that VASP may be a key negative regulator of platelet function in the cGMP-mediated pathways.

Elevation in intracellular cGMP can also increase cAMP levels via inhibition of PDE activity.[1798] This crosstalk between cGMP and cAMP-dependent pathways may synergize to contribute to the inhibitory effects of NO on platelet function.

### CD39 (ATP Diphosphohydrolase; Ecto-ADPase)

Vascular endothelium regulates platelet function by producing prostacyclin and NO, as well as by expressing CD39 NTPDase1, a plasma membrane-associated ectonucleotide (ATP diphosphohydrolase; ATPDase; ecto-ADPase; EC 3.6.1.5) that converts extracellular ATP to ADP, and ADP to AMP.[1799-1801] CD39 limits the platelet-activating effects of ADP released by damaged tissues, RBCs, and activated platelets; furthermore, AMP generated by CD39 is degraded by an ecto-5'-nucleotidase (CD73; EC 3.1.3.5) to adenosine, an inhibitor of ADP-induced platelet activation, that increases cAMP binding to the A2a adenosine receptor on platelets.[1802] Adenosine deaminase (EC 3.5.4.4) degrades adenosine to inosine. CD39 is an Mr 95,000 cell-surface glycoprotein expressed on endothelial cells, subsets of activated natural killer (NK) cells, B cells, monocytes, and T cells. Small amounts may also be on platelets and erythrocytes. It is present in the lymphocytes in chronic lymphocytic leukemia, which may partially account for the thromboprotection noted in that disorder.[1803] CD39 is localized to lipid raft-like caveolae in the plasma membrane, and the cholesterol content may control enzymatic activity. It contains two putative transmembrane regions separated by an extracellular domain with six glycosylation sites and apyrase-like regions that confer the ecto-ADPase activity. A related molecule, ATP-and ATPase 2, which is found on the basolateral surface of endothelial cells, the adventitia of some blood vessels, and microvascular pericytes, is relatively selective for ATP, and thus it has the capacity to increase platelet aggregation by enhancing the production of ADP from ATP.[1799] The physiologic roles of the NTPDases are complex because of their production of variably prothrombotic and antithrombotic agents. It has been postulated that recruitment of microparticles enriched in monocyte CD39/NTPDase1 to thrombi could contribute to the limitation of the size of platelet thrombi. A role for CD39/NTPDase1 in ischemia reperfusion and allograft rejection has also been proposed. Mouse models support the potential of modulating graft rejection and thrombosis by using gene therapy to increase CD39/NTPDase1. A soluble recombinant form of CD39 inhibits platelet aggregation and recruitment *in vitro* and may have potential as an antithrombotic agent *in vivo*.[1804]

# REFERENCES

1. Ruggeri ZM: Platelets in atherothrombosis. *Nat Med* 8(11):1227–1234, 2002.
2. Goldsmith HL, Turitto VT: Rheological aspects of thrombosis and haemostasis: Basic principles and applications. ICTH-Report—Subcommittee on Rheology of the International Committee on Thrombosis and Haemostasis. *Thromb Haemost* 55(3):415–435, 1986.
3. de Groot PG, Sixma JJ: Perfusion chambers, in *Platelets*, edited by AD Michelson, pp 575–586. Academic Press, San Diego, 2007.
4. Savage B, Ruggeri ZM: Platelet thrombus formation in flowing blood, in *Platelets*, edited by AD Michelson, pp 359–376. Academic Press, San Diego, 2007.
5. Coller B: Platelets in cardiovascular thrombosis and thrombolysis, in *The Heart and Cardiovascular System*, edited by HA Fozzard, AM Katz, HE Morgan, E Haber, pp 219–273. Raven Press, New York, 1991.
6. Jackson SP, Nesbitt WS, Westein E: Dynamics of platelet thrombus formation. *J Thromb Haemost* 7(Suppl 1):17–20, 2009.
7. Roth GJ: Developing relationships: Arterial platelet adhesion, glycoprotein Ib, and leucine-rich glycoproteins. *Blood* 77(1):5–19, 1991.
8. Ruggeri ZM: Structure and function of von Willebrand factor. *Thromb Haemost* 82(2):576–584, 1999.
9. Andrews RK, et al: The glycoprotein Ib-IX-V complex in platelet adhesion and signaling. *Thromb Haemost* 82(2):357–364, 1999.
10. Ruggeri ZM: Von Willebrand factor, platelets and endothelial cell interactions. *J Thromb Haemost* 1(7):1335–1342, 2003.
11. Savage B, Ruggeri ZM: Platelet thrombus formation in flowing blood, in *Platelets*, edited by AD Michelson, p 215. Academic Press, San Diego, 2002.
12. Mailhac A, et al: Effect of an eccentric severe stenosis on fibrin(ogen) deposition on severely damaged vessel wall in arterial thrombosis. Relative contribution of fibrin(ogen) and platelets. *Circulation* 90(2):988–996, 1994.
13. Moake JL, et al: Involvement of large plasma von Willebrand factor (VWF) multimers and unusually large VWF forms derived from endothelial cells in shear stress-induced platelet aggregation. *J Clin Invest* 78(6):1456–1461, 1986.
14. Ikeda Y, et al: The role of von Willebrand factor and fibrinogen in platelet aggregation under varying shear stress. *J Clin Invest* 87(4):1234–1240, 1991.
15. Ruggeri ZM: Mechanisms of shear-induced platelet adhesion and aggregation. *Thromb Haemost* 70(1):119–123, 1993.
16. Andrews RK, Lopez JA, Berndt MC: The GPIb-IX-V complex, in *Platelets*, edited by AD Michelson, pp 145–164. Academic Press, San Diego, 2007.
17. Chiang TM, Rinaldy A, Kang AH: Cloning, characterization, and functional studies of a nonintegrin platelet receptor for type I collagen, *J Clin Invest* 100(3):514–521, 1997.
18. Clemetson JM, et al: The platelet collagen receptor glycoprotein VI is a member of the immunoglobulin superfamily closely related to FcalphaR and the natural killer receptors. *J Biol Chem* 274(41):29019–29024, 1999.
19. Clemetson KJ: Platelet collagen receptors: A new target for inhibition? *Haemostasis* 29(1):16–26, 1999.
20. Coller BS, et al: Collagen-platelet interactions: Evidence for a direct interaction of collagen with platelet GPIa/IIa and an indirect interaction with platelet GPIIb/IIIa mediated by adhesive proteins. *Blood* 74(1):182–192, 1989.
21. Gruner S, et al: Multiple integrin-ligand interactions synergize in shear-resistant platelet adhesion at sites of arterial injury in vivo. *Blood* 102(12):4021–4027, 2003.
22. Kato K, et al: The contribution of glycoprotein VI to stable platelet adhesion and thrombus formation illustrated by targeted gene deletion. *Blood* 102(5):1701–1707, 2003.
23. Kuijpers MJ, et al: Complementary roles of glycoprotein VI and alpha2beta1 integrin in collagen-induced thrombus formation in flowing whole blood ex vivo. *FASEB J* 17(6):685–687, 2003.
24. Matsuno K, et al: Inhibition of platelet adhesion to collagen by monoclonal anti-CD36 antibodies. *Br J Haematol* 92(4):960–967, 1996.
25. Nakamura T, et al: Activation of the GP IIb-IIIa complex induced by platelet adhesion to collagen is mediated by both alpha2beta1 integrin and GP VI. *J Biol Chem* 274(17):11897–11903, 1999.
26. Nieswandt B, Watson SP: Platelet-collagen interaction: Is GPVI the central receptor? *Blood* 102(2):449–461, 2003.
27. Saelman EU, et al: Platelet adhesion to collagen types I through VIII under conditions of stasis and flow is mediated by GPIa/IIa (alpha 2 beta 1-integrin). *Blood* 83(5):1244–1250, 1994.
28. Savage B, Almus-Jacobs F, Ruggeri ZM: Specific synergy of multiple substrate-receptor interactions in platelet thrombus formation under flow. *Cell* 94(5):657–666, 1998.
29. Watson SP: Collagen receptor signaling in platelets and megakaryocytes. *Thromb Haemost* 82(2):365–376, 1999.
30. Coller BS, Shattil SJ: The GPIIb/IIIa (integrin alphaIIbbeta3) odyssey: A technology-driven saga of a receptor with twists, turns, and even a bend. *Blood* 112(8):3011–3025, 2008.
31. Naik UP, Naik MU: Association of CIB with GPIIb/IIIa during outside-in signaling is required for platelet spreading on fibrinogen. *Blood* 102(4):1355–1362, 2003.
32. Patel D, et al: Dynamics of GPIIb/IIIa-mediated platelet-platelet interactions in platelet adhesion/thrombus formation on collagen in vitro as revealed by videomicroscopy. *Blood* 101(3):929–936, 2003.
33. Shattil SJ: Regulation of platelet anchorage and signaling by integrin alpha IIb beta 3. *Thromb Haemost* 70(1):224–228, 1993.
34. Shattil SJ: Signaling through platelet integrin alpha IIb beta 3: Inside-out, outside-in, and sideways. *Thromb Haemost* 82(2):318–325, 1999.
35. Shattil SJ, Newman PJ: Integrins: Dynamic scaffolds for adhesion and signaling in platelets. *Blood* 104(6):1606–1615, 2004.
36. Weiss HJ, Turitto VT, Baumgartner HR: Further evidence that glycoprotein IIb-IIIa mediates platelet spreading on subendothelium. *Thromb Haemost* 65(2):202–205, 1991.
37. Santos MT, et al: Enhancement of platelet reactivity and modulation of eicosanoid production by intact erythrocytes. A new approach to platelet activation and recruitment. *J Clin Invest* 87(2):571–580, 1991.
38. Dubois C, Atkinson B, Furie B, Furie B: Real-time imaging of platelets during thrombus formation, in *Platelets*, edited by AD Michelson, pp 611–626. Academic Press, San Diego, 2007.
39. Celi A, et al: Thrombus formation: Direct real-time observation and digital analysis of thrombus assembly in a living mouse by confocal and widefield intravital microscopy. *J Thromb Haemost* 1(1):60–68, 2003.
40. Denis C, et al: A mouse model of severe von Willebrand disease: Defects in hemostasis and thrombosis. *Proc Natl Acad Sci U S A* 95(16):9524–9529, 1998.
41. Ni H, et al: Persistence of platelet thrombus formation in arterioles of mice lacking both von Willebrand factor and fibrinogen. *J Clin Invest* 106(3):385–392, 2000.
42. Peerschke EI: The platelet fibrinogen receptor. *Semin Hematol* 22(4):241–259, 1985.
43. Phillips DR, et al: The platelet membrane glycoprotein IIb-IIIa complex. *Blood* 71(4):831–843, 1988.
44. Plow EF, Ginsberg MH: Cellular adhesion: GPIIb-IIIa as a prototypic adhesion receptor. *Prog Hemost Thromb* 9:117–156, 1989.
45. Plow EF, Pesho MM, Ma YQ: Integrin αIIβ3, in *Platelets*, edited by AD Michelson, pp 165–178. Academic Press, San Diego, 2007.
46. Peerschke EI: Ca+2 mobilization and fibrinogen binding of platelets refractory to adenosine diphosphate stimulation. *J Lab Clin Med* 106(2):111–122, 1985.
47. Steen VM, Holmsen H: Synergism between thrombin and epinephrine in human platelets: Different dose-response relationships for aggregation and dense granule secretion. *Thromb Haemost* 54(3):680–683, 1985.
48. Ware JA, Smith M, Salzman EW: Synergism of platelet-aggregating agents. Role of elevation of cytoplasmic calcium. *J Clin Invest* 80(1):267–271, 1987.
49. Giandomenico G, et al: The leptin receptor system of human platelets. *J Thromb Haemost* 3(5):1042–1049, 2005.
50. Konstantinides S, et al: Leptin-dependent platelet aggregation and arterial thrombosis suggests a mechanism for atherothrombotic disease in obesity. *J Clin Invest* 108(10):1533–1540, 2001.
51. Konstantinides S, et al: Inhibition of endogenous leptin protects mice from arterial and venous thrombosis. *Arterioscler Thromb Vasc Biol* 24(11):2196–2201, 2004.
52. Andre P, et al: CD40L stabilizes arterial thrombi by a beta3 integrin—Dependent mechanism. *Nat Med* 8(3):247–252, 2002.
53. Angelillo-Scherrer A, et al: Role of Gas6 receptors in platelet signaling during thrombus stabilization and implications for antithrombotic therapy. *J Clin Invest* 115(2):237–246, 2005.
54. Balogh I, et al: Analysis of Gas6 in human platelets and plasma. *Arterioscler Thromb Vasc Biol* 25(6):1280–1286, 2005.
55. Gould WR, et al: Gas6 receptors Axl, Sky and Mer enhance platelet activation and regulate thrombotic responses. *J Thromb Haemost* 3(4):733–741, 2005.
56. Maree AO, et al: Growth arrest specific gene (GAS) 6 modulates platelet thrombus formation and vascular wall homeostasis and represents an attractive drug target. *Curr Pharm Des* 13(26):2656–2661, 2007.

57. Saller F, et al: Role of the growth arrest-specific gene 6 (gas6) product in thrombus stabilization. *Blood Cells Mol Dis* 36(3):373–378, 2006.

58. Prevost N, et al: Eph kinases and ephrins support thrombus growth and stability by regulating integrin outside-in signaling in platelets. *Proc Natl Acad Sci U S A* 102(28):9820–9825, 2005.

59. Renne T, et al: Defective thrombus formation in mice lacking coagulation factor XII. *J Exp Med* 202(2):271–281, 2005.

60. Jirouskova M, et al: Antibody blockade or mutation of the fibrinogen gamma-chain C-terminus is more effective in inhibiting murine arterial thrombus formation than complete absence of fibrinogen. *Blood* 103(6):1995–2002, 2004.

61. Loscalzo J, Inbal A, Handin RI: Von Willebrand protein facilitates platelet incorporation in polymerizing fibrin. *J Clin Invest* 78(4):1112–1119, 1986.

62. Deckmyn H, et al: Inhibitors of the interactions between collagen and its receptors on platelets. *Handb Exp Pharmacol* 210:311–337, 2012.

63. George JN, et al: Platelet surface glycoproteins. Studies on resting and activated platelets and platelet membrane microparticles in normal subjects, and observations in patients during adult respiratory distress syndrome and cardiac surgery. *J Clin Invest* 78(2):340–348, 1986.

64. Michelson AD: Thrombin-induced down-regulation of the platelet membrane glycoprotein Ib-IX complex. *Semin Thromb Hemost* 18(1):18–27, 1992.

65. Michelson AD, Barnard MR: Thrombin-induced changes in platelet membrane glycoproteins Ib, IX, and IIb-IIIa complex. *Blood* 70(5):1673–1678, 1987.

66. McEver RP: Properties of GMP-140, an inducible granule membrane protein of platelets and endothelium. *Blood Cells* 16(1):73–80; discussion 80–83, 1990.

67. McEver RP, et al: GMP-140, a platelet alpha-granule membrane protein, is also synthesized by vascular endothelial cells and is localized in Weibel-Palade bodies. *J Clin Invest* 84(1):92–99, 1989.

68. McEver R: P-selectin/PSGL-1 and other interactions between platelets, leukocytes, and endothelium, in *Platelets*, edited by AD Michelson, p 231. Academic Press, San Diego, 2007.

69. Loscalzo J: Nitric oxide insufficiency, platelet activation, and arterial thrombosis. *Circ Res* 88(8):756–762, 2001.

70. Luscher TF: Platelet-vessel wall interaction: Role of nitric oxide, prostaglandins and endothelins. *Baillieres Clin Haematol* 6(3):609–627, 1993.

71. Mitchell JA, et al: Role of nitric oxide and prostacyclin as vasoactive hormones released by the endothelium. *Exp Physiol* 93(1):141–147, 2008.

72. Rex S, Freedman JE: Inhibition of platelet function by the endothelium, in *Platelets*, edited by AD Michelson, pp 251–280. Academic Press, San Diego, 2007.

73. Marcus AJ, et al: The endothelial cell ecto-ADPase responsible for inhibition of platelet function is CD39. *J Clin Invest* 99(6):1351–1360, 1997.

74. Marcus AJ, et al: Inhibition of platelet function by an aspirin-insensitive endothelial cell ADPase. Thromboregulation by endothelial cells. *J Clin Invest* 88(5):1690–1696, 1991.

75. Holme S, et al: Light scatter and total protein signal distribution of platelets by flow cytometry as parameters of size. *J Lab Clin Med* 112(2):223–231, 1988.

76. White J: Anatomy and structural organization of the platelet, in *Hemostasis and Thrombosis: Basic Principles and Clinical Practice*, edited by RW Colman, VJ Marder, EW Salzman, p 397. JB Lippincott, Philadelphia, 1993.

77. Coller BS: Biochemical and electrostatic considerations in primary platelet aggregation. *Ann N Y Acad Sci* 416:693–708, 1983.

78. van Joost T, et al: Purpuric contact dermatitis to benzoyl peroxide. *J Am Acad Dermatol* 22(2 Pt 2):359–361, 1990.

79. Schick P: Megakaryocyte and platelet lipids, in *Hemostasis and Thrombosis: Basic Principles and Clinical Practice*, edited by RW Colman, VJ Marder, EW Salzman, p 574. JB Lippincott, Philadelphia, 1993.

80. Heemskerk JW, Bevers EM, Lindhout T: Platelet activation and blood coagulation. *Thromb Haemost* 88(2):186–193, 2002.

81. Solum NO: Procoagulant expression in platelets and defects leading to clinical disorders. *Arterioscler Thromb Vasc Biol* 19(12):2841–2846, 1999.

82. Sims PJ, et al: Complement proteins C5b-9 cause release of membrane vesicles from the platelet surface that are enriched in the membrane receptor for coagulation factor Va and express prothrombinase activity. *J Biol Chem* 263(34):18205–18212, 1988.

83. Sims PJ, et al: Assembly of the platelet prothrombinase complex is linked to vesiculation of the platelet plasma membrane. Studies in Scott syndrome: An isolated defect in platelet procoagulant activity. *J Biol Chem* 264(29):17049–17057, 1989.

84. Bevers EM, et al: Exposure of endogenous phosphatidylserine at the outer surface of stimulated platelets is reversed by restoration of aminophospholipid translocase activity. *Biochemistry* 28(6):2382–2387, 1989.

85. Comfurius P, Bevers EM, Zwaal RF: The involvement of cytoskeleton in the regulation of transbilayer movement of phospholipids in human blood platelets. *Biochim Biophys Acta* 815(1):143–148, 1985.

86. Tuszynski GP, et al: The platelet cytoskeleton contains elements of the prothrombinase complex. *J Biol Chem* 259(11):6947–6951, 1984.

87. Bodin S, Tronchere H, Payrastre B: Lipid rafts are critical membrane domains in blood platelet activation processes. *Biochim Biophys Acta* 1610(2):247–257, 2003.

88. Locke D, et al: Lipid rafts orchestrate signaling by the platelet receptor glycoprotein VI. *J Biol Chem* 277(21):18801–18809, 2002.

89. Shrimpton CN, et al: Localization of the adhesion receptor glycoprotein Ib-IX-V complex to lipid rafts is required for platelet adhesion and activation. *J Exp Med* 196(8):1057–1066, 2002.

90. Heijnen HF, et al: Concentration of rafts in platelet filopodia correlates with recruitment of c-Src and CD63 to these domains. *J Thromb Haemost* 1(6):1161–1173, 2003.

91. Bodin S, et al: Production of phosphatidylinositol 3,4,5-trisphosphate and phosphatidic acid in platelet rafts: Evidence for a critical role of cholesterol-enriched domains in human platelet activation. *Biochemistry* 40(50):15290–15299, 2001.

92. Baglia FA, et al: The glycoprotein Ib-IX-V complex mediates localization of factor XI to lipid rafts on the platelet membrane. *J Biol Chem* 278(24):21744–21750, 2003.

93. Brownlow SL, et al: A role for hTRPC1 and lipid raft domains in store-mediated calcium entry in human platelets. *Cell Calcium* 35(2):107–113, 2004.

94. Lopez JA, del Conde I, Shrimpton CN: Receptors, rafts, and microvesicles in thrombosis and inflammation. *J Thromb Haemost* 3(8):1737–1744, 2005.

95. White JG: Anatomy and structural organization of the platelet, in *Hemostasis and Thrombosis: Basic Principles and Clinical Practice*, edited by RW Colman, VJ Marder, EW Salzman, pp 397–413. JB Lippincott, Philadelphia, 1993.

96. Behnke O: The morphology of blood platelet membrane systems. *Ser Haematol* 3(4):3–16, 1970.

97. White JG: Electron microscopic studies of platelet secretion. *Prog Hemost Thromb* 2:49, 1974.

98. Suzuki H, Yamazaki H, Tanoue K: Immunocytochemical studies on co-localization of alpha-granule membrane alphaIIbbeta3 integrin and intragranular fibrinogen of human platelets and their cell-surface expression during the thrombin-induced release reaction. *J Electron Microsc (Tokyo)* 52(2):183–195, 1970.

99. Stenberg PE, Shuman MA, Levine SP, Bainton DF: Redistribution of α granules and their contents in thrombin-stimulated platelets. *J Cell Biol* 98:748–760, 1984.

100. Ginsberg MH, Taylor L, Painter RG: The mechanism of thrombin-induced platelet factor 4 secretion. *Blood* 55:661, 1980.

101. Nurden P, Heilmann E, Paponneau A, Nurden A: Two-way trafficking of membrane glycoproteins on thrombin-activated human platelets. *Semin Hematol* 31(3):240–250, 1994.

102. Michelson AD, Barnard MR: Plasmin-induced redistribution of platelet glycoprotein Ib. *Blood* 76(10):2005–2010, 1990.

103. Suzuki H, Nakamura S, Itoh Y, et al: Immunocytochemical evidence for the translocation of α-granule membrane glycoprotein IIb/IIIa (integrin αIIbβ3) of human platelets to the surface membrane during the release reaction. *Histochemistry* 97:381–388, 1992.

104. Suzuki H, Murasaki K, Kodama K, Takayama H: Intracellular localization of glycoprotein VI in human platelets and its surface expression upon activation. *Br J Haematol* 121(6):904–912, 2003.

105. Nurden P, Poujol C, Winckler J, et al: Immunolocalization of P2Y1 and TPalpha receptors in platelets showed a major pool associated with the membranes of alpha-granules and the open canalicular system. *Blood* 101(4):1400–1408, 2003.

106. Breton-Gorius J, Guichard J: Ultrastructural localization of peroxidase activity in human platelets and megakaryocytes. *Am J Pathol* 66:277, 1986.

107. Cramer EM: Platelets and megakaryocytes: Anatomy and structural organization, in *Hemostasis and Thrombosis: Basic Principles in Clinical Practice*, edited by RW Colman, J Hirsh, VJ Marder, AW Clowes, and JN George, pp 411–428. Lippincott, Williams & Wilkins, Philadelphia, 2001.

108. White JG: Interaction of membrane systems in blood platelets. *Am J Pathol* 66(2):295–312, 1972.

109. Menashi S, Davis C, Crawford N: Calcium uptake associated with an intracellular membrane fraction prepared from human blood platelets by high-voltage, free-flow electrophoresis. *FEBS Lett* 140:298, 1982.

110. Robblee LS, Shepro D, Belamarich FA: Calcium uptake and associated adenosine triphosphate activity of isolated platelet membranes. *J Gen Physiol* 61:462, 1973.

111. Hartwig JH: Platelet morphology, in *Thrombosis and Hemorrhage*, edited by J Loscalzo, AI Schafer, pp 207–228. Williams & Wilkins, Baltimore, 1999.

112. Michalak M, Mariani P, Opas M: Calreticulin, a multifunctional Ca2+ binding chaperone of the endoplasmic reticulum. *Biochem Cell Biol* 76(5):779–785, 1998.

113. Brownlow SL, Sage SO: Rapid agonist-evoked coupling of type II Ins(1,4,5)P3 receptor with human transient receptor potential (hTRPC1) channels in human platelets. *Biochem J* 375(Pt 3):697–704, 2003.

114. van Gorp RM, et al: Irregular spiking in free calcium concentration in single, human platelets. Regulation by modulation of the inositol trisphosphate receptors. *Eur J Biochem* 269(5):1543–1552, 2002.

115. Käser-Glanzmann R, Jakábová M, George JN, Lüscher EF: Further characterization of calcium accumulating vesicles from human blood platelets. *Biochim Biophys Acta* 542:357, 1978.

116. Tertyshnikova S, Fein A: Inhibition of inositol 1,4,5-trisphosphate-induced Ca2+ release by cAMP-dependent protein kinase in a living cell. *Proc Natl Acad Sci U S A* 95(4):1613–1617, 1998.

117. Pernollet MG, Lantoine F, Devynck MA: Nitric oxide inhibits ATP-dependent Ca$^{2+}$ uptake into platelet membrane vesicles. *Biochem Biophys Res Commun* 222(3):780–785, 1996.

118. Teijeiro RG, et al: Calcium efflux from platelet vesicles of the dense tubular system. Analysis of the possible contribution of the Ca$^{2+}$ pump. *Mol Cell Biochem* 199(1–2):7–14, 1999.

119. Bergmeier W, Stefanini L: Novel molecules in calcium signaling in platelets. *J Thromb Haemost* 7(Suppl 1):187–190, 2009.

120. Dziadek MA, Johnstone LS: Biochemical properties and cellular localisation of STIM proteins. *Cell Calcium* 42(2):123–132, 2007.

121. Grosse J, et al: An EF hand mutation in Stim1 causes premature platelet activation and bleeding in mice. *J Clin Invest* 117(11):3540–3550, 2007.

122. Varga-Szabo D, et al: The calcium sensor STIM1 is an essential mediator of arterial thrombosis and ischemic brain infarction. *J Exp Med* 205(7):1583–1591, 2008.

123. Bergmeier W, et al: R93W mutation in Orai1 causes impaired calcium influx in platelets. *Blood* 113(3):675–678, 2009.

124. Braun A, et al: Orai1 (CRACM1) is the platelet SOC channel and essential for pathological thrombus formation. *Blood* 113(9):2056–2063, 2009.

125. Feske S, et al: A mutation in Orai1 causes immune deficiency by abrogating CRAC channel function. *Nature* 441(7090):179–185, 2006.

126. Feske S, et al: Severe combined immunodeficiency due to defective binding of the nuclear factor of activated T cells in T lymphocytes of two male siblings. *Eur J Immunol* 26(9):2119–2126, 1996.

127. Picard C, et al: STIM1 mutation associated with a syndrome of immunodeficiency and autoimmunity. *N Engl J Med* 360(19):1971–1980, 2009.

128. Redondo PC, et al: Intracellular Ca2+ store depletion induces the formation of macromolecular complexes involving hTRPC1, hTRPC6, the type II IP3 receptor and SERCA3 in human platelets. *Biochim Biophys Acta* 1783(6):1163–1176, 2008.

129. Sage SO, Brownlow SL, Rosado JA: TRP channels and calcium entry in human platelets. *Blood* 100(12):4245–4246, 2002.

130. Varga-Szabo D, et al: Store-operated Ca(2+) entry in platelets occurs independently of transient receptor potential (TRP) C1. *Pflugers Arch* 457(2):377–387, 2008.

131. Gerrard JM, White JG, Rao GH, Townsend D: Localization of platelet prostaglandin production in the platelet dense tubular system. *Am J Pathol* 83(2):283–298, 1976.

132. Picot D, Loll PJ, Garavito RM: The X-ray crystal structure of the membrane protein prostaglandin H2 synthase-1. *Nature* 367(6460):243–249, 1994.

133. Fox JE: The platelet cytoskeleton. *Thromb Haemost* 70(6):884–893, 1993.

134. Fox JE, et al: Identification of a membrane skeleton in platelets. *J Cell Biol* 106(5):1525–1538, 1988.

135. Fox JE, et al: Spectrin is associated with membrane-bound actin filaments in platelets and is hydrolyzed by the Ca2+-dependent protease during platelet activation. *Blood* 69(2):537–545, 1987.

136. Hartwig JH, DeSisto M: The cytoskeleton of the resting human blood platelet: Structure of the membrane skeleton and its attachment to actin filaments. *J Cell Biol* 112(3):407–425, 1991.

137. Barkalow KL, et al: Alpha-adducin dissociates from F-actin and spectrin during platelet activation. *J Cell Biol* 161(3):557–570, 2003.

138. Kaiser HW, O'Keefe E, Bennett V: Adducin: Ca++-dependent association with sites of cell-cell contact. *J Cell Biol* 109(2):557–569, 1989.

139. Kuhlman PA, et al: A new function for adducin. Calcium/calmodulin-regulated capping of the barbed ends of actin filaments. *J Biol Chem* 271(14):7986–7991, 1996.

140. Matsuoka Y, Li X, Bennett V: Adducin: Structure, function and regulation. *Cell Mol Life Sci* 57(6):884–895, 2000.

141. Calderwood DA, et al: Increased filamin binding to beta-integrin cytoplasmic domains inhibits cell migration. *Nat Cell Biol* 3(12):1060–1068, 2001.

142. Ithychanda SS, et al: Migfilin, a molecular switch in regulation of integrin activation. *J Biol Chem* 284(7):4713–4722, 2009.

143. Kiema T, et al: The molecular basis of filamin binding to integrins and competition with talin. *Mol Cell* 21(3):337–347, 2006.

144. Tadokoro S, et al: Talin binding to integrin beta tails: A final common step in integrin activation. *Science* 302(5642):103–106, 2003.

145. Tremuth L, et al: A fluorescence cell biology approach to map the second integrin-binding site of talin to a 130-amino acid sequence within the rod domain. *J Biol Chem* 279(21):22258–22266, 2004.

146. Ulmer TS, et al: NMR analysis of structure and dynamics of the cytosolic tails of integrin alpha IIb beta 3 in aqueous solution. *Biochemistry* 40(25):7498–7508, 2001.

147. Vinogradova O, et al: A structural mechanism of integrin alpha(IIb)beta(3) "inside-out" activation as regulated by its cytoplasmic face. *Cell* 110(5):587–597, 2002.

148. Yan B, et al: Calpain cleavage promotes talin binding to the beta 3 integrin cytoplasmic domain. *J Biol Chem* 276(30):28164–28170, 2001.

149. Zhu J, et al: Structure of a complete integrin ectodomain in a physiologic resting state and activation and deactivation by applied forces. *Mol Cell* 32(6):849–861, 2008.

150. Podor TJ, et al: Vimentin exposed on activated platelets and platelet microparticles localizes vitronectin and plasminogen activator inhibitor complexes on their surface. *J Biol Chem* 277(9):7529–7539, 2002.

151. Cramer EM, et al: Ultrastructure of platelet formation by human megakaryocytes cultured with the Mpl ligand. *Blood* 89(7):2336–2346, 1997.

152. Italiano JE Jr, et al: Blood platelets are assembled principally at the ends of proplatelet processes produced by differentiated megakaryocytes. *J Cell Biol* 147(6):1299–1312, 1999.

153. Italiano JE, Hartwig JH: Megakaryocyte development and platelet formation, in *Platelets*, edited by A Michelson, p 23. Academic Press, San Diego, 2007.

154. Hartwig J: Platelet structure, in *Platelets*, edited by A Michelson, p 75. Academic Press, San Diego, 2007.

155. Crawford N, Scrutton MC: Biochemistry of the blood platelet, in *Haemostasis and Thrombosis*, edited by AL Bloom, DP Thomas, EGD Tuddenham, p 89. Churchill Livingstone, London, England, 1994.

156. Miki H, Okada Y, Hirokawa N: Analysis of the kinesin superfamily: Insights into structure and function. *Trends Cell Biol* 15(9):467–476, 2005.

157. Pfister KK, et al: Genetic analysis of the cytoplasmic dynein subunit families. *PLoS Genet* 2(1):e1, 2006.

158. Sheetz MP: Microtubule motor complexes moving membranous organelles. *Cell Struct Funct* 21(5):369–373, 1996.

159. Patel-Hett S, et al: Visualization of microtubule growth in living platelets reveals a dynamic marginal band with multiple microtubules. *Blood* 111(9):4605–4616, 2008.

160. Kenney DM, Linck RW: The cytoskeleton of unstimulated blood platelets: Structure and composition of the isolated marginal microtubular band. *J Cell Sci* 78:1–22, 1985.

161. Aslan JE, et al: Histone deacetylase 6-mediated deacetylation of alpha-tubulin coordinates cytoskeletal and signaling events during platelet activation. *Am J Physiol Cell Physiol* 305(12):C1230–C1239, 2013.

162. Sadoul K, et al: HDAC6 controls the kinetics of platelet activation. *Blood* 120(20):4215–4218, 2012.

163. Italiano JE Jr, et al: Mechanisms and implications of platelet discoid shape. *Blood* 101(12):4789–4796, 2003.

164. Freson K, et al: The TUBB1 Q43P functional polymorphism reduces the risk of cardiovascular disease in men by modulating platelet function and structure. *Blood* 106(7):2356–2362, 2005.

165. Kunishima S, et al: Mutation of the beta1-tubulin gene associated with congenital macrothrombocytopenia affecting microtubule assembly. *Blood* 113(2):458–461, 2009.

166. Navarro-Nunez L, et al: Rare homozygous status of P43 beta1-tubulin polymorphism causes alterations in platelet ultrastructure. *Thromb Haemost* 105(5):855–863, 2011.

167. Kunishima S, et al: TUBB1 mutation disrupting microtubule assembly impairs proplatelet formation and results in congenital macrothrombocytopenia. *Eur J Haematol* 92(4):276–282, 2014.

168. Kunishima S, et al: Mutation of the beta1-tubulin gene associated with congenital macrothrombocytopenia affecting microtubule assembly. *Blood* 113(2):458–461, 2009.

169. Nachmias VT, Yoshida K: The cytoskeleton of the blood platelet: A dynamic structure. *Adv Cell Biol* 2:181–211, 1988.

170. Safer D, Nachmias VT: Beta thymosins as actin binding peptides. *Bioessays* 16(8):590, 1994.

171. Rosenberg S, Stracher A: Effect of actin-binding protein on the sedimentation properties of actin. *J Cell Biol* 94(1):51–55, 1982.

172. Rosenberg S, Stracher A, Burridge K: Isolation and characterization of a calcium-sensitive alpha-actinin-like protein from human platelet cytoskeletons. *J Biol Chem* 256(24):12986–12991, 1981.

173. Rosenberg S, Stracher A, Lucas RC: Isolation and characterization of actin and actin-binding protein from human platelets. *J Cell Biol* 91(1):201–211, 1981.

174. Fucini P, et al: The repeating segments of the F-actin cross-linking gelation factor (ABP-120) have an immunoglobulin-like fold. *Nat Struct Biol* 4(3):223–230, 1997.

175. Gorlin JB, et al: Human endothelial actin-binding protein (ABP-280, nonmuscle filamin): A molecular leaf spring. *J Cell Biol* 111(3):1089–1105, 1990.

176. Gorlin JB, et al: Actin-binding protein (ABP-280) filamin gene (FLN) maps telomeric to the color vision locus (R/GCP) and centromeric to G6PD in Xq28. *Genomics* 17(2):496–498, 1993.

177. Takafuta T, et al: Human beta-filamin is a new protein that interacts with the cytoplasmic tail of glycoprotein Ibalpha. *J Biol Chem* 273(28):17531–17538, 1998.

178. Ohta Y, et al: The small GTPase RalA targets filamin to induce filopodia. *Proc Natl Acad Sci U S A* 96(5):2122–2128, 1999.

179. Stossel TP, et al: Filamins as integrators of cell mechanics and signalling. *Nat Rev Mol Cell Biol* 2(2):138–145, 2001.

180. Kovacsovics TJ, Hartwig JH: Thrombin-induced GPIb-IX centralization on the platelet surface requires actin assembly and myosin II activation. *Blood* 87(2):618–629, 1996.

181. Meyer SC, et al: Identification of the region in actin-binding protein that binds to the cytoplasmic domain of glycoprotein IBalpha. *J Biol Chem* 272(5):2914–2919, 1997.

182. Karpatkin S, Langer RM: Biochemical energetics of simulated platelet plug formation. Effect of thrombin, adenosine diphosphate, and epinephrine on intra- and extracellular adenine nucleotide kinetics. *J Clin Invest* 47(9):2158–2168, 1968.

183. Akkerman JW, et al: A novel technique for rapid determination of energy consumption in platelets. Demonstration of different energy consumption associated with three secretory responses. *Biochem J* 210(1):145–155, 1983.

184. Akkerman JW, Holmsen H: Interrelationships among platelet responses: Studies on the burst in proton liberation, lactate production, and oxygen uptake during platelet aggregation and Ca2+ secretion. *Blood* 57(5):956–966, 1981.

185. Guppy M, et al: Fuel choices by human platelets in human plasma. *Eur J Biochem* 244(1):161–167, 1997.

186. Holmsen H, Farstad M: Energy metabolism, in *Platelet Responses and Metabolism*, edited by H Holmsen, p 245. CRC Press, Boca Raton, FL, 1987.

187. Akkerman JWN, Verhgoeven AJM: Energy metabolism and function, in *Platelet Responses and Metabolism*, edited by H Holmsen, p 69. CRC Press, Boca Raton, FL, 1987.

188. Shimizu T, Murphy S: Roles of acetate and phosphate in the successful storage of platelet concentrates prepared with an acetate-containing additive solution. *Transfusion* 33(4):304–310, 1993.

189. Dean WL: Structure, function and subcellular localization of a human platelet Ca2+-ATPase. *Cell Calcium* 10(5):289–297, 1989.

190. Simons ER, Greenberg-Sperssky SM: Transmembrane monovalent cation gradients, in *Platelet Responses and Metabolism*, edited by H Holmsen, p 31. CRC Press, Boca Raton, FL, 1987.

191. Daniel JL, et al: Nucleotide exchange between cytosolic ATP and F-actin-bound ADP may be a major energy-utilizing process in unstimulated platelets. *Eur J Biochem* 156(3):677–684, 1986.

192. Verhoeven AJ, et al: Turnover of the phosphomonoester groups of polyphosphoinositol lipids in unstimulated human platelets. *Eur J Biochem* 166(1):3–9, 1987.

193. Akkerman JW, Holmsen H, Driver HA: Platelet aggregation and Ca2+ secretion are independent of simultaneous ATP production. *FEBS Lett* 100(2):286–290, 1979.

194. van den Bosch H, de Vet EC, Zomer AW: The role of peroxisomes in ether lipid synthesis. Back to the roots of PAF. *Adv Exp Med Biol* 416:33–40, 1996.

195. van den Bosch H, et al: Ether lipid synthesis and its deficiency in peroxisomal disorders. *Biochimie* 75(3–4):183–189, 1993.

196. Wanders RJ, et al: Deficiency of acyl-CoA:dihydroxyacetone phosphate acyltransferase in thrombocytes of Zellweger patients: A simple postnatal diagnostic test. *Clin Chim Acta* 151(3):217–221, 1985.

197. Holmsen H: Platelet secretion and energy metabolism, in *Hemostasis and Thrombosis: Basic Principles and Clinical Practice*, edited by RW Colman, VJ Marder, EW Salzman, p 524. JB Lippincott, Philadelphia, 1993.

198. Shuster RC, Rubenstein AJ, Wallace DC: Mitochondrial DNA in anucleate human blood cells. *Biochem Biophys Res Commun* 155(3):1360–1365, 1988.

199. Boudreau LH, et al: Platelets release mitochondria serving as substrate for bactericidal group IIA-secreted phospholipase A2 to promote inflammation. *Blood* 124(14):2173–2183, 2014.

200. Mason KD, et al: Programmed anuclear cell death delimits platelet life span. *Cell* 128(6):1173–1186, 2007.

201. Cardoso SM, et al: Cytochrome c oxidase is decreased in Alzheimer's disease platelets. *Neurobiol Aging* 25(1):105–110, 2004.

202. Dror N, et al: State-dependent alterations in mitochondrial complex I activity in platelets: A potential peripheral marker for schizophrenia. *Mol Psychiatry* 7(9):995–1001, 2002.

203. Lenaz G, et al: Mitochondrial complex I defects in aging. *Mol Cell Biochem* 174(1–2):329–333, 1997.

204. Lenaz G, et al: Mitochondrial bioenergetics in aging. *Biochim Biophys Acta* 1459(2–3):397–404, 2000.

205. Mancuso M, et al: Decreased platelet cytochrome c oxidase activity is accompanied by increased blood lactate concentration during exercise in patients with Alzheimer disease. *Exp Neurol* 182(2):421–426, 2003.

206. Schapira AH: Mitochondrial dysfunction in neurodegenerative disorders. *Biochim Biophys Acta* 1366(1–2):225–233, 1998.

207. Yamagishi SI, et al: Hyperglycemia potentiates collagen-induced platelet activation through mitochondrial superoxide overproduction. *Diabetes* 50(6):1491–1494, 2001.

208. Dale GL, Friese P: Bax activators potentiate coated-platelet formation. *J Thromb Haemost* 4(12):2664–2669, 2006.

209. Jobe SM, et al: Critical role for the mitochondrial permeability transition pore and cyclophilin D in platelet activation and thrombosis. *Blood* 111(3):1257–1265, 2008.

210. Leung R, et al: Persistence of procoagulant surface expression on activated human platelets: Involvement of apoptosis and aminophospholipid translocase activity. *J Thromb Haemost* 5(3):560–570, 2007.

211. Remenyi G, et al: Role of mitochondrial permeability transition pore in coated-platelet formation. *Arterioscler Thromb Vasc Biol* 25(2):467–471, 2005.

212. Nachmias VT: Platelet and megakaryocyte shape change: Triggered alterations in the cytoskeleton. *Semin Hematol* 20(4):261–281, 1983.

213. Maurer-Spurej E, Devine DV: Platelet aggregation is not initiated by platelet shape change. *Lab Invest* 81(11):1517–1525, 2001.

214. Born GV, et al: Quantification of the morphological reaction of platelets to aggregating agents and of its reversal by aggregation inhibitors. *J Physiol* 280:193–212, 1978.

215. Coller BS: Biochemical and electrostatic considerations in primary platelet aggregation. *Ann N Y Acad Sci* 416:693–708, 1983.

216. Hartwig JH, et al: The elegant platelet: Signals controlling actin assembly. *Thromb Haemost* 82:392–398, 1999.

217. Falet H, et al: Importance of free actin filament barbed ends for Arp2/3 complex function in platelets and fibroblasts. *Proc Natl Acad Sci U S A* 99(26):16782–16787, 2002.

218. Carlier MF, et al: Tbeta 4 is not a simple G-actin sequestering protein and interacts with F-actin at high concentration. *J Biol Chem* 271(16):9231–9239, 1996.

219. Lind SE, Yin HL, Stossel TP: Human platelets contain gelsolin. A regulator of actin filament length. *J Clin Invest* 69(6):1384–1387, 1982.

220. Barkalow K, Hartwig JH: The role of actin filament barbed-end exposure in cytoskeletal dynamics and cell motility. *Biochem Soc Trans* 23(3):451–456, 1995.

221. Barkalow K, et al: A-Adducin dissociates from F-actin filaments and spectrin during platelet activation. *J Cell Biol* 161:557–570, 2003.

222. Machesky LM, Gould KL: The Arp2/3 complex: A multifunctional actin organizer. *Curr Opin Cell Biol* 11(1):117–121, 1999.

223. Mullins RD, Heuser JA, Pollard TD: The interaction of Arp2/3 complex with actin: Nucleation, high affinity pointed end capping, and formation of branching networks of filaments. *Proc Natl Acad Sci U S A* 95(11):6181–6186, 1998.

224. Heemskerk JW, et al: Collagen but not fibrinogen surfaces induce bleb formation, exposure of phosphatidylserine, and procoagulant activity of adherent platelets:

Evidence for regulation by protein tyrosine kinase-dependent Ca2+ responses. *Blood* 90(7):2615–2625, 1997.

225. Watson SP: Collagen receptor signaling in platelets and megakaryocytes. *Thromb Haemost* 82(2):365–376, 1999.

226. Jirouskova M, Jaiswal JK, Coller BS: Ligand density dramatically affects integrin alpha IIb beta 3-mediated platelet signaling and spreading. *Blood* 109(5260):5269, 2007.

227. Coller BS, et al: Studies of activated GPIIb/IIIa receptors on the luminal surface of adherent platelets. Paradoxical loss of luminal receptors when platelets adhere to high density fibrinogen. *J Clin Invest* 92:2796–2806, 1993.

228. Patel D, et al: The dynamics of GPIIb/IIIa-mediated platelet-platelet interactions in platelet adhesion/thrombus formation on collagen in vitro as revealed by videomicroscopy. *Blood* 101:929–936, 2003.

229. Fox JE: On the role of calpain and Rho proteins in regulating integrin-induced signaling. *Thromb Haemost* 82(2):385–391, 1999.

230. Hartwig JH, et al: Thrombin receptor ligation and activated Rac uncap actin filament barbed ends through phosphoinositide synthesis in permeabilized human platelets. *Cell* 82(4):643–653, 1995.

231. Lemmon MA, Ferguson KM, Abrams CS: Pleckstrin homology domains and the cytoskeleton. *FEBS Lett* 513(1):71–76, 2002.

232. Ma AD, Abrams CS: Pleckstrin homology domains and phospholipid-induced cytoskeletal reorganization. *Thromb Haemost* 82(2):399–406, 1999.

233. Lian L, Wang Y, Flick M, et al: Loss of pleckstrin defines a novel pathway for PKC-mediated exocytosis. *Blood* 113(15):3577–3584, 2009.

234. Hitchcock IS, et al: Roles of focal adhesion kinase (FAK) in megakaryopoiesis and platelet function: Studies using a megakaryocyte lineage specific FAK knockout. *Blood* 111(2):596–604, 2008.

235. Coller BS, Shattil SJ: The GPIIb/IIIa (integrin alphaIIbbeta3) odyssey: A technology-driven saga of a receptor with twists, turns, and even a bend. *Blood* 112(8):3011–3025, 2008.

236. Pabla R, et al: Integrin-dependent control of translation: Engagement of integrin alphaIIbbeta3 regulates synthesis of proteins in activated human platelets. *J Cell Biol* 144(1):175–184, 1999.

237. Shattil SJ: Signaling through platelet integrin αIIbβ3: Inside-out, outside-in and sideways. *Thromb Haemost* 82(2):318–325, 1999.

238. Shattil SJ, Newman PJ: Integrins: Dynamic scaffolds for adhesion and signaling in platelets. *Blood* 104(6):1606–1615, 2004.

239. Kulkarni S, et al: Conversion of platelets from a proaggregatory to a proinflammatory adhesive phenotype: Role of PAF in spatially regulating neutrophil adhesion and spreading. *Blood* 110(6):1879–1886, 2007.

240. Cho J, Mosher DF: Role of fibronectin assembly in platelet thrombus formation. *J Thromb Haemost* 4(7):1461–1469, 2006.

241. George JN, et al: Platelet surface glycoproteins. Studies on resting and activated platelets and platelet membrane microparticles in normal subjects, and observations in patients during adult respiratory distress syndrome and cardiac surgery. *J Clin Invest* 78:340–348, 1986.

242. Michelson AD: Thrombin-induced down-regulation of the platelet membrane glycoprotein Ib-IX complex. *Semin Thromb Hemost* 18:18–27, 1992.

243. Bennett JS, et al: The platelet cytoskeleton regulates the affinity of the integrin alpha(IIb)beta(3) for fibrinogen. *J Biol Chem* 274(36):25301–25307, 1999.

244. Patil S, et al: Identification of a talin-binding site in the integrin beta(3) subunit distinct from the NPLY regulatory motif of post-ligand binding functions. The talin n-terminal head domain interacts with the membrane-proximal region of the beta(3) cytoplasmic tail. *J Biol Chem* 274(40):28575–28583, 1999.

245. Tadokoro S, et al: Talin binding to integrin beta tails: A final common step in integrin activation. *Science* 302(5642):103–106, 2003.

246. Yan B, et al: Calpain cleavage promotes talin binding to the beta 3 integrin cytoplasmic domain. *J Biol Chem* 276(30):28164–28170, 2001.

247. Shattil SJ, Brugge JS: Protein tyrosine phosphorylation and the adhesive functions of platelets. *Curr Opin Cell Biol* 3:869–879, 1991.

248. Fox JE: The platelet cytoskeleton. *Thromb Haemost* 70(6):884–893, 1993.

249. Fox JE: Platelet cytoskeleton, in *Hemostasis and Thrombosis: Basic Principles and Clinical Practice*, edited by RW Colman, J Hirsh, VJ Marder, AW Clowes, JN George, pp 429–446. Lippincott, Williams & Wilkins, Philadelphia, 2001.

250. Zhu J, Luo BH, Xiao T, et al: Structure of a complete integrin ectodomain in a physiologic resting state and activation and deactivation by applied forces. *Mol Cell* 32(6):849–861, 2008.

251. Li R, et al: Activation of integrin alphaIIbbeta3 by modulation of transmembrane helix associations. *Science* 300(5620):795–798, 2003.

252. Olorundare OE, Simmons SR, Albrecht RM: Cytochalasin D and E: Effects on fibrinogen receptor movement and cytoskeletal reorganization in fully spread, surface-activated platelets: A correlative light and electron microscopic investigation. *Blood* 79(1):99–109, 1992.

253. White JG: Induction of patching and its reversal on surface-activated human platelets. *Br J Haematol* 76(1):108–115, 1990.

254. Fox JE, et al: Identification of two proteins (actin-binding protein and P235) that are hydrolyzed by endogenous Ca++-dependent protease during platelet aggregation. *J Biol Chem* 260:1060–1066, 1985.

255. Fox JE, Reynolds CC, Phillips DR: Calcium-dependent proteolysis occurs during platelet aggregation. *J Biol Chem* 258(16):9973–9981, 1983.

256. Fox JE, et al: Evidence that activation of platelet calpain is induced as a consequence of binding of adhesive ligand to the integrin, glycoprotein IIb-IIIa. *J Cell Biol* 120(6):1501–1507, 1993.

257. Xi X, et al: Critical roles for the COOH-terminal NITY and RGT sequences of the integrin beta3 cytoplasmic domain in inside-out and outside-in signaling. *J Cell Biol* 162(2):329–339, 2003.

258. Flevaris P, et al: A molecular switch that controls cell spreading and retraction. *J Cell Biol* 179(3):553–565, 2007.

259. Dachary-Prigent J, et al: Annexin V as a probe of aminophospholipid exposure and platelet membrane vesiculation: A flow cytometry study showing a role for free sulfhydryl groups. *Blood* 81:2554–2565, 1993.

260. Azam M, et al: Disruption of the mouse mu-calpain gene reveals an essential role in platelet function. *Mol Cell Biol* 21(6):2213–2220, 2001.

261. Furman MI, Gardner TM, Goldschmidt-Clermont PJ: Mechanisms of cytoskeletal reorganization during platelet activation. *Thromb Haemost* 70(1):229–232, 1993.

262. McNicol A, Israels SJ: Platelet dense granules: Structure, function and implications for haemostasis. *Thromb Res* 95(1):1–18, 1999.

263. Leon C, et al: Megakaryocyte-restricted MYH9 inactivation dramatically affects hemostasis while preserving platelet aggregation and secretion. *Blood* 110(9):3183–3191, 2007.

264. Escolar G, Krumwiede M, White JG: Organization of the actin cytoskeleton of resting and activated platelets in suspension. *Am J Pathol* 123:86–94, 1986.

265. Fox JE, et al: Actin filament content and organization in unstimulated platelets. *J Cell Biol* 98:1985–1991, 1984.

266. Hartwig JH: Platelet structure, in *Platelets*, edited by AD Michelson, pp 75–97. Academic Press, San Diego, 2007.

267. Nachmias VT, Yoshida K: The cytoskeleton of the blood platelets: A dynamic structure. *Adv Cyclic Nucleotide Res* 2:181–211, 1999.

268. Weber A, et al: Interaction of thymosin-$\beta$-4 with muscle and platelet actin. Implications for actin sequestration in resting platelets. *Biochemistry* 31(27):6179–6185, 1992.

269. Gonnella PA, Nachmias VT: Platelet activation and microfilament bundling. *J Biol Chem* 89:146, 1981.

270. Nachmias VT: Cytoskeleton of human platelets at rest and after spreading. *J Cell Biol* 86:795, 1980.

271. Budtz-Olsen OE: *Clot Retraction*. Charles C Thomas, Springfield, 1951.

272. Stalker TJ, et al: A systems approach to hemostasis: 3. Thrombus consolidation regulates intrathrombus solute transport and local thrombin activity. *Blood* 124(11):1824–1831, 2014.

273. Kunitada S, FitzGerald GA, Fitzgerald DJ: Inhibition of clot lysis and decreased binding of tissue-type plasminogen activator as a consequence of clot retraction. *Blood* 79(6):1420–1427, 1992.

274. Cohen I, Gerrard JM, White JG: Ultrastructure of clots during isometric contraction. *J Cell Biol* 93:775-787, 1982.

275. Pollard TD, et al: Contractile proteins in platelet activation and contraction. *Ann N Y Acad Sci* 283:218, 1977.

276. Vaiyapuri S, et al: EphB2 regulates contact-dependent and contact-independent signaling to control platelet function. *Blood* 125(4):720–730, 2015.

277. Khatlani T, et al: The beta isoform of the catalytic subunit of protein phosphatase 2B restrains platelet function by suppressing outside-in alphaII b beta3 integrin signaling. *J Thromb Haemost* 12(12):2089–2101, 2014.

278. Yi W, Li Q, Shen J, et al: Modulation of platelet activation and thrombus formation using a pan-PI3K inhibitor S14161. *PLoS One* 9(8):e102394, 2014.

279. Cohen I: The mechanism of clot retraction, in *Platelet Membrane Glycoproteins*, edited by JN George, AT Nurden, DR Phillips, pp 299–323. Plenum Press, New York, 1985.

280. Carr ME Jr, et al: Glycoprotein IIb/IIIa blockade inhibits platelet-mediated force development and reduces gel elastic modulus. *Thromb Haemost* 73:499–505, 1995.

281. Leistikow EA: Platelet internalization in early thrombogenesis. *Semin Thromb Hemost* 22(3):289–294, 1996.

282. Morgenstern E, Daub M, Dierichs R: A new model for *in vitro* clot formation that considers the mode of the fibrin(ogen) contacts to platelets and the arrangement of the platelet cytoskeleton. *Ann N Y Acad Sci* 936:449–455, 2001.

283. Braaten JV, Jerome WG, Hantgan RR: Uncoupling fibrin from integrin receptors hastens fibrinolysis at the platelet-fibrin interface. *Blood* 83:982–993, 1994.

284. Coller BS, et al: A murine monoclonal antibody that completely blocks the binding of fibrinogen to platelets produces a thrombasthenic-like state in normal platelets and binds to glycoproteins IIb and/or IIIa. *J Clin Invest* 72:325–338, 1983.

285. Collet JP, et al: A structural and dynamic investigation of the facilitating effect of glycoprotein IIb/IIIa inhibitors in dissolving platelet-rich clots. *Circ Res* 90(4):428–434, 2002.

286. Huang TC, et al: Differential effects of c7E3 Fab on thrombus formation and rt-PA-mediated thrombolysis under flow conditions. *Thromb Res* 102(5):411–425, 2001.

287. Mousa SA, Khurana S, Forsythe MS: Comparative *in vitro* efficacy of different platelet glycoprotein IIb/IIIa antagonists on platelet-mediated clot strength induced by tissue factor with use of thromboelastography: Differentiation among glycoprotein IIb/IIIa antagonists. *Arterioscler Thromb Vasc Biol* 20(4):1162–1167, 2000.

288. Seiffert D, et al: Regulation of clot retraction by glycoprotein IIb/IIIa antagonists. *Thromb Res* 108(2–3):181–189, 2002.

289. Jirouskova M, et al: A hamster antibody to the mouse fibrinogen gamma chain inhibits platelet-fibrinogen interactions and FXIIIa-mediated fibrin cross-linking, and facilitates thrombolysis. *Thromb Haemost* 86(4):1047–1056, 2001.

290. Mor-Cohen R, et al: Disulfide bond exchanges in integrins alphaIIbbeta3 and alphavbeta3 are required for activation and post-ligation signaling during clot retraction. *Thromb Res* 133(5):826–836, 2014.

291. Law DA, et al: Integrin cytoplasmic tyrosine motif is required for outside-in alphaIIbbeta3 signalling and platelet function. *Nature* 401:808–811, 1999.

292. Osdoit S, Rosa JP: Fibrin clot retraction by human platelets correlates with alpha(IIb) beta(3) integrin-dependent protein tyrosine dephosphorylation. *J Biol Chem* 276(9): 6703–6710, 2001.

293. Flevaris P, et al: Two distinct roles of mitogen-activated protein kinases in platelets and a novel Rac1-MAPK-dependent integrin outside-in retractile signaling pathway. *Blood* 113(4):893–901, 2009.

294. Weyrich AS, et al: MTOR-dependent synthesis of Bcl-3 controls the retraction of fibrin clots by activated human platelets. *Blood* 109(5):1975–1983, 2007.

295. Ward CM, Kestin AS, Newman PJ: A Leu262Pro mutation in the integrin beta(3) subunit results in an alpha(IIb)-beta(3) complex that binds fibrin but not fibrinogen. *Blood* 96(1):161–169, 2000.

296. Rooney MM, et al: The contribution of the three hypothesized integrin-binding sites in fibrinogen to platelet-mediated clot retraction. *Blood* 92(7):2374–2381, 1998.

297. Rooney MM, Parise LV, Lord ST: Dissecting clot retraction and platelet aggregation. Clot retraction does not require an intact fibrinogen gamma chain C terminus. *J Biol Chem* 271(15):8553–8555, 1996.

298. Podolnikova NP, et al: Identification of a novel binding site for platelet integrins alpha IIb beta 3 (GPIIbIIIa) and alpha 5 beta 1 in the gamma C-domain of fibrinogen. *J Biol Chem* 278(34):32251–32258, 2003.

299. Remijn JA, Ijsseldijk MJ, de Groot PG: Role of the fibrinogen gamma-chain sequence gamma316–322 in platelet-mediated clot retraction. *J Thromb Haemost* 1(10): 2245–2246, 2003.

300. Podolnikova NP, et al: The interaction of integrin alphaIIbbeta3 with fibrin occurs through multiple binding sites in the alphaIIb beta-propeller domain. *J Biol Chem* 289(4):2371–2383, 2014.

301. Kasahara K, et al: Clot retraction is mediated by factor XIII-dependent fibrin-alphaIIbbeta3-myosin axis in platelet sphingomyelin-rich membrane rafts. *Blood* 122(19):3340–3348, 2013.

302. Munday AD, Lopez JA: Factor XIII: Sticking it to platelets. *Blood* 122(19):3246–3247, 2013.

303. Dubois C, et al: Thrombin binding to GPIbalpha induces platelet aggregation and fibrin clot retraction supported by resting alphaIIbbeta3 interaction with polymerized fibrin. *Thromb Haemost* 89(5):853–865, 2003.

304. Keuren JF, et al: Von Willebrand factor C1C2 domain is involved in platelet adhesion to polymerized fibrin at high shear rate. *Blood* 103(5):1741–1746, 2004.

305. Huizing M, et al: Disorders of lysosome-related organelle biogenesis: Clinical and molecular genetics. *Annu Rev Genomics Hum Genet* 9:359–386, 2008.

306. Holmsen H, Kaplan KL, Dangelmaier CA: Differential energy requirements for platelet responses. A simultaneous study of aggregation, three secretory processes, arachidonate liberation, phosphatidylinositol breakdown and phosphatidate production. *Biochem J* 208(1):9–18, 1982.

307. Verhoeven AJ, Mommersteeg ME, Akkerman JW: Quantification of energy consumption in platelets during thrombin-induced aggregation and secretion. Tight coupling between platelet responses and the increment in energy consumption. *Biochem J* 221(3):777–787, 1984.

308. Ciferri S, et al: Platelets release their lysosomal content *in vivo* in humans upon activation. *Thromb Haemost* 83(1):157–164, 2000.

309. Abrams C, Shattil SJ: Immunological detection of activated platelets in clinical disorders. *Thromb Haemost* 65(5):467–473, 1991.

310. Nieuwenhuis HK, et al: Studies with a monoclonal antibody against activated platelets: Evidence that a secreted 53,000-molecular weight lysosome-like granule protein is exposed on the surface of activated platelets in the circulation. *Blood* 70(3):838–845, 1987.

311. Zhang ZG, et al: Dynamic platelet accumulation at the site of the occluded middle cerebral artery and in downstream microvessels is associated with loss of microvascular integrity after embolic middle cerebral artery occlusion. *Brain Res* 912(2):181–194, 2001.

312. Castellot JJ Jr, et al: Inhibition of vascular smooth muscle cell growth by endothelial cell-derived heparin. Possible role of a platelet endoglycosidase. *J Biol Chem* 257(19):11256–11260, 1982.

313. Ugurbil K, Fukami MH, Holmsen H: 31P NMR studies of nucleotide storage in the dense granules of pig platelets. *Biochemistry* 23(3):409–416, 1984.

314. Ugurbil K, Holmsen H, Shulman RG: Adenine nucleotide storage and secretion in platelets as studied by 31P nuclear magnetic resonance. *Proc Natl Acad Sci U S A* 76(5):2227–2231, 1979.

315. Lesurtel M, et al: Platelet-derived serotonin mediates liver regeneration. *Science* 312(5770):104–107, 2006.

316. Gunay-Aygun M, Huizing M, Gahl WA: Molecular defects that affect platelet dense granules. *Semin Thromb Hemost* 30(5):537–547, 2004.

317. Youssefian T, Cramer EM: Megakaryocyte dense granule components are sorted in multivesicular bodies. *Blood* 95(12):4004–4007, 2000.

318. Nagle DL, et al: Identification and mutation analysis of the complete gene for Chediak-Higashi syndrome. *Nat Genet* 14(3):307–311, 1996.

319. FitzGerald GA: Dipyridamole. *N Engl J Med* 316(20):1247–1257, 1987.

320. Hatmi M, et al: Evidence for cAMP-dependent platelet ectoprotein kinase activity that phosphorylates platelet glycoprotein IV (CD36). *J Biol Chem* 271(40):24776–24780, 1996.

321. Kalafatis M, et al: Phosphorylation of factor Va and factor VIIIa by activated platelets. *Blood* 81(3):704–719, 1993.

322. Naik UP, Kornecki E, Ehrlich YH: Phosphorylation and dephosphorylation of human platelet surface proteins by an ecto-protein kinase/phosphatase system. *Biochim Biophys Acta* 1092(2):256–264, 1991.

323. Harrison P, Cramer EM: Platelet alpha-granules. *Blood Rev* 7(1):52–62, 1993.

324. Reed G: Platelet secretion, in *Platelets*, edited by A Michelson A, p 309. Academic Press, San Diego, 2007.

325. Hayward CP, et al: Factor V is complexed with multimerin in resting platelet lysates and colocalizes with multimerin in platelet alpha-granules. *J Biol Chem* 270(33):19217–19224, 1995.

326. Coppinger JA, et al: Characterization of the proteins released from activated platelets leads to localization of novel platelet proteins in human atherosclerotic lesions. *Blood* 103(6):2096–2104, 2004.

327. Maynard DM, et al: Proteomic analysis of platelet alpha-granules using mass spectrometry. *J Thromb Haemost* 5(9):1945–1955, 2007.

328. McRedmond JP, et al: Integration of proteomics and genomics in platelets: A profile of platelet proteins and platelet-specific genes. *Mol Cell Proteomics* 3(2):133–144, 2004.

329. Italiano JE Jr, Richardson JL, Patel-Hett S, et al: Angiogenesis is regulated by a novel mechanism: Pro- and antiangiogenic proteins are organized into separate platelet alpha granules and differentially released. *Blood* 111(3):1227–1233, 2008.

330. Sehgal S, Storrie B: Evidence that differential packaging of the major platelet granule proteins von Willebrand factor and fibrinogen can support their differential release. *J Thromb Haemost* 5(10):2009–2016, 2007.

331. George JN: Platelet immunoglobulin G: Its significance for the evaluation of thrombocytopenia and for understanding the origin of alpha-granule proteins. *Blood* 76(5):859–870, 1990.

332. George JN, Platelet IgG: Measurement, interpretation, and clinical significance. *Prog Hemost Thromb* 10:97–126, 1991.

333. Heijnen HF, et al: Multivesicular bodies are an intermediate stage in the formation of platelet alpha-granules. *Blood* 91(7):2313–2325, 1998.

334. Niewiarowski S: Secreted platelet proteins, in *Haemostasis and Thrombosis*, edited by AL Bloom, DP Thomas, EGD Tuddenham, p 167. Churchill Livingstone, London, England, 1994.

335. Niewiarowski S, Holt JC, Cook JJ: Biochemistry and physiology of secreted platelet proteins, in *Hemostasis and Thrombosis: Basic Principles and Clinical Practice*, edited by RW Colman, VJ Marder, EW Salzman, p 546. JB Lippincott, Philadelphia, 1993.

336. Brown KD, et al: A family of small inducible proteins secreted by leukocytes are members of a new superfamily that includes leukocyte and fibroblast-derived inflammatory agents, growth factors, and indicators of various activation processes. *J Immunol* 142(2):679–687, 1989.

337. Kawahara RS, Deuel TF: Platelet-derived growth factor-inducible gene JE is a member of a family of small inducible genes related to platelet factor 4. *J Biol Chem* 264(2):679–682, 1989.

338. Oppenheim JJ, et al: Properties of the novel proinflammatory supergene "intercrine" cytokine family. *Annu Rev Immunol* 9:617–648, 1991.

339. Gear AR, Camerini D: Platelet chemokines and chemokine receptors: Linking hemostasis, inflammation, and host defense. *Microcirculation* 10(3–4):335–350, 2003.

340. Rollins BJ: Chemokines. *Blood* 90(3):909–928, 1997.

341. Handin RI, Cohen HJ: Purification and binding properties of human platelet factor four. *J Biol Chem* 251(14):4273–4282, 1976.

342. Loscalzo J, Melnick B, Handin RI: The interaction of platelet factor four and glycosaminoglycans. *Arch Biochem Biophys* 240(1):446–455, 1985.

343. Rucinski B, et al: Human platelet factor 4 and its C-terminal peptides: Heparin binding and clearance from the circulation. *Thromb Haemost* 63(3):493–498, 1990.

344. Barber AJ, Käser-Glanzmann R, Jakábová M, Lüscher EF: Chromatography of chondroitin sulfate proteoglycan carrier for heparin neutralizing activity (platelet factor 4) released from human blood platelets. *Biochim Biophys Acta* 286(2):312–329, 1972.

345. Huang SS, Huang JS, Deuel TF: Proteoglycan carrier of human platelet factor 4. Isolation and characterization. *J Biol Chem* 257(19):11546–11550, 1982.

346. Busch C, et al: Binding of platelet factor 4 to cultured human umbilical vein endothelial cells. *Thromb Res* 19(1–2):129–137, 1980.

347. Clore GM, Gronenborn AM: Three-dimensional structures of alpha and beta chemokines. *FASEB J* 9(1):57–62, 1995.

348. Cowan SW, et al: Binding of heparin to human platelet factor 4. *Biochem J* 234(2):485–488, 1986.

349. Visentin GP, et al: Antibodies from patients with heparin-induced thrombocytopenia/thrombosis are specific for platelet factor 4 complexed with heparin or bound to endothelial cells. *J Clin Invest* 93(1):81–88, 1994.

350. Warkentin TE: Heparin-induced thrombocytopenia. *Curr Hematol Rep* 1(1):63–72, 2002.

351. Rucinski B, et al: Uptake and processing of human platelet factor 4 by hepatocytes. *Proc Soc Exp Biol Med* 186(3):361–367, 1987.

352. Deuel TF, et al: Platelet factor 4 is chemotactic for neutrophils and monocytes. *Proc Natl Acad Sci U S A* 78(7):4584–4587, 1981.

353. Maione TE, et al: Inhibition of angiogenesis by recombinant human platelet factor-4 and related peptides. *Science* 247(4938):77–79, 1990.

354. Brindley LL, Sweet JM, Goetzl EJ: Stimulation of histamine release from human basophils by human platelet factor 4. *J Clin Invest* 72(4):1218–1223, 1983.

355. Gewirtz AM, et al: Inhibition of human megakaryocytopoiesis in vitro by platelet factor 4 (PF4) and a synthetic COOH-terminal PF4 peptide. *J Clin Invest* 83(5):1477–1486, 1989.

356. Han ZC, et al: Platelet factor 4 inhibits human megakaryocytopoiesis *in vitro*. *Blood* 75(6):1234–1239, 1990.

357. Lambert MP, et al: Platelet factor 4 is a negative autocrine *in vivo* regulator of megakaryopoiesis: Clinical and therapeutic implications. *Blood* 110(4):1153–1160, 2007.

358. Katz IR, et al: Protease-induced immunoregulatory activity of platelet factor 4. *Proc Natl Acad Sci U S A* 83(10):3491–3495, 1986.

359. Beyth RJ, Culp LA: Complementary adhesive responses of human skin fibroblasts to the cell-binding domain of fibronectin and the heparan sulfate-binding protein, platelet factor-4. *Exp Cell Res* 155(2):537–548, 1984.

360. Capitanio AM, et al: Interaction of platelet factor 4 with human platelets. *Biochim Biophys Acta* 839(2):161–173, 1985.

361. Dumenco LL, et al: Inhibition of the activation of Hageman factor (factor XII) by platelet factor 4. *J Lab Clin Med* 112(3):394–400, 1988.

362. Aziz KA, Cawley JC, Zuzel M: Platelets prime PMN via released PF4: Mechanism of priming and synergy with GM-CSF. *Br J Haematol* 91(4):846–853, 1995.

363. Engstad CS, et al: A novel biological effect of platelet factor 4 (PF4): Enhancement of LPS-induced tissue factor activity in monocytes. *J Leukoc Biol* 58(5):575–581, 1995.

364. Castor CW, Miller JW, Walz DA: Structural and biological characteristics of connective tissue activating peptide (CTAP-III), a major human platelet-derived growth factor. *Proc Natl Acad Sci U S A* 80(3):765–769, 1983.

365. Holt JC, et al: Characterization of human platelet basic protein, a precursor form of low-affinity platelet factor 4 and beta-thromboglobulin. *Biochemistry* 25(8):1988–1996, 1986.

366. Walz A, et al: Effects of the neutrophil-activating peptide NAP-2, platelet basic protein, connective tissue-activating peptide III and platelet factor 4 on human neutrophils. *J Exp Med* 170(5):1745–1750, 1989.

367. Bastl CP, et al: Role of kidney in the catabolic clearance of human platelet antiheparin proteins from rat circulation. *Blood* 57(2):233–238, 1981.

368. Hayward CP: Multimerin: A bench-to-bedside chronology of a unique platelet and endothelial cell protein—From discovery to function to abnormalities in disease. *Clin Invest Med* 20(3):176–187, 1997.

369. Polgar J, et al: Platelet glycoprotein Ia* is the processed form of multimerin—Isolation and determination of N-terminal sequences of stored and released forms. *Thromb Haemost* 80(4):645–648, 1998.

370. Hayward CP, et al: Studies of multimerin in human endothelial cells. *Blood* 91(4):1304–1317, 1998.

371. Harrison P: Platelet alpha-granular fibrinogen. *Platelets* 3(1):1–10, 1992.

372. Harrison P, Wilbourn BR, Saundry RH, et al: Absence of the γ-Leu 427 (γ') variant in the platelet alpha-granular fibrinogen pool supports the role of glycoprotein IIb/IIIa in mediating fibrinogen uptake into platelets/megakaryocytes. *Blood* 79(12):3394–3395, 1992.

373. Reheman A, et al: Plasma fibronectin depletion enhances platelet aggregation and thrombus formation in mice lacking fibrinogen and von Willebrand factor. *Blood* 113(8):1809–1817, 2009.

374. Cho J, Mosher DF: Role of fibronectin assembly in platelet thrombus formation. *J Thromb Haemost* 4(7):1461–1469, 2006.

375. Coller BS, et al: Platelet fibrinogen and vitronectin in Glanzmann thrombasthenia: Evidence consistent with specific roles for glycoprotein IIb/IIIA and alpha v beta 3 integrins in platelet protein trafficking. *Blood* 78(10):2603–2610, 1991.

376. Eitzman DT, et al: Plasminogen activator inhibitor-1 and vitronectin promote vascular thrombosis in mice. *Blood* 95(2):577–580, 2000.

377. Fay WP, et al: Vitronectin inhibits the thrombotic response to arterial injury in mice. *Blood* 93(6):1825–1830, 1999.

378. Konstantinides S, et al: Plasminogen activator inhibitor-1 and its cofactor vitronectin stabilize arterial thrombi after vascular injury in mice. *Circulation* 103(4):576–583, 2001.

379. Adams JC, Lawler J: The thrombospondins. *Int J Biochem Cell Biol* 36(6):961–968, 2004.

380. Baenziger NL, Brodie GN, Majerus PW: A thrombin-sensitive protein of human platelet membranes. *Proc Natl Acad Sci U S A* 68(1):240–243, 1971.

381. Lawler J, Hynes RO: The structure of human thrombospondin, an adhesive glycoprotein with multiple calcium-binding sites and homologies with several different proteins. *J Cell Biol* 103(5):1635–1648, 1986.

382. Mosher DF, Doyle MJ, Jaffe EA: Synthesis and secretion of thrombospondin by cultured human endothelial cells. *J Cell Biol* 93(2):343–348, 1982.

383. Schwartz BS: Monocyte synthesis of thrombospondin. The role of platelets. *J Biol Chem* 264(13):7512–7517, 1989.

384. Aiken ML, et al: Effects of OKM5, a monoclonal antibody to glycoprotein IV, on platelet aggregation and thrombospondin surface expression. *Blood* 76(12):2501–2509, 1990.

385. Asch AS, et al: Analysis of CD36 binding domains: Ligand specificity controlled by dephosphorylation of an ectodomain. *Science* 262(5138):1436–1440, 1993.

386. Chung J, Gao AG, Frazier WA: Thrombospondin acts via integrin-associated protein to activate the platelet integrin alphaIIbbeta3. *J Biol Chem* 272(23):14740–14746, 1997.

387. Chung J, et al: Thrombospondin-1 acts via IAP/CD47 to synergize with collagen in alpha2beta1-mediated platelet activation. *Blood* 94(2):642–648, 1999.

388. Jurk K, et al: Thrombospondin-1 mediates platelet adhesion at high shear via glycoprotein Ib (GPIb): An alternative/backup mechanism to von Willebrand factor. *FASEB J* 17(11):1490–1492, 2003.

389. Lawler J, Hynes RO: An integrin receptor on normal and thrombasthenic platelets that binds thrombospondin. *Blood* 74(6):2022–2027, 1989.

390. Plow EF, et al: Related binding mechanisms for fibrinogen, fibronectin, von Willebrand factor, and thrombospondin on thrombin-stimulated human platelets. *Blood* 66(3): 724–727, 1985.

391. Gao AG, et al: Integrin-associated protein is a receptor for the C-terminal domain of thrombospondin. *J Biol Chem* 271(1):21–24, 1996.

392. Lawler J, Hynes RO: The structure of human thrombospondin, an adhesive glycoprotein with multiple calcium binding sites and homologies with several different proteins. *J Cell Biol* 103:1635–1648, 1986.

393. Elzie CA, Murphy-Ullrich JE: The N-terminus of thrombospondin: The domain stands apart. *Int J Biochem Cell Biol* 36(6):1090–1101, 2004.

394. Tuszynski GP, et al: The interaction of human platelet thrombospondin with fibrinogen. Thrombospondin purification and specificity of interaction. *J Biol Chem* 260(22):12240–12245, 1985.

395. Dardik R, Lahav J: Functional changes in the conformation of thrombospondin-1 during complexation with fibronectin or heparin. *Exp Cell Res* 248(2):407–414, 1999.

396. Leung LL: Role of thrombospondin in platelet aggregation. *J Clin Invest* 74(5): 1764–1772, 1984.

397. Schultz-Cherry S, Murphy-Ullrich JE: Thrombospondin causes activation of latent transforming growth factor-beta secreted by endothelial cells by a novel mechanism. *J Cell Biol* 122(4):923–932, 1993.

398. Silverstein RL, et al: Complex formation of platelet thrombospondin with plasminogen. Modulation of activation by tissue activator. *J Clin Invest* 74(5):1625–1633, 1984.

399. Bouchard BA, et al: Interactions between platelets and the coagulation system, in *Platelets*, edited by AD Michelson, p 229. Academic Press, San Diego, 2002.

400. Chesney CM, Pifer D, Colman RW: Subcellular localization and secretion of factor V from human platelets. *Proc Natl Acad Sci U S A* 78:5180–5184, 1981.

401. Tracy PB, Eide LL, Bowie EJ, et al: Radioimmunoassay of factor V in human plasma and platelets. *Blood* 60(1):59–63, 1982.

402. Camire RM, et al: Secretable human platelet-derived factor V originates from the plasma pool. *Blood* 92(9):3035–3041, 1998.

403. Yang TL, et al: Biosynthetic origin and functional significance of murine platelet factor V. *Blood* 102(8):2851–2855, 2003.

404. Gould WR, Silveira JR, Tracy PB: Unique in vivo modifications of coagulation factor V produce a physically and functionally distinct platelet-derived cofactor: Characterization of purified platelet-derived factor V/Va. *J Biol Chem* 279(4):2383–2393, 2004.

405. Kane WH, Mruk JS, Majerus PW: Activation of coagulation factor V by a platelet protease. *J Clin Invest* 70:1092–1100, 1982.

406. Tracy PB, Nesheim ME, Mann KG: Proteolytic alterations of factor Va bound to platelets. *J Biol Chem* 662:669, 1983.

407. Nesheim ME, et al: Isolation and study of an acquired inhibitor of human coagulation factor V. *J Clin Invest* 405:415, 1986.

408. Tracy PB, et al: Factor V (Quebec): A bleeding diathesis associated with a qualitative platelet factor V deficiency. *J Clin Invest* 74:1221–1228, 1984.

409. Bode AP, et al: Association of factor V activity with membranous vesicles released from human platelets: Requirement for platelet stimulation. *Thromb Res* 39:49–61, 1985.

410. Manfioletti G, et al: The protein encoded by a growth arrest-specific gene (gas6) is a new member of the vitamin K-dependent proteins related to protein S, a negative coregulator in the blood coagulation cascade. *Mol Cell Biol* 13(8):4976–4985, 1993.

411. Melaragno MG, Fridell YW, Berk BC: The Gas6/Axl system: A novel regulator of vascular cell function. *Trends Cardiovasc Med* 9(8):250–253, 1999.

412. Angelillo-Scherrer A, et al: Deficiency or inhibition of Gas6 causes platelet dysfunction and protects mice against thrombosis. *Nat Med* 7(2):215–221, 2001.

413. Chen C, et al: Mer receptor tyrosine kinase signaling participates in platelet function. *Arterioscler Thromb Vasc Biol* 24(6):1118–1123, 2004.

414. Gould WR, et al: Gas6 receptors Axl, Sky and Mer enhance platelet activation and regulate thrombotic responses. *J Thromb Haemost* 3(4):733–741, 2005.

415. Angelillo-Scherrer A, et al: Role of Gas6 receptors in platelet signaling during thrombus stabilization and implications for antithrombotic therapy. *J Clin Invest* 115(2):237–246, 2005.

416. Maree AO, et al: Growth arrest specific gene (GAS) 6 modulates platelet thrombus formation and vascular wall homeostasis and represents an attractive drug target. *Curr Pharm Des* 13(26):2656–2661, 2007.

417. Saller F, et al: Role of the growth arrest-specific gene 6 (gas6) product in thrombus stabilization. *Blood Cells Mol Dis* 36(3):373–378, 2006.

418. Deuel TF, Huang SS, Huang JS: Platelet derived growth factor: Purification, characterization and role in normal and abnormal cell growth, in *Biochemistry of Platelets*, edited by DR Phillips, MA Shuman, pp 347–375. Academic, London, 1986.

419. Heldin CH, Westermark B: Platelet-derived growth factor: Three isoforms and two receptor types. *Trends Genet* 5(4):108–111, 1989.

420. Berk BC, Alexander RW: Vasoactive effects of growth factors. *Biochem Pharmacol* 38:219, 1989.

421. Madtes DK, Raines EW, Ross R: Modulation of local concentrations of platelet-derived growth factor. *Am Rev Respir Dis* 140:1118, 1989.

422. Ross R: Peptide regulatory factors. Platelet-derived growth factor. *Lancet* 1:1179, 1989.

423. Doolittle RF, et al: Simian sarcoma virus onc gene, v-sis, is derived from the gene (or genes) encoding a platelet-derived growth factor. *Science* 22:275, 1983.

424. Waterfield MD, et al: Platelet-derived growth factor is structurally related to the putative transforming protein p28-sis of simian sarcoma virus. *Nature* 304:35, 1983.

425. Williams LT: Signal transduction by the platelet-derived growth factor receptor. *Science* 243:1564–1570, 1989.

426. Nagai MK, Embil JM: Becaplermin: Recombinant platelet derived growth factor, a new treatment for healing diabetic foot ulcers. *Expert Opin Biol Ther* 2(2):211–218, 2002.

427. Maloney JP, Silliman CC, Ambruso DR, et al: In vitro release of vascular endothelial growth factor during platelet aggregation. *Am J Physiol* 275(3 Pt 2):H1054–H1061, 1998.

428. Webb NJ, et al: Vascular endothelial growth factor (VEGF) is released from platelets during blood clotting: Implications for measurement of circulating VEGF levels in clinical disease. *Clin Sci (Lond)* 94(4):395–404, 1998.

429. Weltermann A, et al: Large amounts of vascular endothelial growth factor at the site of hemostatic plug formation in vivo. *Arterioscler Thromb Vasc Biol* 19(7):1757–1760, 1999.

430. Mohle R, et al: Constitutive production and thrombin-induced release of vascular endothelial growth factor by human megakaryocytes and platelets. *Proc Natl Acad Sci U S A* 94(2):663–668, 1997.

431. Amirkhosravi A, et al: Blockade of GPIIb/IIIa inhibits the release of vascular endothelial growth factor (VEGF) from tumor cell-activated platelets and experimental metastasis. *Platelets* 10:285–292, 1999.

432. Katoh O, et al: Expression of the vascular endothelial growth factor (VEGF) receptor gene, KDR, in hematopoietic cells and inhibitory effect of VEGF on apoptotic cell death caused by ionizing radiation. *Cancer Res* 55(23):5687–5692, 1995.

433. Wartiovaara U, et al: Peripheral blood platelets express VEGF-C and VEGF which are released during platelet activation. *Thromb Haemost* 80(1):171–175, 1998.

434. Italiano JE Jr, et al: Angiogenesis is regulated by a novel mechanism: Pro- and anti-angiogenic proteins are organized into separate platelet alpha granules and differentially released. *Blood* 111(3):1227–1233, 2008.

435. Salven P, Orpana A, Joensuu H: Leukocytes and platelets of patients with cancer contain high levels of vascular endothelial growth factor. *Clin Cancer Res* 5(3):487–491, 1999.

436. Verheul HM, Pinedo HM: Tumor growth: A putative role for platelets? *Oncologist* 3(2):II, 1998.

437. Cao J, et al: Angiogenic factors in human proliferative sickle cell retinopathy. *Br J Ophthalmol* 83(7):838–846, 1999.

438. Solovey A, et al: Sickle cell anemia as a possible state of enhanced anti-apoptotic tone: Survival effect of vascular endothelial growth factor on circulating and unanchored endothelial cells. *Blood* 93(11):3824–3830, 1999.

439. Kiuru J, et al: Cytoskeleton-dependent release of human platelet epidermal growth factor. *Life Sci* 49(26):1997–2003, 1991.

440. Bush AI, Martins RN, Rumble B, et al: The amyloid precursor protein of Alzheimer's disease is released by human platelets. *J Biol Chem* 265(26):15977–15983, 1990.

441. Li Q, Beyreuther K, Masters CL: Alzheimer's disease, in *Platelets*, edited by AD Michelson, pp 779–789. Academic Press, San Diego, 2007.

442. Li Q, et al: Products of the Alzheimer's disease amyloid precursor protein generated by β-secretase are present in human platelets, and secreted upon degranulation. *Am J Alzheimer's Dis* 13:236–244, 1998.

443. Li QX, et al: Secretion of Alzheimer's disease Abeta amyloid peptide by activated human platelets. *Lab Invest* 78(4):461–469, 1998.

444. Li QX, et al: Proteolytic processing of Alzheimer's disease beta A4 amyloid precursor protein in human platelets. *J Biol Chem* 270(23):14140–14147, 1995.

445. Li QX, et al: Membrane-associated forms of the beta A4 amyloid protein precursor of Alzheimer's disease in human platelet and brain: Surface expression on the activated human platelet. *Blood* 84(1):133–142, 1994.

446. Van Nostrand WE, et al: Protease nexin-2/amyloid beta-protein precursor in blood is a platelet-specific protein. *Biochem Biophys Res Commun* 175(1):15–21, 1991.

447. Scandura JM, et al: Progress curve analysis of the kinetics with which blood coagulation factor XIa is inhibited by protease nexin-2. *Biochemistry* 36(2):412–420, 1997.

448. Schmaier AH, et al: Factor IXa inhibition by protease nexin-2/amyloid beta-protein precursor on phospholipid vesicles and cell membranes. *Biochemistry* 34(4):1171–1178, 1995.

449. Schmaier AH, et al: Protease nexin-2/amyloid β protein precursor. A tight-binding inhibitor of coagulation factor IXa. *J Clin Invest* 92(5):2540–2545, 1993.

450. Baskin F, et al: Platelet APP isoform ratios correlate with declining cognition in AD. *Neurology* 54(10):1907–1909, 2000.

451. Borroni B, et al: Microvascular damage and platelet abnormalities in early Alzheimer's disease. *J Neurol Sci* 203–204:189–193, 2002.

452. Davies TA, et al: Non-age related differences in thrombin responses by platelets from male patients with advanced Alzheimer's disease. *Biochem Biophys Res Commun* 194(1):537–543, 1993.

453. Davies TA, et al: Moderate and advanced Alzheimer's patients exhibit platelet activation differences. *Neurobiol Aging* 18(2):155–162, 1997.

454. Di Luca M, et al: Differential level of platelet amyloid beta precursor protein isoforms: An early marker for Alzheimer disease. *Arch Neurol* 55(9):1195–1200, 1998.

455. Rosenberg RN, et al: Altered amyloid protein processing in platelets of patients with Alzheimer disease. *Arch Neurol* 54(2):139–144, 1997.

456. Devine DV, Bishop PD: Platelet-associated factor XIII in platelet activation, adhesion, and clot stabilization. *Semin Thromb Hemost* 22(5):409–413, 1996.

457. McDonagh J, et al: Factor XIII in human plasma and platelets. *J Clin Invest* 48(5):940–946, 1969.

458. Adany R, Bardos H: Factor XIII subunit A as an intracellular transglutaminase. *Cell Mol Life Sci* 60(6):1049–1060, 2003.

459. Lorand L, Graham RM: Transglutaminases: Crosslinking enzymes with pleiotropic functions. *Nat Rev Mol Cell Biol* 4(2):140–156, 2003.

460. Inbal A, et al: Platelets but not monocytes contribute to the plasma levels of factor XIII subunit A in patients undergoing autologous peripheral blood stem cell transplantation. *Blood Coagul Fibrinolysis* 15(3):249–253, 2004.

461. Serrano K, Devine DV: Intracellular factor XIII crosslinks platelet cytoskeletal elements upon platelet activation. *Thromb Haemost* 88(2):315–320, 2002.

462. Huff T, et al: Thymosin beta4 is released from human blood platelets and attached by factor XIIIa (transglutaminase) to fibrin and collagen. *FASEB J* 16(7):691–696, 2002.

463. Kulkarni S, Jackson SP: Platelet factor XIII and calpain negatively regulate integrin alpha IIbbeta3 adhesive function and thrombus growth. *J Biol Chem* 279(29):30697–30706, 2004.

464. Szasz R, Dale GL: Thrombospondin and fibrinogen bind serotonin-derivatized proteins on COAT-platelets. *Blood* 100(8):2827–2831, 2002.

465. Szasz R, Dale GL: COAT platelets. *Curr Opin Hematol* 10(5):351–355, 2003.

466. Leask A: TGFbeta, cardiac fibroblasts, and the fibrotic response. *Cardiovasc Res* 74(2):207–212, 2007.

467. Massague J: TGFbeta in Cancer. *Cell* 134(2):215–230, 2008.

468. Rubtsov YP, Rudensky AY: TGFbeta signalling in control of T-cell-mediated self-reactivity. *Nat Rev Immunol* 7(6):443–453, 2007.

469. ten Dijke P, Arthur HM: Extracellular control of TGFbeta signalling in vascular development and disease. *Nat Rev Mol Cell Biol* 8(11):857–869, 2007.

470. Sakamaki S, et al: Transforming growth factor-beta1 (TGF-beta1) induces thrombopoietin from bone marrow stromal cells, which stimulates the expression of TGF-beta receptor on megakaryocytes and, in turn, renders them susceptible to suppression by TGF-beta itself with high specificity. *Blood* 94(6):1961–1970, 1999.

471. Shi Y, Massague J: Mechanisms of TGF-beta signaling from cell membrane to the nucleus. *Cell* 113(6):685–700, 2003.

472. Hoying JB, et al: Transforming growth factor beta1 enhances platelet aggregation through a non-transcriptional effect on the fibrinogen receptor. *J Biol Chem* 274(43):31008–31013, 1999.

473. Kronemann N, et al: Aggregating human platelets stimulate expression of vascular endothelial growth factor in cultured vascular smooth muscle cells through a synergistic effect of transforming growth factor-beta(1) and platelet-derived growth factor(AB). *Circulation* 100(8):855–860, 1999.

474. Koda Y, et al: Protein kinase C subtypes in tissues derived from neural crest. *Brain Res* 518(1–2):334–336, 1990.

475. Annes JP, Munger JS, Rifkin DB: Making sense of latent TGFbeta activation. *J Cell Sci* 116(Pt 2):217–224, 2003.

476. Lawler J, Hynes RO: The structure of human thrombospondin, an adhesive glycoprotein with multiple calcium-binding sites and homologies with several different proteins. *J Cell Biol* 103:1635–1648, 1986.

477. Schultz-Cherry S, Murphy-Ullrich JE: Thrombospondin causes activation of latent transforming growth factor- beta secreted by endothelial cells by a novel mechanism. *J Cell Biol* 1993;122(4):923–932, 1986.

478. Ahamed J, Janczak CA, Wittkowski KM, Coller BS: *In vitro* and *in vivo* evidence that thrombospondin-1 (TSP-1) contributes to stirring- and shear-dependent activation of platelet-derived TGF-β1. *PLoS One* 4(8):e6608, 2009.

479. Blakytny R, Ludlow A, Martin GE, et al: Latent TGF-beta1 activation by platelets. *J Cell Physiol* 199(1):67–76, 2004.

480. Yang Z, et al: Absence of integrin-mediated TGFbeta1 activation *in vivo* recapitulates the phenotype of TGFbeta1-null mice. *J Cell Biol* 176(6):787–793, 2007.

481. Abdelouahed M, et al: Activation of platelet-transforming growth factor beta-1 in the absence of thrombospondin-1. *J Biol Chem* 275(24):17933–17936, 2000.

482. Ahamed J, et al: *In vitro* and *in vivo* evidence for shear-induced activation of latent transforming growth factor-beta1. *Blood* 112(9):3650–3660, 2008.

483. Crawford SE, et al: Thrombospondin-1 is a major activator of TGF-beta1 *in vivo*. *Cell* 93(7):1159–1170, 1998.

484. Slivka SR, Loskutoff DJ: Platelets stimulate endothelial cells to synthesize type 1 plasminogen activator inhibitor. Evaluation of the role of transforming growth factor beta. *Blood* 77(5):1013–1019, 1991.

485. Labelle M, Begum S, Hynes RO: Direct signaling between platelets and cancer cells induces an epithelial-mesenchymal-like transition and promotes metastasis. *Cancer Cell* 20(5):576–590, 2011.

486. Meyer A, et al: Platelet TGF-beta1 contributions to plasma TGF-beta1, cardiac fibrosis, and systolic dysfunction in a mouse model of pressure overload. *Blood* 119(4):1064–1074, 2012.

487. Wang W, et al: Association between shear stress and platelet-derived transforming growth factor-beta1 release and activation in animal models of aortic valve stenosis. *Arterioscler Thromb Vasc Biol* 34(9):1924–1932, 2014.

488. Lin HY, et al: Expression cloning of the TGF-beta type II receptor, a functional transmembrane serine/threonine kinase. *Cell* 68(4):775–785, 1992.

489. Fuhrman B, Brook GJ, Aviram M: Proteins derived from platelet alpha granules modulate the uptake of oxidized low density lipoprotein by macrophages. *Biochim Biophys Acta* 1127(1):15–21, 1992.

490. Heijnen HF, et al: Activated platelets release two types of membrane vesicles: Microvesicles by surface shedding and exosomes derived from exocytosis of multivesicular bodies and alpha-granules. *Blood* 94(11):3791–3799, 1999.

491. Janiszewski M, et al: Platelet-derived exosomes of septic individuals possess proapoptotic NAD(P)H oxidase activity: A novel vascular redox pathway. *Crit Care Med* 32(3):818–825, 2004.

492. Ren Q, Ye S, Whiteheart SW: The platelet release reaction: Just when you thought platelet secretion was simple. *Curr Opin Hematol* 15(5):537–541, 2008.

493. Tolmachova T, et al: Rab27b regulates number and secretion of platelet dense granules. *Proc Natl Acad Sci U S A* 104(14):5872–5877, 2007.

494. Shirakawa R, et al: Small GTPase Rab4 regulates Ca2+-induced alpha-granule secretion in platelets. *J Biol Chem* 275(43):33844–33849, 2000.

495. Fitzgerald ML, Reed GL: Rab6 is phosphorylated in thrombin-activated platelets by a protein kinase C-dependent mechanism: Effects on GTP/GDP binding and cellular distribution. *Biochem J* 342(Pt 2):353–360, 1999.

496. Sudhof TC, Rothman JE: Membrane fusion: Grappling with SNARE and SM proteins. *Science* 323(5913):474–477, 2009.

497. Weber T, et al: SNAREpins: Minimal machinery for membrane fusion. *Cell* 92(6):759–772, 1998.

498. Bernstein AM, Whiteheart SW: Identification of a cellubrevin/vesicle associated membrane protein 3 homologue in human platelets. *Blood* 93(2):571–579, 1999.

499. Graham GJ, Ren Q, Dilks JR, et al: Endobrevin/VAMP-8-dependent dense granule release mediates thrombus formation *in vivo*. *Blood* 114(5):1083–1090, 2009.

500. Lemons PP, et al: Regulated secretion in platelets: Identification of elements of the platelet exocytosis machinery. *Blood* 90(4):1490–1500, 1997.

501. Polgar J, Chung SH, Reed GL: Vesicle-associated membrane protein 3 (VAMP-3) and VAMP-8 are present in human platelets and are required for granule secretion. *Blood* 100(3):1081–1083, 2002.

502. Ren Q, et al: Endobrevin/VAMP-8 is the primary v-SNARE for the platelet release reaction. *Mol Biol Cell* 18(1):24–33, 2007.

503. Flaumenhaft R, et al: Proteins of the exocytotic core complex mediate platelet alpha-granule secretion. Roles of vesicle-associated membrane protein, SNAP-23, and syntaxin 4. *J Biol Chem* 274(4):2492–2501, 1999.

504. Polgar J, et al: Phosphorylation of SNAP-23 in activated human platelets. *J Biol Chem* 278(45):44369–44376, 2003.

505. Chen D, et al: Molecular mechanisms of platelet exocytosis: Role of SNAP-23 and syntaxin 2 in dense core granule release. *Blood* 95(3):921–929, 2000.

506. Chen D, et al: Molecular mechanisms of platelet exocytosis: Role of SNAP-23 and syntaxin 2 and 4 in lysosome release. *Blood* 96(5):1782–1788, 2000.

507. Flaumenhaft R, Furie B, Furie BC: Alpha-granule secretion from alpha-toxin permeabilized, MgATP-exposed platelets is induced independently by H+ and Ca2+. *J Cell Physiol* 179(1):1–10, 1999.

508. Lemons PP, Chen D, Whiteheart SW: Molecular mechanisms of platelet exocytosis: Requirements for alpha-granule release. *Biochem Biophys Res Commun* 267(3):875–880, 2000.

509. Houng A, Polgar J, Reed GL: Munc18-syntaxin complexes and exocytosis in human platelets. *J Biol Chem* 278(22):19627–19633, 2003.

510. Reed GL, Houng AK, Fitzgerald ML: Human platelets contain SNARE proteins and a Sec1p homologue that interacts with syntaxin 4 and is phosphorylated after thrombin activation: Implications for platelet secretion. *Blood* 93(8):2617–2626, 1999.

511. Schraw TD, et al: A role for Sec1/Munc18 proteins in platelet exocytosis. *Biochem J* 374(Pt 1):207–217, 2003.

512. Shirakawa R, et al: Munc13-4 is a GTP-Rab27-binding protein regulating dense core granule secretion in platelets. *J Biol Chem* 279(11):10730–10737, 2004.

513. Shirakawa R, et al: Purification and functional analysis of a Rab27 effector munc 13–4 using a semi-intact platelet dense-granule secretion assay. *Methods Enzymol* 403:778–788, 2005.

514. Vu TK, Hung DT, Wheaton VI, Coughlin SR: Molecular cloning of a functional thrombin receptor reveals a novel proteolytic mechanism of receptor activation. *Cell* 64:1057–1068, 1991.

515. Feldmann J, et al: Munc13–4 is essential for cytolytic granules fusion and is mutated in a form of familial hemophagocytic lymphohistiocytosis (FHL3). *Cell* 115(4):461–473, 2003.

516. Neeft M, et al: Munc13–4 is an effector of rab27a and controls secretion of lysosomes in hematopoietic cells. *Mol Biol Cell* 16(2):731–741, 2005.

517. Jahn R, Fasshauer D: Molecular machines governing exocytosis of synaptic vesicles. *Nature* 490(7419):201–207, 2012.

518. Rizo J, Sudhof TC: The membrane fusion enigma: SNAREs, Sec1/Munc18 proteins, and their accomplices—Guilty as charged? *Annu Rev Cell Dev Biol* 28:279–308, 2012.

519. Weber T, et al: SNAREpins: Minimal machinery for membrane fusion. *Cell* 92(6):759–772, 1998.

520. Bernstein AM, Whiteheart SW: Identification of a cellubrevin/vesicle associated membrane protein 3 homologue in human platelets. *Blood* 93(2):571–579, 1999.

521. Burkhart JM, et al: Systematic and quantitative comparison of digest efficiency and specificity reveals the impact of trypsin quality on MS-based proteomics. *J Proteomics* 75(4):1454–1462, 2012.

522. Graham GJ, et al: Endobrevin/VAMP-8-dependent dense granule release mediates thrombus formation in vivo. *Blood* 114(5):1083–1090, 2009.

523. Lemons PP, et al: Regulated secretion in platelets: Identification of elements of the platelet exocytosis machinery. *Blood* 90(4):1490–1500, 1997.

524. Golebiewska EM, et al: Syntaxin 8 regulates platelet dense granule secretion, aggregation, and thrombus stability. *J Biol Chem* 290(3):1536–1545, 2015.

525. Flaumenhaft R, et al: Proteins of the exocytotic core complex mediate platelet alpha-granule secretion. Roles of vesicle-associated membrane protein, SNAP-23, and syntaxin 4. *J Biol Chem* 274(4):2492–2501, 1999.

526. Polgar J, et al: Phosphorylation of SNAP-23 in activated human platelets. *J Biol Chem* 278(45):44369–44376, 2003.

527. Ye S, et al: Syntaxin-11, but not syntaxin-2 or syntaxin-4, is required for platelet secretion. *Blood* 120(12):2484–2492, 2012.

528. Lemons PP, Chen D, Whiteheart SW: Molecular mechanisms of platelet exocytosis: Requirements for alpha-granule release. *Biochem Biophys Res Commun* 267(3):875–880, 2000.

529. Karim ZA, et al: IkappaB kinase phosphorylation of SNAP-23 controls platelet secretion. *Blood* 121(22):4567–4574, 2013.

530. Al Hawas R, et al: Munc18b/STXBP2 is required for platelet secretion. *Blood* 120(12):2493–2500, 2012.

531. Houng A, Polgar J, Reed GL: Munc18-syntaxin complexes and exocytosis in human platelets. *J Biol Chem* 278(22):19627–19633, 2003.

532. Schraw TD, et al: Platelets from Munc18c heterozygous mice exhibit normal stimulus-induced release. *Thromb Haemost* 92(4):829–837, 2004.

533. Schraw TD, et al: A role for Sec1/Munc18 proteins in platelet exocytosis. *Biochem J* 374(Pt 1):207–217, 2003.

534. Sandrock K, et al: Platelet secretion defect in patients with familial hemophagocytic lymphohistiocytosis type 5 (FHL-5). *Blood* 116(26):6148–6150, 2010.

535. Suzuki T, et al: The mouse organellar biogenesis mutant buff results from a mutation in Vps33a, a homologue of yeast vps33 and *Drosophila* carnation. *Proc Natl Acad Sci U S A* 100(3):1146–1150, 2003.

536. Urban D, et al: The VPS33B-binding protein VPS16B is required in megakaryocyte and platelet alpha-granule biogenesis. *Blood* 120(25):5032–5040, 2012.

537. Ye S, et al: Platelet secretion and hemostasis require syntaxin-binding protein STXBP5. *J Clin Invest* 124(10):4517–4528, 2014.

538. Lillicrap D: Syntaxin-binding protein 5 exocytosis regulation: Differential role in endothelial cells and platelets. *J Clin Invest* 124(10):4231–4233, 2014.

539. Zhu Q, et al: STXBP5 regulates endothelial exocytosis, plasma VWF levels, and platelet endothelial interactions. *Clin Invest* 124(10):4503–4516, 2014.

540. James DJ, Martin TF: CAPS and Munc13: CATCHRs that SNARE vesicles. *Front Endocrinol (Lausanne)* 4:187, 2013.

541. Ren Q, et al: Munc13-4 is a limiting factor in the pathway required for platelet granule release and hemostasis. *Blood* 116(6):869–877, 2010.

542. Nakamura L, et al: First characterization of platelet secretion defect in patients with familial hemophagocytic lymphohistiocytosis type 3 (FHL-3). *Blood* 125(2):412–414, 2015.

543. Barral DC, et al: Functional redundancy of Rab27 proteins and the pathogenesis of Griscelli syndrome. *J Clin Invest* 110(2):247–257, 2002.

544. Hampson A, O'Connor A, Smolenski A: Synaptotagmin-like protein 4 and Rab8 interact and increase dense granule release in platelets. *J Thromb Haemost* 11(1):161–168, 2013.

545. Janka GE: Familial and acquired hemophagocytic lymphohistiocytosis. *Annu Rev Med* 63:233–246, 2012.

546. Lindemann S, et al: Platelets, inflammation and atherosclerosis. *J Thromb Haemost* 5(Suppl 1):203–211, 2007.

547. Bray PF: Platelet glycoprotein polymorphisms as risk factors for thrombosis. *Curr Opin Hematol* 7(5):284–289, 2000.

548. Deloukas P, et al: Large-scale association analysis identifies new risk loci for coronary artery disease. *Nat Genet* 45(1):25–33, 2013.

549. Bray PF, Jones CI, Soranzo N, Ouwehand WH: Platelet genomics, in *Platelets*, edited by A Michelson. Academic Press, San Diego, 2012.

550. Albers CA, et al: Exome sequencing identifies NBEAL2 as the causative gene for gray platelet syndrome. *Nat Genet* 43(8):735–737, 2011.

551. Gunay-Aygun M, et al: NBEAL2 is mutated in gray platelet syndrome and is required for biogenesis of platelet alpha-granules. *Nat Genet* 43(8):732–734, 2011.

552. Hulot JS, et al: Cytochrome P450 2C19 loss-of-function polymorphism is a major determinant of clopidogrel responsiveness in healthy subjects. *Blood* 108(7):2244–2247, 2006.

553. Shuldiner AR, et al: Association of cytochrome P450 2C19 genotype with the antiplatelet effect and clinical efficacy of clopidogrel therapy. *JAMA* 302(8):849–857, 2009.

554. Mega JL, et al: Reduced-function CYP2C19 genotype and risk of adverse clinical outcomes among patients treated with clopidogrel predominantly for PCI: A meta-analysis. *JAMA* 304(16):1821–1830, 2010.

555. Holmes MV, et al: CYP2C19 genotype, clopidogrel metabolism, platelet function, and cardiovascular events: A systematic review and meta-analysis. *JAMA* 306(24):2704–2714, 2011.

556. Yee D, et al: Platelet hyperreactivity to submaximal epinephrine: Biologic and clinical correlates. *Blood* 106(8):2723–2729, 2005.

557. Bray PF, et al: Heritability of platelet function in families with premature coronary artery disease. *J Thromb Haemost* 5(8):1617–1623, 2007.

558. Newman PJ, Derbes RS, Aster RH: The human platelet alloantigens, PlA1 and PlA2, are associated with a leucine33/proline33 amino acid polymorphism in membrane glycoprotein IIIa, and are distinguishable by DNA typing. *J Clin Invest* 83(5):1778–1781, 1989.

559. Vijayan KV, et al: Fibrinogen and prothrombin binding is enhanced to the Pro33 isoform of purified integrin alphaIIbbeta3. *J Thromb Haemost* 4(4):905–906, 2006.

560. Vijayan KV, et al: The Pl(A2) polymorphism of integrin beta(3) enhances outside-in signaling and adhesive functions. *J Clin Invest* 105(6):793–802, 2000.

561. Sajid M, et al: PlA polymorphism of integrin beta 3 differentially modulates cellular migration on extracellular matrix proteins. *Arterioscler Thromb Vasc Biol* 22(12):1984–1989, 2002.

562. Vijayan KV, et al: Shear stress augments the enhanced adhesive phenotype of cells expressing the Pro33 isoform of integrin beta3. *FEBS Lett* 540(1–3):41–46, 2003.

563. Vijayan KV, et al: Enhanced activation of mitogen-activated protein kinase and myosin light chain kinase by the Pro33 polymorphism of integrin beta 3. *J Biol Chem* 278(6):3860–3867, 2003.

564. Vijayan KV, et al: The Pro33 isoform of integrin beta3 enhances outside-in signaling in human platelets by regulating the activation of serine/threonine phosphatases. *J Biol Chem* 280(23):21756–21762, 2005.

565. Johnson AD, et al: Genome-wide meta-analyses identifies seven loci associated with platelet aggregation in response to agonists. *Nat Genet* 42(7):608–613, 2010.

566. Oliver KH, et al: Pro32Pro33 mutations in the integrin beta3 PSI domain result in alphaIIbbeta3 priming and enhanced adhesion: Reversal of the hypercoagulability phenotype by the Src inhibitor SKI-606. *Mol Pharmacol* 85(6):921–931, 2014.

567. Kritzik M, et al: Nucleotide polymorphisms in the alpha2 gene define multiple alleles that are associated with differences in platelet alpha2 beta1 density. *Blood* 92(7):2382–2388, 1998.

568. Roest M, et al: Platelet adhesion to collagen in healthy volunteers is influenced by variation of both alpha(2)beta(1) density and von Willebrand factor. *Blood* 96(4):1433–1437, 2000.

569. Joutsi-Korhonen L, et al: The low-frequency allele of the platelet collagen signaling receptor glycoprotein VI is associated with reduced functional responses and expression. *Blood* 101(11):4372–4379, 2003.

570. Jones CI, et al: A functional genomics approach reveals novel quantitative trait loci associated with platelet signaling pathways. *Blood* 114(7):1405–1416, 2009.

571. Musunuru K, et al: Association of single nucleotide polymorphisms on chromosome 9p21.3 with platelet reactivity: A potential mechanism for increased vascular disease. *Circ Cardiovasc Genet* 3(5):445–453, 2010.

572. Edelstein LC, et al: Human genome-wide association and mouse knockout approaches identify platelet supervillin as an inhibitor of thrombus formation under shear stress. *Circulation* 125(22):2762–2771, 2012.

573. Gieger C, et al: New gene functions in megakaryopoiesis and platelet formation. *Nature* 480(7376):201–208, 2011.

574. Weyrich AS, et al: Protein synthesis by platelets: Historical and new perspectives. *J Thromb Haemost* 7(2):241–246, 2009.

575. Denis MM, et al: Escaping the nuclear confines: Signal-dependent pre-mRNA splicing in anucleate platelets. *Cell* 122(3):379–391, 2005.

576. Edelstein LC, et al: MicroRNAs in platelet production and activation. *J Thromb Haemost* 11(Suppl 1):340–350, 2013.

577. Gnatenko DV, et al: Transcript profiling of human platelets using microarray and serial analysis of gene expression. *Blood* 101(6):2285–2293, 2003.

578. Bugert P, et al: Messenger RNA profiling of human platelets by microarray hybridization. *Thromb Haemost* 90(4):738–748, 2003.

579. Schubert S, Weyrich AS, Rowley JW: A tour through the transcriptional landscape of platelets. *Blood* 124(4):493–502, 2014.

580. Rowley JW, et al: Genome-wide RNA-seq analysis of human and mouse platelet transcriptomes. *Blood* 118(14):e101–e111, 2011.

581. Bray PF, McKenzie SE, Edelstein LC, et al: The complex transcriptional landscape of the anucleate human platelet. *BMC Genomics* 14(1):1, 2013.

582. Simon LM, Edelstein LC, Nagalla S, et al: Human platelet microRNA-mRNA networks associated with age and gender revealed by integrated plateletomics. *Blood* 123(16):e37–e45, 2014.

583. Wang Z, et al: The role of mitochondria-derived reactive oxygen species in hyperthermia-induced platelet apoptosis. *PLoS One* 8(9):e75044, 2013.

584. Hayashi T, Tanaka S, Hori Y, et al: Role of mitochondria in the maintenance of platelet function during in vitro storage. *Transfus Med* 21(3):166–174, 2011.

585. Shim MH, et al: Gene expression profile of primary human CD34+CD38lo cells differentiating along the megakaryocyte lineage. *Exp Hematol* 32(7):638–648, 2004.

586. Tenedini E, et al: Gene expression profiling of normal and malignant CD34-derived megakaryocytic cells. *Blood* 104(10):3126–3135, 2004.

587. Healy AM, et al: Platelet expression profiling and clinical validation of myeloid-related protein-14 as a novel determinant of cardiovascular events. *Circulation* 113(19):2278–2284, 2006.

588. Morrow DA, et al: Myeloid-related protein 8/14 and the risk of cardiovascular death or myocardial infarction after an acute coronary syndrome in the Pravastatin or Atorvastatin Evaluation and Infection Therapy: Thrombolysis in Myocardial Infarction (PROVE IT-TIMI 22) trial. *Am Heart J* 155(1):49–55, 2008.

589. Gnatenko DV, et al: Platelets express steroidogenic 17beta-hydroxysteroid dehydrogenases. Distinct profiles predict the essential thrombocythemic phenotype. *Thromb Haemost* 94(2):412–421, 2005.

590. Gnatenko DV, et al: Class prediction models of thrombocytosis using genetic biomarkers. *Blood* 115(1):7–14, 2010.

591. Sun L, et al: Decreased platelet expression of myosin regulatory light chain polypeptide (MYL9) and other genes with platelet dysfunction and CBFA2/RUNX1 mutation: Insights from platelet expression profiling. *J Thromb Haemost* 5(1):146–154, 2007.

592. Kahr WH, et al: Mutations in NBEAL2, encoding a BEACH protein, cause gray platelet syndrome. *Nat Genet* 43(8):738–740, 2011.

593. Nanda N, et al: Platelet endothelial aggregation receptor 1 (PEAR1), a novel epidermal growth factor repeat-containing transmembrane receptor, participates in platelet contact-induced activation. *J Biol Chem* 280(26):24680–24689, 2005.

594. Kondkar AA, et al: VAMP8/endobrevin is overexpressed in hyperreactive human platelets: Suggested role for platelet microRNA. *J Thromb Haemost* 8(2):369–378, 2010.

595. Goodall AH, et al: Transcription profiling in human platelets reveals LRRFIP1 as a novel protein regulating platelet function. *Blood* 116(22):4646–4656, 2010.

596. Edelstein LC, Simon LM, Montoya RT, et al: Racial differences in human platelet PAR4 reactivity reflect expression of PCTP and miR-376c. *Nat Med* 19(12):1609–1616, 2013.

597. Carninci P, et al: The transcriptional landscape of the mammalian genome. *Science* 309(5740):1559–1563, 2005.

598. Bartel DP: MicroRNAs: Target recognition and regulatory functions. *Cell* 136(2):215–233, 2009.

599. Nagalla S, et al: Platelet microRNA-mRNA coexpression profiles correlate with platelet reactivity. *Blood* 117(19):5189–5197, 2011.

600. Edelstein LC, Bray PF: MicroRNAs in platelet production and activation. *Blood* 117(20):5289–5296, 2011.

601. Georgantas RW 3rd, et al: CD34+ hematopoietic stem-progenitor cell microRNA expression and function: A circuit diagram of differentiation control. *Proc Natl Acad Sci U S A* 104(8):2750–2755, 2007.

602. Lu J, et al: MicroRNA-mediated control of cell fate in megakaryocyte-erythrocyte progenitors. *Dev Cell* 14(6):843–853, 2008.

603. Klusmann JH, et al: MiR-125b-2 is a potential oncomiR on human chromosome 21 in megakaryoblastic leukemia. *Genes Dev* 24(5):478–490, 2010.

604. Kumar MS, et al: Coordinate loss of a microRNA and protein-coding gene cooperate in the pathogenesis of 5q- syndrome. *Blood* 118(17):4666–4673, 2011.

605. Bruchova H, Merkerova M, Prchal JT: Aberrant expression of microRNA in polycythemia vera. *Haematologica* 93(7):1009–1016, 2008.

606. Girardot M, et al: MiR-28 is a thrombopoietin receptor targeting microRNA detected in a fraction of myeloproliferative neoplasm patient platelets. *Blood* 116(3):437–445, 2010.

607. Xu X, et al: Systematic analysis of microRNA fingerprints in thrombocythemic platelets using integrated platforms. *Blood* 120(17):3575–3585, 2012.

608. Zampetaki A, et al: Prospective study on circulating MicroRNAs and risk of myocardial infarction. *J Am Coll Cardiol* 60(4):290–299, 2012.

609. Gidlof O, et al: Platelets activated during myocardial infarction release functional miRNA, which can be taken up by endothelial cells and regulate ICAM1 expression. *Blood* 121(19):3908–3917, S1–S26, 2013.

610. Willeit P, et al: Circulating MicroRNAs as novel biomarkers for platelet activation. *Circ Res* 112(4):595–600, 2013.

611. de Boer HC, et al: Aspirin treatment hampers the use of plasma microRNA-126 as a biomarker for the progression of vascular disease. *Eur Heart J* 34(44):3451–3457, 2013.

612. Garcia A, et al: Extensive analysis of the human platelet proteome by two-dimensional gel electrophoresis and mass spectrometry. *Proteomics* 4(3):656–668, 2004.

613. Garcia A, Senis YA: *Platelet Proteomics: Principles, Analysis, and Applications.* John Wiley & Sons, Hoboken, NJ, 2011.

614. Thon JN, Devine DV: Translation of glycoprotein IIIa in stored blood platelets. *Transfusion* 47(12):2260–2270, 2007.

615. Burkhart JM, et al: The first comprehensive and quantitative analysis of human platelet protein composition allows the comparative analysis of structural and functional pathways. *Blood* 120(15):e73–e82, 2012.

616. Smith MC, Schwertz H, Zimmerman GA, Weyrich AS: The platelet proteome, in *Platelets*, edited by A Michelson. Academic Press, San Diego, 2012.

617. Booyse F, Rafelson ME Jr: *in vitro* incorporation of amino-acids into the contractile protein of human blood platelets. *Nature* 215(5098):283–284, 1967.

618. Cecchetti L, et al: Megakaryocytes differentially sort mRNAs for matrix metalloproteinases and their inhibitors into platelets: A mechanism for regulating synthetic events. *Blood* 118(7):1903–1911, 2011.

619. Hottz ED, Lopes JF, Freitas C, et al: Platelets mediate increased endothelium permeability in dengue through NLRP3-inflammasome activation. *Blood* 122(20):3405–3414, 2013.

620. Martens L, et al: The human platelet proteome mapped by peptide-centric proteomics: A functional protein profile. *Proteomics* 5(12):3193–3204, 2005.

621. Zufferey A, et al: Characterization of the platelet granule proteome: Evidence of the presence of MHC1 in alpha-granules. *J Proteomics* 101:130–140, 2014.

622. Hernandez-Ruiz L, et al: Organellar proteomics of human platelet dense granules reveals that 14–3–3zeta is a granule protein related to atherosclerosis. *J Proteome Res* 6(11):4449–4457, 2007.

623. Senis YA, et al: A comprehensive proteomics and genomics analysis reveals novel transmembrane proteins in human platelets and mouse megakaryocytes including G6b-B, a novel immunoreceptor tyrosine-based inhibitory motif protein. *Mol Cell Proteomics* 6(3):548–564, 2007.

624. Lewandrowski U, et al: Platelet membrane proteomics: A novel repository for functional research. *Blood* 114(1):e10–e19, 2009.

625. Maguire PB, et al: Identification of the phosphotyrosine proteome from thrombin activated platelets. *Proteomics* 2(6):642–648, 2002.

626. Garcia A, et al: A global proteomics approach identifies novel phosphorylated signaling proteins in GPVI-activated platelets: Involvement of G6f, a novel platelet Grb2-binding membrane adapter. *Proteomics* 6(19):5332–5343, 2006.

627. Dowal L, et al: Proteomic analysis of palmitoylated platelet proteins. *Blood* 118(13):e62–e73, 2011.

628. Lewandrowski U, et al: Enhanced N-glycosylation site analysis of sialoglycopeptides by strong cation exchange prefractionation applied to platelet plasma membranes. *Mol Cell Proteomics* 6(11):1933–1941, 2007.

629. Coppinger JA, et al: Characterization of the proteins released from activated platelets leads to localization of novel platelet proteins in human atherosclerotic lesions. *Blood* 103(6):2096–2104, 2004.

630. Piersma SR, et al: Proteomics of the TRAP-induced platelet releasate. *J Proteomics* 72(1):91–109, 2009.

631. Garcia BA, et al: The platelet microparticle proteome. *J Proteome Res* 4(5):1516–1521, 2005.

632. Capriotti AL, et al: Proteomic characterization of human platelet-derived microparticles. *Anal Chim Acta* 776:57–63, 2013.

633. Maurer-Spurej E, et al: The value of proteomics for the diagnosis of a platelet-related bleeding disorder. *Platelets* 19(5):342–351, 2008.

634. Frobel J, et al: Platelet proteome analysis reveals integrin-dependent aggregation defects in patients with myelodysplastic syndromes. *Mol Cell Proteomics* 12(5):1272–1280, 2013.

635. Snyder EL, et al: Protein changes occurring during storage of platelet concentrates. A two-dimensional gel electrophoretic analysis. *Transfusion* 27(4):335–341, 1987.

636. Thiele T, et al: Profiling of alterations in platelet proteins during storage of platelet concentrates. *Transfusion* 47(7):1221–1233, 2007.

637. Thon JN, et al: Comprehensive proteomic analysis of protein changes during platelet storage requires complementary proteomic approaches. *Transfusion* 48(3):425–435, 2008.

638. Parguina AF, Grigorian-Shamajian L, Agra RM, et al: Proteins involved in platelet signaling are differentially regulated in acute coronary syndrome: A proteomic study. *PLoS One* 5(10):e13404, 2010.

639. Londin ER, Hatzimichael E, Loher P, et al: The human platelet: Strong transcriptome correlations among individuals associate weakly with the platelet proteome. *Biol Direct* 9:3, 2014.

640. Handagama PJ, Shuman MA, Bainton DF: Incorporation of intravenously injected albumin, immunoglobulin G, and fibrinogen in guinea pig megakaryocyte granules. *J Clin Invest* 84(1):73–82, 1989.

641. Voora D, et al: Aspirin exposure reveals novel genes associated with platelet function and cardiovascular events. *J Am Coll Cardiol* 62(14):1267–1276, 2013.

642. Bevers EM, et al: Lipid translocation across the plasma membrane of mammalian cells. *Biochim Biophys Acta* 1439(3):317–330, 1999.

643. Pomorski T, Menon AK: Lipid flippases and their biological functions. *Cell Mol Life Sci* 63(24):2908–2921, 2006.

644. Yang H, et al: TMEM16F Forms a Ca(2+)-activated cation channel required for lipid scrambling in platelets during blood coagulation. *Cell* 151(1):111–122, 2012.

645. Barry OP, FitzGerald GA: Mechanisms of cellular activation by platelet microparticles. *Thromb Haemost* 82:794–800, 1999.

646. Thiagarajan P, Tait JF: Collagen-induced exposure of anionic phospholipid in platelets and platelet-derived microparticles. *J Biol Chem* 266:24302–24307, 1991.

647. Bouchard BA, et al: Effector cell protease receptor-1, a platelet activation-dependent membrane protein, regulates prothrombinase-catalyzed thrombin generation. *J Biol Chem* 272(14):9244–9251, 1997.

648. Enjeti AK, Lincz LF, Seldon M: Microparticles in health and disease. *Semin Thromb Hemost* 34(7):683–691, 2008.

649. Hultin MB: Modulation of thrombin-mediated activation of factor VIII:C by calcium ions, phospholipid, and platelets. *Blood* 66(1):53–58, 1985.

650. Miyazaki Y, et al: High shear stress can initiate both platelet aggregation and shedding of procoagulant containing microparticles. *Blood* 88(9):3456–3464, 1996.

651. Nesheim ME, et al: On the existence of platelet receptors for factors V(a) and factor VIII (a). *Thromb Haemost* 70:80–85, 1993.

652. Piccin A, Murphy WG, Smith OP: Circulating microparticles: Pathophysiology and clinical implications. *Blood Rev* 21(3):157–171, 2007.

653. George JN, et al: Platelet surface glycoproteins. Studies on resting and activated platelets and platelet membrane microparticles in normal subjects, and observations in patients during adult respiratory distress syndrome and cardiac surgery. *J Clin Invest* 78(2):340–348, 1986.

654. Siljander P, Carpen O, Lassila R: Platelet-derived microparticles associate with fibrin during thrombosis. *Blood* 87(11):4651–4663, 1996.

655. Dahlback B, Wiedmer T, Sims PJ: Binding of anticoagulant vitamin K-dependent protein S to platelet-derived microparticles. *Biochemistry* 31(51):12769–12777, 1992.

656. Tans G, et al: Comparison of anticoagulant and procoagulant activities of stimulated platelets and platelet-derived microparticles. *Blood* 77(12):2641–2648, 1991.

657. Toti F, et al: Scott syndrome, characterized by impaired transmembrane migration of procoagulant phosphatidylserine and hemorrhagic complications, is an inherited disorder. *Blood* 87(4):1409–1415, 1996.

658. Weiss HJ: Scott syndrome: A disorder of platelet coagulant activity. *Semin Hematol* 31(4):312–319, 1994.

659. Weiss HJ, Lages B: Platelet prothrombinase activity and intracellular calcium responses in patients with storage pool deficiency, glycoprotein IIb-IIIa deficiency, or impaired platelet coagulant activity—A comparison with Scott syndrome. *Blood* 89(5):1599–1611, 1997.

660. Panes O, et al: Human platelets synthesize and express functional tissue factor. *Blood* 109(12):5242–5250, 2007.

661. Schwertz H, et al: Signal-dependent splicing of tissue factor pre-mRNA modulates the thrombogenicity of human platelets. *J Exp Med* 203(11):2433–2440, 2006.

662. Freedman JE, et al: Deficient platelet-derived nitric oxide and enhanced hemostasis in mice lacking the NOSIII gene. *Circ Res* 84(12):1416–1421, 1999.

663. Iafrati MD, Vitseva O, Tanriverdi K, et al: Compensatory mechanisms influence hemostasis in setting of eNOS deficiency. *Am J Physiol Heart Circ Physiol* 288(4): H1627–H1632, 2005.

664. Marjanovic JA, et al: Stimulatory roles of nitric-oxide synthase 3 and guanylyl cyclase in platelet activation. *J Biol Chem* 280(45):37430–37438, 2005.

665. Ozuyaman B, et al: Endothelial nitric oxide synthase plays a minor role in inhibition of arterial thrombus formation. *Thromb Haemost* 93(6):1161–1167, 2005.

666. Osterud B: The role of platelets in decrypting monocyte tissue factor. *Semin Hematol* 38(4 Suppl 12):2–5, 2001.

667. Reinhardt C, et al: Protein disulfide isomerase acts as an injury response signal that enhances fibrin generation via tissue factor activation. *J Clin Invest* 118(3):1110–1122, 2008.

668. Smith SA, et al: Polyphosphate modulates blood coagulation and fibrinolysis. *Proc Natl Acad Sci U S A* 103(4):903–908, 2006.

669. Smith SA, Morrissey JH: Polyphosphate enhances fibrin clot structure. *Blood* 112(7):2810–2816, 2008.

670. Bouchard BA, et al: Interactions between platelets and the coagulation system, in *Platelets*, edited by AD Michelson, pp 377–402. Academic Press, San Diego, 2007.

671. Swords NA, Tracy PB, Mann KG: Intact platelet membranes, not platelet-released microvesicles, support the procoagulant activity of adherent platelets. *Arterioscler Thromb* 13(11):1613–1622, 1993.

672. Zwaal RFA, Comfurius P, Bevers EM: Platelet procoagulant activity and microvesicle formation. Its putative role of hemostasis and thrombosis. *Biochim Biophys Acta* 1180:1–8, 1992.

673. Alberio L, et al: Surface expression and functional characterization of alpha-granule factor V in human platelets: Effects of ionophore A23187, thrombin, collagen, and convulxin. *Blood* 95(5):1694–1702, 2000.

674. Scandura JM, Ahmad SS, Walsh PN: A binding site expressed on the surface of activated human platelets is shared by factor X and prothrombin. *Biochemistry* 35(27):8890–8902, 1996.

675. Byzova TV, Plow EF: Networking in the hemostatic system. Integrin alphaiibbeta3 binds prothrombin and influences its activation. *J Biol Chem* 272(43):27183–27188, 1997.

676. Baglia FA, Walsh PN: Thrombin-mediated feedback activation of factor XI on the activated platelet surface is preferred over contact activation by factor XIIa or factor XIa. *J Biol Chem* 275(27):20514–20519, 2000.

677. Oliver JA, et al: Thrombin activates factor XI on activated platelets in the absence of factor XII. *Arterioscler Thromb Vasc Biol* 19(1):170–177, 1999.

678. Gailani D, et al: Model for a factor IX activation complex on blood platelets: Dimeric conformation of factor XIa is essential. *Blood* 97(10):3117–3122, 2001.

679. Walsh PN: Platelets and factor XI bypass the contact system of blood coagulation. *Thromb Haemost* 82:234–242, 1999.

680. Coller BS: Platelets and thrombolytic therapy. *N Engl J Med* 322:33–42, 1990.

681. Coller BS: Augmentation of thrombolysis with antiplatelet drugs. Overview. *Coron Artery Dis* 6:911–914, 1995.

682. Kolev K, Machovich R: Molecular and cellular modulation of fibrinolysis. *Thromb Haemost* 89(4):610–621, 2003.

683. Korbut R, Gryglewski RJ: Platelets in fibrinolytic system. *J Physiol Pharmacol* 46(4):409–418, 1995.

684. Maron BA, Loscalzo J: The role of platelets in fibrinolysis, in *Platelets*, edited by AD Michelson, pp 415–430. Academic Press, San Diego, 2007.

685. Carroll RC, et al: Plasminogen, plasminogen activator and platelets in the regulation of clot lysis. *J Lab Clin Med* 100:986–996, 1982.

686. de Haan J, van Oeveren W: Platelets and soluble fibrin promote plasminogen activation causing downregulation of platelet glycoprotein Ib/IX complexes: Protection by aprotinin. *Thromb Res* 92(4):171–179, 1998.

687. Jeanneau C, Sultan Y: Tissue plasminogen activator in human megakaryocytes and platelets: Immunocytochemical localization, immunoblotting and zymographic analysis. *Thromb Haemost* 19:529–534, 1988.

688. Miles LA, et al: Plasminogen interacts with human platelets through two distinct mechanisms. *J Clin Invest* 77:2001–2009, 1986.

689. Miles LA, Plow EF: Binding and activation of plasminogen on the platelet surface. *J Biol Chem* 260:4303–4311, 1985.

690. Park S, et al: Demonstration of single chain urokinase-type plasminogen activator on human platelet membrane. *Blood* 73:1421–1425, 1989.

691. Stricker RB, et al: Activation of plasminogen by tissue plasminogen activator on normal and thrombasthenic platelets: Effects on surface proteins and platelet aggregation. *Blood* 68:275–280, 1986.

692. Thorsen S, Brakman P, Astrup T: Influence of platelets on fibrinolysis: A critical review, in *Hematologic Reviews*, edited by JL Ambrole, pp 123–179. Marcel Dekker, New York, 1972.

693. Binder BR, et al: Plasminogen activator inhibitor 1: Physiological and pathophysiological roles. *News Physiol Sci* 17:56–61, 2002.

694. Cox AD, Devine DV: Factor XIIIa binding to activated platelets is mediated through activation of glycoprotein IIb-IIIa. *Blood* 83:1006–1016, 1994.

695. Erickson LA, Ginsberg MH, Loskutoff DJ: Detection and partial characterization of an inhibitor of plasminogen activator in human platelets. *J Clin Invest* 74:1465–1472, 1984.

696. Fay WP, et al: Platelets inhibit fibrinolysis in vitro by both plasminogen activator inhibitor-1 dependent and independent mechanisms. *Blood* 83:351–356, 1994.

697. Francis CW, Marder VJ: Rapid formation of large molecular weight alpha-polymers in cross-linked fibrin induced by high factor XIII concentrations: Role of platelet factor XIII. *J Clin Invest* 80:1459–1465, 1987.

698. Kawasaki T, et al: Vascular release of plasminogen activator inhibitor-1 impairs fibrinolysis during acute arterial thrombosis in mice. *Blood* 96(1):153–160, 2000.

699. Kruithof EKO, Tran-Thang C, Bachmann F: Studies on the release of plasminogen activator inhibitor from human platelets. *Thromb Haemost* 55:201–205, 1986.

700. Plow EF, Collen D: The presence and release of α2-antiplasmin from human platelets. *Blood* 58:1069–1074, 1981.

701. Smariga PE, Maynard JR: Purification of a platelet protein which stimulates fibrinolytic inhibition and tissue factor in human fibroblasts. *J Biol Chem* 257:11960–11965, 1982.

702. Jang IK, et al: Differential sensitivity of erythrocyte-rich and platelet-rich arterial thrombi to lysis with recombinant tissue-type plasminogen activator. A possible explanation for resistance to coronary thrombolysis. *Circulation* 79:920–928, 1989.

703. Fitzgerald DJ, et al: Marked platelet activation *in vivo* after intravenous streptokinase in patients with acute myocardial infarction. *Circulation* 77:142–150, 1988.

704. Fitzgerald DJ, Wright F, FitzGerald GA: Increased thromboxane biosynthesis during coronary thrombolysis: Evidence that platelet activation and thromboxane A2 modulate the response to tissue-type plasminogen activator *in vivo*. *Circ Res* 65:83–94, 1989.

705. Kerins DM, et al: Platelet and vascular function during coronary thrombolysis with tissue-type plasminogen activator. *Circulation* 80:1718–1725, 1990.

706. Ohlstein EH, et al: Tissue-type plasminogen activator and streptokinase induce platelet hyperaggregability in the rabbit. *Thromb Res* 46:575–585, 1987.

707. Penny WF, Ware JA: Platelet activation and subsequent inhibition by plasmin and recombinant tissue-type plasminogen activator. *Blood* 79(1):91–98, 1992.

708. Rudd MA, et al: Temporal effects of thrombolytic agents on platelet function in vivo and their modulation by prostaglandins. *Circ Res* 67(5):1175–1181, 1990.

709. Shebuski RJ: Principles underlying the use of conjunctive agents with plasminogen activators. *Ann N Y Acad Sci* 667:382–394, 1992.

710. Ervin AL, Peerschke EI: Platelet activation by sustained exposure to low-dose plasmin. *Blood Coagul Fibrinolysis* 12(6):415–425, 2001.

711. Ishii-Watabe A, et al: On the mechanism of plasmin-induced platelet aggregation. Implications of the dual role of granule ADP. *Biochem Pharmacol* 59(11):1345–1355, 2000.

712. Niewiarowski S, Senyi AF, Gillies P: Plasmin-induced platelet aggregation and platelet release reaction. *J Clin Invest* 52:1647–1659, 1973.

713. Schafer AI, et al: Platelet protein phosphorylation, elevation of cytosolic calcium, and inositol phospholipid breakdown in platelet activation induced by plasmin. *J Clin Invest* 78:73–79, 1986.

714. Quinton TM, et al: Plasmin-mediated activation of platelets occurs by cleavage of protease-activated receptor 4. *J Biol Chem* 279(18):18434–18439, 2004.

715. Eisenberg PR, Sherman LA, Jaffe AS: Paradoxic elevation of fibrinopeptide A after streptokinase: Evidence for continued thrombosis despite intense fibrinolysis. *J Am Coll Cardiol* 10:527–529, 1987.

716. Leopold JA, Loscalzo J: Platelet activation by fibrinolytic agents: A potential mechanism for resistance to thrombolysis and reocclusion after successful thrombolysis. *Coron Artery Dis* 6(12):923–929, 1995.

717. Owen J, et al: Thrombolytic therapy with tissue plasminogen activator or streptokinase induces transient thrombin activity. *Blood* 72:616–620, 1988.

718. Szczeklik A: Thrombin generation in myocardial infarction and hypercholesterolemia: Effects of aspirin. *Thromb Haemost* 74(1):77–80, 1995.

719. Weitz JI, et al: Human tissue-type plasminogen activator releases fibrinopeptides A and B from fibrinogen. *J Clin Invest* 82:1700–1707, 1988.

720. Coller BS: Platelets in cardiovascular thrombosis and thrombolysis, in *The Heart and Cardiovascular System*, edited by HA Fozzard, Jennings RB, Katz AM, Morgan HE, Haber E, pp 219–273. Raven Press, New York, 1991.

721. Coller BS: Inhibitors of the platelet glycoprotein IIb/IIIa receptor as conjunctive therapy for coronary artery thrombolysis. *Coron Artery Dis* 3:1016–1029, 1992.

722. Eccleston D, Topol EJ: Inhibitors of platelet glycoprotein IIb/IIIa as augmenters of thrombolysis. *Coron Artery Dis* 6(12):947–955, 1995.

723. O'Donnell CJ, Jonas MA, Hennekens CH: Aspirin augmentation of the efficacy of thrombolysis. *Coron Artery Dis* 6(12):936–939, 1995.

724. Topol EJ: Reperfusion therapy for acute myocardial infarction with fibrinolytic therapy or combination reduced fibrinolytic therapy and platelet glycoprotein IIb/IIIa inhibition: The GUSTO V randomised trial. *Lancet* 357(9272):1905–1914, 2001.

725. Di Mario C, Dudek D, Piscione F, et al: Immediate angioplasty versus standard therapy with rescue angioplasty after thrombolysis in the Combined Abciximab REteplase Stent Study in Acute Myocardial Infarction (CARESS-in-AMI): An open, prospective, randomised, multicentre trial. *Lancet* 371(9612):559–568, 2008.

726. Ellis SG, et al: Facilitated PCI in patients with ST-elevation myocardial infarction. *N Engl J Med* 358(21):2205–2217, 2008.

727. Lapchak PA, et al: The nonpeptide glycoprotein IIb/IIIa platelet receptor antagonist SM-20302 reduces tissue plasminogen activator-induced intracerebral hemorrhage after thromboembolic stroke. *Stroke* 33(1):147–152, 2002.

728. Zhang L, et al: Adjuvant treatment with a glycoprotein IIb/IIIa receptor inhibitor increases the therapeutic window for low-dose tissue plasminogen activator administration in a rat model of embolic stroke. *Circulation* 107(22):2837–2843, 2003.

729. Zhang ZG, et al: Dynamic platelet accumulation at the site of the occluded middle cerebral artery and in downstream microvessels is associated with loss of microvascular integrity after embolic middle cerebral artery occlusion. *Brain Res* 912(2):181–194, 2001.

730. Adams HP Jr, et al: Emergency administration of abciximab for treatment of patients with acute ischemic stroke: Results of an international phase III trial: Abciximab in Emergency Treatment of Stroke Trial (AbESTT-II). *Stroke* 39(1):87–99, 2008.

731. Mandava P, Thiagarajan P, Kent TA: Glycoprotein IIb/IIIa antagonists in acute ischaemic stroke: Current status and future directions. *Drugs* 68(8):1019–1028, 2008.

732. Adelman B, et al: Plasmin effect on platelet glycoprotein Ib-von Willebrand factor interactions. *Blood* 64:32–40, 1985.

733. Adnot S, et al: Plasmin: A possible physiological modulator of human platelet adenylate cyclase system. *Clin Sci* 72:467–473, 1987.

734. Federici AB, et al: Proteolysis of von Willebrand factor in patients undergoing thrombolytic therapy. *Circulation* 78(Suppl II):II–120, 1992.

735. Gimple LW, et al: Correlation between template bleeding times and spontaneous bleeding during treatment of acute myocardial infarction with recombinant tissue-type plasminogen activator. *Circulation* 80:581–588, 1989.

736. Johnstone MT, et al: Bleeding time prolongation with streptokinase and its reduction with 1-desamino-8-D-arginine vasopressin. *Circulation* 82(6):2142–2151, 1990.

737. Kamat SG, Schafer AI: Antiplatelet effects of fibrinolytic agents: A potential contributor to the hemostatic defect after thrombolysis. *Coron Artery Dis* 6(12):930–935, 1995.

738. Kowalski E, Kopec M, Wegrzynowicz Z: Influence of fibrinogen degradation products (FDP) on platelet aggregation, adhesiveness and viscous metamorphosis. *Thromb Diath Haemorrh* 10:406–423, 1963.

739. Loscalzo J, Vaughan DE: Tissue plasminogen activator promotes platelet disaggregation in plasma. *J Clin Invest* 79:1749–1754, 1987.

740. Michelson AD, et al: Effect of in vivo infusion of recombinant tissue-type plasminogen activator on platelet glycoprotein Ib. *Thromb Res* 60(5):421–424, 1990.

741. Schafer AL, Adelman B: Plasmin inhibition of platelet function and of arachidonic acid metabolism. *J Clin Invest* 75:456–461, 1985.

742. Schafer AL, et al: Synergistic inhibition of platelet activation by plasmin and prostaglandin I2. *Blood* 69:1504–1507, 1987.

743. Shin Y, et al: Binding of von Willebrand factor cleaving protease ADAMTS13 to Lys-plasmin(ogen). *J Biochem* 152(3):251–258, 2012.

744. Tersteeg C, et al: Plasmin cleavage of von Willebrand factor as an emergency bypass for ADAMTS13 deficiency in thrombotic microangiopathy. *Circulation* 129(12):1320–1331, 2014.

745. Coller BS: Binding of abciximab to $\alpha_V\beta_3$ and activated $\alpha_M\beta_2$ receptors: With a review of platelet-leukocyte interactions. *Thromb Haemost* 82(2):326–336, 1999.

746. Farb A, et al: Pathology of acute and chronic coronary stenting in humans. *Circulation* 99(1):44–52, 1999.

747. Merhi Y, et al: Selectin blockade reduces neutrophil interaction with platelets at the site of deep arterial injury by angioplasty in pigs. *Arterioscler Thromb Vasc Biol* 19(2):372–377, 1999.

748. Smyth SS, et al: β3-integrin-deficient mice, but not P-selectin-deficient mice, develop intimal hyperplasia after vascular injury: Correlation with leukocyte recruitment to adherent platelets 1 hour after injury. *Circulation* 103:2501–2507, 2001.

749. Wehner J, et al: Antibody and complement in transplant vasculopathy. *Circ Res* 100(2):191–203, 2007.

750. Nishimura S, et al: in vivo imaging in mice reveals local cell dynamics and inflammation in obese adipose tissue. *J Clin Invest* 118(2):710–721, 2008.

751. Bozza FA, et al: Amicus or adversary: Platelets in lung biology, acute injury, and inflammation. *Am J Respir Cell Mol Biol* 40(2):123–134, 2009.

752. Schober A, et al: Deposition of platelet RANTES triggering monocyte recruitment requires P-selectin and is involved in neointima formation after arterial injury. *Circulation* 106(12):1523–1529, 2002.

753. von Hundelshausen P, et al: RANTES deposition by platelets triggers monocyte arrest on inflamed and atherosclerotic endothelium. *Circulation* 103(13):1772–1777, 2001.

754. Huo Y, et al: Circulating activated platelets exacerbate atherosclerosis in mice deficient in apolipoprotein E. *Nat Med* 9(1):61–67, 2003.

755. Diacovo TG, et al: Neutrophil rolling, arrest, and transmigration across activated, surface-adherent platelets via sequential action of P-selectin and the beta 2-integrin CD11b/CD18. *Blood* 88(1):146–157, 1996.

756. Hamburger SA, McEver RP: GMP-140 mediates adhesion of stimulated platelets to neutrophils. *Blood* 75(3):550–554, 1990.

757. Kirchhofer D, Riederer MA, Baumgartner HR: Specific accumulation of circulating monocytes and polymorphonuclear leukocytes on platelet thrombi in a vascular injury model. *Blood* 89(4):1270–1278, 1997.

758. Konstantopoulos K, et al: Venous levels of shear support neutrophil-platelet adhesion and neutrophil aggregation in blood via P-selectin and beta2-integrin. *Circulation* 98(9):873–882, 1998.

759. Larsen E, et al: PADGEM protein: A receptor that mediates the interaction of activated platelets with neutrophils and monocytes. *Cell* 59(2):305–312, 1989.

760. Sheikh S, Nash GB: Continuous activation and deactivation of integrin CD11b/CD18 during de novo expression enables rolling neutrophils to immobilize on platelets. *Blood* 87(12):5040–5050, 1996.

761. Yeo EL, Sheppard JA, Feuerstein IA: Role of P-selectin and leukocyte activation in polymorphonuclear cell adhesion to surface adherent activated platelets under physiologic shear conditions (an injury vessel wall model). *Blood* 83(9):2498–2507, 1994.

762. Gear AR, Camerini D: Platelet chemokines and chemokine receptors: Linking hemostasis, inflammation, and host defense. *Microcirculation* 10(3–4):335–350, 2003.

763. Weber C, Springer TA: Neutrophil accumulation on activated, surface-adherent platelets in flow is mediated by interaction of Mac-1 with fibrinogen bound to alphaIIbbeta3 and stimulated by platelet-activating factor. *J Clin Invest* 100(8):2085–2093, 1997.

764. Romo GM, et al: The glycoprotein Ib-IX-V complex is a platelet counterreceptor for P-selectin. *J Exp Med* 190(6):803–814, 1999.

765. Altieri DC, Plescia J, Plow EF: The structural motif glycine 190-valine 202 of the fibrinogen gamma chain interacts with CD11b/CD18 integrin (alpha M beta 2, Mac-1) and promotes leukocyte adhesion. *J Biol Chem* 268(3):1847–1853, 1993.

766. Silverstein RL, Asch AS, Nachman RL: Glycoprotein IV mediates thrombospondin-dependent platelet-monocyte and platelet-U937 cell adhesion. *J Clin Invest* 84:546–552, 1989.

767. Santoso S, et al: The junctional adhesion molecule 3 (JAM-3) on human platelets is a counterreceptor for the leukocyte integrin Mac-1. *J Exp Med* 196(5):679–691, 2002.

768. Marcus AJ, Safier LB: Thromboregulation: Multicellular modulation of platelet reactivity in hemostasis and thrombosis. *FASEB J* 7(6):516–522, 1993.

769. Lindemann S, et al: Activated platelets mediate inflammatory signaling by regulated interleukin 1beta synthesis. *J Cell Biol* 154(3):485–490, 2001.

770. Alderson MR, et al: CD40 expression by human monocytes: Regulation by cytokines and activation of monocytes by the ligand for CD40. *J Exp Med* 178(2):669–674, 1993.

771. Henn V, et al: CD40 ligand on activated platelets triggers an inflammatory reaction of endothelial cells. *Nature* 391(6667):591–594, 1998.

772. Yellin MJ, et al: Functional interactions of T cells with endothelial cells: The role of CD40L-CD40-mediated signals. *J Exp Med* 182(6):1857–1864, 1995.

773. Slupsky JR, et al: Activated platelets induce tissue factor expression on human umbilical vein endothelial cells by ligation of CD40. *Thromb Haemost* 80(6):1008–1014, 1998.

774. Del PD, et al: The plasma membrane redox system in human platelet functions and platelet-leukocyte interactions. *Thromb Haemost* 101(2):284–289, 2009.

775. Goel MS, Diamond SL: Neutrophil enhancement of fibrin deposition under flow through platelet-dependent and -independent mechanisms. *Arterioscler Thromb Vasc Biol* 21(12):2093–2098, 2001.

776. Goel MS, Diamond SL: Neutrophil cathepsin G promotes prothrombinase and fibrin formation under flow conditions by activating fibrinogen-adherent platelets. *J Biol Chem* 278(11):9458–9463, 2003.

777. Giesen PL, et al: Blood-borne tissue factor: Another view of thrombosis. *Proc Natl Acad Sci U S A* 96(5):2311–2315, 1999.

778. Furie B, Furie BC: Role of platelet P-selectin and microparticle PSGL-1 in thrombus formation. *Trends Mol Med* 10(4):171–178, 2004.

779. Pluskota E, et al: Expression, activation, and function of integrin alphaMbeta2 (Mac-1) on neutrophil-derived microparticles. *Blood* 112(6):2327–2335, 2008.

780. Andre P, et al: Pro-coagulant state resulting from high levels of soluble P-selectin in blood. *Proc Natl Acad Sci U S A* 97(25):13835–13840, 2000.

781. Hrachovinova I, et al: Interaction of P-selectin and PSGL-1 generates microparticles that correct hemostasis in a mouse model of hemophilia A. *Nat Med* 9(8):1020–1025, 2003.

782. Ott I, et al: Increased neutrophil-platelet adhesion in patients with unstable angina. *Circulation* 94(6):1239–1246, 1996.

783. Mickelson JK, et al: Leukocyte activation with platelet adhesion after coronary angioplasty: A mechanism for recurrent disease? *J Am Coll Cardiol* 28(2):345–353, 1996.

784. Michelson AD, et al: Circulating monocyte-platelet aggregates are a more sensitive marker of in vivo platelet activation than platelet surface P-selectin: Studies in baboons, human coronary intervention, and human acute myocardial infarction. *Circulation* 104(13):1533–1537, 2001.

785. Bugert P, et al: The variable number of tandem repeat polymorphism in the P-selectin glycoprotein ligand-1 gene is not associated with coronary heart disease. *J Mol Med (Berl)* 81(8):495–501, 2003.

786. Diz-Kucukkaya R, et al: P-selectin glycoprotein ligand-1 VNTR polymorphisms and risk of thrombosis in the antiphospholipid syndrome. *Ann Rheum Dis* 66(10):1378–1380, 2007.

787. Lozano ML, et al: Polymorphisms of P-selectin glycoprotein ligand-1 are associated with neutrophil-platelet adhesion and with ischaemic cerebrovascular disease. *Br J Haematol* 115(4):969–976, 2001.

788. Ozben B, et al: The association of P-selectin glycoprotein ligand-1 VNTR polymorphisms with coronary stent restenosis. *J Thromb Thrombolysis* 23(3):181–187, 2007.

789. Roldan V, et al: Short alleles of P-selectin glycoprotein ligand-1 protect against premature myocardial infarction. *Am Heart J* 148(4):602–605, 2004.

790. Tauxe C, et al: P-selectin glycoprotein ligand-1 decameric repeats regulate selectin-dependent rolling under flow conditions. *J Biol Chem* 283(42):28536–28545, 2008.

791. Wang Y, et al: Platelet-derived S100 family member myeloid-related protein-14 regulates thrombosis. *J Clin Invest* 124(5):2160–2171, 2014.

792. Clark SR, et al: Platelet TLR4 activates neutrophil extracellular traps to ensnare bacteria in septic blood. *Nat Med* 13(4):463–469, 2007.

793. Geddings JE, Mackman N: New players in haemostasis and thrombosis. *Thromb Haemost* 111(4):570–574, 2014.

794. Martinod K, Wagner DD: Thrombosis: Tangled up in NETs. *Blood* 123(18):2768–2776, 2014.

795. Arman M, et al: Amplification of bacteria-induced platelet activation is triggered by FcgammaRIIA, integrin alphaIIbbeta3, and platelet factor 4. *Blood* 123(20):3166–3174, 2014.

796. Boudreau LH, et al: Platelets release mitochondria serving as substrate for bactericidal group IIA-secreted phospholipase A2 to promote inflammation. *Blood* 124(14):2173–2183, 2014.

797. Sun H, et al: Reduced thrombin generation increases host susceptibility to group A streptococcal infection. *Blood* 113(6):1358–1364, 2009.

798. Li N: Platelet-lymphocyte cross-talk. *J Leukoc Biol* 83(5):1069–1078, 2008.

799. McMorran BJ, et al: Platelets kill intraerythrocytic malarial parasites and mediate survival to infection. *Science* 323(5915):797–800, 2009.

800. Boulaftali Y, et al: Platelet immunoreceptor tyrosine-based activation motif (ITAM) signaling and vascular integrity. *Circ Res* 114(7):1174–1184, 2014.

801. Lopez JA: The platelet glycoprotein Ib-IX complex. *Blood Coagul Fibrinolysis* 5(1):97–119, 1994.

802. Wu G, et al: Human endothelial cells in culture and in vivo express on their surface all four components of the glycoprotein Ib/IX/V complex. *Blood* 90(7):2660–2669, 1997.

803. Hynes RO: Integrins: Bidirectional, allosteric signaling machines. *Cell* 110(6):673–687, 2002.

804. Kasirer-Friede A, Kahn ML, Shattil SJ: Platelet integrins and immunoreceptors. *Immunol Rev* 218:247–264, 2007.

805. Bennett JS, Berger BW, Billings PC: The structure and function of platelet integrins. *J Thromb Haemost* 7(Suppl 1):200–205, 2009.

806. Bledzka K, Smyth SS, Plow EF: Integrin alphaIIbbeta3: From discovery to efficacious therapeutic target. *Circ Res* 112(8):1189–1200, 2013.

807. Phillips DR, et al: The platelet membrane glycoprotein IIb-IIIa complex. *Blood* 71:831–843, 1988.

808. Plow EF, Ginsberg MH: Cellular adhesion: GPIIb-IIIa as a prototypic adhesion receptor. *Prog Hemost Thromb* 9:117–156, 1989.

809. Ruggeri ZM: Structure and function of von Willebrand factor. *Thromb Haemost* 82:576–584, 1999.

810. Savage B, Ruggeri ZM: Platelet thrombus formation in flowing blood, in *Platelets*, edited by AD Michelson, p 215. Academic Press, San Diego, 2002.

811. Wagner CL, et al: Analysis of GPIIb/IIIa receptor number by quantification of 7E3 binding to human platelets. *Blood* 88:907–914, 1996.

812. Zhou YF, et al: Sequence and structure relationships within von Willebrand factor. *Blood* 120(2):449–458, 2012.

813. Cramer ER, et al: α Granule pool of glycoprotein IIb-IIIa in normal and pathologic platelets and megakaryocytes. *Blood* 75:1220–1227, 1990.

814. Woods VL Jr, Wolff LE, Keller DM: Resting platelets contain a substantial centrally located pool of glycoprotein IIb-IIIa complexes which may be accessible to some but not other extracellular proteins. *J Biol Chem* 261:15242–15251, 1986.

815. Youssefian T, et al: Platelet and megakaryocyte dense granules contain glycoproteins Ib and IIb-IIIa. *Blood* 89(11):4047–4057, 1997.

816. Peerschke EI: The platelet fibrinogen receptor. *Semin Hematol* 22(4):241–259, 1985.

817. Wencel-Drake JD: Plasma membrane GPIIb/IIIa. Evidence for a cycling receptor pool. *Am J Clin Pathol* 136:61–70, 1990.

818. Harrison P: Platelet α-granular fibrinogen. *Platelets* 3:1–10, 1992.

819. Hynes RO: Integrins: A family of cell surface receptors. *Cell* 48:549–554, 1987.

820. Ruoslahti E: Fibronectin and its receptors. *Annu Rev Biochem* 57:375–413, 1988.

821. Doolittle RF, et al: The amino acid sequence of the alpha-chain of human fibrinogen. *Nature* 280:464, 1979.

822. Cheresh DA, et al: Recognition of distinct adhesive sites on fibrinogen by related integrins on platelets and endothelial cells. *Cell* 58:945–953, 1989.

823. Farrell DH, Thiagarajan P: Binding of recombinant fibrinogen mutants to platelets. *J Biol Chem* 269(1):226–231, 1994.

824. Farrell DH, et al: Role of fibrinogen α and γ chain sites in platelet aggregation. *Proc Natl Acad Sci U S A* 89(22):10729–10732, 1992.

825. Savage B, Ruggeri ZM: Selective recognition of adhesive sites in surface-bound fibrinogen by glycoprotein IIb-IIIa on nonactivated platelets. *J Biol Chem* 266(17):11227–11233, 1991.

826. Springer TA, Zhu J, Xiao T: Structural basis for distinctive recognition of fibrinogen gammaC peptide by the platelet integrin alphaIIbbeta3. *J Cell Biol* 182(4):791–800, 2008.

827. Xiao T, et al: Structural basis for allostery in integrins and binding to fibrinogen-mimetic therapeutics. *Nature* 432:59–67, 2004.

828. Goldsmith HL, et al: Time and force dependence of the rupture of glycoprotein IIb-IIIa-fibrinogen bonds between latex spheres. *Biophys J* 78(3):1195–1206, 2000.

829. Hsieh CF, et al: Stepped changes of monovalent ligand-binding force during ligand-induced clustering of integrin alphaIIb beta3. *J Biol Chem* 281(35):25466–25474, 2006.

830. Huber W, et al: Determination of kinetic constants for the interaction between the platelet glycoprotein IIb-IIIa and fibrinogen by means of surface plasmon resonance. *Eur J Biochem* 227(3):647–656, 1995.

831. Litvinov RI, et al: Multi-step fibrinogen binding to the integrin (alpha)IIb(beta)3 detected using force spectroscopy. *Biophys J* 89(4):2824–2834, 2005.

832. Muller B, et al: Two-step binding mechanism of fibrinogen to alpha IIb beta 3 integrin reconstituted into planar lipid bilayers. *J Biol Chem* 268(9):6800–6808, 1993.

833. Peerschke EI: Reversible and irreversible binding of fibrinogen to platelets. *Platelets* 8(5):311–317, 1997.

834. Wencel-Drake JD, et al: Internalization of bound fibrinogen modulates platelet aggregation. *Blood* 87(2):602–612, 1996.

835. Peerschke EIB: Events occurring after thrombin-induced fibrinogen binding to platelets. *Semin Thromb Hemost* 18:34–43, 1992.

836. Ugarova TP, et al: Conformational changes in fibrinogen elicited by its interaction with platelet membrane glycoprotein GPIIb-IIIa. *J Biol Chem* 268:21080–21087, 1993.

837. Zamarron C, Ginsberg MH, Plow EF: A receptor-induced binding site in fibrinogen elicited by its interaction with platelet membrane glycoprotein IIb-IIIa. *J Biol Chem* 266:17106–17111, 1991.

838. Hato T, Pampori N, Shattil SJ: Complementary roles for receptor clustering and conformational change in the adhesive and signaling functions of integrin alphaIIb beta3. *J Cell Biol* 141(7):1685–1695, 1998.

839. Carrell NA, et al: Structure of human platelet membrane glycoproteins IIb and IIIa as determined by electron microscopy. *J Biol Chem* 260:1743–1749, 1985.

840. Weisel JW, et al: Examination of the platelet membrane glycoprotein IIb-IIIa complex and its interaction with fibrinogen and other ligands by electron microscopy. *J Biol Chem* 267(23):16637–16643, 1992.

841. Arnaout M, Goodman S, Xiong J: Coming to grips with integrin binding to ligands. *Curr Opin Cell Biol* 14(5):641–651, 2002.

842. Arnaout MA: Integrin structure: New twists and turns in dynamic cell adhesion. *Immunol Rev* 186(1):125–140, 2002.

843. Takagi J, et al: Global conformational rearrangements in integrin extracellular domains in outside-in and inside-out signaling. *Cell* 110:599–607, 2002.

844. Xiong JP, et al: Crystal structure of the extracellular segment of integrin alphaVbeta3. *Science* 294(5541):339–345, 2001.

845. Xiong JP, et al: Crystal structure of the extracellular segment of integrin alpha Vbeta3 in complex with an Arg-Gly-Asp ligand. *Science* 296(5565):151–155, 2002.

846. Blue R, et al: Effects of limiting extension at the alphaIIb genu on ligand binding to integrin alphaIIbbeta3. *J Biol Chem* 285(23):17604–17613, 2010.

847. Cheng M, Li J, Negri A, Coller BS: Swing-out of the beta3 hybrid domain is required for alphaIIbbeta3 priming and normal cytoskeletal reorganization, but not adhesion to immobilized fibrinogen. *PLoS One* 8(12):e81609, 2013.

848. Choi WS, et al: Three-dimensional reconstruction of intact human integrin alphaIIbbeta3: New implications for activation-dependent ligand binding. *Blood* 122(26):4165–4171, 2013.

849. Eng ET, et al: Intact alphaIIbbeta3 integrin is extended after activation as measured by solution X-ray scattering and electron microscopy. *J Biol Chem* 286(40):35218–35226, 2011.

850. Kamata T, et al: Structural requirements for activation in alphaIIb beta3 integrin. *J Biol Chem* 285(49):38428–38437, 2010.

851. Nogales A, et al: Three-dimensional model of human platelet integrin alphaIIb beta3 in solution obtained by small angle neutron scattering. *J Biol Chem* 285(2):1023–1031, 2010.

852. Ye F, et al: Recreation of the terminal events in physiological integrin activation. *J Cell Biol* 188(1):157–173, 2010.

853. Zhu J, et al: Structure-guided design of a high affinity platelet integrin αIIbβ3 receptor antagonist that disrupts Mg2+ binding to the MIDAS. *Sci Transl Med* 4:1–12, 2012.

854. Poncz M, et al: Structure of the platelet membrane glycoprotein IIb. Homology to the alpha subunits of the vitronectin and fibronectin membrane receptors. *J Biol Chem* 262(18):8476–8482, 1987.

855. Fitzgerald LA, et al: Protein sequence of endothelial glycoprotein IIIa derived from a cDNA clone. Identity with platelet glycoprotein IIIa and similarity to "integrin." *J Biol Chem* 262(9):3936–3939, 1987.

856. Bray PF, et al: Physical linkage of the genes for platelet membrane glycoproteins IIb and IIIa. *Proc Natl Acad Sci U S A* 85(22):8683–8687, 1988.

857. Thornton MA, et al: The human platelet alphaIIb gene is not closely linked to its integrin partner beta3. *Blood* 94(6):2039–2047, 1999.

858. Steiner B, et al: Ca+2 dependent structural transitions of the platelet glycoprotein IIb-IIIa complex. Preparation of stable glycoprotein IIb and IIIa monomers. *J Biol Chem* 266:14986–14991, 1991.

859. Mitchell WB, et al: AlphaIIbbeta3 biogenesis is controlled by engagement of alphaIIb in the calnexin cycle via the N15-linked glycan. *Blood* 107(7):2713–2719, 2006.

860. Duperray A, et al: Biosynthesis and assembly of platelet GPIIb-IIIa in human megakaryocytes: Evidence that assembly between pro-GPIIb and GPIIIa is a prerequisite for expression of the complex on the cell surface. *Blood* 74:1603–1611, 1989.

861. O'Toole TE, et al: Efficient surface expression of platelet GPIIb-IIIa requires both subunits. *Blood* 74(1):14–18, 1989.

862. McEver RP, Baenziger JU, Majerus PW: Isolation and structural characterization of the polypeptide subunits of membrane glycoprotein IIb-IIIa from human platelets. *Blood* 59:80–85, 1982.

863. Haas TA, Plow EF: The cytoplasmic domain of alphaIIb beta3. A ternary complex of the integrin alpha and beta subunits and a divalent cation. *J Biol Chem* 271(11): 6017–6026, 1996.

864. Kim C, Lau TL, Ulmer TS, Ginsberg MH: Interactions of platelet integrin alphaIIb and beta3 transmembrane domains in mammalian cell membranes and their role in integrin activation. *Blood* 113(19):4747–4753, 2009.

865. Muir TW, et al: Design and chemical synthesis of a neoprotein structural model for the cytoplasmic domain of a multisubunit cell-surface receptor: Integrin alpha IIb beta 3 (platelet GPIIb-IIIa). *Biochemistry* 33(24):7701–7708, 1994.

866. Vallar L, et al: Divalent cations differentially regulate integrin alphaIIb cytoplasmic tail binding to beta3 and to calcium- and integrin-binding protein. *J Biol Chem* 274(24):17257–17266, 1999.

867. Hughes PE, et al: Breaking the integrin hinge. A defined structural constraint regulates integrin signaling. *J Biol Chem* 271(12):6571–6574, 1996.

868. Li A, et al: Integrin alphaII b tail distal of GFFKR participates in inside-out alphaII b beta3 activation. *J Thromb Haemost* 12(7):1145–1155, 2014.

869. O'Toole TE, et al: Integrin cytoplasmic domains mediate inside-out signal transduction. *J Cell Biol* 124(6):1047–1059, 1994.

870. O'Toole TE, et al: Modulation of the affinity of integrin αIIbβ3 (GPIIb-IIIa) by the cytoplasmic domain of alpha IIb. *Science* 254(5033):845–847, 1991.

871. Zhu J, et al: The structure of a receptor with two associating transmembrane domains on the cell surface: Integrin alphaIIbbeta3. *Mol Cell* 34(2):234–249, 2009.

872. Kim M, Carman CV, Springer TA: Bidirectional transmembrane signaling by cytoplasmic domain separation in integrins. *Science* 301(5640):1720–1725, 2003.

873. Li W, et al: A push-pull mechanism for regulating integrin function. *Proc Natl Acad Sci U S A* 102(5):1424–1429, 2005.

874. Luo BH, et al: Disrupting integrin transmembrane domain heterodimerization increases ligand binding affinity, not valency or clustering. *Proc Natl Acad Sci U S A* 102(10):3679–3684, 2005.

875. Partridge AW, et al: Transmembrane domain helix packing stabilizes integrin alphaIIbbeta3 in the low affinity state. *J Biol Chem* 280(8):7294–7300, 2005.

876. Leisner TM, et al: Bidirectional transmembrane modulation of integrin alphaIIb-beta3 conformations. *J Biol Chem* 274(18):12945–12949, 1999.

877. Vinogradova O, et al: A structural mechanism of integrin alpha(IIb)beta(3) "inside-out" activation as regulated by its cytoplasmic face. *Cell* 110(5):587–597, 2002.

878. Xiong JP, Stehle T, Goodman SL, Arnaout MA: A novel adaptation of the integrin PSI domain revealed from its crystal structure. *J Biol Chem* 279(39):40252–40254, 2004.

879. Du X, et al: Long range propagation of conformational changes in integrin alpha IIb beta 3. *J Biol Chem* 268(31):23087–23092, 1993 [published erratum appears in *J Biol Chem* 269(15):11673, 1994].

880. Frelinger AL 3rd, Du XP, Plow EF, Ginsberg MH: Monoclonal antibodies to ligand-occupied conformers of integrin alpha IIb beta 3 (glycoprotein IIb-IIIa) alter receptor affinity, specificity, and function. *J Biol Chem* 266:17106–17111, 1991.

881. Kamata T, et al: Critical cysteine residues for regulation of integrin alphaIIbbeta3 are clustered in the epidermal growth factor domains of the beta3 subunit. *Biochem J* 378(Pt 3):1079–1082, 2004.

882. Kashiwagi H, et al: A mutation in the extracellular cysteine-rich repeat region of the beta3 subunit activates integrins alphaIIbbeta3 and alphaVbeta3. *Blood* 93(8): 2559–2568, 1999.

883. Essex DW: The role of thiols and disulfides in platelet function. *Antioxid Redox Signal* 6(4):736–746, 2004.

884. Zucker MB, Masiello NC: Platelet aggregation caused by dithiothreitol. *Thromb Haemost* 51(1):119–124, 1984.

885. Chen K, Detwiler TC, Essex DW: Characterization of protein disulfide isomerase released from activated platelets. *Br J Haematol* 90(2):425–431, 1995.

886. Essex DW, Chen K, Swiatkowska M: Localization of protein disulfide isomerase to the external surface of the platelet plasma membrane. *Blood* 86(6):2168–2173, 1995.

887. Essex DW, Li M: Redox control of platelet aggregation. *Biochemistry* 42(1):129–136, 2003.

888. Mor-Cohen R, et al: Disulfide bond exchanges in integrins alphaIIbbeta3 and alphavbeta3 are required for activation and post-ligation signaling during clot retraction. *Thromb Res* 133(5):826–836, 2014.

889. O'Neill S, et al: The platelet integrin alpha IIbbeta 3 has an endogenous thiol isomerase activity. *J Biol Chem* 275(47):36984–36990, 2000.

890. Furie B, Flaumenhaft R: Thiol isomerases in thrombus formation. *Circ Res* 114(7): 1162–1173, 2014.

891. Wang L, et al: Platelet-derived ERp57 mediates platelet incorporation into a growing thrombus by regulation of the alphaIIbbeta3 integrin. *Blood* 122(22):3642–3650, 2013.

892. Provasi D, Negri A, Coller BS, Filizola M: Talin-driven inside-out activation mechanism of platelet αIIbβ3 integrin probed by multimicrosecond, all-atom molecular dynamics simulations. *Proteins* 82(12):3231–3240, 2014.

893. Gottschalk KE: A coiled-coil structure of the alphaIIbbeta3 integrin transmembrane and cytoplasmic domains in its resting state. *Structure* 13(5):703–712, 2005.

894. Lau TL, Kim C, Ginsberg MH, Ulmer TS: The structure of the integrin alphaIIb-beta3 transmembrane complex explains integrin transmembrane signalling. *EMBO J* 28(9):1351–1361, 2009.

895. Luo BH, Springer TA, Takagi J: A specific interface between integrin transmembrane helices and affinity for ligand. *PLoS Biol* 2(6):776–786, 2004.

896. Wegener KL, et al: Structural basis of integrin activation by talin. *Cell* 128(1):171–182, 2007.

897. Hernandez-Campo PM, et al: Comparative analysis of different flow cytometry-based immunophenotypic methods for the analysis of CD59 and CD55 expression on major peripheral blood cell subsets. *Cytometry* 50(3):191–201, 2002.

898. Robb L, et al: Molecular characterisation of mouse and human TSSC6: Evidence that TSSC6 is a genuine member of the tetraspanin superfamily and is expressed specifically in haematopoietic organs. *Biochim Biophys Acta* 1522(1):31–41, 2001.

899. Hughes PE, et al: Breaking the integrin hinge. A defined structural constraint regulates integrin signaling. *J Biol Chem* 271(12):6571–6574, 1996.

900. Anthis NJ, Wegener KL, Ye F, et al: The structure of an integrin/talin complex reveals the basis of inside-out signal transduction. *EMBO J* 28(22):3623–3632, 2009.

901. Ithychanda SS, Das M, Ma YQ, et al: Migfilin, a molecular switch in regulation of integrin activation. *J Biol Chem* 284(7):4713–4722, 2009.

902. Jenkins AL, et al: Tyrosine phosphorylation of the beta3 cytoplasmic domain mediates integrin-cytoskeletal interactions. *J Biol Chem* 273(22):13878–13885, 1998.

903. Jones CI, et al: Integrin-linked kinase regulates the rate of platelet activation and is essential for the formation of stable thrombi. *J Thromb Haemost* 12(8):1342–1352, 2014.

904. Calderwood DA, Shattil SJ, Ginsberg MH: Integrins and actin filaments: Reciprocal regulation of cell adhesion and signaling. *J Biol Chem* 275(30):22607–22610, 2000.

905. Calderwood DA, et al: The talin head domain binds to integrin beta subunit cytoplasmic tails and regulates integrin activation. *J Biol Chem* 274:28071–28074, 1999.

906. Cowan KJ, Law DA, Phillips DR: Identification of shc as the primary protein binding to the tyrosine-phosphorylated beta 3 subunit of alpha IIbbeta 3 during outside-in integrin platelet signaling. *J Biol Chem* 275(46):36423–36429, 2000.

907. Eigenthaler M, et al: A conserved sequence motif in the integrin beta3 cytoplasmic domain is required for its specific interaction with beta3-endonexin. *J Biol Chem* 272(12):7693–7698, 1997.

908. Hannigan GE, et al: Regulation of cell adhesion and anchorage-dependent growth by a new beta 1-integrin-linked protein kinase. *Nature* 379(6560):91–96, 1996.

909. Loh E, Qi W, Vilaire G, Bennett JS: Effect of cytoplasmic domain mutations on the agonist-stimulated ligand binding activity of the platelet integrin alphaIIbbeta3. *J Biol Chem* 271(47):30233–30241, 1996.

910. Law DA, Nannizzi-Alaimo L, Phillips DR: Outside-in integrin signal transduction. Alpha IIb beta 3-(GP IIb IIIa) tyrosine phosphorylation induced by platelet aggregation. *J Biol Chem* 271(18):10811–10815, 1996.

911. Leung-Hagesteijn CY, et al: Cell attachment to extracellular matrix substrates is inhibited upon downregulation of expression of calreticulin, an intracellular integrin alpha-subunit-binding protein. *J Cell Sci* 107(Pt 3):589–600, 1994.

912. Naik UP, Patel PM, Parise LV: Identification of a novel calcium-binding protein that interacts with the integrin alphaIIb cytoplasmic domain. *J Biol Chem* 272(8): 4651–4654, 1997.

913. Otey CA, Pavalko FM, Burridge K: An interaction between alpha-actinin and the beta 1 integrin subunit *in vitro. J Cell Biol* 111(2):721–729, 1990.

914. Reddy KB, et al: Identification of an interaction between the m-band protein skelemin and beta-integrin subunits. Colocalization of a skelemin-like protein with beta1- and beta3-integrins in non-muscle cells. *J Biol Chem* 273(52):35039–35047, 1998.

915. Rojiani MV, et al: *In vitro* interaction of a polypeptide homologous to human Ro/SS-A antigen (calreticulin) with a highly conserved amino acid sequence in the cytoplasmic domain of integrin alpha subunits. *Biochemistry* 30(41):9859–9866, 1991.

916. Schaller MD, et al: Focal adhesion kinase and paxillin bind to peptides mimicking beta integrin cytoplasmic domains. *J Cell Biol* 130(5):1181–1187, 1995.

917. Shattil SJ, et al: Beta 3-endonexin, a novel polypeptide that interacts specifically with the cytoplasmic tail of the integrin beta 3 subunit. *J Cell Biol* 131(3):807–816, 1995.

918. Shock DD, et al: Calcium-dependent properties of CIB binding to the integrin alphaIIb cytoplasmic domain and translocation to the platelet cytoskeleton. *Biochem J* 342(Pt 3):729–735, 1999.

919. Zent R, et al: Class- and splice variant-specific association of CD98 with integrin beta cytoplasmic domains. *J Biol Chem* 275(7):5059–5064, 2000.

920. Naik UP, Eckfeld K: Junctional adhesion molecule 1 (JAM-1). *J Biol Regul Homeost Agents* 17(4):341–347, 2003.

921. Ming Z, et al: Lyn and PECAM-1 function as interdependent inhibitors of platelet aggregation. *Blood* 117(14):3903–3906, 2011.

922. Tourdot BE, et al: Immunoreceptor tyrosine-based inhibitory motif (ITIM)-mediated inhibitory signaling is regulated by sequential phosphorylation mediated by distinct nonreceptor tyrosine kinases: A case study involving PECAM-1. *Biochemistry* 52(15):2597–2608, 2013.

923. Scarborough RM, et al: Design of potent and specific integrin antagonists. Peptide antagonists with high specificity for glycoprotein IIb-IIIa. *J Biol Chem* 268:1066–1073, 1993.

924. Beer JH, Springer KT, Coller BS: Immobilized Arg-Gly-Asp (RGD) peptides of varying lengths as structural probes of the platelet GPIIb/IIIa receptor. *Blood* 79:117–128, 1992.

925. Luo BH, Springer TA, Takagi J: Stabilizing the open conformation of the integrin headpiece with a glycan wedge increases affinity for ligand. *Proc Natl Acad Sci U S A* 100(5):2403–2408, 2003.

926. Heilmann E, et al: Thrombin-induced platelet aggregates have a dynamic structure: Time-dependent redistribution of GPIb/IIIa complexes and secreted adhesive proteins. *Arterioscler Thromb* 11:704–718, 1991.

927. Isenberg WM, McEver RP, Phillips DR, et al: The platelet fibrinogen receptor: An immunogold-surface replica study of agonist-induced ligand binding and receptor clustering. *J Cell Biol* 104(6):1655–1663, 1987.

928. Prevost N, Shattil SJ: Outside-in signaling by integrin αIIbβ3, in *Platelets*, edited by AD Michelson, pp 347–350. Academic Press, San Diego, 2007.

929. Asch E, Podack E: Vitronectin binds to activated human platelets and plays a role in platelet aggregation. *J Clin Invest* 85(5):1372–1378, 1990.

930. Haverstick DM, et al: Inhibition of platelet adhesion to fibronectin, fibrinogen, and von Willebrand factor substrates by a synthetic tetrapeptide derived from the cell-binding domain of fibronectin. *Blood* 66:946–952, 1985.

931. Plow EF, D'Souza SE, Ginsberg MH: Ligand binding to GPIIb-IIIa: A status report. *Semin Thromb Hemost* 18(3):324–332, 1992.

932. Weiss HJ, et al: Fibrinogen-independent platelet adhesion and thrombus formation on subendothelium mediated by glycoprotein IIb-IIIa complex at high shear rate. *J Clin Invest* 83:288–297, 1989.

933. Schullek J, Jordan J, Montgomery RR: Interaction of von Willebrand factor with human platelets in the plasma milieu. *J Clin Invest* 73:421–428, 1984.

934. Ni H, et al: Persistence of platelet thrombus formation in arterioles of mice lacking both von Willebrand factor and fibrinogen. *J Clin Invest* 106(3):385–392, 2000.

935. Ni H, et al: Control of thrombus embolization and fibronectin internalization by integrin alpha IIb beta 3 engagement of the fibrinogen gamma chain. *Blood* 102(10):3609–3614, 2003.

936. Ni H, et al: Plasma fibronectin promotes thrombus growth and stability in injured arterioles. *Proc Natl Acad Sci U S A* 100(5):2415–2419, 2003.

937. Coller BS: Interaction of normal, thrombasthenic, and Bernard-Soulier platelets with immobilized fibrinogen: Defective platelet-fibrinogen interaction in thrombasthenia. *Blood* 55:169–178, 1980.

938. Moskowitz KA, Kudryk B, Coller BS: Fibrinogen coating density affects the conformation of immobilized fibrinogen: Implications for platelet adhesion and spreading. *Thromb Haemost* 79(4):824–831, 1998.

939. Hatton MW, Moar SL, Richardson M: Deendothelialization *in vivo* initiates a thrombogenic reaction at the rabbit aorta surface. Correlation of uptake of fibrinogen and antithrombin III with thrombin generation by the exposed subendothelium. *Am J Pathol* 135(3):499–508, 1989.

940. Savage B, Ruggeri ZM: Selective recognition of adhesive sites in surface-bound fibrinogen by glycoprotein IIb-IIIa on nonactivated platelets. *J Biol Chem* 266:11227–11233, 1991.

941. Goto S, et al: Distinct mechanisms of platelet aggregation as a consequence of different shearing flow conditions. *J Clin Invest* 101(2):479–486, 1998.

942. Ruggeri ZM, Dent JA, Saldivar E: Contribution of distinct adhesive interactions to platelet aggregation in flowing blood. *Blood* 94(1):172–178, 1999.

943. Weiss HJ, Turitto VT, Baumgartner HR: Further evidence that glycoprotein IIb-IIIa mediates platelet spreading on subendothelium. *Thromb Haemost* 65(2):202–205, 1991.

944. Coller BS, et al: Platelet fibrinogen and vitronectin in Glanzmann thrombasthenia: Evidence consistent with specific roles for glycoprotein IIb/IIIA and αVβ3 integrins in platelet protein trafficking. *Blood* 78:2603–2610, 1991.

945. Peerschke EI, Grant RA, Zucker MB: Decreased association of 45-calcium with platelets unable to aggregate due to thrombasthenia or prolonged calcium deprivation. *Br J Haematol* 46:247–256, 1980.

946. Powling MJ, Hardisty RM: Glycoprotein IIb-IIIa complex and Ca++ influx into stimulated platelets. *Blood* 66(3):731–734, 1985.

947. Rybak ME, Renzulli LA: Effect of calcium channel blockers on platelet GPIIb-IIIa as a calcium channel in liposomes: Comparison with effects on the intact platelet. *Thromb Haemost* 67:131–136, 1992.

948. Ameisen JC, et al: A role for glycoprotein IIb-IIIa complexes in the binding of IgE to human platelets and platelet IgE-dependent cytolytic function. *Br J Haematol* 64:21–32, 1986.

949. Coburn J, Barthold SW, Leong JM: Diverse Lyme disease spirochetes bind integrin alpha IIb beta 3 on human platelets. *Infect Immun* 62(12):5559–5567, 1994.

950. Gavrilovskaya IN, et al: Cellular entry of hantaviruses which cause hemorrhagic fever with renal syndrome is mediated by beta3 integrins. *J Virol* 73(5):3951–3959, 1999.

951. Kulkarni S, Jackson SP: Platelet factor XIII and calpain negatively regulate integrin alphaIIbbeta3 adhesive function and thrombus growth. *J Biol Chem* 279(29):30697–30706, 2004.

952. Madamanchi A, Santoro SA, Zutter MM: Alpha2beta1 integrin. *Adv Exp Med Biol* 819:41–60, 2014.

953. Barnes MJ, Knight CG, Farndale RW: The collagen-platelet interaction. *Curr Opin Hematol* 5(5):314–320, 1998.

954. Kunicki DJ, Nugent DJ, Staats SJ, et al: The human fibroblast II extracellular matrix receptor mediates platelet adhesion to collagen and is identical to the platelet glycoprotein Ia-IIa complex. *J Biol Chem* 263(10):4516–4519, 1988.

955. Pischel KD, et al: Use of the monoclonal antibody 12F1 to characterize the differentiation antigen VLA-2. *J Immunol* 138:226–233, 1987.

956. Saelman EU, et al: Platelet adhesion to collagen types I through VIII under conditions of stasis and flow is mediated by GPIa/IIa (α2β1-integrin). *Blood* 83(5):1244–1250, 1994.

957. Staatz WD, et al: The membrane glycoprotein Ia-IIa (VLA-2) complex mediates the Mg++-dependent adhesion of platelets to collagen. *J Cell Biol* 108:1917–1924, 1989.

958. Takada Y, Hemler ME: The primary structure of the VLA-2/collagen receptor α2 subunit (platelet GPIa): Homology to other integrins and the presence of a possible collagen-binding domain. *J Cell Biol* 109:397–407, 1987.

959. Clemetson KJ: Platelet receptors, in *Platelets*, edited by AD Michelson, pp 65–84. Academic Press, San Diego, 2002.

960. Emsley J, et al: Crystal structure of the I domain from integrin alpha2beta1. *J Biol Chem* 272(45):28512–28517, 1997.

961. Emsley J, et al: Structural basis of collagen recognition by integrin alpha2beta1. *Cell* 101(1):47–56, 2000.

962. Tulla M, et al: Effects of conformational activation of integrin alpha 1I and alpha 2I domains on selective recognition of laminin and collagen subtypes. *Exp Cell Res* 314(8):1734–1743, 2008.

963. Barnes MJ: The collagen platelet interaction, in *Collagen in Health and Disease*, edited by J Weiss, MJV Jayson, pp 179–197. Churchill Livingstone, Edinburgh, London, 1982.

964. Nieuwenhuis HK, et al: Human blood platelets showing no response to collagen fail to express surface glycoprotein Ia. *Nature* 318:470–472, 1985.

965. Sarratt KL, et al: GPVI and alpha2beta1 play independent critical roles during platelet adhesion and aggregate formation to collagen under flow. *Blood* 106(4):1268–1277, 2005.

966. Nissinen L, et al: Novel alpha2beta1 integrin inhibitors reveal that integrin binding to collagen under shear stress conditions does not require receptor preactivation. *J Biol Chem* 287(53):44694–44702, 2012.

967. Zou Z, Schmaier AA, Cheng L, et al: Negative regulation of activated alpha2 integrins during thrombopoiesis. *Blood* 113(25):6428–6439, 2009.

968. Cruz MA, et al: The platelet glycoprotein Ib-von Willebrand factor interaction activates the collagen receptor alpha2beta1 to bind collagen: Activation-dependent conformational change of the alpha2-I domain. *Blood* 105(5):1986–1991, 2005.

969. Pula G, Poole AW: Critical roles for the actin cytoskeleton and cdc42 in regulating platelet integrin alpha2beta1. *Platelets* 19(3):199–210, 2008.

970. Schoolmeester A, et al: Monoclonal antibody IAC-1 is specific for activated alpha-2beta1 and binds to amino acids 199 to 201 of the integrin alpha2 I-domain. *Blood* 104(2):390–396, 2004.

971. He L, et al: The contributions of the alpha 2 beta 1 integrin to vascular thrombosis *in vivo*. *Blood* 102(10):3652–3657, 2003.

972. Kuijpers MJ, et al: Complementary roles of glycoprotein VI and alpha2beta1 integrin in collagen-induced thrombus formation in flowing whole blood *ex vivo*. *FASEB J* 17(6):685–687, 2003.

973. Lahav J, et al: Enzymatically catalyzed disulfide exchange is required for platelet adhesion to collagen via integrin alpha2beta1. *Blood* 102(6):2085–2092, 2003.

974. Savage B, Ginsberg MH, Ruggeri ZM: Influence of fibrillar collagen structure on the mechanisms of platelet thrombus formation under flow. *Blood* 94(8):2704–2715, 1999.

975. Coller BS, et al: Collagen-platelet interactions: Evidence for a direct interaction of collagen with platelet GPIa/IIa and an indirect interaction with platelet GPIIb/IIa mediated by adhesive proteins. *Blood* 74:182–192, 1989.

976. Deckmyn H, De Meyer SF, Broos K, Vanhoorelbeke K: Inhibitors of the interactions between collagen and its receptors on platelets. *Handb Exp Pharmacol* 210:311–337, 2012.

977. Miller MW, et al: Small-molecule inhibitors of integrin alpha2beta1 that prevent pathological thrombus formation via an allosteric mechanism. *Proc Natl Acad Sci U S A* 106(3):719–724, 2009.

978. Nissinen L, et al: A small-molecule inhibitor of integrin alpha2 beta1 introduces a new strategy for antithrombotic therapy. *Thromb Haemost* 103(2):387–397, 2010.

979. Staatz WD, et al: The α2β1 integrin cell surface collagen receptor binds to the α1(I)-CB3 peptide of collagen. *J Biol Chem* 265:4778–4781, 1990.

980. Knight CG, et al: Identification in collagen type I of an integrin alpha2 beta1-binding site containing an essential GER sequence. *J Biol Chem* 273(50):33287–33294, 1998.

981. Santoro SA: Distinct determinants on collagen support α2β1 integrin-mediated platelet adhesion and platelet activation. *Cell Regul* 2(11):905–913, 1991.

982. Verkleij MW, et al: Adhesive domains in the collagen III fragment alpha1(III)CB4 that support alpha2b. *Thromb Haemost* 82(3):1137–1144, 1999.

983. Yee DL, Bray PF: Clinical and functional consequences of platelet membrane glycoprotein polymorphisms. *Semin Thromb Hemost* 30(5):591–600, 2004.

984. Bray PF: Integrin polymorphisms as risk factors for thrombosis. *Thromb Haemost* 82:337–344, 1999.

985. Kritzik M, et al: Nucleotide polymorphisms in the alpha2 gene define multiple alleles that are associated with differences in platelet alpha2 beta1 density. *Blood* 92(7):2382–2388, 1998.

986. Moshfegh K, et al: Association of two silent polymorphisms of platelet glycoprotein Ia/IIa receptor with risk of myocardial infarction: A case-control study. *Lancet* 353(9150):351–354, 1999.

987. Santoso S, et al: Association of the platelet glycoprotein Ia C807T gene polymorphism with nonfatal myocardial infarction in younger patients. *Blood* 93(8):2449–2453, 1999.

988. Carlsson LE: The alpha2 gene coding sequence T807/A873 of the platelet collagen receptor integrin alpha2beta1 might be a genetic risk factor for the development of stroke in younger patients. *Blood* 93(11):3583–3586, 1999.

989. Matsubara Y, et al: Association between diabetic retinopathy and genetic variations in alpha2beta1 integrin, a platelet receptor for collagen. *Blood* 95(5):1560–1564, 2000.

990. Roest M, et al: Homozygosity for 807 T polymorphism in alpha(2) subunit of platelet alpha(2)beta(1) is associated with increased risk of cardiovascular mortality in high-risk women. *Circulation* 102(14):1645–1650, 2000.

991. Vijayan KV, Bray PF: Molecular mechanisms of prothrombotic risk due to genetic variations in platelet genes: Enhanced outside-in signaling through the Pro33 variant of integrin beta3. *Exp Biol Med (Maywood)* 231(5):505–513, 2006.

992. von Beckerath N, et al: Glycoprotein Ia gene C807T polymorphism and risk for major adverse cardiac events within the first 30 days after coronary artery stenting. *Blood* 95(11):3297–3301, 2000.

993. Fox JE: Linkage of a membrane skeleton to integral membrane glycoproteins in human platelets. Identification of one of the glycoproteins as glycoprotein Ib. *J Clin Invest* 76:1673–1683, 1985.

994. Elices MJ, Hemler ME: The human integrin VLA-2 is a collagen receptor on some cells and a collagen/laminin receptor on others. *Proc Natl Acad Sci U S A* 86(24):9906–9910, 1989.

995. Kirchhofer D, Languino LR, Ruoslahti E, Pierschbacher MD: Alpha 2 beta 1 integrins from different cell types show different binding specificities. *J Biol Chem* 265(2):615–618, 1990.

996. Habart D, Cheli Y, Nugent DJ: Conditional knockout of integrin alpha2beta1 in murine megakaryocytes leads to reduced mean platelet volume. *PLoS One* 8(1):e55094, 2013.

997. Piotrowicz RS, et al: Glycoprotein Ic-IIa functions as an activation-independent fibronectin receptor on human platelets. *J Cell Biol* 106:1359–1364, 1988.

998. Wayner EA, Carter WG, Piotrowicz RS, Kunicki TJ: The function of multiple extracellular matrix receptors in mediating cell adhesion to extracellular matrix: Preparation of monoclonal antibodies to the fibronectin receptor that specifically inhibit cell adhesion of fibronectin and react with platelet glycoproteins Ic-IIa. *J Cell Biol* 107(5):1881–1891, 1988.

999. Garcia AJ, Huber F, Boettiger D: Force required to break alpha5beta1 integrin-fibronectin bonds in intact adherent cells is sensitive to integrin activation state. *J Biol Chem* 273(18):10988–10993, 1998.

1000. Matsunaga T, et al: Potentiated activation of VLA-4 and VLA-5 accelerates proplatelet-like formation. *Ann Hematol* 91(10):1633–1643, 2012.

1001. Plow EF, et al: Related binding mechanisms for fibrinogen, fibronectin, von Willebrand factor and thrombospondin on thrombin-stimulated human platelets. *Blood* 66:724–727, 1985.

1002. Schaff M, et al: Integrin alpha6beta1 is the main receptor for vascular laminins and plays a role in platelet adhesion, activation, and arterial thrombosis. *Circulation* 128(5):541–552, 2013.

1003. Hindriks G, et al: Platelet adhesion to laminin: Role of Ca2+ and Mg2+ ions, shear rate, and platelet membrane glycoproteins. *Blood* 79(4):928–935, 1992.

1004. Sonnenberg A, Modderman PW, Hogervorst F: Laminin receptor on platelets is the integrin VLA-6. *Nature* 336:487–489, 1988.

1005. Chang JC, et al: The integrin alpha6beta1 modulation of PI3K and Cdc42 activities induces dynamic filopodium formation in human platelets. *J Biomed Sci* 12(6):881–898, 2005.

1006. Tandon NN, et al: Interaction of human platelets with laminin and identification of the 67 kDa laminin receptor on platelets. *Biochem J* 274:535–542, 1991.

1007. Arnaout MA, Goodman SL, Xiong JP: Structure and mechanics of integrin-based cell adhesion. *Curr Opin Cell Biol* 19(5):495–507, 2007.

1008. Hynes RO: Integrins. Bidirectional, allosteric signaling machines. *Cell* 110(6):673–687, 2002.

1009. Luo BH, Carman CV, Springer TA: Structural basis of integrin regulation and signaling. *Annu Rev Immunol* 25:619–647, 2007.

1010. Fitzgerald LA, et al: Comparison of cDNA-derived protein sequences of the human fibronectin and vitronectin receptor α subunits and platelet glycoprotein IIb. *Biochemistry* 26:8158–8165, 1987.

1011. Coller BS, et al: Platelet vitronectin receptor expression differentiates Iraqi-Jewish from Arab patients with Glanzmann thrombasthenia in Israel. *Blood* 77:75–83, 1991.

1012. Byzova TV, Plow EF: Activation of alphaVbeta3 on vascular cells controls recognition of prothrombin. *J Cell Biol* 143(7):2081–2092, 1998.

1013. Charo IF, Bekeart LS, Phillips DR: Platelet glycoprotein IIb-IIIa-like proteins mediate endothelial cell attachment to adhesive proteins and the extracellular matrix. *J Biol Chem* 262:9935–9938, 1987.

1014. Kieffer N, et al: Adhesive properties of the β3 integrins. Comparison of GPIIb-IIIa and the vitronectin receptor individually expressed in human melanoma cells. *J Cell Biol* 113:451–461, 1991.

1015. Lam SC, et al: Isolation and characterization of a platelet membrane protein related to the vitronectin receptor. *J Biol Chem* 264:3742–3749, 1989.

1016. Bennett JS, et al: Agonist-activated alphavbeta3 on platelets and lymphocytes binds to the matrix protein osteopontin. *J Biol Chem* 272(13):8137–8140, 1997.

1017. Reverter JC, et al: Inhibition of platelet-mediated, tissue factor-induced thrombin generation by the mouse/human chimeric 7E3 antibody. Potential implications for the effect of c7E3 Fab treatment on acute thrombosis and "clinical restenosis." *J Clin Invest* 98(3):863–874, 1996.

1018. Beckstead JH, Stenberg PE, McEver RP, et al: Immunohistochemical localization of membrane and alpha-granule proteins in human megakaryocytes: Application to plastic-embedded bone marrow biopsy specimens. *Blood* 67(2):285–293, 1986.

1019. Davies J, et al: The osteoclast functional antigen, implicated in the regulation of bone resorption is biochemically related to the vitronectin receptor. *J Cell Biol* 109:1817, 1989.

1020. Feng X, et al: A Glanzmann's mutation in beta 3 integrin specifically impairs osteoclast function. *J Clin Invest* 107(9):1137–1144, 2001.

1021. McHugh KP, et al: Mice lacking beta3 integrins are osteosclerotic because of dysfunctional osteoclasts. *J Clin Invest* 105(4):433–440, 2000.

1022. Savill J, et al: Vitronectin receptor-mediated phagocytosis of cells undergoing apoptosis. *Nature* 343(6254):170–173, 1990.

1023. Brooks PC, Clark RA, Cheresh DA: Requirement of vascular integrin αVβ3 for angiogenesis. *Science* 264(5158):569–571, 1994.

1024. Trikha M, et al: CNTO 95, a fully human monoclonal antibody that inhibits alphav integrins, has antitumor and antiangiogenic activity *in vivo. Int J Cancer* 110(3):326–335, 2004.

1025. Varner JA, Cheresh DA: Integrins and cancer. *Curr Opin Cell Biol* 8:724–730, 1996.

1026. Choi ET: Inhibition of neointimal hyperplasia by blocking αVβ3 integrin with a small peptide antagonist GpenGRGDSPCA. *J Vasc Surg* 19:125–134, 1994.

1027. Sajid M, Stouffer GA: The role of alpha(v)beta3 integrins in vascular healing. *Thromb Haemost* 87(2):187–193, 2002.

1028. Stouffer GA, Smyth SS: Effects of thrombin on interactions between beta3-integrins and extracellular matrix in platelets and vascular cells. *Arterioscler Thromb Vasc Biol* 23(11):1971–1978, 2003.

1029. Kaul DK: Sickle red cell adhesion: Many issues and some answers. *Transfus Clin Biol* 15(1–2):51–55, 2008.

1030. Kaul DK, et al: Monoclonal antibodies to alphaVbeta3 (7E3 and LM609) inhibit sickle red blood cell-endothelium interactions induced by platelet-activating factor. *Blood* 95(2):368–374, 2000.

1031. Belcher JD, et al: Heme triggers TLR4 signaling leading to endothelial cell activation and vaso-occlusion in murine sickle cell disease. *Blood* 123(3):377–390, 2014.

1032. Amann K, et al: Beneficial effects of integrin alphavbeta3-blocking RGD peptides in early but not late phase of experimental glomerulonephritis. *Nephrol Dial Transplant* 27(5):1755–1768, 2012.

1033. Reiser J: Circulating permeability factor suPAR: From concept to discovery to clinic. *Trans Am Clin Climatol Assoc* 124:133–138, 2013.

1034. Gerber EE, et al: Integrin-modulating therapy prevents fibrosis and autoimmunity in mouse models of scleroderma. *Nature* 503(7474):126–130, 2013.

1035. Andrews RK, Lopez JA, Berndt MC: The GPIb-IX-V complex, in *Platelets*, edited by AD Michelson, pp 145–164. Academic Press, San Diego, 2007.

1036. Clemetson KJ, Clemetson JM: Platelet GPIb complex as a target for anti-thrombotic drug development. *Thromb Haemost* 99(3):473–479, 2008.

1037. Li R, Emsley J: The organizing principle of the platelet glycoprotein Ib-IX-V complex. *J Thromb Haemost* 11(4):605–614, 2013.

1038. Lopez JA, et al: Bernard-Soulier syndrome. *Blood* 91(12):4397–4418, 1998.

1039. Lopez JH, et al: The α and β chains of human platelet glycoprotein Ib are both transmembrane proteins containing a leucine-rich amino acid sequence. *Proc Natl Acad Sci U S A* 85:2135–2139, 1988.

1040. McEwan PA, et al: Quaternary organization of GPIb-IX complex and insights into Bernard-Soulier syndrome revealed by the structures of GPIbbeta and a GPIbbeta/GPIX chimera. *Blood* 118(19):5292–5301, 2011.

1041. Ozaki Y, et al: Platelet GPIb-IX-V-dependent signaling. *J Thromb Haemost* 3(8):1745–1751, 2005.

1042. Roth GJ: Developing relationships: Arterial platelet adhesion, glycoprotein Ib, and leucine-rich glycoproteins. *Blood* 77:5–19, 1991.

1043. Zhou L, Yang W, Li R: Analysis of inter-subunit contacts reveals the structural malleability of extracellular domains in platelet glycoprotein Ib-IX complex. *J Thromb Haemost* 12(1):82–89, 2014.

1044. Du X, Beutler L, Ruan C, et al: Glycoprotein Ib and glycoprotein IX are fully complexed in the intact platelet membrane. *Blood* 69(5):1524–1527, 1987.

1045. Hickey MJ, Deaven LL, Roth GJ: Human platelet glycoprotein IX. Characterization of cDNA and localization of the gene to chromosome 3. *FEBS Lett* 274:189–192, 1990.

1046. Hickey MJ, Williams SA, Roth GJ: Human platelet GPIX: An adhesive prototype of leucine-rich glycoproteins with flank-center-flank structures. *Proc Natl Acad Sci U S A* 86:6773–6777, 1989.

1047. Lopez JA, et al: Efficient plasma membrane expression of a functional platelet glycoprotein Ib-IX complex requires the presence of its three subunits. *J Biol Chem* 267:12851–12859, 1992.

1048. Bastian LS, et al: Analysis of the megakaryocyte glycoprotein IX promoter identifies positive and negative regulatory domains and functional GATA and Ets sites. *J Biol Chem* 271(31):18554–18560, 1996.

1049. Block KL, Poncz M: Platelet glycoprotein IIb gene expression as a model of megakaryocyte-specific expression. *Stem Cells* 13(2):135–145, 1995.

1050. Hashimoto Y, Ware J: Identification of essential GATA and Ets binding motifs within the promoter of the platelet glycoprotein Ib alpha gene. *J Biol Chem* 270(41):24532–24539, 1995.

1051. Krause DS, Perkins AS: Gotta find GATA a friend. *Nat Med* 3(9):960–961, 1997.

1052. Lemarchandel V, et al: GATA and Ets cis-acting sequences mediate megakaryocyte-specific expression. *Mol Cell Biol* 13(1):668–676, 1993.

1053. Martin F, et al: The transcription factor GATA-1 regulates the promoter activity of the platelet glycoprotein IIb gene. *J Biol Chem* 268(29):21606–21612, 1993.

1054. Prandini MH, et al: Characterization of a specific erythromegakaryocytic enhancer within the glycoprotein IIb promoter. *J Biol Chem* 267(15):10370–10374, 1992.

1055. Tsang AP, et al: FOG, a multitype zinc finger protein, acts as a cofactor for transcription factor GATA-1 in erythroid and megakaryocytic differentiation. *Cell* 90(1):109–119, 1997.

1056. Uzan G, et al: Tissue-specific expression of the platelet GPIIb gene. *J Biol Chem* 266(14):8932–8939, 1991.

1057. Lopez JA, Ludwig EW, McCarthy BJ: Polymorphism of human glycoprotein Ibα results from a variable number of repeats of a 13-amino acid sequence in the mucin-like macroglycopeptide region. Structure function implications. *J Biol Chem* 267:10055–10061, 1992.

1058. Carlsson LE, et al: Polymorphisms of the human platelet antigens HPA-1, HPA-2, HPA-3, and HPA-5 on the platelet receptors for fibrinogen (GPIIb/IIIa), von Willebrand factor (GPIb/IX), and collagen (GPIa/IIa) are not correlated with an increased risk for stroke. *Stroke* 28(7):1392–1395, 1997.

1059. Shanker J, et al: Platelet function and antiplatelet therapy in cardiovascular disease: Implications of genetic polymorphisms. *Curr Vasc Pharmacol* 9(4):479–489, 2011.

1060. Kaski S, Kekomaki R, Partanen J: Systematic screening for genetic polymorphism in human platelet glycoprotein Ibalpha. *Immunogenetics* 44(3):170–176, 1996.

1061. Suzuki K, et al: StyI polymorphism at nucleotide 1610 in the human platelet glyco-protein Ib alpha gene. *Jpn J Hum Genet* 41(4):419–421, 1996.

1062. Afshar-Kharghan V, et al: Kozak sequence polymorphism of the glycoprotein (GP) Ibalpha gene is a major determinant of the plasma membrane levels of the platelet GP Ib- IX-V complex. *Blood* 94(1):186–191, 1999.

1063. Baker RI, et al: Platelet glycoprotein Ibalpha Kozak polymorphism is associated with an increased risk of ischemic stroke. *Blood* 98(1):36–40, 2001.

1064. Carlsson LE, et al: Platelet receptor and clotting factor polymorphisms as genetic risk factors for thromboembolic complications in heparin-induced thrombocytopenia. *Pharmacogenetics* 13(5):253–258, 2003.

1065. Douglas H, et al: Platelet membrane glycoprotein Ibalpha gene-5T/C Kozak sequence polymorphism as an independent risk factor for the occurrence of coronary thrombosis. *Heart* 87(1):70–74, 2002.

1066. Jilma-Stohlawetz P, et al: Glycoprotein Ib polymorphisms influence platelet plug formation under high shear rates. *Br J Haematol* 120(4):652–655, 2003.

1067. Kenny D, et al: Platelet glycoprotein Ib alpha receptor polymorphisms and recurrent ischaemic events in acute coronary syndrome patients. *J Thromb Thrombolysis* 13(1):13–19, 2002.

1068. Meisel C, et al: Role of Kozak sequence polymorphism of platelet glycoprotein Ibalpha as a risk factor for coronary artery disease and catheter interventions. *J Am Coll Cardiol* 38(4):1023–1027, 2001.

1069. Ozelo MC, et al: Platelet glycoprotein Ibα polymorphisms modulate the risk for myocardial infarction. *Thromb Haemost* 92(2):384–386, 2004.

1070. Rosenberg N, et al: Effects of platelet membrane glycoprotein polymorphisms on the risk of myocardial infarction in young males. *Isr Med Assoc J* 4(6):411–414, 2002.

1071. Tsuji T, et al: The carbohydrate moiety of human platelet glycocalicin. *J Biol Chem* 258(10):6335–6339, 1983.

1072. Fox JEB, Aggerbeck LP, Berndt MC: Structure of the glycoprotein Ib-IX complex from platelet membranes. *J Biol Chem* 263:4882–4890, 1988.

1073. Solum NO, et al: Platelet glycocalicin: Its membrane association in solvent and aqueous media. *Biochim Biophys Acta* 597:235–246, 1990.

1074. Coller BS, et al: Evidence that glycocalicin circulates in normal plasma. *J Clin Invest* 73:794–799, 1984.

1075. Liang X, et al: Specific inhibition of ectodomain shedding of glycoprotein Ibalpha by targeting its juxtamembrane shedding cleavage site. *J Thromb Haemost* 11(12):2155–2162, 2013.

1076. Bergmeier W, et al: Tumor necrosis factor-alpha-converting enzyme (ADAM17) mediates GPIbalpha shedding from platelets *in vitro* and *in vivo*. *Circ Res* 95(7):677–683, 2004.

1077. Mo X, et al: Transmembrane and trans-subunit regulation of ectodomain shedding of platelet glycoprotein Ibalpha. *J Biol Chem* 285(42):32096–32104, 2010.

1078. Wang Z, et al: The role of calpain in the regulation of ADAM17-dependent GPIbalpha ectodomain shedding. *Arch Biochem Biophys* 495(2):136–143, 2010.

1079. Zhang P, et al: The role of intraplatelet reactive oxygen species in the regulation of platelet glycoprotein Ibalpha ectodomain shedding. *Thromb Res* 132(6):696–701, 2013.

1080. Beer JH, Buchi L, Steiner B, Glycocalicin: A new assay—The normal plasma levels and its potential usefulness in selected diseases. *Blood* 83:691–702, 1994.

1081. Himmelfarb J, et al: Elevated plasma glycocalicin levels and decreased ristocetin-induced platelet agglutination in hemodialysis patients. *Am J Kidney Dis* 32(1):132–138, 1998.

1082. Kunishima S, et al: Rapid detection of plasma glycocalicin by a latex agglutination test. A useful adjunct in the differential diagnosis of thrombocytopenia. *Am J Clin Pathol* 100(5):579–584, 1993.

1083. Kurata Y, et al: Diagnostic value of tests for reticulated platelets, plasma glycocalicin, and thrombopoietin levels for discriminating between hyperdestructive and hypoplastic thrombocytopenia. *Am J Clin Pathol* 115(5):656–664, 2001.

1084. Steffan A, et al: Glycocalicin in the diagnosis and management of immune thrombocytopenia. *Eur J Haematol* 61(2):77–83, 1998.

1085. Steinberg MH, Kelton JG, Coller BS: Plasma glycocalicin. An aid in the classification of thrombocytopenic disorders. *N Engl J Med* 317(17):1037–1042, 1987.

1086. Kalomiris EL, Coller BS: Thiol-specific probes indicate that the alpha chain of platelet glycoprotein Ib is a transmembrane protein with a reactive endofacial sulfhydryl group. *Biochemistry* 24:5430–5436, 1985.

1087. Muszbek L, Laposata M: Glycoprotein Ib and glycoprotein IX in human platelets are acylated with palmitic acid through thioester linkages. *J Biol Chem* 264(17):9716–9719, 1989.

1088. Du X, Fox JE, Pei S: Identification of a binding sequence for the 14-3-3 protein within the cytoplasmic domain of the adhesion receptor, platelet glycoprotein Ib alpha. *J Biol Chem* 271(13):7362–7367, 1996.

1089. Andrews RK: Binding of purified 14-3-3 zeta signaling protein to discrete amino acid sequences within the cytoplasmic domain of the platelet membrane glycoprotein Ib-IX-V complex. *Biochemistry* 37(2):638–647, 1998.

1090. Calverley DC, Kavanagh TJ, Roth GJ: Human signaling protein 14–3–3zeta interacts with platelet glycoprotein Ib subunits Ibalpha and Ibbeta. *Blood* 91(4):1295–1303, 1998.

1091. Wardell MR, et al: Platelet glycoprotein Ib beta is phosphorylated on serine 166 by cyclic AMP-dependent protein kinase. *J Biol Chem* 264(26):15656–15661, 1989.

1092. Andrews RK, Fox JE: Identification of a region in the cytoplasmic domain of the platelet membrane glycoprotein Ib-IX complex that binds to purified actin- binding protein. *J Biol Chem* 267(26):18605–18611, 1992.

1093. Andrews RK, et al: The glycoprotein Ib-IX-V complex in platelet adhesion and signaling. *Thromb Haemost* 82:357–364, 1999.

1094. Falet H: New insights into the versatile roles of platelet FlnA. *Platelets* 24(1):1–5, 2013.

1095. Kanaji T, et al: GPIbalpha regulates platelet size by controlling the subcellular localization of filamin. *Blood* 119(12):2906–2913, 2012.

1096. Coller BS: Inhibition of von Willebrand factor-dependent platelet function by increased platelet cyclic AMP and its prevention by cytoskeleton-disrupting agents. *Blood* 57:846–855, 1981.

1097. Coller BS: Effects of tertiary amine local anesthetics on von Willebrand factor-dependent platelet function: Alteration of membrane reactivity and degradation of GPIb by a calcium-dependent protease(s). *Blood* 248:1355–1357, 1982.

1098. Dong JF, et al: The cytoplasmic domain of glycoprotein (GP) Ibalpha constrains the lateral diffusion of the GP Ib-IX complex and modulates von Willebrand factor binding. *Biochemistry* 36(41):12421–12427, 1997.

1099. Delaney MK, et al: The role of Rac1 in glycoprotein Ib-IX-mediated signal transduction and integrin activation. *Arterioscler Thromb Vasc Biol* 32(11):2761–2768, 2012.

1100. Estevez B, et al: LIM kinase-1 selectively promotes glycoprotein Ib-IX-mediated TXA2 synthesis, platelet activation, and thrombosis. *Blood* 121(22):4586–4594, 2013.

1101. Munday AD, Berndt MC, Mitchell CA: Phosphoinositide 3-kinase forms a complex with platelet membrane glycoprotein Ib-IX-V complex and 14–3–3zeta. *Blood* 96(2):577–584, 2000.

1102. Falati S, Edmead CE, Poole AW: Glycoprotein Ib-V-IX, a receptor for von Willebrand factor, couples physically and functionally to the Fc receptor γ-chain, Fyn, and Lyn to activate human platelets. *Blood* 94(5):1648–1656, 1999.

1103. Sullam PM, et al: Physical proximity and functional interplay of the glycoprotein Ib-IX-V complex and the Fc receptor FcgammaRIIA on the platelet plasma membrane. *J Biol Chem* 273(9):5331–5336, 1998.

1104. Watson SP, et al: The role of ITAM- and ITIM-coupled receptors in platelet activation by collagen. *Thromb Haemost* 86(1):276–288, 2001.

1105. Wu Y, et al: Role of Fc receptor gamma-chain in platelet glycoprotein Ib-mediated signaling. *Blood* 97(12):3836–3845, 2001.

1106. Ozaki Y, Suzuki-Inoue K, Inoue O: Platelet receptors activated via mulitmerization: Glycoprotein VI, GPIb-IX-V, and CLEC-2. *J Thromb Haemost* 11(Suppl 1):330–339, 2013.

1107. Blenner MA, Dong X, Springer TA: Structural basis of regulation of von Willebrand factor binding to glycoprotein Ib. *J Biol Chem* 289(9):5565–5579, 2014.

1108. Dumas JJ, et al: Crystal structure of the wild-type von Willebrand factor A1-glycoprotein Ibalpha complex reveals conformation differences with a complex bearing von Willebrand disease mutations. *J Biol Chem* 279(22):23327–23334, 2004.

1109. Huizinga EG, et al: Structures of glycoprotein Ibalpha and its complex with von Willebrand factor A1 domain. *Science* 297(5584):1176–1179, 2002.

1110. Uff S, et al: Crystal structure of the platelet glycoprotein Ib(alpha) N-terminal domain reveals an unmasking mechanism for receptor activation. *J Biol Chem* 277(38):35657–35663, 2002.

1111. Shen Y, et al: Leucine-rich repeats 2–4 (Leu60-Glu128) of platelet glycoprotein Ibalpha regulate shear-dependent cell adhesion to von Willebrand factor. *J Biol Chem* 281(36):26419–26423, 2006.

1112. Shen Y, et al: Requirement of leucine-rich repeats of glycoprotein (GP) Ibalpha for shear-dependent and static binding of von Willebrand factor to the platelet membrane GP Ib-IX-V complex. *Blood* 95(3):903–910, 2000.

1113. Springer TA: von Willebrand factor, Jedi knight of the bloodstream. *Blood* 124(9):1412–1425, 2014.

1114. Tang J, et al: Mutation in the leucine-rich repeat C-flanking region of platelet glycoprotein Ibbeta impairs assembly of von Willebrand factor receptor. *Thromb Haemost* 92(1):75–88, 2004.

1115. Berndt MC, et al: Identification of aspartic acid 514 through glutamic acid 542 as a glycoprotein Ib-IX complex receptor recognition sequence in von Willebrand factor. Mechanism of modulation of von Willebrand factor by ristocetin and botrocetin. *Biochemistry* 31(45):11144–11151, 1992.

1116. Coller BS: Platelet von Willebrand factor interactions, in *Platelet Glycoproteins*, edited by J George, D Phillips, A Nurden, pp 215–244. Plenum, New York, 1985.

1117. Papi M, et al: Ristocetin-induced self-aggregation of von Willebrand factor. *Eur Biophys J* 39(12):1597–1603, 2010.

1118. Scott JP, Montgomery RR, Retzinger GS: Dimeric ristocetin flocculates proteins, binds to platelets, mediates von Willebrand factor-dependent agglutination of platelets. *J Biol Chem* 266(13):8149–8155, 1991.

1119. Andrews RK, et al: Purification of botrocetin from *Bothrops jararaca* venom. Analysis of the botrocetin-mediated interaction between von Willebrand factor and the human platelet membrane glycoprotein Ib-IX complex. *Biochemistry* 28(21):8317–8326, 1989.

1120. Olson JD, et al: Adhesion of platelets to purified solid-phase von Willebrand factor: Effect of wall shear rate, ADP, thrombin, and ristocetin. *J Lab Clin Med* 114:6–18, 1989.

1121. Ruggeri ZM: Von Willebrand factor, platelets and endothelial cell interactions. *J Thromb Haemost* 1(7):1335–1342, 2003.

1122. Sixma JJ: Interaction of blood platelets with the vessel wall, in *Haemostasis and Thrombosis*, edited by AL Bloom, CD Forbes, DP Thomas, EGD Tuddenham, pp 259–285. Churchill Livingstone, London, England, 1994.

1123. Parker RI, Gralnick HR: Fibrin monomer induces binding of endogenous VWF to the glycocalicin portion of platelet glycoprotein Ib. *Blood* 70:1589–1594, 1987.

1124. Sakariassen KS, et al: Role of platelet membrane glycoproteins and von Willebrand factor in adhesion of platelets to subendothelium and collagen. *Ann N Y Acad Sci* 516:52–65, 1987.

1125. Sakariassen KS, et al: The role of platelet membrane glycoproteins Ib and IIb-IIIa in platelet adherence to human artery subendothelium. *Br J Haematol* 63:681–691, 1986.

1126. Ikeda Y, et al: Importance of fibrinogen and platelet membrane glycoprotein IIb/IIIa in shear-induced platelet aggregation. *Thromb Res* 51:157–163, 1988.

1127. Siediecki CA, et al: Shear-dependent changes in the three-dimensional structure of human von Willebrand factor. *Blood* 88(8):2939–2950, 1996.

1128. Yago T, et al: Platelet glycoprotein Ibalpha forms catch bonds with human WT VWF but not with type 2B von Willebrand disease VWF. *J Clin Invest* 118(9):3195–3207, 2008.

1129. Jamieson GA: The activation of platelets by thrombin: A model for activation by high and moderate affinity receptor pathways. *Prog Clin Biol Res* 283:137–158, 1988.

1130. Ruggeri Z: The platelet glycoprotein Ib-IX complex. *Prog Hemost Thromb* 10:35–68, 1991.

1131. Katagiri Y, et al: Localization of von Willebrand factor and thrombin-interactive domains in human platelet glycoprotein Ib. *Thromb Haemost* 63:122–126, 1990.

1132. Zarpellon A, et al: Binding of alpha-thrombin to surface-anchored platelet glycoprotein Ib(alpha) sulfotyrosines through a two-site mechanism involving exosite I. *Proc Natl Acad Sci U S A* 108(21):8628–8633, 2011.

1133. Harmon JT, Jamieson GA: The glycocalicin portion of platelet glycoprotein Ib expresses both high and moderate affinity receptor sites of thrombin. A soluble radioreceptor assay for the injection of thrombin with platelets. *J Biol Chem* 261: 13224–13229, 1986.

1134. Shrimpton CN, et al: Localization of the adhesion receptor glycoprotein Ib-IX-V complex to lipid rafts is required for platelet adhesion and activation. *J Exp Med* 196(8):1057–1066, 2002.

1135. Adam F, et al: Thrombin-induced platelet PAR4 activation: Role of glycoprotein Ib and ADP. *J Thromb Haemost* 1(4):798–804, 2003.

1136. De Candia E, et al: Binding of thrombin to glycoprotein Ib accelerates the hydrolysis of Par-1 on intact platelets. *J Biol Chem* 276(7):4692–4698, 2001.

1137. Frenette PS, et al: Platelet-endothelial interactions in inflamed mesenteric venules. *Blood* 91(4):1318–1325, 1998.

1138. Frenette PS, et al: P-Selectin glycoprotein ligand 1 (PSGL-1) is expressed on platelets and can mediate platelet-endothelial interactions *in vivo*. *J Exp Med* 191(8):1413–1422, 2000.

1139. Bradford HN, et al: Human kininogens regulate thrombin binding to platelets through the glycoprotein Ib-IX-V complex. *Blood* 90(4):1508–1515, 1997.

1140. Bradford HN, Pixley RA, Colman RW: Human factor XII binding to the glycoprotein Ib-IX-V complex inhibits thrombin-induced platelet aggregation. *J Biol Chem* 275(30):22756–22763, 2000.

1141. Baglia FA, et al: Factor XI binding to the platelet glycoprotein Ib-IX-V complex promotes factor XI activation by thrombin. *J Biol Chem* 277(3):1662–1668, 2002.

1142. Simon DI, et al: Platelet glycoprotein Ibα is a counterreceptor for the leukocyte integrin Mac-1 (CD11b/CD18). *J Exp Med* 192(2):193–204, 2000.

1143. Corken A, et al: Platelet glycoprotein Ib-IX as a regulator of systemic inflammation. *Arterioscler Thromb Vasc Biol* 34(5):996–1001, 2014.

1144. Yin H, et al: Role for platelet glycoprotein Ib-IX and effects of its inhibition in endotoxemia-induced thrombosis, thrombocytopenia, and mortality. *Arterioscler Thromb Vasc Biol* 33(11):2529–2537, 2013.

1145. Jain S, et al: Platelet glycoprotein Ib alpha supports experimental lung metastasis. *Proc Natl Acad Sci U S A* 104(21):9024–9028, 2007.

1146. Mo X, et al: Transmembrane domains are critical to the interaction between platelet glycoprotein V and glycoprotein Ib-IX complex. *J Thromb Haemost* 10(9):1875–1886, 2012.

1147. Modderman PW, et al: Glycoproteins V and Ib-IX form a noncovalent complex in the platelet membrane. *J Biol Chem* 267:364–369, 1992.

1148. Dong JF, Gao S, Lopez JA: Synthesis, assembly, and intracellular transport of the platelet glycoprotein Ib-IX-V complex. *J Biol Chem* 273(47):31449–31454, 1998.

1149. McGowan EB, Ding A, Detwiler TC: Correlation of thrombin-induced glycoprotein V hydrolysis and platelet activation. *J Biol Chem* 258:11243–11248, 1983.

1150. Ramakrishnan V, et al: Increased thrombin responsiveness in platelets from mice lacking glycoprotein V. *Proc Natl Acad Sci U S A* 96(23):13336–13341, 1999.

1151. Ramakrishnan V, et al: A thrombin receptor function for platelet glycoprotein Ib-IX unmasked by cleavage of glycoprotein V. *Proc Natl Acad Sci U S A* 98(4):1823–1828, 2001.

1152. Jones CI, Moraes LA, Gibbins JM: Regulation of platelet biology by platelet endothelial cell adhesion molecule-1. *Platelets* 23(5):331–335, 2012.

1153. Newman PJ, et al: PECAM-1 (CD31) cloning and relation to adhesion molecules of the immunoglobulin gene superfamily. *Science* 247:1219–1222, 1990.

1154. Novinska MS, et al: PECAM-1, in *Platelets*, edited by AD Michelson, pp 221–230. Academic Press, San Diego, 2002.

1155. Privratsky JR, Newman DK, Newman PJ: PECAM-1: Conflicts of interest in inflammation. *Life Sci* 87(3–4):69–82, 2010.

1156. Metzelaar MJ, et al: Biochemical characterization of PECAM-1 (CD31 antigen) on human platelets. *Thromb Haemost* 66(6):700–707, 1991.

1157. Paddock C, et al: Residues within a lipid-associated segment of the PECAM-1 cytoplasmic domain are susceptible to inducible, sequential phosphorylation. *Blood* 117(22):6012–6023, 2011.

1158. Jackson DE, et al: The protein-tyrosine phosphatase SHP-2 binds platelet/endothelial cell adhesion molecule-1 (PECAM-1) and forms a distinct signaling complex during platelet aggregation. Evidence for a mechanistic link between PECAM-1- and integrin-mediated cellular signaling. *J Biol Chem* 272(11):6986–6993, 1997.

1159. Crockett J, Newman DK, Newman PJ: PECAM-1 functions as a negative regulator of laminin-induced platelet activation. *J Thromb Haemost* 8(7):1584–1593, 2010.

1160. Jones CI, et al: PECAM-1 expression and activity negatively regulate multiple platelet signaling pathways. *FEBS Lett* 583(22):3618–3624, 2009.

1161. Varon D, et al: Platelet/endothelial cell adhesion molecule-1 serves as a costimulatory agonist receptor that modulates integrin-dependent adhesion and aggregation of human platelets. *Blood* 91(2):500–507, 1998.

1162. Wee JL, Jackson DE: The Ig-ITIM superfamily member PECAM-1 regulates the "outside-in" signaling properties of integrin alpha(IIb)beta3 in platelets. *Blood* 106(12):3816–3823, 2005.

1163. Jones CI, et al: Platelet endothelial cell adhesion molecule-1 inhibits platelet response to thrombin and von Willebrand factor by regulating the internalization of glycoprotein Ib via AKT/glycogen synthase kinase-3/dynamin and integrin alphaIIbbeta3. *Arterioscler Thromb Vasc Biol* 34(9):1968–1976, 2014.

1164. Albelda SM, et al: Molecular and cellular properties of PECAM-1 (endoCAM/CD31): A novel vascular cell-cell adhesion molecule. *J Cell Biol* 114(5):1059–1068, 1991.

1165. DeLisser HM, et al: Platelet/endothelial cell adhesion molecule-1 (CD31)-mediated cellular aggregation involves cell surface glycosaminoglycans. *J Biol Chem* 268(21): 16037–16046, 1993.

1166. Washington AV, et al: A TREM family member, TLT-1, is found exclusively in the alpha-granules of megakaryocytes and platelets. *Blood* 104(4):1042–1047, 2004.

1167. Kahn ML, Platelet-collagen responses: Molecular basis and therapeutic promise. *Semin Thromb Hemost* 30(4):419–425, 2004.

1168. Moroi M, Jung SM: Platelet glycoprotein VI: Its structure and function. *Thromb Res* 114(4):221–233, 2004.

1169. Schulz C, et al: EMMPRIN (CD147/basigin) mediates platelet-monocyte interactions in vivo and augments monocyte recruitment to the vascular wall. *J Thromb Haemost* 9(5):1007–1019, 2011.

1170. Arthur JF, et al: Platelet receptor redox regulation. *Platelets* 19(1):1–8, 2008.

1171. Jung SM, et al: Constitutive dimerization of glycoprotein VI (GPVI) in resting platelets is essential for binding to collagen and activation in flowing blood. *J Biol Chem* 287(35):30000–30013, 2012.

1172. Matus V, et al: An adenine insertion in exon 6 of human GP6 generates a truncated protein associated with a bleeding disorder in four Chilean families. *J Thromb Haemost* 11(9):1751–1759, 2013.

1173. Arthur JF, Dunkley S, Andrews RK: Platelet glycoprotein VI-related clinical defects. *Br J Haematol* 139(3):363–372, 2007.

1174. Dumont B, et al: Absence of collagen-induced platelet activation caused by compound heterozygous GPVI mutations. *Blood* 114(9):1900–1903, 2009.

1175. Hermans C, et al: A compound heterozygous mutation in glycoprotein VI in a patient with a bleeding disorder. *J Thromb Haemost* 7(8):1356–1363, 2009.

1176. Nurden P, et al: An acquired inhibitor to the GPVI platelet collagen receptor in a patient with lupus nephritis. *J Thromb Haemost* 7(9):1541–1549, 2009.

1177. Ezumi Y, Uchiyama T, Takayama H: Molecular cloning, genomic structure, chromosomal localization, and alternative splice forms of the platelet collagen receptor glycoprotein VI. *Biochem Biophys Res Commun* 277(1):27–36, 2000.

1178. Kotulicova D, et al: Variability of GP6 gene in patients with sticky platelet syndrome and deep venous thrombosis and/or pulmonary embolism. *Blood Coagul Fibrinolysis* 23(6):543–547, 2012.

1179. Gibbins J, et al: Tyrosine phosphorylation of the Fc receptor gamma-chain in collagen-stimulated platelets. *J Biol Chem* 271(30):18095–18099, 1996.

1180. Tsuji M, et al: A novel association of Fc receptor gamma-chain with glycoprotein VI and their co-expression as a collagen receptor in human platelets. *J Biol Chem* 272(38):23528–23531, 1997.

1181. Chacko GW, et al: Clustering of the platelet Fc gamma receptor induces noncovalent association with the tyrosine kinase p72syk. *J Biol Chem* 269(51): 32435–32440, 1994.

1182. Qiu WQ, et al: Organization of the human and mouse low-affinity Fc gamma R genes: Duplication and recombination. *Science* 248(4956):732–735, 1990.

1183. Boylan B, et al: Identification of FcgammaRIIa as the ITAM-bearing receptor mediating alphaIIbbeta3 outside-in integrin signaling in human platelets. *Blood* 112(7):2780–2786, 2008.

1184. Zhi H, et al: Cooperative integrin/ITAM signaling in platelets enhances thrombus formation in vitro and in vivo. *Blood* 121(10):1858–1867, 2013.

1185. Yeung J, et al: Platelet 12-LOX is essential for FcgammaRIIa-mediated platelet activation. *Blood* 124(14):2271–2279, 2014.

1186. Berlacher MD, et al: FcgammaRIIa ligation induces platelet hypersensitivity to thrombotic stimuli. *Am J Pathol* 182(1):244–254, 2013.

1187. Rosenfeld SI, et al: Human platelet Fc receptor for immunoglobulin G. Identification as a 40,000-molecular-weight membrane protein shared by monocytes. *J Clin Invest* 76(6):2317–2322, 1985.

1188. Rosenfeld SI, et al: Human Fc gamma receptors: Stable inter-donor variation in quantitative expression on platelets correlates with functional responses. *J Immunol* 138(9):2869–2873, 1987.

1189. Anderson GP, van de Winkel JG, Anderson CL: Anti-GPIIb/IIIa (CD41) monoclonal antibody-induced platelet activation requires Fc receptor-dependent cell-cell interaction. *Br J Haematol* 79(1):75–83, 1991.

1190. Gratacap MP, et al: Phosphatidylinositol 3,4,5-trisphosphate-dependent stimulation of phospholipase C-gamma2 is an early key event in FcgammaRIIA-mediated activation of human platelets. *J Biol Chem* 273(38):24314–24321, 1998.

1191. Hildreth JE, Derr D, Azorsa DO: Characterization of a novel self-associating Mr 40,000 platelet glycoprotein. *Blood* 77(1):121–132, 1991.

1192. Nazi I, Arnold DM, Smith JW, et al: FcgammaRIIa proteolysis as a diagnostic biomarker for heparin-induced thrombocytopenia. *J Thromb Haemost* 11(6):1146–1153, 2013.

1193. Nazi I, et al: The association between platelet activation and FcgammaRIIa proteolysis. *J Thromb Haemost* 9(4):885–887, 2011.

1194. Peerschke EI, Ghebrehiwet B: C1q augments platelet activation in response to aggregated Ig. *J Immunol* 159(11):5594–5598, 1997.

1195. Boilard E, et al: Influenza virus H1N1 activates platelets through FcgammaRIIA signaling and thrombin generation. *Blood* 123(18):2854–2863, 2014.

1196. Tilley DO, et al: Glycoprotein Ialpha and FcgammaRIIa play key roles in platelet activation by the colonizing bacterium, *Streptococcus oralis. J Thromb Haemost* 11(5):941–950, 2013.

1197. Mitrugno A, et al: A novel and essential role for FcgammaRIIa in cancer cell-induced platelet activation. *Blood* 123(2):249–260, 2014.

1198. Chong BH, et al: Increased expression of platelet IgG Fc receptors in immune heparin- induced thrombocytopenia. *Blood* 81(4):988–993, 1993.

1199. Parren PW, et al: On the interaction of IgG subclasses with the low affinity Fc gamma RIIa (CD32) on human monocytes, neutrophils, and platelets. Analysis of a functional polymorphism to human IgG2. *J Clin Invest* 90(4):1537–1546, 1992.

1200. Warmerdam PA, et al: Polymorphism of the human Fc gamma receptor II (CD32): Molecular basis and functional aspects. *Immunobiology* 185(2–4):175–182, 1992.

1201. Chen J, et al: Platelet FcgammaRIIA His131Arg polymorphism and platelet function: Antibodies to platelet-bound fibrinogen induce platelet activation. *J Thromb Haemost* 1(2):355–362, 2003.

1202. Carlsson LE, et al: Heparin-induced thrombocytopenia: New insights into the impact of the FcgammaRIIa-R-H131 polymorphism. *Blood* 92(5):1526–1531, 1998.

1203. Denomme GA, et al: Activation of platelets by sera containing IgG1 heparin-dependent antibodies: An explanation for the predominance of the Fc gammaRIIa "low responder" (his131) gene in patients with heparin-induced thrombocytopenia. *J Lab Clin Med* 130(3):278–284, 1997.

1204. Gruel Y, et al: The homozygous FcgammaRIIIa-158V genotype is a risk factor for heparin-induced thrombocytopenia in patients with antibodies to heparin-platelet factor 4 complexes. *Blood* 104(9):2791–2793, 2004.

1205. Kannan M, et al: An update on the prevalence and characterization of H-PF4 antibodies in Asian-Indian patients. *Semin Thromb Hemost* 35(3):337–343, 2009.

1206. Trikalinos TA, Karassa FB, Ioannidis JP: Meta-analysis of the association between low-affinity Fcgamma receptor gene polymorphisms and hematologic and autoimmune disease. *Blood* 98(5):1634–1635, 2001.

1207. Williams Y, et al: Correlation of platelet Fc gammaRIIA polymorphism in refractory idiopathic (immune) thrombocytopenic purpura. *Br J Haematol* 101(4):779–782, 1998.

1208. Diacovo TG, et al: A functional integrin ligand on the surface of platelets: Intercellular adhesion molecule-2. *J Clin Invest* 94(3):1243–1251, 1994.

1209. Hasegawa S, et al: Functional expression of the high affinity receptor for IgE (FcepsilonRI) in human platelets and its' intracellular expression in human megakaryocytes. *Blood* 93(8):2543–2551, 1999.

1210. Joseph M, et al: Expression and functions of the high-affinity IgE receptor on human platelets and megakaryocyte precursors. *Eur J Immunol* 27(9):2212–2218, 1997.

1211. Kasperska-Zajac A, Rogala B: Platelet function in anaphylaxis. *J Investig Allergol Clin Immunol* 16(1):1–4, 2006.

1212. Gupta SK, Pillarisetti K, Ohlstein EH: Platelet agonist F11 receptor is a member of the immunoglobulin superfamily and identical with junctional adhesion molecule (JAM): Regulation of expression in human endothelial cells and macrophages. *IUBMB Life* 50(1):51–56, 2000.

1213. Kornecki E, et al: Activation of human platelets by a stimulatory monoclonal antibody. *J Biol Chem* 265(17):10042–10048, 1990.

1214. Naik UP, et al: Characterization and chromosomal localization of JAM-1, a platelet receptor for a stimulatory monoclonal antibody. *J Cell Sci* 114(Pt 3):539–547, 2001.

1215. Sobocka MB, et al: Cloning of the human platelet F11 receptor: A cell adhesion molecule member of the immunoglobulin superfamily involved in platelet aggregation. *Blood* 95(8):2600–2609, 2000.

1216. Sobocki T, et al: Genomic structure, organization and promoter analysis of the human F11R/F11 receptor/junctional adhesion molecule-1/JAM-A. *Gene* 366(1):128–144, 2006.

1217. Naik MU, et al: JAM-A protects from thrombosis by suppressing integrin alphaIIb-beta3-dependent outside-in signaling in platelets. *Blood* 119(14):3352–3360, 2012.

1218. Naik MU, Caplan JL, Naik UP: Junctional adhesion molecule-A suppresses platelet integrin alphaIIbbeta3 signaling by recruiting Csk to the integrin-c-Src complex. *Blood* 123(9):1393–1402, 2014.

1219. Stellos K, et al: Expression of junctional adhesion molecule-C on the surface of platelets supports adhesion, but not differentiation, of human CD34 cells *in vitro. Cell Physiol Biochem* 29(1–2):153–162, 2012.

1220. McEver RP: Properties of GMP-140, an inducible granule membrane protein of platelets and endothelium. *Blood Cells* 16:73–83, 1990.

1221. McEver RP, P-selectin/PSGL-1 and other interactions between platelets, leukocytes, and endothelium, in *Platelets*, edited by AD Michelson, p 231. Academic Press, San Diego, 2007.

1222. McEver RP, Beckstead JH, Moore KL, et al: GMP-140, a platelet -granule membrane protein, is also synthesized by vascular endothelial cells and is localized in Weibel-Palade bodies. *J Clin Invest* 84(1):92–99, 1989.

1223. Yong AS, et al: Intracoronary shear-related up-regulation of platelet P-selectin and platelet-monocyte aggregation despite the use of aspirin and clopidogrel. *Blood* 117(1):11–20, 2011.

1224. Abrams C, Shattil SJ: Immunological detection of activated platelets in clinical disorders. *J Thromb Haemost* 65(5):467–473, 1991.

1225. Haskard DO: Adhesive proteins, in *Haemostasis and Thrombosis*, edited by AL Bloom, CD Forbes, DP Thomas, EGD Tuddenham, pp 233–257. Churchill Livingstone, England, 1994.

1226. Ishiwata N, et al: Alternatively spliced isoform of P-selectin is present *in vivo* as a soluble molecule. *J Biol Chem* 269(38):23708–23715, 1994.

1227. Hartwell DW, et al: Role of P-selectin cytoplasmic domain in granular targeting in vivo and in early inflammatory responses. *J Cell Biol* 143(4):1129–1141, 1998.

1228. Geng JG, et al: Rapid neutrophil adhesion to activated endothelium mediated by GMP-140. *Nature* 343:757–760, 1990.

1229. Handa K, et al: Selectin GMP-140 (CD62;PADGEM) binds to sialosyl-Le(a) and sialosyl-Le(x), and sulfated glycans modulate this binding. *Biochem Biophys Res Commun* 181:1223–1230, 1991.

1230. Polley MJ, et al: CD62 and endothelial cell-leukocyte adhesion molecule I (ELAM-1) recognize the same carbohydrate ligand, sialyl-Lewisx. *Proc Natl Acad Sci U S A* 88:6224–6228, 1991.

1231. Aruffo A, et al: CD62/P-selectin recognition of myeloid and tumor cell sulfatides. *Cell* 67:35–44, 1991.

1232. Stone JP, Wagner DD: P-selectin mediates adhesion of platelets to neuroblastoma and small cell lung cancer. *J Clin Invest* 92:804–813, 1993.

1233. McEver RP, Cummings RD: Perspectives series: Cell adhesion in vascular biology. Role of PSGL-1 binding to selectins in leukocyte recruitment. *J Clin Invest* 100(3):485–491, 1997.

1234. Sako D, et al: Expression cloning of a functional glycoprotein ligand for P-selectin. *Cell* 75(6):1179–1186, 1993.

1235. Yang J, Furie BC, Furie B: The biology of P-selectin glycoprotein ligand-1: Its role as a selectin counterreceptor in leukocyte-endothelial and leukocyte-platelet interaction. *Thromb Haemost* 81(1):1–7, 1999.

1236. Falati S, et al: Accumulation of tissue factor into developing thrombi in vivo is dependent upon microparticle P-selectin glycoprotein ligand 1 and platelet P-selectin. *J Exp Med* 197(11):1585–1598, 2003.

1237. Celi A, et al: P-selectin induces the expression of tissue factor on monocytes. *Proc Natl Acad Sci U S A* 91(19):8767–8771, 1994.

1238. Theoret JF, et al: P-selectin ligation induces platelet activation and enhances microaggregate and thrombus formation. *Thromb Res* 128(3):243–250, 2011.

1239. Ridker PM, Buring JE, Rifai N: Soluble P-selectin and the risk of future cardiovascular events. *Circulation* 103(4):491–495, 2001.

1240. Mayadas TN, et al: Leukocyte rolling and extravasation are severely compromised in P-selectin-deficient mice. *Cell* 74(3):541–554, 1993.

1241. Frenette PS, et al: Platelets roll on stimulated endothelium *in vivo*: An interaction mediated by endothelial P-selectin. *Proc Natl Acad Sci U S A* 92(16):7450–7454, 1995.

1242. Padilla A, et al: P-selectin anchors newly released ultralarge von Willebrand factor multimers to the endothelial cell surface. *Blood* 103(6):2150–2156, 2004.

1243. Cambien B, Wagner DD: A new role in hemostasis for the adhesion receptor P-selectin. *Trends Mol Med* 10(4):179–186, 2004.

1244. Ludwig RJ, Schon MP, Boehncke WH: P-selectin: A common therapeutic target for cardiovascular disorders, inflammation and tumour metastasis. *Expert Opin Ther Targets* 11(8):1103–1117, 2007.

1245. Polanowska-Grabowska R, et al: P-selectin-mediated platelet-neutrophil aggregate formation activates neutrophils in mouse and human sickle cell disease. *Arterioscler Thromb Vasc Biol* 30(12):2392–2399, 2010.

1246. Polgar J, Matuskova J, Wagner DD: The P-selectin, tissue factor, coagulation triad. *J Thromb Haemost* 3(8):1590–1596, 2005.

1247. Navarro-Nunez L, et al: The physiological and pathophysiological roles of platelet CLEC-2. *Thromb Haemost* 109(6):991–998, 2013.

1248. Ozaki Y, Suzuki-Inoue K, Inoue O: Novel interactions in platelet biology: CLEC-2/podoplanin and laminin/GPVI. *J Thromb Haemost* 7(Suppl 1):191–194, 2009.

1249. Schacht V, et al: T1alpha/podoplanin deficiency disrupts normal lymphatic vasculature formation and causes lymphedema. *EMBO J* 22(14):3546–3556, 2003.

1250. Tsuruo T, Fujita N: Platelet aggregation in the formation of tumor metastasis. *Proc Jpn Acad Ser B Phys Biol Sci* 84(6):189–198, 2008.

1251. Christou CM, et al: Renal cells activate the platelet receptor CLEC-2 through podoplanin. *Biochem J* 411(1):133–140, 2008.

1252. Gitz E, et al: CLEC-2 expression is maintained on activated platelets and on platelet microparticles. *Blood* 124(14):2262–2270, 2014.

1253. Suzuki-Inoue K, et al: Involvement of the snake toxin receptor CLEC-2, in podoplanin-mediated platelet activation, by cancer cells. *J Biol Chem* 282(36):25993–26001, 2007.

1254. Watson AA, et al: The platelet receptor CLEC-2 is active as a dimer. *Biochemistry* 48(46):10988–10996, 2009.

1255. Gitz E, et al: CLEC-2 expression is maintained on activated platelets and on platelet microparticles. *Blood* 124(14):2262–2270, 2014.

1256. Lowe KL, Navarro-Nunez L, Watson SP: Platelet CLEC-2 and podoplanin in cancer metastasis. *Thromb Res* 129(Suppl 1):S30–S37, 2012.

1257. Bertozzi CC, et al: Platelets regulate lymphatic vascular development through CLEC-2-SLP-76 signaling. *Blood* 116(4):661–670, 2010.

1258. Pollitt AY, et al: Syk and Src family kinases regulate C-type lectin receptor 2 (CLEC-2)-mediated clustering of podoplanin and platelet adhesion to lymphatic endothelial cells. *J Biol Chem* 289(52):35695–35710, 2014.

1259. Suzuki-Inoue K, et al: Essential *in vivo* roles of the C-type lectin receptor CLEC-2: Embryonic/neonatal lethality of CLEC-2-deficient mice by blood/lymphatic misconnections and impaired thrombus formation of CLEC-2-deficient platelets. *J Biol Chem* 285(32):24494–24507, 2010.

1260. Benezech C, et al: CLEC-2 is required for development and maintenance of lymph nodes. *Blood* 123(20):3200–3207, 2014.

1261. Hemler ME: Tetraspanin functions and associated microdomains. *Nat Rev Mol Cell Biol* 6(10):801–811, 2005.

1262. Israels SJ, McMillan-Ward EM: Platelet tetraspanin complexes and their association with lipid rafts. *Thromb Haemost* 98(5):1081–1087, 2007.

1263. Israels SJ, McMillan-Ward EM: Palmitoylation supports the association of tetraspanin CD63 with CD9 and integrin alphaIIbbeta3 in activated platelets. *Thromb Res* 125(2):152–158, 2010.

1264. Goschnick MW, Jackson DE: Tetraspanins-structural and signalling scaffolds that regulate platelet function. *Mini Rev Med Chem* 7(12):1248–1254, 2007.

1265. Goschnick MW, et al: Impaired "outside-in" integrin alphaIIbbeta3 signaling and thrombus stability in TSSC6-deficient mice. *Blood* 108(6):1911–1918, 2006.

1266. Protty MB, et al: Identification of Tspan9 as a novel platelet tetraspanin and the collagen receptor GPVI as a component of tetraspanin microdomains. *Biochem J* 417(1):391–400, 2009.

1267. Boucheix C, et al: Molecular cloning of the CD9 antigen. A new family of cell surface proteins. *J Biol Chem* 266(1):117–122, 1991.

1268. Hato T, et al: Exposure of platelet fibrinogen receptors by a monoclonal antibody to CD9 antigen. *Blood* 72(1):224–229, 1988.

1269. Lanza F, et al: CDNA cloning and expression of platelet p24/CD9. Evidence for a new family of multiple membrane-spanning proteins. *J Biol Chem* 266(16):10638–10645, 1991.

1270. Brisson C, et al: Co-localization of CD9 and GPIb-IIIa (alpha IIb beta 3 integrin) on activated platelet pseudopods and alpha-granule membranes. *Histochem J* 29(2):153–165, 1997.

1271. Hato T, et al: Induction of platelet Ca2+ influx and mobilization by a monoclonal antibody to CD9 antigen. *Blood* 75(5):1087–1091, 1990.

1272. Jennings LK, et al: The activation of human platelets mediated by anti-human platelet p24/CD9 monoclonal antibodies. *J Biol Chem* 265:3815–3822, 1990.

1273. Worthington RE, Carroll RC, Boucheix C: Platelet activation by CD9 monoclonal antibodies is mediated by the Fc gamma II receptor. *Br J Haematol* 74(2):216–222, 1990.

1274. Slupsky JR, et al: Evidence that monoclonal antibodies against CD9 antigen induce specific association between CD9 and the platelet glycoprotein IIb-IIIa complex. *J Biol Chem* 264(21):12289–12293, 1989.

1275. Dale GL, Remenyi G, Friese P: Tetraspanin CD9 is required for microparticle release from coated-platelets. *Platelets* 20(6):361–366, 2009.

1276. Mangin PH, et al: CD9 negatively regulates integrin alphaIIbbeta3 activation and could thus prevent excessive platelet recruitment at sites of vascular injury. *J Thromb Haemost* 7(5):900–902, 2009.

1277. Nishibori M, et al: The protein CD63 is in platelet dense granules, is deficient in a patient with Hermansky-Pudlak syndrome, and appears identical to granulophysin. *J Clin Invest* 91:1775–1782, 1993.

1278. Metzelaar MJ, et al: CD63 antigen. A novel lysosomal membrane glycoprotein, cloned by a screening procedure for intracellular antigens in eukaryotic cells. *J Biol Chem* 266(5):3239–3245, 1991.

1279. Fitter S, et al: Molecular cloning of cDNA encoding a novel platelet-endothelial cell tetra-span antigen, PETA-3. *Blood* 86(4):1348–1355, 1995.

1280. Roberts JJ, et al: Platelet activation induced by a murine monoclonal antibody directed against a novel tetra-span antigen. *Br J Haematol* 89(4):853–860, 1995.

1281. Sincock PM, Mayrhofer G, Ashman LK: Localization of the transmembrane 4 superfamily (TM4SF) member PETA-3 (CD151) in normal human tissues: Comparison with CD9, CD63, and alpha5beta1 integrin. *J Histochem Cytochem* 45(4):515–525, 1997.

1282. Lau LM, et al: The tetraspanin superfamily member, CD151 regulates outside-in integrin alphaIIbbeta3 signalling and platelet function. *Blood* 104(8):2368–2375, 2004.

1283. Orlowski E, et al: A platelet tetraspanin superfamily member, CD151, is required for regulation of thrombus growth and stability in vivo. *J Thromb Haemost* 7(12):2074–2084, 2009.

1284. Polgar J, et al: Additional GPI-anchored glycoproteins on human platelets that are absent or deficient in paroxysmal nocturnal haemoglobinuria. *FEBS Lett* 327(1):49–53, 1993.

1285. Hwang SM, Kim MJ, Chang HE, et al: Human platelet antigen genotyping and expression of CD109 (human platelet antigen 15) mRNA in various human cell types. *Biomed Res Int* 2013:946403, 2013.

1286. Kelton JG, et al: ABH antigens on human platelets: Expression on the glycosyl phosphatidylinositol-anchored protein CD109. *J Lab Clin Med* 132(2):142–148, 2013.

1287. Grunewald M, et al: The platelet function defect of paroxysmal nocturnal haemoglobinuria. *Platelets* 15(3):145–154, 2004.

1288. Jin JY, et al: Glycosylphosphatidyl-inositol (GPI)-linked protein deficiency on the platelets of patients with aplastic anaemia and paroxysmal nocturnal haemoglobinuria: Two distinct patterns correlating with expression on neutrophils. *Br J Haematol* 96(3):493–496, 1997.

1289. Barclay GR, et al: Distribution of cell-associated prion protein in normal adult blood determined by flow cytometry. *Br J Haematol* 107(4):804–814, 1999.

1290. Holada K, et al: Increased expression of phosphatidylinositol-specific phospholipase C resistant prion proteins on the surface of activated platelets. *Br J Haematol* 103(1):276–282, 1998.

1291. MacGregor I, et al: Application of a time-resolved fluoroimmunoassay for the analysis of normal prion protein in human blood and its components. *Vox Sang* 77(2):88–96, 1999.

1292. Starke R, Cramer E, Harrison P: Expression of cell-associated prion protein on normal human platelets. *Br J Haematol* 110(3):748–750, 2000.

1293. Prevost N, et al: Interactions between Eph kinases and ephrins provide a mechanism to support platelet aggregation once cell-to-cell contact has occurred. *Proc Natl Acad Sci U S A* 99(14):9219–9224, 2002.

1294. Prevost N, et al: Signaling by ephrinB1 and Eph kinases in platelets promotes Rap1 activation, platelet adhesion, and aggregation via effector pathways that do not require phosphorylation of ephrinB1. *Blood* 103(4):1348–1355, 2004.

1295. Prevost N, et al: Eph kinases and ephrins support thrombus growth and stability by regulating integrin outside-in signaling in platelets. *Proc Natl Acad Sci U S A* 102(28):9820–9825, 2005.

1296. dem Borne AE, et al: Thrombopoietin and its receptor: Structure, function and role in the regulation of platelet production. *Baillieres Clin Haematol* 11(2):409–426, 1998.

1297. Fielder PJ, et al: Human platelets as a model for the binding and degradation of thrombopoietin. *Blood* 89(8):2782–2788, 1997.

1298. Kaushansky K: Thrombopoietin: A tool for understanding thrombopoiesis. *J Thromb Haemost* 1(7):1587–1592, 2003.

1299. Kaushansky K: Historical review: Megakaryopoiesis and thrombopoiesis. *Blood* 111(3):981–986, 2008.

1300. Chen J, et al: Regulation of platelet activation *in vitro* by the c-Mpl ligand, thrombopoietin. *Blood* 86(11):4054–4062, 1995.

1301. Ezumi Y, Takayama H, Okuma M: Thrombopoietin, c-Mpl ligand, induces tyrosine phosphorylation of Tyk2, JAK2, and STAT3, and enhances agonists-induced aggregation in platelets *in vitro*. *FEBS Lett* 374(1):48–52, 1995.

1302. Kojima H, et al: Modulation of platelet activation *in vitro* by thrombopoietin. *Thromb Haemost* 74(6):1541–1545, 1995.

1303. Kubota Y, et al: Thrombopoietin modulates platelet activation *in vitro* through protein-tyrosine phosphorylation. *Stem Cells* 14(4):439–444, 1996.

1304. Oda A, et al: Thrombopoietin primes human platelet aggregation induced by shear stress and by multiple agonists. *Blood* 87(11):4664–4670, 1996.

1305. Rodriguez-Linares B, Watson SP: Thrombopoietin potentiates activation of human platelets in association with JAK2 and TYK2 phosphorylation. *Biochem J* 316(Pt 1):93–98, 1996.

1306. Fox NE, et al: Compound heterozygous c-Mpl mutations in a child with congenital amegakaryocytic thrombocytopenia: Functional characterization and a review of the literature. *Exp Hematol* 37(4):495–503, 2009.

1307. Kilpivaara O, Levine RL: JAK2 and MPL mutations in myeloproliferative neoplasms: Discovery and science. *Leukemia* 22(10):1813–1817, 2008.

1308. Aiken ML, et al: Effects of OKM5, a monoclonal antibody to glycoprotein IV, on platelet aggregation and thrombospondin surface expression. *Blood* 76(12):2501–2509, 1990.

1309. Daviet L, McGregor JL: Vascular biology of CD36: Roles of this new adhesion molecule family in different disease states. *Thromb Haemost* 78(1):65–69, 1997.

1310. Febbraio M, Silverstein RL: CD36: Implications in cardiovascular disease. *Int J Biochem Cell Biol* 39(11):2012–2030, 2007.

1311. Legrand C, Pidard D, Beiso P, et al: Interaction of a monoclonal antibody to glycoprotein IV (CD36) with human platelets and its effect on platelet function. *Platelets* 2(2):99–105, 1991.

1312. Tandon NN, et al: Isolation and characterization of platelet glycoprotein IV (CD36). *J Biol Chem* 1989;264(13):7570–7575, 1991.

1313. Valiyaveettil M, Podrez EA: Platelet hyperreactivity, scavenger receptors and atherothrombosis. *J Thromb Haemost* 7(Suppl 1):218–221, 2009.

1314. Oquendo P, Hundt E, Lawler J, Seed B: CD36 directly mediates cytoadherence of *Plasmodium falciparum* infected erythrocytes. *Cell* 58(1):95–101, 1989.

1315. Huang MM, et al: Membrane glycoprotein IV (CD36) is physically associated with the Fyn, Lyn, and Yes protein-tyrosine kinases in human platelets. *Proc Natl Acad Sci U S A* 88(17):7844–7848, 1991.

1316. Taketani T, et al: Neonatal isoimmune thrombocytopenia caused by type I CD36 deficiency having novel splicing isoforms of the CD36 gene. *Eur J Haematol* 81(1):70–74, 2008.

1317. Thorne RF, et al: CD36 forms covalently associated dimers and multimers in platelets and transfected COS-7 cells. *Biochem Biophys Res Commun* 240(3):812–818, 1997.

1318. Thibert V, et al: Increased platelet CD36 constitutes a common marker in myeloproliferative disorders. *Br J Haematol* 91(3):618–624, 1995.

1319. Asch AS, et al: Analysis of CD36 binding domains: Ligand specificity controlled by dephosphorylation of an ectodomain. *Science* 262(5138):1436–1440, 1993.

1320. Aiken JW, Ginsberg MH, Plow EF: Mechanisms for expression of thrombospondin on the platelet surface. *Semin Thromb Hemost* 13:307–316, 1987.

1321. Collot-Teixeira S, et al: CD36 and macrophages in atherosclerosis. *Cardiovasc Res* 75(3):468–477, 2007.

1322. Yamashita S, et al: Physiological and pathological roles of a multi-ligand receptor CD36 in atherogenesis; insights from CD36-deficient patients. *Mol Cell Biochem* 299(1–2):19–22, 2007.

1323. Chen K, et al: A specific CD36-dependent signaling pathway is required for platelet activation by oxidized low-density lipoprotein. *Circ Res* 102(12):1512–1519, 2008.

1324. Korporaal SJ, et al: Platelet activation by oxidized low density lipoprotein is mediated by CD36 and scavenger receptor-A. *Arterioscler Thromb Vasc Biol* 27(11):2476–2483, 2007.

1325. Podrez EA, et al: Platelet CD36 links hyperlipidemia, oxidant stress and a prothrombotic phenotype. *Nat Med* 13(9):1086–1095, 2007.

1326. Ma Y, Ashraf MZ, Podrez EA: Scavenger receptor BI modulates platelet reactivity and thrombosis in dyslipidemia. *Blood* 116(11):1932–1941, 2010.

1327. Ghosh A, et al: Platelet CD36 mediates interactions with endothelial cell-derived microparticles and contributes to thrombosis in mice. *J Clin Invest* 118(5):1934–1943, 2008.

1328. Hajjar DP, Gotto AM: Targeting CD36: Modulating inflammation and atherogenesis. *Curr Atheroscler Rep* 5(3):155–156, 2003.

1329. Hirano K, et al: Pathophysiology of human genetic CD36 deficiency. *Trends Cardiovasc Med* 13(4):136–141, 2003.

1330. Pravenec M, Kurtz TW: Genetics of Cd36 and the hypertension metabolic syndrome. *Semin Nephrol* 22(2):148–153, 2002.

1331. Su X, Abumrad NA: Cellular fatty acid uptake: A pathway under construction. *Trends Endocrinol Metab* 20(2):72–77, 2009.

1332. Asch AS, et al: Isolation of the thrombospondin membrane receptor. *J Clin Invest* 79:1054–1061, 1987.

1333. Diaz-Ricart M, et al: Antibodies to CD36 (GPIV) inhibit platelet adhesion to subendothelial surfaces under flow conditions. *Arterioscler Thromb Vasc Biol* 16(7):883–888, 1996.

1334. Tandon NN, Kralisz U, Jamieson GA: Identification of glycoprotein IV (CD36) as a primary receptor for platelet-collagen adhesion. *J Biol Chem* 264:7576–7583, 1989.

1335. Saelman EU, et al: Platelet adhesion to collagen and endothelial cell matrix under flow conditions is not dependent on platelet glycoprotein IV. *Blood* 83(11):3240–3244, 1994.

1336. Wun T, et al: Platelet-erythrocyte adhesion in sickle cell disease. *J Investig Med* 47(3):121–127, 1999.

1337. Valiyaveettil M, et al: Oxidized high-density lipoprotein inhibits platelet activation and aggregation via scavenger receptor BI. *Blood* 111(4):1962–1971, 2008.

1338. Chadwick AC, Sahoo D: Functional genomics of the human high-density lipoprotein receptor scavenger receptor BI: An old dog with new tricks. *Curr Opin Endocrinol Diabetes Obes* 20(2):124–131, 2013.

1339. Choi WS, Jeon OH, Kim DS: CD40 ligand shedding is regulated by interaction between matrix metalloproteinase-2 and platelet integrin alpha(IIb)beta(3). *J Thromb Haemost* 8(6):1364–1371, 2010.

1340. Heeschen C, et al: Soluble CD40 ligand in acute coronary syndromes. *N Engl J Med* 348(12):1104–1111, 2003.

1341. Andre P, et al: Platelet-derived CD40L: The switch-hitting player of cardiovascular disease. *Circulation* 106(8):896–899, 2002.

1342. Aukrust P, Damas JK, Solum NO: Soluble CD40 ligand and platelets: Self-perpetuating pathogenic loop in thrombosis and inflammation? *J Am Coll Cardiol* 43(12):2326–2328, 2004.

1343. Jin R, Yu S, Song Z, et al: Soluble CD40 ligand stimulates CD40-dependent activation of the β2 integrin Mac-1 and protein kinase C zeda (PKCζ) in neutrophils: Implications for neutrophil-platelet interactions and neutrophil oxidative burst. *PLoS One* 8(6):e64631, 2013.

1344. Varo N, deLemos JA, Libby P, et al: Soluble CD40L: Risk prediction after acute coronary syndromes. *Circulation* 108(9):1049–1052, 2003.

1345. Cipollone F, et al: Preprocedural level of soluble CD40L is predictive of enhanced inflammatory response and restenosis after coronary angioplasty. *Circulation* 108(22):2776–2782, 2003.

1346. Lievens D, et al: Platelet CD40L mediates thrombotic and inflammatory processes in atherosclerosis. *Blood* 116(20):4317–4327, 2010.

1347. Pamukcu B, et al: The CD40-CD40L system in cardiovascular disease. *Ann Med* 43(5):331–340, 2011.

1348. Andre P, et al: CD40L stabilizes arterial thrombi by a beta3 integrin-dependent mechanism. *Nat Med* 8(3):247–252, 2002.

1349. Inwald DP, et al: CD40 is constitutively expressed on platelets and provides a novel mechanism for platelet activation. *Circ Res* 92(9):1041–1048, 2003.

1350. Prasad KS, et al: Soluble CD40 ligand induces beta3 integrin tyrosine phosphorylation and triggers platelet activation by outside-in signaling. *Proc Natl Acad Sci U S A* 100(21):12367–12371, 2003.

1351. Urbich C, et al: CD40 ligand inhibits endothelial cell migration by increasing production of endothelial reactive oxygen species. *Circulation* 106(8):981–986, 2002.

1352. Czapiga M, Kirk AD, Lekstrom-Himes J: Platelets deliver costimulatory signals to antigen-presenting cells: A potential bridge between injury and immune activation. *Exp Hematol* 32(2):135–139, 2004.

1353. Elzey BD, et al: Platelet-mediated modulation of adaptive immunity. A communication link between innate and adaptive immune compartments. *Immunity* 19(1):9–19, 2003.

1354. Ahmad R, et al: Activated human platelets express Fas-L and induce apoptosis in Fas-positive tumor cells. *J Leukoc Biol* 69(1):123–128, 2001.

1355. Crist SA, et al: Expression of TNF-related apoptosis-inducing ligand (TRAIL) in megakaryocytes and platelets. *Exp Hematol* 32(11):1073–1081, 2004.

1356. Otterdal K, et al: Platelet-derived LIGHT induces inflammatory responses in endothelial cells and monocytes. *Blood* 108(3):928–935, 2006.

1357. Saftig P, Schroder B, Blanz J: Lysosomal membrane proteins: Life between acid and neutral conditions. *Biochem Soc Trans* 38(6):1420–1423, 2010.

1358. Silverstein RL, Febbraio M: Identification of lysosome-associated membrane protein-2 as an activation-dependent platelet surface glycoprotein. *Blood* 80(6):1470–1475, 1992.

1359. Ghebrehiwet B, et al: GC1q-R/p33, a member of a new class of multifunctional and multicompartment cellular proteins, is involved in inflammation and infection. *Immunol Rev* 180:65–77, 2001.

1360. Peerschke EI, Ghebrehiwet B: Platelet receptors for the complement component C1q: Implications for hemostasis and thrombosis. *Immunobiology* 199(2):239–249, 1998.

1361. Peerschke EIB, Ghebrehiwet B: Human blood platelets possess specific binding sites for C1q. *J Immunol* 138:1537–1541, 1987.

1362. Ghebrehiwet B, et al: Isolation, cDNA cloning, and overexpression of a 33-kD cell surface glycoprotein that binds to the globular "heads" of C1q. *J Exp Med* 179(6):1809–1821, 1994.

1363. Herwald H, et al: Isolation and characterization of the kininogen-binding protein p33 from endothelial cells. Identity with the gC1q receptor. *J Biol Chem* 271(22):13040–13047, 1996.

1364. Nepomuceno RR, Tenner AJ: C1qRP, the C1q receptor that enhances phagocytosis, is detected specifically in human cells of myeloid lineage, endothelial cells, and platelets. *J Immunol* 160(4):1929–1935, 1998.

1365. Peerschke EI, Reid KB, Ghebrehiwet B: Platelet activation by C1q results in the induction of alpha IIb/beta 3 integrins (GPIIb-IIIa) and the expression of P-selectin and procoagulant activity. *J Exp Med* 178(2):579–587, 1993.

1366. Skoglund C, et al: C1q induces a rapid up-regulation of P-selectin and modulates collagen- and collagen-related peptide-triggered activation in human platelets. *Immunobiology* 215(12):987–995, 2010.

1367. Peerschke EIB: Platelet membrane receptors for the complement component C1q. *Semin Hematol* 31:320–328, 1994.

1368. Peerschke EIB, et al: Platelet activation by C1q results in the induction of αIIbβ3 integrins (GPIIb-IIIa) and the expression of P-selectin and procoagulant activity. *J Exp Med* 178:579–587, 1993.

1369. Jiang J, et al: Crystal structure of human p32, a doughnut-shaped acidic mitochondrial matrix protein. *Proc Natl Acad Sci U S A* 96(7):3572–3577, 1999.

1370. Metzelaar MJ, et al: Identification of a 33-Kd protein associated with the alpha-granule membrane (GMP-33) that is expressed on the surface of activated platelets. *Blood* 79(2):372–379, 1992.

1371. Damas C, et al: The 33-kDa platelet alpha-granule membrane protein (GMP-33) is an N-terminal proteolytic fragment of thrombospondin. *Thromb Haemost* 86(3):887–893, 2001.

1372. Rosenstein Y, et al: CD43, a molecule defective in Wiskott-Aldrich syndrome, binds ICAM-1. *Nature* 354(6350):233–235, 1991.

1373. Koupenova M, Mick E, Mikhalev E, et al: Sex differences in platelet toll-like receptors and their association with cardiovascular risk factors. *Arterioscler Thromb Vasc Biol* 35(4):1030–1037, 2015.

1374. Panigrahi S, et al: Engagement of platelet toll-like receptor 9 by novel endogenous ligands promotes platelet hyperreactivity and thrombosis. *Circ Res* 112(1):103–112, 2013.

1375. Rivadeneyra L, et al: Regulation of platelet responses triggered by Toll-like receptor 2 and 4 ligands is another non-genomic role of nuclear factor-kappaB. *Thromb Res* 133(2):235–243, 2014.

1376. Semple JW, et al: Platelet-bound lipopolysaccharide enhances Fc receptor-mediated phagocytosis of IgG-opsonized platelets. *Blood* 109(11):4803–4805, 2007.

1377. Zhang G, et al: Lipopolysaccharide stimulates platelet secretion and potentiates platelet aggregation via TLR4/MyD88 and the cGMP-dependent protein kinase pathway. *J Immunol* 182(12):7997–8004, 2009.

1378. Stahl AL, et al: Lipopolysaccharide from enterohemorrhagic *Escherichia coli* binds to platelets through TLR4 and CD62 and is detected on circulating platelets in patients with hemolytic uremic syndrome. *Blood* 108(1):167–176, 2006.

1379. Cognasse F, et al: Toll-like receptor 4 ligand can differentially modulate the release of cytokines by human platelets. *Br J Haematol* 141(1):84–91, 2008.

1380. Scott T, Owens MD: Thrombocytes respond to lipopolysaccharide through Toll-like receptor-4, and MAP kinase and NF-kappaB pathways leading to expression of interleukin-6 and cyclooxygenase-2 with production of prostaglandin E2. *Mol Immunol* 45(4):1001–1008, 2008.

1381. Stark RJ, Aghakasiri N, Rumbaut RE: Platelet-derived Toll-like receptor 4 (Tlr-4) is sufficient to promote microvascular thrombosis in endotoxemia. *PLoS One* 7(7):e41254, 2012.

1382. Ren MP, et al: Endothelial cells but not platelets are the major source of Toll-like receptor 4 in the arterial thrombosis and tissue factor expression in mice. *Am J Physiol Regul Integr Comp Physiol* 307(7):R901–R907, 2014.

1383. Gould TJ, Vu TT, Swystun LL, et al: Neutrophil extracellular traps promote thrombin generation through platelet-dependent and platelet-independent mechanisms. *Arterioscler Thromb Vasc Biol* 34(9):1977–1984, 2014.

1384. Akbiyik F, et al: Human bone marrow megakaryocytes and platelets express PPARgamma, and PPARgamma agonists blunt platelet release of CD40 ligand and thromboxanes. *Blood* 104(5):1361–1368, 2004.

1385. Ray DM, et al: Peroxisome proliferator-activated receptor gamma and retinoid X receptor transcription factors are released from activated human platelets and shed in microparticles. *Thromb Haemost* 99(1):86–95, 2008.

1386. Ali FY, et al: Role of nuclear receptor signaling in platelets: Antithrombotic effects of PPARbeta. *FASEB J* 20(2):326–328, 2006.

1387. Borchert M, et al: Review of the pleiotropic effects of peroxisome proliferator-activated receptor gamma agonists on platelet function. *Diabetes Technol Ther* 9(5):410–420, 2007.

1388. Santos-Martinez MJ, et al: Matrix metalloproteinases in platelet function: Coming of age. *J Thromb Haemost* 6(3):514–516, 2008.

1389. Soslau G, et al: Intracellular matrix metalloproteinase-2 (MMP-2) regulates human platelet activation via hydrolysis of talin. *Thromb Haemost* 111(1):140–153, 2014.

1390. Trivedi V, et al: Platelet matrix metalloprotease-1 mediates thrombogenesis by activating PAR1 at a cryptic ligand site. *Cell* 137(2):332–343, 2009.

1391. Choi WS, et al: MMP-2 regulates human platelet activation by interacting with integrin alphaIIbbeta3. *J Thromb Haemost* 6(3):517–523, 2008.

1392. Gresele P, et al: Platelets release matrix metalloproteinase-2 in the coronary circulation of patients with acute coronary syndromes: Possible role in sustained platelet activation. *Eur Heart J* 32(3):316–325, 2011.

1393. Rahman M, et al: Platelet shedding of CD40L is regulated by matrix metalloproteinase-9 in abdominal sepsis. *J Thromb Haemost* 11(7):1385–1398, 2013.

1394. Stalker TJ, et al: Platelet signaling. *Handb Exp Pharmacol* 210:59–85, 2012.

1395. Pawelczyk T: Isozymes delta of phosphoinositide-specific phospholipase C. *Acta Biochim Pol* 46(1):91–98, 1999.

1396. Hirata T, et al: Two thromboxane A2 receptor isoforms in human platelets. Opposite coupling to adenylyl cyclase with different sensitivity to Arg60 to Leu mutation. *J Clin Invest* 97(4):949–956, 1996.

1397. Murphy CT, Westwick J: Selective inhibition of protein kinase C. Effect on platelet-activating-factor-induced platelet functional responses. *Biochem J* 283(Pt 1):159–164, 1992.

1398. Cattaneo M: The platelet P2 receptors, in *Platelets*, edited by AD Michelson, pp 201–220. Academic Press, San Diego, 2007.

1399. Kunapuli SP: Funcional characterization of platelet ADP. *Platelets* 9:343–351, 1998.

1400. Murugappa S, Kunapuli SP: The role of ADP receptors in platelet function. *Front Biosci* 11:1977–1986, 2006.

1401. Moheimani F, Jackson DE: P2Y12 receptor: Platelet thrombus formation and medical interventions. *Int J Hematol* 96(5):572–587, 2012.

1402. Conley PB, Delaney SM: Scientific and therapeutic insights into the role of the platelet P2Y12 receptor in thrombosis. *Curr Opin Hematol* 10(5):333–338, 2003.

1403. Dorsam RT, Kunapuli SP: Central role of the P2Y12 receptor in platelet activation. *J Clin Invest* 113(3):340–345, 2004.

1404. Hollopeter G, et al: Identification of the platelet ADP receptor targeted by antithrombotic drugs. *Nature* 409(6817):202–207, 2001.

1405. Jin J, Daniel JL, Kunapuli SP: Molecular basis for ADP-induced platelet activation. II. The P2Y1 receptor mediates ADP-induced intracellular calcium mobilization and shape change in platelets. *J Biol Chem* 273(4):2030–2034, 1998.

1406. Mills DC, et al: Clopidogrel inhibits the binding of ADP analogues to the receptor mediating inhibition of platelet adenylate cyclase. *Arterioscler Thromb* 12(4):430–436, 1992.

1407. Cunningham MR, Nisar SP, Mundell SJ: Molecular mechanisms of platelet P2Y(12) receptor regulation. *Biochem Soc Trans* 41(1):225–230, 2013.

1408. Andre P, et al: P2Y12 regulates platelet adhesion/activation, thrombus growth, and thrombus stability in injured arteries. *J Clin Invest* 112(3):398–406, 2003.

1409. Foster CJ, et al: Molecular identification and characterization of the platelet ADP receptor targeted by thienopyridine antithrombotic drugs. *J Clin Invest* 107(12):1591–1598, 2001.

1410. Fontana P, et al: Adenosine diphosphate-induced platelet aggregation is associated with P2Y12 gene sequence variations in healthy subjects. *Circulation* 108(8):989–995, 2003.

1411. Staritz P, et al: Platelet reactivity and clopidogrel resistance are associated with the H2 haplotype of the P2Y(12)-ADP receptor gene. *Int J Cardiol* 133(3):341–345, 2009.

1412. Zhang D, Gao ZG, Zhang K, et al: Two disparate ligand-binding sites in the human P2Y1 receptor. *Nature* 520(7547):317–321, 2015.

1413. Fabre JE, et al: Decreased platelet aggregation, increased bleeding time and resistance to thromboembolism in P2Y1-deficient mice. *Nat Med* 5(10):1199–1202, 1999.

1414. Leon C, et al: Defective platelet aggregation and increased resistance to thrombosis in purinergic P2Y(1) receptor-null mice. *J Clin Invest* 104(12):1731–1737, 1999.

1415. Offermanns S, et al: Defective platelet activation in G alpha(q)-deficient mice. *Nature* 389(6647):183–186, 1997.

1416. MacKenzie AB, Mahaut-Smith MP, Sage SO: Activation of receptor-operated cation channels via P2X1 not P2T purinoceptors in human platelets. *J Biol Chem* 271(6):2879–2881, 1996.

1417. Valera S, et al: A new class of ligand-gated ion channel defined by P2x receptor for extracellular ATP. *Nature* 371(6497):516–519, 1994.

1418. Oury C, et al: Does the P(2X1del) variant lacking 17 amino acids in its extracellular domain represent a relevant functional ion channel in platelets? *Blood* 99(6):2275–2277, 2002.

1419. Vial C, et al: Lack of evidence for functional ADP-activated human P2X1 receptors supports a role for ATP during hemostasis and thrombosis. *Blood* 102(10):3646–3651, 2003.

1420. Oury C, et al: P2X(1)-mediated activation of extracellular signal-regulated kinase 2 contributes to platelet secretion and aggregation induced by collagen. *Blood* 100(7):2499–2505, 2002.

1421. Vial C, et al: A study of P2X1 receptor function in murine megakaryocytes and human platelets reveals synergy with P2Y receptors. *Br J Pharmacol* 135(2):363–372, 2002.

1422. Hechler B, et al: A role of the fast ATP-gated P2X1 cation channel in thrombosis of small arteries in vivo. *J Exp Med* 198(4):661–667, 2003.

1423. Oury C, et al: Overexpression of the platelet P2X1 ion channel in transgenic mice generates a novel prothrombotic phenotype. *Blood* 101(10):3969–3976, 2003.

1424. Greco NJ, et al: Novel structurally altered P(2X1) receptor is preferentially activated by adenosine diphosphate in platelets and megakaryocytic cells. *Blood* 98(1):100–107, 2001.

1425. Raju NC, Eikelboom JW, Hirsh J: Platelet ADP-receptor antagonists for cardiovascular disease: Past, present and future. *Nat Clin Pract Cardiovasc Med* 5(12):766–780, 2008.

1426. Herbert JM, Savi P: P2Y12, a new platelet ADP receptor, target of clopidogrel. *Semin Vasc Med* 3(2):113–122, 2013.

1427. Banga HS, et al: Activation of phospholipases A and C in human platelets exposed to epinephrine: Role of glycoproteins IIb/IIIa and dual role of epinephrine. *Proc Natl Acad Sci U S A* 83(23):9197–9201, 1986.

1428. Lanza F, et al: Epinephrine potentiates human platelet activation but is not an aggregating agent. *Am J Physiol* 255(6 Pt 2):1276–1288, 1988.

1429. Shattil SJ, Budzynski A, Scrutton MC: Epinephrine induces platelet fibrinogen receptor expression, fibrinogen binding, and aggregation in whole blood in the absence of other excitatory agonists. *Blood* 73(1):150–158, 1989.

1430. Kobilka BK, et al: Cloning, sequencing, and expression of the gene coding for the human platelet alpha 2-adrenergic receptor. *Science* 238(4827):650–656, 1987.

1431. Regan JW, et al: Purification and characterization of the human platelet alpha 2- adrenergic receptor. *J Biol Chem* 261(8):3894–3900, 1986.

1432. Yang J, et al: Loss of signaling through the G protein, Gz, results in abnormal platelet activation and altered responses to psychoactive drugs. *Proc Natl Acad Sci U S A* 97(18):9984–9989, 2000.

1433. Haslam RJ, et al: Cyclic nucleotides in platelet function. *Thromb Haemost* 40(2):232–240, 1978.

1434. Homcy CJ, Graham RM: Molecular characterization of adrenergic receptors. *Circ Res* 56(5):635–650, 1985.

1435. Salzman EW, Ware JA: Ionized calcium as an intracellular messenger in blood platelets. *Prog Hemost Thromb* 9:177–202, 1989.

1436. Yang J, et al: Signaling through Gi family members in platelets. Redundancy and specificity in the regulation of adenylyl cyclase and other effectors. *J Biol Chem* 277(48):46035–46042, 2002.

1437. Patel YM, et al: Evidence for a role for Galphai1 in mediating weak agonist-induced platelet aggregation in human platelets: Reduced Galphai1 expression and defective Gi signaling in the platelets of a patient with a chronic bleeding disorder. *Blood* 101(12):4828–4835, 2003.

1438. Freeman K, et al: Genetic polymorphism of the alpha 2-adrenergic receptor is associated with increased platelet aggregation, baroreceptor sensitivity, and salt excretion in normotensive humans. *Am J Hypertens* 8(9):863–869, 1995.

1439. Small KM, et al: An asn to lys polymorphism in the third intracellular loop of the human alpha 2A-adrenergic receptor imparts enhanced agonist-promoted Gi coupling. *J Biol Chem* 275(49):38518–38523, 2000.

1440. von KR, Dimsdale JE: Effects of sympathetic activation by adrenergic infusions on hemostasis *in vivo. Eur J Haematol* 65(6):357–369, 2000.

1441. Bertha BG, Folts JD: Inhibition of epinephrine-exacerbated coronary thrombus formation by prostacyclin in the dog. *J Lab Clin Med* 103:204–214, 1984.

1442. Folts JD, Rowe GG: Epinephrine potentiation of *in vivo* stimuli reverses aspirin inhibition of platelet thrombus formation in stenosed canine coronary arteries. *Thromb Res* 50:507–516, 1988.

1443. Sibbing D, et al: Platelet function in clopidogrel-treated patients with acute coronary syndrome. *Blood Coagul Fibrinolysis* 18(4):335–339, 2007.

1444. Marcus A: Platelet eicosanoid metabolism, in *Hemostasis and Thrombosis: Basic Principles and Clinical Practice*, edited by RW Colman, J Hirsch, VJ Marder, EW Salzman, pp 676–688. JB Lippincott, Philadelphia, 1987.

1445. Puri RN: Phospholipase A2: Its role in ADP- and thrombin-induced platelet activation mechanisms. *Int J Biochem Cell Biol* 30(10):1107–1122, 1998.

1446. Wong DA, et al: Discrete role for cytosolic phospholipase A(2)alpha in platelets: Studies using single and double mutant mice of cytosolic and group IIA secretory phospholipase A(2). *J Exp Med* 196(3):349–357, 2002.

1447. Adler DH, Cogan JD, Phillips JA 3rd, et al: Inherited human cPLA(2alpha)deficiency is associated with impaired eicosanoid biosynthesis, small intestinal ulceration, and platelet dysfunction. *J Clin Invest* 118(6):2121–2131, 2008.

1448. Prevost N, et al: Group IVA cytosolic phospholipase A2 (cPLA2alpha) and integrin alphaIIbbeta3 reinforce each other's functions during alphaIIbbeta3 signaling in platelets. *Blood* 113(2):447–457, 2009.

1449. Crofford LJ: COX-1 and COX-2 tissue expression: Implications and predictions. *J Rheumatol* 24(Suppl 49):15–19, 1997.

1450. Warner TD, Mitchell JA: Cyclooxygenases: New forms, new inhibitors, and lessons from the clinic. *FASEB J* 18(7):790–804, 2004.

1451. Dubois RN, et al: Cyclooxygenase in biology and disease. *FASEB J* 12(12):1063–1073, 1998.

1452. Smith JB, Willis AL: Aspirin selectively inhibits prostaglandin production in human platelets. *Nat New Biol* 231(25):235–237, 1971.

1453. Svensson J, Hamberg M, Samuelsson B: On the formation and effects of thromboxane A2 in human platelets. *Acta Physiol Scand* 98(3):285–294, 1976.

1454. Rocca B, et al: Cyclooxygenase-2 expression is induced during human megakaryopoiesis and characterizes newly formed platelets. *Proc Natl Acad Sci U S A* 99(11):7634–7639, 2002.

1455. Weber AA, Zimmermann KC, Meyer-Kirchrath J, Schrör K: Cyclooxygenase-2 in human platelets as a possible factor in aspirin resistance. *Lancet* 353(9156):900, 1999.

1456. Funk CD, FitzGerald GA: COX-2 inhibitors and cardiovascular risk. *J Cardiovasc Pharmacol* 50(5):470–479, 2007.

1457. Parent JL, et al: Internalization of the TXA2 receptor alpha and beta isoforms. Role of the differentially spliced COOH terminus in agonist-promoted receptor internalization. *J Biol Chem* 274(13):8941–8948, 1999.

1458. Habib A, FitzGerald GA, Maclouf J: Phosphorylation of the thromboxane receptor alpha, the predominant isoform expressed in human platelets. *J Biol Chem* 274(5):2645–2651, 1999.

1459. Kim SO, et al: Purification of the human blood platelet thromboxane A2/prostaglandin H2 receptor protein. *Biochem Pharmacol* 43(2):313–322, 1992.

1460. Ushikubi F, et al: Purification of the thromboxane A2/prostaglandin H2 receptor from human blood platelets. *J Biol Chem* 264(28):16496–16501, 1989.

1461. Takahara K, et al: The response to thromboxane A2 analogues in human platelets. Discrimination of two binding sites linked to distinct effector systems. *J Biol Chem* 265(12):6836–6844, 1990.

1462. Thomas DW, et al: Coagulation defects and altered hemodynamic responses in mice lacking receptors for thromboxane A2. *J Clin Invest* 102(11):1994–2001, 1998.

1463. Gabbeta J, et al: Platelet signal transduction defect with Gα subunit dysfunction and diminished Gαq in a patient with abnormal platelet responses. *Proc Natl Acad Sci U S A* 94(16):8750–8755, 1997.

1464. Allan CJ, et al: Characterization of the cloned HEL cell thromboxane A2 receptor: Evidence that the affinity state can be altered by G alpha 13 and G alpha q. *J Pharmacol Exp Ther* 277(2):1132–1139, 1996.

1465. Djellas Y, et al: Identification of Galpha13 as one of the G-proteins that couple to human platelet thromboxane A2 receptors. *J Biol Chem* 274(20):14325–14330, 1999.

1466. Nakahata N, et al: Gq/11 communicates with thromboxane A2 receptors in human astrocytoma cells, rabbit astrocytes and human platelets. *Res Commun Mol Pathol Pharmacol* 87(3):243–251, 1995.

1467. Paul BZ, Jin J, Kunapuli SP: Molecular mechanism of thromboxane A(2)-induced platelet aggregation. Essential role for p2t(ac) and alpha(2a) receptors. *J Biol Chem* 274(41):29108–29114, 1999.

1468. Ushikubi F, Nakamura K, Narumiya S: Functional reconstitution of platelet thromboxane A2 receptors with Gq and Gi2 in phospholipid vesicles. *Mol Pharmacol* 46(5):808–816, 1994.

1469. Dorsam RT, et al: Coordinated signaling through both G12/13 and G(i) pathways is sufficient to activate GPIIb/IIIa in human platelets. *J Biol Chem* 277(49):47588–47595, 2002.

1470. Klages B, et al: Activation of G12/G13 results in shape change and Rho/Rho-kinase-mediated myosin light chain phosphorylation in mouse platelets. *J Cell Biol* 144(4):745–754, 1999.

1471. Nieswandt B, et al: Costimulation of Gi- and G12/G13-mediated signaling pathways induces integrin alpha IIbbeta 3 activation in platelets. *J Biol Chem* 277(42):39493–39498, 2002.

1472. Pulcinelli FM, et al: Protein kinase C activation is not a key step in ADP-mediated exposure of fibrinogen receptors on human platelets. *FEBS Lett* 364(1):87–90, 1995.

1473. Knezevic I, Dieter JP, Le Breton GC: Mechanism of inositol 1,4,5-trisphosphate-induced aggregation in saponin-permeabilized platelets. *J Pharmacol Exp Ther* 260(3):947–955, 1992.

1474. Nugteren DH: Arachidonate lipoxygenase in blood platelets. *Biochim Biophys Acta* 380(2):299–307, 1975.

1475. Johnson EN, Brass LF, Funk CD: Increased platelet sensitivity to ADP in mice lacking platelet-type 12-lipoxygenase. *Proc Natl Acad Sci U S A* 95(6):3100–3105, 1998.

1476. Coffey MJ, et al: Platelet 12-lipoxygenase activation via glycoprotein VI: Involvement of multiple signaling pathways in agonist control of H(P)ETE synthesis. *Circ Res* 94(12):1598–1605, 2004.

1477. Dasari VR, Jin J, Kunapuli SP: Distribution of leukotriene B4 receptors in human hematopoietic cells. *Immunopharmacology* 48(2):157–163, 2000.

1478. Maclouf JA, Murphy RC: Transcellular metabolism of neutrophil-derived leukotriene A4 by human platelets. A potential cellular source of leukotriene C4. *J Biol Chem* 263(1):174–181, 1988.

1479. Maugeri N, et al: Polymorphonuclear leukocyte-platelet interaction: Role of P-selectin in thromboxane B2 and leukotriene C4 cooperative synthesis. *Thromb Haemost* 72(3):450–456, 1994.

1480. Levy BD, et al: Agonist-induced lipoxin A4 generation: Detection by a novel lipoxin A4-ELISA. *Lipids* 28(12):1047–1053, 1993.

1481. Ofosu FA, Liu L, Freedman J: Control mechanisms in thrombin generation. *Semin Thromb Hemost* 22(4):303–308, 1996.

1482. Phillips DR: Thrombin interaction with human platelets. Potentiation of thrombin-induced aggregation and release by inactivated thrombin. *Thromb Diath Haemorrh* 32(1):207–215, 1974.

1483. Bahou W: Thrombin receptors, in *Platelets*, edited by AD Michelson, pp 179–200. Academic Press, San Diego, 2007.

1484. Hung DT, et al: Cloned platelet thrombin receptor is necessary for thrombin-induced platelet activation. *J Clin Invest* 89(4):1350–1353, 1992.

1485. Furman MI, et al: The cleaved peptide of the thrombin receptor is a strong platelet agonist. *Proc Natl Acad Sci U S A* 95(6):3082–3087, 1998.

1486. Cho JR, et al: Unmet needs in the management of acute myocardial infarction: Role of novel protease-activated receptor-1 antagonist vorapaxar. *Vasc Health Risk Manag* 10:177–188, 2014.

1487. Zhang C, et al: High-resolution crystal structure of human protease-activated receptor 1. *Nature* 492(7429):387–392, 2012.

1488. Ishihara H, et al: Antibodies to protease-activated receptor 3 inhibit activation of mouse platelets by thrombin. *Blood* 91(11):4152–4157, 1998.

1489. Kahn ML, et al: A dual thrombin receptor system for platelet activation. *Nature* 394(6694):690–694, 1998.

1490. Kahn ML, et al: Protease-activated receptors 1 and 4 mediate activation of human platelets by thrombin. *J Clin Invest* 103(6):879–887, 1999.

1491. Andrade-Gordon P, et al: Design, synthesis, and biological characterization of a peptide-mimetic antagonist for a tethered-ligand receptor. *Proc Natl Acad Sci U S A* 96(22):12257–12262, 1999.

1492. Covic L, Gresser AL, Kuliopulos A: Biphasic kinetics of activation and signaling for PAR1 and PAR4 thrombin receptors in platelets. *Biochemistry* 39(18):5458–5467, 2000.

1493. Shapiro MJ, et al: Protease-activated receptors 1 and 4 are shut off with distinct kinetics after activation by thrombin. *J Biol Chem* 275(33):25216–25221, 2000.

1494. Sambrano GR, et al: Role of thrombin signalling in platelets in haemostasis and thrombosis. *Nature* 413(6851):74–78, 2001.

1495. Nakanishi-Matsui M, et al: PAR3 is a cofactor for PAR4 activation by thrombin. *Nature* 404(6778):609–613, 2000.

1496. Weiss EJ, et al: Protection against thrombosis in mice lacking PAR3. *Blood* 100(9):3240–3244, 2002.

1497. Hoxie JA, et al: Internalization and recycling of activated thrombin receptors. *J Biol Chem* 268(18):13756–13763, 1993.

1498. Trejo J, Coughlin SR: The cytoplasmic tails of protease-activated receptor-1 and substance P receptor specify sorting to lysosomes versus recycling. *J Biol Chem* 274(4):2216–2224, 1999.

1499. Antoniak S, et al: PAR-1 contributes to the innate immune response during viral infection. *J Clin Invest* 123(3):1310–1322, 2013.

1500. Khoufache K, et al: PAR1 contributes to influenza A virus pathogenicity in mice. *J Clin Invest* 123(1):206–214, 2013.

1501. Berri F, et al: Switch from protective to adverse inflammation during influenza: Viral determinants and hemostasis are caught as culprits. *Cell Mol Life Sci* 71(5):885–898, 2014.

1502. Ruggeri ZM, et al: Unravelling the mechanism and significance of thrombin binding to platelet glycoprotein Ib. *Thromb Haemost* 104(5):894–902, 2010.

1503. Celikel R, et al: Modulation of alpha-thrombin function by distinct interactions with platelet glycoprotein Ibalpha. *Science* 301(5630):218–221, 2003.

1504. Dumas JJ, et al: Crystal structure of the GpIbalpha-thrombin complex essential for platelet aggregation. *Science* 301(5630):222–226, 2003.

1505. Lova P, et al: Thrombin induces platelet activation in the absence of functional protease activated receptors 1 and 4 and glycoprotein Ib-IX-V. *Cell Signal* 22(11):1681–1687, 2010.

1506. Gibbins JM: Tweaking the gain on platelet regulation: The tachykinin connection. *Atherosclerosis* 206(1):1-7, 2009.

1507. Graham GJ, et al: Tachykinins regulate the function of platelets. *Blood* 104(4):1058–1065, 2004.

1508. Gleissner CA, von HP, Ley K: Platelet chemokines in vascular disease. *Arterioscler Thromb Vasc Biol* 28(11):1920–1927, 2008.

1509. McIntyre TM, Zimmerman GA, Prescott SM: Biologically active oxidized phospholipids. *J Biol Chem* 274(36):25189–25192, 1999.

1510. Honda Z, et al: Cloning by functional expression of platelet-activating factor receptor from guinea-pig lung. *Nature* 349(6307):342–346, 1991.

1511. Nakamura M, et al: Molecular cloning and expression of platelet-activating factor receptor from human leukocytes. *J Biol Chem* 266(30):20400–20405, 1991.

1512. Carlson SA, Chatterjee TK, Fisher RA: The third intracellular domain of the platelet-activating factor receptor is a critical determinant in receptor coupling to phosphoinositide phospholipase C-activating G proteins. Studies using intracellular domain minigenes and receptor chimeras. *J Biol Chem* 271(38):23146–23153, 1996.

1513. Chao W, et al: Protein tyrosine phosphorylation and regulation of the receptor for platelet-activating factor in rat Kupffer cells. Effect of sodium vanadate. *Biochem J* 288(Pt 3):777–784, 1992.

1514. Stafforini DM: Biology of platelet-activating factor acetylhydrolase (PAF-AH, lipoprotein associated phospholipase A2). *Cardiovasc Drugs Ther* 23(1):73–83, 2009.

1515. Eitzman DT, et al: Hyperlipidemia promotes thrombosis after injury to atherosclerotic vessels in apolipoprotein E-deficient mice. *Arterioscler Thromb Vasc Biol* 20(7):1831–1834, 2000.

1516. Sano T, et al: Multiple mechanisms linked to platelet activation result in lysophosphatidic acid and sphingosine 1-phosphate generation in blood. *J Biol Chem* 277(24):21197–21206, 2002.

1517. Smyth SS, et al: Roles of lysophosphatidic acid in cardiovascular physiology and disease. *Biochim Biophys Acta* 1781(9):563–570, 2008.

1518. Umezu-Goto M, et al: Autotaxin has lysophospholipase D activity leading to tumor cell growth and motility by lysophosphatidic acid production. *J Cell Biol* 158(2):227–233, 2002.

1519. Leblanc R, et al: Interaction of platelet-derived autotaxin with tumor integrin alphaVbeta3 controls metastasis of breast cancer cells to bone. *Blood* 124(20):3141–3150, 2014.

1520. Siess W, et al: Lysophosphatidic acid mediates the rapid activation of platelets and endothelial cells by mildly oxidized low density lipoprotein and accumulates in human atherosclerotic lesions. *Proc Natl Acad Sci U S A* 96(12):6931–6936, 1999.

1521. Retzer M, Essler M: Lysophosphatidic acid-induced platelet shape change proceeds via Rho/Rho kinase-mediated myosin light-chain and moesin phosphorylation. *Cell Signal* 12(9–10):645–648, 2000.

1522. Haseruck N, et al: The plaque lipid lysophosphatidic acid stimulates platelet activation and platelet-monocyte aggregate formation in whole blood: Involvement of P2Y1 and P2Y12 receptors. *Blood* 103(7):2585–2592, 2004.

1523. Olorundare OE, et al: Assembly of a fibronectin matrix by adherent platelets stimulated by lysophosphatidic acid and other agonists. *Blood* 98(1):117–124, 2001.

1524. Maschberger P, et al: Mildly oxidized low density lipoprotein rapidly stimulates via activation of the lysophosphatidic acid receptor Src family and Syk tyrosine kinases and Ca2+ influx in human platelets. *J Biol Chem* 275(25):19159–19166, 2000.

1525. Siess W: Athero- and thrombogenic actions of lysophosphatidic acid and sphingosine-1-phosphate. *Biochim Biophys Acta* 1582(1–3):204–215, 2002.

1526. Motohashi K, et al: Identification of lysophospholipid receptors in human platelets: The relation of two agonists, lysophosphatidic acid and sphingosine 1-phosphate. *FEBS Lett* 468(2–3):189–193, 2000.

1527. Siess W, Tigyi G: Thrombogenic and atherogenic activities of lysophosphatidic acid. *J Cell Biochem* 92(6):1086–1094, 2004.

1528. Yatomi Y, et al: Sphingosine-1-phosphate: A platelet-activating sphingolipid released from agonist-stimulated human platelets. *Blood* 86(1):193–202, 1995.

1529. Nugent D, Xu Y: Sphingosine-1-phosphate: Characterization of its inhibition of platelet aggregation. *Platelets* 11(4):226–232, 2000.

1530. Hoyer D, et al: International Union of Pharmacology classification of receptors for 5-hydroxytryptamine (Serotonin). *Pharmacol Rev* 46(2):157–203, 1994.

1531. Allen JA, Yadav PN, Roth BL: Insights into the regulation of 5-HT2A serotonin receptors by scaffolding proteins and kinases. *Neuropharmacology* 55(6):961–968, 2008.

1532. Cook EH Jr, et al: Primary structure of the human platelet serotonin 5-HT2A receptor: Identify with frontal cortex serotonin 5-HT2A receptor. *J Neurochem* 63(2):465–469, 1994.

1533. De Clerck F, et al: Evidence for functional 5-HT2 receptor sites on human blood platelets. *Biochem PharmacolAm Rev Respir Dis* 33(17):2807–2811, 1984.

1534. Roth BL, et al: 5-Hydroxytryptamine2-family receptors (5-hydroxytryptamine2A, 5- hydroxytryptamine2B, 5-hydroxytryptamine2C): Where structure meets function. *Pharmacol Ther* 79(3):231–257, 1998.

1535. Leysen JE, et al: Identification of nonserotonergic [3H]ketanserin binding sites associated with nerve terminals in rat brain and with platelets; relation with release of biogenic amine metabolites induced by ketans. *J Pharmacol Exp Ther* 244(1):310–321, 1988.

1536. Ozaki N, et al: A naturally occurring amino acid substitution of the human serotonin 5- HT2A receptor influences amplitude and timing of intracellular calcium mobilization. *J Neurochem* 68(5):2186–2193, 1997.

1537. Shimizu M, et al: Serotonin-2A receptor gene polymorphisms are associated with serotonin-induced platelet aggregation. *Thromb Res* 112(3):137–142, 2003.

1538. Arora RC, Meltzer HY: Serotonin2 receptor binding in blood platelets of schizophrenic patients. *Psychiatry Res* 47(2):111–119, 1993.

1539. Coccaro EF, et al: Impulsive aggression in personality disorder correlates with platelet 5-HT2A receptor binding. *Neuropsychopharmacology* 16(3):211–216, 1997.

1540. Pandey GN: Altered serotonin function in suicide. Evidence from platelet and neuroendocrine studies. *Ann N Y Acad Sci* 836:182–200, 1997.

1541. Tomiyoshi R, et al: Serotonin-induced platelet intracellular Ca2+ responses in untreated depressed patients and imipramine responders in remission. *Biol Psychiatry* 45(8):1042–1048, 1999.

1542. Wolfe BE, Metzger E, Jimerson DC: Research update on serotonin function in bulimia nervosa and anorexia nervosa. *Psychopharmacol Bull* 33(3):345–354, 1997.

1543. Cho R, et al: Relationship between central and peripheral serotonin 5-HT2A receptors: A positron emission tomography study in healthy individuals. *Neurosci Lett* 261(3):139–142, 1999.

1544. Schins A, et al: Increased coronary events in depressed cardiovascular patients: 5-HT2A receptor as missing link? *Psychosom Med* 65(5):729–737, 2003.

1545. de Chaffoy de Courcelles D, Leysen JE, De Clerck F, et al: Evidence that phospholipid turnover is the signal transducing system coupled to serotonin-S2 receptor sites. *J Biol Chem* 260(12):7603–7608, 1985.

1546. Erne P, Pletscher A: Rapid intracellular release of calcium in human platelets by stimulation of 5-HT2-receptors. *Br J Pharmacol* 84(2):545–549, 1985.

1547. Li N, et al: Effects of serotonin on platelet activation in whole blood. *Blood Coagul Fibrinolysis* 8(8):517–523, 1997.

1548. Houston DS, Shepherd JT, Vanhoutte PM: Aggregating human platelets cause direct contraction and endothelium-dependent relaxation of isolated canine coronary arteries. Role of serotonin, thromboxane A2, and adenine nucleotides. *J Clin Invest* 78(2):539–544, 1986.

1549. Golino P, et al: Mediation or reocclusion by thromboxane A2 and serotonin after thrombolysis with tissue-type plasminogen activator in a canine preparation of coronary thrombosis. *Circulation* 77:678–684, 1988.

1550. Alberio LJ, Clemetson KJ: All platelets are not equal: COAT platelets. *Curr Hematol Rep* 3(5):338–343, 2004.

1551. Dale GL, et al: Stimulated platelets use serotonin to enhance their retention of procoagulant proteins on the cell surface. *Nature* 415(6868):175–179, 2002.

1552. Walther DJ, et al: Serotonylation of small GTPases is a signal transduction pathway that triggers platelet alpha-granule release. *Cell* 115(7):851–862, 2003.

1553. Carneiro AM, et al: Interactions between integrin alphaIIbbeta3 and the serotonin transporter regulate serotonin transport and platelet aggregation in mice and humans. *J Clin Invest* 118(4):1544–1552, 2008.

1554. McCloskey DJ, et al: Selective serotonin reuptake inhibitors: Measurement of effect on platelet function. *Transl Res* 151(3):168–172, 2008.

1555. Lesurtel M, et al: Platelet-derived serotonin mediates liver regeneration. *Science* 312(5770):104–107, 2006.

1556. Haslam RJ, Rosson GM: Aggregation of human blood platelets by vasopressin. *Am J Physiol* 223(4):958–967, 1972.

1557. Pollock WK, MacIntyre DE: Desensitization and antagonism of vasopressin-induced phosphoinositide metabolism and elevation of cytosolic free calcium concentration in human platelets. *Biochem J* 234(1):67–73, 1986.

1558. Thomas ME, Osmani AH, Scrutton MC: Some properties of the human platelet vasopressin receptor. *Thromb Res* 32(6):557–566, 1983.

1559. Thibonnier M, Roberts JM: Characterization of human platelet vasopressin receptors. *J Clin Invest* 76(5):1857–1864, 1985.

1560. Siess W, et al: Activation of V1-receptors by vasopressin stimulates inositol phospholipid hydrolysis and arachidonate metabolism in human platelets. *Biochem J* 233(1):83–91, 1986.

1561. Thibonnier M, Goraya T, Berti-Mattera L: G protein coupling of human platelet V1 vascular vasopressin receptors. *Am J Physiol* 264(5 Pt 1):C1336–C1344, 1993.

1562. Berrettini WH, et al: Human platelet vasopressin receptors. *Life Sci* 30(5):425–432, 1982.

1563. Siess W: Molecular mechanisms of platelet activation. *Physiol Rev* 69(1):58–178, 1989.

1564. Wun T, Paglieroni T, Lachant NA: Physiologic concentrations of arginine vasopressin activate human platelets *in vitro*. *Br J Haematol* 92(4):968–972, 1996.

1565. Gunnet JW, et al: Pharmacological characterization of RWJ-676070, a dual vasopressin V(1A)/V(2) receptor antagonist. *Eur J Pharmacol* 590(1–3):333–342, 2008.

1566. Serradeil-Le Gal C, et al: Nonpeptide vasopressin receptor antagonists: Development of selective and orally active V1a, V2 and V1b receptor ligands. *Prog Brain Res* 139:197–210, 2002.

1567. Crabos M, Bertschin S, Bühler FR, et al: Identification of AT1 receptors on human platelets and decreased angiotensin II binding in hypertension. *J Hypertens Suppl* 11(Suppl 5):S230–S231, 1993.

1568. Jagroop IA, Mikhailidis DP: Angiotensin II can induce and potentiate shape change in human platelets: Effect of losartan. *J Hum Hypertens* 14(9):581–585, 2000.

1569. Lopez-Farre A, et al: Angiotensin II AT(1) receptor antagonists and platelet activation. *Nephrol Dial Transplant* 16(Suppl 1):45–49, 2001.

1570. Larsson PT, Schwieler JH, Wallen NH: Platelet activation during angiotensin II infusion in healthy volunteers. *Blood Coagul Fibrinolysis* 11(1):61–69, 2000.

1571. Li P, et al: Novel angiotensin II AT(1) receptor antagonist irbesartan prevents thromboxane A(2)-induced vasoconstriction in canine coronary arteries and human platelet aggregation. *J Pharmacol Exp Ther* 292(1):238–246, 2000.

1572. Monton M, et al: Comparative effects of angiotensin II AT-1-type receptor antagonists in vitro on human platelet activation. *J Cardiovasc Pharmacol* 35(6):906–913, 2000.

1573. Kalinowski L, et al: Angiotensin II AT1 receptor antagonists inhibit platelet adhesion and aggregation by nitric oxide release. *Hypertension* 40(4):521–527, 2002.

1574. Jimenez AM, et al: Inhibition of platelet activation in stroke-prone spontaneously hypertensive rats: Comparison of losartan, candesartan, and valsartan. *J Cardiovasc Pharmacol* 37(4):406–412, 2001.

1575. Owens P, et al: Comparison of antihypertensive and metabolic effects of losartan and losartan in combination with hydrochlorothiazide—A randomized controlled trial. *J Hypertens* 18(3):339–345, 2000.

1576. Schieffer B, et al: Comparative effects of AT1-antagonism and angiotensin-converting enzyme inhibition on markers of inflammation and platelet aggregation in patients with coronary artery disease. *J Am Coll Cardiol* 44(2):362–368, 2004.

1577. Serebruany VL, et al: Valsartan inhibits platelet activity at different doses in mild to moderate hypertensives: Valsartan Inhibits Platelets (VIP) trial. *Am Heart J* 151(1): 92–99, 2006.

1578. Yamada K, Hirayama T, Hasegawa Y: Antiplatelet effect of losartan and telmisartan in patients with ischemic stroke. *J Stroke Cerebrovasc Dis* 16(5):225–231, 2007.

1579. Dorahy DJ, et al: Stimulation of platelet activation and aggregation by a carboxyl-terminal peptide from thrombospondin binding to the integrin-associated protein receptor. *J Biol Chem* 272(2):1323–1330, 1997.

1580. Lindberg FP, et al: Molecular cloning of integrin-associated protein: An immunoglobulin family member with multiple membrane-spanning domains implicated in alpha v beta 3-dependent ligand binding. *J Cell Biol* 123(2):485–496, 1993.

1581. Wang XQ, Frazier WA: The thrombospondin receptor CD47 (IAP) modulates and associates with alpha2 beta1 integrin in vascular smooth muscle cells. *Mol Biol Cell* 9(4):865–874, 1998.

1582. Frazier WA, et al: The thrombospondin receptor integrin-associated protein (CD47) functionally couples to heterotrimeric Gi. *J Biol Chem* 274(13):8554–8560, 1999.

1583. Chung J, Gao AG, Frazier WA: Thrombospondin acts via integrin-associated protein to activate the platelet integrin alphaIIbbeta3. *J Biol Chem* 272(23):14740–14746, 1997.

1584. Isenberg JS, et al: Thrombospondin-1 stimulates platelet aggregation by blocking the antithrombotic activity of nitric oxide/cGMP signaling. *Blood* 111(2):613–623, 2008.

1585. Lagadec P, et al: Involvement of a CD47-dependent pathway in platelet adhesion on inflamed vascular endothelium under flow. *Blood* 101(12):4836–4843, 2003.

1586. Pimanda JE, et al: The von Willebrand factor-reducing activity of thrombospondin-1 is located in the calcium-binding/C-terminal sequence and requires a free thiol at position 974. *Blood* 100(8):2832–2838, 2002.

1587. Pimanda JE, et al: Role of thrombospondin-1 in control of von Willebrand factor multimer size in mice. *J Biol Chem* 279(20):21439–21448, 2004.

1588. van Zanten GH, et al: Increased platelet deposition on atherosclerotic coronary arteries. *J Clin Invest* 93(2):615–632, 1994.

1589. van der Rest, M, Garrone R: Collagen family of proteins. *FASEB J* 5(13):2814–2823, 1991.

1590. Ruggeri ZM, Mendolicchio GL: Adhesion mechanisms in platelet function. *Circ Res* 100(12):1673–1685, 2007.

1591. Clemetson JM, et al: The platelet collagen receptor glycoprotein VI is a member of the immunoglobulin superfamily closely related to FcalphaR and the natural killer receptors. *J Biol Chem* 274(41):29019–29024, 1999.

1592. Ichinohe T, et al: Collagen-stimulated activation of Syk but not c-Src is severely compromised in human platelets lacking membrane glycoprotein VI. *J Biol Chem* 272(1):63–68, 1997.

1593. Ishibashi T, et al: Functional significance of platelet membrane glycoprotein p62 (GPVI), a putative collagen receptor. *Int J Hematol* 62(2):107–115, 1995.

1594. Kehrel B, et al: Glycoprotein VI is a major collagen receptor for platelet activation: It recognizes the platelet-activating quaternary structure of collagen, whereas CD36, glycoprotein IIb/IIIa, and von Willebrand factor do not. *Blood* 91(2):491–499, 1998.

1595. Clemetson KJ, Clemetson JM: Platelet receptors, in *Platelets*, edited by AD Michelson, pp 117–143. Academic Press, San Diego, 2007.

1596. Horii K, Kahn ML, Herr AB: Structural basis for platelet collagen responses by the immune-type receptor glycoprotein VI. *Blood* 108(3):936–942, 2006.

1597. Poole A, et al: The Fc receptor gamma-chain and the tyrosine kinase Syk are essential for activation of mouse platelets by collagen. *EMBO J* 16(9):2333–2341, 1997.

1598. Smethurst PA, et al: Identification of the primary collagen-binding surface on human glycoprotein VI by site-directed mutagenesis and by a blocking phage antibody. *Blood* 103(3):903–911, 2004.

1599. Chiang TM, Collagen-platelet interaction: Platelet non-integrin receptors. *Histol Histopathol* 14(2):579–585, 1999.

1600. Keely PJ, Parise LV: The alpha2beta1 integrin is a necessary co-receptor for collagen-induced activation of Syk and the subsequent phosphorylation of phospholipase Cgamma2 in platelets. *J Biol Chem* 271(43):26668–26676, 1996.

1601. Sugiyama T, et al: A novel platelet aggregating factor found in a patient with defective collagen-induced platelet aggregation and autoimmune thrombocytopenia. *Blood* 69:1712–1720, 1987.

1602. Briddon SJ, Watson SP: Evidence for the involvement of p59fyn and p53/56lyn in collagen receptor signalling in human platelets. *Biochem J* 338(Pt 1):203–209, 1999.

1603. Fujii C, et al: Involvement of protein-tyrosine kinase p72syk in collagen-induced signal transduction in platelets. *Eur J Biochem* 226(1):243–248, 1994.

1604. Shattil SJ, Ginsberg MH, Brugge JS: Adhesive signaling in platelets. *Curr Opin Cell Biol* 6(5):695–704, 1994.

1605. Soriano P, et al: Targeted disruption of the c-src proto-oncogene leads to osteopetrosis in mice. *Cell* 64(4):693–702, 1991.

1606. Daniel JL, Dangelmaier C, Smith JB: Evidence for a role for tyrosine phosphorylation of phospholipase Cg2 in collagen-induced platelet cytosolic calcium mobilization. *Biochem J* 302:617–622, 1994.

1607. Keely PJ, Parise LV: The alpha2beta1 integrin is a necessary co-receptor for collagen-induced activation of Syk and the subsequent phosphorylation of phospholipase Cgamma2 in platelets. *J Biol Chem* 271(43):26668–26676, 1996.

1608. Quek LS, Bolen J, Watson SP: A role for Bruton's tyrosine kinase (Btk) in platelet activation by collagen. *Curr Biol* 8(20):1137–1140, 1998.

1609. Jung SM, Moroi M: Platelet collagen receptor integrin alpha2beta1 activation involves differential participation of ADP-receptor subtypes P2Y1 and P2Y12 but not intracellular calcium change. *Eur J Biochem* 268(12):3513–3522, 2001.

1610. Wang Z, Leisner TM, Parise LV: Platelet alpha2beta1 integrin activation: Contribution of ligand internalization and the alpha2-cytoplasmic domain. *Blood* 102(4):1307–1315, 2003.

1611. Bertoni A, et al: Relationships between Rap1b, affinity modulation of integrin alpha IIbbeta 3, and the actin cytoskeleton. *J Biol Chem* 277(28):25715–25721, 2002.

1612. Larson MK, et al: Identification of P2Y12-dependent and -independent mechanisms of glycoprotein VI-mediated Rap1 activation in platelets. *Blood* 101(4):1409–1415, 2003.

1613. Auger JM, et al: C-Cbl negatively regulates platelet activation by glycoprotein VI. *J Thromb Haemost* 1(11):2419–2426, 2003.

1614. Locke D, et al: Fc Rgamma-independent signaling by the platelet collagen receptor glycoprotein VI. *J Biol Chem* 278(17):15441–15448, 2003.

1615. Qiao J, et al: An acquired defect associated with abnormal signaling of the platelet collagen receptor glycoprotein VI. *Acta Haematol* 128(4):233–241, 2012.

1616. Inoue O, et al: Integrin alpha2beta1 mediates outside-in regulation of platelet spreading on collagen through activation of Src kinases and PLCgamma2. *J Cell Biol* 160(5):769–780, 2003.

1617. Chen H, Kahn ML: Reciprocal signaling by integrin and nonintegrin receptors during collagen activation of platelets. *Mol Cell Biol* 23(14):4764–4777, 2003.

1618. Galt SW, et al: Outside-in signals delivered by matrix metalloproteinase-1 regulate platelet function. *Circ Res* 90(10):1093–1099, 2002.

1619. Best D, et al: GPVI levels in platelets: Relationship to platelet function at high shear. *Blood* 102(8):2811–2818, 2003.

1620. Chen H, et al: The platelet receptor GPVI mediates both adhesion and signaling responses to collagen in a receptor density-dependent fashion. *J Biol Chem* 277(4): 3011–3019, 2002.

1621. Furihata K, et al: Variation in human platelet glycoprotein VI content modulates glycoprotein VI-specific prothrombinase activity. *Arterioscler Thromb Vasc Biol* 21(11): 1857–1863, 2001.

1622. Suzuki H, et al: Intracellular localization of glycoprotein VI in human platelets and its surface expression upon activation. *Br J Haematol* 121(6):904–912, 2003.

1623. Matsuno K, et al: Inhibition of platelet adhesion to collagen by monoclonal anti-CD36 antibodies. *Br J Haematol* 92(4):960–967, 1996.

1624. Nakamura T, et al: Platelet adhesion to type I collagen fibrils: Role of GPVI in divalent cation-dependent and -independent adhesion and thromboxane A2 generation. *J Biol Chem* 273:4338–4344, 1998.

1625. Daniel JL, et al: Collagen induces normal signal transduction in platelets deficient in CD36 (platelet glycoprotein IV). *Thromb Haemost* 71:353–356, 1994.

1626. az-Ricart M, et al: Platelets lacking functional CD36 (glycoprotein IV) show reduced adhesion to collagen in flowing whole blood. *Blood* 82(2):491–496, 1993.

1627. Smith JB, et al: Cytosolic calcium as a second messenger for collagen-induced platelet responses. *Biochem J* 288(Pt 3):925–929, 1992.

1628. Greenwalt DE, Tandon NN: Platelet shape change and Ca2+ mobilization induced by collagen, but not thrombin or ADP, are inhibited by phenylarsine oxide. *Br J Haematol* 88(4):830–838, 1994.

1629. Chow TW, et al: Shear stress-induced von Willebrand factor binding to platelet glycoprotein Ib initiates calcium influx associated with aggregation. *Blood* 80(1):113–120, 1992.

1630. Gu M, et al: Analysis of the roles of 14-3-3 in the platelet glycoprotein Ib-IX-mediated activation of integrin alpha(IIb)beta(3) using a reconstituted mammalian cell expression model. *J Cell Biol* 147(5):1085–1096, 1999.

1631. Zaffran Y, et al: Signaling across the platelet adhesion receptor glycoprotein Ib-IX induces alpha IIbbeta 3 activation both in platelets and a transfected Chinese hamster ovary cell system. *J Biol Chem* 275(22):16779–16787, 2000.

1632. Sullam PM, et al: Physical proximity and functional interplay of the glycoprotein Ib-IX-V complex and the Fc receptor FcgammaRIIA on the platelet plasma membrane. *J Biol Chem* 273(9):5331–5336, 1998.

1633. Kasirer-Friede A, et al: Signaling through GP Ib-IX-V activates alphaIIbbeta3 independently of other receptors. *Blood* 103(9):3403–3411, 2004.

1634. Marshall SJ, et al: GPIb-dependent platelet activation is dependent on Src kinases but not MAP kinase or cGMP-dependent kinase. *Blood* 103(7):2601–2609, 2004.

1635. Mangin P, et al: Signaling role for phospholipase C gamma 2 in platelet glycoprotein Ib alpha calcium flux and cytoskeletal reorganization. Involvement of a pathway distinct from FcR gamma chain and Fc gamma RIIA. *J Biol Chem* 278(35):32880–32891, 2003.

1636. Li Z, et al: A stimulatory role for cGMP-dependent protein kinase in platelet activation. *Cell* 112(1):77–86, 2003.

1637. Andrews RK, et al: Interaction of calmodulin with the cytoplasmic domain of the platelet membrane glycoprotein Ib-IX-V complex. *Blood* 98(3):681–687, 2001.

1638. Du X, et al: Association of a phospholipase A2 (14-3-3 protein) with the platelet glycoprotein Ib-IX complex. *J Biol Chem* 269(28):18287–18290, 1994.

1639. Ohtsuka Y, et al: Chronic oral antigen exposure induces lymphocyte migration in anaphylactic mouse intestine. *Pediatr Res* 44(5):791–797, 1998.

1640. Kasirer-Friede A, et al: Lateral clustering of platelet GP Ib-IX complexes leads to up-regulation of the adhesive function of integrin alpha IIbbeta 3. *J Biol Chem* 277(14):11949–11956, 2002.

1641. Fox JE, Berndt MC: Cyclic AMP-dependent phosphorylation of glycoprotein Ib inhibits collagen-induced polymerization of actin in platelets. *J Biol Chem* 264(16):9520–9526, 1989.

1642. Phillips DR, Agin PP: Thrombin-induced alterations in the surface structure of the human platelet plasma membrane. *Ser Haematol* 6(3):292–310, 1973.

1643. Ni H, et al: Increased thrombogenesis and embolus formation in mice lacking glycoprotein V. *Blood* 98(2):368–373, 2001.

1644. Rink TJ: Cytosolic calcium in platelet activation. *Experientia* 44(2):97–100, 1988.

1645. Kovacs T, et al: All three splice variants of the human sarco/endoplasmic reticulum Ca2+-ATPase 3 gene are translated to proteins: A study of their co-expression in platelets and lymphoid cells. *Biochem J* 358(Pt 3):559–568, 2001.

1646. Hassock SR, et al: Expression and role of TRPC proteins in human platelets: Evidence that TRPC6 forms the store-independent calcium entry channel. *Blood* 100(8):2801–2811, 2002.

1647. Roberts DE, McNicol A, Bose R: Mechanism of collagen activation in human platelets. *J Biol Chem* 279:19421–19430, 2004.

1648. Jones GD, Gear AR: Subsecond calcium dynamics in ADP- and thrombin-stimulated platelets: A continuous-flow approach using indo-1. *Blood* 71(6):1539–1543, 1988.

1649. Rybak ME, Renzulli LA: Effect of calcium channel blockers on platelet GPIIb-IIIa as a calcium channel in liposomes: Comparison with effects on the intact platelet. *Thromb Haemost* 67(1):131–136, 1992.

1650. Dessen A, et al: Crystal structure of human cytosolic phospholipase A2 reveals a novel topology and catalytic mechanism. *Cell* 97(3):349–360, 1999.

1651. Khan WA, et al: Selective regulation of protein kinase C isoenzymes by oleic acid in human platelets. *J Biol Chem* 268(7):5063–5068, 1993.

1652. Scholey JM, Taylor KA, and J. Kendrick-Jones, Regulation of non-muscle myosin assembly by calmodulin-dependent light chain kinase. *Nature* 287(5779):233–235, 1980.

1653. Naik MU, Naik UP: Calcium-and integrin-binding protein regulates focal adhesion kinase activity during platelet spreading on immobilized fibrinogen. *Blood* 102(10):3629–3636, 2003.

1654. Barry WT, et al: Molecular basis of CIB binding to the integrin alpha IIb cytoplasmic domain. *J Biol Chem* 277(32):28877–28883, 2002.

1655. Zhang J, et al: Phosphoinositide 3-kinase gamma and p85/phosphoinositide 3-kinase in platelets. Relative activation by thrombin receptor or beta-phorbol myristate acetate and roles in promoting the ligand-binding function of alphaIIbbeta3 integrin. *J Biol Chem* 271(11):6265–6272, 1996.

1656. Rittenhouse SE, Phosphoinositide 3-kinase activation and platelet function. *Blood* 88(12):4401–4414, 1996.

1657. Hartwig JH, et al: D3 phosphoinositides and outside-in integrin signaling by glycoprotein IIb-IIIa mediate platelet actin assembly and filopodial extension induced by phorbol 12-myristate 13-acetate. *J Biol Chem* 271(51):32986–32993, 1996.

1658. Kucera GL, Rittenhouse SE: Human platelets form 3-phosphorylated phosphoinositides in response to α-thrombin, U46619, or GTPgammaS. *J Biol Chem* 265:5345–5348, 1990.

1659. Banfic H, Downes CP, Rittenhouse SE: Biphasic activation of PKBalpha/Akt in platelets. Evidence for stimulation both by phosphatidylinositol 3,4-bisphosphate, produced via a novel pathway, and by phosphatidylinositol 3,4,5-trisphosphate. *J Biol Chem* 273(19):11630–11637, 1998.

1660. Gibbins JM, et al: The p85 subunit of phosphatidylinositol 3-kinase associates with the Fc receptor gamma-chain and linker for activator of T cells (LAT) in platelets stimulated by collagen and convulxin. *J Biol Chem* 273(51):34437–34443, 1998.

1661. Watanabe N, et al: Functional phenotype of phosphoinositide 3-kinase p85alpha-null platelets characterized by an impaired response to GP VI stimulation. *Blood* 102(2):541–548, 2003.

1662. Gratacap MP, et al: Phosphatidylinositol 3,4,5-trisphosphate-dependent stimulation of phospholipase C-gamma2 is an early key event in FcgammaRIIA-mediated activation of human platelets. *J Biol Chem* 273(38):24314–24321, 1998.

1663. Canobbio I, Stefanini L, Cipolla L, et al: Genetic evidence for a predominant role of PI3Kbeta catalytic activity in platelets. *Blood* 114(10):2193–2196, 2009.

1664. Hirsch E, et al: Resistance to thromboembolism in PI3Kgamma-deficient mice. *FASEB J* 15(11):2019–2021, 2001.

1665. Leevers SJ, Vanhaesebroeck B, Waterfield MD: Signalling through phosphoinositide 3-kinases: The lipids take centre stage. *Curr Opin Cell Biol* 11(2):219–225, 1999.

1666. Bae YS, et al: Activation of phospholipase C-gamma by phosphatidylinositol 3,4,5- trisphosphate. *J Biol Chem* 273(8):4465–4469, 1998.

1667. Salim K, et al: Distinct specificity in the recognition of phosphoinositides by the pleckstrin homology domains of dynamin and Bruton's tyrosine kinase. *EMBO J* 15(22):6241–6250, 1996.

1668. Li Z, et al: Phosphatidylinositol 3-kinase-gamma activates Bruton's tyrosine kinase in concert with Src family kinases. *Proc Natl Acad Sci U S A* 94(25):13820–13825, 1997.

1669. Alessi DR, et al: Characterization of a 3-phosphoinositide-dependent protein kinase which phosphorylates and activates protein kinase Balpha. *Curr Biol* 7(4):261–269, 1997.

1670. Stokoe D, et al: Dual role of phosphatidylinositol-3,4,5-trisphosphate in the activation of protein kinase B. *Science* 277(5325):567–570, 1997.

1671. Kroner C, Eybrechts K, Akkerman JW: Dual regulation of platelet protein kinase B. *J Biol Chem* 275(36):27790–27798, 2000.

1672. Li D, August S, Woulfe DS: GSK3beta is a negative regulator of platelet function and thrombosis. *Blood* 111(7):3522–3530, 2008.

1673. Stojanovic A, et al: A phosphoinositide 3-kinase-AKT-nitric oxide-cGMP signaling pathway in stimulating platelet secretion and aggregation. *J Biol Chem* 281(24):16333–16339, 2006.

1674. Zhang W, Colman RW: Thrombin regulates intracellular cyclic AMP concentration in human platelets through phosphorylation/activation of phosphodiesterase 3A. *Blood* 110(5):1475–1482, 2007.

1675. Woulfe D, et al: Defects in secretion, aggregation, and thrombus formation in platelets from mice lacking Akt2. *J Clin Invest* 113(3):441–450, 2004.

1676. Chen J, De S, Damron DS, et al: Impaired platelet response to thrombin and collagen in AKT-1 deficient mice. *Blood* 104(6):1703–1710, 2004.

1677. Bao X, et al: Molecular cloning, bacterial expression and properties of Rab31 and Rab32. *Eur J Biochem* 269(1):259–271, 2002.

1678. Karniguian A, Zahraoui A, Tavitian A: Identification of small GTP-binding rab proteins in human platelets: Thrombin-induced phosphorylation of rab3B, rab6, and rab8 proteins. *Proc Natl Acad Sci U S A* 90(16):7647–7651, 1993.

1679. Richards-Smith B, et al: Analyses of proteins involved in vesicular trafficking in platelets of mouse models of Hermansky Pudlak syndrome. *Mol Genet Metab* 68(1):14–23, 1999.

1680. Wilson SM, et al: A mutation in Rab27a causes the vesicle transport defects observed in ashen mice. *Proc Natl Acad Sci U S A* 97(14):7933–7938, 2000.

1681. Choi W, Karim ZA, Whiteheart SW: Arf6 plays an early role in platelet activation by collagen and convulxin. *Blood* 107(8):3145–3152, 2006.

1682. Bishop AL, Hall A: Rho GTPases and their effector proteins. *Biochem J* 348(Pt 2):241–255, 2000.

1683. Hall A: Rho GTPases and the actin cytoskeleton. *Science* 279(5350):509–514, 1998.

1684. Polakis PG, Snyderman R, Evans T: Characterization of G25K, a GTP-binding protein containing a novel putative nucleotide binding domain. *Biochem Biophys Res Commun* 160(1):25–32, 1989.

1685. Polakis PG, et al: Identification of the ral and rac1 gene products, low molecular mass GTP-binding proteins from human platelets. *J Biol Chem* 264(28):16383–16389, 1989.

1686. Schoenwaelder SM, et al: RhoA sustains integrin alpha IIbbeta 3 adhesion contacts under high shear. *J Biol Chem* 277(17):14738–14746, 2002.

1687. Soulet C, et al: Characterisation of Rac activation in thrombin- and collagen-stimulated human blood platelets. *FEBS Lett* 507(3):253–258, 2001.

1688. Vidal C, et al: Cdc42/Rac1-dependent activation of the p21-activated kinase (PAK) regulates human platelet lamellipodia spreading: Implication of the cortical-actin binding protein cortactin. *Blood* 100(13):4462–4469, 2002.

1689. Moers A, Wettschureck N, Offermanns S: G13-mediated signaling as a potential target for antiplatelet drugs. *Drug News Perspect* 17(8):493–498, 2004.

1690. Soulet C, et al: A differential role of the platelet ADP receptors P2Y1 and P2Y12 in Rac activation. *J Thromb Haemost* 3(10):2296–2306, 2005.

1691. Azim AC, et al: Activation of the small GTPases, rac and cdc42, after ligation of the platelet PAR-1 receptor. *Blood* 95(3):959–964, 2000.

1692. Shock DD, et al: Ras activation in platelets after stimulation of the thrombin receptor, thromboxane A2 receptor or protein kinase C. *Biochem J* 321(Pt 2):525–530, 1997.

1693. Omerovic J, et al: Ras isoform abundance and signalling in human cancer cell lines. *Oncogene* 27(19):2754–2762, 2008.

1694. Omerovic J, Laude AJ, Prior IA: Ras proteins: Paradigms for compartmentalised and isoform-specific signalling. *Cell Mol Life Sci* 64(19–20):2575–2589, 2007.

1695. Tulasne D, Bori T, Watson SP: Regulation of RAS in human platelets. Evidence that activation of RAS is not sufficient to lead to ERK1–2 phosphorylation. *Eur J Biochem* 269(5):1511–1517, 2002.

1696. Shock DD, et al: Ras activation in platelets after stimulation of the thrombin receptor, thromboxane A2 receptor or protein kinase C. *Biochem J* 321(Pt 2):525–530, 1997.

1697. Bauer M, et al: Dichotomous regulation of myosin phosphorylation and shape change by Rho-kinase and calcium in intact human platelets. *Blood* 94(5):1665–1672, 1999.

1698. Morii N, et al: A rho gene product in human blood platelets. II. Effects of the ADP- ribosylation by botulinum C3 ADP-ribosyltransferase on platelet aggregation. *J Biol Chem* 267(29):20921–20926, 1992.

1699. Nemoto Y, et al: A rho gene product in human blood platelets. I. Identification of the platelet substrate for botulinum C3 ADP-ribosyltransferase as rhoA protein. *J Biol Chem* 267(29):20916–20920, 1992.

1700. Klages B, et al: Activation of G12/G13 results in shape change and Rho/Rho-kinase- mediated myosin light chain phosphorylation in mouse platelets. *J Cell Biol* 144(4):745–754, 1999.

1701. Leng L, et al: RhoA and the function of platelet integrin alphaIIbbeta3. *Blood* 91(11):4206–4215, 1998.

1702. Schwartz M: Rho signalling at a glance. *J Cell Sci* 117(Pt 23):5457–5458, 2004.

1703. Akbar H, et al: Genetic and pharmacologic evidence that Rac1 GTPase is involved in regulation of platelet secretion and aggregation. *J Thromb Haemost* 5(8):1747–1755, 2007.

1704. McCarty OJ, et al: Rac1 is essential for platelet lamellipodia formation and aggregate stability under flow. *J Biol Chem* 280(47):39474–39484, 2005.

1705. Pleines I, et al: Rac1 is essential for phospholipase C-gamma2 activation in platelets. *Pflugers Arch* 457(5):1173–1185, 2009.

1706. Falet H, et al: Normal Arp2/3 complex activation in platelets lacking WASp. *Blood* 100(6):2113–2122, 2002.

1707. Kooistra MR, Dube N, Bos JL: Rap1: A key regulator in cell-cell junction formation. *J Cell Sci* 120(Pt 1):17–22, 2007.

1708. Franke B, Akkerman JW, Bos JL: Rapid Ca2+-mediated activation of Rap1 in human platelets. *EMBO J* 16(2):252–259, 1997.

1709. Greco F, et al: Activation of the small GTPase Rap2B in agonist-stimulated human platelets. *J Thromb Haemost* 2(12):2223–2230, 2004.

1710. Chrzanowska-Wodnicka M, et al: Rap1b is required for normal platelet function and hemostasis in mice. *J Clin Invest* 115(3):680–687, 2005.

1711. Eto K, et al: Megakaryocytes derived from embryonic stem cells implicate CalDAG-GEFI in integrin signaling. *Proc Natl Acad Sci U S A* 99(20):12819–12824, 2002.

1712. Crittenden JR, et al: CalDAG-GEFI integrates signaling in platelet aggregation and thrombus formation. *Nat Med* 10(9):982–986, 2004.

1713. Cifuni SM, Wagner DD, Bergmeier W: CalDAG-GEFI and protein kinase C represent alternative pathways leading to activation of integrin alphaIIbbeta3 in platelets. *Blood* 112(5):1696–1703, 2008.

1714. Watanabe N, et al: Mechanisms and consequences of agonist-induced talin recruitment to platelet integrin alphaIIbbeta3. *J Cell Biol* 181(7):1211–1222, 2008.

1715. Cullen PJ, Lockyer PJ: Integration of calcium and Ras signalling. *Nat Rev Mol Cell Biol* 3(5):339–348, 2002.

1716. Bodemann BO, White MA: Ral GTPases and cancer: Linchpin support of the tumorigenic platform. *Nat Rev Cancer* 8(2):133–140, 2008.

1717. Mark BL, Jilkina O, Bhullar RP: Association of Ral GTP-binding protein with human platelet dense granules. *Biochem Biophys Res Commun* 225(1):40–46, 1996.

1718. Wolthuis RM, et al: Activation of the small GTPase Ral in platelets. *Mol Cell Biol* 18(5):2486–2491, 1998.

1719. Kawato M, et al: Regulation of platelet dense granule secretion by the Ral GTPase-exocyst pathway. *J Biol Chem* 283(1):166–174, 2008.

1720. Zerial M, McBride H: Rab proteins as membrane organizers. *Nat Rev Mol Cell Biol* 2(2):107–117, 2001.

1721. Kuchay SM, Chishti AH: Calpain-mediated regulation of platelet signaling pathways. *Curr Opin Hematol* 14(3):249–254, 2007.

1722. Lai KC, Flaumenhaft R: SNARE protein degradation upon platelet activation: Calpain cleaves SNAP-23. *J Cell Physiol* 194(2):206–214, 2003.

1723. Kuchay SM, et al: Double knockouts reveal that protein tyrosine phosphatase 1B is a physiological target of calpain-1 in platelets. *Mol Cell Biol* 27(17):6038–6052, 2007.

1724. Vinogradova O, et al: Membrane-mediated structural transitions at the cytoplasmic face during integrin activation. *Proc Natl Acad Sci U S A* 101(12):4094–4099, 2004.

1725. Haas TA, Plow EF: The cytoplasmic domain of alphaIIb beta3. A ternary complex of the integrin alpha and beta subunits and a divalent cation. *J Biol Chem* 271(11):6017–6026, 1996.

1726. Hughes PE, et al: Breaking the integrin hinge. A defined structural constraint regulates integrin signaling. *J Biol Chem* 271(12):6571–6574, 1996.

1727. Martel V, et al: Conformation, localization, and integrin binding of talin depend on its interaction with phosphoinositides. *J Biol Chem* 276(24):21217–21227, 2001.

1728. Di Paolo G, et al: Recruitment and regulation of phosphatidylinositol phosphate kinase type 1 gamma by the FERM domain of talin. *Nature* 420(6911):85–89, 2002.

1729. Ling K, et al: Type I gamma phosphatidylinositol phosphate kinase targets and regulates focal adhesions. *Nature* 420(6911):89–93, 2002.

1730. Calderwood DA, et al: The phosphotyrosine binding-like domain of talin activates integrins. *J Biol Chem* 277(24):21749–21758, 2002.

1731. Akkerman JW, Holmsen H: Interrelationships among platelet responses: Studies on the burst in protein liberation, lactate production and oxygen uptake during platelet aggregation and Ca2+ secretion. *Blood* 57(5):956–966, 1981.

1732. Garcia-Alvarez B, et al: Structural determinants of integrin recognition by talin. *Mol. Cell* 11(1):49–58, 2003.

1733. van Joost T, et al: Purpuric contact dermatitis to benzoyl peroxide. *J Am Acad Dermatol* 22(2 Pt 2):359–361, 1990.

1734. Wegener KL, Campbell ID: Transmembrane and cytoplasmic domains in integrin activation and protein-protein interactions (review). *Mol Membr Biol* 25(5):376–387, 2008.

1735. Ling K, et al: Tyrosine phosphorylation of type Igamma phosphatidylinositol phosphate kinase by Src regulates an integrin-talin switch. *J Cell Biol* 163(6):1339–1349, 2003.

1736. Xing B, Jedsadayanmata A, Lam SC: Localization of an integrin binding site to the C terminus of talin. *J Biol Chem* 276(48):44373–44378, 2001.

1737. Knezevic I, Leisner TM, Lam SC: Direct binding of the platelet integrin alphaIIbbeta3 (GPIIb-IIIa) to talin. Evidence that interaction is mediated through the cytoplasmic domains of both alphaIIb and beta3. *J Biol Chem* 271(27):16416–16421, 1996.

1738. Ma YQ, et al: Kindlin-2 (Mig-2): A co-activator of beta3 integrins. *J Cell Biol* 181(3):439–446, 2008.

1739. Montanez E, et al: Kindlin-2 controls bidirectional signaling of integrins. *Genes Dev* 22(10):1325–1330, 2008.

1740. Moser M, et al: Kindlin-3 is essential for integrin activation and platelet aggregation. *Nat Med* 14(3):325–330, 2008.

1741. Moser M, et al: Kindlin-3 is essential for integrin activation and platelet aggregation. *Nat Med* 14(3):325–330, 2008.

1742. Kuijpers TW, van de Vijver E, Weterman MA, et al: LAD-1/variant syndrome is caused by mutations in FERMT3. *Blood* 113(19):4740–4746, 2009.

1743. Malinin NL, et al: A point mutation in KINDLIN3 ablates activation of three integrin subfamilies in humans. *Nat Med* 15(3):313–318, 2009.

1744. Mory A, Feigelson SW, Yarali N, et al: Kindlin-3: A new gene involved in the pathogenesis of LAD-III. *Blood* 112(6):2591, 2008.

1745. Svensson L, et al: Leukocyte adhesion deficiency-III is caused by mutations in KINDLIN3 affecting integrin activation. *Nat Med* 15(3):306–312, 2009.

1746. Harburger DS, Bouaouina M, Calderwood DA: Kindlin-1 and -2 directly bind the C-terminal region of beta integrin cytoplasmic tails and exert integrin-specific activation effects. *J Biol Chem* 284(17):11485–11497, 2009.

1747. Li R, et al: Oligomerization of the integrin alphaIIbbeta3: Roles of the transmembrane and cytoplasmic domains. *Proc Natl Acad Sci U S A* 98(22):12462–12467, 2001.

1748. Arias-Salgado EG, et al: Src kinase activation by direct interaction with the integrin beta cytoplasmic domain. *Proc Natl Acad Sci U S A* 100(23):13298–13302, 2003.

1749. Newman DK: The Y's that bind: Negative regulators of Src family kinase activity in platelets. *J Thromb Haemost* 7(Suppl 1):195–199, 2009.

1750. Obergfell A, Eto K, Mocsai A, et al: Coordinate interactions of Csk, Src, and Syk kinases with [alpha]IIb[beta]3 initiate integrin signaling to the cytoskeleton. *J Cell Biol* 157(2):265–275, 2002.

1751. Woodside DG, et al: Activation of Syk protein tyrosine kinase through interaction with integrin beta cytoplasmic domains. *Curr Biol* 11(22):1799–1804, 2001.

1752. Woodside DG, et al: The N-terminal SH2 domains of Syk and ZAP-70 mediate phosphotyrosine-independent binding to integrin beta cytoplasmic domains. *J Biol Chem* 277(42):39401–39408, 2002.

1753. De Virgilio M, Kiosses WB, Shattil SJ: Proximal, selective, and dynamic interactions between integrin alphaIIbbeta3 and protein tyrosine kinases in living cells. *J Cell Biol* 165(3):305–311, 2004.

1754. Falati S, et al: Platelet PECAM-1 inhibits thrombus formation *in vivo*. *Blood* 107(2):535–541, 2006.

1755. Newman EA: New roles for astrocytes: Regulation of synaptic transmission. *Trends Neurosci* 26(10):536–542, 2003.

1756. Newman PJ, Newman DK: Signal transduction pathways mediated by PECAM-1: New roles for an old molecule in platelet and vascular cell biology. *Arterioscler Thromb Vasc Biol* 23(6):953–964, 2003.

1757. Patil S, Newman DK, Newman PJ: Platelet endothelial cell adhesion molecule-1 serves as an inhibitory receptor that modulates platelet responses to collagen. *Blood* 97(6):1727–173, 20012.

1758. Wong C, et al: CEACAM1 negatively regulates platelet-collagen interactions and thrombus growth in vitro and in vivo. *Blood* 113(8):1818–1828, 2009.

1759. Mori J, et al: G6b-B inhibits constitutive and agonist-induced signaling by glycoprotein VI and CLEC-2. *J Biol Chem* 283(51):35419–35427, 2008.

1760. Newland SA, et al: The novel inhibitory receptor G6B is expressed on the surface of platelets and attenuates platelet function *in vitro*. *Blood* 109(11):4806–4809, 2007.

1761. Senis YA, et al: A comprehensive proteomics and genomics analysis reveals novel transmembrane proteins in human platelets and mouse megakaryocytes including G6b-B, a novel immunoreceptor tyrosine-based inhibitory motif protein. *Mol Cell Proteomics* 6(3):548–564, 2007.

1762. Kumar G, et al: The membrane immunoglobulin receptor utilizes a Shc/Grb2/hSOS complex for activation of the mitogen-activated protein kinase cascade in a B-cell line. *Biochem J* 307(Pt 1):215–223, 1995.

1763. Law DA, et al: Integrin cytoplasmic tyrosine motif is required for outside-in alphaIIbbeta3 signalling and platelet function. *Nature* 401(6755):808–811, 1999.

1764. Miranti CK, et al: Identification of a novel integrin signaling pathway involving the kinase Syk and the guanine nucleotide exchange factor Vav1. *Curr Biol* 8(24):1289–1299, 1998.

1765. Prasad KS, et al: The platelet CD40L/GP IIb-IIIa axis in atherothrombotic disease. *Curr Opin Hematol* 10(5):356–361, 2003.

1766. Majerus PW: Arachidonate metabolism in vascular disorders. *J Clin Invest* 72(5):1521–1525, 1983.

1767. Moncada S, Whittle BJ: Biological actions of prostacyclin and its pharmacological use in platelet studies. *Adv Exp Med Biol* 192:337–358, 1985.

1768. Marcus AJ: The role of lipids in platelet function: With particular reference to the arachidonic acid pathway. *J Lipid Res* 19:793–826, 1978.

1769. Katsuyama M, et al: Cloning and expression of a cDNA for the human prostacyclin receptor. *FEBS Lett* 344(1):74–78, 1994.

1770. Kunapuli SP, et al: Cloning and expression of a prostaglandin E receptor EP3 subtype from human erythroleukaemia cells. *Biochem J* 298(Pt 2):263–267, 1994.

1771. Feijge MA, et al: Control of platelet activation by cyclic AMP turnover and cyclic nucleotide phosphodiesterase type-3. *Biochem Pharmacol* 67(8):1559–1567, 2004.

1772. Hung SH, et al: New insights from the structure-function analysis of the catalytic region of human platelet phosphodiesterase 3A: A role for the unique 44-amino acid insert. *J Biol Chem* 281(39):29236–29244, 2006.

1773. Sun B, et al: Role of phosphodiesterase type 3A and 3B in regulating platelet and cardiac function using subtype-selective knockout mice. *Cell Signal* 19(8):1765–1771, 2007.

1774. Chapman TM, Goa KL: Cilostazol: A review of its use in intermittent claudication. *Am J Cardiovasc Drugs* 3(2):117–138, 2003.

1775. Manganello JM, et al: Protein kinase A-mediated phosphorylation of the Galpha13 switch I region alters the Galphabetagamma13-G protein-coupled receptor complex and inhibits Rho activation. *J Biol Chem* 278(1):124–130, 2003.

1776. Bodnar RJ, et al: Regulation of glycoprotein Ib-IX-von Willebrand factor interaction by cAMP-dependent protein kinase-mediated phosphorylation at Ser 166 of glycoprotein Ib(beta). *J Biol Chem* 277(49):47080–47087, 2002.

1777. Cavallini L, et al: Prostacyclin and sodium nitroprusside inhibit the activity of the platelet inositol 1,4,5-trisphosphate receptor and promote its phosphorylation. *J Biol Chem* 271:5545–5551, 1996.

1778. Nishimura T, et al: Antiplatelet functions of a stable prostacyclin analog, SM-10906 are exerted by its inhibitory effect on inositol 1,4,5-trisphosphate production and cytosolic Ca2++ increase in rat platelets stimulated by thrombin. *Thromb Res* 79:307–317, 1995.

1779. Cook SJ, McCormick F: Inhibition by cAMP of Ras-dependent activation of Raf. *Science* 262:1069–1072, 1993.

1780. Dumaz N, Marais R: Protein kinase A blocks Raf-1 activity by stimulating 14-3-3 binding and blocking Raf-1 interaction with Ras. *J Biol Chem* 278(32):29819–29823, 2003.

1781. Fischer TH, et al: The localization of the cAMP-dependent protein kinase phosphorylation site in the platelet rat protein, rap 1B. *FEBS Lett* 2832:173–176, 1991.

1782. Siess W, Grunberg B: Phosphorylation of rap1B by protein kinase A is not involved in platelet inhibition by cyclic AMP. *Cell Signal* 5(2):209–214, 1993.

1783. Lou L, et al: CAMP inhibition of Akt is mediated by activated and phosphorylated Rap1b. *J Biol Chem* 277(36):32799–32806, 2002.

1784. Fabre JE, et al: Activation of the murine EP3 receptor for PGE2 inhibits cAMP production and promotes platelet aggregation. *J Clin Invest* 107(5):603–610, 2001.

1785. Shio H, Ramwell P: Effect of prostaglandin E 2 and aspirin on the secondary aggregation of human platelets. *Nat New Biol* 236(63):45–46, 1972.

1786. Gross S, et al: Vascular wall-produced prostaglandin E2 exacerbates arterial thrombosis and atherothrombosis through platelet EP3 receptors. *J Exp Med* 204(2):311–320, 2007.

1787. Luscher TF, et al: Difference between endothelium-dependent relaxation in arterial and in venous coronary bypass grafts. *N Engl J Med* 319(8):462–467, 1988.

1788. Goretski J, Hollocher TC: Trapping of nitric oxide produced during denitrification by extracellular hemoglobin. *J Biol Chem* 263(5):2316–2323, 1988.

1789. Loscalzo J, Welch G: Nitric oxide and its role in the cardiovascular system. *Prog Cardiovasc Dis* 38(2):87–104, 1995.

1790. Mellion BT, et al: Evidence for the inhibitory role of guanosine 3′,5′-monophosphate in ADP-induced human platelet aggregation in the presence of nitric oxide and related vasodilators. *Blood* 57(5):946–955, 1981.

1791. Radomski MW, Palmer RM, Moncada S: Modulation of platelet aggregation by an L-arginine-nitric oxide pathway. *Trends Pharmacol Sci* 12(3):87–88, 1991.

1792. Wang GR, et al: Mechanism of platelet inhibition by nitric oxide: In vivo phosphorylation of thromboxane receptor by cyclic GMP-dependent protein kinase. *Proc Natl Acad Sci U S A* 95(9):4888–4893, 1998.

1793. Massberg S, et al: Increased adhesion and aggregation of platelets lacking cyclic guanosine 3′,5′-monophosphate kinase I. *J Exp Med* 189(8):1255–1264, 1999.

1794. Aszodi A, et al: The vasodilator-stimulated phosphoprotein (VASP) is involved in cGMP- and cAMP-mediated inhibition of agonist-induced platelet aggregation, but is dispensable for smooth muscle function. *EMBO J* 18(1):37–48, 1999.

1795. Butt E, et al: CAMP- and cGMP-dependent protein kinase phosphorylation sites of the focal adhesion vasodilator-stimulated phosphoprotein (VASP) *in vitro* and in intact human platelets. *J Biol Chem* 269(20):14509–14517, 1994.

1796. Hauser W, et al: Megakaryocyte hyperplasia and enhanced agonist-induced platelet activation in vasodilator-stimulated phosphoprotein knockout mice. *Proc Natl Acad Sci U S A* 96(14):8120–8125, 1999.

1797. Massberg S, et al: Enhanced *in vivo* platelet adhesion in vasodilator-stimulated phosphoprotein (VASP)-deficient mice. *Blood* 103(1):136–142, 2004.

1798. Maurice DH, Haslam RJ: Molecular basis of the synergistic inhibition of platelet function by nitrovasodilators and activators of adenylate cyclase: Inhibition of cyclic AMP breakdown by cyclic GMP. *Mol Pharmacol* 37(5):671–681, 1990.

1799. Atkinson B, et al: Ecto-nucleotidases of the CD39/NTPDase family modulate platelet activation and thrombus formation: Potential as therapeutic targets. *Blood Cells Mol Dis* 36(2):217–222, 2006.

1800. Kaczmarek E, et al: Identification and characterization of CD39/vascular ATP diphosphohydrolase. *J Biol Chem* 271(51):33116–33122, 1996.

1801. Marcus AJ, et al: The endothelial cell ecto-ADPase responsible for inhibition of platelet function is CD39. *J Clin Invest* 99(6):1351–1360, 1997.

1802. Le F, et al: Characterization and chromosomal localization of the human A2a adenosine receptor gene: ADORA2A. *Biochem Biophys Res Commun* 223(2):461–467, 1996.

1803. Pulte D, Olson KE, Broekman MJ, et al: CD39 activity correlates with stage and inhibits platelet reactivity in chronic lymphocytic leukemia. *J Transl Med* 5:23, 2007.

1804. Gayle RB 3rd, Maliszewski CR, Gimpel SD, et al: Inhibition of platelet function by recombinant soluble ecto-ADPase/CD39. *J Clin Invest* 101(9):1851–1859, 1998.

1805. Pollard TD: Actin. *Curr Opin Cell Biol* 2:33–40, 1990.

1806. Vandekerckhove J: Actin-binding proteins. *Curr Opin Cell Biol* 2:41–50, 1990.

1807. Weeds AG, et al: Preparation and characterization of pig plasma and platelet gelsolins. *Eur J Biochem* 161:69–76, 1986.

1808. Smillie LB: Structure and function of tropomyosins from muscle and non-muscle. *Trends Biochem Sci* 4:151, 1979.

1809. Vandekerckhove J: Structural principles of actin-binding proteins. *Curr Opin Cell Biol* 1(1):15–22, 1989.

1810. Chen M, Stracher A: *In situ* phosphorylation of platelet actin-binding protein by cAMP-dependent protein kinase stabilizes it against proteolysis by calpain. *J Biol Chem* 264:14282–14289, 1989.

1811. Lind SE, Stossel TP: The microfilament network of the platelet. *Prog Hemost Thromb* 6:63–84, 1982.

1812. He P, Zhang H, Yun CC: IRBIT, inositol 1,4,5-triphosphate (IP3) receptor-binding protein released with IP3, binds Na+/H+ exchanger NHE3 and activates NHE3 activity in response to calcium. *J Biol Chem* 283(48):33544–33553, 2008.

1813. Beckerle MC, et al: Activation-dependent redistribution of the adhesion plaque protein, talin, in intact human platelets. *J Cell Biol* 109:3333–3346, 1989.

1814. O'Halloran T, Beckerle MC, Burridge K: Identification of talin as a major cytoplasmic protein implicated in platelet activation. *Nature* 317:449–451, 1985.

1815. Koteliansky VE, Gneushev GN, Glukhova MA, et al: Identification and isolation of vinculin from platelets. *FEBS Lett* 165(1):26–30, 1984.

1816. Langer B, Gonnella PA, Nachmias VT: Alpha-actinin and vinculin in normal and thrombasthenic platelets. *Blood* 63(3):606–614, 1984.

1817. Lucas RC, et al: The isolation and characterization of a cytoskeleton and a contractile apparatus from platelets., in *Protides of Biological Fluids*, edited by H Peeters, pp 465–470. Pergamon Press, New York, 1975.

1818. Wang LL, Bryan J: Isolation of calcium-dependent platelet proteins that interact with actin. *Cell* 25(3):637–649, 1981.

1819. Hathaway DR, Adelstein RS: Human platelet myosin light chain kinase requires the calcium binding protein calmodulin for activity. *Proc Natl Acad Sci U S A* 76:1653, 1979.

1820. Wolff DJ, Brostrom CO: Proterties and functions of the calcium-dependent regulator protein. *Adv Cyclic Nucleotide Res* 11:27, 1979.

1821. Daniel JL: Platelet contractile proteins, in *Hemostasis and Thrombosis: Basic Principles and Clinical Practice*, edited by RW Colman, J Hirsh, VJ Marder, EW Salzman, pp 557–573. JB Lippincott, Philadelphia, 1993.

# CHAPTER 3

# MOLECULAR BIOLOGY AND BIOCHEMISTRY OF THE COAGULATION FACTORS AND PATHWAYS OF HEMOSTASIS

Mettine H. A. Bos, Cornelis van't Veer, and Pieter H. Reitsma

## SUMMARY

The coagulation cascade consists of a complex network of reactions that are essential for the conversion of zymogens into enzymes and of inactive pro-cofactors into cofactors. Most of these reactions take place on a membrane surface, which restricts coagulation to the site of injury. Upon initiation, these reactions serve to produce the fibrin that is necessary for the formation of a stable hemostatic plug. In addition, these reactions provide feedback loops that limit and localize thrombus formation and regulate thrombus resolution. This chapter highlights key biochemical characteristics of the individual coagulation factors, essential aspects regarding their synthesis, and the clinical importance of acquired or inherited variations that affect their quantity or function. The coagulation factors are grouped as (1) the vitamin K–dependent zymogens (prothrombin, factor VII, factor IX, factor X, and protein C); (2) the procoagulant cofactors (factor V, factor VIII); (3) the soluble cofactors (protein S, von Willebrand factor); (4) factor XI and the contact system (factor XII, prekallikrein, and high-molecular weight kininogen); (5) the cell-associated cofactors (tissue factor, thrombomodulin, endothelial protein C receptor); (6) the fibrin network (fibrin[ogen], factor XIII, thrombin-activatable fibrinolysis inhibitor); and (7) inhibitors of coagulation (antithrombin, tissue factor pathway inhibitor, protein Z/protein Z–dependent protease inhibitor). Table 3–1 summarizes the major features of the coagulation factors addressed in this chapter. The final sections of this chapter present an overview of the coagulation cascade in which the pathways of hemostasis including the contribution of endothelial cells, blood platelets, and immune cells are described.

**Acronyms and Abbreviations:** APC, activated protein C; ADP, adenosine diphosphate; AT, antithrombin; C4BP, complement 4b–binding protein; COX, cyclooxygenase; EGF, epidermal growth factor; EPCR, endothelial protein C receptor; ER, endoplasmatic reticulum; ERGIC, ER-Golgi intermediate compartment; Gla, γ-carboxyglutamic acid; GP, glycoprotein; HK, high-molecular-weight kininogen; LMAN1, mannose-binding lectin-1; PAI-1, plasminogen activator inhibitor type 1; PAR, protease-activated receptor; PK, prekallikrein; poly-P, polyphosphate; RVV, Russell's viper venom; SHBG, sex hormone–binding globulin; TAFI, thrombin-activatable fibrinolysis inhibitor; TFPI, tissue factor pathway inhibitor; UFH, unfractionated heparin; VWD, von Willebrand disease; VWF, von Willebrand factor; ZPI, protein Z–dependent protease inhibitor.

## ● MOLECULAR BIOLOGY AND BIOCHEMISTRY OF THE COAGULATION FACTORS

### THE VITAMIN K–DEPENDENT ZYMOGENS: PROTHROMBIN, FACTOR VII, FACTOR IX, FACTOR X, AND PROTEIN C

The vitamin K–dependent zymogens circulate in an inactive state and require proteolytic activation to function as a serine protease. All share a similar domain structure of a C-terminal serine protease domain and an N-terminal γ-carboxyglutamic acid (Gla) domain, which are connected by two epidermal growth factor (EGF)-like domains or kringle domains (Fig. 3–1). Each protein domain has a well-defined function and facilitates substrate recognition, interaction with protein cofactors, or binding to a negatively charged lipid surface, such as that of activated platelets or endothelial cells, thereby restricting coagulation to the site of injury. The latter is mediated via the Gla domain, a domain that is characteristic to the vitamin K–dependent proteins.

The high level of protein and gene homology suggests that the vitamin K–dependent zymogens originate from a common ancestral gene as a result of gene duplications.[1] Exon shuffling and tandem duplication may account for the generation of the ancestral gene, in which the functional domains that are encoded by a single exon each were combined and duplicated.[2] This process may also account for the presence of the kringle domains as opposed to EGF-like domains in prothrombin.

The Gla domain refers to the 42-residue region located in the N-terminus of the mature protein that comprises nine to 12 glutamic acid residues that are posttranslationally γ-carboxylated into Gla residues by a specific γ-glutamyl carboxylase in the endoplasmic reticulum of hepatocytes.[3] This γ-carboxylase requires oxygen, carbon dioxide, and the reduced form of vitamin K for its action, hence the name vitamin K–dependent proteins. For each Glu residue that is carboxylated, one molecule of reduced vitamin K is converted to the epoxide form (Fig. 3–2). Vitamin K epoxide reductase converts the epoxide form of vitamin K back to the reduced form.[4] Warfarin and related 4-hydroxycoumarin–containing molecules inhibit the activity of vitamin K epoxide reductase, thereby preventing vitamin K recycling and inhibiting γ-carboxylation. This results in a heterogeneous population of circulating undercarboxylated forms of the vitamin K–dependent proteins with reduced activity. Because warfarin blocks the reductase and not the carboxylase, the inhibitory effect of warfarin can be (temporarily) reversed by administration of vitamin K. Recognition by and interaction with γ-carboxylase is facilitated by the propeptide sequence that is located C-terminal to the signal peptide. The propeptide is highly conserved among the vitamin K–dependent proteins, and amino acids at positions –18, –17, –16, –15, and –10 are critical to recognition by the γ-carboxylase.[5,6] Following γ-carboxylation, the propeptide is removed through limited proteolysis prior to secretion of the mature protein.

A correctly γ-carboxylated Gla domain is essential for interaction of the vitamin K–dependent proteins with phosphatidylserine, a negatively charged phospholipid. Under normal conditions, phosphatidylserine is not exposed on the outer membrane leaflet of cells. However, in activated endothelial cells or platelets, phosphatidylserine is part of the extracellular cell surface where it supports blood coagulation reactions. The Gla domain interacts with the anionic cell surface in a calcium-dependent manner. These calcium ions are coordinated by Gla residues and induce a conformational change in the Gla domain that is characterized by the appearance of a hydrophobic surface loop (Fig. 3–3).

**TABLE 3–1.** Characteristics of Coagulation Proteins

| Protein | Plasma Concentration (μg/mL) | Plasma Concentration (nmol/L) | Mr (kDa) | Plasma Half-Life (hours) |
|---|---|---|---|---|
| **Zymogens** | | | | |
| + Gla domain | | | | |
| Prothrombin (factor II) | 100 | 1400 | 72 | 60 |
| Factor VII | 0.5 | 10 | 50 | 3–6 |
| Factor IX | 5 | 90 | 55 | 18–24 |
| Factor X | 10 | 170 | 59 | 34–40 |
| Protein C | 4 | 65 | 62 | 6–8 |
| – Gla domain | | | | |
| Factor XI | 5 | 30 | 160 | 60–80 |
| Factor XII | 40 | 500 | 80 | 50–70 |
| Prekallikrein | 40 | 490 | 85 | 35 |
| Factor XIIIA[*][†] | – | – | 83 | – |
| Factor XIIIB[*] | 7 | 94 | 76.5 | – |
| Factor XIII | 30 | 94 | 320 | 240 |
| TAFI | 4–15 | 70–275 | 60 | – |
| **Cofactors** | | | | |
| Soluble | | | | |
| Factor V[†] | 5–10 | 20 | 330 | 12–36 |
| Factor VIII | 0.2 | 0.7 | 300 | 8–12 |
| VWF | varies | 10 | 500–20,000 | 8–12 |
| Protein S[‡] | 25 | 350 | 75 | 42 |
| Protein Z[§] | 2.5 | 40 | 62 | 60 |
| HK | 80 | 670 | 120 | 150 |
| Cellular | | | | |
| Tissue factor | – | – | 47 | – |
| Thrombomodulin | – | – | 78 | – |
| EPCR | – | – | 49 | – |
| **Structural Protein** | | | | |
| Fibrinogen | 2500 | 7400 | 340 | 72–120 |
| Aα chain | – | – | 66.5 | – |
| Bβ chain | – | – | 52 | – |
| γ Chain | – | – | 46.5 | – |
| **Inhibitors** | | | | |
| Antithrombin | 150 | 2500 | 58 | 60–72 |
| TFPIα[¶] | 0.01 | 0.25 | 40 | 0.03 |
| ZPI[§] | 4 | 60 | 72 | 60 |

EPCR, endothelial protein C receptor; HK, high-molecular-weight kininogen; TAFI, thrombin-activatable fibrinolysis inhibitor; TFPI, full-length tissue factor pathway inhibitor; VWF, von Willebrand factor; ZPI, protein Z–dependent protease inhibitor.

[*]All of the factor XIIIA chain is in complex with factor XIIIB chain; only half of factor XIIIB is in complex with factor XIIIA, the rest is free in plasma.

[†]Platelets carry significant amounts of factor XIIIA and factor V (20% of circulating factor V).

[‡]Approximately 60% of protein S is in complex with C4b-binding protein; the remainder circulates as free protein S.

[§]ZPI circulates in complex with protein Z.

[¶]TFPI circulates in plasma at 2.5 nM in multiple forms; only 10% of circulating TFPI is the full-length TFPIα.

Membrane binding by the Gla domain occurs when this hydrophobic surface loop penetrates into the hydrophobic portion of the phospholipid bilayer, which is facilitated by the interaction of the Gla-bound calcium ions with the phosphate head groups of phosphatidylserine.[7,8] It has been shown that the phosphate head groups of exposed phosphatidylethanolamine are also capable of coordinating calcium ions, thereby contributing to the interaction of the Gla domains with the negatively charged membrane surface.[9]

The serine protease domains of the vitamin K–dependent proteins are highly homologous, as they bear a chymotrypsin-like fold and display trypsin-like activity.[10] Once activated, they cleave peptide bonds following a positively charged amino acid (Lys or Arg). Activation proceeds through proteolysis at one or more sites N-terminal to the serine protease domain (see Fig. 3–1). Subsequently, the newly formed N-terminus inserts into the serine protease domain to form a salt bridge with an Asp residue, which is associated with conformational changes

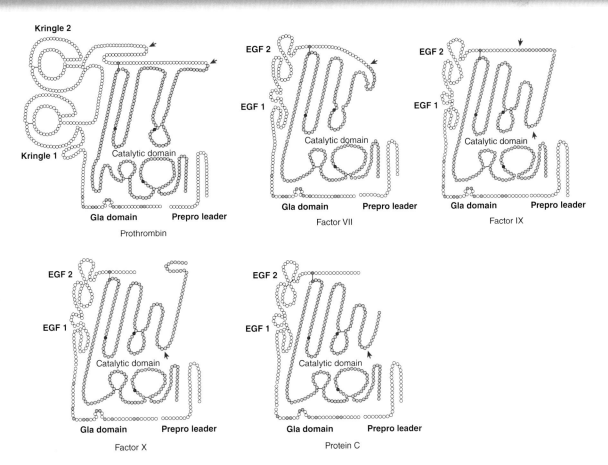

**Figure 3–1.** Vitamin K–dependent schematic of the vitamin K–dependent zymogens. Each circle represents an amino acid. The prepro leader sequence contains the signal peptide as well as the propeptide that directs γ-carboxylation of glutamic acid (Gla) residues. Cleavage of the prepro sequence from the mature protein is indicated by the separation between the two. The Gla domains are indicated with the Gla residues in *blue*. Prothrombin has a finger loop followed by two kringle domains. Factors VII, IX, X, and protein C have epidermal growth factor (EGF)-like domains. Prothrombin, factor VII, and factor IX circulate as single-chain molecules. Factor X and protein C circulate as two chains that are disulfide linked. All have homologous serine protease ("catalytic") domains (shown in *light red*), in which the active site His, Asp, and Ser residues are indicated in *dark red*. Cleavages that convert the zymogen to an active enzyme are indicated by the *red arrows*. In factor IX, factor X, and protein C, the released activation peptide is indicated in *yellow*. After proteolytic activation, all of the molecules are two-chain disulfide-linked molecules, with the cysteines forming a disulfide bridge *(black line)* indicated in *green*. All catalytic domains but that of prothrombin remain attached to the Gla domain following activation.

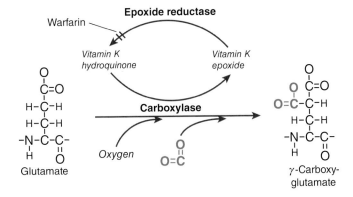

**Figure 3–2.** Vitamin K–dependent γ-carboxylation. Glutamic acid residues are converted to γ-carboxyglutamic acid (Gla) residues by a specific γ-carboxylase. This reaction requires oxygen, carbon dioxide (shown in *green*), and reduced vitamin K in the form of a hydroquinone. Carbon dioxide is incorporated onto the γ-carbon, providing a second carboxylate group on that residue. In the process of this reaction, reduced vitamin K is converted to an epoxide. Reduced vitamin K is recycled by a specific epoxide reductase, a reaction that can be blocked by warfarin and warfarin analogues.

in the serine protease domain. These lead to an optimal configuration of the active site through alignment of the active site residues His, Ser, and Asp, and to formation of the substrate-binding exosites, allowing for substrate conversion. The substrate-binding exosites are unique to each vitamin K–dependent protease and are responsible for their highly specific substrate recognition and associated function in coagulation.

Interaction of the vitamin K–dependent proteases with specific cofactors on a (anionic) membrane surface (Table 3–2) further enhances substrate recognition, as the cofactors interact with both the protease and the substrate, bridging the two together. This results in a dramatic enhancement of the catalytic activity (Table 3–3), thereby making the cofactor–protease complex the physiologic relevant enzyme. The increase in catalytic rate has also been attributed to a cofactor-induced conformational change in the protease.[11] However, whether this molecular mechanism holds true for all cofactor–protease complexes remains to be determined. Tissue factor is the cofactor for factor VIIa, factor VIIIa is the cofactor for factor IXa, and factor Va is the cofactor for factor Xa, while thrombin does not require a cofactor for its procoagulant activity. However, upon association with the cofactor thrombomodulin, thrombin's specificity is changed from procoagulant to anticoagulant (cleaving and activating protein C). The complexes are also named for their physiologic substrate: the factor VIIIa–factor IXa complex is

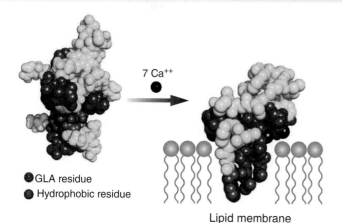

- ● GLA residue
- ● Hydrophobic residue

Lipid membrane

7 Ca⁺⁺

**Figure 3–3.** Calcium-dependent association of the glutamic acid (Gla) domain with the anionic phospholipid surface. Non–calcium bound (Protein Data Bank [PDB] structure 2PF2) and calcium bound (PDB structure 1WHE) molecular models of the Gla domain of prothrombin are shown. Circles represent amino acids, with the Gla (GLA) residues indicated in *red*. Hydrophobic residues involved in membrane insertion are shown in *blue*. In the absence of calcium, the negatively charged Gla residues are exposed to the solution and the hydrophobic residues are buried. Association of calcium ions (in *black*) to the Gla residues provides sufficient energy to alter the overall conformation of the Gla domain and expose the hydrophobic residues. Membrane binding by the Gla domain occurs when this hydrophobic surface loop penetrates into the hydrophobic portion of the phospholipid bilayer (drawn schematically), which is facilitated by interaction of the Gla-bound calcium ions with the negatively charged phosphate head groups.

termed the "tenase" or "intrinsic tenase" complex; the tissue factor–factor VIIa complex is termed the "extrinsic tenase" complex; and the factor Va–factor Xa complex is termed the "prothrombinase" complex.

## PROTHROMBIN (FACTOR II)

Prothrombin, or factor II, which was discovered by Pekelharing in 1894, is one of the four coagulation factors that were described by Paul Morawitz in 1905, in addition to fibrinogen (factor I), thromboplastin (thrombokinase, factor III, now tissue factor), and calcium (factor IV).[12,13] The zymogen prothrombin is primarily synthesized in the liver and circulates in plasma as a single-chain protein of 579 amino acids

**TABLE 3–2.** Protease–Cofactor Complexes

| Protease | Cofactor | Substrate | Cellular Location |
|---|---|---|---|
| Factor VIIa | Tissue factor | Factor IX | Many cells* |
| | | Factor X | |
| Factor IXa | Factor VIIIa | Factor X | Platelets |
| Factor Xa | Factor Va | Prothrombin | Platelets |
| Thrombin | Thrombomodulin | Protein C | Endothelium |
| Activated protein C | Protein S | Factor Va | Endothelium |
| | | Factor VIIIa | |

*Tissue factor is constitutively expressed on many extravascular cells (e.g., stromal cells, epithelial cells, astrocytes) and is induced by inflammatory mediators in many other cells (e.g., monocytes, endothelial cells).

**TABLE 3–3.** Cofactor Enhancement of Serine Protease Activity

| Cofactor-Protease* | Fold Increase† |
|---|---|
| TM-Thrombin | 11,000 |
| TF-VIIa | 31,000 |
| VIIIa-IXa | 9,000,000 |
| Va-Xa | 390,000 |

TF, tissue factor; TM, thrombomodulin.

*Macromolecular enzyme complexes assembled in the presence of anionic phospholipids and calcium.

†Relative rates of enzymatic activity represent fold increase of the reaction rate ($k_{cat}/Km$) observed for the cofactor-protease complex relative to the reaction rate ($k_{cat}/Km$) observed for the protease in absence of the cofactor (see Mann KG, Nesheim ME, Church WR, et al: Surface-dependent reactions of the vitamin K–dependent enzyme complexes. *Blood* 76:1–16, 1990; and Rawala-Sheikh R, Ahmad SS, Ashby B, Walsh PN: Kinetics of coagulation factor X activation by platelet-bound factor IXa. *Biochemistry* 29:2606–2611,1990).

(Mr ≈72,000) at a concentration of 1.4 $\mu$M with a plasma half-life of 60 hours (see Table 3–1).

### Protein Structure

Prothrombin is composed of fragment 1 (F1), fragment 2 (F2), and the serine protease domain. F1 consists of the Gla domain, which comprises 10 Gla residues, and the kringle 1 domain; F2 contains the kringle 2 domain (see Fig. 3–1). The two kringle domains, which replace the EGF-like domains present in most vitamin K–dependent zymogens, are conserved secondary protein structures that fold into large loops that are stabilized by three disulfide bonds and schematically resemble a Danish pastry called a "kringle." Their primary function is to bind other proteins such as the cofactor Va and serine protease factor Xa that activate prothrombin.

Other than $\gamma$-carboxylation of Glu residues, prothrombin is posttranslationally modified via *N*-glycosylation in the kringle 1 (Asn78, Asn143) and serine protease domains (Asn373), which contributes to the stability of the prothrombin precursor during processing in the endoplasmatic reticulum.[14,15]

### Prothrombin Activation and Thrombin Activity

Prothrombin is proteolytically activated by the prothrombinase complex (i.e., factor Va, factor Xa, calcium, and anionic phospholipids) that cleaves at Arg271 and Arg320 (see Fig. 3–1). Cleavage at Arg320 opens the active site of the protease domain, while cleavage at Arg271 removes the activation fragment (F1.2). Both cleavages are necessary to generate procoagulant $\alpha$-thrombin (II$\alpha$) (Fig. 3–4). The composition of the membrane surface directs the cleavage order in prothrombin and the formation of either the zymogen prethrombin 2 (initial cleavage at Arg271) or the proteolytically active intermediate meizothrombin (initial cleavage at Arg320).[16,17] Meizothrombin has impaired procoagulant activity as compared to $\alpha$-thrombin, but superior anticoagulant activity as it displays increased thrombomodulin-dependent protein C activation, which is likely facilitated by membrane binding of meizothrombin through its Gla domain.[18] The snake venom protease Ecarin is capable of generating meizothrombin specifically through proteolysis at Arg323 only. However, this meizothrombin is instable as a result of autocatalysis at Arg155, thereby removing the Gla domain containing F1. The so-formed meizo-des-F1 can be converted to thrombin by prothrombinase,

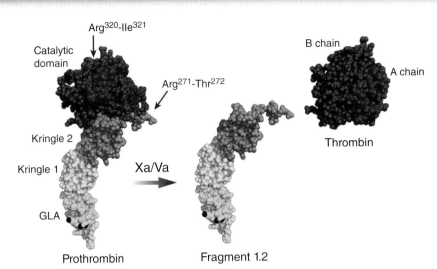

**Figure 3–4.** Prothrombin to thrombin conversion. A molecular model of prothrombin comprising the γ-carboxyglutamic acid (Gla; GLA) domain, both kringle domains, and the catalytic domain is shown (PDB structures 2PF2, 1HAG, 1A0H, 1HAI). Gla domain-bound calcium ions are indicated in *black*. Cleavage by the factor Va-Xa complex at Arg271 and Arg320 releases thrombin (with the A chain and catalytically active B chain) from the rest of the molecule (fragment 1.2).

but at a slower rate as it is incapable of membrane binding. Assessment of F1.2 levels reflects prothrombin activation and is commonly used as a marker for thrombin generation.

Thrombin (IIα) is a two-chain serine protease (Mr ≈37,000) comprising a light chain of 49 residues (A chain; Mr ≈6000) that is covalently linked to the catalytic heavy chain of 259 residues (B chain; Mr ≈31,000). Thrombin's main function is to induce the formation of a fibrin clot by removing fibrinopeptides A and B from fibrinogen to form fibrin monomers, which then spontaneously polymerize. In addition, thrombin is able to cleave a wide variety of substrates with high specificity, which is mediated via its negatively charged, deep active site cleft and via the anion binding exosites I and II that specifically interact with cofactors and/or substrates.[19] The dynamic structural conformation of thrombin allows for binding to diverse ligands, and the subsequent ligand-induced conformational stabilization, known as thrombin allostery, regulates and controls thrombin activity.[20,21]

Thrombin initiates important procoagulant pathways by proteolytic activation of the cofactors V and VIII and zymogen factor XI that collectively amplify thrombin and fibrin formation, and by activating factor XIII that crosslinks and stabilizes the fibrin polymers. Another procoagulant function of thrombin is to inhibit fibrinolysis by proteolytic activation of the thrombin-activatable fibrinolysis inhibitor (TAFI), a reaction enhanced by the endothelial-bound cofactor thrombomodulin. Thrombin also has an anticoagulant function, and upon binding to the cofactor thrombomodulin, it is capable of proteolytically activating protein C, which inactivates the cofactors Va and VIIIa.

Thrombin activates the seven-transmembrane domain, G-protein–coupled protease-activated receptors (PARs) PAR1, PAR3, and PAR4 that are expressed on a wide range of cell types in the vasculature by proteolytic cleavage of their N-terminal extracellular domains.[22–25] Thrombin is one of the strongest platelet activators *in vivo* and activates platelet-expressed PAR1 and PAR4.[25] The platelet glycoprotein (GP) Ib (GPIb) serves as a cofactor for thrombin in PAR1 cleavage (Chap. 2). Thrombin-mediated activation of endothelial-PAR1 triggers release of von Willebrand factor (VWF) and P-selectin, which promote rolling and adhesion of platelets and leukocytes. In addition, this stimulates the endothelial production of platelet-activating factor, a potent platelet and leukocyte activator, as well as the production of chemokines, cyclooxygenase (COX)-2, and prostaglandins.[25] Thrombin-mediated PAR activation is not only critical for coagulation, but also plays an important role in inflammatory and proliferative responses associated with vascular injury, such as in atherosclerosis and cancer.[26]

The physiologic inhibitors of thrombin are the serine protease inhibitors (serpins) antithrombin, heparin cofactor II, protein C inhibitor, and protease nexin 1, with antithrombin being the primary plasma inhibitor. For all four serpins, the rate of thrombin inhibition can be accelerated by glycosaminoglycans, such as heparin (Table 3–4), through mutual binding to the serpin and thrombin (see Fig. 3–2), which ensures rapid inhibition of thrombin at the intact endothelial cell surface where heparin-like glycosaminoglycans are found.

Heparin and heparin derivatives are clinically used as anticoagulants to inhibit thrombin via antithrombin. Hirudin, which originates from the salivary glands of medicinal leeches, and its recombinant and synthetic derivatives are potent and highly specific inhibitors that directly target the active site and exosite I of thrombin.[27] The target-specific oral anticoagulant dabigatran also inhibits thrombin directly with high specificity and reversibly binds the active site of thrombin.[27,28]

**TABLE 3–4.** Antithrombin Inhibition of Coagulation Proteases

| Second-Order Association Rate Constants (M⁻¹s⁻¹) | | | |
|---|---|---|---|
| **Protease** | **– Heparin** | **+ H5** | **+ UFH** |
| Thrombin | $7.7 \times 10^3$ | $1.5 \times 10^4$ | $4.7 \times 10^7$ |
| Factor Xa | $2.6 \times 10^3$ | $7.6 \times 10^5$ | $6.6 \times 10^6$ |
| Factor IXa | 58 | $3.1 \times 10^4$ | $6.2 \times 10^6$ |
| TF-Factor VIIa | 33 | $4.9 \times 10^3$ | $1.5 \times 10^4$ |
| Factor XIa | $3.6 \times 10^2$ | $1.1 \times 10^3$ | $1.8 \times 10^5$ |
| Factor XIIa | 39 | $1.9 \times 10^3$ | $6.6 \times 10^4$ |
| APC | 0.08 | 1.9 | 2.1 |

APC, activated protein C; TF, tissue factor.

The association rate constants characterizing the antithrombin inhibition of coagulation proteases in the absence of heparin or accelerated by H5, the synthetic pentasaccharide fondaparinux, or UFH, unfractionated heparin, which comprises long heparin molecules. *In vivo*, natural glycosaminoglycan molecules on endothelium and other cells accelerate the rate of inhibition. (See Olson et al.[321])

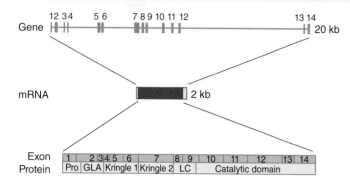

**Figure 3–5.** Relationship of gene structure to protein structure in prothrombin. The exons, introns, mRNA, and protein structure are as indicated. The mRNA is 2 kb with small 5′ and 3′ untranslated regions (shown in *light blue*). In the protein, Pro indicates the prepro leader sequence, GLA indicates the γ-carboxyglutamic acid (Gla) domain, Kringles 1 and 2 are indicated, LC indicates the light chain (also known as the A chain), and the serine protease (catalytic) domain is indicated.

## Gene Structure and Variations

Prothrombin is encoded by a gene (*F2*) on chromosome 11p11.2 that is approximately 20 kb long.[29] The coding sequence is divided over 14 exons that range in size from 25 to 315 bp (Fig. 3–5). The reference sequence of prothrombin mRNA comprises 2018 bases. There are no common, well-characterized, splicing variants with known biology.

Homozygosity or compound heterozygosity for loss-of-function mutations in the prothrombin gene leads to a bleeding tendency. This condition is quite rare, with perhaps one case per 2,000,000 newborns.[30] Heterozygous carriers of loss-of-function mutations are without a bleeding phenotype. Mutations have been characterized in a relatively small number of cases with homozygous or compound heterozygous prothrombin deficiency (consult the Human Gene Mutation Database at http://www.hgmd.org for details). The majority of mutations underlying prothrombin deficiency are missense mutations, but several small deletions/insertions have also been reported.

Gain-of-function mutations in the prothrombin gene increase thrombotic risk. The best known variation is G20210A.[31] This variation of the last nucleotide preceding the poly(A)-tail of the mature mRNA has an effect on 3′-end mRNA processing and increases the level of prothrombin in plasma by approximately 10 to 20 percent in heterozygous individuals.[32] This relatively small increase in the level of prothrombin results in a two- to threefold enhanced risk for venous thrombosis. Homozygotes for the G20210A variation are quite rare, and the risk associated with homozygosity has not been measured with certainty. The G20210A variation is relatively common in whites, with a strong south-north gradient in that the variation is most common in southern Europe.[33]

# FACTOR VII

Factor VII, which was discovered around 1950,[34] is synthesized in the liver and circulates in plasma as a single-chain zymogen of 406 amino acids (Mr ≈50,000) at a concentration of 10 nM with a short plasma half-life of 3 to 6 hours (see Table 3–1).

## Protein Structure

Factor VII consists of a Gla domain with 10 Gla residues, two EGF-like domains, a connecting region, and the serine protease domain (see Fig. 3–1). Calcium coordination in EGF-1 is mediated by partial hydroxylation of Asn63 and *O*-linked fucosylation of Ser60.[35] Further posttranslational modifications of factor VII consist of *O*-linked (Ser52

in EGF-1) and *N*-linked (Asn154 in the connecting region, Asn322 in the serine protease domain) glycosylation.

### Factor VII Activation and Factor VIIa Activity

Factor VII is proteolytically activated once it has formed a high-affinity complex with its cofactor tissue factor. A number of coagulation proteases including thrombin and factors IXa and XIIa are capable of cleaving factor VII at Arg152 to generate factor VIIa (see Fig. 3–1), with factor Xa being considered the most potent and physiologically relevant activator of factor VII.[36] Autoactivation can also occur, which is initiated by minute amounts (approximately 0.1 nM) of preexisting factor VIIa.[37]

Factor VIIa is a two-chain serine protease composed of a light chain (Mr ≈20,000) comprising the Gla and EGF domains and the catalytic heavy chain (Mr ≈30,000), which are covalently linked via a disulfide bond. Factor VIIa activity is only expressed when bound to tissue factor, which induces an active conformation of the factor VIIa serine protease domain (Fig. 3–6).[11] Factor VIIa interacts with tissue factor via its Gla and EGF domains.

The tissue factor–factor VIIa complex activates both coagulation factors IX and X, which is considered to be the main initiating step of the extrinsic pathway of coagulation. In addition, the tissue factor–factor VIIa (–factor Xa) complex is not only critical to processes in coagulation, but also to wound healing, angiogenesis, tissue remodeling, and inflammation through proteolytic activation of PAR2.[38-40]

The ternary tissue factor–factor VIIa–factor Xa complex is inhibited by the tissue factor pathway inhibitor (TFPI). Tissue factor–factor VIIa is also inhibited by antithrombin, but only in the presence of heparin (see Table 3–4).

## Gene Structure and Variations

The gene encoding factor VII (*F7*) is located on chromosome 13q34, is almost 15 kb in length, and comprises 9 exons (Fig. 3–7). The canonical mRNA encoding factor VII comprises 3000 bases.[41] Alternatively spliced transcript variants encoding multiple isoforms have been observed, but their biology is not well characterized.[42]

Inherited factor VII deficiency is a rare autosomal recessive disorder that affects approximately one in 500,000 newborns.[30] Factor VII deficiency is the most common of the inherited rare bleeding disorders,

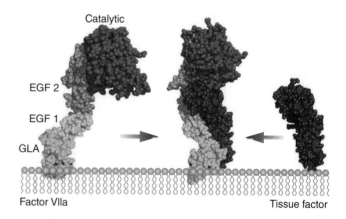

**Figure 3–6.** The tissue factor–factor VIIa complex. A molecular model of factor VIIa (PDB structures 1QHK, 1WHF, 1RFN, 1DAN) and the crystal structures of the tissue factor–factor VIIa complex (PDB structure 1DAN) and the extracellular domain of tissue factor (PDB structure 2HFT) are shown. The γ-carboxyglutamic acid (Gla; GLA) domain, epidermal growth factor (EGF)-like domains 1 and 2, and serine protease (catalytic) domain of factor VIIa are indicated. Binding to tissue factor alters the overall structure of factor VIIa.

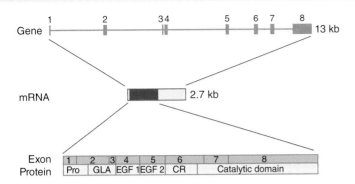

**Figure 3–7.** Relationship of gene structure to protein structure in factor VII. The exons, introns, mRNA, and protein structure are as indicated. The mRNA is 2.7 kb with a small 5′ untranslated region and a relatively large 3′ untranslated region *(light blue)*. In the protein, Pro indicates the prepro leader sequence, GLA indicates the γ-carboxyglutamic acid (Gla) domain, and epidermal growth factor (EGF)-1 and -2, as well as the serine protease (catalytic) domain, are indicated. CR indicates the connecting region that comprises the site of proteolytic activation.

although the reported prevalences vary between countries. Homozygotes and compound heterozygotes develop a hemorrhagic diathesis that may vary from mild to severe.

The Human Gene Mutation Database (http://www.hgmd.org) lists 258 mutations in the factor VII gene. The majority of these are missense mutations, but splicing and regulatory mutations also occur. Small deletions account for almost 10 percent of the documented mutations. Other gross gene abnormalities appear to be uncommon.

The factor VII gene harbors many common polymorphisms of which three are notable: Arg353Gln in the catalytic domain, a 10-bp insertion in the promotor region, and a variable number of 37 bp repeats in intron 7.[43] The minor alleles of these polymorphisms are associated with decreased levels of factor VII and explain up to 30 percent of the variation in activated factor VII levels. Furthermore, the minor alleles have been claimed to lower the risk of myocardial infarction. However, this finding has not led to routine genotyping in the management of this disorder. The relationship between factor VII levels, factor VII polymorphisms, and venous thrombosis has not been established with certainty.

## FACTOR IX

Factor IX was originally reported in 1952 as "Christmas factor," named after one of the first identified hemophilia B patients.[34,44] Factor IX is synthesized in the liver and circulates in plasma as a single-chain zymogen of 415 amino acids (Mr ≈55,000) at a concentration of 90 nM with a half-life of 18 to 24 hours (see Table 3–1).

### Protein Structure

Factor IX consists of a Gla domain, two EGF-like domains, a 35-residue activation peptide, and the serine protease domain (see Fig. 3–1). The Gla domain contains 12 Gla residues, of which the 11th and 12th Gla (Glu36 and Glu40) are not evolutionary conserved in other vitamin K–dependent proteins and are not essential for normal factor IX function.[45]

Factor IX comprises several posttranslational modifications that are not only important for its structure and function, but are also involved in the plasma clearance and distribution of factor IX.[35] Factor IX is sulfated at Tyr155 and phosphorylated at Ser158 in the activation peptide. Hydroxylation of Asp64 in EGF-1 mediates calcium binding, and while only approximately 40 percent of total plasma factor IX carries this modification, complete absence because of a point mutation at this position dramatically reduces factor IX activity resulting in

hemophilia B.[46,47] An *O*-linked fucose (Ser61) and glucose (Ser63) are found in the EGF-1 domain, in addition to several *O*-linked glycans in the activation peptide (Thr159, Thr169, Thr172, and Thr179). Further modification of the activation peptide includes *N*-linked glycosylation of Asn residues 157 and 167, which modulates the circulating levels of factor IX.[48-50]

Factor IX binds with high affinity to the extracellular matrix component collagen IV via residue Lys5 in the Gla domain.[51,52] Although factor IX variants incapable of collagen IV binding exhibit a greater recovery, collagen IV association generates an extravascular reservoir of factor IX that enables prolonged action of factor IX at a hemostatic relevant region.

### Factor IX Activation and Factor IXa Activity

Limited proteolysis of factor IX at both Arg145 and Arg180 by either the tissue factor–factor VIIa complex or factor XIa results in the release of the activation peptide and generation of factor IXa (see Fig. 3–1). Cleavage at Arg180 generates factor IXaα, which displays catalytic activity toward synthetic substrates only, whereas fully active factor IXaβ is formed following cleavage at Arg145.[53,54]

Factor IXa is a two-chain serine protease (Mr ≈45,000) that is composed of a light chain of 145 residues (Mr ≈17,000) and the catalytic heavy chain of 235 residues (Mr ≈28,000), which are covalently linked via a disulfide bond.

Factor IXa has a low catalytic efficiency as a result of impaired access of substrates to the active site that results from steric and electrostatic repulsion.[55] Reversible interaction with the cofactor VIIIa on anionic membranes and subsequent factor X binding leads to rearrangement of the regions surrounding the active site and proteolytic factor X activation.

The primary plasma inhibitor of factor IXa is the serpin antithrombin, and this inhibition is enhanced by heparin (see Table 3–4), which induces a conformational change in antithrombin that is required for simultaneous active site and exosite interactions with factor IXa.[56]

### Gene Structure and Variations

The gene encoding factor IX *(F9)* is located on chromosome Xq27.1 and covers nearly 25 kb.[57] It is divided into eight exons from which a mature mRNA molecule is transcribed with an ultimate length of 2802 bases (Fig. 3–8).

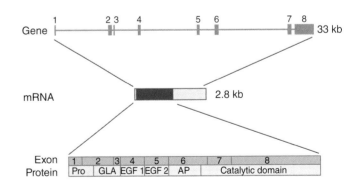

**Figure 3–8.** Relationship of gene structure to protein structure in factor IX. The exons, introns, mRNA, and protein structure are as indicated. The mRNA is 2.8 kb with a small 5′ untranslated region and a relatively large 3′ untranslated region *(light blue)*. In the protein, Pro indicates the prepro leader sequence, GLA indicates the γ-carboxyglutamic acid (Gla) domain, and epidermal growth factor (EGF)-1 and -2, as well as the serine protease (catalytic) domain, are indicated. AP indicates the activation peptide that is released after cleavage of two bonds.

A defect or deficiency in factor IX leads to hemophilia B. Chapter 13 discusses the prevalence, clinical characteristics, and molecular genetics of hemophilia B in detail.

Conversely, increased levels of factor IX are a strong risk factor for venous thrombosis.[58] This is in agreement with a rare gain-of-function mutation (Arg335Leu; factor IX Padua), which renders the protein hyperfunctional and is associated with familial early-onset thrombophilia.[59]

## FACTOR X

Factor X was originally reported in the late 1950s as the "Stuart-Prower factor," named after the first two identified factor X–deficient patients.[60–62] Factor X is primarily synthesized in the liver and circulates in plasma as a two-chain zymogen of 445 amino acids (Mr ≈59,000) at a concentration of 170 nM with a half-life of 34 to 40 hours (see Table 3–1).

### Protein Structure

Factor X is synthesized as a single-chain precursor and during intracellular processing, the three-amino acid peptide Arg140-Lys141-Arg142 is excised. The resulting two-chain zymogen consists of a light chain (Mr ≈16,000), comprising the Gla domain with 11 Gla residues and the EGF domains, that is linked via a disulfide bond to the heavy chain (Mr ≈42,000), which consists of a 52-residue activation peptide and the serine protease domain (see Fig. 3–1).

Hydroxylation of Asp63 mediates calcium binding to the EGF-1 domain and orients the Gla domain, which is essential for factor X clotting activity.[35] N-linked glycosylation of the activation peptide residues Asn181 and Asn191 has been implicated in prolonging the factor X half-life.[63] Further posttranslational modification of factor X consists of O-linked glycosylation at Thr159 and Thr171 in the activation peptide and Thr443 in the serine protease domain. There is some evidence that glycosylation of the human factor X activation peptide may also contribute to substrate recognition by the intrinsic or extrinsic factor X–activating complex.[64,65]

### Factor X Activation and Factor Xa Activity

Factor X is proteolytically activated by either the factor VIIIa–factor IXa ("intrinsic tenase") or the tissue factor–factor VIIa ("extrinsic tenase") enzyme complexes following cleavage at Arg194 in the heavy chain (see Fig. 3–1). This results in the release of the activation peptide and generation of factor Xa, also known as factor Xaα. A snake venom protease from Russell's viper venom (RVV-X) is capable of generating factor Xa in a similar manner.

Factor Xa consists of the Gla and EGF domains comprising light chain (Mr ≈16,000) and the catalytic heavy chain (Mr ≈29,000) that are covalently linked via a disulfide bond. Factor Xa reversibly associates with its cofactor factor Va on an anionic membrane surface in the presence of calcium ions to form prothrombinase, the physiologic activator of prothrombin. Factor Xa is also involved in the proteolytic activation of factors V, VII, and VIII.[66–68]

Similar to thrombin, factor Xa plays a role in other biologic and pathophysiologic processes that are not directly related to coagulation. Factor Xa triggers intracellular signaling via activation of PAR1 and/or PAR2. Factor Xa cleaves PAR2 by itself as well as in complex with tissue factor–factor VIIa. These direct cellular effects of factor Xa contribute to wound healing, tissue remodeling, inflammation, angiogenesis, and atherosclerosis, among others.[26,69]

Further autocatalytic cleavage at Arg429 near the C-terminus of the factor Xa heavy chain leads to release of a 19-residue peptide, yielding the enzymatically active factor Xaβ.[70–72] Plasmin-mediated cleavage

of factor Xa at adjacent C-terminal Arg or Lys residues also results in the generation of factor Xaβ and factor Xaβ derivatives.[73,74] While the coagulation activity is eliminated in the factor Xaβ derivatives, they are capable of interacting with the zymogen plasminogen and enhance its tissue plasminogen activator–mediated conversion to plasmin, thereby promoting fibrinolysis.[75]

A primary plasma inhibitor of factor Xa is the serpin antithrombin, and this inhibition is enhanced by heparin (see Table 3–4), which induces a conformational change in antithrombin that is required for simultaneous active site and exosite interactions with factor Xa.[76] Another potent factor Xa inhibitor is TFPI, which inhibits both the ternary tissue factor–factor VIIa–factor Xa complex as well as free factor Xa, for which protein S functions as a cofactor.[77,78] Free factor Xa is also inhibited by the protein Z/protein Z–dependent protease inhibitor (ZPI) complex on membranes.[79]

Low-molecular-weight heparin and synthetic derivatives (e.g., fondaparinux) are clinically used as anticoagulants to enhance factor Xa inhibition by antithrombin specifically. The target-specific oral anticoagulants rivaroxaban, apixaban, edoxaban, and analogues directly inhibit both free factor Xa and prothrombinase complex–assembled factor Xa with high specificity through a high-affinity, reversible interaction with the factor Xa active site.[80–83]

### Gene Structure and Variations

The gene encoding factor X (F10) is located on chromosome 13q34 and spans almost 27 kb.[84] The eight exons in the factor X gene give rise to a mature mRNA of 1560 bases (Fig. 3–9). There are no common alternative splice variants with known biology.

Loss-of-function mutations in the factor X gene lead to a rare bleeding disorder with a recessive mode of inheritance. Factor X deficiency occurs in approximately one in every 1,000,000 newborns. Most cases of documented factor X deficiency experience serious bleeding problems. In fact, factor X deficiency may be the most severe of the rare congenital bleeding disorders.[30] Well over 100 mutations have been documented in cases with factor X deficiency (http://www.hgmd.org). The majority of these mutations are missense and nonsense mutations.

Gain-of-function mutations in factor X could potentially increase thrombotic risk, but such mutations have not been documented. There

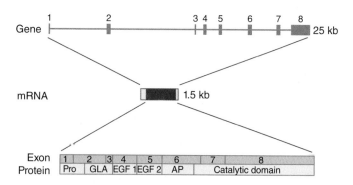

**Figure 3–9.** Relationship of gene structure to protein structure in factor X. The exons, introns, mRNA, and protein structure are as indicated. The mRNA is 1.5 kb with a relatively large 5′ untranslated region and a small 3′ untranslated region. In the protein, Pro indicates the pre-pro leader sequence, GLA indicates the γ-carboxyglutamic acid (Gla) domain, and epidermal growth factor (EGF)-1 and -2, as well as the serine protease (catalytic) domain, are indicated. AP indicates the activation peptide. Before secretion, cleavage in this domain processes factor X to the two-chain mature zymogen. A second cleavage releases the activation peptide and generates factor Xa activity.

is uncertainty about whether common gene variations influence the level of factor X in plasma.[85]

## PROTEIN C

Protein C, which plays a central role in the anticoagulant pathway, was discovered in 1960, and being the third protein peak ("peak C") observed in a vitamin K–dependent plasma protein purification, it was named protein C.[86,87] Protein C is synthesized in the liver and circulates in plasma as a two-chain zymogen of 417 amino acids (Mr ≈62,000) at a concentration of 65 nM with a half-life of 6 to 8 hours (see Table 3–1).

### Protein Structure

Protein C is synthesized as a single-chain precursor, and during intracellular processing, amino acids Lys146-Arg147 are excised. The resulting two-chain zymogen consists of a light chain (Mr ≈21,000) comprising the Gla domain with nine Gla residues and the EGF domains, which is linked via a disulfide bond to the heavy chain (Mr ≈41,000) that consists of the 12-residue activation peptide and the serine protease domain (see Fig. 3–1).

In addition to γ-carboxylation, protein C is hydroxylated at Asp71 in the EGF-1 domain, which coordinates calcium binding.[35] N-linked glycosylation of Asn97 in EGF-1 and Asn248, Asn313, and Asn329 in the serine protease domain are important for efficient protein secretion, proteolytic processing of Lys146-Arg147, and proteolytic activation.[88–90] Some of the total plasma protein C is not glycosylated at either Asn329 (β-protein C) or at both Asn329 and Asn248 (γ-protein C), of which the impact on protein function remains unclear.[91]

### Protein C Activation and Activated Protein C Activity

Protein C is proteolytically activated by α-thrombin in complex with the endothelial cell surface protein thrombomodulin following cleavage at Arg169 (see Fig. 3–1). The activation peptide is released, and the mature serine protease activated protein C (APC) is formed. Activation of protein C is enhanced by its localization on the endothelial surface through association with the endothelial cell protein C receptor (EPCR).[92] Several snake venom proteases (RVV-X and Protac) are also capable of activating protein C.

APC consists of the disulfide-linked light chain comprising the Gla and EGF domains (Mr ≈21,000) and the catalytic heavy chain (Mr ≈32,000). In complex with its cofactor protein S, APC proteolytically inactivates factors Va and VIIIa in a calcium- and membrane-dependent manner. Intact factor V has been reported to function as a cofactor for the inactivation of factor VIIIa in the presence of protein S.[93]

Downregulation of thrombin formation through inactivation of these cofactors seems to occur preferentially on the endothelial cell surface as opposed to that of platelets,[94] where it prevents coagulation and potential thrombosis. However, protein C activation is also accelerated by platelet factor 4 (PF4), which is secreted by activated platelets. Upon interaction with the Gla domain of protein C, PF4 modifies the conformation of protein C, thereby enhancing its affinity for the thrombomodulin-thrombin complex.[95] This ensures APC generation in close proximity of the injury site where platelets are activated, which serves to impede dissemination of coagulation.

APC also plays a major role in the cytoprotective pathway to prevent vascular damage and stress.[96] These activities include antiapoptotic activity, antiinflammatory activity, alterations of gene-expression profiles, and endothelial barrier stabilization. Most of these functions require binding to EPCR and PAR1 cleavage.

APC is primarily inhibited by the heparin-dependent serpin protein C inhibitor and by plasminogen activator inhibitor-1 (PAI-1). Because PAI-1 is the major inhibitor of tissue plasminogen

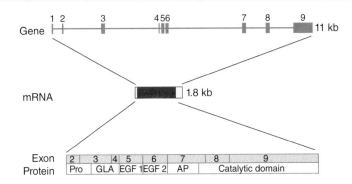

**Figure 3–10.** Relationship of gene structure to protein structure in protein C. The exons, introns, mRNA, and protein structure are as indicated. The mRNA is 1.8 kb with a small 5′ untranslated region coded for by exon 1 and a relatively small 3′ untranslated region (light blue). In the protein, Pro indicates the prepro leader sequence, GLA indicates the γ-carboxyglutamic acid (Gla) domain, and epidermal growth factor (EGF)-1 and -2, as well as the serine protease (catalytic) domain, are indicated. AP indicates the activation peptide. Before secretion, cleavage in this domain processes protein C to the two-chain mature zymogen. A second cleavage releases the activation peptide and generates activated protein C.

activator, inhibition through complex formation with APC contributes to enhanced fibrinolysis. Chapter 4 discusses these and other factors that attenuate the anticoagulant activity of APC.

### Gene Structure and Variations

The protein C gene (PROC) is located on chromosome 2q14.3 and spans almost 11 kb.[97] The gene is divided into nine exons, and the mature mRNA has a length of 1790 bases (Fig. 3–10). There are no alternative mRNA species with known biology.

Loss-of-function mutations cause protein C deficiency. In homozygous or compound heterozygous form, this leads to life-threatening purpura fulminans at birth, which, if left untreated, is fatal.[98] In cases where there is still some protein C activity detectable, symptoms may be much milder.

Heterozygous protein C deficiency increases the risk of venous thrombosis. This is true for most deficiencies of natural anticoagulants and sets them apart from rare bleeding disorders where heterozygosity for loss-of-function mutations is mostly asymptomatic. The risk for venous thrombosis is increased approximately 10-fold in heterozygotes for protein C deficiency, although the risk estimates vary considerably between studies.[99] Family studies in particular suggest a high risk, whereas case-control studies may show markedly lower estimates.[100]

Heterozygous protein C deficiency can be categorized as type I or type II. In type I deficiency, antigen levels are approximately 50 percent of normal, whereas in type II deficiency, antigen levels are (near) normal but activity levels are decreased by 50 percent.

The genetic basis of protein C deficiency, consistent with what is observed in general for congenital loss-of-function disorders, is heterogeneous. In line with this, more than 300 mutations have been documented and are tracked in the Human Gene Mutation Database (http://www.hgmd.org). Two-thirds of these documented mutations are missense or nonsense.

Several common polymorphisms, in particular in the promotor region of the protein C gene, are known to have a small but measurable effect on plasma protein C levels. Alleles of these polymorphisms that are associated with lower protein C levels are also associated with an increased thrombotic risk, albeit the effect is small.[101] Therefore, it is not surprising that measurement of these polymorphisms has not found any clinical application.

# ●THE PROCOAGULANT COFACTORS V AND VIII

Factors V and VIII both function as cofactors in coagulation and dramatically enhance the catalytic rate of their macromolecular enzyme complexes, resulting in the generation of thrombin and factor Xa, respectively. Apart from their functional equivalence, they also share similar gene structures, amino acid sequences, and protein domain structures, which is not surprising considering that factors V and VIII are assumed to descend from the common ancestral A1-A2-A3 domain-containing copper-binding plasma protein ceruloplasmin through a gene duplication event.[102] After acquiring C-type domains as well as the central B domain, a second gene duplication ultimately separated the ancestral genes of factors V and VIII.

Factors V and VIII undergo similar mechanisms of intracellular processing in the endoplasmic reticulum (ER) and Golgi apparatus. Trafficking through this early secretory pathway involves interaction of factors V and VIII with a receptor complex that consists of the mannose-binding lectin-1 gene product LMAN1 (also called ER-Golgi intermediate compartment [ERGIC]-53) and multiple coagulation deficiency protein 2 (MCFD2).[103] Defects or deficiencies in one of the two subunits of the receptor complex can result in a combined deficiency of factors V and VIII (Chap. 14).

## FACTOR V

In 1943, Norwegian physician Paul Owren discovered the fifth coagulation factor thus far known and named it factor V.[104–106] Factor V is synthesized in the liver and circulates in plasma as a large single-chain procofactor of 2196 amino acids ($Mr \approx 330,000$) at a concentration of 20 nM with a half-life of 12 to 36 hours (see Table 3–1).

Approximately 20 percent of the total factor V in blood is stored in the α-granules of platelets. Although it was originally thought that megakaryocytes synthesize factor V, studies in humans indicate that platelet factor V originates from plasma through endocytic uptake.[107–109] Platelet factor V is modified intracellularly such that it is functionally unique compared to its plasma-derived counterpart. It is partially activated, more resistant to inactivation by APC, and has several different posttranslational modifications.[110]

Platelet factor V is associated with the large multimeric protein multimerin.[111] Multimerin has a massive repeating structure, with some of the multimers having molecular weights of several million daltons. Although the function of this platelet factor V–specific multimeric chaperon protein is similar to that of VWF, the multimeric chaperon protein of factor VIII in plasma, multimerin and VWF share no structural homology.

Following platelet activation, platelet factor V becomes available at the site of injury and can reach local concentrations that exceed the factor V plasma concentration by more than 100-fold.[112] Interestingly, the origin of factor V in mouse platelets differs from humans in that it is synthesized in megakaryocytes and stored into the α-granules before platelets are released from the marrow.[113,114]

## Protein Structure

Factor V has an A1-A2-B-A3-C1-C2 domain structure (Fig. 3–11). The three A-type domains share significant homology with those of ancestral ceruloplasmin as well as with the factor VIII A domains (approximately 50 percent sequence identity). The two C-type domains belong to the family of discoidin domains, which are generally involved in cell adhesion, and share approximately 55 percent sequence identity with the factor VIII C domains. The C domains mediate binding to the anionic phospholipid surface, thereby localizing factor V to the site of injury and facilitating interaction with factor Xa and prothrombin.[115–118] In contrast, the large central B domain of factor V shows weak homology to the factor VIII B domain or to any other known protein domain. However, this domain comprises so-called basic and acidic regions that are highly conserved throughout evolution and serve to negatively regulate factor V function and prevent activity of the procofactor.[119,120]

Factor V undergoes extensive posttranslational modifications, including sulfation, phosphorylation, and N-linked glycosylation.[35,121] Sulfation at sites in the A2 and B domain are involved in the thrombin-mediated proteolytic activation of factor V.[122] Phosphorylation at Ser692 in the A2 domain enhances the APC-dependent inactivation of the cofactor Va.[123] N-linked glycosylation occurs throughout the whole protein; however, the majority of carbohydrates are linked to Asn residues within the B domain and play a role in the LMAN1-MCDF2 receptor complex-mediated trafficking of factor V from the ER to the Golgi in the early secretory pathway.[103] Partial glycosylation at Asn2181 in the C2 domain of factor V results in a lower binding affinity for negatively charged membranes of the glycosylated form, thereby reducing the factor V procoagulant activity, particularly at low phospholipid concentrations.[124,125] Furthermore, factor V comprises several disulfide bonds that are important for the three-dimensional structure of the A and C domains.[121]

### Factor V Procofactor Activation and Factor Va Cofactor Function

Sequential proteolytic cleavage of the procofactor factor V at Arg709, Arg1018, and Arg1545 in the B domain results in release of the inhibitory constraints exerted by the B domain and in the generation of the heterodimeric cofactor Va (see Fig. 3–11).[126] Maximal cofactor activity correlates with cleavage at Arg1545, which is consistent with the observation that a snake venom protease from RVV-V, which cleaves only at Arg1545, results in full activation. Thrombin has generally been recognized to be the principal activator of factor V. However, recent findings suggest that in the initiation phase of coagulation factor V is primarily activated by factor Xa.[127] Factor Xa initially cleaves factor V at Arg1018, followed by proteolysis at Arg709 and Arg1545.[128]

Factor Va is composed of a heavy chain ($Mr \approx 105,000$) comprising the A1-A2 domains and the A3-C1-C2 light chain ($Mr \approx 74,000$), which are noncovalently associated via calcium ions. Factor Va is a nonenzymatic cofactor within the prothrombinase complex that greatly accelerates the ability of factor Xa to rapidly convert prothrombin to thrombin.[129] APC catalyzes the inactivation of factor Va by cleavage at the main sites Arg306 and Arg506, upon which the cleaved A2 fragment

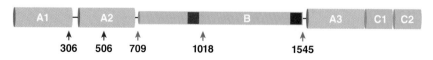

**Figure 3–11.** The domain structure of factor V. Schematic A1-A2-B-A3-C1-C2 domain representation of factor V. Thrombin cleavage sites (Arg709, Arg1018, Arg1545) are indicated by *green arrows*, and activated protein C (APC) cleavage sites (Arg306, Arg506) by *red arrows*. The *blue* and *red* boxes in the B domain represent the basic and acidic regions, respectively, that are highly conserved throughout evolution and serve to negatively regulate factor V function and prevent activity of the procofactor V.

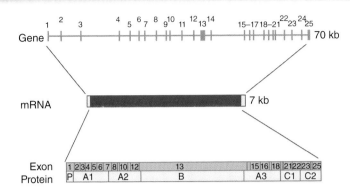

**Figure 3–12.** Relationship of gene structure to protein structure in factor V. The exons, introns, mRNA, and protein structure are as indicated. The mRNA is 7 kb with some 5′ and 3′ untranslated sequences *(light blue)*. In the protein, P indicates the propeptide leader sequence, and the A1-A2-B-A3-C1-C2 domains are indicated.

dissociates and factor Va can no longer associate with factor Xa.[130] A common Arg506Gln mutation in factor V leads to resistance to inactivation by APC (factor V Leiden) and is associated with an increased risk of venous thromboembolism (Chap. 23).[131]

Both factor V and an alternatively spliced isoform of factor V (factor V-short), which lacks the major part of the B domain (residues 756 to 1458) and normally circulates in low abundance, interact with full-length TFPI (TFPIα), most likely through the acidic B domain region.[132,133] The linkage of factor V and TFPIα is considered to attenuate the bleeding phenotype in factor V–deficient patients, as the low TFPIα levels in these patients allow the residual platelet factor V to be sufficient for coagulation.[132,134] Conversely, increased factor V-short expression caused by an A2440G mutation in the factor V gene leads to a dramatic increase in plasma TFPIα, resulting in a bleeding disorder.[133]

### Gene Structure and Variations

The gene for factor V *(F5)* is located on chromosome 1q23. It is located very close to the genes for the selectin family of leukocyte adhesion molecules. The factor V gene spans approximately 70 kb and consists of 25 exons (Fig. 3–12). The gene structure is very similar to that of the factor VIII gene, with exon–intron boundaries occurring at exactly the same location in 21 out of 24 cases.[135]

Homozygosity or compound heterozygosity for loss-of-function mutations in the factor V gene leads to a bleeding disorder (termed *parahemophilia* or *Owren parahemophilia*).[136] At the time of writing, 152 mutations in the factor V gene have been collected in the Human Gene Mutation Database (www.hgmd.org).

Gain-of-function mutations in the factor V gene increase the risk of thrombosis. This is particularly the case for venous thrombosis and not so much for arterial thrombosis. In whites, the most common gain-of-function mutation in the factor V gene is factor V Leiden (Arg506Gln), which leads to a plasma abnormality known as APC resistance (Chap. 23).[137,138]

## FACTOR VIII

Factor VIII (antihemophilic factor) was first discovered in 1937, but it was not until 1979 that its purification by Tuddenham and coworkers led to the molecular identification of the protein.[139,140] Factor VIII is synthesized as a single-chain preprocofactor of 2351 amino acids and, subsequent to intracellular processing, is secreted as a series of metal ion-linked heterodimers due to proteolysis at the A3-B junction and differential processing in the central B domain (Fig. 3–13). The mature factor VIII procofactor comprises 2332 amino acids (Mr ≈300,000) and circulates in a high-affinity complex with its carrier protein VWF at a concentration of approximately 0.7 nM and a circulatory half-life of 8 to 12 hours (see Table 3–1). Complex formation with VWF protects factor VIII from proteolytic degradation, premature ligand binding, and rapid clearance from the circulation.

The primary source of factor VIII is the liver,[141,142] but extrahepatic synthesis of factor VIII also occurs.[143,144] While contradictory evidence exists on the cellular origin of both hepatic and extrahepatic factor VIII synthesis, recent studies in mice support that endothelial cells from many tissues and vascular beds synthesize factor VIII, with a large contribution from hepatic sinusoidal endothelial cells.[145–147] This is consistent with observations on factor VIII expression in human endothelial cells from the liver and lung.[148,149]

Factor VIII is less-efficiently secreted from the cell as compared to factor V, because it interacts with the ER-chaperon proteins calnexin and calreticulin, whereas factor V interacts with calreticulin only.[150] Both chaperons preferentially interact with GPs comprising mono-glucosylated N-linked oligosaccharides and promote correct folding of proteins that enter the secretory pathway and target misfolded proteins for degradation. Factor VIII, but not factor V, also interacts with the ER-chaperon immunoglobulin-binding protein (BiP/GRP78), which appears to enhance the stability of factor VIII but also retards its secretion.[151] Factor VIII trafficking from the ER to the Golgi is mediated via the LMAN1-MCDF2 receptor complex, similar to factor V.[103]

Several clearance receptors are responsible for actively removing factor VIII from the circulation, which include the low-density lipoprotein (LDL) receptor-related protein 1 (LRP1), the LDL receptor, and receptors that specifically interact with carbohydrate structures on factor VIII.[152–156]

### Protein Structure

The A1-A2-B-A3-C1-C2 domain structure of factor VIII shares significant homology with factor V except in the B domain region (see Fig. 3–13). In contrast to factor V, the factor VIII B domain is dispensable for procoagulant activity. The mature factor VIII procofactor comprises a variably sized heavy chain (A1-A2-B; Mr ≈90,000 to 200,000 depending on the extent of proteolysis) and a light chain (A3-C1-C2; Mr ≈80,000). The C-terminal regions of the A1 and A2 domains and the N-terminal portion of the A3 domain contain short segments of 30 to 40 negatively charged residues known as the a1, a2, and a3 regions. Interaction with VWF is facilitated by the a3 region and C1 domain.[157,158] The C domains mediate binding to the anionic phospholipid surface, thereby localizing factor VIII to the site of injury and facilitating interaction with factor IXa and factor X.[159–161]

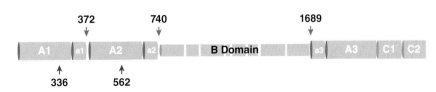

**Figure 3–13.** The domain structure of factor VIII. Schematic A1-a1-A2-a2-B-a3-A3-C1-C2 domain representation of factor VIII. The acidic regions denoted by a1, a2, and a3 are indicated, thrombin cleavage sites (Arg372, Arg740, Arg1689) are indicated by *green arrows*, and activated protein C (APC) cleavage sites (Arg336, Arg562) by *red arrows*. The variably sized B domain as a result of differential proteolytic processing is indicated.

Factor VIII is heavily glycosylated, and the majority of the *N*-linked glycosylation sites are found in the B domain, which mediate interaction with the chaperons calnexin and calreticulin and, in part, with the LMAN1–MCDF2 receptor complex.[103,150,162] Sulfation of tyrosine residues is required for optimal activation by thrombin, maximal activity in complex with factor IXa, and maximal affinity of factor VIIIa for VWF.[35,163] Factor VIII comprises two phosphorylation sites that are located in the A1 (Thr351) and B (Ser1657) domains.

### Factor VIII Procofactor Activation and Factor VIIIa Cofactor Function

Thrombin and factor Xa are the principal activators of the procofactor VIII and generate the cofactor VIIIa through sequential proteolysis at Arg740, Arg372, and Arg1689.[126,164–166] The heterotrimeric factor VIIIa is composed of the A1 (Mr ≈50,000), A2 (Mr ≈43,000), and the A3-C1-C2 light chain (Mr ≈73,000) subunits (see Fig. 3–13). The A1 and A3-C1-C2 subunits are noncovalently linked through calcium ions, whereas A2 is associated with weak affinity primarily by electrostatic interactions.[167,168] Once activated, factor VIIIa functions as a cofactor for factor IXa in the phospholipid-dependent conversion of factor X to factor Xa. The rapid and spontaneous loss of factor VIIIa cofactor activity is attributed to A2 domain dissociation from the heterotrimer.[167,168] Additional proteolysis by APC, factor Xa, or factor IXa also results in the downregulation of factor VIIIa cofactor activity.[169]

### Gene Structure and Variations

The factor VIII encoding gene (*F8*) is situated at chromosome Xq28. The factor VIII gene contains 26 exons (Fig. 3–14), one more than factor V, because exon 5 of factor V corresponds to exons 5 and 6 of the factor VIII gene.[170] In addition, the gene for factor VIII is much larger than that of factor V, spanning approximately 190 kb. This is largely because six of the introns in the factor VIII gene are much larger than the corresponding *F5* introns. The mRNA for factor VIII is also much larger than the factor V mRNA because of a 1.8-kb 3'-untranslated region.

A defect or deficiency in factor VIII leads to hemophilia A. Chapter 13 discusses the prevalence, clinical characteristics, and molecular genetics of hemophilia A in detail.

High levels of factor VIII are a common and strong risk factor for venous thrombosis. It has been suspected that certain genetic variations in the factor VIII gene might play a role in determining the level of factor VIII; however, such variations have not been identified.[171] The ABO blood group does play a role in determining the level of factor VIII, but probably indirectly through an effect on the level of VWF.[172,173]

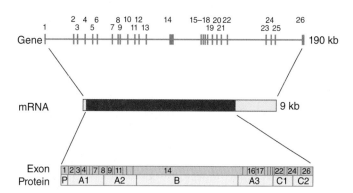

**Figure 3–14.** Relationship of gene structure to protein structure in factor VIII. The exons, introns, mRNA, and protein structure are as indicated. The mRNA is 9 kb with some 5' untranslated sequence and a large 3' untranslated region (*light blue*). In the protein, P indicates the propeptide leader sequence, and the A1-A2-B-A3-C1-C2 domains are indicated.

# THE SOLUBLE COFACTORS PROTEIN S AND VON WILLEBRAND FACTOR

## PROTEIN S

Protein S, which is named after the city (Seattle) where it was discovered by the group of Earl Davie in 1977, is a vitamin K–dependent single-chain GP of 635 amino acids (Mr ≈75,000) that circulates with a plasma half-life of 42 hours (see Table 3–1). Part of the total protein S pool circulates in a free form at a concentration of 150 nM, whereas the majority (approximately 60 percent; 200 nM) circulates bound to the complement regulatory protein C4b–binding protein (C4BP). Protein S is primarily synthesized in the liver by hepatocytes, in addition to endothelial cells, megakaryocytes, testicular Leydig cells, and osteoblasts.[174–178]

### Protein Structure

The protein structure of protein S differs from the other vitamin K–dependent proteins as it lacks a serine protease domain and, consequently, is not capable of catalytic activity. Protein S is composed of a Gla domain comprising 11 Gla residues, a thrombin-sensitive region (TSR), four EGF domains, and a C-terminal sex hormone–binding globulin (SHBG)-like region that consists of two laminin G-type domains (Fig. 3–15). The SHBG-like domain is involved in the interaction with the β-subunit of C4BP.

Apart from γ-carboxylation of Glu residues, protein S is post-translationally modified via *N*-glycosylation in the second laminin G-type domain of the SHBG-like region (Asn458, Asn468, Asn489). β-Hydroxylation of Asp95 or Asn residues (Asn136, Asn178, Asn217) in each EGF domain allows for calcium binding that orients the four EGF domains relative to each other.[35]

### Protein S Cofactor Function

Free protein S serves as a cofactor for APC in the proteolytic inactivation of factors Va and VIIIa.[179,180] Interaction of protein S with APC on a negatively charged membrane surface alters the location of the APC active site relative to factor Va,[181] which accounts for the selective protein S–dependent rate enhancement of APC cleavage at Arg306 in factor Va.[182] C4BP-bound protein S also exerts a similar stimulatory effect on Arg306 cleavage, albeit to lower extent, whereas it inhibits the initial APC-mediated factor Va cleavage at Arg506, resulting in an overall inhibition of factor Va inactivation.[183] Cleavage of the TSR by thrombin and/or factor Xa results in a loss of APC-cofactor activity.[184] Protein S also functions as a cofactor for TFPIα in the inhibition of factor Xa, which is mediated by the SHBG-like region in protein S.[77,185]

Protein S has been implied to play a role in phagocytosis of apoptotic cells, cell survival, activation of innate immunity, vessel integrity and angiogenesis, and local invasion and metastasis through interaction with a family of protein tyrosine kinase receptors referred to as Tyro-3, Axl and Mer (TAM) receptors.[186,107]

### Gene Structure and Variations

The gene encoding protein S (*PROS1*) is located on the long arm of chromosome 3 (3q11.1), very close to the centromere. A highly homologous protein S pseudogene (*PROSP*) is located on the other side of the centromere. This pseudogene is inactive, as it is not transcribed into mRNA.[188] The active protein S gene encompasses 15 exons and covers a little more than 100 kb (Fig. 3–16). The mRNA sequence consists of 3560 bases. Several alternative transcripts have been identified, but none of these have known biology.

Loss-of-function mutations in *PROS1* lead to protein S deficiency. Several cases of homozygous and compound heterozygous

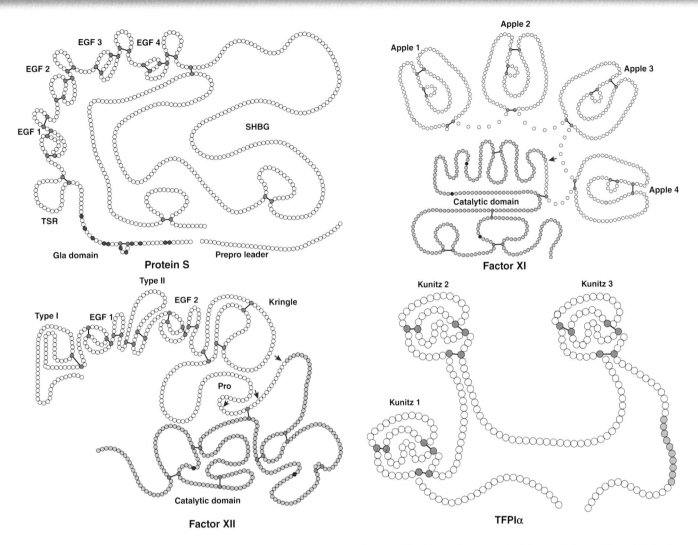

**Figure 3–15.** Protein S, factor XI, factor XII, and tissue factor pathway inhibitor (TFPI). Schematic of protein S, factor XI, factor XII, and TFPIα. Each *circle* represents an amino acid. For protein S: the prepro leader sequence comprising the signal peptide as well as the propeptide is indicated, the γ-carboxyglutamic acid (Gla) domain is indicated with the Gla residues in *blue*, TSR represents the thrombin-sensitive region, the four epidermal growth factor (EGF) domains are indicated, and SHBG represents the sex hormone–binding globulin-like region. For factor XI: the four apple domains are indicated, and the serine protease (catalytic) domain is shown. Cys321 in the apple 4 domain that forms a disulfide link with Cys321 in the other factor XI subunit, thereby mediating dimerization, is indicated in *yellow*. For factor XII: types I and II represent the fibronectin types I and II domains, the two EGF-like domains are indicated, the kringle domain is indicated, Pro indicates the proline-rich region, and the serine protease (catalytic) domain is indicated. For TFPIα: the three Kunitz domains are indicated and the C-terminal sequence of basic residues is indicated in *light blue*. Factors XI and XII have homologous serine protease ("catalytic") domains (shown in *light red*), in which the active site His, Asp, and Ser residues are indicated in *dark red*. Cleavages that convert the zymogens factor XI and factor XII to an active enzyme are indicated by the *red arrows*. Cysteine residues that form a disulfide bridge *(black line)* are indicated in *green*.

protein S deficiency have been described with extremely low protein S levels. These very rare cases suffer from life-threatening purpura fulminans at birth.[189]

Much more common are heterozygous deficiencies of protein S, which can be categorized into three types of deficiency. Type I deficiency is characterized by antigen levels that are approximately 50 percent of normal. In type II deficiency, antigen levels are (near) normal while activity levels are decreased by 50 percent. Type III deficiency is defined by a low level of free protein S. In keeping with this classification, clinical chemistry laboratories may offer a protein S activity assay, free antigen assay, or total antigen assay (or a combination thereof). These assays are not without problems, and the evaluation of protein S levels is fraught with complications that need careful attention before a final diagnosis can be made.[190]

The genetic basis of protein S deficiency is highly heterogeneous, and there are more than 200 entries in the Human Gene Mutation Database (www.hgmd.org). Most of these are missense mutations. However, protein S deficiency is often characterized by gross gene deletions that sometimes even involve neighboring genes.[191] The reason for this preponderance of gross gene abnormalities remains unknown.

It is commonly assumed that protein S deficiency increases venous thrombotic risk by 10-fold.[100] This assertion is mainly based on studies in thrombophilic families. In population-based case-control studies, however, the risk increase appears to be much more modest, if present at all.[192] The reason for this discrepancy between family and population-based studies remains enigmatic. The findings argue against including tests for protein S deficiency in a thrombophilia workup of venous thrombosis cases with a negative family history.

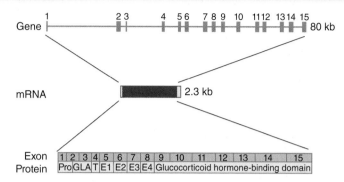

**Figure 3–16.** Relationship of gene structure to protein structure in protein S. The exons, introns, mRNA, and protein structure are as indicated. The mRNA is 2.3 kb with small 5′ and 3′ untranslated regions *(light blue)*. In the protein, Pro indicates the prepro leader sequence, GLA indicates the γ-carboxyglutamic acid (Gla) domain, T indicates the thrombin-sensitive region, E indicates the epidermal growth factor (EGF)-like domains, and the glucocorticoid hormone–binding domain represents the sex hormone–binding globulin (SHBG)-like domain.

## VON WILLEBRAND FACTOR

Chapter 16 discusses the structure, function, and molecular biology of VWF in detail. VWF is a large multimeric GP that is required for normal platelet adhesion to components of the vessel wall and that serves as a carrier for factor VIII. It is exclusively synthesized in megakaryocytes and endothelial cells and stored in specialized organelles in platelets and endothelial cells. Release of VWF multimers from these organelles follows upon a stimulus or via unstimulated basal secretion from endothelial cells.[193] VWF multimers circulate at a concentration of 10 nM with a half-life of 8 to 12 hours (see Table 3–1). Clearance of VWF multimers is mainly mediated by macrophages from the liver and spleen.[194]

Large VWF multimers are cleaved by the plasma protease ADAMTS-13 (a disintegrin and metalloproteinase with thrombospondin motifs 13).[195] This cleavage produces the smaller size VWF multimers that circulate in plasma. Reduced ADAMTS-13 activity is linked to various microangiopathies with increased platelet activity.

### Protein Structure

The precursor protein of VWF is composed of a 22-residue signal peptide and of a proVWF protein comprising 2791 amino acids that has 14 distinct domains in the order of D1-D2-D′-D3-A1-A2-A3-D4-B1-B2-B3-C1-C2-CK.[196] Upon translocation to the ER, the signal peptide is cleaved off, and the proVWF dimerizes in a tail-to-tail fashion through cysteines in its cysteine knot (CK) domain. During transit through the Golgi apparatus, proVWF dimers multimerize in a head-to-head fashion through the formation of disulfide bonds between cysteine residues in the D3 domain. At the same time, D1 and D2 domains are cleaved off as a single fragment to form the VWF propeptide (741 amino acids), while the remaining domains comprising 2050 amino acid residues and up to 22 carbohydrate chains form mature VWF. In the *trans*-Golgi network, the VWF propeptide promotes mature VWF to assemble into high-molecular-weight multimers (Mr ≈500,000 to 20,000,000). These multimers subsequently aggregate into tubular structures that are packaged into α-granules in megakaryocytes and into Weibel-Palade bodies in endothelial cells.

### von Willebrand Factor Function

Upon exocytosis from Weibel-Palade bodies and at high shear rates, multimeric VWF unrolls from a globular to a filamental conformation (often called *VWF strings*), up to many microns long, which becomes a high-affinity surface for the platelet GPIb–V–IX complex. Large VWF multimers are more active than smaller multimers, which is explained by the fact that the former contain multiple domains that support the interactions between platelets, endothelial cells, and subendothelial collagen.

VWF binds to matrix collagens via its A1 and A3 domains. The A1 domain also mediates binding to platelet GPIb, which is required for the fast capture of platelets.[197] Platelet adhesion to VWF is further supported by VWF immobilization on a surface (collagen, other platelets) and by high shear stress.

VWF complexes with factor VIII through the first 272 residues in the N-terminal region of the mature VWF protein subunit,[198] thereby protecting factor VIII from proteolytic degradation, premature ligand binding, and rapid clearance from the circulation.

### Gene Structure and Variations

The VWF gene (*VWF*) is located on chromosome 12p13.3, spans approximately 180 kb, and contains 52 exons.[199] The VWF mRNA is 8.7 kb long. There are no alternative transcripts with known biology. A partially inactive pseudogene that includes exons 23 to 34 is located on chromosome 22p11–13.[199] The VWF gene is very polymorphic, which makes it sometimes difficult to distinguish between disease causing mutations and neutral gene variations.

Qualitative or quantitative deficiencies in VWF cause von Willebrand disease (VWD), a mild to severe bleeding disorder. Quantitative deficiency of VWF leads to type 1 or type 3 VWD, whereas functional defects lead to type 2 VWD. Type 1 VWD is the most common form, but type 3 VWD is the most severe. Chapter 16 discusses VWD in detail.

High levels of VWF are a risk factor for venous and arterial thrombosis. Genome-wide association studies led to the identification of several genomic loci that influence the level of VWF, including the VWF gene itself, the ABO blood group, *STXB5*, and *SCARA5*.[200] Polymorphisms in several of these loci are also associated with thrombotic risk.[201]

## ⬤ FACTOR XI AND THE CONTACT SYSTEM

### FACTOR XI

Factor XI, which was discovered in the early 1950s,[202,203] is synthesized in the liver and secreted as a single-chain zymogen of 607 amino acids (Mr ≈80,000). In the circulation, factor XI is found as a homodimer (Mr ≈160,000) at a concentration of 30 nM with a plasma half-life of 60 to 80 hours (see Table 3–1). All factor XI homodimers circulate in complex with high-molecular-weight kininogen (HK).[204] HK is thought to mediate binding of factor XI to negatively charged surfaces, thereby facilitating factor XI activation.[205] There is conflicting evidence suggesting that HK may be also involved in the interaction of factor XI with the activated platelet surface via GPIb.[206]

### Protein Structure

Each factor XI subunit comprises four apple domains and a serine protease domain (see Fig. 3–15). The apple domains are structured by three disulfide bonds and form a disk-like platform on which the serine protease domain rests.[207] The dimerization of two factor XI subunits is mediated by interactions between the two apple 4 domains that involve a disulfide bond between the Cys321 residues, hydrophobic interactions, and a salt bridge, of which only the latter two are required for dimerization.[206] The domain structure of factor XI is highly similar to that of the monomer prekallikrein (PK), the zymogen of the protease kallikrein, which also circulates in complex with HK.[206]

Factor XI does not bear a Gla domain and thus does not require γ-carboxylation to exert its procoagulant activity. *N*-linked glycosylation occurs at three sites in the apple 1, 2, and 4 domains (Asn82, Asn114, Asn335) and at two sites in the serine protease domain (Asn432, Asn473).

### Factor XI Activation and Activity

Activation of a factor XI subunit to factor XIa proceeds through proteolysis at Arg369 in the N-terminal region of the serine protease domain and yields two-chain activated factor XIa. There are several catalysts capable of factor XI activation, which include the contact factor XIIa, thrombin, or factor XIa itself in the presence of negatively charged surfaces.[208,209] However, their mechanisms differ as factor XI must be a dimer to be activated by factor XIIa, whereas thrombin and factor XIa lack this requirement.[210] An activated factor XI dimer may comprise either one (1/2-factor XIa) or two factor XIa subunits.[211]

Following activation of factor XI, binding sites for the substrate factor IX become available in the apple 3 domain and serine protease domain of factor XIa.[212,213] Factor XIa proteolytically activates factor IX to factor IXa in a calcium-dependent but phospholipid-independent manner. Both forms of the factor XIa dimer as well as monomeric factor XIa activate factor IX in a similar manner.[211]

Accumulating evidence supports the notion that factor XIa–dependent activation of factor XI is not essential to normal hemostasis but is important in pathologic thrombus formation.[214-216] Thrombin-mediated activation of factor XI, on the other hand, seems most significant under conditions of low tissue factor and is assumed to enhance clot stability through thrombin activation of TAFI.[217,218]

Factor XI has been reported to interact with platelet GPIb, which is mediated through a site within the apple 3 domain, and to platelet apolipoprotein E receptor 2 (ApoER2).[219,220] It has been proposed that the dimeric structure allows for simultaneous interaction with the platelet by one subunit, thereby localizing factor XI to the site of clot formation, while binding to factor IX with the other subunit.[221]

Factor XIa function is regulated by the serpins protease nexin 1, antithrombin, C1-inhibitor, $\alpha_1$-protease inhibitor, protein Z–dependent protease inhibitor, and $\alpha_2$-antiplasmin.[216,222] Platelets also contain a factor XIa inhibitor, the Kunitz-type inhibitor protease nexin 2.[223]

### Gene Structure and Variations

The human factor XI gene *(F11)* is 23 kb in length and is localized to chromosome 4q35. It consists of 15 exons and 14 introns (Fig. 3–17). Each of the four apple domains is encoded by two exons. The serine protease domain is encoded by five exons, with an organization similar to the homologous protein PK.

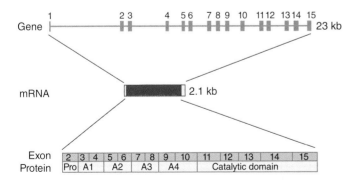

**Figure 3–17.** Relationship of gene structure to protein structure in factor XI. The exons, introns, mRNA, and protein structure are as indicated. The mRNA is 2.1 kb with small 5′ and 3′ untranslated regions (*light blue*). In the protein, Pro indicates the prepro leader sequence, A1 to A4 indicate apple domains 1 to 4, and the serine protease (catalytic) domain is indicated.

Deficiencies of factor XI in humans can lead to a bleeding tendency, although not as severe as in hemophilia A or B.[224] Deficiency of factor XI is relatively common among Ashkenazi Jews in Israel.[225] The Human Gene Mutation Database lists 232 mutations in the factor XI gene (www.hgmd.org).

Increased levels of factor XI are a risk factor for venous thrombosis.[226] Genetic variations in the form of common single nucleotide polymorphisms (SNPs) seem to play a role in determining the level of factor XI and contribute to thrombotic risk.[227]

## ● THE CONTACT SYSTEM: FACTOR XII, PREKALLIKREIN, AND HIGH-MOLECULAR-WEIGHT KININOGEN

Factor XII, HK, and PK are part of the contact system in blood coagulation, which is triggered following contact activation of factor XII mediated via a negatively charged surface. PK is synthesized in the liver, circulates as a zymogen, and is highly homologous to factor XI (see Table 3–1). Conversion into the serine protease proceeds through limited proteolysis by activated factor XII, and the generated kallikrein reciprocally activates more factor XII. HK, which is also synthesized in the liver, is a nonenzymatic cofactor that circulates in complex with factor XI or PK (see Table 3–1). HK is cleaved at two sites by kallikrein to release the bioactive nonapeptide bradykinin, a potent vasodilator.

The contact system is at the basis of the activated partial thromboplastin time (APTT) assay that is widely used in clinical practice. In this clinical laboratory test, the negatively charged surface is provided by reagents such as glass, kaolin, celite, or ellagic acid. Factor XIIa activates factor XI, which then activates factor IX. Despite HK and PK being required for a normal APTT, they appear to be dispensable for coagulation *in vivo*.[228] Individuals who are deficient in any of these factors do not have a bleeding tendency, even after significant trauma or surgery. However, factor XII, HK, and PK do participate in bacteremia or inflammatory responses in acute-phase reactions that do not involve the coagulation, but the classical complement system.[228]

### FACTOR XII

Factor XII was originally reported in 1955 as the "Hageman factor," named after the first identified factor XII–deficient patient.[229] Factor XII is synthesized in the liver and circulates in plasma as a single-chain zymogen of 596 amino acids (Mr ≈80,000) at a concentration of 500 nM with a half-life of 50 to 70 hours (see Table 3–1).

### Protein Structure

Factor XII, which is homologous to plasminogen activators, consists of an N-terminal fibronectin type I domain, an EGF-like domain, a fibronectin type II domain, a second EGF-like domain, a kringle domain, a proline-rich region, and a C-terminal serine protease domain (see Fig. 3–15). The proline-rich region is unique to factor XII, as it is not found in any of the other serine proteases.

Factor XII comprises an O-linked fucose in EGF-1 (Thr90), N-linked glycosylation sites in the kringle domain (Asn230) and the serine protease domain (Asn414), and several O-linked glycosylation sites in the kringle domain and proline-rich region.[230,231]

### Factor XII Activation and Activity

Limited proteolysis by kallikrein at Arg353 in factor XII yields the activated two-chain α-factor XIIa, in which the heavy chain (the fibronectin types I and II domains, both EGF domains, the kringle domain, and proline-rich region; Mr ≈52,000) and light chain (serine protease domain; Mr ≈28,000) are linked via a Cys340–Cys467 disulfide bond (see Fig. 3–15). Once activated, α-factor XIIa activates factor XI to factor XIa. Furthermore, α-factor XIIa activates PK, thereby contributing to its own feedback activation.[232]

Factor XII is also known to acquire α-factor XIIa activity upon contact with a negatively charged surface, the latter inducing a conformational change in factor XII.[233] This conformational change induces a limited amount of proteolytic activity in factor XII, known as autoactivation.[234,235] Furthermore, the surface-induced active conformation of factor XII is suggested to enhance the proteolytic conversion to α-factor XIIa.[236] The fibronectin types I and II domains, EGF-2, the kringle domain, and the proline-rich region are reported to contribute to interaction with a negatively charged surface.[237–240] These naturally occurring surfaces include platelet polyphosphate (poly-P), microparticles derived from platelets and erythrocytes, RNA, and collagen.[241–244]

Further cleavage of α-factor XIIa by kallikrein at Arg334 and Arg343 in the light chain (proline-rich region) results in the generation of β-factor XIIa, which comprises a nine-residue heavy-chain fragment that is disulfide-linked to the light chain.[230] Given the absence of the heavy chain, β-factor XIIa does not interact with anionic surfaces. Even though β-factor XIIa is still capable of activating PK, it no longer activates factor XI.[245]

Despite its contribution to fibrin formation *in vitro*, factor XII has long been considered to be dispensable for coagulation *in vivo*, because factor XII deficiency is not associated with a bleeding.[229,246] However, newer *in vivo* studies indicate that factor XII contributes to surface-induced pathologic thrombosis via activation of factor XI.[215,242,247,248]

The serpin C1 inhibitor is the main plasma inhibitor of α-factor XIIa and β-factor XIIa. In addition, antithrombin (AT) and PAI-1 also inhibit factor XIIa activity. Conditions in which the factor XIIa activity is not properly controlled, such as in C1 inhibitor deficiency states or in case of a constitutively active form of factor XIIa, can result in the disorder hereditary angioedema.[249]

### Gene Structure and Variations

The gene for factor XII is located on chromosome 5q35.3, spans approximately 12 kb, and contains 14 exons.[250] The intron–exon structure of the gene is similar to the plasminogen activator family of serine proteases. Portions of the gene are homologous to domains found in fibronectin and tissue-type plasminogen activator.

Loss-of-function mutations in the factor XII gene do not cause clinical symptoms in the form of a bleeding tendency in homozygous or compound heterozygous individuals, although they have a prolonged APTT.

Several common allelic variations in the factor XII gene have been examined to determine whether these variations influence plasma factor XII levels and whether these are associated with thrombotic risk. Best studied is a 46C>T transition four nucleotides upstream of the start codon. TT homozygotes have lower plasma factor XII levels than CC homozygotes, but there was no relationship with risk for venous thrombosis or myocardial infarction.[251]

## ● THE CELL-ASSOCIATED COFACTORS TISSUE FACTOR, THROMBOMODULIN, AND ENDOTHELIAL PROTEIN C RECEPTOR

### TISSUE FACTOR

Tissue factor, also known as thromboplastin or CD142, is the cellular receptor and cofactor for factors VII and VIIa (see Fig. 3–6) and was first described in 1905.[12] Tissue factor is expressed in extravascular tissue, particularly fibroblasts and smooth muscle cells, where it serves as a hemostatic "envelope," poised to activate coagulation upon vascular damage. Generally, tissue factor is not exposed to the blood, but endothelial cells and adhered leukocytes may express tissue factor in response to injury or stimuli such as endotoxin or cytokines.

### Protein Structure

Although many of the coagulation factors share some degree of homology, the structure of tissue factor is unique. It is the only procoagulant protein that is an integral membrane protein and shares structural homology with class II interferon receptors. Tissue factor consists of 263 amino acids (Mr ≈47,000) and comprises a 219-residue extracellular domain, a 23-residue hydrophobic transmembrane portion, and a short 21-residue intracellular tail.[252] The extracellular domain is made up of two fibronectin type III domains, which each comprise a disulfide bond (Cys49–Cys57, Cys186–Cys209). Elimination of the second disulfide link distorts the coagulant activity of tissue factor.

### Tissue Factor Activation and Cofactor Function

The tissue factor–factor VIIa complex is generally acknowledged to be the major physiologic initiator of blood coagulation. The process of coagulation is initiated when an injury ruptures a vessel and allows blood to come into contact with extravascular tissue factor. Escape of blood from the vessel allows factor VII to bind to extravascular tissue factor and initiate coagulation. However, it is very likely that in the absence of injury, tissue factor located in close proximity of the vessels is already associated with factor VIIa.[253] An injury allows the extravascular tissue factor–factor VIIa complexes to come into contact with blood and initiate thrombin generation on activated platelet surfaces. Interaction of tissue factor with factor VII induces conformational changes in the serine protease domain of factor VIIa (see Fig. 3–6), thereby allowing the latter to proteolytically activate factors IX and X.[11]

Tissue factor does not require proteolytic activation to express its activity. However, it appears that tissue factor can occur in an inactive or "encrypted" state, and procoagulant activity follows after an appropriate stimulus. Even though the exact nature of the molecular mechanism remains to be identified, several models explaining tissue factor decryption have been put forward.

Originally, it was assumed that tissue factor encryption–decryption depends on the phospholipid environment, with decryption following upon expression of negatively charged phosphatidylserine on the membrane surface. Interaction of tissue factor with phosphatidylserine restricts the orientation of the tissue factor–factor VIIa complex, thereby ensuring correct alignment of the factor VIIa active site with the membrane-bound substrates factors X and IX.[254] Encryption of tissue factor has been proposed to occur upon localization into lipid rafts, which are known to be poor in phosphatidylserine. In endothelial cells, assembly of the ternary tissue factor–factor VIIa–factor X complex does result in tissue factor translocation to caveolae, which renders tissue factor inactive.[255] In addition, cell-membrane anchoring of tissue factor via acylation of palmitic and stearic acids may serve to target tissue factor to specific lipid domains.[256]

In a second model, the tissue factor–dependent procoagulant activity is explained by oxidation and reduction of the Cys186–Cys209 bond. This disulfide bond is less stable because of its strained conformation, and disruption of this link may cause conformational changes that alter the affinity of tissue factor for factor VIIa.[257,258] The breaking and formation of this disulfide link is suggested to be modulated by protein disulfide isomerases.[255]

A final model assumes that decryption relies on the dimerization of tissue factor. Like other members of the class II interferon receptors, tissue factor is capable of dimerization in a manner determined by the

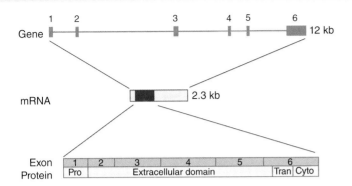

**Figure 3–18.** Relationship of gene structure to protein structure in tissue factor. The exons, introns, mRNA, and protein structure are as indicated. The mRNA is 2.3 kb with a 5′ untranslated region and a large 3′ untranslated region (light blue). Pro indicates the prepro leader sequence, the extracellular domain is indicated, Tran indicates the transmembrane region, and Cyto indicates the cytoplasmic domain.

redox (oxidation-reduction) environment and the exposure of phosphatidylserine. However, both monomeric and dimeric forms of tissue factor appear to possess procoagulant activity.[255]

Tissue factor is not only the primary initiator of the extrinsic pathway of coagulation, it also supports activation of PAR2 on endothelial cells and smooth muscle cells. Activation of PAR2 by the tissue factor–factor VIIa(–factor Xa) complex is not necessarily directly relevant for coagulation, but it is currently speculated that this event is important for wound healing, angiogenesis, tissue remodeling, and inflammation.[38-40]

### Gene Structure and Variations

The human tissue factor gene is located on chromosome 1p21-p22. The DNA sequence of the tissue factor gene has been determined and consists of six exons and five introns that span approximately 12 kb (Fig. 3–18).

The primary transcript encoding full-length tissue factor contains six exons, but an alternatively spliced form of tissue factor (asTF) also exists in which exon 5 is spliced out. Because of a 3′ frameshift mutation, the full-length tissue factor transmembrane and cytoplasmic tail are replaced with a hydrophobic C-terminal domain, which renders the asTF soluble. asTF is expressed in lung, pancreas, placenta, heart, endothelium, and monocytes.[259-261] Although the level of asTF in human plasma may be substantial and amounts to 10 to 30 percent of total tissue factor,[262] it remains a matter of debate whether asTF contributes to coagulation.

In theory, variations in the tissue factor gene could influence thrombotic and bleeding risk. There are claims that polymorphisms in the tissue factor gene influence thrombotic risk, but these claims have not been sufficiently confirmed.[263]

No relationship between loss-of-function mutations and bleeding has been described. This is perhaps not surprising in view of the fact that mice lacking tissue factor die early in gestation.

## THROMBOMODULIN

Thrombomodulin, which was first identified by Esmon and colleagues in the early 1980s,[264,265] is a predominantly endothelial transmembrane protein and functions as an endothelial receptor for thrombin. In addition to endothelium, thrombomodulin has also been detected on a number of other cell types, including megakaryocytes, monocytes, and neuthrophils.[266]

### Protein Structure

Mature single-chain thrombomodulin comprises 557 residues (Mr ≈78,000) and is composed of a lectin-like domain, a hydrophobic region, six EGF-like domains, a serine- and threonine-rich region, a transmembrane domain, and a 23-residue cytoplasmic tail. The highly charged lectin-like domains bear homology to the C-type lectins. Post-translational modifications include five N-linked glycosylation sites that are located in the lectin-like and EGF-4 and 5 domains. O-linked glycosylation in the serine- and threonine-rich region (Ser474) supports attachment of a glycosaminoglycan, a chondroitin sulfate moiety, which forms a low-affinity binding site for thrombin.

### Thrombomodulin Cofactor Function

Thrombomodulin interacts with thrombin through its EGF-5 and -6 domains in a calcium-dependent manner.[267] As a result, thrombin's procoagulant exosite I is shielded, which causes thrombin's specificity to switch to the anticoagulant substrate protein C, requiring EGF domains 4 to 6 of thrombomodulin, and to TAFI, requiring EGF-3 to -6.[268] Thrombomodulin enhances the thrombin-dependent activation of protein C more than 1000-fold.

As a result of the relatively large endothelial surface area in capillary beds, the thrombomodulin-dependent activation of protein C proceeds efficiently in the microcirculation, which serves a major role in preventing thrombosis from occurring on intact endothelium.[269] In larger vessels where the endothelial surface area-blood volume ration is low, the presence of EPCR aids in the interaction with and presentation of protein C to the thrombomodulin-thrombin complex.[270]

Thrombomodulin also enhances the thrombin-mediated conversion of single-chain urokinase-type plasminogen activator to thrombin-cleaved two-chain urokinase-type plasminogen activator, which interferes with the generation of plasmin. Furthermore, thrombomodulin is a negative regulator of PAR signaling, as thrombomodulin-bound thrombin is incapable of PAR activation.[271] Based on this and because thrombomodulin is the cofactor responsible for APC generation, thrombomodulin plays an important role, albeit indirect, as an antiinflammatory protein. A direct contribution to suppress inflammation has been attributed to the lectin-like domains and hydrophobic region of thrombomodulin, independent of its anticoagulant activity.[272]

Protein C inhibitor is an effective inhibitor of the thrombomodulin–thrombin complex.[273]

Proteolysis of thrombomodulin by neutrophil-derived metalloproteinases and possibly rhomboids results in the generation of soluble thrombomodulin.[274] Normal plasma levels of soluble thrombomodulin are 3 to 50 ng/mL, but may increase as a result of vascular damage associated with infection, sepsis, or inflammation.[274]

### Gene Structure and Variations

The human thrombomodulin gene (THBD) is located on chromosome 20p11.2, spans approximately 3.5 kb, and consists of a single exon (Fig. 3–19). Intronless genes are uncommon in eukaryotes and include rhodopsin, angiogenin, mitochondrial genes, interferon α, and β-adrenergic receptors. Intronless genes represent recent additions to the genome, created mostly by retroposition of processed mRNAs with retained functionality. Genetic variation in thrombomodulin has been studied in conjunction with venous thrombosis, bleeding, and atypical hemolytic uremic syndrome (aHUS).

There are early reports that mutations in thrombomodulin are present in patients with venous thrombosis, but it was difficult to prove causality.[275] More recent work that made use of thrombomodulin sequencing in relatively large studies supports the putative relationship between thrombomodulin function and venous thrombosis.[276] Such

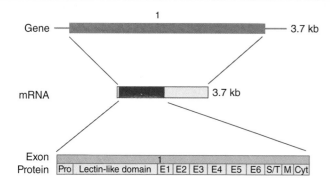

**Figure 3–19.** Relationship of gene structure to protein structure in thrombomodulin. The thrombomodulin gene has no introns. The exon, mRNA, and protein structure are as indicated. The mRNA is 3.7 kb, with a small 5' untranslated region and a large 3' untranslated region (*light blue*). In the protein, Pro indicates the prepro leader sequence, the lectin-like domain is indicated, E indicates the epidermal growth factor (EGF)-like domains, S/T indicates the serine- and threonine-rich region, M indicates the transmembrane region, and Cyt indicates the cytoplasmic domain.

mutations, however, do not explain a large proportion of the heritability of venous thrombosis as they seem to be quite rare.

Recently a novel thrombomodulin mutation, p.Cys537Stop, was described in a family with a history of posttraumatic bleeding.[277] The endogenous thrombin potential was markedly reduced at low tissue factor concentrations in heterozygous carriers. Plasma thrombomodulin levels were elevated (433 to 845 ng/mL, normal range 2 to 8 ng/mL), and the addition of exogenous protein C further decreased thrombin generation. It was surmised that as a consequence of the premature stop codon, the truncated thrombomodulin is shed from the endothelial surface into the blood plasma, which would promote systemic protein C activation, thereby explaining the bleeding phenotype.

Missense mutations in thrombomodulin were also reported in patients with aHUS, and this involvement in aHUS is probably related to the role of thrombomodulin in the complement system.[278] Thrombomodulin binds to C3b and factor H and negatively regulates complement by accelerating factor I–mediated inactivation of C3b. In addition, by promoting activation of TAFI, thrombomodulin also accelerates the inactivation of C3a and C5a. Thrombomodulin variants associated with aHUS had diminished capacity to inactivate C3b and to activate TAFI and were thus less protected from activated complement, thereby providing an explanation for their involvement in aHUS.

## ENDOTHELIAL PROTEIN C RECEPTOR

The EPCR, a single-chain transmembrane receptor discovered in 1995 by Fukodome and Esmon,[279] binds both protein C and APC. EPCR increases the rate of activation of protein C[92] and alters the function of APC from anticoagulant to cytoprotective.[280] EPCR is mainly expressed by endothelial cells but also by leukocytes and other cell types.

### Protein Structure

EPCR is homologous to CD1 and major histocompatibility class I proteins and folds with a β-sheet platform supporting two α-helical regions that form the potential binding pocket for protein C and APC. The mature protein (Mr ≈49,000) consists of 223 amino acids and is glycosylated through four N-linked glycosylation sites (Asn30, Asn47, Asn119, Asn155). EPCR contains a 25-residue long C-terminal transmembrane region with a short 3-residue cytoplasmic tail.

### Endothelial Protein C Receptor Function

EPCR enhances the activation of membrane-bound protein C by the thrombomodulin–thrombin complex,[92] thereby enhancing the APC-mediated anticoagulant pathway.

APC bound to membrane-associated or soluble EPCR is disabled in its anticoagulant capacity. Instead, EPCR-bound APC activates PAR1 in an alternative manner by noncanonical cleavage at a Arg46,[281] resulting in an increased barrier function of endothelial cells mediated via the β-arrestin/PI3K (phosphatidylinositide 3'-kinase)/AKT/Rac1 pathway. This is in contrast to the barrier-disruptive Arg41 cleavage of PAR1 by thrombin that activates the G-protein/ERK (extracellular regulated kinase) 1.2/RhoA pathway.[281]

EPCR is essential at the maternal–embryonic interface on trophoblast giant cells where it prevents fibrin formation. Consequently, complete EPCR deficiency leads to embryonic lethality. EPCR-deficient embryos rescued by the presence of EPCR in the trophoblast are viable and thrive, which seems to indicate that EPCR is not essential to blood circulation, at least in mice.[282] Additional ligands for EPCR have been discovered such as factor VIIa, *Plasmodium falciparum* erythrocyte membrane protein, and the V(γ)4V(δ)5 T-cell receptor.[283] These additional ligands indicate potential involvement of EPCR in the therapeutic effect of factor VIIa in hemophilia patients, and roles for EPCR in malaria, cytomegalovirus infection, and cancer.

### Gene Structure and Variations

The chromosomal location of the EPCR gene (*PROCR*) is 20q11.2, and it contains four exons and spans 6 kb. Exon 1 encodes for the 5'-untranslated region and the signal peptide; exons 2 and 3 encode for almost the entire extracellular region; and exon 4 encodes for the transmembrane domain and cytoplasmic tail. One single mRNA encodes the centrosomal protein CCD41 and EPCR. Deletion of the signal sequence confers the centrosomal location of CCD41, while the unprocessed protein is incorporated into cell membranes as EPCR.

Variants of EPCR with reduced protein C affinity or increased cellular shedding are reported to be associated with unprovoked venous thromboembolism.[284]

## ● THE FIBRIN NETWORK: FIBRIN(OGEN), FACTOR XIII, AND THROMBIN-ACTIVATABLE FIBRINOLYSIS INHIBITOR

### FIBRINOGEN

Fibrinogen, when converted to fibrin, forms the structural meshwork that consolidates an initial platelet plug into a solid hemostatic clot. Fibrinogen is synthesized in the liver and circulates in a concentration of approximately 7.4 μM. The plasma half-life of fibrinogen is 3 to 5 days, with only a small proportion of the catabolism caused by consumption.[285] Fibrinogen is also found in the α-granules of platelets. It was initially assumed that megakaryocytes synthesized fibrinogen. However, although some γ-chain transcripts are present in marrow precursors, it appears that most of the fibrinogen found within platelets is taken up from the plasma by endocytosis.[286,287]

### Protein Structure

Chapter 25 provides a detailed description of the biochemistry of fibrinogen and of fibrin formation and degradation. Fibrinogen is a dimeric GP (Mr ≈340,000), and each of the two subunits contains three disulfide-linked polypeptide chains that are referred to as the Aα (Mr ≈66,500), Bβ (Mr ≈52,000), and γ (Mr ≈46,500) chains. A trinodular model of fibrinogen structure has been established from the crystal structure of fibrinogen (Fig. 3–20).[288]

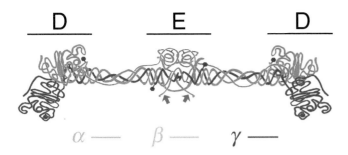

**Figure 3–20.** Structure of fibrinogen. Fibrinogen is a dimer. Each monomer consists of three chains: Aα shown in *light blue*, Bβ shown in *pink*, and γ shown in *dark blue*. The disulfides that link the two monomers are in the central E domain. The D domains consist primarily of the C-terminal regions of the Bβ and γ chains. The helical region connecting the two domains consists of all three chains intertwined. *(Reproduced with permission from Côté HC, Lord ST, Pratt KP: gamma-Chain dysfibrinogenemias: Molecular structure-function relationships of naturally occurring mutations in the gamma chain of human fibrinogen, Blood 1998 Oct 1;92(7):2195–2212.)*

Because human fibrinogen is subject to modification at a number of different sites both during and after biosynthesis, the fibrinogen present in the circulation is a heterogeneous mixture of molecules. These normal variants are caused by alternative splicing, modification of certain amino acids by sulfation, phosphorylation, and hydroxylation, different degrees of glycosylation, and proteolysis. It has been estimated that the number of nonidentical fibrinogen molecules that can be produced by these mechanisms is in excess of 1 million.[289] Some of these variations may have significant functional consequences. For example, the level of one variant of fibrinogen with an alternatively spliced γ-chain (fibrinogen-γ′) is associated with a risk of venous thrombosis.[290]

### Fibrinogen Activation and Fibrin Function

Thrombin binds to the central domain of fibrinogen and proteolytically releases two fibrinopeptides A (Aα, residues 1 to 16) and two fibrinopeptides B (Bβ, residues 1 to 14) from each fibrinogen molecule.[291] Release of the fibrinopeptides exposes binding sites in the E domain that have complementary sites in the D domains of other fibrin monomers.[292,293] These complementary binding sites lead to the initial formation of two-stranded protofibrils with a half-staggered overlap configuration (Fig. 3–21). Protofibrils then aggregate into thick fibers that branch into a meshwork of interconnected thick fibers.[294] The half-staggered overlap of the fibrin monomers gives a characteristic cross-banded pattern on electron micrographs.[295]

During fibrin monomer polymerization, other plasma proteins also bind to the surface of the developing meshwork. These include elements of the fibrinolytic system and a variety of adhesive proteins, such as fibronectin, thrombospondin, and VWF. These surface proteins influence the generation, crosslinking, and lysis of fibrin. Fibrin(ogen) also has specific integrin-binding sites that are essential for platelet binding. The thrombin that initiates fibrin polymerization also activates factor XIII, which stabilizes the fibrin polymer by crosslinking. Factor XIIIa also crosslinks other bound proteins, for example, PAI-1, vitronectin, fibronectin, and α2-antiplasmin, to the fibrin network.

Once formed, the fibrin mesh can be degraded by the fibrinolytic system. Plasmin cleaves fibrin and fibrinogen in an ordered sequence at arginyl and lysyl bonds, giving rise to a series of soluble degradation products.[296] In this process, the crosslink between two D fragments remains intact, resulting in the formation of a fragment consisting of two D domains and one E domain, called D-dimer. Circulating D-dimer concentrations are often measured as a surrogate marker of activated coagulation.

In addition to its obvious procoagulant role in stabilizing the initial platelet hemostatic plug, fibrin can also act as an important inhibitor of thrombin generation. Fibrin functions as "antithrombin I" by sequestering thrombin in the developing fibrin clot, and also by reducing the catalytic activity of fibrin-bound thrombin.[297]

### Gene Structure and Variations

The genes for the three chains of fibrinogen are found within a 50-kb region on chromosome 4 at q23-q32 (Fig. 3–22). The genomic sequences show a high degree of homology, suggesting they were derived through duplication of a common ancestral gene. The homology extends to sites upstream of the gene, suggesting that common regulatory elements may reside in these areas, thus helping to coordinate synthesis of the three chains.

The physiologic importance of fibrinogen is underscored by the bleeding diathesis associated with afibrinogenemia and some dysfibrinogenemias (Chap. 15). Other dysfibrinogenemias are associated with thromboembolic disease. Although afibrinogenemia is associated with a bleeding tendency, it is usually not as severe as classical hemophilia.

## FACTOR XIII

The GP factor XIII is a protransglutaminase that, upon activation, crosslinks and stabilizes fibrin clots.[298] Plasma factor XIII is a heterotetramer consisting of two factor XIIIA subunits (731 amino acids; Mr ≈83,000) bound to two factor XIIIB subunits (641 amino acids; Mr ≈76,500) that

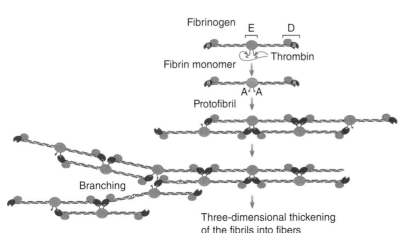

**Figure 3–21.** Cleavage of fibrinogen and polymerization of fibrin. The structure of fibrinogen is indicated schematically. Cleavage sites for fibrinopeptide A by thrombin are shown. Cleavage of the B peptide is not shown in this figure. Release of fibrinopeptide A exposes binding sites in the E domain that match complementary sites in the D domain. Fibrin monomers polymerize by half-staggered overlaps. Polymerization can also lead to branched structures. *(Reproduced with permission from Côté HC, Lord ST, Pratt KP: gamma-Chain dysfibrinogenemias: Molecular structure-function relationships of naturally occurring mutations in the gamma chain of human fibrinogen, Blood 1998 Oct 1; 92(7):2195–2212.)*

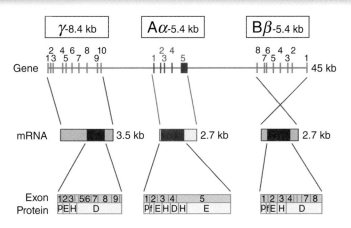

Gene

mRNA

Exon
Protein

**Figure 3–22.** Relationship of gene structure to protein structure in fibrinogen. The exons, introns, mRNA, and protein structure for the three chains of fibrinogen are shown. The Bβ chain is translated in the opposite direction from the Aα and γ chains. Lighter colors in the mRNA indicate 5′ and 3′ untranslated regions. In the proteins, P designates the prepro leader sequence, f designates fibrinopeptide (A in Aα and B in Bβ), E designates residues in the E domain, H designates residues in the helical connecting region, and D designates residues in the D domain.

circulates in plasma as an A2B2 complex (Mr ≈320,000) at a concentration of 94 nM with a plasma half-life of 10 days (Fig. 3–23; see Table 3–1). Factor XIII circulates in plasma associated to fibrinogen via interaction of the factor XIIIB subunit with the fibrinogen γ′-chain.

The A and B subunits of factor XIII are synthesized and expressed separately and assemble in the circulation to the heterotetramer factor XIII-A2B2.[299] Factor XIIIA is synthesized in monocytes/macrophages, megakaryocytes, and hepatocytes, whereas factor XIIIB is synthesized exclusively in the liver and kidney.

### Protein Structure

The factor XIIIA subunit consists of an activation peptide, a β-sandwich, a catalytic transglutaminase, and two β-barrel domains.[298] Factor XIIIB

acts as a carrier protein providing the long plasma half-life of factor XIII. Factor XIIIB consists of 10 Sushi domains in tandem, of which the first two Sushi domains are crucial for the binding to factor XIIIA.

### Factor XIII Activation and Factor XIIIa Activity

Factor XIIIA is a proenzyme that is proteolytically activated by thrombin via cleavage at Arg37 (see Fig. 3–23), resulting in release of the activation peptide and dissociation of the factor XIIIB subunit from factor XIII-A2B2, thereby exposing the active site Cys314 of factor XIIIA. Cofactors for the activation of factor XIIIA by thrombin are calcium and fibrin(ogen). Platelets only contain the factor XIIIA (cofactor XIII-A2) dimer that is activated intracellularly in a proteolytic-independent manner through a rise in cytosolic calcium and subsequent conformational change before secretion by the stimulated platelet (see Fig. 3–23).[300]

Activation of factor XIII by thrombin is not a late event in blood coagulation, as it is activated with the same velocity by thrombin as the cleavage of the fibrinopeptides of fibrinogen.[301] Factor XIII can also be alternatively activated and inactivated by neutrophil elastase.[302]

Factor XIIIa consists of a factor XIII-A2 dimer comprising two activated factor XIIIA subunits that result from either thrombin-activation (factor XIIIa*) or conformational-activation (factor XIIIa°). The transglutaminase activity of factor XIIIa crosslinks a γ-carbon of glutamine in one protein chain to the ε-amino group of lysine in another protein chain in a reaction named transamidation. The specificity of factor XIIIa crosslinking of proteins stems mainly from the recognition by factor XIIIa of specific glutamines, while the crosslink to lysine appears to be random and limited to the ones that are in the vicinity.

When thrombin cleaves the fibrinopeptides A and B of fibrinogen molecules, the binding site on the central E domain for the D domain of other fibrin molecules is uncovered. This initiates lateral aggregation of protofibrils and fiber formation. Factor XIIIa stabilizes the forming of protofibrils by linking two γ-chains in adjacent D domains in fibrin polymers. Binding of Arg158 in one subunit of the factor XIIIa dimer to the αC region residue AαGlu396 of fibrin facilitates crosslinking via αC chains to a next fibrin molecule by the other activated factor XIIIA subunit in factor XIIIa.[303]

The crosslinking of fibrin γ-chains or α-chains by factor XIIIa has independent and specific effects on clot formation and structure.

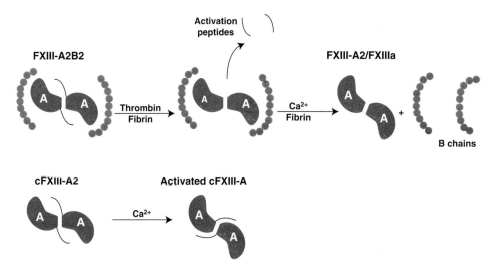

**Figure 3–23.** Factor XIII (FXIII) activation. The structures of the FXIIIA and FXIIIB subunits are indicated schematically. Plasma FXIII (FXIII-A2B2) consists of two FXIIIA (*A*, in *red*) subunits bound to two FXIIIB (in *green*) subunits. Cleavage of the activation peptides from FXIIIA by thrombin releases the FXIIIB subunits (B chains) and induces a conformational change in the FXIIIA subunits that opens the active site. This thrombin cleaved form of FXIIIA is known as FXIIIa or FXIIIa. Cellular FXIII (cFXIII-A2) found in platelets and macrophages consists only of the FXIIIA2 (cFXIII-A2) dimer. Before release by activated platelets, the cFXIII-A2 dimer becomes activated by an increase in intracellular calcium ions (Ca²⁺) that induces the active conformation without proteolysis of the activation peptide. This calcium-activated form of cFXIIIA (cFXIII-A) is known as FXIIIa.

Crosslinks stabilize a clot by incorporation of the plasmin inhibitor $\alpha_2$-antiplasmin, which makes it resistant to fibrinolytic attack by plasmin.[304]

Several other processes during clotting are factor XIII dependent, including red blood cell incorporation in clots,[305] complement factor 3 (C3) crosslinking to fibrin,[306] and clot retraction by platelets.[307] Factor XIII also plays a role in the functioning of multiple adhesive and contractile proteins and in angiotensin type I receptor crosslinking.[308] Fetal specific crosslinking of Fas by factor XIII dampens apoptosis, suggesting that factor XIII may play a role in cell survival prenatally.[309] Related to its expression by monocytes/macrophages, factor XIII levels may drop after inhibition of interleukin-6 receptor signaling by tocilizumab.[310] Besides its crucial role in hemostasis, factor XIII has important functions during tissue regeneration and infection.[311] Factor XIII is necessary to prevent bleeding/stroke and maintain pregnancy and aids in wound healing.[298]

### Gene Structure and Function

The factor XIIIA chain gene *(F13A1)* has been localized to chromosome 6 p25.1.[312] It contains 15 exons and is larger than 160 kb (Fig. 3–24). The fibrin-binding domain is encoded by exons 2 to 12. The active site, with its reactive thiol at Cys314, is present in exon 7. The gene encoding the factor XIIIB *(F13B)* chain has been localized to chromosome 1q31.3. It has 12 exons and is approximately 28 kb (Fig. 3–25).[313] Each Sushi domain is encoded by a single exon. The regulation of factor XIIIB expression is poorly understood. A total of 30 potential start sites are located upstream of the initial methionine.

Homozygosity or compound heterozygosity for loss-of-function mutations in the factor XIIIA or XIIIB genes leads to a severe bleeding disorder that is rare (1 in 2,000,000 of the population).[314] Factor XIII–deficient newborns often present with bleeding from the umbilical cord. The natural course is characterized by a life-long bleeding tendency and spontaneous miscarriages in affected women. Acquired factor XIII deficiency by development of an inhibitory antibody may lead to fatal bleeding if not treated.[315]

Mutations underlying factor XIII deficiency are more commonly found in the gene encoding factor XIIIA than the one encoding factor XIIIB. In accordance with this, the Human Gene Mutation Database lists 107 mutations in the factor XIIIA gene and 19 mutations in the factor XIIIB gene. Mutations in the gene encoding factor XIIIB often lead low levels of both factor XIII subunits. This is probably because free factor XIIIA has a short plasma half-life.

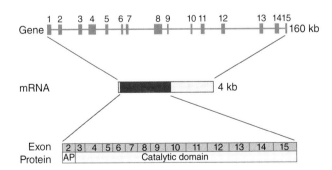

**Figure 3–24.** Relationship of gene structure to protein structure in the factor XIIIA chain. The exons, mRNA, and protein structure of the factor XIIIA chain are shown. The mRNA is 4 kb with some 5′ untranslated sequence coded in exon 1 and a large 3′ untranslated region (*light blue*). In the protein, AP indicates the activation peptide, and the catalytic domain is indicated.

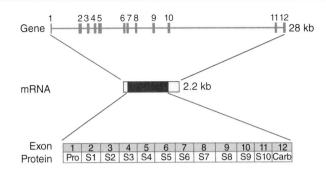

**Figure 3–25.** Relationship of gene structure to protein structure in the factor XIIIB chain. The exons, introns, mRNA, and protein structure are as indicated. The mRNA is 2.2 kb with small 3′ and 5′ untranslated noncoding regions (*light blue*). In the protein, Pro indicates the propeptide, S1 to S10 indicates the Sushi 1 to 10 domains, and the C-terminal region is indicated by Carb.

A Val34Leu polymorphism associated with fatal atherothrombotic ischemic stroke results in a faster factor XIIIA activation rate by thrombin, which affects clot structure.[316]

## THROMBIN-ACTIVATABLE FIBRINOLYSIS INHIBITOR

TAFI is the zymogen of a zinc-bound metalloprotease and is also known as carboxypeptidase B, R, or U. TAFI is synthesized in the liver. Most TAFI present in the blood is in the plasma compartment, which circulates at 70 to 275 nM (see Table 3–1).

### Protein Structure

TAFI is a 401-amino-acid proenzyme (Mr $\approx$60,000) and consists of an N-terminal activation peptide (residues 1 to 76), a linker region (residues 77 to 92), and a catalytic domain (residues 93 to 401). Twenty percent of the protein mass of TAFI is accounted for by carbohydrate side chains that are attached to four sites within the activation peptide (Asn22, Asn51, Asn63) and linker region (Asn86). The active site residues (Glu271, Arg125) and zinc-binding residues (His67, Glu70, His196) in TAFI are conserved between other members of the carboxypeptidase A family.

### Thrombin-Activatable Fibrinolysis Inhibitor Activation and Thrombin-Activatable Fibrinolysis Inhibitor-a Activity

TAFI is proteolytically activated by plasmin or thrombin, reactions that are accelerated 1000-fold when thrombin is bound to thrombomodulin. Both enzymes cleave TAFI at Arg92 to give rise to activated TAFI (TAFIa; Mr $\approx$37,000) upon release of the activation peptide. TAFIa catalyzes removal of C-terminal lysine and arginine residues from fibrin and fibrin cleavage products. These residues are important for binding and activation of plasminogen, and removal of these residues by TAFIa reduces formation of plasmin on clots resulting in decreased clot lysis.

TAFIa may also have an antiinflammatory role as it can efficiently cleave C-terminal arginines of anaphylatoxins such as bradykinin and the complement activation peptides C3a and C5a.

Inhibitors of TAFIa have not been identified. Rather, the primary regulatory mechanism of TAFI activity involves its intrinsic thermal instability with a half-life of less than 15 minutes at 37°C.

### Gene Structure and Variations

The gene for TAFI *(CPB2)* has been localized to 13q14.13. The gene contains 11 exons with 10 introns and spans 48 kb. Homozygosity or compound heterozygosity for mutations in the gene encoding TAFI has not been described.

In total, 19 SNPs have been identified in the gene encoding TAFI, of which six are in the coding region. Of the latter SNPs, two lead to an amino acid substitution: an Ala/Thr substitution at position 147 and a Thr/Ile substitution at position 325.[317] There appears to be a strong correlation between plasma levels of TAFI and polymorphisms in the promoter and 3′-region, but their clinical significance is unclear.

Epidemiologic studies have indicated that elevated TAFI levels are correlated with an increased risk of venous thrombosis, albeit the methods to quantify TAFI or TAFIa have limitations.[318]

# ●INHIBITORS OF COAGULATION: ANTITHROMBIN, TISSUE FACTOR PATHWAY INHIBITOR, AND PROTEIN Z/PROTEIN Z–DEPENDENT PROTEASE INHIBITOR

## ANTITHROMBIN

AT was previously known as AT III as a result of a classification of several AT activities in plasma discovered in the 1950s.[319] AT is mainly synthesized in the liver and circulates in plasma as a single-chain GP of 432 amino acids (Mr ≈58,000) at a concentration of 2.5 $\mu$M with a half-life of 60 to 70 hours (see Table 3–1). AT is a member of the large serpin family and is known as SERPINC1 in the systematic nomenclature.

### Protein Structure

AT consists of an N-terminal heparin-binding domain, a carbohydrate-rich domain, and a C-terminal serine protease-binding region that comprises the long, flexible, and surface-exposed reactive center loop. Structural stability is provided by three disulfide bonds, two of which are located in the N-terminal region and one in the serine protease-binding region. Posttranslational modifications comprise four N-glycosylation sites, with three in the carbohydrate-rich domain (Asn96, Asn135, Asn155) and one in the serine protease-binding region (Asn192).

### Antithrombin Function

The primary proteases targeted by AT are thrombin, factor Xa, and factor IXa. In addition, AT also inhibits factors XIa and XIIa, as well as tissue factor–factor VIIa; however, the latter is only inhibited in the presence of heparin.

Similar to other serpins, AT acts as a "suicide" substrate for its target proteases. These cleave at site Arg393 in the reactive center loop of AT, upon which AT is, unlike normal substrates, not released, but forms a 1:1 covalent complex with the protease, thereby blocking the active site. This complex is facilitated by a conformational change of the reactive center loop that folds into the N-terminal region of AT. By doing so, the covalently attached protease is dragged along, resulting in distortion of its serine protease domain and effectively converting the protease back into a zymogen-like state.[320]

Heparin and related molecules, such as endothelial-bound glycosaminoglycans, dramatically accelerate the rate of protease inhibition by AT (see Table 3–4) through two distinct mechanisms that characterize inhibition of either factors IXa and Xa or thrombin (Fig. 3–26). In case of the former, binding of a specific pentasaccharide sequence in heparin results in a conformational change in the reactive center loop of AT, which allows for enhanced access by the target protease and is known as allosteric activation of AT (Fig. 3–26, middle panel).[320] This results in a 500-fold acceleration of inhibition of factors IXa and Xa.[321] The pentasaccharide sequence is present in all forms of heparin including low-molecular-weight heparin and fondaparinux, a synthetic pentasaccharide. Heparin-accelerated thrombin inhibition involves bridging of AT to the protease, which serves to align the two molecules and enhances the rate of complex formation (Fig. 3–26, right panel).[322,323] This mechanism, also known as the template mechanism, requires longer heparin molecules found in unfractionated heparin (UFH).

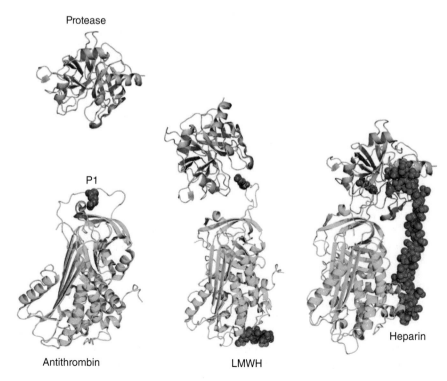

Protease

P1

Antithrombin          LMWH          Heparin

**Figure 3–26.** Effect of glycosaminoglycans on antithrombin inhibition. *Left panel:* Structures of thrombin (PDB structure 1TB6, *cyan*) and antithrombin (PDB structure 1T1F, *green*) with Arg393 (P1 residue, *red*) in the reactive center loop of antithrombin are shown. *Middle panel:* Binding of a specific pentasaccharide sequence (low-molecular-weight heparin [LMWH], *blue*) to antithrombin (PDB structure 2GD4) alters the conformation of the reactive center loop, thereby increasing exposure of the P1 residue and allowing for access of the target protease (allosteric activation). *Right panel:* A long heparin molecule *(blue)* interacts with both thrombin and antithrombin (PDB structure 1TB6), which aligns the two molecules and enhances the rate of complex formation (template mechanism).

Heparin-bridging of AT also contributes to some extent to the AT-mediated inhibition of factors IXa and Xa, but the majority of rate enhancement is provided by the allosteric activation of AT.

Protease–AT complexes are cleared from the circulation by lipoprotein receptor-related protein (LRP)-1–mediated endocytosis in the liver.[324,325]

### Gene Structure and Variations

The 13.5-kb AT gene *(SERPINC1)* is localized on chromosome 1q25.1 and consists of seven exons. The cDNA is 1395 bp long, whereas the mRNA is approximately 1.4 kb.

Because of its essential role as an inhibitor of coagulation, individuals who are heterozygous for loss-of-function mutations are at increased risk for thrombosis. The prevalence of this condition in the general population is approximately one in 5000 individuals,[326] while it occurs in approximately 5 percent of patients with a history of thromboembolic disease.[327] AT deficiency can be categorized into type I and type II deficiencies.[328] Type I deficiency is characterized by reduced plasma levels of AT; however, homozygous type I deficiency is not compatible with life. Type II deficiency covers all functional AT defects.

The Human Gene Mutation Database (www.hgmd.org) lists 274 mutations. Mutations resulting in type I deficiency consist of large deletions, frameshift mutations, premature stop codons, splice-site mutations, and missense mutations. Mutations observed in type II deficiency impair heparin binding or affect the overall protein structure. Chapters 20 and 23 provide a more detailed description of the clinical significance of AT deficiency.

## TISSUE FACTOR PATHWAY INHIBITOR

TFPI is a Kunitz-type protease inhibitor that inhibits factor Xa and tissue factor–factor VIIa activity and was discovered by Broze and Miletich in 1987.[329] TFPI circulates in plasma at 2.5 nM in multiple forms of which the majority is either truncated at the C-terminus or lipoprotein associated. Only 10 percent of the circulating TFPI is the full-length TFPIα form of 276 amino acids (Mr ≈40,000; see Table 3–1).[330] The half-life of TFPIα in the circulation is only 2 minutes because it readily associates with the vessel wall endothelium.

### Protein Structure

Full-length TFPIα consists of three tandem Kunitz domains and a C-terminus that contains a basic region (see Fig. 3–15).[331] However, TFPI is very heterogeneous as a result of proteolysis and alternative splicing. The latter gives rise to TFPIβ that lacks the third Kunitz domain and C-terminus, but instead includes a sequence that facilitates anchorage to the endothelial cell membrane via GPI linkage.[332]

Endothelial cells and platelets are the main producers of TFPI, with endothelial cells expressing both TFPIα and β, while platelets only produce TFPIα that is secreted upon platelet activation. Although a significant fraction of TFPIβ is GPI-linked to the endothelial cells, it is also found in plasma. *In vivo*, most of the full-length TFPIα appears to be bound to endothelial heparan sulphate proteoglycans through its positively charged C-terminus. This is because total plasma TFPI levels rise by approximately threefold upon heparin treatment, which is completely attributable to an increase in TFPIα. In addition, TFPIα also circulates in complex with factor V.

### Tissue Factor Pathway Inhibitor Function

The physiologic relevance of TFPI stems from its ability to regulate tissue factor–dependent coagulation as well as its direct inhibition of factor Xa. TFPI inhibits the tissue factor–factor VIIa complex in a two-step mechanism. TFPI will bind via its second Kunitz domain to the active site of factor Xa, thereby inhibiting the proteolytic capacity of factor Xa.[331] This step is accelerated profoundly via protein S through interactions with the third Kunitz domain of TFPI.[333,334] The following step is the inhibition of the catalytic activity of tissue factor–factor VIIa complexes by formation of the quaternary tissue factor–factor VIIa–factor Xa–TFPI complex. This complex formation depends on the binding of Kunitz 1 to the factor VIIa active site. Overall, the effects of TFPI as regulator of tissue factor–initiated thrombin generation appear to depend on the fast protein S–dependent TFPI interaction with factor Xa.[333]

TFPI that is truncated at the C-terminus is effective in inhibiting tissue factor–factor VIIa activity; however, this seems to occur too slow to control thrombin generation at least *in vitro*. In contrast, inhibition of tissue factor–factor VIIa activity by GPI-anchored TFPIβ is effective and independent of protein S.[332] GPI-anchored TFPIβ also acts as an inhibitor of tissue factor–factor VIIa signaling by PARs, a function that TFPIα seems to lack.

TFPI may prevent prothrombinase formation by factor Xa in the presence of the procofactor factor V, factor V that is partially activated by factor Xa, or platelet factor V.[335] However, the factor Va–factor Xa prothrombinase complex is not inhibited by TFPI as a result of competition by prothrombin.

The heterogeneity and different activities of the multiple forms of TFPI have frustrated the measurement of TFPI for clinical purposes. However, tests that estimate the free full-length form in plasma indicate an association of low TFPIα levels with venous thrombosis.[336] Low levels of TFPIα are observed in protein S–deficient patients, which may be the result of a lack of association of TFPI with protein S in the circulation and faster clearance of free TFPIα.[337] High TFPIα levels have been observed in patients with increased expression of a splice variant of factor V, known as *factor V-short*. Factor V-short, which lacks the major part of the B domain, interacts with the basic C-terminus of TFPIα, most likely through the acidic B domain region in factor V.[132,133] Increased factor V-short levels lead to a dramatic increase in plasma TFPIα, resulting in a bleeding disorder.[133]

TFPI activity is downregulated by proteolysis at the C-terminus, upon which the basic C-terminal region or the third Kunitz domain is removed, thereby impairing inhibition of factor Xa and tissue factor–factor VIIa. Complete inactivation of TFPI is observed after proteolysis by the neutrophil-derived proteases elastase and cathepsin G, which also cleave in between Kunitz 1 and 2. In this way, tissue factor–factor VIIa activity may be protected or reactivated during inflammatory processes.[338]

The *in vivo* relevance of TFPI was shown by the sensitization of rabbits to tissue factor–triggered disseminated intravascular coagulation after immunodepletion of TFPI.[339] Furthermore, mice lacking the first Kunitz domain of TFPI are not viable.[340]

### Gene Structure and Variations

The human TFPI gene *(TFPI)* is located on chromosome 2q31-q32.1 and has nine exons that span 70 kb. TFPI is synthesized in two alternatively spliced forms, α and β.[332] TFPIβ is formed by an alternative splice event after exon 7 such that TFPIβ lacks the third Kunitz domain and instead has a unique C-terminus. Exon 2 appears to downregulate translation of the TFPIβ splice variant by a unique interaction with a sequence in the 3′-end of the TFPIβ mRNA.

Homozygosity or compound heterozygosity for loss-of-function mutations in the gene encoding TFPI has not been described. Several genetic polymorphisms have been identified, and their relationship with venous thrombosis has been investigated. There is one report describing that a T33C polymorphism in intron 7 is highly associated with total TFPI antigen and protects against venous thrombosis,[341] but this relationship with thrombosis was not confirmed in a subsequent study.[342]

# PROTEIN Z/PROTEIN Z–DEPENDENT PROTEASE INHIBITOR

ZPI is a serine protease inhibitor (Mr ≈72,000; SERPINA10 in the systematic nomenclature) that inhibits coagulation factors Xa and XIa. ZPI circulates in plasma at 60 nM with a half-life of 60 hours (see Table 3–1).[343] The ZPI-dependent inhibition of factor Xa is enhanced in the presence of protein Z.[79] Protein Z is a vitamin K–dependent plasma GP (Mr ≈62,000) that circulates at 40 nM (see Table 3–1). In normal plasma, which has a molar excess of ZPI over protein Z, all protein Z circulates in complex with ZPI.[344]

## Protein Structure

ZPI displays 25 to 30 percent homology with other serpins such as AT. Based on this homology, Tyr387 was predicted and confirmed as P1 residue in the reactive center loop of ZPI and shown as pivotal for inhibition of factor Xa.[345] Unlike other serpins, the N-terminal region of ZPI contains a very acidic domain.

Protein Z consists of a Gla domain, a hydrophobic region, and two EGF-like domains. Even though the C-terminal region of protein Z contains a domain that is homologous to the serine protease domains of the other Gla-containing proteins, it lacks the His and Ser active site residues characteristic for trypsin-like serine proteases.[346] Thus, protein Z has no protease activity.

## Protein Z/Protein Z–Dependent Protease Inhibitor Function

The protein Z–ZPI complex associates with anionic phospholipid membranes in a calcium-dependent manner mediated by the Gla domain of protein Z, which facilitates formation of the ternary protein Z–ZPI–factor Xa complex. Furthermore, protein Z has also been suggested to induce conformational changes in ZPI, resulting in alignment of the reactive center loop and P1 site of ZPI with the factor Xa active site.[347] Together, these effects of protein Z enhance the inhibitory activity of ZPI to factor Xa by 1000-fold. In contrast, ZPI inactivation of factor XIa is protein Z–independent.[79] Similar to other serpins, ZPI acts as a "suicide" substrate. However, factors Xa and XIa eventually cleave ZPI at the P1 residue Tyr387, which results in release of a 4.2-kDa C-terminal ZPI peptide.[79]

The combination of protein Z and ZPI dramatically delays the initiation and reduces the ultimate rate of thrombin generation in mixtures containing prothrombin, factor V, phospholipids, and calcium. However, in similar mixtures containing factor Va, protein Z and ZPI do not inhibit thrombin generation.[79] Thus, the major effect of protein Z and ZPI is to dampen the coagulation response prior to the formation of the prothrombinase complex.

In mice, protein Z and ZPI deficiency is associated with a prothrombotic phenotype, and both deficiencies dramatically increase mortality in animals with the factor V Leiden mutation. This indicates that protein Z and ZPI deficiency may be a risk factor for thrombotic disease in humans.[348] Indeed, low protein Z levels appear weakly associated with thrombosis and ischemic stroke in subgroups of some small studies. However, these studies lack power to show a definite interaction with vascular disease.[349] Other studies demonstrate a possible association of protein Z and ZPI mutations with thrombosis and pregnancy complications.[350]

## Gene Structure and Variations

The chromosomal location of the ZPI gene (SERPINA10) is 14q32.13. The gene encodes six exons and spans almost 10 kb. The gene for protein Z (PROZ) is on the long arm of chromosome 13 (q34) in close proximity to the genes for factor X and factor VII. The protein Z gene spans 14 kb and consists of nine exons. The intron/exon boundaries are identical to the other Gla-containing coagulation proteins. There is an alternative exon that codes for a unique peptide of 22 amino acids in the prepro leader sequence. The gene is transcribed into a 1.6-kb mRNA.

Several mutations and polymorphisms have been described for the gene encoding ZPI,[351] but the association between such gene variations and risk of venous thrombosis has not been established with certainty.[352]

The Human Gene Mutation Database lists nine loss-of-function mutations in the protein Z gene. The relationship between these mutations and disease is uncertain at best, but a relationship with ischemic stroke and recurrent fetal loss cannot be excluded.[353–355]

# PATHWAYS OF HEMOSTASIS

## Early Coagulation Schemes

With the accumulated knowledge of the biochemistry of hemophilia, it was recognized in the 1960s that blood coagulation was regulated by a sequential series of steps in which activation of one clotting factor led to the activation of another, finally leading to a burst of thrombin generation.[356,357] Each clotting factor was thought to exist as a proenzyme that could be converted to an active enzyme.

Since then, the original waterfall reaction scheme of enzymes has been modified extensively. Factors V and VIII were identified as nonenzymatic procofactors for factors Xa and IXa, respectively, and the subsequent clotting events were divided into so-called extrinsic and intrinsic systems (Fig. 3–27). The extrinsic system was shown to consist of factor VIIa and tissue factor, the latter being viewed as extrinsic to the circulating blood. The tissue factor pathway could be activated in clotting tests by a brain tissue extract. The factor XII–dependent intrinsic system could even be activated by china clay (kaolin) and was viewed as being intravascular. Both pathways activate factor X, which, in complex with the activated cofactor Va, converts prothrombin to thrombin.

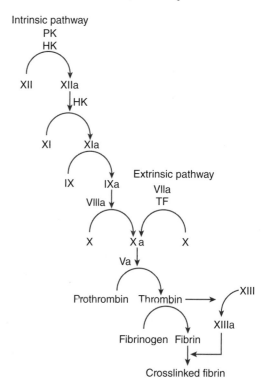

**Figure 3–27.** Cascade model of coagulation. This model shows successive activation of coagulation factors proceeding from the top of the schematic to thrombin generation and fibrin formation at the bottom of the schematic. The intrinsic and extrinsic pathways are indicated. HK, high-molecular-weight kininogen; PK, prekallikrein; TF, tissue factor.

Although these earlier concepts of coagulation were extremely valuable, investigators recognized that the intrinsic and extrinsic systems could not operate independently. The pivotal role of factor XII for the initiation of intrinsic thrombin generation and lack of bleeding tendency of factor XII–deficient individuals were inconsistent with the extreme bleeding associated with a deficiency in factor VIII or IX, participants of the same intrinsic pathway, which urged investigators to search for additional links in the cascades.

### Revision of the Coagulation Scheme

Key to the revision of the coagulation model was the purification and characterization of the transmembrane protein tissue factor.[358,359] A crucial observation was that the tissue factor–factor VIIa complex not only activates factor X, but also factor IX.[360] This showed that factor VIII or IX deficiencies, which result in hemophilia A or B, respectively, are in fact abnormalities of the tissue factor–factor VIIa pathway, even though factors VIII and IX are components of the intrinsic system. With the notion that traces of tissue factor–factor VIIa are rapidly inactivated by TFPI, it became clear that factor VIIIa–factor IXa activity is necessary to sustain hemostatic factor Xa and thrombin generation.[361-364] The embryonic lethality caused by both tissue factor as well as TFPI deficiency in mice underscores the importance of tissue factor–mediated thrombin generation and the control thereof.[340,365] Finally, it was observed that thrombin could directly activate factor XI,[366] thus providing an amplification loop once thrombin generation has been initiated: thrombin

→ factor XIa → factor IXa → FXa → thrombin. This model explains the mild bleeding tendency observed in factor XI–deficient patients and the absence of bleeding in factor XII–deficient individuals. A revised coagulation scheme is depicted in Fig. 3-28. This scheme builds on the conclusion that the major initiating event in hemostasis *in vivo* is the formation of the tissue factor–factor VIIa complex at the site of injury.[367]

It was also recognized that *in vivo* coagulation is regulated by control mechanisms, one of which is the localization of the coagulation reactions to cell surfaces. In addition, earlier and more recent observations emphasized the importance of plasma inhibitors targeting each step of the coagulation process. These include (1) TFPI, which controls tissue factor–factor VIIa and factor Xa activity in cooperation with protein S[331,333]; (2) thrombomodulin and APC, which inactivate thrombin and factors Va and VIIIa, the latter also in cooperation with protein S[368]; (3) AT, which inhibits thrombin and other coagulation proteases[369]; and (4) ZPI, which inhibits factor Xa on phospholipid surfaces in cooperation with protein Z prior to incorporation of factor Xa into the prothrombinase complex.[79] See also Fig. 3-28 for an overview of the inhibitory mechanisms of coagulation.

Most of the essential pathways of tissue factor–dependent thrombin generation and inhibitory control have been captured in a mathematical model based on the empirically derived rate constants of the individual reactions.[370] Completion and refinement of such models will aid our understanding of the biochemistry of the coagulation reactions on artificial membranes, given that the enzymatic events on

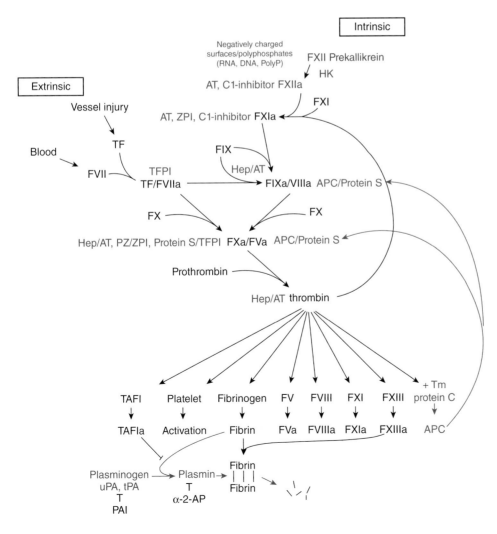

**Figure 3–28.** Revised model of coagulation. Schematic overview of the coagulation reactions in which several revisions have been made as compared to the classic cascade model of coagulation. The tissue factor–factor VIIa complex of the extrinsic pathway also activates factor IX, and thrombin activates factor XI, in a positive feedback loop. The factor IX–dependent amplification of factor Xa generation is necessary for hemostatic fibrin formation at low tissue factor concentrations, because tissue factor–factor VIIa–mediated factor X activation is inhibited by tissue factor pathway inhibitor (TFPI). Procoagulant extrinsic pathway components are indicated in *black*; the part of the intrinsic coagulation pathway that is not necessary for hemostasis is indicated in *gray*. Anticoagulant mediators are indicated in *red*. AP, antiplasmin; APC, activated protein C; AT, antithrombin; Hep, heparin; HK, high-molecular-weight kininogen; PAI, plasminogen activator inhibitor; PZ, protein Z; TAFI, thrombin-activatable fibrinolysis inhibitor; TF, tissue factor; Tm, thrombomodulin; tPA, tissue plasminogen activator; uPA, urokinase plasminogen activator; ZPI, protein Z–dependent protease inhibitor.

cellular membranes under (reduced) flow are still complicated, which hampers their incorporation into a mathematical model.[370]

### A Cell-Based Scheme of Coagulation

The goal of coagulation is to produce a fibrin clot that seals the site of injury in the vessel wall. This process is initiated when tissue factor–bearing cells are exposed to blood at the damaged site. Tissue factor is anchored to cells via a transmembrane domain and acts as a receptor for plasma factor VII. Both trace amounts of factor VIIa as well as zymogen factor VII that is rapidly converted to factor VIIa by factor Xa and/or autoactivation bind to tissue factor. Tissue factor is expressed around vessels and in the epithelium, where it forms a "hemostatic envelope." The tissue factor surrounding the vessels may already be in complex with factor VIIa, even in the absence of an injury.[253]

The tissue factor–factor VIIa complex catalyzes two very important reactions: (1) activation of factor X to factor Xa and (2) activation of factor IX to IXa. The initial factors Xa and IXa formed on tissue factor–bearing cells may have distinct functions in initiating the process of blood coagulation.[371] When a vessel is damaged, the blood delivers platelets to the site of injury. These bind to extravascular matrix components to produce the primary hemostatic plug and become partially activated in the process. The platelets are consequently localized in close proximity to active tissue factor–factor VIIa complexes.

The factor Xa formed on the tissue factor–bearing cell interacts with factor Va to form prothrombinase complexes that generate small amounts of thrombin (Fig. 3–29). Although this amount of thrombin may not be sufficient to clot fibrinogen, it is sufficient to initiate events that "prime" the clotting system for a subsequent burst of thrombin generation. Experiments using tissue factor–activated whole blood and cell-based systems have shown that platelets can be activated by thrombin that is generated by direct tissue factor–factor VIIa activation of factor Xa.[371-373] The small amounts of factor Va required for prothrombinase assembly are likely provided by activated platelets, by factor Xa activation, or potentially by noncoagulation proteases secreted by the tissue factor–bearing cells.[335,374,375]

The small amounts of thrombin generated are capable of accomplishing the following: (1) activating platelets; (2) activating factor V; (3) activating factor VIII and dissociating factor VIII from VWF; and (4) activating factor XI (see Fig. 3–29).[366,372,373] The activity of the factor Xa formed by the tissue factor–factor VIIa complex will be mostly restricted to the tissue factor–bearing surface because free factor Xa that diffuses off the cell surface is rapidly inhibited by TFPI, AT, and/or the protein Z–ZPI complex. Factor IXa, on the other hand, will most likely act on activated platelets in close proximity to the tissue factor–bearing cell. This is because factor IXa can diffuse to adjacent cell surfaces as it is not inhibited by TFPI and ZPI, while the rate of factor IXa inhibition by AT is much lower than that of factor Xa (see Table 3–4).

### The Role of Activated Platelets

Platelets also play a major role in localizing clotting reactions to the site of injury, as they adhere and aggregate at the same location where tissue factor is exposed to blood. Platelet localization and activation are mediated by VWF, thrombin, platelet receptors, and vessel wall components such as collagen (Chap. 2). Once platelets are activated, the cofactors Va and VIIIa are rapidly localized to the platelet membrane surface (see Fig. 3–29). Cofactor binding is mediated in part by the exposure of phosphatidylserine on the platelet membrane, a process resulting from a flip-flop mechanism whereby phosphatidylserine on the inner leaflet of the membrane bilayer flips to the outer membrane leaflet.[376] Endothelial cells, platelets, and leukocytes also generate procoagulant microvesicles that sustain thrombin generation. While the procoagulant characteristics of microvesicles have been studied in detail *in vitro*, their relative contribution to coagulation *in vivo* is still subject of debate.

Factor Xa generation is amplified on platelets by localization of factors IXa and XIa through specific binding sites,[377,378] and thrombin-mediated factor XI activation is enhanced by poly-P that is released by activated platelets (see Fig. 3–29).[379] Once formed, factor Xa associates with factor Va on the platelet surface to generate a burst of thrombin that is sufficient to clot fibrinogen and form a hemostatic plug. Subsequently, thrombin-activated factor XIII crosslinks fibrin and stabilizes the hemostatic plug, thereby rendering it impermeable. Thrombin also activates TAFI, which helps to stabilize the fibrin clot. The factor XIa–mediated feedback loop has been implicated to generate ample thrombin required for TAFI activation.[380]

It should be noted that the balance between the pro- and anticoagulant reactions, the pro- and antifibrinolytic potential, as well as stress on the local vasculature vary greatly in different organs, muscles, joints, and other sites in the body. This is probably fundamental to the variation in bleeding phenotypes observed in various coagulation factor deficiencies.[381] The notion that factors XI and XII are not crucial to hemostasis, but are involved in thrombosis, has led to their identification as new targets to improve the safety of anticoagulant therapy by reducing the risk of bleeding complications.[382,383]

### The Role of Immune Cells

It has become clear that thrombi may have a major physiologic role in immune defense. This so-called immunothrombosis may aid in the recognition, containment, and killing of pathogens.[384] However, if not

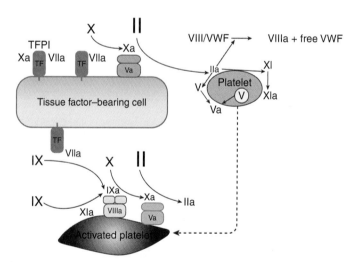

**Figure 3–29.** Cellular model of tissue factor–factor VIIa–mediated thrombin generation on tissue factor–bearing cells and propagation on platelets. After the initial generation of factor Xa on tissue factor–bearing cells, subsequent factor Xa generation is shutdown when tissue factor pathway inhibitor (TFPI) reacts with factor Xa to inactivate the tissue factor–factor VIIa complex. The small amount of thrombin generated on the tissue factor–bearing cell plays a critical role in priming platelets for subsequent coagulation steps. This thrombin activates platelets, releases factor V from platelet *a*-granules, activates factor V, activates factor VIII and releases it from von Willebrand factor (VWF), and activates factor XI. Factor IXa, generated on tissue factor–bearing cells, is only slowly inhibited by plasma inhibitors and can therefore make its way to the primed platelet surface where it binds to factor VIIIa. This factor VIIIa–IXa complex activates factor X on the platelet surface. The generated factor Xa complexes with factor Va and subsequently activates prothrombin, which leads to the burst of thrombin generation responsible for cleaving fibrinogen. Additional factor IXa is supplied by factor XIa on the platelet surface.

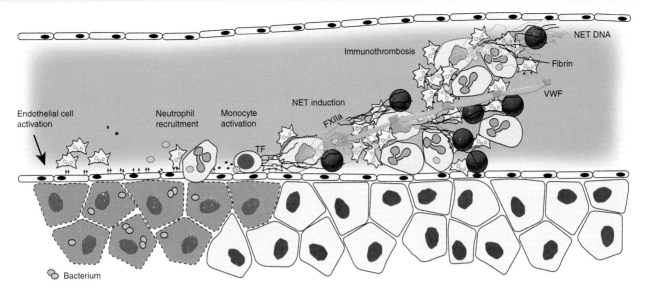

**Figure 3–30.** The role of immune cells: immunothrombosis. Endothelial cell activation by perturbation or infection causes neutrophil adhesion and monocyte activation. Induced tissue factor (TF) expression causes initial fibrin formation, while neutrophil activation by platelet interactions results in depolymerization of the DNA that bursts out the neutrophil as a mesh-generating neutrophil extracellular trap (NET). NETs may trap bacteria as innate immune defense, but also cause thrombosis by DNA-dependent factor XII activation and histone-dependent platelet activation. Furthermore, von Willebrand factor (VWF) may interact with DNA, which enhances platelet interaction with NETs.

controlled, it may contribute to thrombosis.[385] Figure 3–30 provides an overview of immunothrombosis.

The tight link between immune host defense and thrombosis is further demonstrated by the fact that immune cells play an active role in clot formation through several processes. First, monocytes express tissue factor upon activation by pathogens, which leads to thrombin generation by the extrinsic pathway.[386] Second, activated endothelium recruits neutrophils and, as a result of platelet–neutrophil interplay, neutrophil extracellular traps (NETs) can be formed,[387] which consist of decondensed chromatin fibers and DNA released by neutrophils.[388] NET-related proteins, such as histones and neutrophil elastase, activate platelets and inactivate TFPI, respectively, with both processes driving clot formation.[338,389] Moreover, NET DNA activates factor XII, resulting in enhanced thrombus formation mediated by the intrinsic pathway.[385] NETs also interact with VWF, which facilitates platelet binding to NETs.

The decondensation of chromatin that contributes to NET formation is caused by PAD4 relocalization to the neutrophil nucleus where it citrullinates histones. This results in unwinding of the DNA, which subsequently bursts out of the neutrophil.[388] The crucial role that PAD4-mediated NET formation may play in thrombosis has been shown in a physiologically relevant inferior vena cava thrombosis model in mice.[385,390] Consistent with this, NETs have been shown to be an integral component of human thrombi.[391] The notion that DNA is involved in pathologic thrombus formation opens doors to alternative ways of anticoagulation.

### The Role of Endothelial Cells

Once a blood clot is formed to seal the injury, the clotting process must be terminated to avoid thrombotic occlusion in the adjacent, nonperturbed vascular bed. If the coagulation reactions are not controlled, clotting could occur throughout the entire vasculature, even after a modest procoagulant stimulus.

Endothelial cells play a major role in confining the coagulation reactions to the site of injury and preventing clot extension to areas where the endothelium is intact (Chap. 5). Endothelial cells have two major types of anticoagulant/antithrombotic activities, as illustrated in Fig. 3–31.

First, the protein C/protein S/thrombomodulin/EPCR system is activated in response to thrombin generation. This was demonstrated by Hanson and colleagues, who showed that thrombin infusion *in vivo* is anticoagulant in a protein C–dependent manner.[392] This indicates that thrombin present at sites other than that of vascular damage is able to generate APC, which subsequently inactivates the cofactors Va and VIIIa, thereby terminating or preventing downstream thrombin generation.

Second, the protease inhibitors AT and TFPI are bound to heparan sulfates expressed on the endothelial surface, where they can inactivate proteases.[393] GPI-anchored TFPIβ may also play a role in controlling intravascular thrombin generation.[332] Furthermore, endothelial cells inhibit platelet activation by releasing the inhibitors prostacyclin (PGI$_2$) and nitric oxide (NO), as well as degrading adenosine diphosphate (ADP) by their membrane ecto-ADPase, CD39.[394]

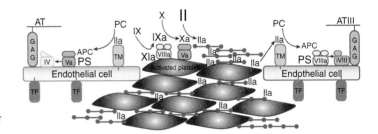

**Figure 3–31.** The role of endothelial cells. Activated coagulation proteins generated on platelets localized to the site of injury need to be confined to the site of injury. Activated coagulation factors that move to an endothelial cell surface are rapidly inhibited by antithrombin (AT), which is associated with glycosaminoglycans (GAG) on the endothelial surface. Furthermore, thrombin that reaches the endothelial cell surface binds to thrombomodulin (TM). Once bound, thrombin can no longer cleave fibrinogen. Instead, this thrombin activates protein C (APC), leading to the formation of APC–protein S (PS) complexes on the endothelial cell surface. APC-PS on the endothelial cell surface inactivates the procoagulant cofactors Va (to IV) and VIIIa (to iVIII). PC, protein C; TF, tissue factor.

## Role of Plasma Protease Inhibitors

Circulating protease inhibitors are also critical for localizing the coagulation reactions to specific cell surfaces by directly inhibiting proteases that diffuse away from the site of clot formation. Not only are the plasma protease inhibitors key players in confining a clot to the proper location, but also their synergistic action imposes a threshold effect on the coagulation process.[363,395,396] Thus, in the presence of inhibitors, coagulation does not proceed unless procoagulant factors are generated in sufficient amounts to overcome the inhibitory mechanisms. In case the triggering event is inadequate, the system returns to baseline rather than continuing through the coagulation process. Under pathologic conditions, the trigger for clotting may be so strong as to overwhelm the control mechanisms, leading to disseminated intravascular coagulation or thrombosis (Chaps. 19 and 23).

## ROLE OF FIBRINOLYSIS

Once a hemostatic clot has been formed and protected from fibrinolysis by the action of factor XIII and TAFI, some provision must be made for its eventual removal as wound healing takes place. Dissolution of clots is accomplished by the fibrinolytic system, as discussed in detail in Chap. 25.

## The Concept of Basal Coagulation and Anticoagulation

The coagulation process only proceeds when enough thrombin is generated on or near the tissue factor–bearing cell to trigger activation of platelets and cofactors. One may wonder, however, if minute hemostatic plugs are not constantly formed throughout the body to maintain the integrity of the vasculature. Indeed, a low level of coagulation factor activation probably occurs at all times.[397] More than 30 years ago, it was shown that fibrinopeptides are continuously cleaved from fibrinogen at low levels in normal individuals.[398] Minute amounts of factor VIIa as well as the activation peptides of factors IX and X have also been demonstrated to circulate in the bloodstream of normal individuals.[399–401] This is known as basal coagulation or idling. Basal activation of coagulation factors likely results from minor injuries that occur during normal daily activities. The basal coagulation must be balanced by basal activity of the anticoagulation and fibrinolytic systems. This is evidenced by the presence of low levels of the protein C activation peptide and tissue plasminogen activator activity in normal individuals.[402]

## REFERENCES

1. Davidson CJ, Hirt RP, Lal K, et al: Molecular evolution of the vertebrate blood coagulation network. *Thromb Haemost* 89:420–428, 2003.
2. Patthy L: Evolution of the proteases of blood coagulation and fibrinolysis by assembly from modules. *Cell* 41:657–663, 1985.
3. Wu SM, Cheung WF, Frazier D, Stafford DW: Cloning and expression of the cDNA for human gamma-glutamyl carboxylase. *Science* 254:1634–1636, 1991.
4. Li T, Chang C-Y, Jin D-Y, et al: Identification of the gene for vitamin K epoxide reductase. *Nature* 427:541–544, 2004.
5. Jorgensen MJ, Cantor AB, Furie BC, et al: Recognition site directing vitamin K-dependent gamma-carboxylation resides on the propeptide of factor IX. *Cell* 48:185–191, 1987.
6. Huber P, Schmitz T, Griffin J, et al: Identification of amino acids in the gamma-carboxylation recognition site on the propeptide of prothrombin. *J Biol Chem* 265:12467–12473, 1990.
7. Falls LA, Furie BC, Jacobs M, et al: The omega-loop region of the human prothrombin gamma-carboxyglutamic acid domain penetrates anionic phospholipid membranes. *J Biol Chem* 276:23895–23902, 2001.
8. Huang M, Rigby AC, Morelli X, et al: Structural basis of membrane binding by Gla domains of vitamin K-dependent proteins. *Nat Struct Biol* 10:751–756, 2003.
9. Tavoosi N, Davis-Harrison RL, Pogorelov TV, et al: Molecular determinants of phospholipid synergy in blood clotting. *J Biol Chem* 286:23247–23253, 2011.
10. Bode W, Mayr I, Baumann U, et al: The refined 1.9 A crystal structure of human alpha-thrombin: Interaction with D-Phe-Pro-Arg chloromethylketone and significance of the Tyr-Pro-Pro-Trp insertion segment. *EMBO J* 8:3467–3475, 1989.
11. Persson E, Olsen OH: Allosteric activation of coagulation factor VIIa. *Front Biosci (Landmark Ed)* 16:3156–3163, 2011.
12. Morawitz P: Die Chemie der Blutgerinnung. *Ergeb Physiol* 4:307–422, 1905.
13. Quick AJ: *Hemorrhagic Diseases*, pp 451–490. Lea and Febiger, Philadelphia, 1957.
14. Degen SJ: The prothrombin gene and its liver-specific expression. *Semin Thromb Hemost* 18:230–242, 1992.
15. Wu W, Suttie JW: N-glycosylation contributes to the intracellular stability of prothrombin precursors in the endoplasmic reticulum. *Thromb Res* 96:91–98, 1999.
16. Bradford HN, Orcutt SJ, Krishnaswamy S: Membrane binding by prothrombin mediates its constrained presentation to prothrombinase for cleavage. *J Biol Chem* 288:27789–27800, 2013.
17. Krishnaswamy S: The transition of prothrombin to thrombin. *J Thromb Haemost* 11(Suppl 1):265–276, 2013.
18. Bradford HN, Krishnaswamy S: Meizothrombin is an unexpectedly zymogen-like variant of thrombin. *J Biol Chem* 287:30414–30425, 2012.
19. Bode W, Turk D, Karshikov A: The refined 1.9-A X-ray crystal structure of D-Phe-Pro-Arg chloromethylketone-inhibited human alpha-thrombin: Structure analysis, overall structure, electrostatic properties, detailed active-site geometry, and structure-function relationships. *Protein Sci* 1:426–471, 1992.
20. Lechtenberg BC, Freund SM, Huntington JA: An ensemble view of thrombin allostery. *Biol Chem* 393:889–898, 2012.
21. Lechtenberg BC, Johnson DJ, Freund SM, Huntington JA: NMR resonance assignments of thrombin reveal the conformational and dynamic effects of ligation. *Proc Natl Acad Sci U S A* 107:14087–14092, 2010.
22. Vu TK, Hung DT, Wheaton VI, Coughlin SR: Molecular cloning of a functional thrombin receptor reveals a novel proteolytic mechanism of receptor activation. *Cell* 64:1057–1068, 1991.
23. Ishihara H, Connolly AJ, Zeng D, et al: Protease-activated receptor 3 is a second thrombin receptor in humans. *Nature* 386:502–506, 1997.
24. Xu WF, Andersen H, Whitmore TE, et al: Cloning and characterization of human protease-activated receptor 4. *Proc Natl Acad Sci U S A* 95:6642–6646, 1998.
25. Coughlin SR: Protease-activated receptors in hemostasis, thrombosis and vascular biology. *J Thromb Haemost* 3:1800–1814, 2005.
26. Spronk HM, de Jong AM, Crijns HJ, et al: Pleiotropic effects of factor Xa and thrombin: What to expect from novel anticoagulants. *Cardiovasc Res* 101:344–351, 2014.
27. Coppens M, Eikelboom JW, Gustafsson D, et al: Translational success stories: Development of direct thrombin inhibitors. *Circ Res* 111:920–929, 2012.
28. Hauel NH, Nar H, Priepke H, et al: Structure-based design of novel potent nonpeptide thrombin inhibitors. *J Med Chem* 45:1757–1766, 2002.
29. Royle NJ, Irwin DM, Koschinsky ML, et al: Human genes encoding prothrombin and ceruloplasmin map to 11p11-q12 and 3q21–24, respectively. *Somat Cell Mol Genet* 13:285–292, 1987.
30. Peyvandi F, Bolton-Maggs PH, Batorova A, De Moerloose P: Rare bleeding disorders. *Haemophilia* 18(Suppl 4):148–153, 2012.
31. Poort SR, Rosendaal FR, Reitsma PH, Bertina RM: A common genetic variation in the 3′-untranslated region of the prothrombin gene is associated with elevated plasma prothrombin levels and an increase in venous thrombosis. *Blood* 88:3698–3703, 1996.
32. Gehring NH, Frede U, Neu-Yilik G, et al: Increased efficiency of mRNA 3′ end formation: A new genetic mechanism contributing to hereditary thrombophilia. *Nat Genet* 28:389–392, 2001.
33. Rosendaal FR, Doggen CJ, Zivelin A, et al: Geographic distribution of the 20210 G to A prothrombin variant. *Thromb Haemost* 79:706–708, 1998.
34. Giangrande PLF: Six characters in search of an author: The history of the nomenclature of coagulation factors. *Br J Haematol* 121:703–712, 2003.
35. Hansson K, Stenflo J: Post-translational modifications in proteins involved in blood coagulation. *J Thromb Haemost* 3:2633–2648, 2005.
36. Butenas S, Mann KG: Kinetics of human factor VII activation. *Biochemistry* 35:1904–1910, 1996.
37. Neuenschwander PF, Fiore MM, Morrissey JH: Factor VII autoactivation proceeds via interaction of distinct protease-cofactor and zymogen-cofactor complexes. Implications of a two-dimensional enzyme kinetic mechanism. *J Biol Chem* 268:21489–21492, 1993.
38. Camerer E, Huang W, Coughlin SR: Tissue factor- and factor X-dependent activation of protease-activated receptor 2 by factor VIIa. *Proc Natl Acad Sci U S A* 97:5255–5260, 2000.
39. Hoffman M, Monroe DM: The multiple roles of tissue factor in wound healing. *Front Biosci (Schol Ed)* 4:713–721, 2012.
40. Riewald M, Ruf W: Mechanistic coupling of protease signaling and initiation of coagulation by tissue factor. *Proc Natl Acad Sci U S A* 98:7742–7747, 2001.
41. O'Hara PJ, Grant FJ: The human factor VII gene is polymorphic due to variation in repeat copy number in a minisatellite. *Gene* 66:147–158, 1988.
42. Berkner K, Busby S, Davie E, et al: Isolation and expression of cDNAs encoding human factor VII. *Cold Spring Harb Symp Quant Biol* 51(Pt 1):531–541, 1986.
43. Girelli D, Russo C, Ferraresi P, et al: Polymorphisms in the factor VII gene and the risk of myocardial infarction in patients with coronary artery disease. *N Engl J Med* 343:774–780, 2000.
44. Biggs R, Douglas AS, MacFarlane RG, et al: Christmas disease: A condition previously mistaken for haemophilia. *Br Med J* 2:1378–1382, 1952.
45. Gillis S, Furie BC, Furie B, et al: gamma-Carboxyglutamic acids 36 and 40 do not contribute to human factor IX function. *Protein Sci* 6:185–196, 1997.

46. Winship PR, Dragon AC: Identification of haemophilia B patients with mutations in the two calcium binding domains of factor IX: Importance of a beta-OH Asp 64–Asn change. *Br J Haematol* 77:102–109, 1991.

47. Rallapalli PM, Kemball-Cook G, Tuddenham EG, et al: An interactive mutation database for human coagulation factor IX provides novel insights into the phenotypes and genetics of hemophilia B. *J Thromb Haemost* 11:1329–1340, 2013.

48. Begbie ME, Mamdani A, Gataiance S, et al: An important role for the activation peptide domain in controlling factor IX levels in the blood of haemophilia B mice. *Thromb Haemost* 94:1138–1147, 2005.

49. Bolt G, Bjelke JR, Hermit MB, et al: Hyperglycosylation prolongs the circulation of coagulation factor IX. *J Thromb Haemost* 10:2397–2398, 2012.

50. Brooks AR, Sim D, Gritzan U, et al: Glycoengineered factor IX variants with improved pharmacokinetics and subcutaneous efficacy. *J Thromb Haemost* 11:1699–1706, 2013.

51. Cheung WF, Hamaguchi N, Smith KJ, Stafford DW: The binding of human factor IX to endothelial cells is mediated by residues 3–11. *J Biol Chem* 267:20529–20531, 1992.

52. Cheung WF, van den Born J, Kühn K, et al: Identification of the endothelial cell binding site for factor IX. *Proc Natl Acad Sci U S A* 93:11068–11073, 1996.

53. Lenting PJ, ter Maat H, Clijsters PP, et al: Cleavage at arginine 145 in human blood coagulation factor IX converts the zymogen into a factor VIII binding enzyme. *J Biol Chem* 270:14884–14890, 1995.

54. Lindquist PA, Fujikawa K, Davie EW: Activation of bovine factor IX (Christmas factor) by factor XIa (activated plasma thromboplastin antecedent) and a protease from Russell's viper venom. *J Biol Chem* 253:1902–1909, 1978.

55. Zögg T, Brandstetter H: Activation mechanisms of coagulation factor IX. *Biol Chem* 390:391–400, 2009.

56. Johnson DJD, Langdown J, Huntington JA: Molecular basis of factor IXa recognition by heparin-activated antithrombin revealed by a 1.7-A structure of the ternary complex. *Proc Natl Acad Sci U S A* 107:645–650, 2010.

57. Camerino G, Grzeschik KH, Jaye M, et al: Regional localization on the human X chromosome and polymorphism of the coagulation factor IX gene (hemophilia B locus). *Proc Natl Acad Sci U S A* 81:498–502, 1984.

58. van Hylckama Vlieg A, van der Linden IK, Bertina RM, Rosendaal FR: High levels of factor IX increase the risk of venous thrombosis. *Blood* 95:3678–3682, 2000.

59. Simioni P, Tormene D, Tognin G, et al: X-linked thrombophilia with a mutant factor IX (factor IX Padua). *N Engl J Med* 361:1671–1675, 2009.

60. Denson K: Electrophoretic studies of the Prower factor: A blood coagulation factor which differs from factor VII. *Br J Haematol* 4:313–325, 1957.

61. Telfer TP, Denson KW, Wright DR: A new coagulation defect. *Br J Haematol* 2:308–316, 1956.

62. Hougie C, Barrow EM, Graham JB: Stuart clotting defect. I. Segregation of an hereditary hemorrhagic state from the heterogeneous group heretofore called stable factor (SPCA, proconvertin, factor VII) deficiency. *J Clin Invest* 36:485–496, 1957.

63. Gueguen P, Cherel G, Badirou I, et al: Two residues in the activation peptide domain contribute to the half-life of factor X *in vivo*. *J Thromb Haemost* 8:1651–1653, 2010.

64. Rudolph AE, Mullane MP, Porche-Sorbet R, et al: The role of the factor X activation peptide: A deletion mutagenesis approach. *Thromb Haemost* 88:756–762, 2002.

65. Yang L, Manithody C, Rezaie AR: Functional role of O-linked and N-linked glycosylation sites present on the activation peptide of factor X. *J Thromb Haemost* 7:1696–1702, 2009.

66. Rao LV, Rapaport SI: Activation of factor VII bound to tissue factor: A key early step in the tissue factor pathway of blood coagulation. *Proc Natl Acad Sci U S A* 85:6687–6691, 1988.

67. Monkovic DD, Tracy PB: Activation of human factor V by factor Xa and thrombin. *Biochemistry* 29:1118–1128, 1990.

68. Neuenschwander PF, Jesty J: Thrombin-activated and factor Xa-activated human factor VIII: Differences in cofactor activity and decay rate. *Arch Biochem Biophys* 296:426–434, 1992.

69. Borensztajn K, Peppelenbosch MP, Spek CA: Factor Xa: At the crossroads between coagulation and signaling in physiology and disease. *Trends Mol Med* 14:429–440, 2008.

70. Jesty J, Spencer AK, Nemerson Y: The mechanism of activation of factor X. Kinetic control of alternative pathways leading to the formation of activated factor X. *J Biol Chem* 249:5614–5622, 1974.

71. Fujikawa K, Titani K, Davie EW: Activation of bovine factor X (Stuart factor): Conversion of factor Xaalpha to factor Xabeta. *Proc Natl Acad Sci U S A* 72:3359–3363, 1975.

72. Pryzdial EL, Kessler GE: Kinetics of blood coagulation factor Xaalpha autoproteolytic conversion to factor Xabeta. Effect on inhibition by antithrombin, prothrombinase assembly, and enzyme activity. *J Biol Chem* 271:16621–16626, 1996.

73. Pryzdial EL, Kessler GE: Autoproteolysis or plasmin-mediated cleavage of factor Xaalpha exposes a plasminogen binding site and inhibits coagulation. *J Biol Chem* 271:16614–16620, 1996.

74. Grundy JE, Lavigne N, Hirama T, et al: Binding of plasminogen and tissue plasminogen activator to plasmin-modulated factor X and factor Xa. *Biochemistry* 40:6293–6302, 2001.

75. Talbot K, Meixner SC, Pryzdial ELG: Enhanced fibrinolysis by proteolysed coagulation factor Xa. *Biochim Biophys Acta* 1804:723–730, 2010.

76. Johnson DJD, Li W, Adams TE, Huntington JA: Antithrombin-S195A factor Xa-heparin structure reveals the allosteric mechanism of antithrombin activation. *EMBO J* 25:2029–2037, 2006.

77. Hackeng TM, Seré KM, Tans G, Rosing J: Protein S stimulates inhibition of the tissue factor pathway by tissue factor pathway inhibitor. *Proc Natl Acad Sci U S A* 103:3106–3111, 2006.

78. Ndonwi M, Broze G: Protein S enhances the tissue factor pathway inhibitor inhibition of factor Xa but not its inhibition of factor VIIa-tissue factor. *J Thromb Haemost* 6:1044–1046, 2008.

79. Han X, Fiehler R, Broze GJ Jr: Characterization of the protein Z-dependent protease inhibitor. *Blood* 96:3049–3055, 2000.

80. Roehrig S, Straub A, Pohlmann J, et al: Discovery of the novel antithrombotic agent 5-chloro-N-({(5S)-2-oxo-3-[4-(3-oxomorpholin-4-yl)phenyl]-1,3-oxazolidin-5-yl} methyl) thiophene- 2-carboxamide (BAY 59-7939): An oral, direct factor Xa inhibitor. *J Med Chem* 48:5900–5908, 2005.

81. Pinto DJ, Orwat MJ, Koch S, et al: Discovery of 1-(4-methoxyphenyl)-7-oxo-6-(4-(2-oxopiperidin-1-yl)phenyl)-4,5,6,7-tetrahydro-1H-pyrazolo[3,4-c]pyridine-3-carboxamide (apixaban, BMS-562247), a highly potent, selective, efficacious, and orally bioavailable inhibitor of blood coagulation factor Xa. *J Med Chem* 50:5339–5356, 2007.

82. Furugohri T, Isobe K, Honda Y, et al: DU-176b, a potent and orally active factor Xa inhibitor: *In vitro* and *in vivo* pharmacological profiles. *J Thromb Haemost* 6:1542–1549, 2008.

83. Perzborn E, Roehrig S, Straub A, et al: The discovery and development of rivaroxaban, an oral, direct factor Xa inhibitor. *Nat Rev Drug Discov* 10:61–75, 2011.

84. Scambler PJ, Williamson R: The structural gene for human coagulation factor X is located on chromosome 13q34. *Cytogenet Cell Genet* 39:231–233, 1985.

85. de Visser MC, Poort SR, Vos HL, et al: Factor X levels, polymorphisms in the promoter region of factor X, and the risk of venous thrombosis. *Thromb Haemost* 85:1011–1017, 2001.

86. Mammen EF, Thomas WH, Seegers WH: Activation of purified prothrombin to autoprothrombin I or autoprothrombin II (platelet cofactor II or autoprothrombin II-A). *Thromb Diath Haemorrh* 5:218–249, 1960.

87. Stenflo J: A new vitamin K-dependent protein. *J Biol Chem* 251:355–363, 1976.

88. Foster DC, Yoshitake S, Davie EW: The nucleotide sequence of the gene for human protein C. *Proc Natl Acad Sci U S A* 82:4673–4677, 1985.

89. Grinnell BW, Walls JD, Gerlitz B: Glycosylation of human protein C affects its secretion, processing, functional activities, and activation by thrombin. *J Biol Chem* 266:9778–9785, 1991.

90. McClure DB, Walls JD, Grinnell BW: Post-translational processing events in the secretion pathway of human protein C, a complex vitamin K-dependent antithrombotic factor. *J Biol Chem* 267:19710–19717, 1992.

91. Preston R, Rawley O: Elucidating the role of carbohydrate determinants in regulating hemostasis: Insights and opportunities. *Blood* 121:3801–3810, 2013.

92. Stearns-Kurosawa DJ, Kurosawa S, Mollica JS, Ferrell GL, Esmon CT: The endothelial cell protein C receptor augments protein C activation by the thrombin-thrombomodulin complex. *Proc Natl Acad Sci U S A* 93:10212–10216, 1996.

93. Shen L, Dahlback B: Factor V and protein S as synergistic cofactors to activated protein C in degradation of factor VIIIa. *J Biol Chem* 269:18735–18738, 1994.

94. Oliver JA, Monroe DM, Church FC, et al: Activated protein C cleaves factor Va more efficiently on endothelium than on platelet surfaces. *Blood* 100:539–546, 2002.

95. Slungaard A, Fernandez JA, Griffin JH, et al: Platelet factor 4 enhances generation of activated protein C *in vitro* and *in vivo*. *Blood* 102:146–151, 2003.

96. Bouwens EA, Stavenuiter F, Mosnier LO: Mechanisms of anticoagulant and cytoprotective actions of the protein C pathway. *J Thromb Haemost* 11(Suppl 1):242–253, 2013.

97. Foster DC, Yoshitake S, Davie EW: The nucleotide sequence of the gene for human protein C. *Proc Natl Acad Sci U S A* 82:4673–4677, 1985.

98. Branson HE, Katz J, Marble R, Griffin JH: Inherited protein C deficiency and coumarin-responsive chronic relapsing purpura fulminans in a newborn infant. *Lancet* 2:1165–1168, 1983.

99. Reitsma PH: Protein C deficiency: From gene defects to disease. *Thromb Haemost* 78:344–350, 1997.

100. Lijfering WM, Christiansen SC, Rosendaal FR, Cannegieter SC: Contribution of high factor VIII, IX and XI to the risk of recurrent venous thrombosis in factor V Leiden carriers. *J Thromb Haemost* 7:1944–1946, 2009.

101. Spek CA, Koster T, Rosendaal FR, et al: Genotypic variation in the promoter region of the protein C gene is associated with plasma protein C levels and thrombotic risk. *Arterioscler Thromb Vasc Biol* 15:214–218, 1995.

102. Davidson CJ, Tuddenham EG, McVey JH: 450 Million years of hemostasis. *J Thromb Haemost* 1:1487–1494, 2003.

103. Zheng C, Zhang B: Combined deficiency of coagulation factors V and VIII: An update. *Semin Thromb Hemost* 39:613–620, 2013.

104. Owren PA: The coagulation of blood: Investigations on a new clotting factor. *Acta Med Scand* 128 (Suppl 194), 1947.

105. Owren PA: Parahaemophilia. Haemorrhagic diathesis due to absence of a previously unknown clotting factor. *Lancet* 1:446–448, 1947.

106. Stormorken H: The discovery of factor V: A tricky clotting factor. *J Thromb Haemost* 1:206–213, 2003.

107. Camire RM, Pollak ES, Kaushansky K, Tracy PB: Secretable human platelet-derived factor V originates from the plasma pool. *Blood* 92:3035–3041, 1998.

108. Thomassen MC, Castoldi E, Tans G, et al: Endogenous factor V synthesis in megakaryocytes contributes negligibly to the platelet factor V pool. *Haematologica* 88:1150–1156, 2003.

109. Bouchard BA, Williams JL, Meisler NT, et al: Endocytosis of plasma-derived factor V by megakaryocytes occurs via a clathrin-dependent, specific membrane binding event. *J Thromb Haemost* 3:541–551, 2005.

110. Gould WR, Silveira JR, Tracy PB: Unique *in vivo* modifications of coagulation factor V produce a physically and functionally distinct platelet-derived cofactor: Characterization of purified platelet-derived factor V/Va. *J Biol Chem* 279:2383–2393, 2004.

111. Hayward CP: Multimerin: A bench-to-bedside chronology of a unique platelet and endothelial cell protein—From discovery to function to abnormalities in disease. *Clin Invest Med* 20:176–187, 1997.

112. Nesheim ME, Nichols WL, Cole TL, et al: Isolation and study of an acquired inhibitor of human coagulation factor V. *J Clin Invest* 77:405–415, 1986.

113. Sun H, Yang TL, Yang A, et al: The murine platelet and plasma factor V pools are biosynthetically distinct and sufficient for minimal hemostasis. *Blood* 102:2856–2861, 2003.

114. Yang TL, Pipe SW, Yang A, Ginsburg D: Biosynthetic origin and functional significance of murine platelet factor V. *Blood* 102:2851–2855, 2003.

115. Ortel TL, Devore-Carter D, Quinn-Allen M, Kane WH: Deletion analysis of recombinant human factor V. Evidence for a phosphatidylserine binding site in the second C-type domain. *J Biol Chem* 267:4189–4198, 1992.

116. Adams TE, Hockin MF, Mann KG, Everse SJ: The crystal structure of activated protein C-inactivated bovine factor Va: Implications for cofactor function. *Proc Natl Acad Sci U S A* 101:8918–8923, 2004.

117. Peng W, Quinn-Allen Ma, Kane WH: Mutation of hydrophobic residues in the factor Va C1 and C2 domains blocks membrane-dependent prothrombin activation. *J Thromb Haemost* 3:351–354, 2005.

118. Stoilova-McPhie S, Parmenter CD, Segers K, et al: Defining the structure of membrane-bound human blood coagulation factor Va. *J Thromb Haemost* 6:76–82, 2008.

119. Bos MH, Camire RM: A bipartite autoinhibitory region within the B-domain suppresses function in factor V. *J Biol Chem* 287:26342–26351, 2012.

120. Bunce MW, Bos MH, Krishnaswamy S, Camire RM: Restoring the procofactor state of factor Va-like variants by complementation with B-domain peptides. *J Biol Chem* 288:30151–30160, 2013.

121. Mann KG, Kalafatis M: Factor V: A combination of Dr Jekyll and Mr Hyde. *Blood* 101:20–30, 2003.

122. Pittman DD, Tomkinson KN, Michnick D, et al: Posttranslational sulfation of factor V is required for efficient thrombin cleavage and activation and for full procoagulant activity. *Biochemistry* 33:6952–6959, 1994.

123. Kalafatis M: Identification and partial characterization of factor Va heavy chain kinase from human platelets. *J Biol Chem* 273:8459–8466, 1998.

124. Kim SW, Ortel TL, Quinn-Allen MA, et al: Partial glycosylation at asparagine-2181 of the second C-type domain of human factor V modulates assembly of the prothrombinase complex. *Biochemistry* 38:11448–11454, 1999.

125. Nicolaes GA, Villoutreix BO, Dahlbäck B: Partial glycosylation of Asn2181 in human factor V as a cause of molecular and functional heterogeneity. Modulation of glycosylation efficiency by mutagenesis of the consensus sequence for N-linked glycosylation. *Biochemistry* 38:13584–13591, 1999.

126. Camire RM, Bos MH: The molecular basis of factor V and VIII procofactor activation. *J Thromb Haemost* 7:1951–1961, 2009.

127. Schuijt TJ, Bakhtiari K, Daffre S, et al: Factor Xa activation of factor V is of paramount importance in initiating the coagulation system: Lessons from a tick salivary protein. *Circulation* 128:919–966, 2013.

128. Thorelli E, Kaufman RJ, Dahlback B: Cleavage requirements for activation of factor V by factor Xa. *Eur J Biochem* 247:12–20, 1997.

129. Mann KG, Nesheim ME, Church WR, et al: Surface-dependent reactions of the vitamin K-dependent enzyme complexes. *Blood* 76:1–16, 1990.

130. Mann KG, Hockin MF, Begin KJ, Kalafatis M: Activated protein C cleavage of factor Va leads to dissociation of the A2 domain. *J Biol Chem* 272:20678–20683, 1997.

131. Bertina RM, Koeleman BP, Koster T, et al: Mutation in blood coagulation factor V associated with resistance to activated protein C. *Nature* 369:64–67, 1994.

132. Duckers C, Simioni P, Spiezia L, et al: Low plasma levels of tissue factor pathway inhibitor in patients with congenital factor V deficiency. *Blood* 112:3615, 2008.

133. Vincent L, Tran S: Coagulation factor V A2440G causes east Texas bleeding disorder via TFPIα. *J Clin Invest* 123:3777–3787, 2013.

134. Duckers C, Simioni P, Spiezia L, et al: Residual platelet factor V ensures thrombin generation in patients with severe congenital factor V deficiency and mild bleeding symptoms. *Blood* 115:879–886, 2010.

135. Cripe LD, Moore KD, Kane WH: Structure of the gene for human coagulation factor V. *Biochemistry* 31:3777–3785, 1992.

136. Owren PA: Parahaemophilia; haemorrhagic diathesis due to absence of a previously unknown clotting factor. *Lancet* 1:446–448, 1947.

137. Dahlbäck B, Carlsson M, Svensson PJ: Familial thrombophilia due to a previously unrecognized mechanism characterized by poor anticoagulant response to activated protein C: Prediction of a cofactor to activated protein C. *Proc Natl Acad Sci U S A* 90:1004–1008, 1993.

138. Bertina RM, Koeleman BP, Koster T, et al: Mutation in blood coagulation factor V associated with resistance to activated protein C. *Nature* 369:64–67, 1994.

139. Patek AJ, Taylor FH: Hemophilia. II. Some properties of a substance obtained from normal human plasma effective in accelerating the coagulation of hemophilic blood. *J Clin Invest* 16:113–124, 1937.

140. Tuddenham EG, Trabold NC, Collins JA, Hoyer LW: The properties of factor VIII coagulant activity prepared by immunoadsorbent chromatography. *J Lab Clin Med* 93:40–53, 1979.

141. Shaw E, Giddings JC, Peake IR, Bloom AL: Synthesis of procoagulant factor VIII, factor VIII related antigen and other coagulation factors by the isolated perfused rat liver. *Br J Haematol* 41:585–596, 1979.

142. Bontempo FA, Lewis JH, Gorenc TJ, et al: Liver transplantation in hemophilia A. *Blood* 69:1721–1724, 1987.

143. Lamont PA, Ragni MV: Lack of desmopressin (DDAVP) response in men with hemophilia A following liver transplantation. *J Thromb Haemost* 3:2259–2263, 2005.

144. Madeira C, Layman R, de Vera M, et al: Extrahepatic factor VIII production in transplant recipient of hemophilia donor liver. *Blood* 113:5364–5366, 2009.

145. Kumaran V, Benten D, Follenzi A, et al: Transplantation of endothelial cells corrects the phenotype in hemophilia A mice. *J Thromb Haemost* 3:2022–2031, 2005.

146. Everett L, Cleuren A: Murine coagulation factor VIII is synthesized in endothelial cells. *Blood* 123:3697–3706, 2014.

147. Fahs SA, Hille MT, Shi Q, et al: A conditional knockout mouse model reveals endothelial cells as the principal and possibly exclusive source of plasma factor VIII. *Blood* 123:3706–3714, 2014.

148. Jacquemin M, Neyrinck A, Hermanns M, et al: FVIII production by human lung microvascular endothelial cells. *Blood* 108:515–518, 2006.

149. Shahani T, Covens K, Lavend'homme R, et al: Human liver sinusoidal endothelial cells but not hepatocytes contain factor VIII. *J Thromb Haemost* 12:36–42, 2014.

150. Pipe SW, Morris JA, Shah J, Kaufman RJ: Differential interaction of coagulation factor VIII and factor V with protein chaperones calnexin and calreticulin. *J Biol Chem* 273:8537–8544, 1998.

151. Swaroop M, Moussalli M, Pipe SW, Kaufman RJ: Mutagenesis of a potential immunoglobulin-binding protein-binding site enhances secretion of coagulation factor VIII. *J Biol Chem* 272:24121–24124, 1997.

152. Lenting PJ, Neels JG, van den Berg BM, et al: The light chain of factor VIII comprises a binding site for low density lipoprotein receptor-related protein. *J Biol Chem* 274:23734–23739, 1999.

153. Saenko EL, Yakhyaev AV, Mikhailenko I, et al: Role of the low density lipoprotein-related protein receptor in mediation of factor VIII catabolism. *J Biol Chem* 274:37685–37692, 1999.

154. Bovenschen N, Rijken DC, Havekes LM, et al: The B domain of coagulation factor VIII interacts with the asialoglycoprotein receptor. *J Thromb Haemost* 3:1257–1265, 2005.

155. Bovenschen N, Mertens K, Hu L, et al: LDL receptor cooperates with LDL receptor-related protein in regulating plasma levels of coagulation factor VIII *in vivo*. *Blood* 106:906–912, 2005.

156. Pegon JN, Kurdi M, Casari C, et al: Factor VIII and von Willebrand factor are ligands for the carbohydrate-receptor Siglec-5. *Haematologica* 97:1855–1863, 2012.

157. Leyte A, Verbeet MP, Brodniewicz-Proba T, et al: The interaction between human blood-coagulation factor VIII and von Willebrand factor. Characterization of a high-affinity binding site on factor VIII. *Biochem J* 257:679–683, 1989.

158. Saenko EL, Scandella D: The acidic region of the factor VIII light chain and the C2 domain together form the high affinity binding site for von Willebrand factor. *J Biol Chem* 272:18007–18014, 1997.

159. Gilbert GE, Kaufman RJ, Arena AA, et al: Four hydrophobic amino acids of the factor VIII C2 domain are constituents of both the membrane-binding and von Willebrand factor-binding motifs. *J Biol Chem* 277:6374–6381, 2002.

160. Meems H, Meijer A, Cullinan D, et al: Factor VIII C1 domain residues Lys 2092 and Phe 2093 contribute to membrane binding and cofactor activity. *Blood* 114:3938–3947, 2009.

161. Bloem E, van den Biggelaar M, Wroblewska A, et al: Factor VIII C1 domain spikes 2092–2093 and 2158–2159 comprise regions that modulate cofactor function and cellular uptake. *J Biol Chem* 288:29670–29679, 2013.

162. Cunningham MA, Pipe SW, Zhang B, et al: LMAN1 is a molecular chaperone for the secretion of coagulation factor VIII. *J Thromb Haemost* 1:2360–2367, 2003.

163. Michnick DA, Pittman DD, Wise RJ, Kaufman RJ: Identification of individual tyrosine sulfation sites within factor VIII required for optimal activity and efficient thrombin cleavage. *J Biol Chem* 269:20095–20102, 1994.

164. Vehar GA, Keyt B, Eaton D, et al: Structure of human factor VIII. *Nature* 312:337–342, 1983.

165. Eaton D, Rodriguez H, Vehar GA: Proteolytic processing of human factor VIII. Correlation of specific cleavages by thrombin, factor Xa, and activated protein C with activation and inactivation of factor VIII coagulant activity. *Biochemistry* 25:505–512, 1986.

166. Newell JL, Fay PJ: Proteolysis at Arg740 facilitates subsequent bond cleavages during thrombin-catalyzed activation of factor VIII. *J Biol Chem* 282:25367–25375, 2007.

167. Fay PJ, Haidaris PJ, Smudzin TM: Human factor VIIIa subunit structure. Reconstruction of factor VIIIa from the isolated A1/A3-C1-C2 dimer and A2 subunit. *J Biol Chem* 266:8957–8962, 1991.

168. Lollar P, Parker ET: Structural basis for the decreased procoagulant activity of human factor VIII compared to the porcine homolog. *J Biol Chem* 266:12481–12486, 1991.

169. Fay PJ: Activation of factor VIII and mechanisms of cofactor action. *Blood Rev* 18:1–15, 2004.

170. Gitschier J, Wood WI, Goralka TM, et al: Characterization of the human factor VIII gene. *Nature* 312:326–330, 1984.

171. Kamphuisen PW, Eikenboom JC, Rosendaal FR, et al: High factor VIII antigen levels increase the risk of venous thrombosis but are not associated with polymorphisms in the von Willebrand factor and factor VIII gene. *Br J Haematol* 115:156–158, 2001.

172. Preston AE, Barr A: The plasma concentration of factor VIII in the normal population. II. The effects of age, sex and blood group. *Br J Haematol* 10:238–245, 1964.

173. Morelli VM, De Visser MC, Vos HL, et al: ABO blood group genotypes and the risk of venous thrombosis: Effect of factor V Leiden. *J Thromb Haemost* 3:183–185, 2005.

174. Fair DS, Marlar RA: Biosynthesis and secretion of factor VII, protein C, protein S, and the protein C inhibitor from a human hepatoma cell line. *Blood* 67:64–70, 1986.

175. Fair DS, Marlar RA, Levin EG: Human endothelial cells synthesize protein S. *Blood* 67:1168–1171, 1986.

176. Ogura M, Tanabe N, Nishioka J, et al: Biosynthesis and secretion of functional protein S by a human megakaryoblastic cell line (MEG-01). *Blood* 70:301–306, 1987.

177. Dahlbäck B: Protein S and C4b-binding protein: Components involved in the regulation of the protein C anticoagulant system. *Thromb Haemost* 66:49–61, 1991.

178. Maillard C, Berruyer M, Serre CM, et al: Protein-S, a vitamin K-dependent protein, is a bone matrix component synthesized and secreted by osteoblasts. *Endocrinology* 130:1599–1604, 1992.

179. Walker FJ: Regulation of activated protein C by a new protein. A possible function for bovine protein S. *J Biol Chem* 255:5521–5524, 1980.

180. van de Poel RH, Meijers JC, Bouma BN: C4b-binding protein inhibits the factor V-dependent but not the factor V-independent cofactor activity of protein S in the activated protein C-mediated inactivation of factor VIIIa. *Thromb Haemost* 85:761–765, 2001.

181. Yegneswaran S, Wood GM, Esmon CT, Johnson AE: Protein S alters the active site location of activated protein C above the membrane surface. A fluorescence resonance energy transfer study of topography. *J Biol Chem* 272:25013–25021, 1997.

182. Rosing J, Hoekema L, Nicolaes GA, et al: Effects of protein S and factor Xa on peptide bond cleavages during inactivation of factor Va and factor VaR506Q by activated protein C. *J Biol Chem* 270:27852–27858, 1995.

183. Maurissen LF, Thomassen MC, Nicolaes GA, et al: Re-evaluation of the role of the protein S-C4b binding protein complex in activated protein C-catalyzed factor Va-inactivation. *Blood* 111:3034–3041, 2008.

184. Dahlback B: The tale of protein S and C4b-binding protein, a story of affection. *Thromb Haemost* 98:90–96, 2007.

185. Reglińska-Matveyev N, Andersson H, Rezende S, et al: TFPI cofactor function of protein S: Essential role of the protein S SHBG-like domain. *Blood* 123:3979–3988, 2014.

186. Suleiman L, Négrier C, Boukerche H: Protein S: A multifunctional anticoagulant vitamin K-dependent protein at the crossroads of coagulation, inflammation, angiogenesis, and cancer. *Crit Rev Oncol Hematol* 88:637–654, 2013.

187. van der Meer JH, van der Poll T, van't Veer C: TAM receptors, Gas6, and protein S: Roles in inflammation and hemostasis. *Blood* 123:2460–2470, 2014.

188. Ploos van Amstel HK, Reitsma PH, van der Logt CP, Bertina RM: Intron-exon organization of the active human protein S gene PS alpha and its pseudogene PS beta: Duplication and silencing during primate evolution. *Biochemistry* 29:7853–7861, 1990.

189. Gómez E, Ledford MR, Pegelow CH, et al: Homozygous protein S deficiency due to a one base pair deletion that leads to a stop codon in exon III of the protein S gene. *Thromb Haemost* 71:723–726, 1994.

190. Marlar RA, Gausman JN: Protein S abnormalities: A diagnostic nightmare. *Am J Hematol* 86:418–421, 2011.

191. Pintao MC, Garcia AA, Borgel D, et al: Gross deletions/duplications in PROS1 are relatively common in point mutation-negative hereditary protein S deficiency. *Hum Genet* 126:449–456, 2009.

192. Pintao MC, Ribeiro DD, Bezemer ID, et al: Protein S levels and the risk of venous thrombosis: Results from the MEGA case-control study. *Blood* 122:3210–3219, 2013.

193. Giblin JP, Hewlett LJ, Hannah MJ: Basal secretion of von Willebrand factor from human endothelial cells. *Blood* 112:957–964, 2008.

194. van Schooten CJ, Shahbazi S, Groot E, et al: Macrophages contribute to the cellular uptake of von Willebrand factor and factor VIII *in vivo*. *Blood* 112:1704–1712, 2008.

195. Furlan M, Robles R, Lammle B: Partial purification and characterization of a protease from human plasma cleaving von Willebrand factor to fragments produced by *in vivo* proteolysis. *Blood* 87:4223–4234, 1996.

196. Bonthron DT, Handin RI, Kaufman RJ, et al: Structure of pre-pro-von Willebrand factor and its expression in heterologous cells. *Nature* 324:270–273, 1986.

197. Huizinga EG, Tsuji S, Romijn RA, et al: Structures of glycoprotein Ibalpha and its complex with von Willebrand factor A1 domain. *Science* 297:1176–1179, 2002.

198. Foster PA, Fulcher CA, Marti T, et al: A major factor VIII binding domain resides within the amino-terminal 272 amino acid residues of von Willebrand factor. *J Biol Chem* 262:8443–8446, 1987.

199. Mancuso DJ, Tuley EA, Westfield LA, et al: Human von Willebrand factor gene and pseudogene: Structural analysis and differentiation by polymerase chain reaction. *Biochemistry* 30:253–269, 1991.

200. Smith NL, Chen MH, Dehghan A, et al: Novel associations of multiple genetic loci with plasma levels of factor VII, factor VIII, and von Willebrand factor: The CHARGE (Cohorts for Heart and Aging Research in Genome Epidemiology) Consortium. *Circulation* 121:1382–1392, 2010.

201. Smith NL, Rice KM, Bovill EG, et al: Genetic variation associated with plasma von Willebrand factor levels and the risk of incident venous thrombosis. *Blood* 117:6007–6011, 2011.

202. Aggeler PM, White SG, Glendening MB, et al: Plasma thromboplastin component (PTC) deficiency; a new disease resembling hemophilia. *Proc Soc Exp Biol Med* 79:692–694, 1952.

203. Rosenthal RL, Dreskin OH, Rosenthal N: New hemophilia-like disease caused by deficiency of a third plasma thromboplastin factor. *Proc Soc Exp Biol Med* 82:171–174, 1953.

204. Thompson RE, Mandle R, Kaplan AP: Association of factor XI and high molecular weight kininogen in human plasma. *J Clin Invest* 60:1376–1380, 1977.

205. Kurachi K, Fujikawa K, Davie EW: Mechanism of activation of bovine factor XI by factor XII and factor XIIa. *Biochemistry* 19:1330–1338, 1980.

206. Emsley J, McEwan PA, Gailani D: Structure and function of factor XI. *Blood* 115:2569–2577, 2010.

207. Papagrigoriou E, McEwan PA, Walsh PN, Emsley J: Crystal structure of the factor XI zymogen reveals a pathway for transactivation. *Nat Struct Mol Biol* 13:557–558, 2006.

208. Bouma B, Griffin JH: Human blood coagulation factor XI. Purification, properties, and mechanism of activation by activated factor XII. *J Biol Chem* 252:6432, 1977.

209. Naito K, Fujikawa K: Activation of human blood coagulation factor XI independent of factor XII. Factor XI is activated by thrombin and factor XIa in the presence of negatively charged surfaces. *J Biol Chem* 266:7353–7358, 1991.

210. Geng Y, Verhamme I, Smith S: The dimeric structure of factor XI and zymogen activation. *Blood* 121:3962–3970, 2013.

211. Smith SB, Verhamme IM, Sun M-F, et al: Characterization of novel forms of coagulation factor XIa: Independence of factor XIa subunits in factor IX activation. *J Biol Chem* 283:6696–6705, 2008.

212. Sun Y, Gailani D: Identification of a factor IX binding site on the third apple domain of activated factor XI. *J Biol Chem* 271:29023–29028, 1996.

213. Sinha D, Marcinkiewicz M, Navaneetham D, Walsh PN: Macromolecular substrate-binding exosites on both the heavy and light chains of factor XIa mediate the formation of the Michaelis complex required for factor IX-activation. *Biochemistry* 46:9830–9839, 2007.

214. Kravtsov DV, Matafonov A, Tucker EI, et al: Factor XI contributes to thrombin generation in the absence of factor XII. *Blood* 114:452–458, 2009.

215. Cheng Q, Tucker E, Pine M, et al: A role for factor XIIa–mediated factor XI activation in thrombus formation in vivo. *Blood* 116:3981–3990, 2010.

216. He R, Chen D, He S: Factor XI: Hemostasis, thrombosis, and antithrombosis. *Thromb Res* 129:541–550, 2012.

217. von dem Borne PA, Cox LM, Bouma BN: Factor XI enhances fibrin generation and inhibits fibrinolysis in a coagulation model initiated by surface-coated tissue factor. *Blood Coagul Fibrinolysis* 17:251–257, 2006.

218. von dem Borne PA, Meijers JC, Bouma BN: Feedback activation of factor XI by thrombin in plasma results in additional formation of thrombin that protects fibrin clots from fibrinolysis. *Blood* 86:3035–3042, 1995.

219. Baglia FA, Gailani D, López JA, Walsh PN: Identification of a binding site for glycoprotein Ibalpha in the Apple 3 domain of factor XI. *J Biol Chem* 279:45470–45476, 2004.

220. White-Adams TC, Berny MA, Tucker EI, et al: Identification of coagulation factor XI as a ligand for platelet apolipoprotein E receptor 2 (ApoER2). *Arterioscler Thromb Vasc Biol* 29:1602–1607, 2009.

221. Gailani D, Ho D, Sun MF, et al: Model for a factor IX activation complex on blood platelets: Dimeric conformation of factor XIa is essential. *Blood* 97:3117–3122, 2001.

222. Knauer DJ, Majumdar D, Fong PC, Knauer MF: SERPIN regulation of factor XIa. The novel observation that protease nexin 1 in the presence of heparin is a more potent inhibitor of factor XIa than C1 inhibitor. *J Biol Chem* 275:37340–37346, 2000.

223. Cronlund AL, Walsh PN: A low molecular weight platelet inhibitor of factor XIa: Purification, characterization, and possible role in blood coagulation. *Biochemistry* 31:1685–1694, 1992.

224. Ragni MV, Sinha D, Seaman F, et al: Comparison of bleeding tendency, factor XI coagulant activity, and factor XI antigen in 25 factor XI-deficient kindreds. *Blood* 65:719–724, 1985.

225. Asakai R, Chung DW, Davie EW, Seligsohn U: Factor XI deficiency in Ashkenazi Jews in Israel. *N Engl J Med* 325:153–158, 1991.

226. Meijers JC, Tekelenburg WL, Bouma BN, et al: High levels of coagulation factor XI as a risk factor for venous thrombosis. *N Engl J Med* 342:696–701, 2000.

227. Bezemer ID, Bare LA, Doggen CJ, et al: Gene variants associated with deep vein thrombosis. *JAMA* 299:1306–1314, 2008.

228. Maas C, Oschatz C, Renne T: The plasma contact system 2.0. *Semin Thromb Hemost* 37:375–381, 2011.

229. Ratnoff O, Colopy J: A familial hemorrhagic trait associated with a deficiency of a clot-promoting fraction of plasma. *J Clin Invest* 34:602–613, 1955.

230. McMullen BA, Fujikawa K: Amino acid sequence of the heavy chain of human alpha-factor XIIa (activated Hageman factor). *J Biol Chem* 260:5328–5341, 1985.

231. Harris RJ, Ling VT, Spellman W: O-linked fucose is present in the first epidermal growth factor domain of factor XI1 but not protein C. *J Biol Chem* 15:5102–5107, 1992.

232. Cochrane CG, Revak SD, Wuepper KD: Activation of Hageman factor in solid and fluid phases. A critical role of kallikrein. *J Exp Med* 138:1564–1583, 1973.

233. Samuel M, Pixley RA, Villanueva MA, et al: Human factor XII (Hageman factor) auto-activation by dextran sulfate. Circular dichroism, fluorescence, and ultraviolet difference spectroscopic studies. *J Biol Chem* 267:19691–19697, 1992.

234. Engel R, Brain CM, Paget J, et al: Single-chain factor XII exhibits activity when complexed to polyphosphate. *J Thromb Haemost* 12:1513–1522, 2014.

235. Ratnoff OD, Saito H: Amidolytic properties of single-chain activated Hageman factor. *Proc Natl Acad Sci U S A* 76:1461–1463, 1979.

236. Griffin JH: Role of surface in surface-dependent activation of Hageman factor (blood coagulation factor XII). *Proc Natl Acad Sci U S A* 75:1998–2002, 1978.

237. Clarke BJ, Côté HC, Cool DE, et al: Mapping of a putative surface-binding site of human coagulation factor XII. *J Biol Chem* 264:11497–11502, 1989.

238. Citarella F, Ravon DM, Pascucci B, et al: Structure/function analysis of human factor XII using recombinant deletion mutants. Evidence for an additional region involved in the binding to negatively charged surfaces. *Eur J Biochem* 238:240–249, 1996.

239. Citarella F, te Velthuis H, Helmer-Citterich M, Hack CE: Identification of a putative binding site for negatively charged surfaces in the fibronectin type II domain of human factor XII—An immunochemical and homology modeling approach. *Thromb Haemost* 84:1057–1065, 2000.

240. Beringer DX, Kroon-Batenburg LMJ. The structure of the FnI-EGF-like tandem domain of coagulation factor XII solved using SIRAS. *Acta Crystallogr Sect F Struct Biol Cryst Commun* 69:94–102, 2013.

241. Kannemeier C, Shibamiya A, Nakazawa F, et al: Extracellular RNA constitutes a natural procoagulant cofactor in blood coagulation. *Proc Natl Acad Sci U S A* 104:6388–6393, 2007.

242. van der Meijden PE, Munnix IC, Auger JM, et al: Dual role of collagen in factor XII–dependent thrombus formation. *Blood* 114:881–891, 2014.

243. Muller F, Mutch NJ, Schenk WA, et al: Platelet polyphosphates are proinflammatory and procoagulant mediators in vivo. *Cell* 139:1143–1156, 2009.

244. van der Meijden PE, van Schilfgaarde M, van Oerle R, et al: Platelet- and erythrocyte-derived microparticles trigger thrombin generation via factor XIIa. *J Thromb Haemost* 10:1355–1362, 2012.

245. Revak SD, Cochrane CG, Bouma BN, Griffin JH: Surface and fluid phase activities of two forms of activated Hageman factor produced during contact activation of plasma. *J Exp Med* 147:719–729, 1978.

246. Lämmle B, Wuillemin WA, Huber I, et al: Thromboembolism and bleeding tendency in congenital factor XII deficiency—A study on 74 subjects from 14 Swiss families. *Thromb Haemost* 65:117–121, 1991.

247. Renne T, Pozgajova M, Gruner S, et al: Defective thrombus formation in mice lacking coagulation factor XII. *J Exp Med* 202:271–281, 2005.

248. Matafonov A, Leung PY, Gailani AE, et al: Factor XII inhibition reduces thrombus formation in a primate thrombosis model. *Blood* 123:1739–1747, 2014.

249. Cichon S, Martin L, Hennies HC, et al: Increased activity of coagulation factor XII (Hageman factor) causes hereditary angioedema type III. *Am J Hum Genet* 79:1098–1104, 2006.

250. Cool DE, MacGillivray RT: Characterization of the human blood coagulation factor XII gene. Intron/exon gene organization and analysis of the 5′-flanking region. *J Biol Chem* 262:13662–13673, 1987.

251. Johnson CY, Tuite A, Morange PE, et al: The factor XII 4C>T variant and risk of common thrombotic disorders: A HuGE review and meta-analysis of evidence from observational studies. *Am J Epidemiol* 173:136–144, 2011.

252. Morrissey JH, Gregory SA, Mackman N, Edgington TS: Tissue factor regulation and gene organization. *Oxf Surv Eukaryot Genes* 6:67–84, 1989.

253. Hoffman M, Colina CM, McDonald AG, et al: Tissue factor around dermal vessels has bound factor VII in the absence of injury. *J Thromb Haemost* 5:1403–1408, 2007.

254. Banner DW, D'Arcy A, Chene C, et al: The crystal structure of the complex of blood coagulation factor VIIa with soluble tissue factor. *Nature* 380:41–46, 1996.

255. Versteeg HH, Heemskerk JW, Levi M, Reitsma PH: New fundamentals in hemostasis. *Physiol Rev* 93:327–358, 2013.

256. Dorfleutner A, Ruf W: Regulation of tissue factor cytoplasmic domain phosphorylation by palmitoylation. *Blood* 102:3998–4005, 2003.

257. van den Hengel LG, Kocaturk B, Reitsma PH, et al: Complete abolishment of coagulant activity in monomeric disulfide-deficient tissue factor. *Blood* 118:3446–3448, 2011.

258. Rehemtulla A, Ruf W, Edgington TS: The integrity of the cysteine 186-cysteine 209 bond of the second disulfide loop of tissue factor is required for binding of factor VII. *J Biol Chem* 266:10294–10299, 1991.

259. Bogdanov VY, Balasubramanian V, Hathcock J, et al: Alternatively spliced human tissue factor: A circulating, soluble, thrombogenic protein. *Nat Med* 9:458–462, 2003.

260. Szotowski B, Antoniak S, Poller W, et al: Procoagulant soluble tissue factor is released from endothelial cells in response to inflammatory cytokines. *Circ Res* 96:1233–1239, 2005.

261. Szotowski B, Goldin-Lang P, Antoniak S, et al: Alterations in myocardial tissue factor expression and cellular localization in dilated cardiomyopathy. *J Am Coll Cardiol* 45:1081–1089, 2005.

262. Goldin-Lang P, Tran QV, Fichtner I, et al: Tissue factor expression pattern in human non-small cell lung cancer tissues indicate increased blood thrombogenicity and tumor metastasis. *Oncol Rep* 20:123–128, 2008.

263. Luyendyk JP, Tilley RE, Mackman N: Genetic susceptibility to thrombosis. *Curr Atheroscler Rep* 8:193–197, 2006.

264. Esmon NL, Owen WG, Esmon CT: Isolation of a membrane-bound cofactor for thrombin-catalyzed activation of protein C. *J Biol Chem* 257:859–864, 1982.

265. Esmon CT, Owen WG: The discovery of thrombomodulin. *J Thromb Haemost* 2:209–213, 2004.

266. Conway EM: Thrombomodulin and its role in inflammation. *Semin Immunopathol* 34:107–125, 2012.

267. Light DR, Glaser CB, Betts M, et al: The interaction of thrombomodulin with Ca2+. *Eur J Biochem* 262:522–533, 1999.

268. Adams TE, Huntington JA: Thrombin-cofactor interactions: Structural insights into regulatory mechanisms. *Arterioscler Thromb Vasc Biol* 26:1738–1745, 2006.

269. Cadroy Y, Diquelou A, Dupouy D, et al: The thrombomodulin/protein C/protein S anticoagulant pathway modulates the thrombogenic properties of the normal resting and stimulated endothelium. *Arterioscler Thromb Vasc Biol* 17:520–527, 1997.

270. Laszik Z, Mitro A, Taylor FB Jr, et al: Human protein C receptor is present primarily on endothelium of large blood vessels: Implications for the control of the protein C pathway. *Circulation* 96:3633–3640, 1997.

271. Lafay M, Laguna J, Le Bonniec BF, et al: Thrombomodulin modulates the mitogenic response to thrombin of human umbilical vein endothelial cells. *Thromb Haemost* 79:848–852, 1998.

272. Van de Wouwer M, Conway EM: Novel functions of thrombomodulin in inflammation. *Crit Care Med* 32(Suppl 5):S254–S261, 2004.

273. Rezaie AR, Cooper ST, Church FC, Esmon CT: Protein C inhibitor is a potent inhibitor of the thrombin-thrombomodulin complex. *J Biol Chem* 270:25336–25339, 1995.

274. Martin FA, Murphy RP, Cummins PM: Thrombomodulin and the vascular endothelium: Insights into functional, regulatory, and therapeutic aspects. *Am J Physiol Heart Circ Physiol* 304:H1585–H1597, 2013.

275. Ohlin AK, Norlund L, Marlar RA: Thrombomodulin gene variations and thromboembolic disease. *Thromb Haemost* 78:396–400, 1997.

276. Tang L, Wang HF, Lu X, et al: Common genetic risk factors for venous thrombosis in the Chinese population. *Am J Hum Genet* 92:177–187, 2013.

277. Langdown J, Luddington RJ, Huntington JA, Baglin TP: A hereditary bleeding disorder resulting from a premature stop codon in thrombomodulin (p.Cys537Stop). *Blood* 124:1951–1956, 2014.

278. Delvaeye M, Noris M, De Vriese A, et al: Thrombomodulin mutations in atypical hemolytic-uremic syndrome. *N Engl J Med* 361:345–357, 2009.

279. Fukudome K, Esmon CT: Molecular cloning and expression of murine and bovine endothelial cell protein C/activated protein C receptor (EPCR). The structural and functional conservation in human, bovine, and murine EPCR. *J Biol Chem* 270:5571–5577, 1995.

280. Mosnier LO, Zlokovic BV, Griffin JH: The cytoprotective protein C pathway. *Blood* 109:3161–3172, 2007.

281. Mosnier LO, Sinha RK, Burnier L, et al: Biased agonism of protease-activated receptor 1 by activated protein C caused by noncanonical cleavage at Arg46. *Blood* 120:5237–5246, 2012.

282. Li W, Zheng X, Gu JM, et al: Extraembryonic expression of EPCR is essential for embryonic viability. *Blood* 106:2716–2722, 2005.

283. Mohan Rao LV, Esmon CT, Pendurthi UR: Endothelial cell protein C receptor: A multiliganded and multifunctional receptor. *Blood* 124:1553–1562, 2014.

284. Wu C, Dwivedi DJ, Pepler L, et al: Targeted gene sequencing identifies variants in the protein C and endothelial protein C receptor genes in patients with unprovoked venous thromboembolism. *Arterioscler Thromb Vasc Biol* 33:2674–2681, 2013.

285. Collen D, Tytgat GN, Claeys H, Piessens R: Metabolism and distribution of fibrinogen. I. Fibrinogen turnover in physiological conditions in humans. *Br J Haematol* 22:681–700, 1972.

286. Handagama PJ, Shuman MA, Bainton DF: *In vivo* defibrination results in markedly decreased amounts of fibrinogen in rat megakaryocytes and platelets. *Am J Pathol* 137:1393–1399, 1990.

287. Louache F, Debili N, Cramer E, et al: Fibrinogen is not synthesized by human megakaryocytes. *Blood* 77:311–316, 1991.

288. Côté HC, Lord ST, Pratt KP: Gamma-chain dysfibrinogenemias: Molecular structure-function relationships of naturally occurring mutations in the gamma chain of human fibrinogen. *Blood* 92:2195–2212, 1998.

289. Henschen AH: Human fibrinogen—Structural variants and functional sites. *Thromb Haemost* 70:42–47, 1993.

290. Uitte de Willige S, de Visser MC, Houwing-Duistermaat JJ, et al: Genetic variation in the fibrinogen gamma gene increases the risk for deep venous thrombosis by reducing plasma fibrinogen gamma levels. *Blood* 106:4176–4183, 2005.

291. Blomback B: Studies on fibrinogen: Its purification and conversion into fibrin. *Acta Physiol Scand Suppl* 43:1–51, 1958.

292. Olexa SA, Budzynski AZ: Evidence for four different polymerization sites involved in human fibrin formation. *Proc Natl Acad Sci U S A* 77:1374–1378, 1980.

293. Kaczmarek E, McDonagh J: Thrombin binding to the A alpha-, B beta-, and gamma-chains of fibrinogen and to their remnants contained in fragment E. *J Biol Chem* 263:13896–13900, 1988.

294. Weisel JW, Phillips GN Jr, Cohen C: The structure of fibrinogen and fibrin: II. Architecture of the fibrin clot. *Ann N Y Acad Sci* 408:367–379, 1983.

295. Hantgan R, Fowler W, Erickson H, Hermans J: Fibrin assembly: A comparison of electron microscopic and light scattering results. *Thromb Haemost* 44:119–124, 1980.

296. Marder VJ, Budzynski AZ: The structure of the fibrinogen degradation products. *Prog Hemost Thromb* 2:141–174, 1974.

297. Mosesson MW: Update on antithrombin I (fibrin). *Thromb Haemost* 98:105–108, 2007.

298. Komaromi I, Bagoly Z, Muszbek L: Factor XIII: Novel structural and functional aspects. *J Thromb Haemost* 9:9–20, 2011.

299. Souri M, Koseki-Kuno S, Takeda N, et al: Administration of factor XIII B subunit increased plasma factor XIII A subunit levels in factor XIII B subunit knock-out mice. *Int J Hematol* 87:60–68, 2008.

300. Muszbek L, Haramura G, Polgar J: Transformation of cellular factor XIII into an active zymogen transglutaminase in thrombin-stimulated platelets. *Thromb Haemost* 73:702–705, 1995.

301. Brummel KE, Paradis SG, Butenas S, Mann KG: Thrombin functions during tissue factor-induced blood coagulation. *Blood* 100:148–152, 2002.

302. Bagoly Z, Fazakas F, Komaromi I, et al: Cleavage of factor XIII by human neutrophil elastase results in a novel active truncated form of factor XIII A subunit. *Thromb Haemost* 99:668–674, 2008.

303. Smith KA, Pease RJ, Avery CA, et al: The activation peptide cleft exposed by thrombin cleavage of FXIII-A(2) contains a recognition site for the fibrinogen alpha chain. *Blood* 121:2117–2126, 2013.

304. Fraser SR, Booth NA, Mutch NJ: The antifibrinolytic function of factor XIII is exclusively expressed through alpha(2)-antiplasmin cross-linking. *Blood* 117:6371–6374, 2011.

305. Aleman MM, Byrnes JR, Wang JG, et al: Factor XIII activity mediates red blood cell retention in venous thrombi. *J Clin Invest* 124:3590–3600, 2014.

306. Hoppe B: Fibrinogen and factor XIII at the intersection of coagulation, fibrinolysis and inflammation. *Thromb Haemost* 112:649–658, 2014.

307. Kasahara K, Souri M, Kaneda M, et al: Impaired clot retraction in factor XIII A subunit-deficient mice. *Blood* 115:1277–1279, 2010.

308. Richardson VR, Cordell P, Standeven KF, Carter AM: Substrates of factor XIII-a: Roles in thrombosis and wound healing. *Clin Sci (Lond)* 124:123–137, 2013.

309. Kikuchi H, Kuribayashi F, Imajoh-Ohmi S: Down-regulation of Fas-mediated apoptosis by plasma transglutaminase factor XIII that catalyzes fetal-specific cross-link of the Fas molecule. *Biochem Biophys Res Commun* 443:13–17, 2014.

310. Mokuda S, Murata Y, Sawada N, et al: Tocilizumab induced acquired factor XIII deficiency in patients with rheumatoid arthritis. *PLoS One* 8:e69944, 2013.

311. Soendergaard C, Kvist PH, Seidelin JB, Nielsen OH: Tissue-regenerating functions of coagulation factor XIII. *J Thromb Haemost* 11:806–816, 2013.

312. Weisberg LJ, Shiu DT, Greenberg CS, et al: Localization of the gene for coagulation factor XIII a-chain to chromosome 6 and identification of sites of synthesis. *J Clin Invest* 79:649–652, 1987.

313. Bottenus RE, Ichinose A, Davie EW: Nucleotide sequence of the gene for the b subunit of human factor XIII. *Biochemistry* 29:11195–11209, 1990.

314. Muszbek L, Bagoly Z, Cairo A, Peyvandi F: Novel aspects of factor XIII deficiency. *Curr Opin Hematol* 18:366–372, 2011.

315. Ichinose A: Factor XIII is a key molecule at the intersection of coagulation and fibrinolysis as well as inflammation and infection control. *Int J Hematol* 95:362–370, 2012.

316. Shemirani AH, Antalfi B, Pongracz E, et al: Factor XIII-A subunit Val34Leu polymorphism in fatal atherothrombotic ischemic stroke. *Blood Coagul Fibrinolysis* 25:364–368, 2014.

317. Foley JH, Kim PY, Mutch NJ, Gils A: Insights into thrombin activatable fibrinolysis inhibitor function and regulation. *J Thromb Haemost* 11(Suppl 1):306–315, 2013.

318. van Tilburg NH, Rosendaal FR, Bertina RM: Thrombin activatable fibrinolysis inhibitor and the risk for deep vein thrombosis. *Blood* 95:2855–2859, 2000.

319. Seegers WH, Johnson JF, Fell C: An antithrombin reaction to prothrombin activation. *Am J Physiol* 176:97–103, 1954.

320. Huntington JA: Serpin structure, function and dysfunction. *J Thromb Haemost* 9(Suppl 1):26–34, 2011.

321. Olson ST, Swanson R, Raub-Segall E, et al: Accelerating ability of synthetic oligosaccharides on antithrombin inhibition of proteinases of the clotting and fibrinolytic systems. Comparison with heparin and low-molecular-weight heparin. *Thromb Haemost* 92:929–939, 2004.

322. Olson ST, Bjork I: Predominant contribution of surface approximation to the mechanism of heparin acceleration of the antithrombin-thrombin reaction. Elucidation from salt concentration effects. *J Biol Chem* 266:6353–6364, 1991.

323. Li W, Johnson DJ, Esmon CT, Huntington JA: Structure of the antithrombin-thrombin-heparin ternary complex reveals the antithrombotic mechanism of heparin. *Nat Struct Mol Biol* 11:857–862, 2004.

324. Pizzo SV: Serpin receptor 1: A hepatic receptor that mediates the clearance of antithrombin III-proteinase complexes. *Am J Med* 87(3B):10S–14S, 1989.

325. Kounnas MZ, Church FC, Argraves WS, Strickland DK: Cellular internalization and degradation of antithrombin III-thrombin, heparin cofactor II-thrombin, and alpha 1-antitrypsin-trypsin complexes is mediated by the low density lipoprotein receptor-related protein. *J Biol Chem* 271:6523–6529, 1996.

326. Tait RC, Walker ID, Perry DJ, et al: Prevalence of antithrombin deficiency in the healthy population. *Br J Haematol* 87:106–112, 1994.

327. Harper PL, Luddington RJ, Daly M, et al: The incidence of dysfunctional antithrombin variants: Four cases in 210 patients with thromboembolic disease. *Br J Haematol* 77:360–364, 1991.

328. Lane DA, Bayston T, Olds RJ, et al: Antithrombin mutation database: 2nd (1997) update. For the Plasma Coagulation Inhibitors Subcommittee of the Scientific and Standardization Committee of the International Society on Thrombosis and Haemostasis. *Thromb Haemost* 77:197–211, 1997.

329. Broze GJ Jr, Miletich JP: Isolation of the tissue factor inhibitor produced by HepG2 hepatoma cells. *Proc Natl Acad Sci U S A* 84:1886–1890, 1987.

330. Novotny WF, Girard TJ, Miletich JP, Broze GJ Jr: Purification and characterization of the lipoprotein-associated coagulation inhibitor from human plasma. *J Biol Chem* 264:18832–18837, 1989.

331. Girard TJ, Warren LA, Novotny WF, et al: Functional significance of the Kunitz-type inhibitory domains of lipoprotein-associated coagulation inhibitor. *Nature* 338:518–520, 1989.

332. Wood JP, Ellery PE, Maroney SA, Mast AE: Biology of tissue factor pathway inhibitor. *Blood* 123:2934–2943, 2014.

333. Hackeng TM, Sere KM, Tans G, Rosing J: Protein S stimulates inhibition of the tissue factor pathway by tissue factor pathway inhibitor. *Proc Natl Acad Sci U S A* 103:3106–3111, 2006.

334. Ndonwi M, Tuley EA, Broze GJ Jr: The Kunitz-3 domain of TFPI-alpha is required for protein S-dependent enhancement of factor Xa inhibition. *Blood* 116:1344–1351, 2010.

335. Wood JP, Bunce MW, Maroney SA, et al: Tissue factor pathway inhibitor-alpha inhibits prothrombinase during the initiation of blood coagulation. *Proc Natl Acad Sci U S A* 110:17838–17843, 2013.

336. Dahm A, Van Hylckama Vlieg A, Bendz B, et al: Low levels of tissue factor pathway inhibitor (TFPI) increase the risk of venous thrombosis. *Blood* 101:4387–4392, 2003.

337. Castoldi E, Simioni P, Tormene D, et al: Hereditary and acquired protein S deficiencies are associated with low TFPI levels in plasma. *J Thromb Haemost* 8:294–300, 2010.

338. Massberg S, Grahl L, von Bruehl ML, et al: Reciprocal coupling of coagulation and innate immunity via neutrophil serine proteases. *Nat Med* 16:887–896, 2010.

339. Sandset PM, Warn-Cramer BJ, Rao LV, et al: Depletion of extrinsic pathway inhibitor (EPI) sensitizes rabbits to disseminated intravascular coagulation induced with tissue factor: Evidence supporting a physiologic role for EPI as a natural anticoagulant. *Proc Natl Acad Sci U S A* 88:708–712, 1991.

340. Huang ZF, Higuchi D, Lasky N, Broze GJ Jr: Tissue factor pathway inhibitor gene disruption produces intrauterine lethality in mice. *Blood* 90:944–951, 1997.

341. Ameziane N, Seguin C, Borgel D, et al: The 33T—>C polymorphism in intron 7 of the TFPI gene influences the risk of venous thromboembolism, independently of the factor V Leiden and prothrombin mutations. *Thromb Haemost* 88:195–199, 2002.

342. Opstad TB, Eilertsen AL, Hoibraaten E, et al: Tissue factor pathway inhibitor polymorphisms in women with and without a history of venous thrombosis and the effects of postmenopausal hormone therapy. *Blood Coagul Fibrinolysis* 21:516–521, 2010.

343. Han X, Fiehler R, Broze GJ Jr: Isolation of a protein Z-dependent plasma protease inhibitor. *Proc Natl Acad Sci U S A* 95:9250–9255, 1998.

344. Tabatabai A, Fiehler R, Broze GJ Jr: Protein Z circulates in plasma in a complex with protein Z-dependent protease inhibitor. *Thromb Haemost* 85:655–660, 2001.

345. Han X, Huang ZF, Fiehler R, Broze GJ Jr: The protein Z-dependent protease inhibitor is a serpin. *Biochemistry* 38:11073–11078, 1999.

346. Sejima H, Hayashi T, Deyashiki Y, et al: Primary structure of vitamin K-dependent human protein Z. *Biochem Biophys Res Commun* 171:661–668, 1990.

347. Huang X, Yan Y, Tu Y, et al: Structural basis for catalytic activation of protein Z-dependent protease inhibitor (ZPI) by protein Z. *Blood* 120:1726–1733, 2012.

348. Zhang J, Tu Y, Lu L, et al: Protein Z-dependent protease inhibitor deficiency produces a more severe murine phenotype than protein Z deficiency. *Blood* 111:4973–4978, 2008.

349. Al-Shanqeeti A, van Hylckama Vlieg A, Berntorp E, et al: Protein Z and protein Z-dependent protease inhibitor. Determinants of levels and risk of venous thrombosis. *Thromb Haemost* 93:411–413, 2005.

350. Almawi WY, Al-Shaikh FS, Melemedjian OK, Almawi AW: Protein Z, an anticoagulant protein with expanding role in reproductive biology. *Reproduction* 146:R73–R80, 2013.

351. Van de Water N, Tan T, Ashton F, et al: Mutations within the protein Z-dependent protease inhibitor gene are associated with venous thromboembolic disease: A new form of thrombophilia. *Br J Haematol* 127:190–194, 2004.

352. Young LK, Birch NP, Browett PJ, et al: Two missense mutations identified in venous thrombosis patients impair the inhibitory function of the protein Z dependent protease inhibitor. *Thromb Haemost* 107:854–863, 2012.

353. McQuillan AM, Eikelboom JW, Hankey GJ, et al: Protein Z in ischemic stroke and its etiologic subtypes. *Stroke* 34:2415–2419, 2003.

354. Dossenbach-Glaninger A, van Trotsenburg M, Helmer H, et al: Association of the protein Z intron F G79A gene polymorphism with recurrent pregnancy loss. *Fertil Steril* 90:1155–1160, 2008.

355. Grandone E, Colaizzo D, Cappucci F, et al: Protein Z levels and unexplained fetal losses. *Fertil Steril* 82:982–983, 2004.

356. Macfarlane RG: An enzyme cascade in the blood clotting mechanism, and its function as a biochemical amplifier. *Nature* 202:498–499, 1964.

357. Davie EW, Ratnoff OD: Waterfall sequence for intrinsic blood clotting. *Science* 145:1310–1312, 1964.

358. Pitlick FA, Nemerson Y: Purification and characterization of tissue factor apoprotein. *Methods Enzymol* 45:37–48, 1976.

359. Mackman N, Morrissey JH, Fowler B, Edgington TS: Complete sequence of the human tissue factor gene, a highly regulated cellular receptor that initiates the coagulation protease cascade. *Biochemistry* 28:1755–1762, 1989.

360. Osterud B, Rapaport SI: Activation of factor IX by the reaction product of tissue factor and factor VII: Additional pathway for initiating blood coagulation. *Proc Natl Acad Sci U S A* 74:5260–5264, 1977.

361. Repke D, Gemmell CH, Guha A, et al: Hemophilia as a defect of the tissue factor pathway of blood coagulation: Effect of factors VIII and IX on factor X activation in a continuous-flow reactor. *Proc Natl Acad Sci U S A* 87:7623–7627, 1990.

362. van't Veer C, Hackeng TM, Delahaye C, et al: Activated factor X and thrombin formation triggered by tissue factor on endothelial cell matrix in a flow model: Effect of the tissue factor pathway inhibitor. *Blood* 84:1132–1142, 1994.

363. van't Veer C, Mann KG: Regulation of tissue factor initiated thrombin generation by the stoichiometric inhibitors tissue factor pathway inhibitor, antithrombin-III, and heparin cofactor-II. *J Biol Chem* 272:4367–4377, 1997.

364. Hilden I, Lauritzen B, Sorensen BB, et al: Hemostatic effect of a monoclonal antibody mAb 2021 blocking the interaction between FXa and TFPI in a rabbit hemophilia model. *Blood* 119:5871–5878, 2012.

365. Carmeliet P, Mackman N, Moons L, et al: Role of tissue factor in embryonic blood vessel development. *Nature* 383:73–75, 1996.

366. Gailani D, Broze GJ Jr: Factor XI activation in a revised model of blood coagulation. *Science* 253:909–912, 1991.

367. Nemerson Y: The tissue factor pathway of blood coagulation. *Semin Hematol* 29:170–176, 1992.

368. Esmon CT: The protein C pathway. *Chest* 124(Suppl 3):26S–32S, 2003.

369. Holmer E, Kurachi K, Soderstrom G: The molecular-weight dependence of the rate-enhancing effect of heparin on the inhibition of thrombin, factor Xa, factor IXa, factor XIa, factor XII a and kallikrein by antithrombin. *Biochem J* 193:395–400, 1981.

370. Brummel-Ziedins KE, Everse SJ, Mann KG, Orfeo T: Modeling thrombin generation: Plasma composition based approach. *J Thromb Thrombolysis* 37:32–44, 2014.

371. Monroe DM, Hoffman M, Roberts HR: Platelets and thrombin generation. *Arterioscler Thromb Vasc Biol* 22:1381–1389, 2002.

372. Cawthern KM, van't Veer C, Lock JB, et al: Blood coagulation in hemophilia A and hemophilia C. *Blood* 91:4581–4592, 1998.

373. Monroe DM, Roberts HR, Hoffman M: Platelet procoagulant complex assembly in a tissue factor-initiated system. *Br J Haematol* 88:364–371, 1994.

374. Schuijt TJ, Bakhtiari K, Daffre S, et al: Factor Xa activation of factor V is of paramount importance in initiating the coagulation system: Lessons from a tick salivary protein. *Circulation* 128:254–266, 2013.

375. Allen DH, Tracy PB: Human coagulation factor V is activated to the functional cofactor by elastase and cathepsin G expressed at the monocyte surface. *J Biol Chem* 270:1408–1415, 1995.

376. Williamson P, Bevers EM, Smeets EF, et al: Continuous analysis of the mechanism of activated transbilayer lipid movement in platelets. *Biochemistry* 34:10448–10455, 1995.

377. Yang X, Walsh PN: An ordered sequential mechanism for factor IX and factor IXa binding to platelet receptors in the assembly of the Factor X-activating complex. *Biochem J* 390(Pt 1):157–167, 2005.

378. White-Adams TC, Berny MA, Tucker EI, et al: Identification of coagulation factor XI as a ligand for platelet apolipoprotein E receptor 2 (ApoER2). *Arterioscler Thromb Vasc Biol* 29:1602–1607, 2009.

379. Choi SH, Smith SA, Morrissey JH: Polyphosphate is a cofactor for the activation of factor XI by thrombin. *Blood* 118:6963–6970, 2011.

380. von dem Borne PA, Bajzar L, Meijers JC, et al: Thrombin-mediated activation of factor XI results in a thrombin-activatable fibrinolysis inhibitor-dependent inhibition of fibrinolysis. *J Clin Invest* 99:2323–2327, 1997.

381. Mackman N: Tissue-specific hemostasis in mice. *Arterioscler Thromb Vasc Biol* 25:2273–2281, 2005.

382. Kenne E, Renne T: Factor XII: A drug target for safe interference with thrombosis and inflammation. *Drug Discov Today* 19:1459–1464, 2014.

383. Buller HR, Bethune C, Bhanot S, et al: Factor XI antisense oligonucleotide for prevention of venous thrombosis. *N Engl J Med* 372:232–240, 2015.

384. Engelmann B, Massberg S: Thrombosis as an intravascular effector of innate immunity. *Nat Rev Immunol* 13:34–45, 2013.

385. von Bruhl ML, Stark K, Steinhart A, et al: Monocytes, neutrophils, and platelets cooperate to initiate and propagate venous thrombosis in mice *in vivo*. *J Exp Med* 209:819–835, 2012.

386. Broze GJ Jr: Binding of human factor VII and VIIa to monocytes. *J Clin Invest* 70:526–535, 1982.

387. Clark SR, Ma AC, Tavener SA, et al: Platelet TLR4 activates neutrophil extracellular traps to ensnare bacteria in septic blood. *Nat Med* 13:463–469, 2007.

388. Wang Y, Li M, Stadler S, et al: Histone hypercitrullination mediates chromatin decondensation and neutrophil extracellular trap formation. *J Cell Biol* 184:205–213, 2009.

389. Semeraro F, Ammollo CT, Morrissey JH, et al: Extracellular histones promote thrombin generation through platelet-dependent mechanisms: Involvement of platelet TLR2 and TLR4. *Blood* 118:1952–1961, 2011.

390. Martinod K, Demers M, Fuchs TA, et al: Neutrophil histone modification by peptidyl-larginine deiminase 4 is critical for deep vein thrombosis in mice. *Proc Natl Acad Sci U S A* 110:8674–8679, 2013.

391. Savchenko AS, Martinod K, Seidman MA, et al: Neutrophil extracellular traps form predominantly during the organizing stage of human venous thromboembolism development. *J Thromb Haemost* 12:860–870, 2014.

392. Hanson SR, Griffin JH, Harker LA, et al: Antithrombotic effects of thrombin-induced activation of endogenous protein C in primates. *J Clin Invest* 92:2003–2012, 1993.

393. de Agostini AI, Watkins SC, Slayter HS, et al: Localization of anticoagulantly active heparan sulfate proteoglycans in vascular endothelium: Antithrombin binding on cultured endothelial cells and perfused rat aorta. *J Cell Biol* 111:1293–1304, 1990.

394. Marcus AJ, Broekman MJ, Drosopoulos JH, et al: The endothelial cell ecto-ADPase responsible for inhibition of platelet function is CD39. *J Clin Invest* 99:1351–1360, 1997.

395. van't Veer C, Golden NJ, Kalafatis M, Mann KG: Inhibitory mechanism of the protein C pathway on tissue factor-induced thrombin generation. Synergistic effect in combination with tissue factor pathway inhibitor. *J Biol Chem* 272:7983–7994, 1997.

396. Jesty J, Beltrami E: Positive feedbacks of coagulation: Their role in threshold regulation. *Arterioscler Thromb Vasc Biol* 25:2463–2469, 2005.

397. Brakman P, Albrechtsen OK, Astrup T: A comparative study of coagulation and fibrinolysis in blood from normal men and women. *Br J Haematol* 12:74–85, 1966.

398. Nossel HL, Yudelman I, Canfield RE, et al: Measurement of fibrinopeptide A in human blood. *J Clin Invest* 54:43–53, 1974.

399. Bauer KA, Kass BL, ten Cate H, et al: Detection of factor X activation in humans. *Blood* 74:2007–2015, 1989.

400. Bauer KA, Kass BL, ten Cate H, et al: Factor IX is activated in vivo by the tissue factor mechanism. *Blood* 76:731–736, 1990.

401. Morrissey JH: Tissue factor modulation of factor VIIa activity: Use in measuring trace levels of factor VIIa in plasma. *Thromb Haemost* 74:185–188, 1995.

402. Conard J, Bauer KA, Gruber A, et al: Normalization of markers of coagulation activation with a purified protein C concentrate in adults with homozygous protein C deficiency. *Blood* 82:1159–1164, 1993.

# CHAPTER 4
# CONTROL OF COAGULATION REACTIONS

Laurent O. Mosnier and John H. Griffin

## SUMMARY

The blood coagulation system, like a powerful idling engine, is always active and generating thrombin at very low levels, poised for explosive thrombin generation. Positive feedback activation of factors V, VII, VIII, and XI imparts special threshold properties to blood coagulation, making the coagulant response nonlinearly responsive to stimuli. Overt blood coagulation represents a threshold system with apparent all-or-none responses to various levels of stimuli, and an ensemble of opposing reactions determines the ultimate upregulation and downregulation of thrombin generation both locally and systemically. Cellular and humoral anticoagulant mechanisms synergize with plasma coagulation inhibitors to prevent massive thrombin generation in the absence of a substantial procoagulant stimulus. This chapter highlights mechanisms that inhibit blood coagulation, with an emphasis on defects of plasma proteins that cause hereditary thrombophilias. Major thrombophilic defects involve the anticoagulant protein C pathway, comprising multiple cofactors or effectors that additionally include thrombomodulin, endothelial protein C receptor, protein S, high-density lipoprotein, and factor V. Activated protein C exerts multiple protective homeostatic actions, including proteolytic inactivation of factors Va and VIIIa, as well as direct cell-signaling activities involving protease activated receptors 1 and 3, endothelial cell protein C receptor, integrin CD11b/CD18, and apolipoprotein E receptor 2. The factor V Leiden variant causes hereditary activated protein C resistance by impairing the ability of the protein C pathway to inhibit coagulation because it cannot properly cleave factor Va Leiden. Plasma protease inhibitors are also key to block coagulation. Antithrombin inhibits thrombin and factors Xa, IXa, XIa, and XIIa in reactions stimulated by physiologic heparan sulfate or pharmacologic heparins. Tissue factor pathway inhibitor neutralizes the extrinsic coagulation pathway factors VIIa and Xa. Other plasma protease inhibitors can also neutralize various coagulation proteases.

Control of coagulation reactions is essential for normal hemostasis. As part of the tangled web of host defense systems that respond to vascular injury, the blood coagulation factors (Chap. 3) act in concert with the endothelium and blood cells, especially platelets, to generate a protective fibrin-platelet clot, forming a hemostatic plug. Pathologic thrombosis occurs when the protective clot is extended beyond its beneficial size, when a clot occurs inappropriately at sites of vascular disease, or when a clot embolizes to other sites in the

circulatory bed. For normal hemostasis, both procoagulant and anticoagulant factors must interact with the vascular components and cell surfaces, including the vessel wall (Chap. 5) and platelets (Chap. 2). Moreover, the action of the fibrinolytic system must be integrated with coagulation reactions for timely formation and dissolution of blood clots (Chap. 25). This chapter on control of coagulation highlights the major physiologic mechanisms for downregulation of blood coagulation reactions and the plasma proteins that inhibit blood coagulation, with an emphasis on those mechanisms whose defects are clinically significant based on insights gleaned from consideration of the hereditary thrombophilias (Chap. 20). Chapter 3 provides a complete description of blood coagulation factors and hemostatic pathways.

## ● BLOOD COAGULATION PATHWAYS AND THE PROTEIN C PATHWAYS

Although decades have elapsed since the elaboration of the cascade model[1,2] for blood coagulation (see Chap. 3, Fig. 3–27), the basic outline of sequential conversions of protease zymogens to active serine proteases is still useful, albeit with important modifications (see Chap. 3, Fig. 3–28), to represent blood coagulation reactions. The major conceptual advances for procoagulant pathways in the past two decades emphasize both positive and negative feedback reactions affecting thrombin generation as depicted in Fig. 4–1.

In positive feedback reactions, procoagulant thrombin activates platelets and factors V, VIII, and XI (Chap. 3).[3–5] Small amounts of thrombin can be generated by trace amounts of tissue factor via the extrinsic pathway. Subsequently, thrombin can activate factors XI, VIII, and V, thereby stimulating each of the steps in the intrinsic pathway and amplifying thrombin generation (see Fig. 4–1).

In negative feedback reactions, anticoagulant activated protein C (APC) that is generated on endothelial cell surfaces[6–8] (Fig. 4–2) downregulates coagulation (see Figs. 4–1 and 4–3). Furthermore, APC can exert direct cytoprotective effects on cells via reactions that involve certain receptors, including endothelial cell protein C receptor (EPCR) and protease-activated receptor-1 (PAR-1) (Fig. 4–4), PAR-3, integrin CD11b/CD18, and possibly apolipoprotein E receptor 2 (apoER2).[7,8] APC's cytoprotective effects include antiinflammatory and antiapoptotic activities, as well as alterations of gene-expression profiles and stabilization of endothelial barriers (see "Activated Protein C Activities" below). Because inflammation, apoptosis, and vascular barrier breakdown contribute significantly to reactions that promote thrombin generation, such direct cytoprotective effects of APC on cells indirectly downregulate thrombin generation.[7,8]

For APC generation by the protein C cellular pathway, binding of thrombin to thrombomodulin converts the bound thrombin from a procoagulant enzyme to an anticoagulant enzyme that converts the protein C zymogen to an anticoagulant serine protease, APC (see Figs. 4–1 and 4–2). This surface-dependent reaction is enhanced by the EPCR that binds protein C.[6,9,10] With the aid of its nonenzymatic cofactor, protein S, as well as other potential lipid and protein cofactors, APC inactivates factors Va and VIIIa by highly selective proteolysis, yielding inactive (i) cofactors, that is, factors $V_i$ and $VIII_i$ (see Fig. 4–3 and Chap. 3, Figs. 3–11 and 3–13). Protein S also can directly inhibit factors VIIIa, Xa, and Va.[11–13] Thus, APC and protein S inhibit multiple steps in the intrinsic coagulation pathway.

At each step in the coagulation pathways, each clotting protease can be inhibited by one or more plasma protease inhibitors in reactions stimulated by negatively charged glycosaminoglycans such as heparan sulfate or heparin (see "Inhibition of Coagulation Proteases by Protease Inhibitors" below). Given the highly nonlinear nature of the coagulation

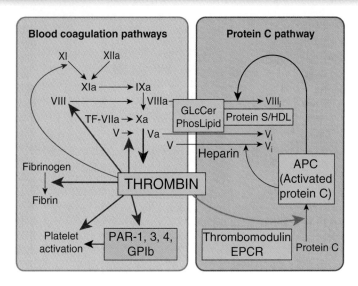

**Figure 4–1.** Blood coagulation pathways and protein C anticoagulant pathway. Thrombin can be either a procoagulant *(left)* or an anticoagulant *(right)*, depending on cofactors and surfaces. Coagulant thrombin clots fibrinogen and activates platelets and factors V, VIII, XI, and XIII. Conversion of zymogen protein C to the active protease, APC, by thrombomodulin-bound thrombin is enhanced by endothelial protein C receptor (EPCR). APC with its nonenzymatic cofactor, protein S, inactivates factors Va and VIIIa by highly selective proteolysis (e.g., at Arg506 and Arg306 in factor Va), yielding inactivated (i) factors $V_i$ and $VIII_i$. This anticoagulant action may be enhanced by phospholipid (PhosLipid) surfaces on platelets, endothelial cells, or their microparticles. High-density lipoprotein (HDL) can also provide protein S–dependent anticoagulant APC-cofactor activity. Similarly, neutral glycosphingolipids such as glucosylceramide (GLcCer) can enhance APC anticoagulant activity. GPIb, glycoprotein Ib; PAR, protease-activated receptor. *(Adapted with permission from Griffin JH: Blood coagulation. The thrombin paradox, Nature 1995 Nov 23;378(6555):337–338.)*

pathways with both positive and negative feedback reactions, synergy between the protein C pathway and plasma protease inhibitors is important for regulating thrombin generation.

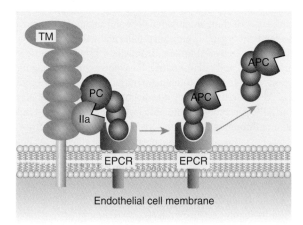

**Figure 4–2.** Protein C activation on endothelial cell surface. On an endothelial surface, activated protein C (APC) generation follows binding of protein C (PC) to endothelial protein C receptor (EPCR) where PC is activated by limited proteolysis by the thrombin (IIa)–thrombomodulin (TM) complex. This action of thrombin liberates a dodecapeptide (residues 158 to 169) from protein C to generate the multifunctional protease APC. *(Adapted with permission from Mosnier LO, Zlokovic BV, Griffin JH: cytoprotective protein C pathway, Blood 2007 Apr 15;109(8):3161–3172.)*

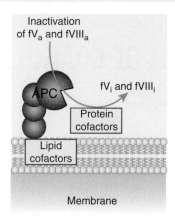

**Figure 4–3.** Activated protein C (APC) exerts its anticoagulant activity by proteolytic inactivation of factors Va and VIIIa on membrane surfaces containing phospholipids that are derived from cells, lipoproteins, or cellular microparticles. A variety of lipid and protein cofactors (see Fig. 4–1 legend and text) accelerate the inactivation of factors Va and VIIIa to yield the irreversibly inactivated factors Vi and VIIIi. *(Adapted with permission from Mosnier LO, Zlokovic BV, Griffin JH: The cytoprotective protein C pathway, Blood 2007 Apr 15;109(8):3161–3172.)*

There is continuous activation of coagulation factors at a basal physiologic low level. Plasma from all normal subjects contains circulating active enzymes, factor VIIa,[14] and APC,[15] as well as various polypeptide fragments generated by the action of clotting proteases, namely fibrinopeptides,[16,17] prothrombin fragment 1+2,[18] and activation peptides for factors IX and X.[19,20] The presence of multiple clotting factors that require positive feedback activation (e.g., factors V, VIII, XI, and VII) imparts special threshold properties to the blood coagulation pathways, making the coagulant response nonlinearly responsive to stimuli. Theoretical analysis of blood coagulation as a threshold system suggests

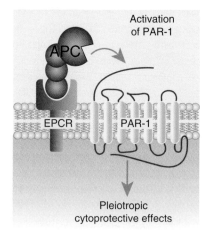

**Figure 4–4.** Paradigm for activated protein C (APC)'s initiation of cell signaling and multiple cytoprotective effects. Direct effects of APC on cells are initiated by activation of the G-protein–coupled receptor, protease-activated receptor-1 (PAR-1), by endothelial protein C receptor (EPCR)-bound APC. The γ-carboxyglutamic acid (GLA) domain of APC binds to EPCR to help position APC's protease domain for efficient cleavage of the extracellular N-terminal tail of PAR-1, which results in G-protein–coupled receptor activation and subsequent antiinflammatory and antiapoptotic effects, alterations of gene expression profiles, and stabilization of endothelial junctions. *(Adapted with permission from Mosnier LO, Zlokovic BV, Griffin JH: The cytoprotective protein C pathway, Blood 2007 Apr 15;109(8):3161–3172.)*

there can be an all-or-none response to various levels of stimulation, depending on the ensemble of activating and inhibitory reactions that defines upregulation and downregulation of thrombin generation.[21,22] The coagulation system is active, but idling, and is poised for extensive and explosive generation of thrombin. Because of synergy among various cellular and humoral anticoagulant mechanisms that establish a threshold system, the presence of multiple coagulation inhibitors with complementary modes of action prevents massive thrombin generation in the absence of a substantial procoagulant stimulus.

## HEREDITARY DEFICIENCIES ASSOCIATED WITH THROMBOTIC DISEASE

Evidence for the physiologic importance of specific factors for controlling coagulation reactions comes from clinical observations and animal model studies. Major identified genetic risk factors for venous thrombosis involve protein structural defects in factor V, protein C, protein S, and antithrombin (Chap. 20). There are also gene regulatory defects associated with thrombotic disease, such as the G20210A polymorphism in the prothrombin gene that causes elevated levels of prothrombin, and defects in protein C gene regulatory elements that decrease the expression of protein C. Deficiencies of thrombomodulin might also be associated with increased risk of arterial thrombosis. Association of hereditary abnormalities of EPCR with increased risks of thrombosis has been suggested, but this remains somewhat controversial.

## PROTEIN C PATHWAY COMPONENTS

Figure 4–5 is a schematic of the structures of protein C, protein S, thrombomodulin, and EPCR. These proteins contain multiple domains,

each of which may mediate different molecular functions. Values for the molecular weight, normal plasma concentration, chromosomal location, and gene structures of these factors are given in Table 4–1. Factors Va and VIIIa, as substrates of APC, are also participants in the reactions of the anticoagulant protein C pathway. Moreover, factor V, but not factor V Leiden, appears to act as an APC cofactor for the inactivation of factor VIIIa (see "Factor V as Activated Protein C Cofactor" below).[23]

## PROTEIN C

In 1976, Stenflo designated a bovine plasma vitamin K–dependent protein that eluted in the third peak (peak C) from an anion exchange column as bovine "protein C."[24] Protein C, actually previously described as the anticoagulant factor autoprothrombin II-A,[25] is a plasma serine protease zymogen that can be converted to an active serine protease by the action of thrombin.

Protein C is synthesized in the liver as a polypeptide precursor of 461 residues, with a prepropeptide of 42 amino acids that contains the signal for carboxylation of Glu residues by a carboxylase that forms nine $\gamma$-carboxyglutamic acid (GLA) residues and secretion of the mature protein.[26-28] The mature glycoprotein of Mr 62,000 contains 419 residues (see Chap. 3, Fig. 3–1 and Fig. 4–5) and N-linked carbohydrate, and the majority of the secreted protein C molecules are cleaved by a furin-like endoprotease that releases Lys156-Arg157 and generates a two-chain zymogen that circulates in plasma at 65 nM (4 mcg/mL).[29] The heavy and light chains of plasma protein C are covalently linked by a disulfide bond that keeps the serine protease globular domain (residues 170 to 419) covalently tethered to the N-terminal string of three domains, the GLA domain and the epidermal growth factor (EGF)-like domains EGF-1 and EGF-2.[26-30]

The GLA domain of protein C (residues 1 to 42) and APC is important for a number of functions, including binding to

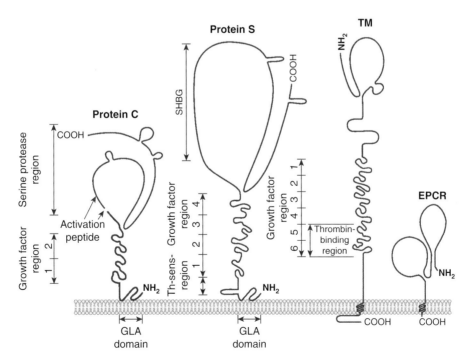

**Figure 4–5.** Membrane-bound protein C, protein S, thrombomodulin (TM) and endothelial cell protein C receptor (EPCR). Each protein is a multidomain protein that extends above the surface of cell membranes, and different domains mediate different functions of each protein. Protein C and protein S can bind reversibly to phospholipid membranes through their NH$_2$-terminal $\gamma$-carboxyglutamic acid (GLA) domains, which contain nine or 11 GLA residues that bind four to six Ca$^{2+}$ ions. TM and EPCR are integral membrane proteins that are embedded in cell membranes by a single hydrophobic transmembrane sequence. *(Adapted with permission from Esmon CT: The roles of protein C and thrombomodulin in the regulation of blood coagulation, J Biol Chem 1989 Mar 25;264(9):4743–4746.)*

**TABLE 4–1.** Characteristics of Blood Coagulation Regulatory Molecules

| | Molecular Weight (kDa) | Plasma Concentration (mcg/mL) | Half-Life (h) | Chromosome | Gene (kb) | Exon (N) | Function |
|---|---|---|---|---|---|---|---|
| Protein C | 62 | 4 | 6 | 2q13–14 | 11 | 9 | Anticoagulant protease |
| Protein S | 75 | 26 | 42 | 3p11.1–11.2 | 80 | 15 | Activated protein C (APC)-cofactor and coagulation inhibitor |
| Thrombomodulin | 60–105 | 0.020 | ND | 20p11.2–cen | 3.7 | 1 | Receptor for thrombin/ protein C |
| Endothelial protein C receptor (EPCR) | 46 | 0.098 | ND | 20q11.2 | 6 | 4 | Receptor for protein C/ APC |
| Protease-activated receptor-1 (PAR-1) | 68 | NA | NA | 5q13 | 27 | 2 | G-protein–coupled receptor |
| Antithrombin | 58 | 150 | 70 | 1q23–25 | 14 | 7 | Protease inhibitor |
| Tissue factor pathway inhibitor (TFPI) | 34 | 0.1 | ND | 2q31–32.1 | 85 | 9 | Protease inhibitor |
| Heparin cofactor II | 66 | 70 | 60 | 22q11 | 16 | 5 | Protease inhibitor |
| Protein Z | 70 | 1.7 | 60 | 13q34 | | 9 | Plasma protein |
| Protein Z–dependent protease inhibitor (ZPI) | 72 | 1.5 | | 14q32.13 | | 5 | Protease inhibitor |

NA, not applicable; ND, not determined.

phospholipid-containing membranes (see Chap. 3, Fig. 3–3), thrombomodulin, and EPCR; thus, incomplete carboxylation impairs the functional anticoagulant activity of APC.[31–33] The two EGF modules in the light chain may contribute to interactions of APC with protein S and of protein C with thrombomodulin.

The serine protease domain of protein C is homologous to other trypsin-like proteases, and three-dimensional modeling[34] and X-ray crystallographic structures[30] reflect the structural similarity of APC to members of the serine protease family of which chymotrypsin is the prototype (see Mather and colleagues[30] for conversion of protein C to chymotrypsin numbering). APC's trypsin-like protease domain exerts its anticoagulant activity by highly specific interactions with factors Va and VIIIa followed by cleavage at only two Arg-containing peptide bonds in factors Va and VIIIa (see "Factors Va and VIIIa as Substrates for Activated Protein C" below). These stereo-specific interactions involve both the APC enzymatic active site region and a number of APC residues that are termed *exosites* because they are not located in the immediate vicinity of APC's enzymatic active site. Such APC exosites are essential for specific recognition of the macromolecular substrates, factors Va and VIIIa, as well as recognition of cellular APC receptors.[35–44]

### Protein C and Activated Protein C Therapy
Purified plasma protein C concentrate (Ceprotin) is FDA-approved for treating protein C–deficient patients.[45] Recombinant human APC (Xigris) reduced all-cause 28-day mortality in adult patients with severe sepsis in the PROWESS phase III trial in 2001 and was FDA-approved for this indication.[46] This successful therapy of adult severe sepsis using APC followed preclinical antithrombotic and sepsis studies in baboons.[47,48] However, a decade later, in the PROWESS-SHOCK trial, recombinant APC did not reduce mortality in adult severe sepsis patients,[49–51] and Xigris was withdrawn from the market. Animal injury model studies have also shed light on *in vivo* mechanisms for the beneficial effects of APC in many preclinical injury models, and in many models, the pharmacologic benefits of APC appear to be independent of APC's anticoagulant actions (see "Activated Protein C Direct Cellular Activities" below).[7,8]

### Protein C Gene
The protein C gene, comprising nine exons and eight introns, is located on chromosome 2q14–21 and spans 11 kb (see Chap. 3, Fig. 3–10, and Table 4–1).[52] The protein C gene is homologous to the genes for factors VII, IX, and X (Chap. 3).

### Protein C Mutations
Hereditary protein C deficiency associated with thrombosis is caused by numerous mutations (see protein C mutation databases).[53,54] Based on three-dimensional structures of the protein C, the structural basis for hereditary protein C defects has been rationalized.[34,55,56] Most mutations that cause type I protein C deficiency, characterized by parallel reductions in activity and antigen, involve amino acid residues that form the hydrophobic cores of the two folded globulin-like domains that are characteristic of serine proteases. These mutations destabilize either the process or the product of protein folding, and they result in unstable molecules that are poorly secreted and/or exhibit a very short circulatory half-life. In contrast, most mutations that cause type II defects (reduced anticoagulant or enzymatic activity but normal antigen levels), that is, circulating dysfunctional molecules, involve polar surface residues that do not affect polypeptide folding or thermodynamic stability; these polar residues presumably are involved in protein–protein interactions important for expression of anticoagulant activity.

Rare variants derived from a founder's mutation appear to be distinctive for races. Two protein C mutations, Arg147Trp and a Lys150 deletion, are significant venous thrombosis risk factors in Chinese but not in Americans of European descent or Japanese.[57–59]

Severe protein C deficiency as a consequence of homozygous knockout of the mouse protein C gene showed a similar phenotype as severe human protein C deficiency (Chap. 20), with perinatal consumptive coagulopathy in the brain and liver and either death or massive thrombosis that occurred either in the uterus or shortly after birth.[60]

## PROTEIN S

Plasma "protein S," which was named in honor of Seattle, the city of its discovery, is a vitamin K–dependent glycoprotein[61] that is synthesized by hepatocytes, neuroblastoma cells, kidney cells, testis, megakaryocytes, and endothelial cells, and is also found in platelet α granules.[62]

Protein S is synthesized as a precursor protein of 676 amino acids, which gives rise to a mature secreted single-chain glycoprotein of 635 residues with three N-linked carbohydrate side chains (see Fig. 4–5).[63,64] Eleven GLA residues in the N-terminal region of mature protein S contribute to $Ca^{2+}$-mediated binding of the protein to phospholipid membranes. The thrombin-sensitive region, residues 47 to 72, follows the GLA domain (see Fig. 4–5).

The C-terminal region of protein S, residues 270 to 635, the sex hormone–binding globulin-like (SHBG) region, contains binding sites for C4b-binding protein (see "Activated Protein C–Independent Anticoagulant Activity of Protein S" below)[65] and for factor V, as well as factor Va.[66,67] Protein S, like the homologous gas6, also binds to receptor tyrosine kinases, for example, Axl, and initiates cell signaling, and the SHBG region binds the receptor.[68] Thus, for the expression of its multiple activities, different domains of protein S exhibit a number of different binding sites for different proteins.

### Protein S Gene

The protein S gene, comprising 15 exons and 14 introns, is located on chromosome 3p11.1–11.2 and spans 80 kb (see Chap. 3, Fig. 3–16 and Table 4–1).[69,70] The protein S gene has limited homology with other genes for vitamin K–dependent factors in the GLA and EGF domains and notable homology of the region coding for residues 240 to 635 with genes of the SHBG family. Humans contain a protein S pseudogene that contains several stop codons and is not translated and that is located very near the normal protein S gene on chromosome 3.

### Protein S Mutations

The molecular basis for hereditary protein S deficiency associated with venous thrombosis (Chap. 20) is linked to more than 100 different mutations.[71] A protein S polymorphism that is strongly linked to risk for venous thrombosis in Japanese subjects is known as protein S Tokushima. It involves K155E, which ablates APC-cofactor activity.[57,72] But the K155E apparently is not present in Americans of European ancestry or Chinese populations, thus mirroring the presence of factor V Leiden and prothrombin G20210A, which are risk factors in Americans of European descent but not in the Japanese, Chinese, or Americans of African descent populations.[73] Another single nucleotide polymorphism present in approximately 1 percent of Americans of European descent is S460P, which is designated protein S Heerlen; it results in absence of N-linked carbohydrate on Asn458 but has no accepted significant functional consequence.[74]

## THROMBOMODULIN

Thrombomodulin was discovered as an endothelial cell surface receptor that binds protein C and thrombin, thereby accelerating protein C activation.[75–78] Binding of thrombin to thrombomodulin converts thrombin from a procoagulant enzyme to an anticoagulant enzyme because thrombomodulin-bound thrombin loses its normal ability to clot fibrinogen or activate platelets.[79,80] Thrombomodulin is a multidomain transmembrane protein comprising an N-terminal lectin-like domain, six EGF domains, a Ser/Thr-rich region, a single membrane-spanning sequence, and an intracellular C-terminal tail (see Fig. 4–5).[5–8,75–83] EGF domains 4, 5, and 6 are essential for activation of protein C, with the latter two domains binding thrombin and the first domain binding protein C. The mature protein has 557-amino-acid residues and variable amounts of N- and O-linked carbohydrate modifications that cause variability in molecular size. Glycosaminoglycans, notably chondroitin sulfate, covalently attached to the Ser/Thr-rich region, contribute to the functional properties of thrombomodulin by enhancing either protein C activation by thrombin or by accelerating neutralization of thrombin by protease inhibitors. Modulation of the substrate specificity of thrombin by thrombomodulin involves conformational changes in thrombin caused by binding of thrombomodulin.

Low levels of soluble thrombomodulin circulate in plasma, presumably as a result of limited proteolysis of the protein near its transmembrane cell surface anchor. The functional significance of circulating thrombomodulin is unknown, although variations in its plasma level arise in different clinical conditions.

Recombinant soluble thrombomodulin has been developed for its potential therapeutic value for disseminated intravascular coagulation and has been approved for this indication in Japan.[77,84]

### Thrombomodulin Gene

The thrombomodulin gene, which lacks introns, is located on chromosome 20p11.2 and spans 3.7 kb (see Chap. 3, Fig. 3–19, Fig. 4–5, and Table 4–1).[77,82] Deletion of the thrombomodulin gene in mice is embryonically lethal.[85] Downregulation of thrombomodulin gene expression is promoted by a variety of inflammatory agents, including endotoxin, interleukin-1, and tumor necrosis factor (TNF)-α, whereas its expression is upregulated by retinoic acid.[5–8,86,87] Generally, thrombomodulin is a key member among the counterbalancing factors that contribute to inflammation, thrombin generation, and coagulation in the endothelium.

### Thrombomodulin Mutations

Thrombomodulin mutations are well documented in atypical hemolytic uremic syndrome patients,[78,88] and they may also be associated with an increased risk of arterial thrombosis and myocardial infarction. In contrast, there is less supportive data for association with risk for venous thrombosis (Chap. 20).[89–92] Atypical hemolytic uremic syndrome is strongly linked to excessive complement activation, and thrombomodulin's lectin-like domain inhibits complement activation.[77,93] Furthermore, besides promoting protein C activation by thrombin, thrombomodulin also supports activation of the carboxypeptidase, also known as thrombin-activatable fibrinolysis inhibitor (TAFI), which is a potent inactivator of bradykinin, and of the activated complement components, C3a and C5a.[94–96]

## ENDOTHELIAL PROTEIN C RECEPTOR

EPCR binds both protein C and APC with similar affinities through their GLA domains and mediates multiple activities of this zymogen or its activated protease, APC.[9,10,33,86,97–107] The mature EPCR glycoprotein contains 221-amino-acid residues and N-linked carbohydrate, giving an Mr of 46,000. EPCR is an integral membrane protein that is homologous to CD1/major histocompatibility complex class I molecules. The N-terminus is part of an extracellular domain, which is connected to a single transmembrane sequence that is followed by a short Arg-Arg-Cys-COOH cytoplasmic tail (see Fig. 4–5). The cytoplasmic tail can be palmitoylated, and this modification may help localize EPCR to certain lipid rafts or caveolae. The three-dimensional structure of EPCR determined by X-ray crystallography or inferred by molecular modeling established that the GLA domain of protein C and APC binds to EPCR.[107,108] EPCR on endothelial surfaces enhances by greater than fivefold the rate of activation of protein C by thrombin–thrombomodulin (see Fig. 4–2). EPCR is also required for the cytoprotective activities of APC by promoting the cleavage of PAR-1 by APC to induce cell-signaling pathways (see Fig. 4–4). Notably, the cytoprotective actions of APC are completely independent of its anticoagulant activity and are based on cell signaling actions (see "Activated Protein C Direct Cellular Activities" below).[7,8,109–111]

The presence of functional EPCR on the cell surface is regulated by two mechanisms, namely generation of EPCR and clearance of EPCR. Inflammatory mediators induce EPCR ectodomain shedding from the endothelial cell surface by metalloproteinase TNF-$\alpha$ converting enzyme (known as "TACE").[112] The soluble EPCR ectodomain is found in normal human plasma at 100 ng/mL; however, carriers of the H3 EPCR haplotype that includes a Ser219Gly polymorphism (rs867186) have threefold higher soluble EPCR plasma levels.[113] Higher plasma levels of soluble EPCR are found in patients with disseminated intravascular coagulation or systemic lupus erythematosus, although plasma EPCR levels are not correlated with pathology-related alterations in circulating thrombomodulin levels.[114] Soluble EPCR binds the protein C and APC via their GLA domains with an affinity similar to the membrane-bound receptor. Because binding of the APC GLA domain to negatively charged phospholipid membranes is required for its anticoagulant activity, soluble EPCR at relatively high levels in purified reaction mixtures inhibits the anticoagulant action of APC against factor Va, although it does not block the reaction of APC with protease inhibitors.[10,86,99,115]

The EPCR crystal structure surprisingly revealed a single phospholipid molecule bound in a surface groove on the protein.[107] Secreted phospholipase $A_2$ group V can modify the lipid in EPCR and cause EPCR to lose its ability to bind protein C and APC.[116,117] The presence of functional EPCR on the cell surface has important implications for thrombotic and inflammatory vascular disease because EPCR inactivation *in vivo* increases susceptibility to thrombotic and inflammatory diseases.[10,86,97]

The physiologic requirement for EPCR in mice was established by the embryonic lethality observed for knockout of the murine EPCR gene.[118]

EPCR has functionally important interactions with multiple molecules beyond protein C and APC. It binds factor VII and factor VIIa.[10] Furthermore, EPCR was recently implicated to play a potentially important role in the pathogenesis of severe malaria.[119-122]

### Endothelial Protein C Receptor Gene

The EPCR gene, comprising four exons and three introns, is located on human chromosome 20q11.2 and spans 6 kb (see Table 4–1).[123]

## PROTEASE-ACTIVATED RECEPTOR-1

PAR-1, discovered as a high-affinity human platelet receptor for thrombin,[124] is the prototype of a four-member subfamily of G-protein–coupled receptors that share an unusual mechanism of activation, namely activation by proteases.[124-130] Each PAR contains seven transmembrane helical domains and an extracellular N-terminal tail that is cleaved by an activating protease such that the newly generated aminoterminus is a tethered ligand that triggers activation of the coupled G-protein. Human platelets employ PAR-1 and PAR-4 for activation by thrombin, whereas, curiously, murine platelets that are devoid of PAR-1 require PAR-3 and PAR-4 for thrombin's normal effects.[125,131] PAR-1 is activated by various plasma proteases[132-135] and is generally required for APC's cytoprotective activities (see "Cellular Receptors for Physiologic Effects of Activated Protein C on Cells" below).[7,8,110,111]

### Protease-Activated Receptor-1 Gene

The PAR-1 gene contains only two introns, is located on chromosome 5q13, and spans 25 kb (see Table 4–1).[125] Much is known about many factors that can either upregulate or downregulate the PAR-1 gene.[124-130]

## ● ACTIVATION OF PROTEIN C

Protein C is activated from zymogen to active protease as a result of cleavage by thrombin at the Arg169–Leu170 peptide bond in a reaction that is accelerated by thrombomodulin and EPCR (see Fig. 4–2

and "Thrombomodulin" above).[5,7,8,76,81,86] Thrombin infusions into animals generate anticoagulant activity because of APC.[136,137] Interestingly, thrombin infusion into hyperlipidemic monkeys with atherosclerosis generates less APC and causes a poorer *ex vivo* response to APC compared with normolipidemic control monkeys,[138] showing that hyperlipidemia and vascular disease can affect protein C activation.

Ischemia causes protein C activation *in vivo*. A brief occlusion of the left anterior descending coronary artery in pigs results in APC generation.[139] During cerebral ischemia in humans undergoing routine endarterectomy, APC increases in the venous cerebral blood.[140] Protein C is significantly activated during cardiopulmonary bypass, mainly during the minutes immediately after aortic unclamping in the ischemic vascular beds.[141] Streptokinase therapy for acute myocardial infarction increases circulating APC.[142]

Circulating APC concentration in normal human subjects is highly correlated with circulating levels of protein C zymogen.[143] Based on protein C infusion studies in protein C–deficient subjects, the level of circulating APC is strongly determined by the concentration of protein C.[144] EPCR appears to be required for normal protein C activation in response to thrombin infusions in experimental animals.[145] EPCR and thrombomodulin must be in close proximity on cell surfaces (see Fig. 4–2), although this has yet to be experimentally demonstrated.

Thrombomodulin and EPCR appear to differ markedly in their relative distribution densities on blood vessels as the former is abundantly present in the small blood vessels but less so in large vessels, whereas the latter is more abundant in large vessels than in small vessels.[85,86,146,147] Low levels of thrombomodulin are expressed in brain,[148] and brain-specific activation of protein C in humans occurs during carotid occlusion.[140]

Proteolytic cleavage and activation of protein C can also be effected by meizothrombin, plasmin, or factor Xa.[149-153] On the surface of cultured endothelial cells, negatively charged sulfated polysaccharides in the presence of phospholipid vesicles containing phosphatidylethanolamine can enhance the rate of protein C activation by factor Xa to approach the protein C activation rate of thrombin:thrombomodulin.[152] No data yet indicate whether protein C activation by meizothrombin, plasmin, or factor Xa is physiologically relevant.

Protein C activation is stimulated by platelet factor 4. Both *in vitro* and *in vivo* data imply that platelet factor 4 may play a physiologic role in enhancing APC generation and influencing the activities of the protein C system.[154-157]

## ● ACTIVATED PROTEIN C ACTIVITIES

The clinical phenotype of severe protein C deficiency in neonatal purpura fulminans implies that APC exerts multiple physiologically essential activities, including potent anticoagulant and antiinflammatory actions (Chap. 20). Recent advances establish that APC's antiinflammatory actions are but one manifestation of its ability to interact directly with cell receptors to provide multiple cytoprotective activities.[7,8,110,111] These two distinct types of activities of APC—intravascular anticoagulant activity and initiation of cell signaling—are mediated by different sets of molecular interactions, and both types of activities are clinically relevant.

### ACTIVATED PROTEIN C ANTICOAGULANT ACTIVITY

Mechanisms for APC's direct anticoagulant activity involve factors V and VIII, the two homologous coagulation cofactors that circulate as inactive molecules and that are converted to active cofactors by limited proteolysis (see Chap. 3, Figs. 3–11 and 3–13). APC circulates at 40 pM (picomolars) in normal humans, and there is an inverse correlation between fibrinopeptide A, the product that is cleaved from fibrinogen by thrombin, and APC levels in healthy nonsmoking adults, suggesting APC is a significant regulator of basal thrombin activity.[15,158]

Factors V and VIII are synthesized as large single-chain precursor coagulation cofactors of Mr 330,000, consisting of three homologous A domains (A1, A2, and A3) and two homologous C domains (C1 and C2) with a very large intervening, generally nonhomologous domain, designated the *B domain,* that connects the A2 and A3 domains (Chap. 3). Activation of the inactive precursor form of the two cofactors V and VIII involves limited proteolysis.[23,159-164] Factor V activation involves cleavages at Arg709, Arg1018, and Arg1545 by thrombin, factor Xa, or other proteases.[23,164-168] Cleavage at Arg1545 is the key step for generating factor Va activity because this proteolysis releases the B domain that blocks binding of factor Xa to factor Va.[164,169] The various forms of factor Va (see Chap. 3, Fig. 3–11) are composed of two polypeptide chains, one bearing the A1-A2 domains and the other bearing the A3-C1-C2 domains. Although generally similar to factor V activation, factor VIII activation (see Chap. 3, Fig. 3–13) involves formation of a heterotrimer of polypeptide chains containing the A1 domain, the A2 domain, and the A3-C1-C2 domains, respectively. In contrast to heterodimeric factor Va, heterotrimeric factor VIIIa is intrinsically unstable as a consequence of spontaneous dissociation of the A2 domain.[170]

### Factors Va and VIIIa as Substrates for Activated Protein C

Irreversible proteolytic inactivation of factors Va and VIIIa by APC can be accomplished by proteolysis at Arg506 and Arg306 in factor Va and Arg562 and Arg336 in factor VIIIa (see Chap. 3, Figs. 3–11 and 3–13).[23,171-173] Currently, the most common identifiable venous thrombosis risk factor involves a mutation of Arg506 to Gln in factor V that results in APC resistance (Chap. 20). The complexities of APC-dependent inactivation of factor Va and VIIIa are compounded by the number of different molecular forms of Va and VIIIa that can be generated by limited proteolysis by a variety of proteases and by their differing susceptibilities to APC and to the different APC cofactors.

### Activated Protein C Resistance

APC resistance is defined as an abnormally reduced anticoagulant response of a plasma sample to APC (Chap. 20) and can be caused by many potential abnormalities in the protein C anticoagulant pathway. Such abnormalities could include defective APC cofactors, defective APC substrates, or other molecules that interfere with the normal functioning of the protein C anticoagulant pathway (e.g., autoantibodies against APC, APC cofactors, or APC substrates).

A report of familial venous thrombosis associated with APC resistance without any identifiable defect in four Swedish families[174] led to an intensive search for a genetic explanation that was soon found to involve replacement of G by A at nucleotide 1691 in exon 10 of the factor V gene, which causes the amino acid replacement of Arg506 by Gln.[175-177] This factor V variant, like the prothrombin variant nt G20210A, arose in a single white founder some 18,000 to 29,000 years ago[178,179] and is known as *Gln506-factor V* or *factor V Leiden*. This mutation is currently a common, but not the only, cause of APC resistance (Chap. 20).

The molecular mechanism for APC resistance of Gln506-factor V is based on the fact that the variant molecule is inactivated 10 times slower than normal Arg506-factor Va.[23,177,180-182] The variant factor Va exhibits only a partial resistance to APC because cleavage at Arg306 in factor Va also occurs, causing complete loss of factor Va activity.

Plasma and recombinant factor V can exist in two biochemically distinct forms, designated *factor V1* and *factor V2,* that differ in *N*-linked carbohydrate on Asn2181, near the phospholipid binding region of the C2 domain, as factor V2 has none.[183,184] Because the *N*-linked carbohydrate appears to decrease the apparent affinity of factor V1 or Va1 for phospholipid, it reduces the specific clotting activity and susceptibility to

APC. Normal plasma contains a mixture of factors V1 and V2. Removal of the carbohydrate attached to factor V increases the rate of inactivation of factor Va by APC, although the clinical significance of this phenomenon is unknown.[185]

APC resistance with no identifiable genetic or acquired abnormalities is well described in patients with venous and arterial thrombosis and, at least for research purposes, should be therefore examined in patients with a suspected thrombophilia. Further studies are needed to identify the causes of APC resistance in such patients.[186-188] One major challenge involves defining the normal range for the clotting assays that are actually used to characterize APC resistance and the multiple plasma analytes or nonplasma assay components that are present in the assays. For example, activated partial thromboplastin time–based assays are not as sensitive as dilute tissue factor–based assays to plasma high-density lipoprotein (HDL) levels or oral contraceptive use.[189-191] Plasma variables, such as elevated prothrombin levels,[192,193] may affect the response to APC by inhibiting APC anticoagulant actions. Endogenous thrombin potential assays involving dilute tissue factor as the procoagulant initiator provide additional tools for defining and characterizing APC resistance and extend the tools for shedding light on the gray area of APC resistance found in some thrombosis patients that is not linked to currently known factors.

## ACTIVATED PROTEIN C ANTICOAGULANT COFACTORS

APC anticoagulant activity is enhanced by a number of factors that may be termed *APC anticoagulant cofactors*; these include Ca$^{2+}$ ions; certain, but not all, phospholipids; protein S; factor V; certain glycosphingolipids; and HDL.

### Phospholipids as Activated Protein C Cofactors

Certain phospholipids, such as phosphatidylserine, phosphatidylethanolamine, and cardiolipin, enhance the anticoagulant activity of APC. In addition, phosphatidylethanolamine and cardiolipin stimulate the APC anticoagulant pathway activities much more than they stimulate the procoagulant pathway activities.[194-197]

### Protein S as Activated Protein C Cofactor

Protein S structure–activity relationships are informed by much biochemical work and the large number of mutations.[71,198] Protein S, as an anticoagulant APC cofactor, forms a 1:1 complex with APC and enhances by 10- to 20-fold the rate of APC's cleavage at Arg306 in factor Va but not the Arg506 cleavage.[181,182] Part of the mechanism for this activity of protein S may be related to its ability to bring the active site of APC closer to the plane of the phospholipid membrane on which the APC–protein S complex is located when the complex is formed.[199,200] Protein S also facilitates the action of APC against factor VIIIa.[201] Protein S enhances APC's action, in part at least, by ablating the ability of factor Xa to protect factor Va from APC.[202] The GLA domain, thrombin-sensitive region, and EGF1 and EGF2 domains of protein S are implicated in binding APC for expression of anticoagulant activity by the APC–protein S complex.[198,203-206] Cleavage of the thrombin-sensitive region by thrombin abolishes normal binding of protein S to phospholipid and its normal APC-cofactor anticoagulant activity.[205,207]

### Factor V as Activated Protein C Cofactor

Factor V apparently can have anticoagulant as well as procoagulant properties because it enhances the anticoagulant action of APC against factors VIIIa and Va in a reaction in which protein S acts synergistically with factor V.[23,208-211] Cleavage at Arg1545, which optimizes factor Va procoagulant activity, ablates the molecule's anticoagulant cofactor activity. However, when factor V is cleaved at Arg506 by APC, its APC cofactor activity is increased 10-fold. This suggests that Gln506-factor V has two potential prothrombotic defects, namely, resistance of the variant factor Va to APC inactivation and resistance of the variant factor V to activation of its APC cofactor function.[23,209–211]

### High-Density Lipoprotein as Activated Protein C Cofactor

HDL can exert antithrombotic activity through multiple mechanisms.[212] HDL enhances the anticoagulant activity of APC both in plasma and in purified reaction mixtures, and this APC cofactor activity requires protein S and involves, at least in part, stimulation of APC's cleavage at Arg306 in factor Va.[189,190] HDL is heterogeneous in both protein and lipid composition, and the components responsible for this activity have not been identified, although large HDL, but not small HDL, possesses APC anticoagulant cofactor activity.[190] Venous thrombosis in males and venous thrombosis recurrence are associated with a pattern of dyslipoproteinemia and low HDL, consistent with the hypothesis that deficiency of large HDL is a risk factor for venous thrombosis.[213,214]

### Glycosphingolipids as Activated Protein C Cofactors

Although both procoagulant and anticoagulant reactions are markedly enhanced by the presence of negatively charged phospholipid surfaces *in vitro*, certain lipoproteins, for example, HDL,[189] and certain lipids, for example, glycosphingolipids and sphingosine,[215–218] selectively enhance anticoagulant reactions in plasma. Plasma glucosylceramide deficiency is a biomarker and may be a potential risk factor for venous thrombosis.[215] Sphingosine and several of its common analogues are potent inhibitors of thrombin generation in plasma and on cell surfaces because they inhibit interactions between factors Va and Xa.[218] Further studies are needed to characterize the anticoagulant or procoagulant properties of minor abundance plasma and their significance for clinical thrombotic events.

## ACTIVATED PROTEIN C DIRECT CELLULAR ACTIVITIES

As noted in Chap. 3, control of coagulation reactions does not occur in the absence of an integrated host defense system that involves a number of biologic processes involving multiple overlapping and integrated pathways. Reactions of the innate and acquired immune system including inflammatory processes, blood coagulation reactions, fibrinolysis, and thrombotic processes are intertwined *in vivo* via multiple molecular and cellular mechanisms.[5,7,8,81,86,87,212,219,220] In addition to its anticoagulant activity, APC acts directly on cells to cause multiple cytoprotective effects. Cytoprotective actions of APC include antiapoptotic and antiinflammatory activities, beneficial changes in gene-expression profiles, and endothelial barrier stabilization. These cytoprotective activities of APC generally require EPCR, involve APC's ability to activate PAR-1, and may also require additional receptors such as PAR-3, sphingosine-1-phosphate receptor 1, integrin CD11b/CD18, apoER2, EGF receptor, and/or Tie2.[7,8,86,110,221–227]

Pharmacologic APC infusions showed benefits in numerous animal injury model systems, with the most informative animal studies to date being in sepsis models and in neuroprotection experiments.[7,8,110,111,226,227] Protein engineering permitted the molecular dissection of APC's anticoagulant activity from its cytoprotective activities[7,8,37,40–44,228] and led to proof of principle that APC's cell-signaling activities are both necessary and most likely sufficient for reducing lethality in murine septic shock models[42,229] and for providing neuroprotective effects in ischemic stroke models.[226,227,230–232] Notably, recombinant APC mutants that have little anticoagulant activity (<10 percent) but normal cell-signaling activity are able to convey beneficial effects in multiple injury and disease models with diminished risks for bleeding that would be anticipated with wild-type APC therapy.[8,40–44]

### Activated Protein C Neuroprotective Effects

Neuroprotective effects of APC have been convincingly demonstrated in rodent ischemic stroke models and N-methyl-D-aspartate (NMDA) excitotoxic injury models.[8,223,226,227,231,233–242] APC not only provides direct cytoprotection *in vitro* and *in vivo* for brain endothelium against ischemic injury but also directly protects neurons against NMDA-induced excitotoxic injury both *in vivo* and *in vitro*. APC mutants with reduced anticoagulant activity were as neuroprotective as wild-type APC, and certain cellular receptors were required for APC's neuroprotection, strongly implying that neuroprotection by APC involves its actions directly on the endothelium and on neurons. Remarkably, in the ischemic penumbra in a murine stroke model, APC caused neovascularization and neurogenesis.[223,240,243–245] The extensive preclinical studies on APC's neuroprotective effects paved the pathway for translation of the 3K3A-APC variant to potential neuroprotective therapy for acute ischemic stroke.[246,247] Because of the greatly reduced anticoagulant activity of 3K3A-APC (<10 percent of normal), high-dose bolus dosing in healthy volunteers can achieve circulating APC levels that are 100-fold higher than those used in the PROWESS or PROWESS-SHOCK sepsis trials without notable anticoagulant effects.[46,49,246]

### Cellular Receptors for Physiologic Effects of Activated Protein C on Cells

The ability of exogenously administered APC to alter gene-expression profiles of cultured endothelial cells, to stabilize endothelial barriers, to reduce lethality caused by endotoxin in murine sepsis models, to prevent apoptosis of stressed endothelial cells, and to provide neuroprotection requires EPCR and PAR-1, strongly supporting the EPCR–PAR-1 cell-signaling pathway as key for APC's pharmacologic benefits (see Fig. 4–4).[7,8,40–43,221,225,229,233,234,236,237,244,248–251]

Although few details are known about intracellular mechanisms for APC's multiple cytoprotective actions, some mechanistic details for APC's cell signaling have become clear, as depicted in Fig. 4–6.[8] Multiple considerations help explain how PAR-1 can mediate thrombin's disruption of endothelial barrier leading to vascular leakage while, paradoxically, the same receptor mediates APC's endothelial barrier protection, preventing vascular leakage.[249,250] First, PAR-1–mediated APC signaling occurs in caveolae microdomains that contain EPCR, whereas PAR-1–mediated thrombin signaling is not limited to caveolae (Fig. 4–6).[252,253] Second, different cleavages in the extracellular N-terminus of PAR-1, either at the canonical Arg41 thrombin-cleavage site (i.e., widely recognized as the essential thrombin cleavage site) or at the novel Arg46 APC-cleavage site, result in very different signaling initiated by different tethered N-terminal peptide sequences that begin at either residue 42 or residue 47.[124,254,255] Third, following thrombin cleavage at Arg41, PAR-1 initiates signaling involving G proteins, extracellular signal-regulated kinase (ERK)1/2, and RhoA, whereas, following APC cleavage at Arg46, PAR-1 initiates signaling involving β-arrestin-2, phosphatidylinositide 3′-kinase (PI3K)/Akt, and Rac1.[256] Fourth, peptides mimicking the N-terminus of cleaved PAR-1 are peptide agonists with pharmacologic effects resembling those of the respective proteases that cleave PAR-1 differentially. For example, "thrombin receptor activating peptides (TRAPs)" that begin with Ser 42 promote G-protein–mediated signaling similar to thrombin. In contrast, peptides that begins with Asn 47 (TR47) promote APC-like signaling.[254] TRAP but not TR47 promotes ERK1/2 phosphorylation on endothelial cells, whereas TR47 but not TRAP promotes Akt phosphorylation.[254] The different and opposite

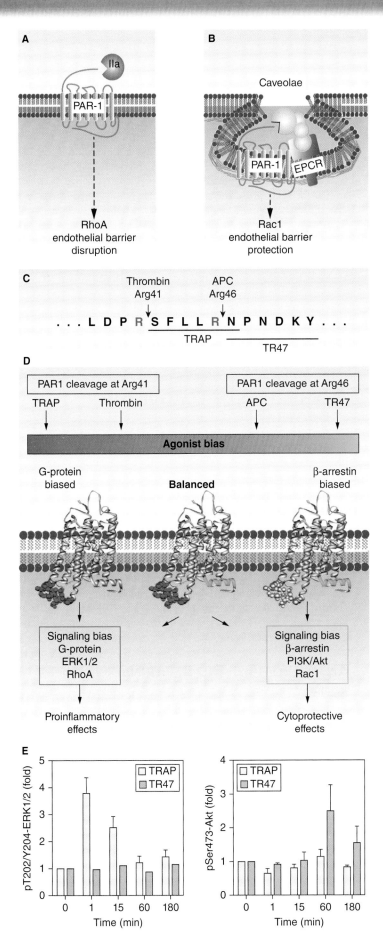

**Figure 4–6.** Biased protease-activated receptor (PAR)-1 signaling dependent on activation by thrombin or activated protein C (APC). Activation of PAR-1 by thrombin results in endothelial barrier-disruptive signaling (**A**) but activation of PAR-1 by APC in caveolae that also contain endothelial cell protein C receptor (EPCR) results in endothelial barrier-protective signaling (**B**).[252,253] The different PAR-1 signaling induced by thrombin and APC is caused by different proteolysis cleavage sites in PAR-1 for thrombin and APC.[254] Thrombin activates PAR-1 by cleavage at Arg41 (**C**). Synthetic agonist peptides with the N-terminal tethered-ligand sequence beginning with residue 42 are known as TRAPs (thrombin receptor-activating peptides) and cause thrombin-like effects on cells. APC activates PAR-1 by cleavage at Arg46 (**C**). A synthetic agonist peptide with the N-terminal tethered-ligand sequence beginning with residue 47 (TR47) causes APC-like effects on cells. Activation of PAR-1 by thrombin or TRAP induces PAR-1 conformations such that the intracellular loops of PAR-1 preferentially interact with G-proteins (termed "G-protein biased") resulting in G-protein–dependent signaling, whereas activation of PAR-1 by APC or TR47 induces PAR-1 conformations that preferentially interact with β-arrestin-2 (termed "β-arrestin biased"), resulting in β-arrestin-2–dependent signaling (**D**).[254,256] The implications of biased PAR-1 signaling are evident by the differences in phosphorylation of extracellular signal-regulated kinase (ERK)1/2 compared to Akt because TRAP, but not TR47, induces phosphorylation of ERK1/2, whereas TR47 but not TRAP induces phosphorylation of Akt (**E**).[254] *(Reproduced with permission of Griffin JH, Zlokovic BV, Mosnier LO: Activated protein C: Biased for translation, Blood 2015 May 7; 125(19):2898–2907.)*

induction of signaling pathways is also mirrored in different and opposite functional effects, as thrombin peptide and TRAP cause endothelial barrier disruption and proinflammatory effects, whereas APC and the TR47 peptide cause barrier-protective and antiinflammatory effects. Thus, PAR-1 displays biased signaling depending on the activation cleavage sites and the generated tethered ligand with absolutely opposing outcomes for the cell, the tissue, and the host depending on which coagulation system protease, thrombin or APC, is cleaving PAR-1.

Other receptors are recognized that may also play key roles for APC's beneficial signaling effects, including PAR-3 and sphingosine-1-phosphate receptor-1.[249,250,257,258] ApoER2 can initiate disabled-1-dependent pathway activation of the PI3K-Akt cell-survival pathway, which may ultimately help explain additional aspects of APC's cytoprotection.[259]

Although most studies demonstrating the cell-signaling activities of APC have focused on pharmacologic levels of APC, several reports of murine injury models demonstrate the physiologic importance of cell signaling by endogenous APC,[260-262] implying that defects in APC's endogenous cytoprotective actions might have pathophysiologic relevance. Future investigations on APC cellular receptors and on intracellular mechanisms involved in the protein C cellular pathway will likely provide novel clinical insights with diagnostic and therapeutic potential.

## INHIBITION OF ACTIVATED PROTEIN C

Blood contains circulating APC in a well-defined normal concentration range that contributes to antithrombotic surveillance mechanisms and possibly to homeostatic cell signaling.[15,142,144] Circulating APC levels are determined by the balance between countervailing mechanisms for APC generation and for APC inhibition and clearance. APC generation is influenced by protein C zymogen levels, endogenous thrombin generation, and the availability of thrombomodulin and EPCR. Clearance of circulating APC is based on inhibition of APC by protease inhibitors and clearance of APC:inhibitor complexes.[263-269] The major plasma inhibitors of APC include $\alpha_1$-antitrypsin, protein C inhibitor, and $\alpha_2$-macroglobulin.

## ACTIVATED PROTEIN C–INDEPENDENT ANTICOAGULANT ACTIVITY OF PROTEIN S

Because hereditary protein S deficiency[270,271] is strongly linked to increased venous thrombosis risk (Chap. 20), protein S is a significant physiologic anticoagulant factor.[71,198] In addition to its anticoagulant cofactor activity for APC, protein S can also inhibit coagulation reactions independently of APC. Several plausible mechanisms have been described for protein S's anticoagulant activity independent of APC. First, protein S can bind directly to procoagulant factors Xa and Va and thereby inhibit directly the activity of the prothrombinase complex.[11-13] The thrombin-sensitive region and the EGF3 domains of protein S (see Fig. 4–5) likely bind factor Xa, contributing to APC-independent anticoagulant activity.[206,272,273] Second, protein S can also bind factor VIIIa and inhibit activation of factor X by factor IXa–factor VIIIa complexes.[274-276] Third, protein S binds tissue factor pathway inhibitor (TFPI) and enhances its ability to inhibit factor Xa.[277-279] Zn$^{2+}$ ions might play a key role for APC-independent protein S activity.[280] It is not easy to decipher the relative importance of each of these or other mechanisms for APC-independent anticoagulant activities of protein S or to establish their physiologic relevance, but infusions of protein S without APC are antithrombotic in baboon thrombosis models.[281]

The activities of protein S can be strongly influenced by C4b-binding protein, a plasma protein that enhances inactivation of the complement cascade by binding to C4b and promoting its proteolytic inactivation by the protease factor I. C4b-binding protein reversibly binds protein S with high affinity,[282-284] and formation of this complex affects some but not all of the anticoagulant activities of protein S.[71,198,271,285] Because of the influence of C4b-binding protein on protein S activities and plasma levels, interpretation of clinical assays for protein S requires evaluation of free and bound protein S as plasma contains approximately 240 nM protein S–C4b-binding protein complexes and 120-nM free protein S.[283] C4b-binding protein is a heteropolymer containing six or seven $\alpha$ chains that are disulfide-linked to a single $\beta$ chain that binds protein S.[286,287] Residues 30 to 45 of the $\beta$ chain bind with high affinity to the C-terminal SHBG domain of protein S.[65,288,289] During an acute-phase reaction, the level of the C4b-binding protein $\alpha$ chain, but not the $\beta$ chain, is increased, so that the acute-phase change in total C4b-binding protein does not alter the level of free and bound protein S.[290]

Another potential mechanism for the antithrombotic actions of protein S is based on its APC-independent direct interactions with cells that might contribute to its antithrombotic actions. Protein S promotes clearance of apoptotic cells,[68,71,198,291-294] and this antiapoptotic activity of protein S might contribute to its antithrombotic activity. Protein S has direct effects on cells by activating one or more transmembrane receptor tyrosine kinases.[68,198,292] Protein S is a potent neuroprotectant as it can protect brain endothelium against ischemic injury in murine stroke models and can protect neurons against NMDA-induced excitotoxic injury, presumably acting via transmembrane receptor tyrosine kinases.[295-299]

## INHIBITION OF COAGULATION PROTEASES BY PROTEASE INHIBITORS

Antithrombin, initially designated *antithrombin III*, is clinically the best known inhibitor of clotting factor proteases. Antithrombin can neutralize all coagulation proteases in reactions that are enhanced by heparin and related glycosaminoglycans (see Chap. 3 and Fig. 3–28).[300] However, antithrombin does not inhibit the anticoagulant protease APC. TFPI can neutralize factors VIIa and Xa, proteases of the extrinsic coagulation pathway.[277,278,301-303] In addition, other plasma protease inhibitors, such as $\alpha_1$-antitrypsin, heparin cofactor II, protein C inhibitor, $\alpha_2$-macroglobulin, or protein Z–dependent protease inhibitor, can neutralize various coagulation proteases, although the ultimate clinical significance of these reactions is less well defined than the clinical relevance of antithrombin for thrombophilia (Chap. 20). Antithrombin is key for anticoagulant therapy based on the heparin-stimulated inhibition of thrombin and factor Xa.

### ANTITHROMBIN AND HEPARINS

Antithrombin is synthesized in the liver and is present in plasma at 150 mcg/mL, and it is a typical member of the serine protease inhibitor (SERPIN) superfamily and is denoted as SERPINC1.[300,304-306] Based on X-ray crystallographic studies,[307-311] models of serpin–protease complexes in various reaction states have emerged, and the mechanism for the effects of heparin on the reaction of thrombin with antithrombin is reasonably clear.

The neutralization of proteases by antithrombin is a result of a stable enzyme–antithrombin complex that is formed by a molecular mechanism characteristic of inhibitory serpins.[304-307,309-312] Following binding of a protease to a "reactive site" loop in a serpin, a single peptide bond in the serpin is cleaved with formation of an acyl-enzyme intermediate via the active site Ser residue. This metastable enzyme–serpin complex can either break apart because of deacylation or form a more stable covalent enzyme–serpin complex. To break apart the enzyme–serpin covalent complex, deacylation liberates the cleaved product and regenerates the active site Ser residue of the protease. However, serpins have an ability to undergo major conformational changes following cleavage at the reactive site residue that can distort that protease's active site region and lock the enzyme into the protease–serpin complex in which both the serpin and the protease are essentially deformed.[304-307,309-312] The dominant structural feature of native serpins is a large five-stranded β-sheet that defines the structure of an ellipsoidal protein. Following cleavage at the reactive residue in the reactive center loop by a protease, this extended loop is able to partially or completely insert itself into the five-stranded β-sheet, forming a very stable six-stranded β-sheet. If this insertion reaction proceeds before deacylation occurs, then the protease remains covalently attached to the reactive center P1 residue through the protease's active site Ser residue, and a stable covalent protease–inhibitor complex with each protein in an altered conformation is formed.[307,308]

Heparin enhancement of the rate of reaction between antithrombin and thrombin or other clotting factors is caused by two distinct effects of heparin, one involving conformational effects on antithrombin and the other involving "approximation" effects on both antithrombin and thrombin.[300,307,308,311-315] For the first effect, a particular pentasaccharide sequence within heparin binds antithrombin and potently causes a conformational change that converts antithrombin from its native state of moderate reactivity to a conformation with relatively high reactivity. This pentasaccharide contains a specific sulfated sequence of glucosamine and iduronic acid residues,[300,307,308,311-315] and when it is present in a large heparin molecule, in low-molecular-weight heparin, or in a synthetic pentasaccharide, it alters antithrombin conformation and greatly accelerates the reaction of antithrombin, especially with factor Xa. Synthetic pentasaccharides, such as fondaparinux, which are analogues of the naturally occurring sequence, are often termed to be indirect factor Xa inhibitors and have significant clinical utility. For the second mechanistic effect, namely the approximation effect, unfractionated heparin or low-molecular-weight heparins simultaneously bind to antithrombin and the target protease to promote frequent and geometrically productive encounters between protease and inhibitor, thus increasing the reaction rate. Heparan sulfates to some extent can also act in this manner.

The mature antithrombin polypeptide chain contains 432-amino-acid residues after cleavage of a propeptide from a 464-amino-acid-residue precursor.[316] It has four sites for N-linked carbohydrate attachment, one of which (Asn135) is variably glycosylated, giving rise to a β-isoform that has higher affinity for heparin.[317,318] Heparin binding to antithrombin is mediated by a number of positively charged Arg and Lys residues in the N-terminal region of the molecule, including Lys11, Arg13, Arg47, Lys114, Lys125, and Arg129, whereas the reactive center loop containing the scissile peptide bond at Arg393-Ser394 is near the C-terminus.[311]

## ANTITHROMBIN GENE

The antithrombin gene comprising seven exons and six introns spans 13.4 kb and is located on chromosome 1q23–25 (see Table 4–1).[319,320]

## ANTITHROMBIN MUTATIONS

Hereditary deficiencies of antithrombin are risk factors for venous thrombosis (Chap. 20). More than 100 different antithrombin mutations are associated with thrombosis. An extensive database of mutations is published[321] and is available at http://www1.imperial.ac.uk/departmentofmedicine/divisions/experimentalmedicine/haematology/coag/antithrombin/.

Mutations that cause antithrombin deficiency are scattered throughout the gene. Molecular defects can be classified as type I, characterized by parallel decreases in antigen and activity, or type II, characterized by circulating dysfunctional molecules such that plasma has decreased functional activity but normal or near-normal antigen levels. Type II defects are further classified based on whether the dysfunction involves only reactive center defects that can be tested in the absence of heparin, only heparin-binding defects that can be tested only in the presence of heparin, or both of these defects (pleiotropic effects). Reactive center defects carry the largest risk of thrombosis, whereas heparin-binding defects are associated with less risk of venous thrombosis (Chap. 20).

## ●TISSUE FACTOR PATHWAY INHIBITOR

TFPI, also known as *lipoprotein-associated coagulation inhibitor* or *extrinsic pathway inhibitor*, has a predicted mature protein sequence of 276 residues and an Mr of 34,000. However, TFPI is a complex protein and has at least three isoforms in blood vessels.[277,301-303,322-327] There are two alternatively spliced forms of TFPI designated TFPIα and TFPIβ (Fig. 4–7).[323,324] TFPIα is the full-length mature protein that contains an acidic N-terminal sequence, three homologous but distinct Kunitz-type

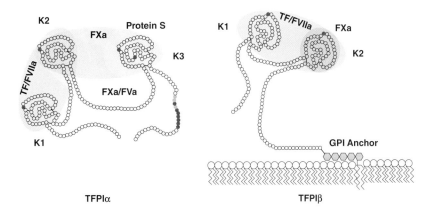

**Figure 4–7.** Tissue factor pathway inhibitor (TFPI) exists in multiple forms, TFPIα and TFPIβ, because of alternative splicing. Mature, full-length TFPIα is a multivalent protease inhibitor containing three Kunitz-type protease inhibitor domains (K1, K2, and K3) and a highly positively charged basic amino acid cluster near the C-terminus *(blue circles)*. TFPIβ contains K1 and K2 but lacks K3 and the basic amino acid cluster, but it can acquire a glycosylphosphatidylinositol (GPI) moiety that anchors it to cell membranes. As indicated by color overlays, K1 and K2 inhibit factor (F) VIIa and FXa, respectively. Both TFPIα and TFPIβ can form a quaternary complex with tissue factor (TF), FVIIa and FXa. However, TFPIα, but not TFPIβ, can interact with protein S or certain forms of FVa/FV via K3 or the positive amino acid cluster, respectively. Via such interactions, protein S or FVa/FV can promote inhibition of FXa with no involvement of FVIIa or tissue factor. TFPIα is the predominant form in plasma, whereas TFPIβ is the predominant form on the endothelium. *(Reproduced with permission from Wood JP, Ellery PE, Maroney SA, Mast AE: Biology of tissue factor pathway inhibitor, Blood 2014 May 8;123(19):2934–2943.)*

protease inhibitor domains (K1, K2, K3), and a C-terminal positively charged basic amino acid sequence (Fig. 4–7). TFPIβ contains K1 and K2, but an unrelated sequence replaces the K3 domain and the C-terminus. TFPIβ can be covalently modified by addition of glycosylphosphatidylinositol (GPI) that localizes TFPIβ to cell membranes (Fig. 4–7). Some TFPI in plasma is present as a disulfide-linked heterodimer of TFPI–apolipoprotein A-II (ApoA-II),[327,328] but the functional significance of the apoA-II appendage is unknown. TFPI in its multiple forms is a significant inhibitor of the coagulation pathways that can function synergistically with the protein C pathway and antithrombin to suppress thrombin generation.

TFPI is synthesized by endothelial cells, megakaryocytes, and smooth muscle cells.[301–303] Free TFPI in plasma is TFPIα, but it is a minor fraction of the amount of TFPI in blood vessels. More than half of TFPIα in plasma is associated with lipoproteins, especially HDL and low-density lipoprotein. TFPIα is also the main form within platelets, and it is secreted by activated platelets. A substantial amount of TFPIα is released from the vessel wall when heparin is infused.[329] TFPIβ is membrane bound, especially to endothelium, because of its GPI anchor.

The interaction of TFPI with lipoproteins reduces its anticoagulant activity measured in vitro, although the physiologic significance of TFPI's binding to various lipoproteins remains uncertain. In addition to binding lipoproteins, TFPIα, but not TFPIβ, binds to protein S and to certain forms of factor Va/factor V.[277–279,330–333] Different regions of TFPIα, namely the K3 domain or the basic amino acid cluster, respectively, are responsible for binding protein S or factors Va/V (see Fig. 4–7). Inhibition of factor Xa by TFPIα is accelerated by protein S and by certain but not all forms of factor Va (see below).

TFPI neutralizes factors Xa and VIIa by multiple complicated mechanisms.[277,301–303] In each mechanism, the K1 domain binds and inhibits factor VIIa, whereas the K2 domain inhibits factor Xa (see Fig. 4–7). No protease has yet been identified as the target of the K3 protease inhibitor domain. In one mechanism, initially the K2 domain of TFPI reacts with and inhibits the enzyme activity of factor Xa. Subsequently, this binary complex reacts with factor VIIa in the tissue factor–factor VIIa complex to form a quaternary protein complex on a membrane with both proteases neutralized. In an alternative proposed scheme, TFPI first reacts with factor VIIa in a tissue factor–factor VIIa complex that has generated factor Xa, and thereafter it rapidly reacts with factor Xa before it can dissociate from the ternary tissue factor–factor VIIa–factor Xa complex. Possibly each proposal is valid. Some argue that because some kinetic studies showed that TFPI requires factor Xa for kinetically favorable reactions with factor VIIa, TFPI does not shut off the initiation of the extrinsic pathway by tissue factor until some significant though small amount of factor Xa is generated, in which case TFPI provides negative feedback inhibition of the generation of factor Xa by the factor VIIa–tissue factor complex. An additional property of TFPIα involves its inhibition of factor Xa in the absence of factor VIIa, and this reaction is accelerated by protein S and by certain forms of factor Va.[277–279,330–333] In contrast to the anticoagulant factors, antithrombin, protein C, and protein S, for which hereditary deficiencies are linked to significantly increased risk for venous thrombosis (Chap. 20), no clear pattern for increased risk of thrombosis has been definitively established for TFPI deficiency in humans. In mice, knockout of TFPI is embryonically lethal.[334] In a highly informative kindred that presented with a serious bleeding diathesis, highly elevated plasma TFPI levels were linked to increased bleeding risk, indicating that TFPI functions in man as a physiologically significant inhibitor of coagulation.[322,332] The genetic mutation causing elevated plasma TFPI levels was in the factor V gene, not the TFPI gene. The mutated factor V, named "factor V-short," has a higher affinity for TFPIα than wild-type factor V, thereby binding more TFPIα and prolonging its half-life. Factor V-short may also enhance

inhibition of factor Xa by TFPI with the effect of increasing bleeding risk. This genetic disorder, as well as previous studies showing that inhibition of TFPI reduced bleeding in preclinical hemophilia models, lends support for ongoing efforts to develop TFPI inhibitors for reducing bleeding in some hemophilia subjects, especially those with anti–factor VIII inhibitors.

### TFPI GENE

The sequence of TFPI was established from cloning of its complementary DNA. The gene contains nine exons, spans 85 kb, and is located on chromosome 2q31–32.1 (see Table 4–1).[335,336]

# ●THER PROTEASE INHIBITORS

## HEPARIN COFACTOR II

Heparin cofactor II, a serpin whose inhibitory activity is enhanced by dermatan sulfate, inhibits thrombin in vivo and in vitro by an approximation mechanism.[337–340] A few reports link heparin cofactor II deficiency to venous thrombosis, but no significant clinical relevance has been established.[341] Curiously, a severe heparin cofactor II deficiency was reported in an asymptomatic subject.[342] Some studies imply that heparin cofactor II may play significant roles in arterial vascular wall processes, but definitive mechanisms remain to be elucidated.

## PROTEIN Z–DEPENDENT PROTEASE INHIBITOR

Protein Z–dependent protease inhibitor (ZPI) is a plasma serpin that inhibits factors Xa, XIa, and IXa, but not factor XIIa or thrombin.[343–350] Protein Z, which is a vitamin K–dependent protein that contains a GLA domain, two EGF-like domains, and a protease-like domain,[351] stimulates factor Xa inhibition by ZPI. Curiously, the protease-like domain of protein Z lacks any protease activity because it has mutations at two of the three active site triad residues. The major hypothesis for stimulation of inhibition of factor Xa by protein Z is based on a structural model in which three proteins assemble on a phospholipid membrane via the two GLA domains (see Fig. 4–7).[351] In this putative ternary complex, the protease-like domain and the second EGF-like domain of protein Z bind ZPI in an alignment that facilitates reaction of factor Xa with the reactive center loop of ZPI.

In plasma, ZPI is in slight protein molar excess over protein Z with which it associates noncovalently, and it has been speculated, but not proven, that almost all plasma protein Z is associated with ZPI.[352–357] If the ZPI is a physiologic coagulation inhibitor, the deficiency of either protein Z or ZPI might be associated with thrombosis. Knocking out the protein Z gene in a mouse does not produce a remarkable phenotype unless protein Z deficiency coexists with factor V Leiden, in which case the mouse exhibits a hypercoagulable, prothrombotic state.[353] This murine observation is mirrored by one clinical report that subnormal levels of protein Z are associated with venous thrombosis in subjects who are heterozygous for factor V Leiden.[354] Some associations between venous thrombosis and defects in protein Z or ZPI have been reported but not uniformly confirmed.[352,354–357] An association with peripheral arterial disease was reported.[358] However, to date, no convincing pattern between thrombosis and defects in either protein Z or ZPI has been firmly established.

## OTHER MINOR PROTEASE INHIBITORS

Thrombin in plasma can be inhibited not only by antithrombin but also by $\alpha_2$-macroglobulin, an acute-phase reactant. No association between defects in bleeding or thrombosis has been confirmed for this inhibitor.

In purified reaction mixtures, protein C inhibitor also efficiently neutralizes thrombin in the presence of thrombomodulin,[359] although no studies show that this is a physiologic reaction or that it is associated with thrombosis.

# REFERENCES

1. MacFarlane RG: An enzyme cascade in the blood clotting mechanism and its function as a biochemical amplifier. *Nature* 202:498–499, 1964.
2. Davie EW, Ratnoff OD: Waterfall sequence for intrinsic blood clotting. *Science* 145(3638):1310–1312, 1964.
3. Furie B, Furie BC: Mechanisms of thrombus formation. *N Engl J Med* 359(9):938–949, 2008.
4. Lammle B, Griffin JH: Formation of the fibrin clot: The balance of procoagulant and inhibitory factors. *Clin Haematol* 14(2):281–342, 1985.
5. van de Wouwer M, Collen D, Conway EM: Thrombomodulin-protein C-EPCR system: Integrated to regulate coagulation and inflammation. *Arterioscler Thromb Vasc Biol* 24(8):1374–1383, 2004.
6. Griffin JH: The thrombin paradox. *Nature* 378(6555):337–338, 1995.
7. Mosnier LO, Zlokovic BV, Griffin JH: The cytoprotective protein C pathway. *Blood* 109(8):3161–3172, 2007.
8. Griffin JH, Zlokovic BV, Mosnier LO: Activated protein C: Biased for translation. *Blood* 125(19):2898–2907, 2015.
9. Fukudome K, Esmon CT: Identification, cloning, and regulation of a novel endothelial cell protein C/activated protein C receptor. *J Biol Chem* 269(42):26486–26491, 1994.
10. Rao LV, Esmon CT, Pendurthi UR: Endothelial cell protein C receptor: A multiliganded and multifunctional receptor. *Blood* 124(10):1553–1562, 2014.
11. Heeb MJ, Mesters RM, Tans G, et al: Binding of protein S to factor Va associated with inhibition of prothrombinase that is independent of activated protein C. *J Biol Chem* 268(4):2872–2877, 1993.
12. Heeb MJ, Rosing J, Bakker HM, et al: Protein S binds to and inhibits factor Xa. *Proc Natl Acad Sci U S A* 91(7):2728–2732, 1994.
13. Hackeng TM, van't Veer C, Meijers JC, Bouma BN: Human protein S inhibits prothrombinase complex activity on endothelial cells and platelets via direct interactions with factors V and Xa. *J Biol Chem* 269(33):21051–21058, 1994.
14. Morrissey JH, Macik BG, Neuenschwander PF, Comp PC: Quantitation of activated factor VII levels in plasma using a tissue factor mutant selectively deficient in promoting factor VII activation. *Blood* 81(3):734–744, 1993.
15. Gruber A, Griffin JH: Direct detection of activated protein C in blood from human subjects. *Blood* 79(9):2340–2348, 1992.
16. Nossel HL, Yudelman I, Canfield RE, et al: Measurement of fibrinopeptide A in human blood. *J Clin Invest* 54(1):43–53, 1974.
17. Nossel HL: Radioimmunoassay of fibrinopeptides in relation to intravascular coagulation and thrombosis. *N Engl J Med* 295(8):428–432, 1976.
18. Bauer KA, Rosenberg RD: The pathophysiology of the prethrombotic state in humans: Insight gained from studies using markers of hemostatic system activation. *Blood* 70(2):343–350, 1987.
19. Bauer KA, Kass BL, ten Cate H, et al: Detection of factor X activation in humans. *Blood* 74(6):2007–2015, 1989.
20. Bauer KA, Kass BL, ten Cate H, et al: Factor IX is activated *in vivo* by the tissue factor mechanism. *Blood* 76(4):731–736, 1990.
21. Jesty J, Beltrami E, Willems G: Mathematical analysis of a proteolytic positive-feedback loop: Dependence of lag time and enzyme yields on the initial conditions and kinetic parameters. *Biochemistry* 32(24):6266–6274, 1993.
22. Beltrami E, Jesty J: Mathematical analysis of activation thresholds in enzyme-catalyzed positive feedbacks: Application to the feedbacks of blood coagulation. *Proc Natl Acad Sci U S A* 92(19):8744–8748, 1995.
23. Nicolaes GAF, Dahlbäck B: Factor V and thrombotic disease: Description of a Janus-faced protein. *Arterioscler Thromb Vasc Biol* 22(4):530–538, 2002.
24. Stenflo J: A new vitamin K-dependent protein. Purification from bovine plasma and preliminary characterization. *J Biol Chem* 251(2):355–363, 1976.
25. Seegers WH, Novoa E, Henry RL, Hassouna HI: Relationship of "new" vitamin K-dependent protein C and "old" autoprothrombin II-a. *Thromb Res* 8(5):543–552, 1976.
26. Kisiel W: Human plasma protein C: Isolation, characterization, and mechanism of activation by alpha-thrombin. *J Clin Invest* 64(3):761–769, 1979.
27. Foster DC, Davie EW: Characterization of a cDNA coding for human protein C. *Proc Natl Acad Sci U S A* 81(15):4766–4770, 1984.
28. Beckmann RJ, Schmidt RJ, Santerre RF, et al: The structure and evolution of a 461 amino acid human protein C precursor and its messenger RNA, based upon the DNA sequence of cloned human liver cDNAs. *Nucleic Acids Res* 13(14):5233–5247, 1985.
29. Griffin JH, Evatt B, Zimmerman TS, et al: Deficiency of protein C in congenital thrombotic disease. *J Clin Invest* 68(5):1370–1373, 1981.
30. Mather T, Oganessyan V, Hof P, et al: The 2.8 Å crystal structure of Gla-domainless activated protein C. *EMBO J* 15(24):6822–6831, 1996.
31. Kurosawa S, Galvin JB, Esmon NL, Esmon CT: Proteolytic formation and properties of functional domains of thrombomodulin. *J Biol Chem* 262(5):2206–2212, 1987.
32. Jhingan A, Zhang L, Christiansen WT, Castellino FJ: The activities of recombinant gamma-carboxyglutamic-acid-deficient mutants of activated human protein C toward human coagulation factor Va and factor VIII in purified systems and in plasma. *Biochemistry* 33(7):1869–1875, 1994.
33. Regan LM, Mollica JS, Rezaie AR, Esmon CT: The interaction between the endothelial cell protein C receptor and protein C is dictated by the gamma-carboxyglutamic acid domain of protein C. *J Biol Chem* 272(42):26279–26284, 1997.
34. Greengard JS, Fisher CL, Villoutreix B, Griffin JH: Structural basis for type I and type II deficiencies of antithrombotic plasma protein C: Patterns revealed by three-dimensional molecular modelling of mutations of the protease domain. *Proteins* 18(4):367–380, 1994.
35. Gale AJ, Heeb MJ, Griffin JH: The autolysis loop of activated protein C interacts with factor Va and differentiates between the Arg506 and Arg306 cleavage sites. *Blood* 96(2):585–593, 2000.
36. Friedrich U, Nicolaes GAF, Villoutreix BO, Dahlbäck B: Secondary substrate-binding exosite in the serine protease domain of activated protein C important for cleavage at Arg-506 but not at Arg-306 in factor Va. *J Biol Chem* 276(25):23105–23108, 2001.
37. Rezaie AR: Exosite-dependent regulation of the protein C anticoagulant pathway. *Trends Cardiovasc Med* 13(1):8–15, 2003.
38. Gale AJ, Griffin JH: Characterization of a thrombomodulin binding site on protein C and its comparison to an activated protein C binding site for factor Va. *Proteins* 54(3):433–441, 2004.
39. Gale AJ, Tsavaler A, Griffin JH: Molecular characterization of an extended binding site for coagulation factor Va in the positive exosite of activated protein C. *J Biol Chem* 277(32):28836–28840, 2002.
40. Mosnier LO, Gale AJ, Yegneswaran S, Griffin JH: Activated protein C variants with normal cytoprotective but reduced anticoagulant activity. *Blood* 104(6):1740–1745, 2004.
41. Mosnier LO, Yang XV, Griffin JH: Activated protein C mutant with minimal anticoagulant activity, normal cytoprotective activity, and preservation of thrombin activable fibrinolysis inhibitor-dependent cytoprotective functions. *J Biol Chem* 282(45):33022–33033, 2007.
42. Mosnier LO, Zampolli A, Kerschen EJ, et al: Hyper-antithrombotic, non-cytoprotective Glu149Ala-activated protein C mutant. *Blood* 113(23):5970–5978, 2009.
43. Bae JS, Yang L, Manithody C, Rezaie AR: Engineering a disulfide bond to stabilize the calcium-binding loop of activated protein C eliminates its anticoagulant but not its protective signaling properties. *J Biol Chem* 282(12):9251–9259, 2007.
44. Yang L, Bae JS, Manithody C, Rezaie AR: Identification of a specific exosite on activated protein C for interaction with protease activated receptor 1. *J Biol Chem* 282(35):25493–25500, 2007.
45. Dreyfus M, Magny JF, Bridey F, et al: Treatment of homozygous protein C deficiency and neonatal purpura fulminans with a purified protein C concentrate. *N Engl J Med* 325(22):1565–1568, 1991.
46. Bernard GR, Vincent JL, Laterre PF, et al: Efficacy and safety of recombinant human activated protein C for severe sepsis. *N Engl J Med* 344(10):699–709, 2001.
47. Gruber A, Griffin JH, Harker LA, Hanson SR: Inhibition of platelet-dependent thrombus formation by human activated protein C in a primate model. *Blood* 73(3):639–642, 1989.
48. Taylor FB Jr, Chang AC, Esmon CT, et al: Protein C prevents the coagulopathic and lethal effects of *Escherichia coli* infusion in the baboon. *J Clin Invest* 79(3):918–925, 1987.
49. Ranieri VM, Thompson BT, Barie PS, et al: Drotrecogin alfa (Activated) in adults with septic shock. *N Engl J Med* 366(22):2055–2064, 2012.
50. Kalil AC, LaRosa SP: Effectiveness and safety of drotrecogin alfa (activated) for severe sepsis: A meta-analysis and metaregression. *Lancet Infect Dis* 12(9):678–686, 2012.
51. Christiaans SC, Wagener BM, Esmon CT, Pittet JF: Protein C and acute inflammation: A clinical and biologic perspective. *Am J Physiol Lung Cell Mol Physiol* 305(7):L455–L466, 2013.
52. Foster DC, Yoshitake S, Davie EW: The nucleotide sequence of the gene for human protein C. *Proc Natl Acad Sci U S A* 82(14):4673–4677, 2013.
53. D'Ursi P, Marino F, Caprera A, et al: ProCMD: A database and 3D web resource for protein C mutants. *BMC Bioinformatics* 8(Suppl 1):S11, 2007.
54. Saunders RE, Perkins SJ: CoagMDB: A database analysis of missense mutations within four conserved domains in five vitamin K-dependent coagulation serine proteases using a text-mining tool. *Hum Mutat* 29(3):333–344, 2008.
55. Greengard JS, Griffin JH, Fisher CL: Possible structural implications of 20 mutations in the protein C protease domain. *Thromb Haemost* 72(6):869–873, 1994.
56. Rovida E, Merati G, D'Ursi P, et al: Identification and computationally-based structural interpretation of naturally occurring variants of human protein C. *Hum Mutat* 28(4):345–355, 2007.
57. Yin T, Miyata T: Dysfunction of protein C anticoagulant system, main genetic risk factor for venous thromboembolism in northeast Asians. *J Thromb Thrombolysis* 37(1):56–65, 2014.
58. Tang L, Lu X, Yu JM, et al: PROC c.574_576del polymorphism: A common genetic risk factor for venous thrombosis in the Chinese population. *J Thromb Haemost* 10(10):2019–2026, 2012.
59. Ding Q, Yang L, Hassanian SM, Rezaie AR: Expression and functional characterisation of natural R147W and K150del variants of protein C in the Chinese population. *Thromb Haemost* 109(4):614–624, 2013.
60. Jalbert LR, Rosen ED, Moons L, et al: Inactivation of the gene for anticoagulant protein C causes lethal perinatal consumptive coagulopathy in mice. *J Clin Invest* 102(8):1481–1488, 1998.
61. DiScipio RG, Davie EW: Characterization of protein S, a gamma-carboxyglutamic acid containing protein from bovine and human plasma. *Biochemistry* 18(5):899–904, 1979.

62. Schwarz HP, Heeb MJ, Wencel-Drake JD, Griffin JH: Identification and quantitation of protein S in human platelets. *Blood* 66(6):1452–1455, 1985.

63. Lundwall A, Dackowski W, Cohen E, et al: Isolation and sequence of the cDNA for human protein S, a regulator of blood coagulation. *Proc Natl Acad Sci U S A* 83(18):6716–6720, 1986.

64. Hoskins J, Norman DK, Beckmann RJ, Long GL: Cloning and characterization of human liver cDNA encoding a protein S precursor. *Proc Natl Acad Sci U S A* 84(2):349–353, 1987.

65. Fernández JA, Heeb MJ, Griffin JH: Identification of residues 413–433 of plasma protein S as essential for binding to C4b-binding protein. *J Biol Chem* 268(22):16788–16794, 1993.

66. Heeb MJ, Kojima Y, Rosing J, et al: C-terminal residues 621–635 of protein S are essential for binding to factor Va. *J Biol Chem* 274(51):36187–36192, 1999.

67. Nyberg P, Dahlback B, Garcia de FP: The SHBG-like region of protein S is crucial for factor V-dependent APC-cofactor function. *FEBS Lett* 433(1–2):28–32, 1998.

68. van der Meer JH, van der Poll T, van't Veer C: TAM receptors, Gas6 and protein S: Roles in inflammation and hemostasis. *Blood* 123(16):2460–2469, 2014.

69. Ploos van Amstel JK, van der Zanden AL, Bakker E, et al: Two genes homologous with human protein S cDNA are located on chromosome 3. *Thromb Haemost* 58(4):982–987, 1987.

70. Schmidel DK, Tatro AV, Phelps LG, et al: Organization of the human protein S genes. *Biochemistry* 29(34):7845–7852, 1990.

71. Garcia de Frutos P, Fuentes-Prior P, Hurtado B, Sala N: Molecular basis of protein S deficiency. *Thromb Haemost* 98(3):543–556, 2007.

72. Kimura R, Honda S, Kawasaki T, et al: Protein S-K196E mutation as a genetic risk factor for deep vein thrombosis in Japanese patients. *Blood* 107(4):1737–1738, 2006.

73. Pecheniuk NM, Elias DJ, Xu X, Griffin JH: Failure to validate association of gene polymorphisms in EPCR, PAR-1, FSAP and protein S Tokushima with venous thromboembolism among Californians of European ancestry. *Thromb Haemost* 99(2):453–455, 2008.

74. Bertina RM, Ploos van Amstel HK, van Wijngaarden A, et al: Heerlen polymorphism of protein S, an immunologic polymorphism due to dimorphism of residue 460. *Blood* 76(3):538–548, 1990.

75. Esmon CT, Owen WG: Identification of an endothelial cell cofactor for thrombin catalyzed activation of protein C. *Proc Natl Acad Sci U S A* 78(4):2249–2252, 1981.

76. Esmon CT, Owen WG: The discovery of thrombomodulin. *J Thromb Haemost* 2(2):209–213, 2004.

77. Morser J: Thrombomodulin links coagulation to inflammation and immunity. *Curr Drug Targets* 13(3):421–431, 2012.

78. Conway EM: Thrombomodulin and its role in inflammation. *Semin Immunopathol* 34(1):107–125, 2012.

79. Esmon CT, Esmon NL, Harris KW: Complex formation between thrombin and thrombomodulin inhibits both thrombin-catalyzed fibrin formation and factor V activation. *J Biol Chem* 257(14):7944–7947, 1982.

80. Esmon NL, Carroll RC, Esmon CT: Thrombomodulin blocks the ability of thrombin to activate platelets. *J Biol Chem* 258(20):12238–12242, 1983.

81. Esmon CT: The roles of protein C and thrombomodulin in the regulation of blood coagulation. *J Biol Chem* 264(9):4743–4746, 1989.

82. Jackman RW, Beeler DL, Fritze L, et al: Human thrombomodulin gene is intron depleted: Nucleic acid sequences of the cDNA and gene predict protein structure and suggest sites of regulatory control. *Proc Natl Acad Sci U S A* 84(18):6425–6429, 1987.

83. Sadler JE, Lentz SR, Sheehan JP, et al: Structure-function relationships of the thrombin-thrombomodulin interaction. *Haemostasis* 23(Suppl 1):183–193, 1993.

84. Saito H, Maruyama I, Shimazaki S, et al: Efficacy and safety of recombinant human soluble thrombomodulin (ART-123) in disseminated intravascular coagulation: Results of a phase III, randomized, double-blind clinical trial. *J Thromb Haemost* 5(1):31–41, 2007.

85. Healy AM, Rayburn HB, Rosenberg RD, Weiler H: Absence of the blood-clotting regulator thrombomodulin causes embryonic lethality in mice before development of a functional cardiovascular system. *Proc Natl Acad Sci U S A* 92(3):850–854, 1995.

86. Esmon CT: Inflammation and the activated protein C anticoagulant pathway. *Semin Thromb Hemost* 32(Suppl 1):49–60, 2006.

87. Schouten M, Wiersinga WJ, Levi M, van der Poll T: Inflammation, endothelium, and coagulation in sepsis. *J Leukoc Biol* 83(3):536–545, 2008.

88. Delvaeye M, Noris M, de Vriese A, et al: Thrombomodulin mutations in atypical hemolytic-uremic syndrome. *N Engl J Med* 361(4):345–357, 2009.

89. Norlund L, Holm J, Zoller B, Ohlin AK: A common thrombomodulin amino acid dimorphism is associated with myocardial infarction. *Thromb Haemost* 77(2):248–251, 1997.

90. Ireland H, Kunz G, Kyriakoulis K, et al: Thrombomodulin gene mutations associated with myocardial infarction. *Circulation* 96(1):15–18, 1997.

91. Doggen CJ, Kunz G, Rosendaal FR, et al: A mutation in the thrombomodulin gene, 127G to A coding for Ala25Thr, and the risk of myocardial infarction in men. *Thromb Haemost* 80(5):743–748, 1998.

92. Wu KK: Soluble thrombomodulin and coronary heart disease. *Curr Opin Lipidol* 14(4):373–375, 2003.

93. van de Wouwer M, Plaisance S, de Vriese A, et al: The lectin-like domain of thrombomodulin interferes with complement activation and protects against arthritis. *J Thromb Haemost* 4(8):1813–1824, 2006.

94. Mosnier LO, Bouma BN: Regulation of fibrinolysis by thrombin activatable fibrinolysis inhibitor, an unstable carboxypeptidase B that unites the pathways of coagulation and fibrinolysis. *Arterioscler Thromb Vasc Biol* 26(11):2445–2453, 2006.

95. Foley JH, Kim PY, Mutch NJ, Gils A: Insights into thrombin activatable fibrinolysis inhibitor function and regulation. *J Thromb Haemost* 11(Suppl 1):306–315, 2013.

96. Myles T, Nishimura T, Yun TH, et al: Thrombin activatable fibrinolysis inhibitor, a potential regulator of vascular inflammation. *J Biol Chem* 278(51):51059–51067, 2003.

97. Bouwens EA, Stavenuiter F, Mosnier LO: Mechanisms of anticoagulant and cytoprotective actions of the protein C pathway. *J Thromb Haemost* 11(Suppl 1):242–253, 2013.

98. Fukudome K, Esmon CT: Molecular cloning and expression of murine and bovine endothelial cell protein C/activated protein C receptor (EPCR). The structural and functional conservation in human, bovine, and murine EPCR. *J Biol Chem* 270(10):5571–5577, 1995.

99. Regan LM, Stearns-Kurosawa DJ, Kurosawa S, et al: The endothelial cell protein C receptor. Inhibition of activated protein C anticoagulant function without modulation of reaction with proteinase inhibitors. *J Biol Chem* 271(29):17499–17503, 1996.

100. Fukudome K, Kurosawa S, Stearns-Kurosawa DJ, et al: The endothelial cell protein C receptor. Cell surface expression and direct ligand binding by the soluble receptor. *J Biol Chem* 271(29):17491–17498, 1996.

101. Stearns-Kurosawa DJ, Kurosawa S, Mollica JS, et al: The endothelial cell protein C receptor augments protein C activation by the thrombin-thrombomodulin complex. *Proc Natl Acad Sci U S A* 93(19):10212–10216, 1996.

102. Xu J, Esmon NL, Esmon CT: Reconstitution of the human endothelial cell protein C receptor with thrombomodulin in phosphatidylcholine vesicles enhances protein C activation. *J Biol Chem* 274(10):6704–6710, 1999.

103. Fukudome K, Ye X, Tsuneyoshi N, et al: Activation mechanism of anticoagulant protein C in large blood vessels involving the endothelial cell protein C receptor. *J Exp Med* 187(7):1029–1035, 1998.

104. Liang Z, Rosen ED, Castellino FJ: Nucleotide structure and characterization of the murine gene encoding the endothelial cell protein C receptor. *Thromb Haemost* 81(4):585–588, 1999.

105. Ye X, Fukudome K, Tsuneyoshi N, et al: The endothelial cell protein C receptor (EPCR) functions as a primary receptor for protein C activation on endothelial cells in arteries, veins, and capillaries. *Biochem Biophys Res Commun* 259(3):671–677, 1999.

106. Simmonds RE, Lane DA: Structural and functional implications of the intron/exon organization of the human endothelial cell protein C/activated protein C receptor (EPCR) gene: Comparison with the structure of CD1/major histocompatibility complex alpha1 and alpha2 domains. *Blood* 94(2):632–641, 1999.

107. Oganesyan V, Oganesyan N, Terzyan S, et al: The crystal structure of the endothelial protein C receptor and a bound phospholipid. *J Biol Chem* 277(28):24851–24854, 2002.

108. Villoutreix BO, Blom AM, Dahlbäck B: Structural prediction and analysis of endothelial cell protein C/activated protein C receptor. *Protein Eng* 12(10):833–840, 1999.

109. Rezaie AR: Protease-activated receptor signalling by coagulation proteases in endothelial cells. *Thromb Haemost* 112(5):876–882, 2014.

110. McKelvey K, Jackson CJ, Xue M: Activated protein C: A regulator of human skin epidermal keratinocyte function. *World J Biol Chem* 5(2):169–179, 2014.

111. Danese S, Vetrano S, Zhang L, et al: The protein C pathway in tissue inflammation and injury: Pathogenic role and therapeutic implications. *Blood* 115(6):1121–1130, 2010.

112. Qu D, Wang Y, Esmon NL, Esmon CT: Regulated endothelial protein C receptor shedding is mediated by tumor necrosis factor-alpha converting enzyme/ADAM17. *J Thromb Haemost* 5(2):395–402, 2007.

113. Qu D, Wang Y, Song Y, et al: The Ser219—>Gly dimorphism of the endothelial protein C receptor contributes to the higher soluble protein levels observed in individuals with the A3 haplotype. *J Thromb Haemost* 4(1):229–235, 2006.

114. Kurosawa S, Stearns-Kurosawa DJ, Carson CW, et al: Plasma levels of endothelial cell protein C receptor are elevated in patients with sepsis and systemic lupus erythematosus: Lack of correlation with thrombomodulin suggests involvement of different pathological processes. *Blood* 91(2):725–727, 1998.

115. Kurosawa S, Stearns-Kurosawa DJ, Hidari N, Esmon CT: Identification of functional endothelial protein C receptor in human plasma. *J Clin Invest* 100(2):411–418, 1997.

116. Lopez-Sagaseta J, Puy C, Tamayo I, et al: SPLA2-V inhibits EPCR anticoagulant and antiapoptotic properties by accommodating lysophosphatidylcholine or PAF in the hydrophobic groove. *Blood* 119(12):2914–2921, 2012.

117. Tamayo I, Velasco SE, Puy C, et al: SPLA2-V impairs EPCR-dependent protein C activation and accelerates thrombosis *in vivo*. *J Thromb Haemost* 12(11):1921–1927, 2014.

118. Gu JM, Crawley JT, Ferrell G, et al: Disruption of the endothelial cell protein C receptor gene in mice causes placental thrombosis and early embryonic lethality. *J Biol Chem* 277(45):43335–43343, 2002.

119. Lau CK, Turner L, Jespersen JS, et al: Structural conservation despite huge sequence diversity allows EPCR binding by the pfemp1 family implicated in severe childhood malaria. *Cell Host Microbe* 17(1):118–129, 2015.

120. Turner L, Lavstsen T, Berger SS, et al: Severe malaria is associated with parasite binding to endothelial protein C receptor. *Nature* 498(7455):502–505, 2013.

121. Moxon CA, Wassmer SC, Milner DA Jr, et al: Loss of endothelial protein C receptors links coagulation and inflammation to parasite sequestration in cerebral malaria in African children. *Blood* 122(5):842–851, 2013.

122. Aird WC, Mosnier LO, Fairhurst RM: *Plasmodium falciparum* picks (on) EPCR. *Blood* 123(2):163–167, 2014.

123. Hayashi T, Nakamura H, Okada A, et al: Organization and chromosomal localization of the human endothelial protein C receptor gene. *Gene* 238(2):367–373, 1999.

124. Vu TK, Hung DT, Wheaton VI, Coughlin SR: Molecular cloning of a functional thrombin receptor reveals a novel proteolytic mechanism of receptor activation. *Cell* 64(6):1057–1068, 1991.

125. Kahn ML, Nakanishi-Matsui M, Shapiro MJ, et al: Protease-activated receptors 1 and 4 mediate activation of human platelets by thrombin. *J Clin Invest* 103(6):879–887, 1999.

126. Coughlin SR: Thrombin signaling and protease-activated receptors. *Nature* 407(6801):258–264, 2000.

127. Macfarlane SR, Seatter MJ, Kanke T, et al: Proteinase-Activated Receptors. *Pharmacol Rev* 53(2):245–282, 2001.

128. Steinhoff M, Buddenkotte J, Shpacovitch V, et al: Proteinase-activated receptors: Transducers of proteinase-mediated signaling in inflammation and immune response. *Endocr Rev* 26(1):1–43, 2005.

129. Leger AJ, Covic L, Kuliopulos A: Protease-activated receptors in cardiovascular diseases. *Circulation* 114(10):1070–1077, 2006.

130. Traynelis SF, Trejo J: Protease-activated receptor signaling: New roles and regulatory mechanisms. *Curr Opin Hematol* 14(3):230–235, 2007.

131. Nakanishi-Matsui M, Zheng YW, Sulciner DJ, et al: PAR3 is a cofactor for PAR4 activation by thrombin. *Nature* 404(6778):609–613, 2000.

132. Sidhu TS, French SL, Hamilton JR: Differential signaling by protease-activated receptors: Implications for therapeutic targeting. *Int J Mol Sci* 15(4):6169–6183, 2014.

133. Hollenberg MD, Mihara K, Polley D, et al: Biased signalling and proteinase-activated receptors (PARs): Targeting inflammatory disease. *Br J Pharmacol* 171(5):1180–1194, 2014.

134. Bahou WF: Protease-activated receptors. *Curr Top Dev Biol* 54:343–369, 2003.

135. Austin KM, Covic L, Kuliopulos A: Matrix metalloproteases and PAR1 activation. *Blood* 121(3):431–439, 2013.

136. Comp PC, Jacocks RM, Ferrell GL, Esmon CT: Activation of protein C *in vivo. J Clin Invest* 70(1):127–134, 1982.

137. Hanson SR, Griffin JH, Harker LA, et al: Antithrombotic effects of thrombin-induced activation of endogenous protein C in primates. *J Clin Invest* 92(4):2003–2012, 1993.

138. Lentz SR, Fernandez JA, Griffin JH, et al: Impaired anticoagulant response to infusion of thrombin in atherosclerotic monkeys associated with acquired defects in the protein C system. *Arterioscler Thromb Vasc Biol* 19(7):1744–1750, 1999.

139. Snow TR, Deal MT, Dickey DT, Esmon CT: Protein C activation following coronary artery occlusion in the in situ porcine heart. *Circulation* 84(1):293–299, 1991.

140. Macko RF, Killewich LA, Fernández JA, et al: Brain-specific protein C activation during carotid artery occlusion in humans. *Stroke* 30(3):542–545, 1999.

141. Petaja J, Pesonen E, Fernandez JA, et al: Cardiopulmonary bypass and activation of antithrombotic plasma protein C. *J Thorac Cardiovasc Surg* 118(3):422–429, 1999.

142. Gruber A, Pal A, Kiss RG, et al: Generation of activated protein C during thrombolysis. *Lancet* 342(8882):1275–1276, 1993.

143. Macko RF, Ameriso SF, Gruber A, et al: Impairments of the protein C system and fibrinolysis in infection-associated stroke. *Stroke* 27(11):2005–2011, 1996.

144. Conard J, Bauer KA, Gruber A, et al: Normalization of markers of coagulation activation with a purified protein C concentrate in adults with homozygous protein C deficiency. *Blood* 82(4):1159–1164, 1993.

145. Taylor FB Jr, Peer GT, Lockhart MS, et al: Endothelial cell protein C receptor plays an important role in protein C activation *in vivo. Blood* 97(6):1685–1688, 2001.

146. Ishii H, Salem HH, Bell CE, et al: Thrombomodulin, an endothelial anticoagulant protein, is absent from the human brain. *Blood* 67(2):362–365, 1986.

147. Bajaj MS, Kuppuswamy MN, Manepalli AN, Bajaj SP: Transcriptional expression of tissue factor pathway inhibitor, thrombomodulin and von Willebrand factor in normal human tissues. *Thromb Haemost* 82:1047–1052, 1999.

148. Wong VL, Hofman FM, Ishii H, Fisher M: Regional distribution of thrombomodulin in human brain. *Brain Res* 556(1):1–5, 1991.

149. Hackeng TM, Tans G, Koppelman SJ, et al: Protein C activation on endothelial cells by prothrombin activation products generated in situ: Meizothrombin is a better protein C activator than alpha-thrombin. *Biochem J* 319(Pt 2):399–405, 1996.

150. Varadi K, Philapitsch A, Santa T, Schwarz HP: Activation and inactivation of human protein C by plasmin. *Thromb Haemost* 71(5):615–621, 1994.

151. Haley PE, Doyle MF, Mann KG: The activation of bovine protein C by factor Xa. *J Biol Chem* 264(27):16303–16310, 1989.

152. Rezaie AR: Rapid activation of protein C by factor Xa and thrombin in the presence of polyanionic compounds. *Blood* 91(12):4572–4580, 1998.

153. Shim K, Zhu H, Westfield LA, Sadler JE: A recombinant murine meizothrombin precursor, prothrombin R157A/R268A, inhibits thrombosis in a model of acute carotid artery injury. *Blood* 104(2):415–419, 2004.

154. Slungaard A, Fernández JA, Griffin JH, et al: Platelet factor 4 enhances generation of activated protein C *in vitro* and *in vivo. Blood* 102(1):146–151, 2003.

155. Slungaard A, Key NS: Platelet factor 4 stimulates thrombomodulin protein C-activating cofactor activity. A structure-function analysis. *J Biol Chem* 269(41):25549–25556, 1994.

156. Kowalska MA, Zhao G, Zhai L, et al: Modulation of protein C activation by histones, platelet factor 4, and heparinoids: New insights into activated protein C formation. *Arterioscler Thromb Vasc Biol* 34(1):120–126, 2014.

157. Kowalska MA, Rauova L, Poncz M: Role of the platelet chemokine platelet factor 4 (PF4) in hemostasis and thrombosis. *Thromb Res* 125(4):292–296, 2010.

158. Fernandez JA, Petaja J, Gruber A, Griffin JH: Activated protein C correlates inversely with thrombin levels in resting healthy individuals. *Am J Hematol* 56(1):29–31, 1997.

159. Pellequer JL, Gale AJ, Griffin JH, Getzoff ED: Homology models of the C domains of blood coagulation factors V and VIII: A proposed membrane binding mode for FV and FVIII C2 domains. *Blood Cells Mol Dis* 24(4):448–461, 1998.

160. Autin L, Steen M, Dahlbäck B, Villoutreix BO: Proposed structural models of the prothrombinase (FXa-FVa) complex. *Proteins* 63(3):440–450, 2006.

161. Adams TE, Hockin MF, Mann KG, Everse SJ: The crystal structure of activated protein C-inactivated bovine factor Va: Implications for cofactor function. *Proc Natl Acad Sci U S A* 101(24):8918–8923, 2004.

162. Lechtenberg BC, Murray-Rust TA, Johnson DJ, et al: Crystal structure of the prothrombinase complex from the venom of *Pseudonaja textilis. Blood* 122(16):2777–2783, 2013.

163. Lee CJ, Wu S, Pedersen LG: A proposed ternary complex model of prothrombinase with prothrombin: Protein-protein docking and molecular dynamics simulations. *J Thromb Haemost* 9(10):2123–2126, 2011.

164. Camire RM, Kalafatis M, Tracy PB: Proteolysis of factor V by cathepsin G and elastase indicates that cleavage at Arg1545 optimizes cofactor function by facilitating factor Xa binding. *Biochemistry* 37(34):11896–11906, 1998.

165. Steen M, Dahlbäck B: Thrombin-mediated proteolysis of factor V resulting in gradual B-domain release and exposure of the factor Xa-binding site. *J Biol Chem* 277(41):38424–38430, 2002.

166. Toso R, Camire RM: Removal of B-domain sequences from factor V rather than specific proteolysis underlies the mechanism by which cofactor function is realized. *J Biol Chem* 279(20):21643–21650, 2004.

167. Thorelli E, Kaufman RJ, Dahlbäck B: Cleavage requirements for activation of factor V by factor Xa. *Eur J Biochem* 247(1):12–20, 1997.

168. Camire RM: A new look at blood coagulation factor V. *Curr Opin Hematol* 18(5):338–342, 2011.

169. Bos MH, Camire RM: A bipartite autoinhibitory region within the B-domain suppresses function in factor V. *J Biol Chem* 287(31):26342–26351, 2012.

170. Fay PJ: Regulation of factor VIIIa in the intrinsic factor Xase. *Thromb Haemost* 82(2):193–200, 1999.

171. Marlar RA, Kleiss AJ, Griffin JH: Mechanism of action of human activated protein C, a thrombin dependent anticoagulant enzyme. *Blood* 59:1067–1072, 1982.

172. Fulcher CA, Gardiner JE, Griffin JH, Zimmerman TS: Proteolytic inactivation of human factor VIII procoagulant protein by activated human protein C and its analogy with factor V. *Blood* 63(2):486–489, 1984.

173. Kalafatis M, Rand MD, Mann KG: The mechanism of inactivation of human factor V and human factor Va by activated protein C. *J Biol Chem* 269(50):31869–31880, 1994.

174. Dahlbäck B, Carlsson M, Svensson PJ: Familial thrombophilia due to a previously unrecognized mechanism characterized by poor anticoagulant response to activated protein C: Prediction of a cofactor to activated protein C. *Proc Natl Acad Sci U S A* 90(3):1004–1008, 1993.

175. Bertina RM, Koeleman BPC, Koster T, et al: Mutations in blood coagulation factor V associated with resistance to activated protein C. *Nature* 369(6475):64–67, 1994.

176. Greengard JS, Sun X, Xu X, et al: Activated protein C resistance caused by Arg506Gln mutation in factor Va. *Lancet* 343(8909):1361–1362, 1994.

177. Sun X, Evatt B, Griffin JH: Blood coagulation factor Va abnormality associated with resistance to activated protein C in venous thrombophilia. *Blood* 83(11):3120–3125, 1994.

178. Zivelin A, Griffin JH, Xu X, et al: A single genetic origin for a common Caucasian risk factor for venous thrombosis. *Blood* 89(2):397–402, 1997.

179. Zivelin A, Mor-Cohen R, Kovalsky V, et al: Prothrombin 20210G>A is an ancestral prothrombotic mutation that occurred in whites approximately 24,000 years ago. *Blood* 107(12):4666–4668, 2006.

180. Heeb MJ, Kojima Y, Greengard JS, Griffin JH: Activated protein C resistance: Molecular mechanisms based on studies using purified Gln506-factor V. *Blood* 85(12):3405–3411, 1995.

181. Rosing J, Hoekema L, Nicolaes GAF, et al: Effects of protein S and factor Xa on peptide bond cleavages during inactivation of factor Va and factor Va R506Q by activated protein C. *J Biol Chem* 270(46):27852–27858, 1995.

182. Gale AJ, Xu X, Pellequer JL, et al: Interdomain engineered disulfide bond permitting elucidation of mechanisms of inactivation of coagulation factor Va by activated protein C. *Protein Sci* 11(9):2091–2101, 2002.

183. Rosing J, Bakker HM, Thomassen MC, et al: Characterization of two forms of human factor Va with different cofactor activities. *J Biol Chem* 268(28):21130–21136, 1993.

184. Nicolaes GAF, Villoutreix BO, Dahlbäck B: Partial glycosylation of Asn2181 in human factor V as a cause of molecular and functional heterogeneity. Modulation of glycosylation efficiency by mutagenesis of the consensus sequence for N-linked glycosylation. *Biochemistry* 38(41):13584–13591, 1999.

185. Fernández JA, Hackeng TM, Kojima K, Griffin JH: The carbohydrate moiety of factor V modulates inactivation by activated protein C. *Blood* 89(12):4348–4354, 1997.

186. Fisher M, Fernández JA, Ameriso SF, et al: Activated protein C resistance in ischemic stroke not due to factor V arginine506—>glutamine mutation. *Stroke* 27(7):1163–1166, 1996.

187. de Visser MCH, Rosendaal FR, Bertina RM: A reduced sensitivity for activated protein C in the absence of factor V Leiden increases the risk of venous thrombosis. *Blood* 93(4):1271–1276, 1999.

188. Rodeghiero F, Tosetto A: Activated protein C resistance and factor V Leiden mutation are independent risk factors for venous thromboembolism. *Ann Intern Med* 130(8):643–650, 1999.

189. Griffin JH, Kojima K, Banka CL, et al: High-density lipoprotein enhancement of anticoagulant activities of plasma protein S and activated protein C. *J Clin Invest* 103(2):219–227, 1999.

190. Fernandez JA, Deguchi H, Banka CL, et al: Re-evaluation of the anticoagulant properties of high-density lipoprotein. *Arterioscler Thromb Vasc Biol* 35(3):570–572, 2015.

191. Curvers J, Thomassen MC, Nicolaes GAF, et al: Acquired APC resistance and oral contraceptives: Differences between two functional tests. *Br J Haematol* 105(1):88–94, 1999.

192. Smirnov MD, Safa O, Esmon NL, Esmon CT: Inhibition of activated protein C anticoagulant activity by prothrombin. *Blood* 94(11):3839–3846, 1999.

193. Brugge JM, Tans G, Rosing J, Castoldi E: Protein S levels modulate the activated protein C resistance phenotype induced by elevated prothrombin levels. *Thromb Haemost* 95(2):236–242, 2006.

194. Bakker HM, Tans G, Janssen-Claessen T, et al: The effect of phospholipids, calcium ions and protein S on rate constants of human factor Va inactivation by activated human protein C. *Eur J Biochem* 208(1):171–178, 1992.

195. Smirnov MD, Esmon CT: Phosphatidylethanolamine incorporation into vesicles selectively enhances factor Va inactivation by activated protein C. *J Biol Chem* 269(2):816–819, 1994.

196. Smirnov MD, Triplett DT, Comp PC, et al: On the role of phosphatidylethanolamine in the inhibition of activated protein C activity by antiphospholipid antibodies. *J Clin Invest* 95(1):309–316, 1995.

197. Fernández JA, Kojima K, Petäjä J, et al: Cardiolipin enhances protein C pathway anticoagulant activity. *Blood Cells Mol Dis* 26(2):115–123, 2000.

198. Rezende SM, Simmonds RE, Lane DA: Coagulation, inflammation, and apoptosis: Different roles for protein S and the protein S-C4b binding protein complex. *Blood* 103(4):1192–1201, 2004.

199. Yegneswaran S, Smirnov MD, Safa O, et al: Relocating the active site of activated protein C eliminates the need for its protein S cofactor. A fluorescence resonance energy transfer study. *J Biol Chem* 274(9):5462–5468, 1999.

200. Yegneswaran S, Wood GM, Esmon CT, Johnson AE: Protein S alters the active site location of activated protein C above the membrane surface. A fluorescence resonance energy transfer study of topography. *J Biol Chem* 272(40):25013–25021, 1997.

201. Koedam JA, Meijers JCM, Sixma JJ, Bouma BN: Inactivation of human factor VIII by activated protein C. Cofactor activity of protein S and protective effect of von Willebrand factor. *J Clin Invest* 82(4):1236–1243, 1988.

202. Solymoss S, Tucker MM, Tracy PB: Kinetics of inactivation of membrane-bound factor Va by activated protein C. Protein S modulates factor Xa protection. *J Biol Chem* 263(29):14884–14890, 1988.

203. Dahlbäck B, Hildebrand B, Malm J: Characterization of functionally important domains in human vitamin K-dependent protein S using monoclonal antibodies. *J Biol Chem* 265(14):8127–8135, 1990.

204. Saller F, Villoutreix BO, Amelot A, et al: The gamma-carboxyglutamic acid domain of anticoagulant protein S is involved in activated protein C cofactor activity, independently of phospholipid binding. *Blood* 105(1):122–130, 2005.

205. Saller F, Kaabache T, Aiach M, et al: The protein S thrombin-sensitive region modulates phospholipid binding and the gamma-carboxyglutamic acid-rich (Gla) domain conformation in a non-specific manner. *J Thromb Haemost* 4(3):704–706, 2006.

206. Heeb MJ, Mesters RM, Fernandez JA, et al: Plasma protein S residues 37–50 mediate its binding to factor Va and inhibition of blood coagulation. *Thromb Haemost* 110(2):275–282, 2013.

207. Walker FJ: Regulation of vitamin K-dependent protein S. Inactivation by thrombin. *J Biol Chem* 259:10335–10339, 1984.

208. Varadi K, Rosing J, Tans G, et al: Factor V enhances the cofactor function of protein S in the APC-mediated inactivation of factor VIII: Influence of the factor V^R506Q mutation. *Thromb Haemost* 76(2):208–214, 1996.

209. Thorelli E, Kaufman RJ, Dahlbäck B: Cleavage of factor V at Arg 506 by activated protein C and the expression of anticoagulant activity of factor V. *Blood* 93(8):2552–2558, 1999.

210. Cramer TJ, Gale AJ: The anticoagulant function of coagulation factor V. *Thromb Haemost* 107(1):15–21, 2012.

211. Cramer TJ, Griffin JH, Gale AJ: Factor V Is an anticoagulant cofactor for activated protein C during inactivation of factor Va. *Pathophysiol Haemost Thromb* 37(1):17–23, 2010.

212. Mineo C, Deguchi H, Griffin JH, Shaul PW: Endothelial and antithrombotic actions of HDL. *Circ Res* 98(11):1352–1364, 2006.

213. Deguchi H, Pecheniuk NM, Elias DJ, et al: High-density lipoprotein deficiency and dyslipoproteinemia associated with venous thrombosis in men. *Circulation* 112(6):893–899, 2005.

214. Eichinger S, Pecheniuk NM, Hron G, et al: High-density lipoprotein and the risk of recurrent venous thromboembolism. *Circulation* 115(12):1609–1614, 2007.

215. Deguchi H, Fernández JA, Pabinger I, et al: Plasma glucosylceramide deficiency as potential risk factor for venous thrombosis and modulator of anticoagulant protein C pathway. *Blood* 97(7):1907–1914, 2001.

216. Deguchi H, Fernández JA, Griffin JH: Neutral glycosphingolipid-dependent inactivation of coagulation factor Va by activated protein C and protein S. *J Biol Chem* 277(11):8861–8865, 2002.

217. Yegneswaran S, Deguchi H, Griffin JH: Glucosylceramide, a neutral glycosphingolipid anticoagulant cofactor, enhances the interaction of human- and bovine-activated protein C with negatively charged phospholipid vesicles. *J Biol Chem* 278(17):14614–14621, 2003.

218. Deguchi H, Yegneswaran S, Griffin JH: Sphingolipids as bioactive regulators of thrombin generation. *J Biol Chem* 279(13):12036–12042, 2004.

219. Esmon CT: Interactions between the innate immune and blood coagulation systems. *Trends Immunol* 25(10):536–542, 2004.

220. Levi M, van der Poll T, Buller HR: Bidirectional relation between inflammation and coagulation. *Circulation* 109(22):2698–2704, 2004.

221. Riewald M, Ruf W: Protease-activated receptor-1 signaling by activated protein C in cytokine perturbed endothelial cells is distinct from thrombin signaling. *J Biol Chem* 280(20):19808–19814, 2005.

222. Kerschen EJ, Hernandez I, Zogg M, et al: Activated protein C targets CD8+ dendritic cells to reduce the mortality of endotoxemia in mice. *J Clin Invest* 120(9):3167–3178, 2010.

223. Guo H, Zhao Z, Yang Q, et al: An activated protein C analog stimulates neuronal production by human neural progenitor cells via a PAR1-PAR3-S1PR1-Akt pathway. *J Neurosci* 33(14):6181–6190, 2013.

224. Xue M, Chow SO, Dervish S, et al: Activated protein C enhances human keratinocyte barrier integrity via sequential activation of epidermal growth factor receptor and tie2. *J Biol Chem* 286(8):6742–6750, 2011.

225. Riewald M, Petrovan RJ, Donner A, et al: Activation of endothelial cell protease activated receptor 1 by the protein C pathway. *Science* 296(5574):1880–1882, 2002.

226. Mosnier LO, Zlokovic BV, Griffin JH: Cytoprotective-selective activated protein C therapy for ischaemic stroke. *Thromb Haemost* 112(5):883–892, 2014.

227. Zlokovic BV, Griffin JH: Cytoprotective protein C pathways and implications for stroke and neurological disorders. *Trends Neurosci* 34(4):198–209, 2011.

228. Wildhagen KC, Lutgens E, Loubele ST, et al: The structure-function relationship of activated protein C. Lessons from natural and engineered mutations. *Thromb Haemost* 106(6):1034–1045, 2011.

229. Kerschen EJ, Fernandez JA, Cooley BC, et al: Endotoxemia and sepsis mortality reduction by non-anticoagulant activated protein C. *J Exp Med* 204(10):2439–2448, 2007.

230. Wang Y, Sinha RK, Mosnier LO, et al: Neurotoxicity of the anticoagulant-selective E149A-activated protein C variant after focal ischemic stroke in mice. *Blood Cells Mol Dis* 51(2):104–108, 2013.

231. Guo H, Singh I, Wang Y, et al: Neuroprotective activities of activated protein C mutant with reduced anticoagulant activity. *Eur J Neurosci* 29(6):1119–1130, 2009.

232. Wang Y, Thiyagarajan M, Chow N, et al: Differential neuroprotection and risk for bleeding from activated protein C with varying degrees of anticoagulant activity. *Stroke* 40(5):1864–1869, 2008.

233. Cheng T, Liu D, Griffin JH, et al: Activated protein C blocks p53-mediated apoptosis in ischemic human brain endothelium and is neuroprotective. *Nat Med* 9(3):338–342, 2003.

234. Cheng T, Petraglia AL, Li Z, et al: Activated protein C inhibits tissue plasminogen activator-induced brain hemorrhage. *Nat Med* 12(11):1278–1285, 2006.

235. Griffin JH, Fernández JA, Liu D, et al: Activated protein C and ischemic stroke. *Crit Care Med* 32(5 Suppl):S247–S253, 2004.

236. Guo H, Liu D, Gelbard H, et al: Activated protein C prevents neuronal apoptosis via protease activated receptors 1 and 3. *Neuron* 41(4):563–572, 2004.

237. Liu D, Cheng T, Guo H, et al: Tissue plasminogen activator neurovascular toxicity is controlled by activated protein C. *Nat Med* 10(12):1379–1383, 2004.

238. Shibata M, Kumar SR, Amar A, et al: Anti-inflammatory, antithrombotic, and neuroprotective effects of activated protein C in a murine model of focal ischemic stroke. *Circulation* 103(13):1799–1805, 2001.

239. Wang Y, Zhang Z, Chow N, et al: An activated protein C analog with reduced anticoagulant activity extends the therapeutic window of tissue plasminogen activator for ischemic stroke in rodents. *Stroke* 43(9):2444–2449, 2012.

240. Wang Y, Zhao Z, Chow N, et al: Activated protein C analog promotes neurogenesis and improves neurological outcome after focal ischemic stroke in mice via protease activated receptor 1. *Brain Res* 1507:97–104, 2013.

241. Wang Y, Zhao Z, Chow N, et al: Activated protein C analog protects from ischemic stroke and extends the therapeutic window of tissue-type plasminogen activator in aged female mice and hypertensive rats. *Stroke* 44(12):3529–3536, 2013.

242. Zlokovic BV: Neurodegeneration and the neurovascular unit. *Nat Med* 16(12):1370–1371, 2010.

243. Petraglia AL, Marky AH, Walker C, et al: Activated protein C is neuroprotective and mediates new blood vessel formation and neurogenesis after controlled cortical impact. *Neurosurgery* 66(1):165–171, 2010.

244. Thiyagarajan M, Fernandez JA, Lane SM, et al: Activated protein C promotes neovascularization and neurogenesis in postischemic brain via protease-activated receptor 1. *J Neurosci* 28(48):12788–12797, 2008.

245. Walker CT, Marky AH, Petraglia AL, et al: Activated protein C analog with reduced anti-coagulant activity improves functional recovery and reduces bleeding risk following controlled cortical impact. *Brain Res* 1347:125–131, 2010.

246. Lyden P, Levy H, Weymer S, et al: Phase 1 safety, tolerability and pharmacokinetics of 3K3A-APC in healthy adult volunteers. *Curr Pharm Des* 19(42):7479–7485, 2013.

247. Williams PD, Zlokovic BV, Griffin JH, et al: Preclinical safety and pharmacokinetic profile of 3K3A-APC, a novel, modified activated protein C for ischemic stroke. *Curr Pharm Des* 18(27):4215–4222, 2012.

248. Mosnier LO, Griffin JH: Inhibition of staurosporine-induced apoptosis of endothelial cells by activated protein C requires protease activated receptor-1 and endothelial cell protein C receptor. *Biochem J* 373(Pt 1):65–70, 2003.

249. Feistritzer C, Riewald M: Endothelial barrier protection by activated protein C through PAR1-dependent sphingosine 1-phosphate receptor-1 crossactivation. *Blood* 105(8):3178–3184, 2005.

250. Finigan JH, Dudek SM, Singleton PA, et al: Activated protein C mediates novel lung endothelial barrier enhancement: Role of sphingosine 1-phosphate receptor transactivation. *J Biol Chem* 280(17):17286–17293, 2005.

251. Schuepbach RA, Feistritzer C, Fernandez JA, et al: Protection of vascular barrier integrity by activated protein C in murine models depends on protease-activated receptor-1. *Thromb Haemost* 101(4):724–733, 2009.

252. Bae JS, Yang L, Rezaie AR: Receptors of the protein C activation and activated protein C signaling pathways are colocalized in lipid rafts of endothelial cells. *Proc Natl Acad Sci U S A* 104(8):2867–2872, 2007.

253. Russo A, Soh UJ, Paing MM, et al: Caveolae are required for protease-selective signaling by protease-activated receptor-1. *Proc Natl Acad Sci U S A* 106(15):6393–6397, 2009.

254. Mosnier LO, Sinha RK, Burnier L, et al: Biased agonism of protease-activated receptor 1 by activated protein C caused by non-canonical cleavage at Arg46. *Blood* 120(26):5237–5246, 2012.

255. Scarborough RM, Naughton MA, Teng W, et al: Tethered ligand agonist peptides. Structural requirements for thrombin receptor activation reveal mechanism of proteolytic unmasking of agonist function. *J Biol Chem* 267(19):13146–13149, 1992.

256. Soh UJ, Trejo J: Activated protein C promotes protease-activated receptor-1 cytoprotective signaling through beta-arrestin and dishevelled-2 scaffolds. *Proc Natl Acad Sci U S A* 108(50):E1372–E1380, 2011.

257. Burnier L, Mosnier LO: Novel mechanisms for activated protein C cytoprotective activities involving non-canonical activation of protease-activated receptor 3. *Blood* 122(5):807–816, 2013.

258. Stavenuiter F, Mosnier LO: Non-canonical PAR3 activation by factor Xa identifies a novel pathway for Tie2 activation and stabilization of vascular integrity. *Blood* 124(23):3480–3489, 2014.

259. Yang XV, Banerjee Y, Fernandez JA, et al: Activated protein C ligation of ApoER2 (LRP8) causes Dab1-dependent signaling in U937 cells. *Proc Natl Acad Sci U S A* 106(1):274–279, 2009.

260. Xu J, Ji Y, Zhang X, et al: Endogenous activated protein C signaling is critical to protection of mice from lipopolysaccharide induced septic shock. *J Thromb Haemost* 7(5):851–856, 2009.

261. Alabanza LM, Esmon NL, Esmon CT, Bynoe MS: Inhibition of endogenous activated protein C attenuates experimental autoimmune encephalomyelitis by inducing myeloid-derived suppressor cells. *J Immunol* 191(7):3764–3777, 2013.

262. Kager LM, Joost WW, Roelofs JJ, et al: Endogenous protein C has a protective role during Gram-negative pneumosepsis (melioidosis). *J Thromb Haemost* 11(2):282–292, 2013.

263. Heeb MJ, Gruber A, Griffin JH: Identification of divalent metal ion-dependent inhibition of activated protein C by alpha 2-macroglobulin and alpha 2-antiplasmin in blood and comparisons to inhibition of factor Xa, thrombin, and plasmin. *J Biol Chem* 266(26):17606–17612, 1991.

264. Heeb MJ, Griffin JH: Physiologic inhibition of human activated protein C by alpha 1-antitrypsin. *J Biol Chem* 263(24):11613–11616, 1988.

265. Heeb MJ, Espana F, Griffin JH: Inhibition and complexation of activated protein C by two major inhibitors in plasma. *Blood* 73(2):446–454, 1989.

266. Espana F, Vicente V, Tabernero D, et al: Determination of plasma protein C inhibitor and of two activated protein C-inhibitor complexes in normals and in patients with intravascular coagulation and thrombotic disease. *Thromb Res* 59(3):593–608, 1990.

267. Espana F, Gilabert J, Aznar J, et al: Complexes of activated protein C with alpha 1-anti-trypsin in normal pregnancy and in severe preeclampsia. *Am J Obstet Gynecol* 164(5 Pt 1):1310–1316, 1991.

268. Scully MF, Toh CH, Hoogendoorn H, et al: Activation of protein C and its distribution between its inhibitors, protein C inhibitor, alpha 1-antitrypsin and alpha 2-macroglobulin, in patients with disseminated intravascular coagulation. *Thromb Haemost* 69(5):448–453, 1993.

269. Bhiladvala P, Strandberg K, Stenflo J, Holm J: Early identification of acute myocardial infarction by activated protein C–protein C inhibitor complex. *Thromb Res* 118(2):213–219, 2006.

270. Schwarz HP, Fischer M, Hopmeier P, et al: Plasma protein S deficiency in familial thrombotic disease. *Blood* 64(6):1297–1300, 1984.

271. Comp PC, Nixon RR, Cooper MR, Esmon CT: Familial protein S deficiency is associated with recurrent thrombosis. *J Clin Invest* 74(6):2082–2088, 1984.

272. Stenberg Y, Muranyi A, Steen C, et al: EGF-like module pair 3–4 in vitamin K-dependent protein S: Modulation of calcium affinity of module 4 by module 3, and interaction with factor X. *J Mol Biol* 293(3):653–665, 1999.

273. Yegneswaran S, Hackeng TM, Dawson PE, Griffin JH: The thrombin-sensitive region of protein S mediates phospholipid-dependent interaction with factor Xa. *J Biol Chem* 283(48):33046–33052, 2008.

274. van't Veer C, Hackeng TM, Biesbroeck D, et al: Increased prothrombin activation in protein S-deficient plasma under flow conditions on endothelial cell matrix: An independent anticoagulant function of protein S in plasma. *Blood* 85(7):1815–1821, 1995.

275. Koppelman SJ, Hackeng TM, Sixma JJ, Bouma BN: Inhibition of the intrinsic factor X activating complex by protein S: Evidence for a specific binding of protein S to factor VIII. *Blood* 86:1062–1071, 1995.

276. Koppelman SJ, van't Veer C, Sixma JJ, Bouma BN: Synergistic inhibition of the intrinsic factor X activation by protein S and C4b-binding protein. *Blood* 86(7):2653–2660, 1995.

277. Peraramelli S, Rosing J, Hackeng TM: TFPI-dependent activities of protein S. *Thromb Res* 129(Suppl 2):S23–S26, 2012.

278. Ndonwi M, Tuley EA, Broze GJ Jr: The Kunitz-3 domain of TFPI-alpha is required for protein S-dependent enhancement of factor Xa inhibition. *Blood* 116(8):1344–1351, 2010.

279. Hackeng TM, Sere KM, Tans G, Rosing J: Protein S stimulates inhibition of the tissue factor pathway by tissue factor pathway inhibitor. *Proc Natl Acad Sci U S A* 103(9):3106–3111, 2006.

280. Heeb MJ, Prashun D, Griffin JH, Bouma BN: Plasma protein S contains zinc essential for efficient activated protein C-independent anticoagulant activity and binding to factor Xa, but not for efficient binding to tissue factor pathway inhibitor. *FASEB J* 23(7):2244–2253, 2009.

281. Heeb MJ, Marzec U, Gruber A, Hanson SR: Antithrombotic activity of protein S infused without activated protein C in a baboon thrombosis model. *Thromb Haemost* 107(4):690–698, 2012.

282. Dahlback B: Purification of human C4b-binding protein and formation of its complex with vitamin K-dependent protein S. *Biochem J* 209(3):847–856, 1983.

283. Griffin JH, Gruber A, Fernández JA: Reevaluation of total, free, and bound protein S and C4b-binding protein levels in plasma anticoagulated with citrate or hirudin. *Blood* 79(12):3203–3211, 1992.

284. Schwarz HP, Muntean W, Watzke H, et al: Low total protein S antigen but high protein S activity due to decreased C4b-binding protein in neonates. *Blood* 71(3):562–565, 1988.

285. Maurissen LF, Thomassen MC, Nicolaes GA, et al: Re-evaluation of the role of the protein S-C4b binding protein complex in activated protein C-catalyzed factor Va-inactivation. *Blood* 111(6):3034–3041, 2008.

286. Hillarp A, Dahlbäck B: Novel subunit in C4b-binding protein required for protein S binding. *J Biol Chem* 263(25):12759–12764, 1988.

287. Hillarp A, Hessing M, Dahlbäck B: Protein S binding in relation to the subunit composition of human C4b-binding protein. *FEBS Lett* 259(1):53–56, 1989.

288. Fernandez JA, Griffin JH: A protein S binding site on C4b-binding protein involves beta chain residues 31–45. *J Biol Chem* 269(4):2535–2540, 1994.

289. Fernández JA, Griffin JH, Chang GT, et al: Involvement of amino acid residues 423–429 of human protein S in binding to C4b-binding protein. *Blood Cells Mol Dis* 24(2):101–112, 1998.

290. Garcia de Frutos P, Alim RI, Hardig Y, et al: Differential regulation of alpha and beta chains of C4b-binding protein during acute-phase response resulting in stable plasma levels of free anticoagulant protein S. *Blood* 84(3):815–822, 1994.

291. Anderson HA, Maylock CA, Williams JA, et al: Serum-derived protein S binds to phosphatidylserine and stimulates the phagocytosis of apoptotic cells. *Nat Immunol* 4(1):87–91, 2003.

292. Prasad D, Rothlin CV, Burrola P, et al: TAM receptor function in the retinal pigment epithelium. *Mol Cell Neurosci* 33(1):96–108, 2006.

293. Uehara H, Shacter E: Auto-oxidation and oligomerization of protein S on the apoptotic cell surface is required for Mer tyrosine kinase-mediated phagocytosis of apoptotic cells. *J Immunol* 180(4):2522–2530, 2008.

294. McColl A, Bournazos S, Franz S, et al: Glucocorticoids induce protein S-dependent phagocytosis of apoptotic neutrophils by human macrophages. *J Immunol* 183(3):2167–2175, 2009.

295. Liu D, Guo H, Griffin JH, et al: Protein S confers neuronal protection during ischemic/hypoxic injury in mice. *Circulation* 107(13):1791–1796, 2003.

296. Fernandez JA, Heeb MJ, Xu X, et al: Species-specific anticoagulant and mitogenic activities of murine protein S. *Haematologica* 94(12):1721–1731, 2009.

297. Zhu D, Wang Y, Singh I, et al: Protein S controls hypoxic/ischemic blood-brain barrier disruption through the TAM receptor Tyro3 and sphingosine 1-phosphate receptor. *Blood* 115(23):4963–4972, 2010.

298. Zhong Z, Wang Y, Guo H, et al: Protein S protects neurons from excitotoxic injury by activating the TAM receptor Tyro3-phosphatidylinositol 3-kinase-Akt pathway through its sex hormone-binding globulin-like region. *J Neurosci* 30(46):15521–15534, 2010.

299. Guo H, Barrett TM, Zhong Z, et al: Protein S blocks the extrinsic apoptotic cascade in tissue plasminogen activator/N-methyl D-aspartate-treated neurons via Tyro3-Akt-FKHRL1 signaling pathway. *Mol Neurodegener* 6(1):13, 2011.

300. Gray E, Hogwood J, Mulloy B: The anticoagulant and antithrombotic mechanisms of heparin. *Handb Exp Pharmacol* 207:43–61, 2012.

301. Broze GJ Jr, Girard TJ: Tissue factor pathway inhibitor: Structure-function. *Front Biosci (Landmark Ed)* 17:262–280, 2012.

302. Winckers K, ten Cate H, Hackeng TM: The role of tissue factor pathway inhibitor in atherosclerosis and arterial thrombosis. *Blood Rev* 27(3):119–132, 2013.

303. Wood JP, Ellery PE, Maroney SA, Mast AE: Biology of tissue factor pathway inhibitor. *Blood* 123(19):2934–2943, 2014.

304. Gettins PG: Serpin structure, mechanism, and function. *Chem Rev* 102(12):4751–4804, 2002.

305. Whisstock JC, Bottomley SP: Molecular gymnastics: Serpin structure, folding and misfolding. *Curr Opin Struct Biol* 16(6):761–768, 2006.

306. Rau JC, Beaulieu LM, Huntington JA, Church FC: Serpins in thrombosis, hemostasis and fibrinolysis. *J Thromb Haemost* 5(Suppl 1):102–115, 2007.

307. Huntington JA: Serpin structure, function and dysfunction. *J Thromb Haemost* 9(Suppl 1):26–34, 2011.

308. Huntington JA: Thrombin inhibition by the serpins. *J Thromb Haemost* 11(Suppl 1):254–264, 2013.

309. Schreuder HA, de Boer B, Dijkema R, et al: The intact and cleaved human antithrombin III complex as a model for serpin-proteinase interactions. *Nat Struct Biol* 1(1):48–54, 1994.

310. Skinner R, Abrahams JP, Whisstock JC, et al: The 2.6 A structure of antithrombin indicates a conformational change at the heparin binding site. *J Mol Biol* 266(3):601–609, 1997.

311. Li W, Johnson DJ, Esmon CT, Huntington JA: Structure of the antithrombin-thrombin-heparin ternary complex reveals the antithrombotic mechanism of heparin. *Nat Struct Mol Biol* 11(9):857–862, 2004.

312. Huber R, Carell RW: Implications of the three dimensional structure of $\alpha_1$-antitrypsin for the structure and function of serpins. *Biochemistry* 28:8951–8966, 1989.

313. Choay J, Petitou M, Lormeau JC, et al: Structure-activity relationship in heparin: A synthetic pentasaccharide with high affinity for antithrombin III and eliciting high anti-factor Xa activity. *Biochem Biophys Res Commun* 116(2):492–499, 1983.

314. Bourin MC, Lindahl U: Glycosaminoglycans and the regulation of blood coagulation. *Biochem J* 289(Pt 2):313–330, 1993.

315. Hirsh J, O'Donnell M, Eikelboom JW: Beyond unfractionated heparin and warfarin: Current and future advances. *Circulation* 116(5):552–560, 2007.

316. Olds RJ, Lane DA, Chowdhury V, et al: Complete nucleotide sequence of the antithrombin gene: Evidence for homologous recombination causing thrombophilia. *Biochemistry* 32(16):4216–4224, 1993.

317. Picard V, Ersdal-Badju E, Bock SC: Partial glycosylation of antithrombin III asparagine-135 is caused by the serine in the third position of its N-glycosylation consensus sequence and is responsible for production of the beta-antithrombin III isoform with enhanced heparin affinity. *Biochemistry* 34(26):8433–8440, 1995.

318. Turko IV, Fan B, Gettins PG: Carbohydrate isoforms of antithrombin variant N135Q with different heparin affinities. *FEBS Lett* 335(1):9–12, 1993.

319. Chandra T, Stackhouse R, Kidd VJ, Woo SL: Isolation and sequence characterization of a cDNA clone of human antithrombin III. *Proc Natl Acad Sci U S A* 80(7):1845–1848, 1983.

320. Prochownik EV, Markham AF, Orkin SH: Isolation of a cDNA clone for human antithrombin III. *J Biol Chem* 258(13):8389–8394, 1983.

321. Lane DA, Bayston T, Olds RJ, et al: Antithrombin mutation database: 2nd (1997) update. For the Plasma Coagulation Inhibitors Subcommittee of the Scientific and Standardization Committee of the International Society on Thrombosis and Haemostasis. *Thromb Haemost* 77(1):197–211, 1997.

322. Broze GJ Jr, Girard TJ: Factor V, tissue factor pathway inhibitor, and east Texas bleeding disorder. *J Clin Invest* 123(9):3710–3712, 2013.

323. Chang JY, Monroe DM, Oliver JA, Roberts HR: TFPIbeta, a second product from the mouse tissue factor pathway inhibitor (TFPI) gene. *Thromb Haemost* 81(1):45–49, 1999.

324. Zhang J, Piro O, Lu L, Broze GJ Jr: Glycosyl phosphatidylinositol anchorage of tissue factor pathway inhibitor. *Circulation* 108(5):623–627, 2003.

325. Piro O, Broze GJ Jr: Comparison of cell-surface TFPIalpha and beta. *J Thromb Haemost* 3(12):2677–2683, 2005.

326. Girard TJ, Warren LA, Novotny WF, et al: Functional significance of the Kunitz-type inhibitory domains of lipoprotein-associated coagulation inhibitor. *Nature* 338(6215):518–520, 1989.

327. Lesnik P, Vonica A, Guerin M, et al: Anticoagulant activity of tissue factor pathway inhibitor in human plasma is preferentially associated with dense subspecies of LDL and HDL and with Lp(a). *Arterioscler Thromb* 13(7):1066–1075, 1993.

328. Novotny WF, Girard TJ, Miletich JP, Broze GJ Jr: Purification and characterization of the lipoprotein-associated coagulation inhibitor from human plasma. *J Biol Chem* 264(31):18832–18837, 1989.

329. Sandset PM, Abildgaard U, Larsen ML: Heparin induces release of extrinsic coagulation pathway inhibitor (EPI). *Thromb Res* 50(6):803–813, 1988.

330. Ndonwi M, Girard TJ, Broze GJ Jr: The C-terminus of tissue factor pathway inhibitor alpha is required for its interaction with factors V and Va. *J Thromb Haemost* 10(9):1944–1946, 2012.

331. Castoldi E, Simioni P, Tormene D, et al: Hereditary and acquired protein S deficiencies are associated with low TFPI levels in plasma. *J Thromb Haemost* 8(2):294–300, 2010.

332. Vincent LM, Tran S, Livaja R, et al: Coagulation factor VA2440G causes east Texas bleeding disorder via TFPIalpha. *J Clin Invest* 123(9):3777–3787, 2013.

333. Duckers C, Simioni P, Spiezia L, et al: Low plasma levels of tissue factor pathway inhibitor in patients with congenital factor V deficiency. *Blood* 112(9):3615–3623, 2008.

334. Huang ZF, Broze G Jr: Consequences of tissue factor pathway inhibitor gene-disruption in mice. *Thromb Haemost* 78(1):699–704, 1997.

335. van der Logt CP, Reitsma PH, Bertina RM: Intron-exon organization of the human gene coding for the lipoprotein-associated coagulation inhibitor: The factor Xa dependent inhibitor of the extrinsic pathway of coagulation. *Biochemistry* 30(6):1571–1577, 1991.

336. Girard TJ, Eddy R, Wesselschmidt RL, et al: Structure of the human lipoprotein-associated coagulation inhibitor gene. Intro/exon gene organization and localization of the gene to chromosome 2. *J Biol Chem* 266(8):5036–5041, 1991.

337. Tollefsen DM, Majerus DW, Blank MK: Heparin cofactor II. Purification and properties of a heparin-dependent inhibitor of thrombin in human plasma. *J Biol Chem* 257(5):2162–2169, 1982.

338. Aihara K: Heparin cofactor II attenuates vascular remodeling in humans and mice. *Circ J* 74(8):1518–1523, 2010.

339. Tollefsen DM: Vascular dermatan sulfate and heparin cofactor II. *Prog Mol Biol Transl Sci* 93:351–372, 2010.

340. Rau JC, Mitchell JW, Fortenberry YM, Church FC: Heparin cofactor II: Discovery, properties, and role in controlling vascular homeostasis. *Semin Thromb Hemost* 37(4):339–348, 2011.

341. Bertina RM, van der Linden IK, Engesser L, et al: Hereditary heparin cofactor II deficiency and the risk of development of thrombosis. *Thromb Haemost* 57(2):196–200, 1987.

342. Corral J, Aznar J, Gonzalez-Conejero R, et al: Homozygous deficiency of heparin cofactor II: Relevance of P17 glutamate residue in serpins, relationship with conformational diseases, and role in thrombosis. *Circulation* 110(10):1303–1307, 2004.

343. Broze GJJ: Protein Z-dependent regulation of coagulation. *Thromb Haemost* 86(1):8–13, 2001.

344. Heeb MJ, Cabral KM, Ruan L: Down-regulation of factor IXa in the factor Xase complex by protein Z-dependent protease inhibitor. *J Biol Chem* 280(40):33819–33825, 2005.

345. Choi Q, Kim JE, Hyun J, et al: Contributions of procoagulants and anticoagulants to the international normalized ratio and thrombin generation assay in patients treated with warfarin: Potential role of protein Z as a powerful determinant of coagulation assays. *Thromb Res* 132(1):e70–e75, 2013.

346. Bolkun L, Galar M, Piszcz J, et al: Plasma concentration of protein Z and protein Z-dependent protease inhibitor in patients with haemophilia A. *Thromb Res* 131(3):e110–e113, 2013.

347. Huang X, Yan Y, Tu Y, et al: Structural basis for catalytic activation of protein Z-dependent protease inhibitor (ZPI) by protein Z. *Blood* 120(8):1726–1733, 2012.

348. Vasse M: The protein Z/protein Z-dependent protease inhibitor complex. Systemic or local control of coagulation? *Hamostaseologie* 31(3):155–158, 160–164, 2011.

349. Huang X, Rezaie AR, Broze GJ Jr, Olson ST: Heparin is a major activator of the anticoagulant serpin, protein Z-dependent protease inhibitor. *J Biol Chem* 286(11):8740–8751, 2011.

350. Sofi F, Cesari F, Abbate R, et al: A meta-analysis of potential risks of low levels of protein Z for diseases related to vascular thrombosis. *Thromb Haemost* 103(4):749–756, 2010.

351. Wei Z, Yan Y, Carrell RW, Zhou A: Crystal structure of protein Z-dependent inhibitor complex shows how protein Z functions as a cofactor in the membrane inhibition of factor X. *Blood* 114(17):3662–3667, 2009.

352. Corral J, Gonzalez-Conejero R, Hernandez-Espinosa D, Vicente V: Protein Z/Z-dependent protease inhibitor (PZ/ZPI) anticoagulant system and thrombosis. *Br J Haematol* 137(2):99–108, 2007.

353. Yin ZF, Huang ZF, Cui JS, et al: Prothrombotic phenotype of protein Z deficiency. *Proc Natl Acad Sci U S A* 97(12):6734–6738, 2000.

354. Kemkes-Matthes B, Nees M, Kuhnel G, et al: Protein Z influences the prothrombotic phenotype in factor V Leiden patients. *Thromb Res* 106(4–5):183–185, 2002.

355. Van de Water N, Tan T, Ashton F, et al: Mutations within the protein Z-dependent protease inhibitor gene are associated with venous thromboembolic disease: A new form of thrombophilia. *Br J Haematol* 127(2):190–194, 2004.

356. Vasse M: Protein Z, a protein seeking a pathology. *Thromb Haemost* 100(4):548–556, 2008.

357. Dentali F, Gianni M, Lussana F, et al: Polymorphisms of the Z protein protease inhibitor and risk of venous thromboembolism: A meta-analysis. *Br J Haematol* 143(2):284–287, 2008.

358. Sofi F, Cesari F, Tu Y, et al: Protein Z-dependent protease inhibitor and protein Z in peripheral arterial disease patients. *J Thromb Haemost* 7(5):731–735, 2009.

359. Rezaie AR, Cooper ST, Church FC, Esmon CT: Protein C inhibitor is a potent inhibitor of the thrombin-thrombomodulin complex. *J Biol Chem* 270(43):25336–25339, 1995.

# CHAPTER 5
# VASCULAR FUNCTION IN HEMOSTASIS

Katherine A. Hajjar, Aaron J. Marcus[1], and William Muller

## SUMMARY

Blood vessels, especially their endothelial lining, play a critical role in the maintenance of vascular fluidity, arrest of hemorrhage (hemostasis), prevention of occlusive vascular phenomena (thrombosis), and regulation of inflammatory cell processes. The endothelium extends to all recesses of the body and maintains an intimate association with flowing blood and blood cells. However, endothelial cell morphologies, gene-expression profiles, and functions vary among different vascular beds. For example, in straight arterial segments, but not at branch points or curvatures of the arteries or veins, endothelial cells align themselves in parallel to the direction of blood flow. Similarly, endothelial cells in postcapillary venules are primarily responsible for mediating adhesion and transmigration of leukocytes, whereas arteriolar endothelium is important for regulation of vasomotor tone. Proteomic studies have revealed that endothelial cells have the unique capacity to express and elaborate thromboregulatory molecules, which can be classified according to their chronologic appearance following vascular injury. Early thromboregulators appear prior to thrombin formation, and late thromboregulators arrive after thrombin has formed. This chapter reviews some of the mechanisms by which the vascular wall regulates hemostasis and discusses their implications for vascular health and disease (Table 5–1).

Acronyms and Abbreviations: APC, activated protein C; Apo, apolipoprotein; APS, antiphospholipid syndrome; C5a, complement factor 5a; CAM, cell adhesion molecule; COX, cyclooxygenase; DAG, diacylglycerol; DDAVP, deamino D-arginine vasopressin; EPCR, endothelial protein C receptor; GMP, guanosine monophosphate; IL, interleukin; $IP_3$, inositol triphosphate; Lp(a), lipoprotein(a); NFκB, nuclear factor kappa B; NO, nitric oxide; NOS, nitric oxide synthase; PAF, platelet-activating factor; PDGF, platelet-derived growth factor; PECAM, platelet endothelial cell adhesion molecule; $PGI_2$, prostacyclin; PGIS, prostacyclin synthase; PSGL, P-selectin glycoprotein ligand; scu-PA, single-chain urokinase-type plasminogen activator; TAFI, thrombin-activatable fibrinolysis inhibitor; TF, tissue factor; TFPI, tissue factor pathway inhibitor; TM, thrombomodulin; TNF, tumor necrosis factor; t-PA, tissue-type plasminogen activator; VWF, von Willebrand factor.

[1]Dr. Aaron Marcus died on May 6, 2015.

## ●VASCULAR FUNCTION IN HEMOSTASIS: INTRODUCTION

The endothelium represents a dynamic interface between flowing blood and the vessel wall and produces a variety of factors that regulate blood fluidity (Fig. 5–1). Endothelial cells are subject to unique shear stress forces, to soluble factors in the blood, and to signals emanating from cells in the circulation, vascular wall, and tissues, all of which create region-specific phenotypes.[1–3] In addition to modulating vascular permeability and fragility, the endothelium regulates the fluid state of blood through its thromboresistant nature, profibrinolytic properties, and antiinflammatory potential. These activities maintain vascular patency.[4]

### ENDOTHELIAL CELL HETEROGENEITY

The heterogeneity of endothelial cells is mediated by two mechanisms.[5,6] First, extracellular biochemical and biomechanical signals trigger posttranscriptional and/or posttranslational changes that vary across the vascular tree. Second, certain site-specific properties of the endothelium are genetically programmed, and therefore, independent of the extracellular milieu. This phenotypic variability serves at least two important purposes: (1) It allows endothelial cells to meet the specific metabolic needs of the surrounding tissue. For example, the tight junctions of the blood–brain barrier protect neurons from fluctuations in composition of the aqueous blood supply, whereas the fenestrated discontinuous endothelium of hepatic sinusoids allows ready access of nutrient-rich portal venous blood for the metabolic systems in hepatocytes; and (2) phenotypic variability provides endothelial cells with site-specific mechanisms for thriving within many different microenvironments. For example, endothelial cells in the inner medulla of the kidney must survive the relatively hypoxic and hyperosmolar local environment, whereas endothelial cells in the pulmonary capillary bed have adapted to an oxygen-rich environment.

A rapid endothelial cell response is required for sudden environmental perturbations. Translational control mechanisms, which are more immediate than transcriptional changes, provide regulatory responses for up to 10 percent of genes expressed in endothelial cells.[7] Because of their close association with both flowing blood and solid tissues, endothelial cells are subject to a broad spectrum of agonistic and inhibitory external signals that frequently require rapid functional and phenotypic responses. Clinically, such stimuli are associated with sepsis, inflammation, ischemia–reperfusion injury, and direct mechanical vascular trauma induced clinically by stents, balloon catheters, and graft procedures.

### ENDOTHELIAL PRODUCTION OF THROMBOREGULATORY MOLECULES

Thromboregulatory compounds, such as eicosanoids, nitric oxide, and the ecto-ATP/Dase-1/CD39, control platelet and vascular reactivity during the early stages of thrombus formation (Table 5–2).[8] Eicosanoids are hydrocarbon compounds derived from essential fatty acids in the diet. The most important endothelial eicosanoid is prostacyclin ($PGI_2$), which blocks platelet reactivity, induces vascular relaxation, and stimulates cytokine production.[9] Nitric oxide (NO) is a naturally occurring gas released from vascular endothelial cells in response to binding of vasodilators to endothelial cell membrane receptors. Thus, it is a short-lived vasodilator and inhibitor of platelet reactivity.

**TABLE 5–1.** Chronology of Endothelial Cell Thromboregulators

Early thromboregulators
  Nitric oxide (NO)
  Eicosanoids (prostacyclin and prostaglandin D$_2$)
  Endothelial cell CD39/ENTPDase1
  Endothelin
Late thromboregulators
  Endothelin
  Antithrombin
  Endothelial cell/heparin proteoglycans
  Tissue factor pathway inhibitor
  Thrombomodulin–protein C–protein S pathway
  Fibrinolytic system (plasminogen activators, inhibitors, and receptors)
  Inflammatory thromboregulators
  Thrombomodulin–protein C–protein S pathway
  Cellular adhesion molecules
  Selectins

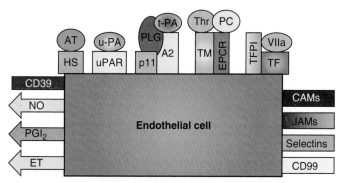

**Figure 5–1.** Schematic of endothelial cell thromboregulatory molecules. Products that are secreted and exert their effects in the fluid phase are represented by *arrows*. Cell-surface–associated molecules are shown as *rectangles*. Metabolites synthesized by endothelial cells are indicated. Thromboregulators that modulate platelet activation, recruitment, and blood vessel contractility are shown on the *left*. Agents that regulate components of the coagulation cascade and/or fibrinolytic system are located at the *top*. Inflammatory molecules whose expression or activity is directed by inflammatory mediators are shown at the *right*. A2, annexin 2; AT, antithrombin; CAMs, cellular adhesion molecules; CD39, endothelial cell ecto-ADPase/CD39; EPCR, endothelial cell protein C receptor; ET, endothelin; FVIIa, factor VIIa; HS, heparan sulfate; JAMs, junctional adhesion molecules; NO, nitric oxide; PC, protein C; PGI$_2$, prostacyclin; PLG, plasminogen; TF, tissue factor; TFPI, tissue factor pathway inhibitor; TM, thrombomodulin; t-PA, tissue plasminogen activator; u-PA, urokinase plasminogen activator; uPAR, urokinase plasminogen activator receptor. These components are discussed further in the text.

By activating guanylate cyclase, the resulting increase in cyclic guanylate monophosphate (GMP) inhibits platelet function and induces vascular relaxation.[10,11] Endothelial cell ecto-ATP/Dase-1/CD39 is a membrane-associated apyrase that metabolizes adenosine diphosphate (ADP) in the primary platelet releasate, preventing further platelet activation and recruitment.[12,13]

Late thromboregulators produced by endothelial cells act either to prevent excessive thrombin generation or to promote lysis of intravascular thrombi (see Table 5–1). Antithrombin, a natural anticoagulant, acts as an inhibitor of thrombin and factor Xa in the circulation. Endothelial cell heparan proteoglycans act as cofactors for antithrombin. The tissue factor pathway inhibitor (TFPI) inhibits the complex between factor VIIa and tissue factor (TF). The thrombomodulin/endothelial cell protein C receptor (EPCR)/protein C system in the vascular wall regulates hemostasis through inactivation of procoagulant cofactors and antiinflammatory activity.[14] The fibrinolytic system is intimately involved with the vascular endothelium because endothelial cells not only synthesize and secrete tissue plasminogen activator (t-PA), but also regulate formation of plasmin from its precursor, plasminogen, through the expression of receptors.[15] Impairment of fibrinolytic potential can play a central role in the etiology of occlusive vascular disease.[16] Finally, endothelial cell adhesion molecules, including the cell adhesion molecules (CAMs: mucosal addressin cell adhesion molecule [MAdCAM]-1, intercellular adhesion molecule [ICAM]-1, vascular cell adhesion molecule [VCAM]-1, and platelet endothelial cell adhesion molecule [PECAM]-1) and the selectins (P- and E-selectin), are glycoproteins that modulate multiple interactions between the endothelium and various classes of circulating leukocytes, thereby modulating vascular patency.[17] Together, these mechanisms define *thromboregulation*, the processes by which blood cells and cells of the vessel wall, through their close proximity, interact to facilitate or inhibit thrombus formation.[18]

The physiologic defense systems that render endothelial surfaces and blood cells antithrombotic can be overwhelmed by excessive shear stress, increased turbulence, injury, inflammation, and severe atherosclerosis.[19] These events transform the endothelial cells into a prothrombotic and antifibrinolytic phenotype,[20] which is accompanied by upregulation of leukocyte and endothelial CAMs, increased expression of TF, and accumulation of monocytes/macrophages in the vessel wall.[21] These events commonly occur at the site of fissured atherosclerotic plaques in the coronary and cerebrovascular circulation.[22] Because the eicosanoids such as PGI$_2$ (prostaglandin [PG]I$_2$), as well as NO, and the ecto-ATP/Dase-1/CD39 group reach peak activity very early in the hemostatic/thrombotic cascade (Figs. 5–2 to 5–4), they represent potential targets for therapeutic intervention in the sequence of events beginning with platelet activation, and leading to coagulation, thrombosis, and atherogenesis.[21,22] Finally, functional and physical contacts between platelets and endothelial cells are of critical importance for the maintenance of vascular integrity and cell permeability.[1,23]

**TABLE 5–2.** Early Pro- and Antithrombotic Thromboregulators Associated with Human Endothelial Cells

| Class | Type | Site of Action | Aspirin Sensitivity | Mode of Action |
|---|---|---|---|---|
| Eicosanoids | PGI$_2$, PGD$_2$ | Fluid phase autacoid | Sensitive | Elevation of platelet cAMP |
| Nitrovasodilators | EDRF/NO | Fluid phase autacoid | Insensitive | Elevation of platelet cGMP |
| Ectonucleotidases | CD39/ENTPD1 | Endothelial cell surface | Insensitive | Enzymatic removal of secreted ADP |
| Thromboxane | TXA$_2$ | Fluid phase vasoconstrictor | Sensitive | Lowers platelet cAMP and platelet agonist |
| Endothelins | ET-1, ET-2 | Fluid phase vasoconstrictor | Insensitive | Direct vasoconstrictor peptide |

ADP, adenosine diphosphate; cAMP, cyclic adenosine monophosphate; cGMP, cyclic guanosine monophosphate; EDRF, endothelium-derived relaxing factor; ET, endothelin; NO, nitric oxide; PGD$_2$, prostaglandin D$_2$; PGI$_2$, prostacyclin; TXA$_2$, thromboxane A$_2$.

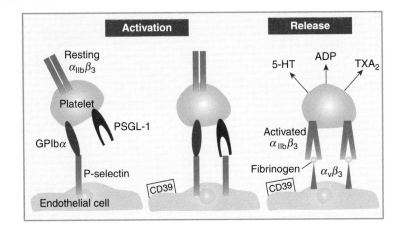

**Figure 5–2.** Following injury to the blood vessel wall, platelets adhere to the damaged surface of the endothelial cell. Concomitant with adhesion, platelets and endothelial cells become activated. P-selectin is expressed on the endothelial cell surface. Platelet surface receptors glycosylphosphatidylinositol (GPI)ba and P-selectin glycoprotein ligand (PSGL)-1 interact with endothelial P-selectin, thereby mediating platelet rolling. Firm adhesion is mediated by the integrin $\alpha_{IIb}\beta_3$. In parallel with these intercellular events, platelet activation and release occur. The enzyme CD39 on the endothelial surface modulates the ambient concentration of adenosine diphosphate (ADP) by metabolizing it.[7,8] 5-HT, 5-hydroxytryptamine; TXA$_2$, thromboxane A$_2$. *(Adapted with permission from Gawaz M, Langer H, May AE: Platelets in inflammation and atherogenesis, J Clin Invest. 2005 Dec;115(12):3378–3384.)*

# ●THE EICOSANOID PATHWAY IN BIOLOGY AND MEDICINE: CELL–CELL INTERACTIONS AND TRANSCELLULAR METABOLISM

Dietary fatty acids give rise to arachidonic acid, the starting point for synthesis of other eicosanoids. Originating from different cells, intermediates in the arachidonic acid pathway can interact with each other to produce new products with new biologic activities. Oxygenation and further enzymatic transformation of arachidonic acid give rise to eicosanoids (formerly classified as PGs) and hydroxy acids, such as the leukotrienes. Eicosanoids are autocoids, an important group of transient, physiologically active endogenous substances, that act within the immediate environment of the cell, where they promote or inhibit a biologic function.[24] These autacoids have a very short life span and may act within a few seconds, a phenomenon that is clinically important but difficult to study experimentally.

In 1975, Hamberg and colleagues discovered that a new eicosanoid, PGI$_2$, was derived from arachidonic acid in endothelial cells.[25] Soon thereafter, Moncada realized that the effects of PGI$_2$ opposed those of

thromboxane, namely vasodilation and inhibition of platelet aggregation.[26,27] The biologic half-life of PGI$_2$ was found to be 10 to 20 seconds. In addition, it was determined that the first step in arachidonic acid oxidation and conversion, which is carried out by cyclooxygenase (COX)-1, is inhibited by aspirin (acetylsalicylic acid), which donates an acetyl group that inactivates COX-1 and inhibits platelet function.[28]

## BIOSYNTHESIS OF PROSTACYCLIN IN ENDOTHELIAL CELLS

PGI$_2$ is the major and most important eicosanoid produced by endothelial cells. A broad range of stimuli, including hormones, biochemicals, or physical forces such as shear stress, can elicit release of PGI$_2$. Kinetic studies revealed two distinct patterns of PGI$_2$ production: (1) rapid release, independent of new COX-1 mRNA or protein synthesis, and (2) slower production reflecting increased COX-2 expression.

In the case of rapid stimulation of PGI$_2$ production, as induced by thrombin, histamine, bradykinin, and ionophore, the response plateaus at 10 minutes.[29] These agonists activate phospholipase C, which generates inositol trisphosphate (IP$_3$) and diacylglycerol (DAG). The released IP$_3$ induces an elevation of intracellular calcium, which translocates phospholipase A to the outer portion of the nuclear envelope and

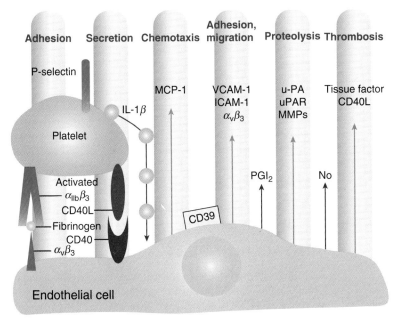

**Figure 5–3.** Adherent activated platelets induce an inflammatory response in endothelial cells. Platelet adhesion involving $\alpha_{IIb}\beta_3$ induces exposure of P-selectin (CD62P) and release of platelet CD40 ligand (CD40L) and interleukin (IL)-1$\beta$ which then stimulate endothelial cells to respond with an inflammatory reaction that supports prothrombotic and proatherogenic alterations in the endothelium. IL-8 and MCP-1 (monocyte chemoattractant protein-1) are the principal chemoattractants for neutrophils and monocytes. ICAM, intercellular adhesion molecule; MMP, matrix metalloproteinase; u-PA, urokinase plasminogen activator; uPAR, urokinase plasminogen activator receptor; VCAM, vascular cell adhesion molecule. *(Adapted with permission from Gawaz M, Langer H, May AE: Platelets in inflammation and atherogenesis, J Clin Invest. 2005 Dec;115(12):3378–3384.)*

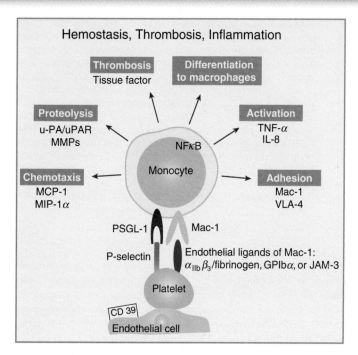

**Figure 5–4.** Adherent/activated platelets promote an inflammatory response in monocytes. The platelets mainly interact with monocyte P-selectin glycoprotein ligand (PSGL)-1 via P-selectin and with monocyte Mac-1 ($\alpha_M\beta_2$) via $\alpha_{IIb}\beta_3$ (and fibrinogen bridging) or glycosylphosphatidylinositol (GPI)b$\alpha$. Through this mechanism, platelets initiate monocyte secretion of chemokines, cytokines, and procoagulant tissue factor. These serve to upregulate and activate adhesion receptors and proteases. In parallel, they induce monocyte differentiation into macrophages. Therefore, platelet–monocyte interactions provide a prothrombotic and atherogenic milieu at the vascular wall, which can eventually support plaque formation. IL, interleukin; JAM, junctional adhesion molecule; MCP, monocyte chemoattractant protein; MIP, macrophage inhibitory protein; MMP, matrix metalloproteinase; NF$\kappa$B, nuclear factor kappa B; u-PA, urokinase plasminogen activator; uPAR, urokinase plasminogen activator receptor; TNF, tumor necrosis factor; VLA, very late antigen. *(Adapted with permission from Gawaz M, Langer H, May AE: Platelets in inflammation and atherogenesis, J Clin Invest. 2005 Dec;115(12):3378–3384.)*

endoplasmic reticulum. Phospholipase A then couples functionally to COX-1, which is located on the luminal membrane. Prostacyclin synthase (PGIS) colocalizes with COX-1 in endothelial cells. Activated phospholipase A2 (cPLA2) catalyzes the release of arachidonic acid from membrane phospholipids, and the free arachidonate interacts with COX-1 and is converted to the endoperoxide $PGH_2$. PGIS converts prostaglandin $H_2$ ($PGH_2$) to $PGI_2$. The half-life of COX-1 is approximately 10 minutes, whereupon it autoinactivates.

Stimulation of $PGI_2$ production by proinflammatory cytokines and growth factors, such as lipopolysaccharide (LPS), interleukin (IL)-1$\beta$, tumor necrosis factor (TNF)-$\alpha$, and platelet-derived growth factor (PDGF), is a slower, more sustained process.[29] In response to these agonists, $PGI_2$ production occurs within 30 to 60 minutes and parallels the time course of production induced by COX-2, but not COX-1.

## THE TWO ISOFORMS OF PROSTACYCLIN G/H SYNTHASE

The recognition that there was a constitutive and an inducible cyclooxygenase (COX-1 and COX-2, respectively) was a major advance.[30] Cloning studies of an immediate to early response gene from 3T3 fibroblasts revealed that the COX-2 complementary DNA was highly homologous

to that of COX-1.[30-34] COX-2 is inducible in endothelial cells by prothrombotic, inflammatory, or mitogenic stimuli and in neutrophils by inflammatory stimuli.[35,36]

Within a specific species, there is approximately 60 percent homology between deduced amino acid sequences of COX-1 (576 residues) and COX-2 (587 residues). The C-terminal sequence of 18 amino acids in COX-2 is absent in COX-1. Therefore, antibodies directed at this C-terminal sequence can identify COX-2 in tissues by immunoblot. The catalytic activity of both COX enzymes is similar, and all amino acids critical for COX-1 activity are conserved in COX-2. The active site in COX-1 is slightly larger than that of COX-2, a fact that has impacted design of COX inhibitors. COX-2 contains mannose, and an *N*-glycosylation site within the 18-amino-acid C-terminal sequence. An *N*-glycosylation site at Asn410 is required for COX-1 to fold into its active conformation.

The gene for COX-1 is located on chromosome 9 and spans 22 kb of genomic DNA, while the gene for COX-2 is located on chromosome 1 and spans 8 kb of DNA. Transcription of COX-2 proceeds via several signaling mechanisms initiated by cyclic adenosine monophosphate (cAMP)/ protein kinase A, protein kinase C, tyrosine kinases, and pathways activated by growth factors, endotoxin, and cytokines.[33,37-39] The discoveries of COX-1 and COX-2 were of great importance and have led to new concepts concerning the structure and function of COX-induced autacoids.[40]

## PROSTACYCLIN AS AN AUTACOID

$PGI_2$ is released from stimulated endothelial cells by a broad range of agonists and plays a critical role in the maintenance of vascular integrity by promoting thromboresistance and inhibiting inflammatory responses in the vasculature. Production of $PGI_2$ is dynamically regulated to meet the challenges arising from frequent prothrombotic and proinflammatory events.[29] As an autacoid, $PGI_2$ has a half-life of 3 minutes, whereupon it undergoes chemical hydrolysis to 6-keto-$PGF_1\alpha$. It acts on the type I platelet PG receptor (IP) by increasing cAMP levels in a paracrine manner.[41] IP is a seven-transmembrane, G-protein– and adenylyl cyclase–coupled receptor. The latter binds to and activates protein kinase A (PKA), resulting in inhibition of platelet activation and recruitment.[42] Physical or chemical perturbation of endothelial cells results in enhanced $PGI_2$ production, which increases platelet cAMP resulting in abolition of platelet shape change, inhibition of platelet secretion and recruitment, and impaired binding of von Willebrand factor (VWF) and fibrinogen to the platelet surface. $PGI_2$ also inhibits platelet adhesion to subendothelium, especially at high shear rates.[43]

The discovery of $PGI_2$ revealed that the vascular endothelium had a protective effect on blood fluidity.[2,8] It also meant that $PGI_2$ released from endothelial cells could counteract the effect of excessive thromboxane formation. In addition, it was appreciated that intermediates in the synthesis of $PGI_2$ from arachidonic acid could interact with other cells and tissues. Thus, $PGI_2$ could be synthesized from platelet-derived endoperoxides by cultured human endothelial cells.[44] Because of a low threshold for toxicity (hypotension and diarrhea), $PGI_2$ does not display a satisfactory therapeutic window. An interesting compendium of eicosanoid-related disorders is described in a review on eicosanoids in health and disease.[45]

## ● NITRIC OXIDE: AN ENDOTHELIAL VASODILATOR AND INHIBITOR OF PLATELET ACTIVATION AND RECRUITMENT

In vascular endothelial cells, NO synthase (NOS) catalyzes formation of NO from L-arginine, in the presence of nicotinamide adenine dinucleotide phosphate (NADPH) and oxygen.[46] The L-arginine is subsequently converted to citrulline and NO. The endothelial cell isoform of NO synthase (eNOS or the *NOS3* gene product) functions constitutively and is further activated by receptor agonists that elevate intracellular calcium. Major stimuli include ADP, thrombin, bradykinin, and shear stress.[43] Shear forces induce transcriptional activation of the eNOS gene because its promoter contains a shear response consensus sequence (GAGACC). The NO that forms activates guanylate cyclase, thereby generating cyclic GMP. NO becomes oxidized to nitrite and then to nitrate, which is measurable in blood samples. NO in the circulation is rapidly inactivated by erythrocytes.[11,47,48] NO has a vasodilatory effect on the pulmonary vasculature, and, in patients with congestive heart failure, its inhalation decreases pulmonary hypertension and increases pulmonary ventilation.[10,11,47-54] Acetylcholine released by activated nerve terminals in the vessel wall activate the endothelial cell to produce and release NO. This NO effect also explains the action of nitroglycerin, which has long been used to treat patients with angina resulting from coronary artery disease.[54]

Importantly, production of NO by endothelial cells is impaired in the presence of the thiol-containing amino acid, homocysteine. Cynomolgus monkeys with diet-induced hyperhomocysteinemia demonstrated reduced blood flow in the lower extremity and an impaired response to endothelial cell–dependent vasodilators.[51] Similarly, production of NO by endothelial cells *in vitro* is significantly inhibited in the presence of homocysteine, possibly by a mechanism involving impairment of the enzyme glutathione peroxidase.[52,53]

## STRUCTURE AND BIOCHEMICAL PROPERTIES OF NITRIC OXIDE SYNTHASE

There are two isoforms of NOS, the constitutive form (eNOS), synthesized by the endothelial cell and regulated by $Ca^{2+}$ and calmodulin, and the cytokine-inducible, posttranscriptionally regulated form (iNOS).[47] Both constitutive and inducible forms are mainly cytosolic, although a membrane-bound constitutive NOS isoform containing a myristoylation consensus sequence has been isolated from bovine aortic endothelial cells.[43] eNOS has a molecular mass of 144 kDa and shares 57 percent amino acid sequence identity with neuronal NOS. The cofactor (6R-tetrahydro-L-biopterin [$H_4B$]) participates in inducible and constitutive NOS isoform reactions. It is thought that $H_4B$ stabilizes the enzyme in a manner allowing for maximum activity of the NOS subunit to which the pterin binds.[10,11,47,54]

## BLOCKADE OF PLATELET AGGREGATION AND SECRETION BY NITRIC OXIDE

Platelet activation and recruitment in response to all agonists, such as ADP, collagen, epinephrine, and thrombin, are blocked by NO. Blockade also occurs *in vivo* via formation of NO from endothelium.[10] Importantly, the inhibitory action of NO is not affected by aspirin either *in vivo* or *ex vivo*. Therefore, NO production is not caused by participation of endothelial cell eicosanoids.

In addition to eNOS, the *NOS3* gene product, endothelial cells stimulated by agonists such as cytokines express the inducible form of NO synthase, iNOS, the *NOS2* gene product. Through this mechanism, NO can further inhibit platelet reactivity and reduce basal vessel tone by inducing relaxation of vascular smooth muscle. The biochemical basis for the reaction is that NO binds to the heme prosthetic group of guanylyl cyclase. The inhibitory effect of NO on platelet activation can be monitored by measuring surface expression of P-selectin. The ability of NO to inhibit mobilization of intracellular platelet calcium results in reduction of the conformational changes in platelet membrane glycoprotein (GP)IIb/IIIa, an absolute requirement for fibrinogen binding

and subsequent platelet aggregation. There is a broad spectrum of other effects of NO, including inhibition of leukocyte adhesion to endothelial cell surfaces, inhibition of smooth muscle migration, and reduction of smooth muscle cell proliferation. These phenomena suggest that secretion of NO into the microenvironment is a major component of the response to vascular injury.[43]

## ● INHIBITION OF PLATELET ACTIVATION AND RECRUITMENT BY ECTO-ATP/DASE-1/CD39

In addition to the platelet inhibition by $PGI_2$ and NO, endothelial cells inhibit platelet function via the action of endothelial cell ecto-ATP/Dase-1/CD39, an ecto-apyrase with ADPase and adenosine triphosphatase (ATPase) activities. The cluster designation symbol for this compound is CD39, the product of *ENTPD1*, the ectonucleotide triphosphate diphosphohydrolase gene.[55] CD39 is localized mainly in endothelial cells and leukocytes. In endothelial cells, CD39 is located on the cell surface with the major portion of the molecule facing the vessel lumen.[12,13,56] The enzyme has both N- and C-terminal transmembrane regions with small cytosolic portions anchoring the molecule.[57] In addition to CD39, CD73 (5'-nucleotidase) is present on vascular cells and converts the adenosine monophosphate (AMP) generated from CD39 metabolism to adenosine (Fig. 5–5). In contrast to all other known platelet inhibitors, acting in concert with CD73, CD39 can convert the local environment from a prothrombotic ADP/ATP-rich entity to an antithrombotic adenosine-rich environment.[58] This phenomenon was evident from observations that platelets became unresponsive to all agonists when in motion or in proximity to endothelial cells, even when eicosanoid and NO production were blocked.[2] Importantly, CD39 and CD73 do not exert their action on the platelet *per se* but act in series to metabolize ATP and ADP secreted from activated platelets to AMP and hence to adenosine.[13,59] ADP released from activated platelets is metabolized by CD39, thereby inhibiting ADP-induced platelet activation, release, and aggregation (Fig. 5–5).

Most platelet agonists initiate secretion of dense granule contents within 15 to 20 seconds. The enhanced metabolism of ATP and ADP by therapeutically administered soluble CD39 would also reduce secondary autoamplification and recruitment and, consequently, thrombus formation.[9,27,60] Because CD39 and CD73 are probably acting together, they will theoretically increase levels of endogenous adenosine and elevate the threshold for platelet activation in the local microenvironment. In a murine model, soluble CD39 administration ameliorates the extent of stroke and reverses excessive platelet reactivity without bleeding complications, even if administered 3 hours following stroke induction.[61] Therapeutic benefit of soluble CD39 has also been demonstrated in animal models of cardiac ischemia,[62] in the development of atherosclerosis,[63] in regulation of leukocyte proinflammatory activity,[64] in inhibition of metastasis,[65] and in transplantation medicine.[66] That the preclinical therapeutic use of soluble CD39 could abrogate thrombosis without inducing the hemorrhage seen with the use of existing antiplatelet therapies[67] could provide a therapeutic advantage over existing therapies for thrombotic disorders, including those that are resistant to existing therapeutic paradigms.[9] CD39 represents a major control system for blood fluidity.[68]

## ● THE PROTEIN C PATHWAY

The protein C pathway[69] plays a critical role in the prevention of thrombosis and is an integral part of the host inflammatory response. This pathway is initiated on the endothelial cell surface when thrombin

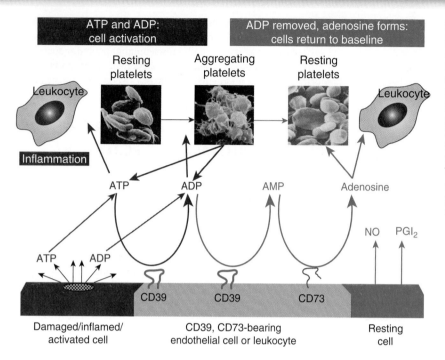

**Figure 5–5.** Released platelet adenosine diphosphate (ADP) is a major control system for hemostasis: ADP → adenosine monophosphate (AMP) → adenosine. Perturbation of endothelial cells, as a consequence of vascular injury, initiates the release of newly synthesized prostacyclin as well as nitric oxide, both of which inhibit platelet reactivity in the fluid phase. The apyrase CD39 is a cell-associated inhibitory thromboregulator. CD39 is substrate activated, and in concert with CD39, CD73 brings the reaction to completion with the formation of adenosine.[309,310] The early metabolic deletion of ADP from the system may serve as a biologic safeguard to avoid excessive platelet accumulation, which would result in thrombosis.[21,22,309,310] NO, nitric oxide; PGI$_2$, prostacyclin.

combines with the endothelial receptor protein thrombomodulin (TM). Although thrombin is capable of slowly activating protein C, this reaction is markedly inhibited in the presence of physiologic concentrations of calcium ions. Upon binding of thrombin to TM, the rate of protein C activation is dramatically enhanced and becomes dependent on the presence of calcium. The detailed biochemistry of this activation reaction has been reviewed elsewhere.[70] Another protein found predominantly in large vessels, the EPCR, can bind protein C and further augment its activation by the thrombin–TM complex.[70] Activated protein C (APC) can dissociate from EPCR and interact with protein S on either the endothelial cell or other membrane surface to exert its anticoagulant function. The function of APC can be found in several reviews.[14,71–73]

By far, the best known function of TM is its role in protein C activation. When thrombin is bound to TM, it is no longer able to clot fibrinogen, activate platelets, activate factors V and VIII,[74] or interact with the protease-activated receptors.[75,76] Instead, thrombin–TM acts as a direct anticoagulant. TM also promotes the activation by thrombin of the plasma thrombin-activatable fibrinolysis inhibitor (TAFI).[77] TAFI inhibits plasmin-mediated fibrinolysis by removing carboxy-terminal lysine residues from fibrin, thereby reducing available binding sites for plasminogen and t-PA. In addition, TAFI is the major enzyme responsible for the removal of a C-terminal arginine from complement factor 5a (C5a),[78,79] leading to the inactivation of this potent anaphylotoxin generated during complement activation. Other vasoactive substances may also be inactivated by this enzyme. TM also accelerates the proteolytic inactivation of prourokinase (also called single-chain urokinase-type plasminogen activator [scu-PA]) by thrombin,[80,81] which may affect both fibrinolysis and tissue remodeling.[82] Despite these antifibrinolytic effects of TM, many in vivo experiments have demonstrated that soluble TM infusion results in a net antithrombotic and/or antiinflammatory effect.[83]

Independent of its effect on hemostasis, TM is essential to normal fetal development. When the TM gene is deleted by homologous recombination in mice, embryos die on day 8.5, prior to the development of a functional cardiovascular system,[84] implying that TM has functions in addition to its anticoagulant and antifibrinolytic properties. Both TM[85]

and EPCR[86] are highly expressed on the giant trophoblast cells of the placenta. If TM expression is maintained on these cells, the TM-null embryos survive past this blockade point.[87,88]

The EPCR is a 220-amino-acid, type 1 transmembrane protein.[89–92] EPCR has two extracellular domains that show structural homology with the α and β domains of major histocompatibility complex (MHC) class I molecules, most notably the CD1d family. Because there are three Cys residues in the extracellular domain, the possibility of crosslinking with another protein exists. The cytoplasmic domain of human EPCR is only three amino acids long, Arg-Arg-Cys. The terminal Cys can be acylated with palmitate, which may have functional consequences.[93] Both protein C and APC bind to EPCR with similar affinity, approximately 30 nM.[89] Binding requires the presence of calcium and is enhanced in the presence of magnesium ions. In addition, a soluble form of EPCR found normally in plasma[94] is also capable of binding both protein C and APC with equivalent affinity.

EPCR augments protein C activation by the thrombin–TM complex in vitro and in vivo, primarily by decreasing the $K_m$ (Michaelis-Menten dissociation constant) for protein C.[70,95,96] Just as thrombin changes its function from procoagulant to anticoagulant when it binds to TM, it appears that APC bound to EPCR undergoes a similar switch from anticoagulant to antiinflammatory molecule.[97,98] Unfortunately, however, early studies that suggested a possible therapeutic role for APC in human sepsis have not been borne out in clinical trials.[99] Deletion of the EPCR gene by homologous recombination leads to early embryonic lethality around day 9.5,[100] at which time EPCR is highly expressed in the giant trophoblasts of the placenta, but not in the embryo itself.[86] In contrast to TM knockout animals,[101] the placentas of EPCR knockout embryos show significant fibrin deposition at the fetal–maternal interface.

# ● VASCULAR FIBRINOLYSIS

Plasmin, the major clot-dissolving protease in humans, is formed upon the cleavage of a single peptide bond within the zymogen plasminogen (Chap. 25). This tightly regulated reaction is strongly influenced by cells of the blood vessel wall, including endothelial cells, smooth muscles cells, and macrophages, which express plasminogen activators, plasminogen activator inhibitors, and fibrinolytic receptors.

## ENDOTHELIAL CELL PRODUCTION OF FIBRINOLYTIC PROTEINS

In 1958, Todd demonstrated that human blood vessels possess fibrinolytic activity that is dependent upon an intact endothelium.[102,103] We now know that the endothelium is the principal source of t-PA *in vivo* where it appears to be highly restricted to small blood vessels in specific anatomic locations, a pattern that likely reflects the heterogeneity of endothelial cells as they respond to a myriad of tissue-specific cues.[104,105] In the baboon, for example, sites of t-PA production include 7- to 30-$\mu$m precapillary arterioles and postcapillary venules, but not large arteries and veins.[106] In the mouse lung, similarly, bronchial, but not pulmonary, endothelial cells express t-PA.[107] Moreover, enhanced expression of t-PA at branch points of pulmonary blood vessels may reflect stimulation by laminar shear stress.[108] In addition, peripheral sympathetic neurons that invest the walls of small arteries may represent a significant source of circulating t-PA.[109]

Although *in vitro* studies suggest that t-PA expression in cultured endothelial cells is regulated by a wide array of factors, only a few of these pathways have been confirmed *in vivo*. Thrombin,[110] histamine,[111,112] oxygen radicals,[113] phorbol myristate acetate,[114] DDAVP (deamino D-arginine vasopressin),[115] and butyric acid liberated from dibutyryl cAMP[116] all increase t-PA mRNA in cultured endothelial cells. Both thrombin and histamine appear to act via receptor-mediated activation of the protein kinase C pathway.[105] Laminar shear stress stimulates both t-PA secretion[117] and steady-state mRNA levels.[118] Hyperosmotic stress and repetitive stretch also enhance t-PA expression.[119,120] In addition, differentiating agents, such as retinoids,[121,122] stimulate transcription of t-PA in endothelial cells *in vitro*.

*In vivo*, the circulating half-life of t-PA is approximately 5 minutes. Infusion of DDAVP, bradykinin, platelet-activating factor (PAF), endothelin, or thrombin is associated with an acute release of t-PA, and a burst of fibrinolytic activity can be detected within minutes.[123] In the mouse lung, exposure to hyperoxia leads to 4.5-fold upregulation of t-PA mRNA in small-vessel endothelial cells.[107] In humans, infusion of TNF into patients with malignancy is associated with an increase in plasma t-PA.[123] Deficient release of t-PA in response to venous occlusion in humans is associated with deep venous thrombosis,[124] as well as atrophie blanche and other cutaneous vasculitides.[125]

*In vivo*, urokinase plasminogen activator (u-PA) is not a product of resting endothelium,[126] but is produced primarily by renal tubular epithelium.[127] Expression of u-PA mRNA in endothelium, however, is strongly stimulated during wound repair and physiologic angiogenesis within ovarian follicles, corpus luteum, and maternal decidua.[128] Endothelial cells passaged in culture do synthesize u-PA,[129] and expression of its mRNA is stimulated by TNF-$\alpha$ by 5- to 30-fold.[130] Small increases in u-PA have also been observed *in vitro* in response to IL-1 and LPS.[131–133]

The association of u-PA with the blood vessel wall appears to reflect its association with the u-PA receptor (uPAR), which may fulfill a variety of nonproteolytic functions ranging from directed cell migration to cellular adhesion, differentiation, and proliferation (Fig. 5–6).[134] In the adult mouse, uPAR mRNA is not normally detected by *in situ* hybridization in the endothelium of either large or small blood vessels.[135] However, upon stimulation with endotoxin, expression is detected in endothelium lining aorta, as well as arteries, veins, and capillaries in heart, kidney, brain, and liver,[135] and in renal tubular epithelial cells.[127]

Plasminogen activator inhibitor (PAI)-1 is likely to function as a major regulator of plasmin generation in the vicinity of the endothelial cell. Thrombin, IL-1, transforming growth factor $\beta$, TNF, lipoprotein(a) (Lp[a]), and LPS all induce dramatic increases in steady-state PAI-1 message levels.[110,131,132,136,137] Heparin-binding growth factor 1 reduces

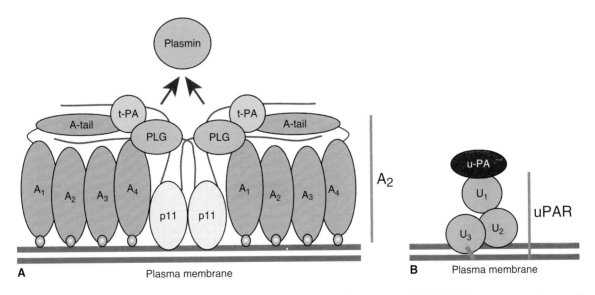

**Figure 5–6.** Schematic of principal endothelial cell fibrinolytic receptors. **A.** The annexin A2/S100A10 heterotetrameric complex. Annexin A2 consists of a hydrophilic aminoterminal tail domain (A-Tail, approximately 3 kDa) and a membrane-oriented carboxyl terminal core domain (approximately 33 kDa).[311,312] The tail domain contains residues required for tissue-type plasminogen activator (t-PA) binding. The core domain is composed of four homologous annexin repeats (A1, A2, A3, and A4), each consisting of five *a*-helical regions that contribute to calcium-dependent phospholipid binding sites. Repeat 2 appears to be most important for the interaction of annexin A2 with the endothelial cell surface. Plasminogen (PLG) binding requires lysine residue 307 within helix C of repeat 4. **B.** Urokinase plasminogen activator receptor (uPAR) is a 55- to 60-kDa, glycosylphosphatidylinositol-linked protein that consists of three disulfide-linked domains (U1, U2, U3).[313] Domain 1 contains sequences required for urokinase plasminogen activator (u-PA) binding, while domains 2 and 3 mediate the receptor's interaction with matrix proteins such as vitronectin. Domain 3 contains glycosylphosphatidylinositol-linked membrane anchor. *(A, adapted with permission from Gerke V, Creutz CE, Moss SE: Annexins: linking Ca2+ signalling to membrane dynamics,* Nat Rev Mol Cell Biol. 2005 Jun;6(6):449–461.)

PAI-1 mRNA production by cultured endothelial cells but has no effect on t-PA.[138] Thus, synthesis and secretion of PAI-1 by the endothelial cell *in vitro* appear to be regulated independently of t-PA.

*In vivo*, elevated levels of circulating PAI-1 have been linked epidemiologically to risk for myocardial infarction.[124] Although the liver is the major source of plasma PAI-1, endothelial expression of PAI-1 is detected near neovascular sprouts during decidual neovascularization in the ovary.[128] In addition, inflammatory cytokines are powerful stimuli for induction of PAI-1 in a variety of tissues including liver, as injection of TNF in both rats and humans with active malignancy results in a striking increase in plasma concentrations of PAI-1.[105,123]

The endothelial cell coreceptor for t-PA and plasminogen, the annexin A2/S100A10 complex (see Fig. 5–6), appears to be expressed constitutively *in vivo* by endothelial cells in a wide variety of tissues in the chicken,[139] mouse,[140] rat,[141] and human.[142] Annexin A2 is upregulated transcriptionally by hypoxia both *in vivo* and in endothelial cells *in vitro*,[143] and by nerve growth factor in neuronal-like PC12 cells.[144] In addition, the *in vitro* transition of human monocyte to macrophage is associated with a several-fold increase in both annexin A2 protein and steady-state mRNA expression.[145]

The evidence that the annexin A2 system plays a role in maintaining vascular patency includes the findings that (1) overexpression of annexin A2 in blast cells in acute promyelocytic leukemia blast cells increases plasmin production and contributes to hyperfibrinolytic bleeding,[146–149] (2) systemic injection of annexin A2 diminishes thrombotic vascular occlusion resulting from vascular injury in experimental animals,[150] (3) annexin A2–deficient mice display fibrin deposition on microvessels and impaired clearance of arterial thrombi following vascular injury,[151] (4) high titer antibodies directed against annexin A2 are associated with thrombosis in antiphospholipid syndrome and in individuals with cerebral venous thrombosis,[152,153] and (5) polymorphisms in the *ANXA2* gene are associated with cerebral vascular occlusion and osteonecrosis of bone in patients with sickle cell disease.[154–156] Whether defects in S100A10, which could serve either as a chaperone for annexin A2 or as a direct binding site for plasminogen,[157] might also be associated with these clinical entities remains to be determined.

## NONFIBRINOLYTIC VASCULAR FUNCTIONS OF PLASMIN

Although not yet demonstrated *in vivo*, plasmin may inactivate factor Va *in vitro* by cleaving both the heavy and light chains of this 168-kDa protein, in a manner that is distinct from the action of activated protein C.[158,159] Plasmin can also inactivate factor VIIIa, a procoagulant cofactor that is structurally related to factor Va.[160] In addition, platelet GPIIb/IIIa and GPIb, the cell surface receptors for fibrinogen and VWF, respectively, are both plasmin substrates.[161,162] Thus, plasmin formation in the vicinity of a hemostatic plug could lead to impaired adhesion and poor aggregation in response to agonists. *In vivo*, prolonged bleeding times were found in patients 90 minutes after t-PA infusion for thrombolysis, suggesting early impairment of platelet function upon plasmin generation.[163] However, there is also evidence that platelets may promote thrombotic reocclusion following successful thrombolytic therapy.[164]

## FIBRINOLYTIC FUNCTION IN VASCULAR INJURY

Transgenic mouse models of vascular disease have helped to elucidate the complex role of the fibrinolytic system in atherosclerosis (Table 5–3).[165,166] In mice, the general effects of plasminogen deficiency include runting, fibrin deposition in intra- and extravascular locations, and premature death.[167,168] In addition, the mice display impaired healing

**TABLE 5–3.** The Fibrinolytic System in Cardiovascular Disease—Transgenic Mouse Models

| Genotype | Result | Reference(s) |
|---|---|---|
| **Atherogenesis:** | | |
| PLG$^{-/-}$ ApoE$^{-/-}$ | Increased atherogenesis | 178 |
| t-PA$^{-/-}$ ApoE$^{-/-}$ | Unchanged atherogenesis | 179 |
| u-PA$^{-/-}$ ApoE$^{-/-}$ | Unchanged atherogenesis | 179 |
| PAI-1$^{-/-}$ ApoE$^{-/-}$ | Decrease in early plaque size; increase in advanced plaque size | 180–182 |
| **Transplant arteriosclerosis:** | | |
| PLG$^{-/-}$ | Reduced leukocyte invasion in transplantation model; reduced extent of disease | 185 |
| **Coronary ligation:** | | |
| u-PA$^{-/-}$ | Protection from ventricular rupture, but poor revascularization and late death from heart failure | 186 |
| t-PA$^{-/-}$ | No protection | 186 |
| uPAR$^{-/-}$ | No protection | 186 |
| **Aortic aneurysm:** | | |
| u-PA$^{-/-}$ ApoE$^{-/-}$ | Protected | 179 |
| t-PA$^{-/-}$ ApoE$^{-/-}$ | Not protected | 179 |
| **Early oxidative injury:** | | |
| PAI-1$^{-/-}$ | Attenuated thrombotic occlusion (Rose Bengal) | 194 |
| PAI-1$^{-/-}$ | Attenuated thrombotic occlusion (FeCl$_3$) | 195 |
| u-PA$^{-/-}$ | Increased thrombosis (FeCl$_3$) | 196 |
| t-PA$^{-/-}$ | Increased thrombosis (FeCl$_3$) | 196 |
| A2$^{-/-}$ | Increased thrombosis (FeCl$_3$) | 155 |
| **Restenosis with prominent thrombosis:** | | |
| PAI-1$^{-/-}$ | No neointima (Cu cuff) | 199 |
| PAI-1$^{-/-}$ | Reduced neointima (ligation) | 314 |
| PAI-1$^{-/-}$ | Reduced neointima (FeCl$_3$) | 314 |
| PAI-1$^{-/-}$ ApoE$^{-/-}$ | Reduced neointima (FeCl$_3$) | 198 |
| **Restenosis without prominent thrombosis:** | | |
| PLG$^{-/-}$ | Reduced neointima (electrical) | 187,188 |
| t-PA$^{-/-}$ | No change (electrical or mechanical) | 187,189 |
| u-PA$^{-/-}$ | Reduced neointima (electrical or mechanical) | 187,189 |
| u-PA$^{-/-}$ t-PA$^{-/-}$ | Reduced neointima (electrical or mechanical) | 187,189 |
| uPAR$^{-/-}$ | No change (electrical) | 190 |
| PAI-1$^{-/-}$ | Increased neointima (ligation) | 315 |
| PAI-1$^{-/-}$ | Increased neointima (electrical or mechanical) | 191 |

A2, annexin A2; ApoE, apolipoprotein E; PAI-1, plasminogen activator inhibitor-1; PLG, plasminogen; t-PA, tissue-type plasminogen activator; u-PA, urokinase plasminogen activator; uPAR, u-PA receptor.

of cutaneous wounds,[169] a response that appears to depend largely on the fibrinolytic action of plasmin as loss of fibrinogen eliminates these defects.[170] Mice doubly deficient in plasminogen and apolipoprotein E (ApoE) showed an increased predisposition to atherosclerosis compared to animals deficient in ApoE alone (Fig. 5–7A).[171] Mice with ApoE deficiency combined with deficiency of either u-PA or t-PA showed the same predilection for early fatty streaks and advanced plaques as was observed in mice with isolated ApoE deficiency, suggesting that complete elimination of plasmin-generating activity is required to exacerbate the proatherogenic state.[172] Finally, mice doubly deficient in ApoE and PAI-1 exhibit no change in early plaque size at the aortic root[173,174] and decreased early plaque size at the carotid bifurcation,[173,174] but increased advanced plaque size with accelerated deposition of matrix.[175]

Once the atherosclerotic plaque is established, plasmin may affect its evolution by mediating invasion of leukocytes (see Table 5–3).[176] In the peritoneal cavity, recruitment of inflammatory cells is profoundly influenced by the presence or absence of plasminogen.[177] In transplant-associated arteriosclerosis, the extent of disease is significantly reduced in plasminogen-deficient mice, reflecting, at least in part, reduced influx of macrophages, with an associated reduction in medial necrosis, fragmentation of elastic laminae, and remodeling of the adventitia.[178] Thus, the role of plasmin in degrading fibrin and other matrix constituents in the early lesion limits atherosclerosis, whereas its ability to promote cellular invasion later on appears to promote atherogenesis.

During aortic aneurysm formation in mice, deficiency of u-PA, but not t-PA, was associated with reduced medial destruction and impaired activation of downstream plasmin-dependent matrix metalloproteinases (Fig. 5–7B and Table 5–3).[172] Similarly, u-PA–, but not t-PA–, deficient mice were protected from cardiac rupture secondary to ventricular aneurysm. In this study, temporary administration of PAI-1 or the general matrix metalloproteinase inhibitor, tissue inhibitor of metalloproteinase (TIMP)-1, completely protected wild-type mice from aortic rupture, reinforcing the concept that plasmin-based protease activity promotes aneurysm progression.[179]

Vascular remodeling may occur following acute arterial injury induced by interventions for vascular compromise, leading to vascular restenosis (Fig. 5–7C and Table 5–3). This process reflects leukocyte invasion, proliferation and migration of smooth muscle cells, deposition of extracellular matrix, and reendothelialization. Electrical or mechanical injury studies in gene-targeted mice indicate that neointima formation, an initial step in restenosis, requires intact expression of plasminogen and u-PA, but not t-PA.[180-182] Interestingly, loss of uPAR has no effect on neointima formation,[183] whereas loss of PAI-1 is associated with increased neointimal stenosis.[184,185] In these injury models, which do not induce severe thrombosis, it is thought that vascular occlusion, reflecting migration of smooth muscle cells and leukocytes, is impaired when fibrinolytic potential is attenuated.[186]

In the ferric chloride, Rose Bengal, and copper cuff models, on the other hand, thrombosis is observed within minutes of arterial injury (see Fig. 5–7 and Table 5–3). In these systems, deficiency of PAI-1 is associated with later and less extensive thrombotic occlusion of the injured artery,[187,188] whereas loss of u-PA is associated with more rapid and more significant thrombotic occlusion.[189] At the same time, the absence of PAI-1 led to reduced vascular stenosis, regardless of whether ApoE was absent[190,191] or present.[192,193] In balloon-injured rat carotid arteries, finally, transduction of a PAI-1–expressing gene led to increased restenosis of the vessel, again suggesting that clearance of the initial thrombus may have long-term effects on vessel patency and neointima formation.[194] In these models, the predominant effect of the fibrinolytic system may be to clear the initial thrombus, which may provide a provisional scaffolding for later restenosis.

## ● FIBRINOLYTIC ASSEMBLY AND VASCULAR DISEASE

Endothelial cells use receptors, primarily uPAR and the annexin A2/S100A10 system, to assemble the fibrinolytic system on their surface (Chap. 25; see Fig. 5–6). Recent evidence suggests that impairment of receptor-mediated fibrinolytic assembly may lead to vascular compromise.

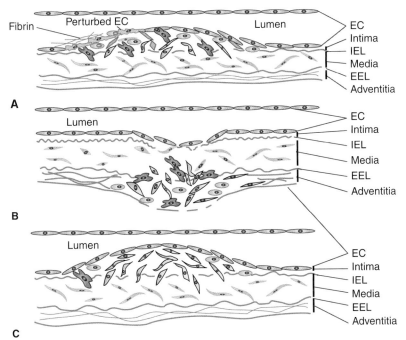

**Figure 5–7.** Working model for the actions of the fibrinolytic system in vascular disease. **A.** Plaque formation. Atheromatous plaque is thought to form in response to endothelial cell (EC) *(orange)* injury or perturbation. Following the initial injury, perturbed endothelial cells may fail to clear fibrin on the blood vessel surface and may also promote adhesion and invasion of leukocytes *(blue)*. In addition, smooth muscle cells arising in the tunica media invade the developing plaque within the intima *(green)*. Endothelial cells may use cell-surface receptors for focal activation of plasmin to maintain a thromboresistant vascular surface. Leukocytes, macrophages, and smooth muscle cells may use plasmin to migrate into the evolving plaque (cells outlined in *red*). **B.** Aneurysm. Fragmentation and dissolution of the elastic laminae of the arterial wall may occur upon matrix metalloproteinase activation via plasmin-dependent pathways, possibly mediated by smooth muscle cells. Cells migrating outward toward the adventitial surface of the vessel induce further matrix degradation and the potential for rupture. **C.** Restenosis. In response to vascular injury, smooth muscle cells proliferate in and, together with leukocytes, invade the subendothelial space establishing a thickened neointima that compromises vascular patency. In all three scenarios, cell migration is thought to require plasmin activity, possibly in association with cell surfaces. EEL, external elastic lamina; IEL, internal elastic lamina.

## LIPOPROTEIN(A)

Lp(a) is a low-density lipoprotein (LDL)-like particle that is an independent risk factor for atherosclerosis.[195–197] In addition to the apolipoprotein B-100 found on LDL, Lp(a) contains a disulfide-linked moiety called apolipoprotein(a) [apo(a)]. Apo(a) shares a remarkable degree of homology with plasminogen, as it possesses multiple tandem repeats of a kringle IV-like domain, a single domain resembling kringle V, and a pseudoprotease domain.[198,199] Plasminogen and apo(a), furthermore, are closely linked on chromosome 6 and appear to have arisen from a common ancestral gene.[200]

Whereas Lp(a) levels are only transiently responsive to diet,[201,202] plasma levels appear to be subject to mendelian inheritance.[203–205] Plasma Lp(a) concentrations correlate inversely with the ratio of kringle IV to kringle V encoding domains within the apo(a) gene,[206,207] such that larger apo(a) gene products are associated with lower plasma concentrations of apo(a). In addition, Lp(a) is an acute-phase reactant in the postsurgical and post–myocardial infarction setting[204] and in patients with cancer,[205] suggesting a role for soluble inflammatory mediators in regulating its synthesis or assembly. Apo(a) possesses a high-affinity lysine-binding site within kringle 4 that closely resembles that of kringle 1 of plasminogen,[208] and kringle 37 of the originally cloned apo(a) resembles the lysine-binding plasminogen kringle 4 of plasminogen.[209] In vivo, Lp(a) colocalizes histologically with fibrin in atheromatous tissue.[210]

When apo(a) is overexpressed in transgenic mice,[211] cell-associated plasmin activity is reduced such that the animals are resistant to t-PA thrombolysis.[212] Three potential explanations for the prothrombotic, proatherogenic effect of Lp(a) include (1) the observation that both Lp(a) and apo(a) inhibit Lys-plasminogen binding to endothelial cells (half-maximal inhibitory dose $[ID_{50}] = 36$-fold excess)[213] and to annexin A2,[214] with affinity similar to that for plasminogen[215–217]; (2) endothelial cell exposure to Lp(a) in vitro enhances expression of PAI-1[137]; and (3) Lp(a) may act as a competitive inhibitor of t-PA in the presence of fibrinogen[218] or as an uncompetitive inhibitor of the fibrin-dependent enhancement of t-PA–induced plasmin generation.[219] Overexpression of Lp(a) in mice receiving a high-fat diet results in atherosclerosis-like lesions containing anti-apo(a) cross-reactive material.[220] Deposition of both lipid and apo(a) was reduced in mice expressing apo(a) in which lysine-binding sites had been mutated.[221] Thus, lysine-binding sites of apo(a) appear to allow it to compete with plasminogen for cell surface receptors, thereby increasing atherogenicity.

## HOMOCYSTEINE

Homocysteine is a thiol-containing amino acid that accumulates in nutritional deficiencies of vitamin $B_6$, vitamin $B_{12}$, or folic acid, or in inherited abnormalities of cystathionine $\beta$-synthase, methylene tetrahydrofolate reductase, or methionine synthase.[222] Multiple studies have shown homocysteine to be an independent risk factor for atherosclerosis,[223] venous thromboembolism, and death.[224] Homocysteine lowering in patients with inborn errors of homocysteine metabolism leads to a striking reduction in cardiovascular morbidity, but supplementation with B vitamins in patients with established cardiovascular disease is of no benefit.[225] In vitro, homocysteine-treated endothelial cells bound approximately 50 percent less t-PA than untreated cells and activated approximately 50 percent less plasminogen.[226] Mass spectrometry studies indicate that homocysteine directly disables the t-PA binding domain of annexin A2 by forming a covalent adduction product with cysteine 9 within the tail domain of purified annexin A2, thus inhibiting its ability to bind t-PA.[227] Mice on a high homocysteine-generating diet, moreover, displayed dysfunctional annexin A2 and loss of both fibrinolytic and angiogenic potential. This phenotype mimicked that of annexin A2–deficient mice and was overcome upon intravenous infusion of unmodified annexin A2.[228]

## ANTIPHOSPHOLIPID SYNDROME

Antiphospholipid syndrome (APS) is an autoimmune disorder characterized by thrombosis, recurrent pregnancy loss, and persistently positive antiphospholipid antibodies.[229,230] Compared to patients with lupus erythematosus, nonimmune thrombosis, or healthy controls, a relatively high proportion of patients with APS and severe thrombosis (22 percent) has antibodies directed against annexin A2. Antiannexin A2 antibodies may block t-PA–dependent cell-surface plasmin generation and also induce expression of procoagulant molecules, such as TF.[152] These events may require crosslinking of $\beta_2$-GPI bound to closely associated cell-surface A2[231,232] and signaling via myeloid differentiation protein 88 (MyD88) and nuclear factor kappa B (NF$\kappa$B)-dependent pathway.[233] Additional evidence shows that A2 is required for the pathogenic effects of antiphospholipid antibodies in mice.[234] High-titer antiannexin A2 antibodies are also associated with cerebral vein thrombosis in patients without the full diagnostic criteria for APS.[153]

## ● ROLE OF ADHESION MOLECULES

A proinflammatory environment is also prothrombotic. Endothelial cells express molecules that regulate binding of leukocytes to their surface during inflammation. These interactions have both direct and indirect roles in hemostasis and thrombosis, and in some cases, interactions of leukocytes and platelets with inflamed endothelial cells feed forward to promote thrombosis.[235] Moreover, the inflammatory response itself results in the expression of adhesion molecules and mediators that secondarily promote hemostasis. In addition, membrane microparticles derived from platelets, leukocytes, and perhaps endothelium provide circulating sources of TF, proinflammatory lipids, and other molecules that have the potential to regulate thrombosis and inflammation at a distance from the primary site.[236–240]

## ● MOLECULAR CHANGES IN AN INFLAMMATORY MILIEU

### IMMEDIATE CHANGES

Either histamine or thrombin produced locally at the site of inflammation by degranulation of resident tissue mast cells stimulates the overlying endothelial cells to express P-selectin on their surfaces.[241] This change occurs within minutes and is caused by the rapid fusion of Weibel-Palade bodies, with the plasma membrane bringing P-selectin to the surface. Along with P-selectin expression, fusion of the Weibel-Palade bodies also results in the release of VWF into the local environment.

P-selectin serves as a leukocyte receptor for P-selectin glycoprotein ligand (PSGL)-1, L-selectin, and other ligands.[242] PSGL-1 is a specific sialomucin-containing sialylated, fucosylated O-linked oligosaccharide as well as an unusual sulfated tyrosine residue motif.[243] Dimerization of PSGL-1 is required for optimal recognition of P-selectin.[244] Adhesive interactions between P-selectin and its ligands result in the tethering of passing leukocytes to, and rolling on, the surface of the endothelial cell as the first step in leukocyte emigration. PSGL-1 also interacts with P-selectin expressed on platelets that have become activated and adherent to endothelium.[45,245] L-selectin, another member of the selectin family, is constitutively expressed on most leukocytes. It binds to sialylated, fucosylated GP ligands expressed by endothelial cells in response to inflammation, as well as to CD34 constitutively expressed by cells of the high endothelial venules.

Adhesion of leukocytes to the endothelium at the site of inflammation results in their rolling along the luminal surface, which slows their movement and brings them into contact with a wide variety of chemical mediators that trigger the next stage of leukocyte emigration—tight adhesion to the endothelial surface. These mediators include surface-bound chemokines,[246] new adhesion molecules expressed by the endothelium in response to inflammatory cytokines,[247] PAF,[248] soluble chemokines,[249] and ligands that crosslink leukocyte CD31[250-252] and seem to work by stimulating the activation of leukocyte integrin adhesion molecules by so-called inside-out signaling. This process involves a conformational change and/or clustering of the two chains of these heterodimeric surface molecules such that the affinity or avidity, respectively, for their ligands on the surfaces of endothelial cells is increased.[253] The ligands identified are members of a third family of adhesion molecules, the immunoglobulin gene superfamily.[254]

Table 5-4 lists some of the more common leukocyte/endothelial CAM pairs participating in the inflammatory response. It is interesting to note that the mucosal addressin MAdCAM-1, a unique molecule expressed by endothelial cells of high endothelial venules of mesenteric lymph nodes and Peyer patches, has structural features of both a mucin and an immunoglobulin superfamily molecule. It can bind both L-selectin and the leukocyte integrin $\alpha_4\beta_7$, expressed by a subset of memory T cells. It is believed to interact with L-selectin through its mucin (carbohydrate) domain and with $\alpha_4\beta_7$ through its immunoglobulin domains. Until recently, identified protein ligands for L-selectin (MAdCAM-1 and CD34) have been demonstrated to bind to L-selectin only in the context of lymphocyte homing, although recent evidence now suggests that they may play a role in rolling during inflammation.[255] Interestingly, intravital microscopy shows that leukocytes may roll on already adherent leukocytes and platelets through the interactions of L-selectin and PSGL-1 to amplify the inflammatory process.[256,257]

PAF is made and secreted acutely by leukocytes, mast cells, and endothelial cells at the site of inflammation. PAF (1-alkyl-2-acetyl-*sn*- glycero-3-phosphocholine) is produced enzymatically from phosphatidyl choline in the plasma membrane. Although its role as an activator of neutrophils in this environment has been established,[248] it appears to be a relatively weak agonist of platelet activation in this location.

Adherent leukocytes migrate to nearby interendothelial junctions by repeated cycles of adhesion in the front and disadhesion in the rear.[254,258] At the junction, additional distinct molecular interactions

**TABLE 5–4.** Common Leukocyte–Endothelial Cell Adhesion Molecule Pairs in Inflammation

| Leukocyte Molecule | CD and Integrin Nomenclature | Leukocytes Expressing | Action | Endothelial Counter Ligand | CD Number |
|---|---|---|---|---|---|
| L-selectin | CD62L | PMN, Mo, T, B, NK | Tethering, rolling | MAdCAM-1* | Pending |
| | | | | GP105–120 | CD34 |
| PSGL-1 | CD162 | PMN, Mo, T, B, NK | Tethering, rolling | P-selectin | CD62P |
| Sialyl LewisX ESL-1†, CLA† | CD15s | PMN, Mo, T, B, NK | Tethering, rolling | E-selectin | CD62E |
| LFA-1 | CD11a/CD18 ($\alpha_L\beta_2$) | PMN, Mo, T, B, NK | Tight adhesion | ICAM-1 | CD54 |
| | | | | ICAM-2 | CD102 |
| | | | | ICAM-3 | CD50 |
| | | | Adhesion, diapedesis | JAM-A | Pending |
| Mac-1 | CD11b/CD18 | PMN, Mo, NK | Tight adhesion | ICAM-1 | CD54 |
| VLA-4 | CD49d/CD29 | Mo, B, Eo‡ > NK, T | Tight adhesion§ Rolling | VCAM-1 | CD106 |
| PECAM-1 | CD31 | PMN, Mo, NK Subsets of T | Diapedesis | PECAM-1 | CD31 |
| CD99 | CD99 | All leukocytes to varying degrees | Diapedesis | CD99 | CD99 |
| JAM-C? | Pending | T | Diapedesis | JAM-C? | Pending |

B, B lymphocytes; CLA, cutaneous lymphocyte antigen; Eo, eosinophils; ESL-1, E-selectin ligand; GP, glycoprotein; ICAM, intercellular adhesion molecule; JAM, junctional adhesion molecule; MAdCAM-1, mucosal addressin cell-adhesion molecule; Mo, monocytes; NK, natural killer cells; PECAM, platelet endothelial adhesion molecule; PMN, polymorphonuclear neutrophils; PSGL, P-selectin glycoprotein ligand; T, T lymphocytes; VCAM, vascular cell adhesion molecule; VLA, very-late antigen.

*MAdCAM-1 and CD34 have been shown to be important for homing of T cells to lymph nodes via high endothelial venules. The protein structures bearing the L-selectin ligands, including CD15s, at sites of inflammation have not been identified.

†ESL-1, a protein with homology to fibroblast growth factor receptor, has been identified in mice. CLA, a molecule on the surface of skin-homing T cells related to PSGL-1, directs them to skin via E-selectin expressed on dermal venules.

‡Expression of VLA-4 on granulocytes is limited to eosinophils and basophils. Adult human neutrophils do not express it under normal circumstances.

§Although VLA-4/VCAM-1 interactions are generally thought to be important for tight adhesion of leukocytes to endothelium, there are reports[316,317] that leukocytes can use VLA-4 to roll on endothelial VCAM-1, as well.

between leukocytes and endothelial cells regulate transendothelial migration for the vast majority of neutrophils, monocytes, and natural killer (NK) cells. Transendothelial migration and the nomenclature of the junctional adhesion molecule (JAM) family are reviewed elsewhere.[17,259,260] PECAM/CD31 on the leukocyte contacts the same molecule concentrated at the endothelial junctions in a homophilic manner.[261-263] Although the relevant signal(s) transduced by this interaction remain unclear, a transient rise in endothelial cell intracellular calcium is required for transmigration.[264] Blocking the function of either leukocyte PECAM or endothelial cell PECAM arrests the leukocyte poised over the junction,[263,265,266] a phenotype very similar to that seen when the rise in intracellular calcium is blocked by the chelator, bis(2-amino-5-methylphenoxy)ethane-$N,N,N',N'$-tetraacetic acid tetraacetoxymethyl ester (MAPTAM).[264]

Because anti-PECAM reagents never block diapedesis completely, PECAM-independent pathways of transendothelial migration must exist. The leukocyte integrins $\alpha_4\beta_1$ (very-late antigen [VLA]-4) and $\alpha_L\beta_2/\alpha_M\beta_2$ (lymphocyte function-associated antigen [LFA]-1/macrophage [Mac]-1) and their endothelial counterreceptors VCAM-1 and ICAM-1 have been implicated in transmigration.[254] Interaction of leukocyte LFA-1 with JAM-A on endothelial cells has also been implicated in leukocyte recruitment.[267] Antibodies directed against JAM-C also blocked migration of lymphocytes across endothelial cell monolayers, implicating its role in lymphocyte migration.[268] In addition, under certain specialized conditions, there appear to be pathways across the endothelial cell that bypass the intercellular junction.[269,270]

CD99 is a GP expressed on leukocytes, platelets, and erythrocytes and concentrated at the endothelial cell borders. CD99 controls a step in diapedesis distal to the step controlled by PECAM both *in vitro* and *in vivo*,[271-273] by interfering with homophilic interaction between leukocyte CD99 and endothelial cell CD99-arrested monocytes. Their leading edges were below the endothelial cell monolayer, while their trailing uropods remained on the apical surface of the endothelial cell.

At the onset of most acute inflammatory responses, vascular permeability transiently increases as a result of histamine release. The endothelial junctions are soon re-established, and the junctions are closed to the leukocytes that arrive at the scene over the next hour. Studies performed both *in vivo* and *in vitro* indicate that, during subsequent diapedesis, leukocytes penetrate the vessel wall without further compromising the vascular permeability barrier.[264,274] Cortactin-deficient mice, for example, have constitutively leaky vascular junctions in the postcapillary venule circulation and an exaggerated response to histamine, yet leukocyte recruitment is diminished because of inefficient clustering of ICAM-1,[275] which prevents exposure of subendothelial collagen and VWF deposits to circulating platelets. Although PECAM-1 has no known role in binding platelets to endothelial cells, it has been hypothesized to maintain the tight apposition of endothelial cells and leukocytes during diapedesis.[263]

## ACUTE CHANGES

In addition to stimulating endothelial cell immediate responses, cytokines and inflammatory mediators released at the site of inflammation activate new endothelial cell genetic programs. Within several hours of exposure to mediator, *de novo* synthesis of mRNA and protein establishes an inflammatory endothelial cell phenotype that is both procoagulant and proadhesive.

Inflammatory cytokines such as TNF-$\alpha$ and IL-1 induce endothelial cell surface expression of several important CAMs. Expression of E-selectin peaks at 4 to 6 hours *in vitro* but may be maintained by interferon (IFN)-$\gamma$ for several days *in vivo*.[276,277] E-selectin mediates the slow rolling of leukocytes bearing sialylated, fucosylated carbohydrate

receptors similar to sialylated Lewis X antigen.[278] Endothelial cell P-selectin stimulated by thrombin or histamine is transient but can be prolonged to hours or days by IL-3, IL-4, or oncostatin M stimulation of human endothelium and by TNF-$\alpha$ stimulation of murine, but not human, endothelium.[279-282]

In general, expression of the immunoglobulin superfamily members ICAM-1 and VCAM-1 is induced by the same stimuli that induce E-selectin. Some specializations exist, at least *in vitro*. For example, IL-4 induces VCAM-1 but not E-selectin or ICAM-1 in microvascular endothelial cells.[283,284] These molecules serve as counter-receptors for the leukocyte integrins in the tight adhesion step.

## CHRONIC CHANGES

Stimulation of endothelial cells over several days with IFN-$\gamma$ leads to surface expression of MHC class II molecules (human leukocyte antigen [HLA]-DR and -DQ). In human tissues such as skin and gut, class II is commonly seen even in the absence of overt inflammation and is thought to be a result of chronic exposure of these sites to subclinical inflammation and antigenic stimulation. When costimulatory molecules such as CD40, ICAM-1, or LFA-3 are induced by inflammatory stimuli, the endothelial cell becomes capable (at least *in vitro*) of acting as an antigen-presenting cell that can stimulate CD4+ memory T cells. This mechanism may stimulate graft rejection by the host when the endothelium belongs to an organ graft with foreign MHC class II.[285-287]

In contrast, the expression of the adhesion molecule ICAM-2 does not change in response to inflammatory mediators. PECAM-1 shows a unique expression pattern in response to IFN-$\gamma$ *in vitro*[288] and *in vivo*,[289] as its distribution becomes diffuse over the surface of the cell, rather than being concentrated at intercellular borders. *In vitro* chronic exposure of human umbilical vein endothelial cells to a combination of IFN-$\gamma$ and TNF-$\alpha$ at relatively high doses leads to a decrease in total PECAM-1 expression.[290] Such a response has not been described to date *in vivo*.

## ADHESION MOLECULES IN A THROMBOTIC MILIEU

Activation of the hemostatic system exposes leukocytes to ligands that promote their adhesion and recruitment to the vessel wall. For example, *in vitro* thrombin induces E-selectin expression and IL-8 secretion by human umbilical vein endothelial cells.[291] These changes are classically induced by inflammatory cytokines such as IL-1 and TNF-$\alpha$. Table 5–5 lists some mediators that could have dual roles in inflammation and hemostasis/thrombosis.

## LEUKOCYTE–PLATELET AND ENDOTHELIAL CELL–PLATELET INTERACTIONS

Activated platelets bind to circulating lymphocytes in a P-selectin–dependent manner. This interaction can facilitate leukocyte rolling on the endothelium[292] and also allows homing of lymphocytes to peripheral lymph nodes in the absence of L-selectin, because P-selectin on the adherent platelets will interact with the peripheral lymph node addressin.[293] *In vitro*, neutrophils are capable of rolling on immobilized platelets via PSGL-1 on the leukocyte interacting with degranulated P-selectin on the platelet membranes.[294] Moreover, $\alpha_M\beta_2$ (CD11b/CD18)-dependent arrest and tight adhesion of neutrophils to bound platelets following P-selectin–dependent rolling has been described.[294,295] The endothelial ligand for this is not known. ICAM-2 has been found on the surface of activated platelets, but it is not a ligand for $\alpha_M\beta_2$.

**TABLE 5–5.** Dual Roles of Inflammatory Mediators in Thrombosis and Hemostasis

| Mediator | Role in Inflammation | Role in Thrombosis or Hemostasis |
|---|---|---|
| Histamine, thrombin | P-selectin expression induced on vascular endothelium | Degranulation of Weibel-Palade bodies; extrusion of VWF |
| Platelet-activating factor | Activation of leukocyte integrins | Activation of platelets |
| Expression of P-selectin glycoprotein ligand 1 (PSGL-1) | Adhesion of leukocytes to endothelial P-selectin | Adhesion of platelets to adherent leukocytes via P-selectin bidirectionally |
| Adherent platelets | Leukocyte rolling on platelet P-selectin; tight adhesion to platelet membrane component | Thrombosis |
| Fibrinogen | Adhesion of leukocytes to fibrinogen via CD11b/CD18 | Bridging of platelets to VWF and matrix via $\alpha_{IIb}/\beta_{III}$ |
| Thrombin | Induction of E-selectin expression and IL-8 secretion by endothelial cells | Fibrinogen formation and platelet aggregation |
| Leukocyte integrin CD11b/CD18 | Adhesion of leukocytes to endothelium; phagocytosis CD11b/CD18 | Binding and activation of factor X, adhesion of platelets via GPIbα; adhesion of platelets via JAM-C |

GP, glycoprotein; IL, interleukin; JAM, junctional adhesion molecule; VWF, von Willebrand factor.

In fact, antibodies against neither ICAM-2 nor its neutrophil receptor $\alpha_L$ (CD11) blocked this adhesion.[295,296] On the other hand, neutrophil $\alpha_M\beta_2$ reportedly binds to fibrinogen, which may be present on the surfaces of activated platelets bound to $\alpha_{IIb}\beta_3$ (GPIIb/IIIa). Two additional platelet surface molecules, GPIbα and JAM-C, have been demonstrated as ligands for leukocyte CD11b/CD18. GPIbα is part of the GP1b–IX–V complex,[297,298] and JAM-C was originally described as a component of epithelial and endothelial cell tight junctions.

Platelets can interact with activated endothelial cells. Platelets express PSGL-1 and can use this expression to interact with P-selectin on the surfaces of activated endothelial cells.[299] Activated platelets can also bind to endothelial cells via fibrinogen, fibrin, or VWF, forming a molecular bridge between platelet GPIIb/IIIa and endothelial cell integrin $\alpha_v\beta_3$ and ICAM-1.

Ultralarge VWF molecules are stored in Weibel-Palade bodies and released upon inflammatory endothelial cell activation. Ultralarge VWF molecules are normally cleaved by endothelial cell-surface proteases, notably the metalloprotease ADAMTS13 (a disintegrin and metalloprotease with thrombospondin repeats 13). Data in mice suggest that ADAMTS13 plays a homeostatic role in dampening inflammation.[300] In ADAMTS13-deficient mice, platelets bound to ultralarge VWF molecules on the endothelial surface and supported slower leukocyte rolling on venules at rest and greater leukocyte extravasation in models of inflammation.[300]

## LEUKOCYTE–ENDOTHELIAL CELL MATRIX INTERACTIONS THAT PROMOTE COAGULATION

The same proinflammatory stimuli that stimulate *de novo* expression of E-selectin and VCAM-1, and augment expression of ICAM-1 for the recruitment of leukocytes, may stimulate synthesis and expression of TF by endothelial cells.[301] Furthermore, adhesion of monocytic cell lines to cytokine-activated endothelial cells in culture leads to rapidly increased TF-related procoagulant activity. This effect is partially blocked by a monoclonal antibody directed against E-selectin on endothelium and is mimicked by crosslinking Le$^X$ on the monocyte cell lines.[302] A similar increase in TF gene expression can be induced by crosslinking $\alpha_4$ or $\beta_1$ integrin chains, the components of VLA-4 on monocytic cell lines.[303]

During prolonged interaction of peripheral blood monocytes with human endothelial cells, monocytes that migrated across endothelial cell monolayers expressed functional cell surface TF.[304] Over the next several days, approximately half of these monocytes differentiated into immature dendritic cells bearing even higher levels of TF and migrated back across the intact endothelial cell monolayer. This migration could be blocked by soluble fragments of TF. Therefore, in this system, TF was hypothesized to support both adhesion and a possible procoagulant role.[304]

Leukocytes that bind to P-selectin exposed on the surfaces of platelets on adherent thrombi promote the conversion of fibrinogen to fibrin.[305] The leukocyte integrin CD11b/CD18 has been shown to bind fibrinogen.[306] The same integrin has a conformational form that binds coagulation factor X.[307] Monocytic cells are capable of activating the bound factor X to factor Xa when activated,[308] defining a pathway for activation of factor X that is independent of TF.

## REFERENCES

1. Nachman RL, Rafii S: Platelets, petechiae, and preservation of the vascular wall. *N Engl J Med* 359:1261–1270, 2008.
2. Marcus AJ, Broekman MJ, Drosopoulos JH, et al: Heterologous cell-cell interactions: Thromboregulation, cerebroprotection and cardioprotection by CD39 (NTPDase-1). *J Thromb Haemost* 1:2497–2509, 2003.
3. Furie B, Furie BC: Mechanisms of thrombus formation. *N Engl J Med* 359:938–949, 2008.
4. Kanthi YM, Sutton NR, Pinsky DJ: CD39: Interface between vascular thrombosis and inflammation. *Curr Atheroscler Rep* 16:425, 2014.
5. Aird WC: Phenotypic heterogeneity of the endothelium: I. Structure, function, and mechanisms. *Circ Res* 100:158–173, 2007.
6. Aird WC: Phenotypic heterogeneity of the endothelium: II. Representative vascular beds. *Circ Res* 100:174–190, 2007.
7. Brant-Zawadzki PB, Schmid DI, Jiang H, et al: Translational control in endothelial cells. *J Vasc Surg* 45(Suppl A):A8–A14, 2007.
8. Marcus AJ, Safier LB, Hajjar KA, et al: Inhibition of platelet function by an aspirin-insensitive endothelial cell ADPase. Thromboregulation by endothelial cells. *J Clin Invest* 88:1690–1696, 1991.
9. Marcus AJ, Broekman MJ, Drosopoulos JH, et al: Role of CD39 (NTPDase-1) in thromboregulation, cerebroprotection, and cardioprotection. *Semin Thromb Hemost* 31:234–246, 2005.
10. Broekman MJ, Eiroa AM, Marcus AJ: Inhibition of human platelet reactivity by endothelium-derived relaxing factor from human umbilical vein endothelial cells in suspension. Blockade of aggregation and secretion by an aspirin-insensitive mechanism. *Blood* 78:1033–1040, 1991.
11. Moncada S, Higgs EA: Molecular mechanisms and therapeutic strategies related to nitric oxide. *FASEB J* 9:1319–1330, 1995.
12. Kaczmarek E, Koziak K, Sevigny J, et al: Identification and characterization of CD39 vascular ATP diphosphohydrolase. *J Biol Chem* 271:33116–33122, 1996.
13. Marcus AJ, Broekman MJ, Drosopoulos JHF, et al: The endothelial cell ecto-ADPase responsible for inhibition of platelet function is CD39. *J Clin Invest* 99:1351–1360, 1997.
14. Esmon CT: Inflammation and the activated protein C anticoagulant pathway. *Semin Thromb Hemost* 32(Suppl 1):49–60, 2006.
15. Flood EC, Hajjar KA: The annexin A2 system and vascular homeostasis. *Vascul Pharmacol* 54:59–67, 2011.
16. Lisman T, De Groot PG, Meijers JC, Rosendaal FR: Reduced plasma fibrinolytic potential is a risk factor for venous thrombosis. *Blood* 105:1102–1105, 2005.

17. Muller WA: Mechanisms of leukocyte transendothelial migration. *Annu Rev Pathol* 6:323–344, 2011.

18. Marcus AJ, Safier LB: Thromboregulation: Multicellular modulation of platelet reactivity in hemostasis and thrombosis. *FASEB J* 7:516–522, 1993.

19. Ross R: Atherosclerosis: An inflammatory disease. *N Engl J Med* 340:115–126, 1999.

20. Garlanda C, Dejana E: Heterogeneity of endothelial cells: Specific markers. *Arterioscler Thromb Vasc Biol* 17:1193–1202, 1999.

21. Gawaz M, Langer H, May AE: Platelets in inflammation and atherogenesis. *J Clin Invest* 115:3378–3384, 2005.

22. May AE, Langer H, Seizer P, et al: Platelet-leukocyte interactions in inflammation and atherothrombosis. *Semin Thromb Hemost* 33:123–127, 2007.

23. Brass LF, Zhu L, Stalker TJ: Novel therapeutic targets at the platelet vascular interface. *Arterioscler Thromb Vasc Biol* 28(3):s43–s50, 2008.

24. Marcus AJ: Transcellular metabolism of eicosanoids. *Prog Hemost Thromb* 8:127–142, 1986.

25. Hamberg M, Svensson J, Samuelsson B: Thromboxanes: A new group of biologically active compounds derived from prostaglandin endoperoxides. *Proc Natl Acad Sci U S A* 72:2994–2998, 1975.

26. Moncada S, Gryglewski R, Bunting S, Vane JR: An enzyme isolated from arteries transforms prostaglandin endoperoxides to an unstable substance that inhibits platelet aggregation. *Nature* 263:663–665, 1976.

27. Woulfe D, Yang J, Brass L: ADP and platelets: The end of the beginning. *J Clin Invest* 107:1503–1505, 2001.

28. Al-Mondhiry H, Marcus AJ, Spaet TH: On the mechanism of platelet function inhibition by acetylsalicylic acid. *Proc Soc Exp Biol Med* 133:632–636, 1970.

29. Wu KK, Aird WC: Endothelial eicosanoids, in *Endothelial Biomedicine*, pp 1004–1014. Cambridge University Press, Cambridge, 2009.

30. McAdam BF, Catella-Lawson F, Mardini IA, et al: Systemic biosynthesis of prostacyclin by cyclooxygenase (COX)-2: The human pharmacology of a selective inhibitor of COX-2. *Proc Natl Acad Sci U S A* 96:272–277, 1999.

31. Herschman HR: Prostaglandin synthase 2. *Biochim Biophys Acta* 1299:125–140, 1996.

32. Maclouf J, Folco G, Patrono C: Eicosanoids and iso-eicosanoids: Constitutive, inducible and transcellular biosynthesis in vascular disease. *Thromb Haemost* 79:691–705, 1998.

33. Smith WL, DeWitt DL: Prostaglandin endoperoxide H synthases-1 and -2. *Adv Immunol* 62:167–215, 1996.

34. Xie WL, Chipman JG, Robertson DL, et al: Expression of a mitogen-responsive gene encoding prostaglandin synthase is regulated by mRNA splicing. *Proc Natl Acad Sci U S A* 88:2692–2696, 1991.

35. Kurumbail RG, Stevens Am, Gierse JK, et al: Structural basis for selective inhibition of cyclooxygenase-2 by anti-inflammatory agents. *Nature* 384:644–648, 1996 [published erratum appears in *Nature* 385(6616):555, 1997].

36. Pouliot M, Gilbert C, Borgeat P, et al: Expression and activity of prostaglandin endoperoxide synthase-2 in agonist-activated human neutrophils. *FASEB J* 12:1109–1123, 1998.

37. DeWitt DL, Smith WL: Cloning of sheep and mouse prostaglandin endoperoxide synthases. *Methods Enzymol* 187:469–479, 1990.

38. Dubois RN, Abramson SB, Crofford L, et al: Cyclooxygenase in biology and disease. *FASEB J* 12:1063–1073, 1998.

39. Lipsky LPE, Abramson SB, Crofford L, et al: The classification of cyclooxygenase inhibitors. *J Rheumatol* 25:2298–2303, 1998.

40. Marnett LJ: The COXIB experience: A look in the rear-view mirror. *Annu Rev Pharmacol Toxicol* 49:265–290, 2008.

41. Moncada S, Vane JR: Pharmacology and endogenous roles of prostaglandin endoperoxides, thromboxane A2, and prostacyclin. *Pharmacol Rev* 30:293–331, 1978.

42. Narumiya S, FitzGerald GA: Genetic and pharmacologic analysis prostanoid receptor function. *J Clin Invest* 108:25–30, 2001.

43. Cines DB, Pollak ES, Buck CA, et al: Endothelial cells in physiology and in the pathophysiology of vascular disorders. *Blood* 91:3527–3561, 1998.

44. Marcus AJ, Weksler BB, Jaffe EA, Broekman MJ: Synthesis of prostacyclin from platelet-derived endoperoxides by cultured human endothelial cells. *J Clin Invest* 66:979–986, 1980.

45. Smyth SS, McEver RP, Weyrich AS, et al: Platelet functions beyond hemostasis. *J Thromb Haemost* 7:1759–1766, 2009.

46. Pepine CJ: Impact of nitric oxide on cardiovascular medicine: Untapped potential utility. *Am J Med* 122:S10–S15, 2009.

47. Marletta MA: Nitric oxide synthase structure and mechanism. *J Biol Chem* 268:12231–12234, 1993.

48. Moncada S, Palmer RMJ, Higgs EA. Nitric oxide: Physiology, pathophysiology, and pharmacology. *Pharmacol Rev* 43:109–142, 1991.

49. Furchgott RF, Zawadzki JV: The obligatory role of endothelial cells in the relaxation of arterial smooth muscle by acetylcholine. *Nature* 288:373–376, 1980.

50. Matsumoto A, Momomura S, Sugiura S, et al: Effect of inhaled nitric oxide on gas exchange in patients with congestive heart failure. *Ann Intern Med* 130:40–44, 1999.

51. Lentz SR, Sobey CG, Piegers DJ, et al: Vascular dysfunction in monkeys with diet-induced hyperhomocyst(e)inemia. *J Clin Invest* 98:24–29, 1996.

52. Stamler JS, Osborne JA, Jaraki O, et al: Adverse vascular effects of homocysteine are modulated by endothelium-derived relaxing factor and related oxides of nitrogen. *J Clin Invest* 91:308–318, 1993.

53. Upchurch GR Jr, Welch GN, Fabian AJ, et al: Homocyst(e)ine decrease bioavailable nitric oxide by a mechanism involving glutathione peroxidase. *J Biol Chem* 272:17012–17017, 1997.

54. Voetsch B, Loscalzo J: Genetic determinants of arterial thrombosis. *Arterioscler Thromb Vasc Biol* 24:216–229, 2004.

55. Robson SC, Sevigny J, Zimmermann H: The E-NTPDase family of ectonucleotidases: Structure function relationships and pathophysiological significance. *Purinergic Signal* 2:409–430, 2006.

56. Gayle RB, Maliszewski CR, Gimpel SD, et al: Inhibition of platelet function by recombinant soluble ecto-ADPase/CD39. *J Clin Invest* 101:1851–1859, 1998.

57. Handa M, Guidotti G: Purification and cloning of a soluble ATP-diphosphohydrolase (apyrase) from potato tubers (Solanum tuberosum). *Biochem Biophys Res Commun* 218:916–923, 1996.

58. Hyman MC, Ptrovic-Djergovic D, Visovatti SH, et al: Self-regulation of inflammatory cell trafficking in mice by the leukocyte surface apyrase CD39. *J Clin Invest* 119:1136–1149, 2009.

59. Colgan S, Eltzschig H, Eckle T, Thompson L: Physiological roles for ecto-5'-nucleotidase (CD73). *Purinergic Signal* 2:351–360, 2006.

60. Atkinson BT, Jarvis GE, Watson SP: Activation of GPVI by collagen is regulated by alpha2beta1 and secondary mediators. *J Thromb Haemost* 1:1278–1287, 2003.

61. Pinsky DJ, Broekman MJ, Peschon JJ, et al: Elucidation of the thromboregulatory role of CD39/ectoapyrase in the ischemic brain. *J Clin Invest* 109:1031–1040, 2002.

62. Marcus AJ, Broekman MJ, Drosopoulos JHF, et al: Metabolic control of excessive extracellular nucleotide accumulation by CD39/ectonucleotidase-1: Implications for ischemic vascular diseases. *J Pharmacol Exp Ther* 305:9–16, 2003.

63. Koziak K, Bojakowska M, Robson SC, et al: Overexpression of CD39/nucleoside triphosphate diphosphohydrolase-1 decreases smooth muscle cell proliferation and prevents neointima formation after angioplasty. *J Thromb Haemost* 6:1191–1197, 2008.

64. Deaglio S, Dwyer KM, Gao W, et al: Adenosine generation catalyzed by CD39 and CD73 expressed on regulatory T cells mediates immune suppression. *J Exp Med* 204:1257–1265, 2007.

65. Uluckan O, Eagleton MC, Floyd DH, et al: APT102, a novel ADPase, cooperates with aspirin to disrupt bone metastasis in mice. *J Cell Biochem* 104:1311–1323, 2008.

66. Dwyer KM, Robson SC, Nandurkar HH, et al: Thromboregulatory manifestations in human CD39 transgenic mice and the implications for thrombotic disease and transplantation. *J Clin Invest* 113:1440–1446, 2004.

67. Serebruany VL, Malinin AI, Ferguson JJ, et al: Bleeding risks of combination vs. single antiplatelet therapy: A meta-analysis of 18 randomized trials comprising 129,314 patients. *Fundam Clin Pharmacol* 22:315–321, 2008.

68. Fung CY, Marcus AJ, Broekman MJ, Mahaut-Smith MP: P2X1 receptor inhibition and soluble CD39 administration as novel approaches to widen the cardiovascular therapeutic window. *Trends Cardiovasc Med* 19:1–5, 2009.

69. Esmon CT, Owen WG: Identification of an endothelial cell cofactor for thrombin-catalyzed activation of protein C. *Proc Natl Acad Sci U S A* 78:2249–2252, 1981.

70. Stearns-Kurosawa DJ, Kurosawa S, Mollica JS, et al: The endothelial cell protein C receptor augments protein C activation by the thrombin-thrombomodulin complex. *Proc Natl Acad Sci U S A* 93:10212–10216, 1996.

71. Esmon CT: Protein C pathway in sepsis. *Ann Med* 34:598–605, 2002.

72. Esmon CT: Inflammation and thrombosis. *J Thromb Haemost* 1:1343–1348, 2003.

73. Esmon CT: The protein C pathway. *Chest* 124(3 Suppl):26S–32S, 2003.

74. Esmon CT: The roles of protein C and thrombomodulin in the regulation of blood coagulation. *J Biol Chem* 264:4743–4746, 1989.

75. Grinnell BW, Berg DT: Surface thrombomodulin modulates thrombin receptor responses on vascular smooth muscle cells. *Am J Physiol* 270:H603–H609, 1996.

76. Lafay M, Laguna R, Le Bonniec BF, et al: Thrombomodulin modulates the mitogenic response to thrombin of human umbilical vein endothelial cells. *Thromb Haemost* 79:848–852, 1998.

77. Bajzar L, Manuel R, Nesheim M: Purification and characterization of TAFI, a thrombin activatable fibrinolysis inhibitor. *J Biol Chem* 270:14477–14484, 1995.

78. Campbell WD, Okada N, Okada H: Carboxypeptidase R is an inactivator of complement-derived inflammatory peptides and an inhibitor of fibrinolysis. *Immunol Rev* 180:162–167, 2001.

79. Ikeguchi H, Fujita Y, Kato T, et al: Effects of human soluble thrombomodulin on experimental glomerulonephritis. *Kidney Int* 61:490–501, 2002.

80. de Munk GA, Groeneveld E, Rijken DC: Acceleration of the thrombin inactivation of single chain urokinase-type plasminogen activator (pro-urokinase) by thrombomodulin. *J Clin Invest* 88:1680–1684, 1991.

81. Molinari A, Giogetti C, Lansen J, et al: Thrombomodulin is a cofactor for thrombin degradation of recombinant single-chain urokinase plasminogen activator *in vitro* and in a perfused rabbit heart model. *Thromb Haemost* 67:226–232, 1992.

82. Preissner KT, May AE, Wohn KD, et al: Molecular crosstalk between adhesion receptors and proteolytic cascades in vascular remodeling. *Thromb Haemost* 78:88–95, 1997.

83. Esmon CT, Scriver CR, Beaudet AL, et al: Anticoagulant protein C/thrombomodulin pathway, in *The Metabolic and Molecular Bases of Inherited Disease*, 8th ed, edited by CR Scriver, AL Beaudet, D Valle, WS Sly, B Childs, KW Kinzler, B Vogelstein, pp 4327–4343. McGraw-Hill, New York, 2001.

84. Healy AM, Hancock WW, Christie PD, et al: Intravascular coagulation activation in a murine model of thrombomodulin deficiency: Effects of lesion size, age, and hypoxia on fibrin deposition. *Blood* 263:15815–15822, 1988.

85. Weiler-Guettler H, Aird WC, Rayburn H, et al: Developmentally regulated gene expression of thrombomodulin in postimplantation mouse embryos. *Development* 122:2271–2281, 1996.

86. Crawley JT, Gu AM, Ferrell G, Esmon CT: Distribution of endothelial cell protein C/activated protein C receptor (EPCR) during mouse embryo development. *Thromb Haemost* 88:259–266, 2002.

87. Isermann B, Hendrickson SB, Hutley K, et al: Tissue-restricted expression of thrombomodulin in the placenta rescues thrombomodulin-deficient mice from early lethality and reveals a secondary developmental block. *Development* 128:827–838, 2001.

88. Isermann B, Hendrickson SB, Zogg M, et al: Endothelium-specific loss of muine thrombomodulin disrupts the protein C anticoagulant pathway and causes juvenile-onset thrombosis. *J Clin Invest* 108:537–546, 2001.

89. Fukodome K, Esmon CT: Identification, cloning, and regulation of a novel endothelial cell protein C/activated protein C receptor. *J Biol Chem* 269:26486–26491, 1994.

90. Esmon CT, Gu J, Xu J, et al: Regulation and functions of the protein C anticoagulant pathway. *Haematologica* 84:363–368, 1999.

91. Esmon CT, Xu J, Gu J, et al: Endothelial protein C receptor. *Thromb Haemost* 82:251–258, 1999.

92. Esmon CT: The endothelial cell protein C receptor. *Curr Opin Hematol* 13:382–385, 2006.

93. Xu J, Liaw PC, Esmon CT: A novel transmembrane domain of the endothelial cell protein C receptor (EPCR) dictates receptor localization of sphingolipid-cholesterol rich regions on plasma membrane while EPCR palmitoylation modulates intracellular trafficking patterns. *Thromb Haemost* 1999.

94. Kurosawa S, Stearns-Kurosawa DJ, Hidari N, Esmon CT: Identification of functional endothelial protein C receptor in human plasma. *J Clin Invest* 100:411–418, 1997.

95. Fukodome K, Ye X, Tsuneyoshi N, et al: Activation mechanism of anticoagulant protein C in large blood vessels involving the endothelial cell protein C receptor. *J Exp Med* 187:1029–1035, 1998.

96. Taylor FB Jr, Peer GT, Lockhart MS: Endothelial cell protein C receptor plays an important role in protein C activation *in vivo*. *Blood* 97:1685–1688, 2001.

97. Esmon CT, Taylor FB, Snow TR: Inflammation and coagulation: Linked processes potentially regulated through a common pathway mediated by protein C. *Thromb Haemost* 66:160–165, 1991.

98. Esmon CT, Schwarz HP: An update on clinical and basic aspects of the protein C anticoagulant pathway. *Trends Cardiovasc Med* 5:141–148, 1995.

99. Ranieri VM, Thompson BT, Barie PS, et al: Drotrecogin alfa (activated) in adults with septic shock. *N Engl J Med* 366:2055–2064, 2012.

100. Gu JM, Crawley JTB, Ferrell G, et al: Disruption of the endothelial cell protein C receptor gene in mice causes placental thrombosis and early embryonic lethality. *J Biol Chem* 277:43335–43343, 2002.

101. Weiler H, Isermann B: Thrombomodulin. *J Thromb Haemost* 1:1515–1524, 2003.

102. Todd AS: Fibrinolysis autographs. *Nature* 181:495–496, 1958.

103. Todd AS: Localization of fibrinolytic activity in tissues. *Br Med Bull* 20:210–212, 1964.

104. Augustin HG, Kozian DH, Johnson RC: Differentiation of endothelial cells: Analysis of the constitutive and activated endothelial cell phenotypes. *Bioessays* 16:901–906, 1994.

105. van Hinsbergh VW, Kooistra T, Emeis JJ, Koolwijk P: Regulation of plasminogen activator production by endothelial cells: Role in fibrinolysis and local proteolysis. *Int J Radiat Biol* 60:261–272, 1991.

106. Levin EG, del Zoppo GJ: Localization of tissue plasminogen activator in the endothelium of a limited number of vessels. *Am J Pathol* 144:855–861, 1994.

107. Levin EG, Santell L, Osborn KG: The expression of endothelial tissue plasminogen activator in vivo: A function defined by vessel size and anatomic location. *J Cell Sci* 110:139–148, 1997.

108. Levin EG, Osborn KG, Schleuning WD: Vessel-specific gene expression in the lung: Tissue plasminogen activator is limited to bronchial arteries and pulmonary vessels of discrete size. *Chest* 114:68S, 1998.

109. O'Rourke J, Jiang X, Hao Z, Cone RE, Hand AR: Distribution of sympathetic tissue plasminogen activator (tPA) to a distant microvasculature. *J Neurosci* 79:727–733, 2005.

110. Dichek D, Quertermous T: Thrombin regulation of mRNA levels of tissue plasminogen activator inhibitor-1 in cultured human umbilical vein endothelial cells. *Blood* 74:222–228, 1989.

111. Hanss M, Collen D: Secretion of tissue-type plasminogen activator and plasminogen activator inhibitor by cultured human endothelial cells: Modulation by thrombin, endotoxin, and histamine. *J Lab Clin Med* 109:97–104, 1987.

112. Levin EG, Santell L: Stimulation and desensitization of tissue plasminogen activator release from human endothelial cells. *J Biol Chem* 263:9360–9365, 1988.

113. Shatos MA, Doherty JM, Orfeo T, et al: Modulation of the fibrinolytic response of cultured human vascular endothelium by extracellularly generated oxygen radicals. *J Biol Chem* 267:597–601, 1992.

114. Levin EG, Marotti KR, Santell L: Protein kinase C and the stimulation of tissue plasminogen activator release from human endothelial cells. *J Biol Chem* 264:16030–16036, 1989.

115. Cugno M, Uziel L, Fabrizi I, et al: Fibrinolytic response in normal subjects to venous occlusion and DDAVP infusion. *Thromb Res* 56:625–634, 1989.

116. Kooistra T, van den Berg J, Tons A, et al: Butyrate stimulates tissue type plasminogen activator synthesis in cultured human endothelial cells. *Biochem J* 247:605–612, 1987.

117. Diamond SL, Eskin SG, McIntire LV: Fluid flow stimulates tissue plasminogen activator secretion by cultured human endothelial cells. *Science* 243:1483–1485, 1989.

118. Diamond SL, Sharefkin JB, Dieffenbach C, et al: Tissue plasminogen activator messenger RNA levels increase in cultured human endothelial cells exposed to laminar shear stress. *J Cell Physiol* 143:364–371, 1990.

119. Levin EG, Santell L, Saljooque F: Hyperosmotic stress stimulates tissue plasminogen activator expression by a PKC-dependent pathway. *Am J Physiol* 265:C387–C396, 1993.

120. Iba T, Shin T, Sonoda T, et al: Stimulation of endothelial secretion of tissue-type plasminogen activator by repetitive stretch. *J Surg Res* 50:457–460, 1991.

121. Thompson EA, Nelles L, Collen D: Effect of retinoic acid on the synthesis of tissue-type plasminogen activator and plasminogen activator inhibitor 1 in human endothelial cells. *Eur J Biochem* 201:627–632, 1991.

122. Bulens F, Ibanez-Tallon I, Van Acker P, et al: Retinoic acid induction of human tissue-type plasminogen activator gene expression via a direct repeat element (DR5) located at −7 kilobases. *J Biol Chem* 270:7167–7175, 1995.

123. van Hinsbergh VW, Bauer KA, Kooistra T, et al: Progress of fibrinolysis during tumor necrosis factor infusions in humans. Concomitant increase in tissue-type plasminogen activator, plasminogen activator inhibitor type-1, and fibrin(ogen) degradation products. *Blood* 76:2284–2289, 1990.

124. Hamsten A, Wiman B, De Faire U, Blomback M: Increased plasma levels of a rapid inhibitor of tissue plasminogen activator in young survivors of myocardial infarction. *N Engl J Med* 313:1557–1563, 1985.

125. Pizzo SV, Murray JC, Gonias SL: Atrophie blanche: A disorder associated with defective release of tissue plasminogen activator. *Arch Pathol Lab Med* 110:517–519, 1986.

126. Kristensen P, Larson LI, Nielsen LS, et al: Human endothelial cells contain one type of plasminogen activator. *FEBS Lett* 168:33–37, 1984.

127. Yamamoto K, Loskutoff DJ: Fibrin deposition in tissues from endotoxin-treated mice correlates with decreases in the expression of urokinase-type but not tissue-type plasminogen activator. *J Clin Invest* 97:2440–2451, 1996.

128. Bacharach E, Itin A, Keshet E: *In vivo* patterns of expression of urokinase and its inhibitor PAI-1 suggest a concerted role in regulating physiological angiogenesis. *Proc Natl Acad Sci U S A* 89:10686–10690, 1992.

129. Booyse FM, Scheinbuks J, Radek J, et al: Immunological identification and comparison of plasminogen activator forms in cultured normal human endothelial cells and smooth muscle cells. *Thromb Res* 24:495–504, 1981.

130. van Hinsbergh VW, van den Berg EA, Fiers W, Dooijewaard G: Tumor necrosis factor induces the production of urokinase-type plasminogen activator by human endothelial cells. *Blood* 75:1991–1998, 1990.

131. Sawdey M, Podor TJ, Loskutoff DJ: Regulation of type-1 plasminogen activator inhibitor gene expression in cultured bovine aortic endothelial cells. *J Biol Chem* 264:10396–10401, 1989.

132. van den Berg EA, Sprengers ED, Jaye M, et al: Regulation of plasminogen activator inhibitor-1 mRNA in human endothelial cells. *Thromb Haemost* 60:63–67, 1988.

133. Ellis V, Scully MF, Kakkar VV: Plasminogen activation by single-chain urokinase in functional isolation. *J Biol Chem* 262:14998–15003, 1987.

134. Blasi F, Carmeliet P: uPAR: A versatile signalling orchestrator. *Nat Rev Mol Cell Biol* 3:932–943, 2002.

135. Almus-Jacobs F, Varki N, Sawdey MS, Loskutoff DJ: Endotoxin stimulates expression of the murine urokinase receptor gene in vivo. *Am J Pathol* 147:688–698, 1995.

136. Medina R, Socher SH, Han JH, Friedman PA: Interleukin-1, endotoxin, or tumor necrosis factor/cachectin enhance the level of plasminogen activator inhibitor messenger RNA in bovine aortic endothelial cells. *Thromb Res* 54:41–52, 1989.

137. Etingin OR, Hajjar DP, Hajjar KA, et al: Lipoprotein(a) regulates plasminogen activator inhibitor-1 expression in endothelial cells. *J Biol Chem* 266:2459–2465, 1990.

138. Konkle B, Ginsburg D: The addition of endothelial cell growth factor and heparin to human endothelial cell cultures decrease plasminogen activator. *J Clin Invest* 82:579, 1988.

139. Greenberg ME, Brackenbury R, Edelman GM: Changes in the distribution of the 34-kdalton tyrosine kinase substrate during differentiation and maturation of chicken tissues. *J Cell Biol* 98:473–486, 1984.

140. Hamre KM, Chepenik KP, Goldowitz D: The annexins: Specific markers of midline structures and sensory neurons in the developing murine central nervous system. *J Comp Neurol* 352:421–435, 1995.

141. Gould KL, Cooper JA, Hunter T: The 46,000-dalton tyrosine kinase substrate is widespread, whereas the 36,000-dalton substrate is only expressed at high levels in certain rodent tissues. *J Cell Biol* 98:487–497, 1984.

142. Dreier R, Schmid KW, Gerke V, Riehemann K: Differential expression of annexins I, II, and IV in human tissues: An immunohistochemical study. *Histochem Cell Biol* 110:137–148, 1998.

143. Huang B, Deora AB, He K, et al: Hypoxia-inducible factor-1 drives annexin A2 system-mediated perivascular fibrin clearance in oxygen-induced retinopathy in mice. *Blood* 118(10):2918–2929, 2011.

144. Jacovina AT, Zhong F, Khazanova E, et al: Neuritogenesis and the nerve growth factor-induced differentiation of PC-12 cells requires annexin II-mediated plasmin generation. *J Biol Chem* 276:49350–49358, 2001.

145. Brownstein C, Deora AB, Jacovina AT, et al: Annexin II mediates plasminogen-dependent matrix invasion by human monocytes: Enhanced expression by macrophages. *Blood* 103:317–324, 2004.

146. Menell JS, Cesarman GM, Jacovina AT, et al: Annexin II and bleeding in acute promyelocytic leukemia. *N Engl J Med* 340:994–1004, 1999.

147. Tallman MS, Abutalib SA, Altman JK: The double hazard of thrombophilia and bleeding in acute promyelocytic leukemia. *Semin Thromb Hemost* 33:330–338, 2007.

148. Stein E, McMahon B, Kwaan H, et al: The coagulopathy of acute promyelocytic leukaemia revisited. *Best Pract Res Clin Haematol* 22:152–163, 2009.

149. Liu Y, Wang Z, Jiang M, et al: The expression of annexin II and its role in the fibrinolytic activity in acute promyelocytic leukemia. *Leuk Res* 35:879–884, 2011.

150. Ishii H, Yoshida M, Hiraoka M, et al: Recombinant annexin II modulates impaired fibrinolytic activity *in vitro* and in rat carotid artery. *Circ Res* 89:1240–1245, 2001.

151. Ling Q, Jacovina AT, Deora AB, et al: Annexin II is a key regulator of fibrin homeostasis and neoangiogenesis. *J Clin Invest* 113:38–48, 2004.

152. Cesarman-Maus G, Rios-Luna NP, Deora AB, et al: Autoantibodies against the fibrinolytic receptor, annexin 2, in antiphospholipid syndrome. *Blood* 107:4375–4382, 2006.

153. Cesarman-Maus G, Cantu-Brito C, Barinagarrementeria F, et al: Autoantibodies against the fibrinolytic receptor, annexin A2, in cerebral venous thrombosis. *Stroke* 42:501–503, 2011.

154. Sebastiani P, Ramoni MF, Nolan V, et al: Genetic dissection and prognostic modeling of overt stroke in sickle cell anemia. *Nat Genet* 37:435–440, 2005.

155. Flanagan JM, Frohlich DM, Howard TA, et al: Genetic predictors for stroke in children with sickle cell anemia. *Blood* 117:6681–6684, 2011.

156. Baldwin CT, Nolan VG, Wyszynski DF, et al: Association of klotho, bone morphogenetic protein 6, and annexin A2 polymorphisms with sickle cell disease. *Blood* 106:372–375, 2005.

157. Surette AP, Madureira PA, Phipps KD, et al: Regulation of fibrinolysis by S100A10 in vivo. *Blood* 118:3172–3181, 2011.

158. Omar MN, Mann KG: Inactivation of factor Va by plasmin. *J Biol Chem* 262:9750–9755, 1987.

159. Esmon CT: The regulation of natural anticoagulant pathways. *Science* 235:1348–1352, 1987.

160. McKee PA, Anderson JC, Switzer ME: Molecular structural studies of human factor VIII. *Ann N Y Acad Sci* 240:8–33, 1975.

161. Stricker RB, Wong D, Shiu DT, et al: Activation of plasminogen by tissue plasminogen activator on normal and thrombasthenic platelets: Effects on surface proteins and platelet aggregation. *Blood* 68:275–280, 1986.

162. Adelman B, Michelson AD, Greenberg J, Handin RI: Proteolysis of platelet glycoprotein by plasmin is facilitated by plasmin lysine-binding regions. *Blood* 68:1280–1284, 1986.

163. Gimple LW, Gold HK, Leinbach RC, et al: Correlation between template bleeding times and spontaneous bleeding during treatment of acute myocardial infarction with recombinant tissue type plasminogen activator. *Blood* 80:581–588, 1989.

164. Coller BS: Platelets and thrombolytic therapy. *N Engl J Med* 322:33–42, 1990.

165. Fay WP, Garg N, Sunkar M: Vascular function of the plasminogen activation system. *Arterioscler Thromb Vasc Biol* 27:1231–1237, 2007.

166. Libby P, Aikawa M, Jain MK: Vascular endothelium and atherosclerosis. *Handb Exp Pharmacol* 176(Part 2):285–306, 2006.

167. Ploplis VA, Carmeliet P, Vazirzadeh S, et al: Effects of disruption of the plasminogen gene on thrombosis, growth, and health in mice. *Circulation* 92:2585–2593, 1995.

168. Bugge TH, Flick MJ, Daugherty CC, Degen JL: Plasminogen deficiency causes severe thrombosis but is compatible with development and reproduction. *Genes Dev* 9:794–807, 1995.

169. Romer J, Bugge TH, Pyke C, et al: Impaired wound healing in mice with a disrupted plasminogen gene. *Nat Med* 2:287–292, 1996.

170. Bugge TH, Kombrinck KW, Flick MJ, et al: Loss of fibrinogen rescues mice from the pleiotropic effects of plasminogen deficiency. *Cell* 87:709–719, 1996.

171. Xiao Q, Danton MJS, Witte DP, et al: Plasminogen deficiency accelerates vessel wall disease in mice predisposed to atherosclerosis. *Proc Natl Acad Sci U S A* 94:10335–10340, 1997.

172. Carmeliet P, Moons L, Lijnen R, et al: Urokinase-generated plasmin activates matrix metalloproteinases during aneurysm formation. *Nat Genet* 17:439–444, 1997.

173. Eitzman DT, Westrick RJ, Xu Z, et al: Plasminogen activator inhibitor-1 deficiency protects against atherosclerosis progression in the mouse carotid artery. *Blood* 96:4212–4215, 2000.

174. Sjoland H, Eitzman DT, Gordon D, et al: Atherosclerosis progression in LDL receptor-deficient and apolipoprotein E-deficient mice is independent of genetic alterations in plasminogen activator inhibitor-1. *Arterioscler Thromb Vasc Biol* 20:846–852, 1999.

175. Luttun A, Lupu F, Storkebaum E, et al: Lack of plasminogen activator inhibitor-1 promotes growth and abnormal remodeling of advanced atherosclerotic plaque in apolipoprotein E-deficient mice. *Arterioscler Thromb Vasc Biol* 22:499–505, 2002.

176. Plow EF, Ploplis VA, Busuttil S, et al: A role of plasminogen in atherosclerosis and restenosis models in mice. *Thromb Haemost* 82(Suppl):4–7, 1999.

177. Ploplis VA, French EL, Carmeliet P, et al: Plasminogen deficiency differentially affects recruitment of inflammatory cell populations in mice. *Blood* 91:2005–2009, 1998.

178. Moons L, Wi C, Ploplis V, et al: Reduced transplant arteriosclerosis in plasminogen-deficient mice. *J Clin Invest* 102:1788–1797, 1998.

179. Heymans S, Luttun A, Nuyens D, et al: Inhibition of plasminogen activators or matrix metalloproteinases prevents cardiac rupture but impairs therapeutic angiogenesis and causes cardiac failure. *Nat Med* 5:1135–1142, 1999.

180. Lijnen HR, Van Hoef B, Lupu F, et al: Function of the plasminogen/plasmin and matrix metalloproteinase systems after vascular injury in mice with targeted inactivation of fibrinolytic system genes. *Arterioscler Thromb Vasc Biol* 18:1035–1045, 1998.

181. Carmeliet P, Moons L, Ploplis VA, et al: Impaired arterial neointima formation in mice with disruption of the plasminogen gene. *J Clin Invest* 99:200–208, 1997.

182. Carmeliet P, Moons L, Herbert JM, et al: Urokinase but not tissue plasminogen activator mediates arterial neointima formation in mice. *Circ Res* 81:829–839, 1997.

183. Carmeliet P, Moons L, Dewerchin M, et al: Receptor-independent role of urokinase-type plasminogen activator in pericellular plasmin and matrix metalloproteinase proteolysis during vascular wound healing in mice. *J Cell Biol* 140:233–245, 1998.

184. Carmeliet P, Moons L, Lijnen R, et al: Inhibitory role of plasminogen activator inhibitor-1 in arterial wound healing and neointima formation. *Circulation* 96:3180–3191, 1997.

185. de Waard V, Armitage RJ, Carmeliet P, et al: Plasminogen activator inhibitor-1 and vitronectin protect against stenosis in a murine carotid ligation model. *Arterioscler Thromb Vasc Biol* 22:1978–1983, 2002.

186. Konstantinides S, Schafer K, Loskutoff DJ: Do PAI-1 and vitronectin promote or inhibit neointima formation? *Arterioscler Thromb Vasc Biol* 22:1943–1945, 2002.

187. Eitzman DT, Westrick RJ, Nabel EG, Ginsburg D: Plasminogen activator inhibitor-1 and vitronectin promote vascular thrombosis in mice. *Blood* 95:577–580, 2000.

188. Konstantinides S, Schafer K, Thinnes T, Loskutoff DJ: Plasminogen activator inhibitor-1 and its cofactor vitronectin stabilize arterial thrombi following vascular injury in mice. *Circulation* 103:576–583, 2001.

189. Schafer K, Konstantinides S, Riedel C, et al: Different mechanisms of increased luminal stenosis after arterial injury in mice deficient for urokinase- or tissue-type plasminogen activator. *Circulation* 106:1847–1852, 2002.

190. Schafer K, Muller K, Hecker A, et al: Enhanced thrombosis in atherosclerosis-prone mice is associated with increased arterial expression of plasminogen activator. *Arterioscler Thromb Vasc Biol* 23:2097–2103, 2003.

191. Zhu Y, Farrehi PM, Fay WP: Plasminogen activator inhibitor type 1 enhances neointima formation after oxidative vascular injury in atherosclerosis-prone mice. *Circulation* 103:3105–3110, 2001.

192. Ploplis VA, Cornelissen I, Sandoval-Cooper MJ, et al: Remodeling of the vessel wall after copper-induced injury is highly attenuated in mice with a total deficiency of plasminogen activator inhibitor-1. *Am J Pathol* 158:107–117, 2001.

193. Peng L, Bhatia N, Parker AC, et al: Endogenous vitronectin and plasminogen activator-1 promote neointima formation in murine carotid arteries. *Arterioscler Thromb Vasc Biol* 22:934–939, 2002.

194. DeYoung MB, Tom C, Dichek DA: Plasminogen activator inhibitor type 1 increases neointima formation in balloon-injured rat carotid arteries. *Circulation* 104:1972–1981, 2001.

195. Scanu AM, Fless GM: Lipoprotein(a) heterogeneity and biologic relevance. *J Clin Invest* 85:1709–1715, 1990.

196. Utermann G: The mysteries of lipoprotein(a). *Science* 246:904–910, 1989.

197. Loscalzo J: Lipoprotein(a), a unique risk factor for atherothrombotic disease. *Arteriosclerosis* 10:672–679, 1990.

198. Hajjar KA, Nachman RL: The role of lipoprotein(a) in atherogenesis and thrombosis. *Annu Rev Med* 47:423–442, 1996.

199. McLean JW, Tomlinson JE, Kuang WJ, et al: CDNA sequence of human apolipoprotein(a) is homologous to plasminogen. *Nature* 330:132–137, 1987.

200. Weitkamp LR, Guttormsen SA, Schultz JS: Linkage between the loci for the Lp(a) lipoprotein (Lp) and plasminogen (PLG). *Hum Genet* 79:80–82, 1988.

201. Neven L, Khalil A, Pfaffinger D, et al: Rhesus monkey model of familial hypercholesterolemia: Relation between plasma Lp(a) levels, apo(a) isoforms and LDL-receptor function. *J Lipid Res* 31:633–643, 1990.

202. Pfaffinger D, Schuelke J, Kim C, et al: Relationship between apo(a) isoforms and Lp(a) density in subjects with different apo(a) phenotype: A study before and after a fatty meal. *J Lipid Res* 32:679–683, 1991.

203. Utermann G, Menzel HJ, Kraft HG, Duba HC, Kemmler HG, Seitz C: Lp(a) glycoprotein phenotypes. *J Clin Invest* 80:458–465, 1987.

204. Maeda S, Abe A, Seishima M, et al: Transient changes of serum lipoprotein(a) as an acute phase protein. *Atherosclerosis* 78:145–150, 1989.

205. Wright LC, Sullivan DR, Muller M, et al: Elevated apolipoprotein(a) levels in cancer patients. *Int J Cancer* 43:241–244, 1989.

206. Gavish D, Azrolan N, Breslow JL: Fish oil reduces plasma Lp(a) levels and affects post-prandial association of apo(a) with triglyceride rich lipoproteins. *J Clin Invest* 84:2021–2027, 1989.

207. Koschinsky ML, Beisiegel U, Henne-Bruns D, et al: Apolipoprotein(a) size heterogeneity is related to variable number of repeat sequences in its mRNA. *Biochemistry* 29:640–644, 1990.

208. Lerch PG, Rickli EE, Lergier W, Gillessen D: Localization of individual lysine-binding regions in human plasminogen and investigations on their complex-forming properties. *Eur J Biochem* 107:7–13, 1980.

209. Armstrong VW, Harrach B, Robenek H, et al: Heterogeneity of human lipoprotein Lp(a): Cytochemical and biochemical studies on the interaction of two Lp(a) species with the LDL receptor. *J Lipid Res* 31:429–441, 1990.

210. Wolf K, Rith M, Niendorf A, et al: Thrombosis: Cellular elements of the vasculature. *Circulation* 80:522, 1989.

211. Grainger DJ, Kemp PR, Liu AC, et al: Activation of transforming growth factor-beta is inhibited in transgenic apolipoprotein(a) mice. *Nature* 370:460–462, 1994.

212. Palabrica TM, Liu AC, Aronovitz MJ, et al: Antifibrinolytic activity of apolipoprotein(a) in vivo: Human apolipoprotein(a) transgenic mice are resistant to tissue plasminogen activator-mediated thrombolysis. *Nat Med* 1:256–259, 1995.

213. Petros AM, Ramesh V, Llinas M: NMR studies of aliphatic ligand binding to human plasminogen kringle 4. *Biochemistry* 28:1368–1376, 1989.

214. Hajjar KA: The endothelial cell tissue plasminogen activator receptor: Specific interaction with plasminogen. *J Biol Chem* 266:21962–21970, 1991.

215. Hajjar KA, Gavish D, Breslow J, Nachman RL: Lipoprotein(a) modulation of endothelial cell surface fibrinolysis and its potential role in atherosclerosis. *Nature* 339:303–305, 1989.

216. Gonzales-Gronow M, Edelberg JM, Pizzo SV: Further characterization of the cellular plasminogen binding site: Evidence that plasminogen 2 and lipoprotein a compete for the same site. *Biochemistry* 28:2374–2377, 1989.

217. Miles LA, Fless GM, Levin EG, et al: A potential basis for the thrombotic risks associated with lipoprotein(a). *Nature* 339:301–303, 1989.

218. Edelberg JM, Gonzalez-Gronow M, Pizzo SV: Lipoprotein(a) inhibition of plasminogen activation by tissue-type plasminogen activator. *Thromb Res* 57:155–162, 1990.

219. Loscalzo J, Weinfeld M, Fless G, Scanu AM: Lipoprotein(a), fibrin binding, and plasminogen activation. *Arteriosclerosis* 10:240–245, 1990.

220. Lawn RM, Wade DP, Hammer RE, et al: Atherogenesis in transgenic mice expressing human apolipoprotein(a). *Nature* 360:670–672, 1992.

221. Boonmark NW, Lou XJ, Schwartz K, et al: Modification of apolipoprotein(a) lysine binding site reduces atherosclerosis in transgenic mice. *J Clin Invest* 100:558–564, 1997.

222. Kraus JP: Molecular basis of phenotype expression in homocystinuria. *J Inherit Metab Dis* 17:383–390, 1994.

223. Boushey CJ, Beresford SAA, Omenn GS, Motulsky AG: A quantitative assessment of plasma homocysteine as a risk factor for vascular disease. *JAMA* 274:1049–1057, 1995.

224. Refsum H, Ueland PM, Nygard O, Vollset SE: Homocysteine and cardiovascular disease. *Annu Rev Med* 49:31–62, 1998.

225. Ueland PM, Loscalzo J: Homocysteine and cardiovascular risk: The perils of reductionism in a complex system. *Clin Chem* 58:1623–1625, 2012.

226. Hajjar KA: Homocysteine-induced modulation of tissue plasminogen activator binding to its endothelial cell membrane receptor. *J Clin Invest* 91:2873–2879, 1993.

227. Hajjar KA, Mauri L, Jacovina AT, et al: Tissue plasminogen activator binding to the annexin II tail domain: Direct modulation by homocysteine. *J Biol Chem* 273:9987–9993, 1998.

228. Jacovina AT, Deora AB, Ling Q, et al: Homocysteine inhibits neoangiogenesis in mice through blockade of annexin A2-dependent fibrinolysis. *J Clin Invest* 119:3384–3394, 2009.

229. Miyakis S, Lockshin MD, Atsumi T, et al: International consensus statement on an update of the classification criteria for definite antiphospholipid syndrome (APS). *J Thromb Haemost* 4:295–306, 2006.

230. Cockrell E, Espinola RG, McCrae KR: Annexin A2: Biology and relevance to the antiphospholipid syndrome. *Lupus* 17:943–951, 2008.

231. Ma K, Simantov R, Zhang JC, et al: High affinity binding of beta 2-glycoprotein I to human endothelial cells is mediated by annexin II. *J Biol Chem* 275:15541–15548, 2000.

232. Zhang J, McCrae KR: Annexin A2 mediates endothelial cell activation by antiphospholipid/anti-beta2 glycoprotein I antibodies. *Blood* 105:1964–1969, 2005.

233. Raschi E, Testoni C, Bosisio D, et al: Role of the My88 transduction signaling pathway in endothelial activation by antiphospholipid antibodies. *Blood* 101:3295–3500, 2003.

234. Romay-Penabad Z, Montiel-Manzano MG, Pappalardo E, et al: Pathogenic effects of antiphospholipid antibodies are ameliorated in annexin A2 deficient mice. *Blood* 114:3074–3083, 2009.

235. von Bruhl ML, Stark K, Steinhart A, et al: Monocytes, neutrophils, and platelets cooperate to initiate and propagate venous thrombosis in mice *in vivo*. *J Exp Med* 209:819–835, 2012.

236. Polgar J, Matuskova J, Wagner DD: The P-selectin, tissue factor, coagulation triad. *J Thromb Haemost* 3:1590–1596, 2005.

237. Ardoin SP, Shanahan JC, Pisetsky DS: The role of microparticles in inflammation and thrombosis. *Scand J Immunol* 66:159–165, 2007.

238. George FD: Microparticles in vascular diseases. *Thromb Res* 122:S55–S59, 2008.

239. Lechner D, Weltermann A: Circulating tissue factor-exposing microparticles. *Thromb Res* 122:S47–S54, 2008.

240. Peerschke EI, Yin W, Ghebrehiwet B: Platelet mediated complement activation. *Adv Exp Med Biol* 632:81–91, 2008.

241. Muller WA: Leukocyte-endothelial cell interactions in leukocyte transmigration and the inflammatory response. *Trends Immunol* 24:326–333, 2003.

242. Angiari S, Donnarumma T, Rossi B, et al: TIM-1 glycoprotein binds the adhesion receptor P-selectin and mediates T cell trafficking during inflammation and autoimmunity. *Immunity* 40:542–553, 2014.

243. Wilkins PP, Moore KL, McEver RP, Cummings RD: Tyrosine sulfation of P-selectin glycoprotein ligand-1 is required for high affinity binding to P-selectin. *J Biol Chem* 270:22677–22680, 1995.

244. Snapp KR, Craig R, Herron M, et al: Dimerization of P-selectin glycoprotein ligand-1 (PSGL-1) required for optimal recognition of P-selectin. *J Cell Biol* 142:263–270, 1998.

245. Lalor P, Nash GB: Adhesion of flowing leucocytes to immobilized platelets. *Br J Haematol* 89:725–732, 1995.

246. Tanaka Y, Adams DH, Hubscher S, et al: T-cell adhesion induced by proteoglycan-immobilized cytokine MIP-1 beta. *Nature* 361:79–82, 1995.

247. Lo SK, Lee S, Ramos RA, et al: Endothelial-leukocyte adhesion molecule 1 stimulates the adhesive activity of leukocyte integrin CD3 (CD11B/CD18, Mac-1, alpha m beta 2) on human neutrophils. *J Exp Med* 173:1493–1500, 1991.

248. Lorant DE, Patel KD, McIntyre TM, et al: Coexpression of GMP-140 and PAF by endothelium stimulated by histamine or thrombin: A juxtacrine system for adhesion and activation of neutrophils. *J Cell Biol* 115:223–234, 1991.

249. Huber AR, Kunkel SL, Todd RF, Weiss SL: Regulation of transendothelial neutrophil migration by endogenous interleukin-8. *Science* 254:99–102, 1991.

250. Tanaka Y, Albelda SM, Horgan KJ, et al: CD31 expressed on distinctive T cell subsets is a preferential amplifier of beta 1 integrin-mediated adhesion. *J Exp Med* 176:245–253, 1992.

251. Piali L, Albelda SM, Baldwin HS, et al: Murine platelet endothelial cell adhesion molecule (PECAM-1/CD31) modulates beta2 integrins on lymphokine-activated killer cells. *Eur J Immunol* 23:2464–2471, 1993.

252. Berman ME, Muller WA: Ligation of platelet/endothelial cell adhesion molecule 1 (PECAM-1/CD31) on monocytes and neutrophils increases binding capacity of leukocyte CR3 (CD11b/CD18). *J Immunol* 154:299–307, 1995.

253. Hynes RO: Integrins: Versatility, modulation, and signalling in cell adhesion. *Cell* 69:11–25, 1992.

254. Carlos TM, Harlan JM: Leukocyte-endothelial cell adhesion molecules. *Blood* 84:2068–2101, 1994.

255. Miles A, Liaskou E, Eksteen B, et al: CCL25 and CCL28 promote alpha4 beta7-integrin-dependent adhesion of lymphocytes to MAdCAM-1 under shear flow. *Am J Physiol Gastrointest Liver Physiol* 294:G1257–G1267, 2008.

256. Bargatze RF, Kurk S, Butcher EC, Jutila MA: Neutrophils roll on adherent neutrophils bound to cytokine-induced endothelial cells via L-selectin on the rolling cells. *J Exp Med* 180:1785–1792, 1994.

257. Walcheck B, Moore KL, McEver RP, Kishimoto TK: Neutrophil-neutrophil interactions under hydrodynamic shear stress involve L-selectin and PSGL-1. *J Clin Invest* 98:1081–1087, 1996.

258. Muller WA: Migration of leukocytes across the vascular intima. Molecules and mechanisms. *Trends Cardiovasc Med* 5:15–20, 1995.

259. Sullivan DP, Muller WA: Neutrophil and monocyte recruitment by PECAM, CD99, and other molecules via the LBRC. *Semin Immunopathol* 36:193–209, 2014.

260. Ley K, Laudanna C, Cybulsky MI, Nourshargh S: Getting to the site of inflammation: The leukocyte adhesion cascade updated. *Nat Rev Immunol* 7:678–689, 2007.

261. Muller WA, Ratti CM, McDonnell SL, Cohn ZA: A human endothelial cell-restricted, externally disposed plasmalemmal protein enriched in intercellular junctions. *J Exp Med* 170:399–414, 1989.

262. Newman PJ, Berndt MC, Gorski J, et al: PECAM-1 (CD31) cloning and relation to adhesion molecules of the immunoglobulin gene superfamily. *Science* 247:1219–1222, 1990.

263. Muller WA, Weigl SA, Deng X, Phillips DM: PECAM-1 is required for transendothelial migration of leukocytes. *J Exp Med* 178:449–460, 1993.

264. Huang AJ, Manning JE, Bandak TM, et al: Endothelial cell cytosolic free calcium regulates neutrophil migration across monolayers of endothelial cells. *J Cell Biol* 120:1371–1380, 1993.

265. Liao F, Ali J, Greene T, Muller WA: Soluble domain 1 of platelet-endothelial cell adhesion molecule (PECAM) is sufficient to block transendothelial migration in vitro and in vivo. *J Exp Med* 185:1349–1357, 1997.

266. Liao F, Huynh HK, Eiroa A, et al: Migration of monocytes across endothelium and passage through extracellular matrix involve separate molecular domains of PECAM-1. *J Exp Med* 182:1337–1343, 1995.

267. Ostermann G, Weber KSC, Zernecke A, et al: JAM-1 is a ligand for the b2 integrin LFA-1 involved in transendothelial migration of leukocytes. *Nat Immunol* 3:151–158, 2002.

268. Johnson-Leger C, Aurrand-Lions M, Beltraminelli N, et al: Junctional adhesion molecule-2 (JAM-2) promotes lymphocyte transendothelial migration. *Blood* 100:2479–2486, 2002.

269. Feng D, Nagy JA, Pyne K, et al: Neutrophils emigrate from venules by a transendothelial cell pathway in response to fMLP. *J Exp Med* 187:903–915, 1999.

270. Carman CV, Springer TA: Trans-cellular migration: Cell-cell contacts get intimate. *Curr Opin Cell Biol* 20:533–540, 2008.

271. Bixel MG, Petri B, Khandoga AG, et al: A CD99-related antigen on endothelial cells mediates neutrophil, but not lymphocyte extravasation *in vivo*. *Blood* 109:5327–5336, 2009.

272. Dufour EM, Deroche A, Bae Y, Muller WA: CD99 is essential for leukocyte diapedesis in vivo. *Cell Commun Adhes* 15:351–363, 2008.

273. Schenkel AR, Mamdouh Z, Chen X, et al: CD99 plays a major role in the migration of monocytes through endothelial junctions. *Nat Immunol* 3:2479–2486, 2002.

274. Marchesi VT, Florey HW: Electron micrographic observations on the emigration of leukocytes. *Q J Exp Physiol Cogn Med Sci* 45:343–347, 1960.

275. Schnoor M, Lai FP, Zarbock A, et al: Cortactin deficiency is associated with reduced neutrophil recruitment but increased vascular permeability *in vivo*. *J Exp Med* 208:1721–1735, 2011.

276. Leeuwenberg JFM, von Asmuth EJ, Jeunhomme TM, Buurman WA: IFN-gamma regulates the expression of the adhesion molecule ELAM-1 and IL-6 production by human endothelial cells in vitro. *J Immunol* 145:2110–2114, 1990.

277. Strindall J, Lundblad A, Pahlsson P: Interferon-gamma enhancement of E-selectin expression on endothelial cells is inhibited by monensin. *Scand J Immunol* 46:338–343, 1997.

278. Ley K, Arbones ML, Bosse R, et al: Sequential contribution of L- and P-selectin to leukocyte rolling *in vivo*. *J Exp Med* 181:669–675, 1995.

279. Khew-Goodall Y, Butcher E, Litwin MS, et al: Chronic expression of P-selectin on endothelial cells stimulated by the T-cell cytokine, interleukin-3. *Blood* 87:1432–1438, 1999.

280. Yao L, Pan J, Setiadi H, et al: Interleukin-4 or oncostatin M induces a prolonged increase in P-selectin mRNA and protein in human endothelial cells. *J Exp Med* 184:81–92, 1996.

281. Jung U, Ley K: Regulation of E-selectin, P-selectin, and intercellular adhesion molecule-1 expression in mouse cremaster vasculature. *Microcirculation* 4:311–319, 1997.

282. Pan J, Xia L, Yao L, McEver RP: Tumor necrosis factor-alpha- or lipopolysaccharide-induced expression of the murine P-selectin gene in endothelial cells involves novel kappaB sites and a variant activating transcription factor/cAMP response element. *J Biol Chem* 273:10067–10077, 1998.

283. Masinovsky B, Urdal D, Gallatin WM: IL-4 acts synergistically with IL-1 beta to promote lymphocyte adhesion to microvascular endothelium by induction of vascular cell adhesion molecule-1. *J Immunol* 145:2886–2895, 1990.

284. Blease K, Seybold J, Adcock IM, et al: Interleukin-4 and lipopolysaccharide synergize to induce vascular cell adhesion molecule-1 expression in human lung microvascular endothelial cells. *Am J Respir Cell Mol Biol* 18:620–630, 1998.

285. Pober JS, Collins T, Gimbrone M, et al: Inducible expression of class II major histocompatibility complex antigens and the immunogenicity of vascular endothelium. *Transplantation* 41:141–146, 1986.

286. Savage CO, Hughes CC, McIntyre BW, et al: Human CD4+ cells proliferate to HLA-DR+ allogeneic vascular endothelium. Identification of accessory interactions. *Transplantation* 56:128–134, 1993.

287. Pober JS, Orosz CG, Rose ML, Savage CO: Can graft endothelial cells initiate a host anti-graft immune response? *Transplantation* 61:343–349, 1996.

288. Romer LH, McLean NV, Horng-Chin Y, et al: IFN-gamma and TNF-alpha induce redistribution of PECAM-1 (CD31) on human endothelial cells. *J Immunol* 154:6582–6592, 1995.

289. Tang Q, Hendricks RL: Interferon gamma regulates platelet endothelial cell adhesion molecule-1 expression and neutrophil infiltration into herpes simplex virus-infected mouse corneas. *J Exp Med* 184:1435–1447, 1996.

290. Rival Y, Del Maschio A, Rabiet MJ, et al: Inhibition of platelet endothelial cell adhesion molecule-1 synthesis and leukocyte transmigration in endothelial cells by the combined action of TNF-alpha and IFN-gamma. *J Immunol* 157:1233–1241, 1996.

291. Kaplanski G, Fabrigoule M, Boulay V, et al: Thrombin induces endothelial type II activation *in vitro*: IL-1 and TNF-alpha-independent IL-8 secretion and E-selectin expression. *J Immunol* 158:5435–5441, 1997.

292. Diacovo TG, Puri KD, Warnock RA, et al: Platelet-mediated lymphocyte delivery to high endothelial venules. *Science* 273:252–255, 1996.

293. Diacovo TG, Catalina MD, Siegelman MH, Von Adrian UH: Circulating activated platelets reconstitute lymphocyte homing and immunity in L-selectin-deficient mice. *J Exp Med* 187:197–204, 1998.

294. Buttrum SM, Hatton R, Nash GB: Selectin-mediated rolling of neutrophils on immobilized platelets. *Blood* 82:1165–1174, 1993.

295. Diacovo TG, Roth SJ, Buccola JM, et al: Neutrophil rolling, arrest, and transmigration across activated, surface-adherent platelets via sequential action of P-selectin and the beta 2-integrin CD11b/CD18. *Blood* 88:146–157, 1996.

296. Diacovo TG, de Fougerolles AR, Bainton DF, Springer TA: A functional integrin ligand on the surface of platelets: Intercellular adhesion molecule-2. *J Clin Invest* 94:1243–1251, 1994.

297. Simon DI, Chen Z, Xu H, et al: Platelet glycoprotein Ibα is a counterreceptor for the leukocyte integrin Mac-1 (CD11b/CD18). *J Exp Med* 192:193–214, 2000.

298. Santoso S, Sachs UJ, Kroll H, et al: The junctional adhesion molecule 3 (JAM-3) on human platelets is a counterreceptor for the leukocyte integrin Mac-1. *J Exp Med* 196:679–691, 2002.

299. Frenette PS, Denis CV, Weiss L, et al: P-selectin glycoprotein ligand 1 (PSGL-1) is expressed on platelets and can mediate platelet-endothelial interactions *in vivo*. *J Exp Med* 191:1413–1422, 2000.

300. Chauhan AK, Kisucka J, Brill A, et al: ADAMTS13: A new link between thrombosis and inflammation. *J Exp Med* 205:2065–2074, 2008.

301. Altieri DC: Coagulation assembly on leukocytes in transmembrane signaling and cell adhesion. *Blood* 81:569–579, 1993.

302. Lo SK, Cheung A, Zheng Q, Silverstein RL: Induction of tissue factor in monocytes by adhesion to endothelial cells. *J Immunol* 154:4768–4777, 1995.

303. Fan ST, Mackman N, Cui MZ, Edgington TS: Integrin regulation of an inflammatory effector gene: Direct induction of the tissue factor promoter by engagement of beta1 or alpha4 integrin chains. *J Immunol* 154:3266–3274, 1995.

304. Randolph GJ, Luther T, Albrecht S, et al: Role of tissue factor adhesion of mononuclear phagocytes to and trafficking through endothelium. *Blood* 92:4167–4177, 1998.

305. Palabrica T, Lobb R, Furie BC, et al: Leukocyte accumulation promoting fibrin deposition is mediated in vivo by P-selectin on adherent platelets. *Nature* 359:848–851, 1992.

306. Wright SD, Weitz JI, Huang AJ, et al: Complement receptor type (CR3, CD11b/CD18) of human polymorphonuclear leukocytes recognizes fibrinogen. *Proc Natl Acad Sci U S A* 85:7734–7738, 1988.

307. Altieri DC, Morrisey JH, Edgington TS: Adhesive receptor Mac-1 coordinates the activation of factor X on stimulated cells of monocytic and myeloid differentiation: An alternative initiation of the coagulation protease cascade. *Proc Natl Acad Sci U S A* 85:7462–7466, 1988.

308. Altieri DC, Edgington TS: The saturable high affinity association of factor X to ADP-stimulated monocytes defines a novel function of the Mac-1 receptor. *J Biol Chem* 263:7007–7015, 1988.

309. Macfarlane RG: An enzyme cascade in the blood clotting mechanism, and its function as a biochemical amplifier. *Nature* 202:498–499, 1964.

310. Davie EW, Ratnoff OD: Waterfall sequence for intrinsic blood clotting. *Science* 145:1310–1312, 1964.

311. Huber R, Berendes R, Burger A, et al: Crystal and molecular structure of human annexin V after refinement: Implications for structure, membrane binding and ion channel formation of the annexin family of proteins. *J Mol Biol* 223:683–704, 1992.

312. Huang KS, Wallner BP, Mattaliano RJ, et al: Two human 35 kd inhibitors of phospholipase A2 are related to substrates of pp60 v-src and of the epidermal growth factor receptor/kinase. *Cell* 46:191–199, 1986.

313. Blasi F, Conese M, Moller LB, et al: The urokinase receptor: Structure, regulation and inhibitor-mediated internalization. *Fibrinolysis* 8:182–188, 1994.

# CHAPTER 6

# CLASSIFICATION, CLINICAL MANIFESTATIONS, AND EVALUATION OF DISORDERS OF HEMOSTASIS

Marcel Levi, Uri Seligsohn, and Kenneth Kaushansky

## SUMMARY

Evaluation of a hemostatic disorder is commonly initiated when (1) a patient or referring physician suspects a bleeding tendency, (2) a bleeding tendency is discovered in one or more family members, (3) an abnormal coagulation assay result is obtained from an individual as part of a routine examination, (4) an abnormal assay result is obtained from a patient during preparation for surgery, or (5) a patient has unexplained diffuse bleeding during or after surgery or following trauma. Evaluation of a possible hemostatic disorder in each of these scenarios is a stepwise process that requires knowledge of the various classes of hemostatic disorders commonly found under the particular circumstances. The patient's history, the results of physical examination, and an initial set of hemostatic tests usually enable a tentative diagnosis. However, more specific tests are commonly necessary to make a definitive diagnosis. This chapter reviews the necessary steps.

## ● CLASSIFICATION OF HEMOSTATIC DISORDERS

Hemostatic disorders can conveniently be classified as either hereditary or acquired (Table 6–1). Alternatively, hemostatic disorders can be classified according to the mechanism of the defect. Of the acquired disorders, the thrombocytopenias are the most frequently encountered entities. Thrombocytopenias can result from reduced production of platelets, excessive destruction caused by antibodies or other consumptive processes, or pooling of platelets in the spleen, as in hypersplenism (Chap. 7); however, if hypersplenism is the sole cause of a hemostatic disorder, it is rarely severe enough to cause pathologic bleeding.

## ● BLEEDING HISTORY

The bleeding history is a crucial element in the evaluation of a patient with a hemorrhagic disorder. The bleeding history helps define the subsequent diagnostic approach and the likelihood of future bleeding.

**Acronyms and Abbreviations:** aPTT, activated partial thromboplastin time; DIC, disseminated intravascular coagulation; ELISA, enzyme-linked immunosorbent assay; PT, prothrombin time; RCF, ristocetin cofactor.

Eliciting and interpreting all of the relevant information requires a systematic and methodical approach. The following points are worth considering:

1. Patients vary in their responses to hemorrhagic symptoms. Some patients ignore significant symptoms, whereas other patients are highly sensitive to even minor symptoms. When asked in standardized questionnaires, many normal, healthy people indicate they have excessive bleeding or bruising.[1,2] Therefore, some experts believe the question "Do you bruise easily?" is virtually worthless. Women are more likely to respond that they have excessive bleeding or bruising than are men.

2. Patients with severe hemorrhagic disorders invariably have very abnormal bleeding histories, for example, severe hemophilia A or hemophilia B, type 3 (homozygous) von Willebrand disease, and Glanzmann thrombasthenia. Importantly, these patients may experience spontaneous bleeding episodes.

3. The diagnostic value of any specific symptom varies in the different disorders. Therefore, recognizing typical patterns of bleeding is important (Table 6–2). Unprovoked hemarthroses and muscle hemorrhages suggest one of the hemophilias, whereas mucocutaneous bleeding (epistaxis, gingival bleeding, menorrhagia) is more characteristic of patients with qualitative platelet disorders, thrombocytopenia, or von Willebrand disease.

4. Assessing the extent of hemorrhage against the background of any trauma or provocation that may have elicited the hemorrhage is important. If a patient has never had a significant hemostatic challenge, such as tooth extraction, surgery, trauma, or childbirth, the lack of a significant bleeding history is much less valuable in excluding a mild hemorrhagic disorder. For example, a significant percentage of patients with mild von Willebrand disease or mild forms of hemophilia may have negative bleeding histories,[1] even though they may be at considerable risk for excessive bleeding after surgery or other interventions. Thus, these diagnoses must be considered even in elderly patients if their first severe hemostatic challenge occurs at that age.

5. Obtaining objective confirmation of the subjective information conveyed in the bleeding history is valuable. Objective data include (1) previous hospital or physician visits for bleeding symptoms, (2) results of previous laboratory evaluations, (3) previous transfusions of blood products for bleeding episodes, and (4) a history of anemia and/or previous treatment with iron.

6. Although self-administered questionnaires may provide useful background information, they cannot substitute for a dialogue between the physician and the patient. Thus, history taking in general, but especially in the often subtle histories related to hemostatic disorders, is an intellectually active process involving data collection, hypothesis development, new question formulation, additional data gathering, and new hypothesis development. However, this iterative procedure has its limitations even when it is carefully pursued.[3,4]

7. A medication history is a crucial component of the bleeding history, with particular attention to nonprescription drugs, such as aspirin and nonsteroidal antiinflammatory agents, which may affect bleeding symptoms. A medication history is especially important in patients with thrombocytopenia, because drug-induced thrombocytopenia is common (Chap. 10 and see Table 6–1). Medication also may affect hemostasis through deleterious effects on the liver or kidney functions. The increased use of herbal and alternative medicines poses particular problems, because patients may not readily share information about what they are taking, and

**TABLE 6–1.** Classification of Disorders of Hemostasis

| Major Types | Disorders | Examples |
|---|---|---|
| Acquired | Thrombocytopenias | Autoimmune and alloimmune, drug-induced, hypersplenism, hypoplastic (primary, myelosuppressive therapy, myelophthisic marrow infiltration), disseminated intravascular coagulation (DIC), thrombotic thrombocytopenic purpura, hemolytic uremic syndrome (Chaps. 7, 19, and 22) |
| | Liver diseases | Cirrhosis, acute hepatic failure, liver transplantation (Chap. 18), thrombopoietin deficiency |
| | Renal failure | |
| | Vitamin K deficiency | Malabsorption syndrome, hemorrhagic disease of the newborn, prolonged antibiotic therapy, malnutrition, prolonged biliary obstruction |
| | Hematologic disorders | Acute leukemias (particularly promyelocytic), myelodysplasias, monoclonal gammopathies, essential thrombocythemia |
| | Acquired antibodies against coagulation factors | Neutralizing antibodies against factors V, VIII, and XIII, accelerated clearance of antibody-factor complexes, e.g., acquired von Willebrand disease, hypoprothrombinemia associated with antiphospholipid antibodies (Chaps. 16, 17, and 21) |
| | DIC | Acute (sepsis, malignancies, trauma, obstetric complications) and chronic (malignancies, giant hemangiomas, retained products of conception) (Chap. 19) |
| | Drugs | Antiplatelet agents, anticoagulants, antithrombins, and thrombolytic, hepatotoxic, and nephrotoxic agents (Chaps. 23–25) |
| | Vascular | Nonpalpable purpura ("senile," solar, and factitious purpura), use of corticosteroids, vitamin C deficiency, child abuse, thromboembolic, purpura fulminans; palpable purpura (Henoch-Schönlein, vasculitis, dysproteinemias; Chap. 12), amyloidosis |
| Inherited | Deficiencies of coagulation factors | Hemophilia A (factor VIII deficiency), hemophilia B (factor IX deficiency), deficiencies of fibrinogen factors II, V, VII, X, XI, and XIII, and von Willebrand disease (Chaps. 13–16) |
| | Platelet disorders | Glanzmann thrombasthenia, Bernard-Soulier syndrome, platelet granule disorders (Chap. 10) |
| | Fibrinolytic disorders | $a_2$-Antiplasmin deficiency, plasminogen activator inhibitor-1 deficiency (Chap. 25) |
| | Vascular | Hemorrhagic telangiectasias (Chap. 12) |
| | Connective tissue disorders | Ehlers-Danlos syndrome (Chap. 12) |

the dose they are taking of any particular active ingredient may be difficult to determine. *Ginkgo biloba* and ginseng are the most commonly used herbals that can cause platelet dysfunction and induce bleeding.[5] Other dietary supplements can display similar effects.[5,6]

8. A nutrition history should be obtained to assess the likelihood of (1) vitamin K deficiency, especially if the patient also is taking broad-spectrum antibiotics; (2) vitamin C deficiency, especially if the patient has skin bleeding consistent with scurvy (perifollicular purpura); and (3) general malnutrition and/or malabsorption.

9. Several tissues have an increased local fibrinolytic activity. Such tissues include the urinary tract, endometrium, and mucous membranes of the nose and oral cavity. These sites are particularly likely to have prolonged oozing of blood after trauma in patients with hemostatic abnormalities. Excessive bleeding following tooth extraction is one of the most common manifestations. Bleeding resulting from defects in fibrin crosslinking (factor XIII deficiency), or fibrinolytic defects may often manifest as delayed bleeding after trauma.

10. Bleeding isolated to a single organ or system (e.g., hematuria, hematemesis, melena, hemoptysis, or recurrent nosebleeds) is less likely to result from a hemostatic abnormality than from a local cause such as neoplasm, ulcer, or angiodysplasia. Thus, careful anatomic evaluation of the involved organ or system should be performed.

11. Bleeding may result from blood vessel disorders such as hereditary hemorrhagic telangiectasias, Cushing disease, scurvy, or Ehlers-Danlos syndrome. Many primary dermatologic disorders also have a purpuric or hemorrhagic component and must also be considered in the differential diagnosis (Chap. 12).

12. A family history is particularly important when hereditary disorders are considered. Patients usually will not spontaneously offer a history of consanguinity, so specific inquiry should be made about this possibility. A diagram of the patient's genealogic tree, extending back at least two generations, should be included to document consideration of genetic disorders. A sex-linked pattern of inheritance is consistent with hemophilia A or B (Chap. 13). An autosomal dominant pattern is characteristic of most forms of von Willebrand disease (Chap. 16). An autosomal recessive pattern is typical for all other coagulation factor deficiencies (Chap. 14), inherited platelet disorders (Chap. 10), and the rare, severe (homozygous), type 3 von Willebrand disease. Population genetic information may be helpful; for example, the higher prevalence of factor XI deficiency in Ashkenazi Jews (Chap. 14).

13. The history should include information on diseases and organs that may affect hemostasis, such as cirrhosis, renal insufficiency, myeloproliferative neoplasms (e.g., essential thrombocythemia), acute leukemia, myelodysplasia, systemic lupus erythematosus, and Gaucher disease.

**TABLE 6-2.** Clinical Manifestations Typically Associated with Specific Hemostatic Disorders

| Clinical Manifestations | Hemostatic Disorders |
| --- | --- |
| Mucocutaneous bleeding | Thrombocytopenias, platelet dysfunction, von Willebrand disease |
| Cephalohematomas in newborns, hemarthroses, hematuria, and intramuscular, intracerebral, and retroperitoneal hemorrhages | Severe hemophilias A and B, severe deficiencies of factor VII, X, or XIII, severe type 3 von Willebrand disease, afibrinogenemia |
| Injury-related bleeding and mild spontaneous bleeding | Mild and moderate hemophilias A and B, severe factor XI deficiency, moderate deficiencies of fibrinogen and factors II, V, VII, or X, combined factors V and VIII deficiency, $\alpha_2$-antiplasmin deficiency |
| Bleeding from stump of umbilical cord and habitual abortions | Afibrinogenemia, hypofibrinogenemia, dysfibrinogenemia, factor XIII deficiency |
| Impaired wound healing | Factor XIII deficiency |
| Facial purpura in newborns | Glanzmann thrombasthenia, severe thrombocytopenia |
| Recurrent severe epistaxis and chronic iron deficiency anemia | Hereditary hemorrhagic telangiectasias |

# ● CLINICAL MANIFESTATIONS

Individual hemorrhagic symptoms often require detailed analysis before the significance of the symptoms and the resulting diagnosis or therapy can be determined. Some of the more common symptoms are discussed below, and Table 6–2 summarizes clinical manifestations that are typical for specific hemostatic disorders.

1. Epistaxis is one of the most common signs of platelet disorders and von Willebrand disease. It also is the most common symptom of hereditary hemorrhagic telangiectasia. In the latter condition, epistaxis almost always becomes more severe with advancing age. Epistaxis is not uncommon in normal children, but it usually resolves before puberty. Dry air heating systems can provoke epistaxis even in otherwise normal individuals. Bleeding confined to a single nostril more likely results from a local vascular problem than a systemic coagulopathy.

2. Gingival hemorrhage is very common in patients with both qualitative and quantitative platelet abnormalities and von Willebrand disease. Occasional gum bleeding occurs in normal individuals, especially if they use a hard bristle tooth brush and dental hygiene procedures. Thus, establishing whether the bleeding is excessive may be difficult. Frequent gingival hemorrhage can occur in individuals with normal hemostasis if they have gingivitis.

3. Oral mucous membrane bleeding in the form of blood blisters is a common manifestation of severe thrombocytopenia. Such bleeding usually has a predilection for sites where teeth can traumatize the inner surface of the cheek.

4. Skin hemorrhage in the form of petechiae and ecchymoses is a common manifestation of hemostatic disorders. However, skin hemorrhage also is common among individuals without hemostatic disorders. Excessive bruising is more common in women than men.

Moreover, women frequently note that the severity of their bruising varies with the phase of their menstrual cycle, although the most severe phase of the cycle may differ in different women. Features that help establish the severity of skin hemorrhage include the size of the bruises, the frequency of bruising, whether the bruises occur spontaneously or only with trauma, and the appearance of bruises on regions of the body that usually are not traumatized, such as the trunk and back. The color of the bruise may yield information. Red bruises on the extensor surfaces of the arms and hands indicate loss of supporting tissues, as occurs in Cushing syndrome, glucocorticoid therapy, senile purpura, and damage from chronic sun exposure. Jet-black bruises may be caused by warfarin-induced skin necrosis and similar disorders. Easy bruising can also occur in patients with Ehlers-Danlos syndrome manifested by distensible skin or extraordinary ligament laxness and in patients with hyperflexibility of the thumb.[7]

5. Tooth extractions are common hemostatic challenges and may be helpful in defining the risk of bleeding. Molar extractions are greater hemostatic challenges than extractions of other teeth. Objective data regarding excessive bleeding based on the need for blood products or the need to pack or suture the extraction site are valuable.

6. Excessive bleeding in response to razor nicks is common in patients with platelet disorders or von Willebrand disease.

7. Hemoptysis almost never is the presenting symptom of a bleeding disorder and is rare even in patients with serious bleeding disorders. However, blood-tinged sputum in association with upper respiratory tract infections may be more common in patients with hemostatic disorders.

8. Hematemesis, like hemoptysis, almost never is the presenting symptom of a hemostatic disorder. However, a hemostatic disorder may lead to hematemesis because of an anatomic abnormality in the upper gastrointestinal tract, and bleeding may be more severe than expected. Some hemostatic disorders more likely result in hematemesis because of a combination of effects, such as liver disease with deficient synthesis of coagulation proteins and with esophageal varices and aspirin ingestion with gastritis.

9. Hematuria is rarely the presenting symptom of a hemostatic disorder except for the hemophilias. However, hemostatic disorders can exacerbate hematuria caused by other disorders, including simple urinary tract infections.

10. Rectal bleeding in individuals with normal hemostasis most often results from hemorrhoids. However, von Willebrand disease and platelet disorders may contribute to repeated episodes of rectal bleeding when associated with a number of different underlying causes, including diverticula, hemorrhoids, or angiodysplasia. Melena is also only rarely the presenting symptom of a hemorrhagic disorder. However, repeated episodes of melena may occur in patients with hemorrhagic disorders.

11. Menorrhagia is common in women with platelet disorders and von Willebrand disease. In general, menstrual bleeding is considered excessive if the patient indicates she has heavy flow for more than 3 days or total flow for more than 7 days. However, an objective distinction between menorrhagia (loss of more than 80 mL blood per period) and normal blood loss can only be made by a visual assessment technique using pictorial charts of towels or tampons.[8]

12. Postpartum hemorrhage. Childbirth poses a considerable hemostatic challenge. Consequently, patients with bleeding disorders commonly manifest excessive bleeding during or after labor necessitating blood transfusion. An exception may be mild and moderate von Willebrand disease due to the vast increase in von Willebrand factor during pregnancy.

13. Habitual spontaneous abortions raise the possibility that the patient has a quantitative or qualitative abnormality of fibrinogen (Chap. 15), factor XIII deficiency (Chap. 14), or the antiphospholipid syndrome (Chap. 21). There is also an association between infertility and spontaneous abortion in patients with inherited thrombophilia (Chap. 20).

14. Hemarthroses are the hallmark abnormality in the hemophiliac; they are rare in other disorders except in severe factor VII deficiency and type 3 von Willebrand disease (Chaps. 14 and 16). Because discoloration of the skin overlying the joint with hemarthroses does not occur, patients may not recognize that their symptoms (pain, swelling, and limitation of motion) are caused by bleeding into their joints.

15. Excessive hemorrhage associated with surgical procedures is common in patients with hemorrhagic disorders. Procedures involving tissues with increased local fibrinolytic activity, such as the urinary tract, nose, tonsils and oral cavity, are particularly prone to bleed.

16. Excessive bleeding following circumcision is common in males with severe hemostatic disorders such as hemophilia A, hemophilia B, or Glanzmann thrombasthenia and often is the patient's first symptom.

17. Bleeding from the umbilical stump is characteristic of factor XIII deficiency (Chap. 14) and afibrinogenemia (Chap. 15).

## ● PHYSICAL EXAMINATION

Physical examination is essential for identifying signs of bleeding or their sequelae and for identifying signs of a possible underlying disorder that can cause the hemostatic derangement (see Table 6–1). Careful examination of the skin is essential for detecting petechiae and ecchymoses. These signs may be prominent on the legs, where the hydrostatic pressure is greatest, or around the hair follicles in vitamin C deficiency.

Telangiectasias may range from pinpoint erythematous dots that blanch with pressure to classic cherry angiomata ranging in size up to several centimeters. Many normal individuals develop increasing numbers of telangiectasias with aging. Patients with hereditary hemorrhagic telangiectasia have more florid lesions that characteristically affect the vermilion border of the lips and the tongue (including the underside of the tongue), but not all patients have these classic features. Thus, a systematic search of the integument is necessary. Spider telangiectasias found in patients with chronic liver disease have a more splotchy and serpiginous appearance than the telangiectasias associated with hereditary hemorrhagic telangiectasia. In addition, the telangiectasias tend to be concentrated on the shoulders, chest, and face.

Chapter 12 details the differential diagnosis of nonpalpable purpuras and palpable purpuras. Hematomas, ecchymoses, and protracted oozing should be sought at venipuncture sites, injection sites, and arterial and venous catheter insertion sites. Joint deformities and limited joint mobility are suggestive of severe hemophilia A or B, severe deficiency of factor VII, or type 3 von Willebrand disease (Chaps. 13, 14, and 16). Hyperelasticity of the skin and hyperextensibility of joints are typical of Ehlers-Danlos syndrome, and hyperextensibility of only the thumb probably is a variant.[7]

## ● EVALUATION BASED ON BLEEDING HISTORY, PHYSICAL EXAMINATION, AND BASIC LABORATORY TESTS

The patient's history and results of physical examination provide important information on the likelihood of the patient having a hemostatic defect and the possible cause of the defect, if one is present. However,

performing an initial set of widely available and inexpensive tests, including prothrombin time (PT), activated partial thromboplastin time (aPTT), and platelet count, is important for the following reasons: (1) The patient's history sometimes is unreliable; (2) the patient may have a mild hemostatic abnormality that has not manifested itself for lack of hemostatic challenge; (3) the patient may have developed an acquired hemostatic defect that has remained asymptomatic; and (4) the tests may reveal more than one abnormality.[9]

Figure 6–1 shows a series of algorithms that integrate the patient's bleeding history and the results of the initial hemostatic tests. A prolonged aPTT as a sole abnormality can be caused by a deficiency of factor VIII, IX, XI, or XII; by presence of heparin; or by an inhibitor, which can be either factor specific, such as an antibody against factor VIII, or factor nonspecific, such as the presence of heparin or a lupus anticoagulant (Fig. 6–1A). A prolonged PT as the sole finding can indicate a factor VII deficiency, a mild vitamin K deficiency, or the presence of an inhibitor (Fig. 6–1B). Abnormalities of both PT and aPTT may indicate a deficiency of fibrinogen, prothrombin, factor V or factor X, an inhibitor to one of these factors, or a combined deficiency of coagulation factors (Fig. 6–1C).

To distinguish between a deficiency state and the presence of an inhibitor, repeating the abnormal test, the PT and/or aPTT, using a 1:1 mixture of the patient's plasma and normal plasma is useful. If the mixture normalizes the prolonged PT or aPTT, a deficiency state is likely, as most coagulation tests are calibrated to produce a normal result if each of the relevant factor levels are 50 percent of normal or greater. If the mixture still yields a significantly prolonged PT or aPTT, an inhibitor probably is present. Some inhibitors, such as antibodies to factor VIII, require time to inhibit the factor VIII activity in the assay, whereas other inhibitors, such as lupus anticoagulant or heparin, do not. Consequently, incubating the mixture for 1 or 2 hours at 37°C before performing the coagulation assay is desirable.

When none of the initial test results (PT, aPTT, and platelet count) is abnormal and the patient exhibits bleeding manifestations, ristocetin cofactor (RCF) or von Willebrand factor activity and examination of the blood film can be helpful for distinguishing among various candidate hemostatic abnormalities. The bleeding time is not used anymore because the test is highly operator and situation (e.g., room temperature, skin circulation) dependent and is not sufficiently reliable to be useful in the diagnostic process. Instead, many laboratories have introduced the platelet function analyzer (PFA) to detect qualitative defects in primary hemostasis. Figure 6–2 shows an algorithm that includes these secondary tests. Patients with type 1 and type 2 von Willebrand disease often have normal findings on initial laboratory tests because factor VIII levels are sufficiently high (>30 U/dL) for a normal aPTT result (Chap. 16). Examination of the blood film is helpful for distinguishing between Bernard-Soulier syndrome and von Willebrand disease because giant platelets are characteristic of the former (Chap. 10). Distinguishing mild-type von Willebrand disease from normal is difficult because levels of von Willebrand factor in the normal population are highly variable, partly accounted for by differing von Willebrand factor levels in individuals with different ABO blood types. In fact, some investigators have questioned whether patients with von Willebrand factor levels as low as 35 percent should be labeled as having von Willebrand disease.[10] The likelihood of having von Willebrand disease is a function of bleeding history, the von Willebrand factor level, and the number of first-degree family members with reduced von Willebrand factor levels.[11]

The ristocetin-induced platelet aggregation test is useful for distinguishing type 2B and platelet-type von Willebrand disease from the other types of von Willebrand disease. In type 2B and platelet-type von Willebrand disease, an enhanced response to low concentrations

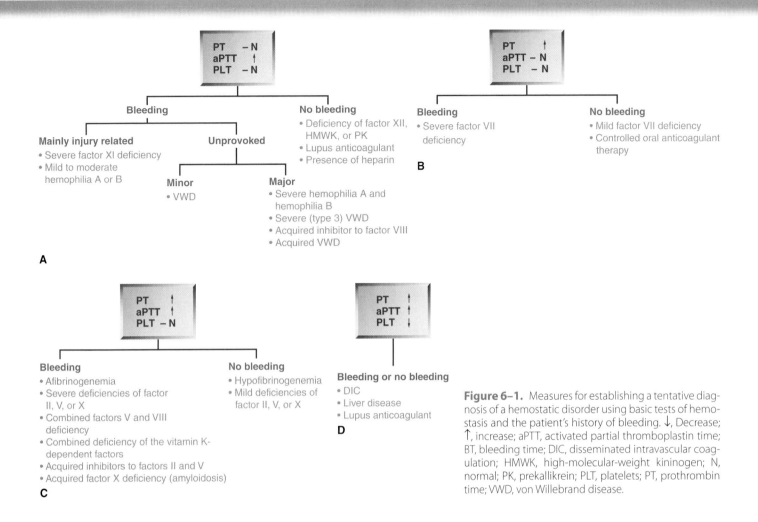

**Figure 6–1.** Measures for establishing a tentative diagnosis of a hemostatic disorder using basic tests of hemostasis and the patient's history of bleeding. ↓, Decrease; ↑, increase; aPTT, activated partial thromboplastin time; BT, bleeding time; DIC, disseminated intravascular coagulation; HMWK, high-molecular-weight kininogen; N, normal; PK, prekallikrein; PLT, platelets; PT, prothrombin time; VWD, von Willebrand disease.

of ristocetin is observed, whereas in the other types of von Willebrand disease, a decreased response is found. Total absence of platelet aggregates in a blood film prepared from non-anticoagulated blood and absent clot retraction are characteristic of Glanzmann thrombasthenia (Chap. 10).

Another simple test that may be useful for distinguishing among hemostatic disorders is the thrombin time (i.e., time for plasma to clot after adding thrombin). The thrombin time is prolonged in (1) afibrinogenemia, hypofibrinogenemia, and dysfibrinogenemias (Chap. 15); (2) the presence of heparin; (3) disseminated intravascular coagulation (DIC) causing increased levels of fibrin(ogen) degradation products, which inhibit fibrin monomer polymerization (see Fig. 6–1D and Chap. 19); and (4) patients with amyloidosis and an immunoglobulin inhibitor of thrombin.[12]

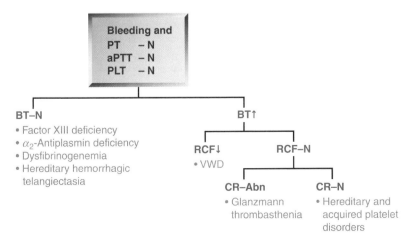

**Figure 6–2.** Tentative diagnoses in patients with bleeding manifestations and normal primary hemostatic tests using secondary tests. ↓, Decrease; ↑, increase; Abn, abnormal; aPTT, activated partial thromboplastin time; BT, bleeding time; CR, clot retraction; N, normal; PK, prekallikrein; PLT, platelets; PT, prothrombin time; RCF, ristocetin cofactor activity; VWD, von Willebrand disease.

# ● PREOPERATIVE ASSESSMENT OF HEMOSTASIS

Because surgical procedures are a great challenge to the hemostatic system, careful assessment of the risk of bleeding in every patient is important. The risk assessment is based on the bleeding history, physical examination, the underlying disorder if any, the type and site of surgery that is planned, and the results of basic hemostatic tests (PT, aPTT, platelet count). Several studies indicate that unselected coagulation tests have no significant predictive value of perioperative bleeding and that patients with a negative bleeding history do not require routine coagulation screening.[13] However, this conclusion does not consider that patients with mild to moderate bleeding disorders who can bleed excessively following surgery may have a negative bleeding history because they have not been challenged; obtaining a good bleeding history is an expertise that is not shared by all physicians; and if bleeding occurs during or after surgery for whatever reason, the basic tests performed preoperatively are an essential reference for determining the cause of bleeding.

Table 6–3 lists low-risk and high-risk conditions. A critical analysis of each potential cause of bleeding should be undertaken for the high-risk conditions. In addition to the extent of the surgical trauma, the magnitude of the fibrinolytic activity at the surgical site must be considered. For example, prostatectomy carries considerable risk of prolonged bleeding because of the presence of high fibrinolytic activity in the urine. Some surgical procedures can be anticipated to cause hemostatic abnormalities, such as operations in which extracorporeal circulation is used (because the extracorporeal circuits and/or the anticoagulation cause platelet dysfunction) and operations on patients with extensive malignancies or brain injury, which can give rise to DIC. Finally, the ability to institute local hemostatic measures should be considered. Thus, liver, lung, and kidney biopsies, although considered minor procedures, have a significant risk of bleeding because local measures, such as direct pressure, cannot be used to control bleeding.

**TABLE 6–3.** Evaluation of Bleeding Risk During Surgery

| Assessed Factor | Risk of Bleeding | |
| --- | --- | --- |
| | Low | High |
| Bleeding history | Negative | Positive* |
| Underlying conditions that compromise hemostasis (see Table 6–1) | Absent | Present |
| Initial hemostatic tests | Normal | Abnormal |
| Type of surgery | Minor | Major |
| | Not expected to induce a hemostatic defect at a site without local fibrinolysis | Expected to induce a hemostatic defect† at a site with local fibrinolysis‡ |
| | Local hemostatic measures effective | Local hemostatic measures ineffective§ |

*Spontaneous bleeding episodes or injury-related hemorrhage.

†Open heart surgery or brain surgery.

‡Prostatectomy, tonsillectomy, oral or nasal surgery.

§Liver, lung, or kidney biopsy.

# ● SPECIFIC ASSAYS FOR ESTABLISHING THE DIAGNOSIS

A tentative diagnosis can be made by following the stepwise process of evaluation outlined in Figs. 6–1 and 6–2. However, further testing usually is required to establish a definitive diagnosis.

## THROMBOCYTOPENIAS

When the laboratory reports an abnormally low platelet count, looking at the blood film to exclude pseudothrombocytopenia as a result of anticoagulant-induced platelet clumping (e.g., induced by ethylenediaminetetraacetic acid [EDTA]) is essential.[14] Examination of the blood film also can reveal the presence of giant platelets, as in some inherited thrombocytopenias; giant platelets and Döhle bodies in leukocytes, as in May-Hegglin and other MYH9 platelet syndromes; moderately enlarged platelets, as in immune thrombocytopenia or other conditions associated with shortened platelet survival; small platelets, as in Wiskott-Aldrich syndrome; schistocytes and burr cells, as in the hemolytic uremic syndrome and thrombotic thrombocytopenic purpura and occasionally in DIC; rouleaux formation, as in monoclonal gammopathies; macrocytosis and/or hypersegmentation, as in vitamin $B_{12}$ or folic acid deficiency; and abnormal white blood cells, as in leukemias and myeloproliferative disorders. Chapter 7 further discusses the evaluation and differential diagnosis of the thrombocytopenias.

## FACTOR DEFICIENCIES

Coagulation factors usually are assayed by measuring their clotting activity. The most common assays analyze the ability of dilutions of the patient's plasma to correct the clotting time of a plasma known to be deficient in the factor being measured (substrate plasma). The results are compared to the ability of dilutions of a normal reference plasma to correct the abnormality in the substrate plasma. The activities of factors II, V, VII, and X usually are determined in PT-based assays, whereas the activities of factors VIII, IX, XI, and XII, prekallikrein, and high-molecular-weight kininogen are measured in aPTT-based assays. The plasma level of fibrinogen most commonly is measured by assessing the time required for thrombin to clot the patient's diluted plasma (Clauss method).[15] Several assays of transglutaminase activity are available for measuring factor XIII activity,[16] but a simple qualitative test based on dissolving a fibrin clot in 5 M urea usually is sufficient (Chap. 14). The RCF function of von Willebrand factor can be measured by the ability of the patient's plasma to support the agglutination of a suspension of formaldehyde-fixed normal platelets by ristocetin.[17] This activity is defined as *RCF activity*. As with the coagulation factor assays, the results using patient plasma are compared to the results obtained with a normal reference plasma.

To determine whether a coagulation factor activity deficiency results from a quantitative decrease in protein or a qualitative abnormality in the protein, immunologic assays can be performed using specific polyclonal or monoclonal antibodies to assess the presence of the protein, independent of its function. Electroimmunoassays, enzyme-linked immunosorbent assays (ELISAs), and immunoradiometric assays all have been used successfully. Crossed immunoelectrophoresis measures both the immunologic reactivity and the mobility of the protein in an electric field; thus, it can detect protein abnormalities that affect electrophoretic migration. The abnormalities include the presence of antibody–antigen complexes that migrate differently from the protein itself, such as antiprothrombin–prothrombin complexes in patients with systemic lupus erythematosus or antiphospholipid syndrome. Diagnosis of the specific type of von Willebrand disease requires additional tests of the multimeric structure of plasma and, perhaps, platelet von Willebrand factor.

## INHIBITORS TO COAGULATION FACTORS

If an inhibitor is suspected as a result of a prolonged PT or aPTT performed on a 1:1 mixture of the patient's plasma and normal plasma, further studies can help define the nature of the inhibitor and its titer. Among inhibitors that do not require incubation (i.e., immediate-type), perhaps the most common cause is the presence of heparin in the sample. This cause can be verified by finding a prolonged thrombin time on a test of the patient's plasma that is corrected with toluidine blue or other agents that neutralize heparin. The lupus anticoagulant also does not require incubation, and several methods for its detection are available (Chap. 21). However, with lupus anticoagulant, the PT usually is less prolonged than is the aPTT, and aPTT reagents have markedly different sensitivity to lupus-type anticoagulant depending on the amount of phosphatidyl serine present in each reagent.

Immunoglobulin inhibitors to specific coagulation factors may develop either after factor replacement therapy in patients with inherited deficiencies of coagulation factors (Chaps. 13 and 14) or spontaneously in patients without factor deficiencies (Chap. 17). Antibodies that neutralize factor activity frequently can be detected by incubating the patient's plasma with normal plasma, usually for 2 hours at 37°C, and then assaying the specific factor. The Bethesda assay originally was designed to quantify factor VIII inhibitors but can be modified to detect other inhibitors of coagulation factors (Chap. 13).[18] Some inhibitors do not directly neutralize clotting activity; instead, they reduce factor levels by forming complexes with coagulation factors, which then are rapidly cleared from the circulation. Such plasmas do not produce prolonged clotting times when mixed 1:1 with normal plasma and thus may be confused with inherited deficiency states. More elaborate assays are required to identify this type of inhibitor, which may, for example, produce severe deficiency of prothrombin in some patients with the antiphospholipid syndrome (Chap. 21) and deficiency of von Willebrand factor in some acquired forms of von Willebrand disease (Chap. 16).[19]

## PLATELET FUNCTION DISORDERS

Some laboratories nowadays routinely use an automated PFA to detect qualitative defects in primary hemostasis. Use of the RCF activity assay, platelet aggregation, and/or clot retraction is useful for assessing whether the patient has von Willebrand disease or a platelet function disorder (see Fig. 6–2). Chapter 10 contains a flow diagram of the steps required to diagnose the different qualitative disorders of platelet function. Additional platelet function assays and glycoprotein analysis may be required to establish the diagnosis.

## REFERENCES

1. Miller CH, Graham JB, Goldin LR, Elston RC: Genetics of classic von Willebrand's disease: II. Optimal assignment of the heterozygous genotype (diagnosis) by discriminant analysis. *Blood* 54:137, 1979.
2. Wahlberg T, Blomback M, Hall P, Axelsson G: Application of indicators, predictors and diagnostic indices in coagulation disorders: I. Evaluation of a self-administered questionnaire with binary questions. *Methods Inf Med* 19:194, 1980.
3. Eikenboom JC, Rosendaal FR, Briet E: Value of the patient interview: All but consensus among haemostasis experts. *Haemostasis* 22:221, 1992.
4. Sramek A, Eikenboom JC, Briet E, et al: Usefulness of patient interview in bleeding disorders. *Arch Intern Med* 155:1409, 1995.
5. Dinehart SM, Henry L: Dietary supplements: Altered coagulation and effects on bruising. *Dermatol Surg* 31:819, 2005.
6. Basila D, Yuan C-S: Effects of dietary supplements on coagulation and platelet function. *Thromb Res* 117:49, 2005.
7. Kaplinsky C, Kenet G, Seligsohn U, Rechavi G: Association between hyperflexibility of the thumb and an unexplained bleeding tendency: Is it a rule of thumb? *Br J Haematol* 101:260, 1998.
8. Janssen CAH, Scholten PC, Heintz APM: A simple visual assessment technique to discriminate between menorrhagia and normal menstrual blood loss. *Obstet Gynecol* 85:977, 1995.
9. Rapaport SI: Preoperative hemostatic evaluation: Which tests, if any? *Blood* 61:229, 1983.
10. Sadler JE: Von Willebrand disease type 1: A diagnosis in search of a disease. *Blood* 101:2089, 2003.
11. Tosetto A, Castaman G, Rodeghiero F: Evidence-based diagnosis of type 1 von Willebrand disease: A Bayes theorem approach. *Blood* 111:3998, 2008.
12. Gastineau DA, Gertz MA, Daniels TM, et al: Inhibitor of the thrombin time in systemic amyloidosis: A common coagulation abnormality. *Blood* 77:2637, 1991.
13. Chee YL, Crawford JC, Watson HG, Greaves M: Guidelines on the assessment of bleeding risk prior to surgery or invasive procedures. *Br J Haematol* 140:496, 2008.
14. Payne BA, Pierre RV: Pseudothrombocytopenia: A laboratory artifact with potentially serious consequences. *Mayo Clin Proc* 59:123, 1984.
15. Clauss A: Gerinnungsphysiologische schnell methodes zur des fibrinogens. *Acta Haematol* 17:327, 1957.
16. Fickenscher K, Aab A, Stuber W: A photometric assay for blood coagulation factor XIII. *Thromb Haemost* 65:535, 1991.
17. McFarlane DE, Stibbe J, Kirby EP, et al: A method for assaying von Willebrand factor (ristocetin cofactor). *Thromb Diath Haemorrh* 34:306, 1975.
18. Kasper CK, Aledort L, Aronson D, et al: Proceedings: A more uniform measurement of factor VIII inhibitors. *Thromb Diath Haemorrh* 34:612, 1975.
19. Inbal A, Bank I, Zivelin A, et al: Acquired von Willebrand disease in a patient with angiodysplasia resulting from immune-mediated clearance of von Willebrand factor. *Br J Haematol* 96:179, 1997.

# CHAPTER 7
# THROMBOCYTOPENIA

Reyhan Diz-Küçükkaya and José A. López

## SUMMARY

Thrombocytopenia is one of the most frequent causes for hematologic consultation in the practice of medicine and may be life threatening. Although the normal platelet count in humans (150 to $400 \times 10^9$/L) far exceeds the minimal level required to avoid pathologic hemorrhage ($<50 \times 10^9$/L), a number of medical conditions either increasing the destruction of platelets or reducing their production enhance the risk of bleeding. This chapter discusses an approach to the diagnosis of thrombocytopenia, grouping various causes by mechanism of action, and describing our current understanding of the pathogenesis, treatment, and prognosis. In the vast majority of patients, a cause for thrombocytopenia can be identified and effective therapy instituted.

## ● DEFINITION AND HISTORY

Platelets are anucleate blood cells produced in the marrow by polyploid cells termed megakaryocytes and were described in the 19th century after the application of the improved compound microscope allowed these very small cellules, approximately 2 $\mu$M in

Acronyms and Abbreviations: ACOG, American College of Obstetricians and Gynecologists; ADP, adenosine diphosphate; AFLP, acute fatty liver of pregnancy; AML, acute myelogenous leukemia; APLA, antiphospholipid antibody; APS, antiphospholipid syndrome; ARC, arthrogryposis–renal dysfunction–cholestasis; ASH, American Society of Hematology; ATG, antithymocyte globulin; ATRUS, amegakaryocytic thrombocytopenia with radioulnar synostosis; CAMT, congenital amegakaryocytic thrombocytopenia; CAPTURE, c7E3 Fab Antiplatelet Therapy in Unstable Refractory Angina; CTP, cyclic thrombocytopenia; CVID, common variable immunodeficiency; DIC, disseminated intravascular coagulation; EDTA, ethylenediaminetetraacetic acid; EPIC, Evaluation of 7E3 for the Prevention of Ischemic Complications; EPILOG, Evaluation of Percutaneous Transluminal Coronary Angioplasty to Improve Long-term Outcome of c7E3 GPIIb-IIIa Receptor Blockade; EPISTENT, Evaluation of Platelet IIb/IIIa Inhibitor for Stenting; Flt1, fms-like tyrosine kinase-1; FPD/AML, familial platelet disorder with propensity to acute myeloid malignancy; GP, glycoprotein; HCV, hepatitis C virus; HELLP, hemolysis, elevated liver enzymes, low platelets; HIT, heparin-induced thrombocytopenia; HPA, human platelet alloantigen; HUS, hemolytic uremic syndrome; ICSH, International Council for Standardization in Hematology; IDA, iron-deficiency anemia; IPD, inherited platelet disorder; ITP, immune thrombocytopenia; IVIG, intravenous immunoglobulin; IWG, International Working Group; LTA, light transmission aggregometry; MACE, modified antigen capture enzyme-linked immunosorbent assay; MAIPA, monoclonal antibody-specific immobilization of platelet antigens; MDS, myelodysplastic syndrome; MHC, major histocompatibility complex; NAIT, neonatal alloimmune thrombocytopenia; PAIgG, platelet-associated immunoglobulin G; sFlt1, soluble Flt1; SLE, systemic lupus erythematosus; TAR, thrombocytopenia with absent radii; TPO, thrombopoietin; Treg, T-regulatory; TTP, thrombotic thrombocytopenic purpura; VEGF, vascular endothelial growth factor; VWD, von Willebrand disease; VWF, von Willebrand factor.

diameter, to be identified. Many early investigators are associated with the discovery of blood platelets, including Donné, Hayem, Bizzozero, and Osler, but it was James Homer Wright who, in 1906, using his special stain (later called Wright stain), described the morphology of platelets with their central granular area and marginal hyaline zone and established that they were the product of the fragmentation of marrow megakaryocytes. Clot retraction was discovered long before platelets, but Hayem, through a series of studies, showed retraction to be dependent on platelets. During the mid-20th century, the aggregation of platelets, their adherence to collagen of damaged tissues, their acceleration of blood coagulation, and their relationship to the bleeding time and the biochemistry underlying several of these processes were described by scientists, among whom were Paul Owren, Kenneth Brinkhaus, Edwin Chargaff, Ernst Lüsher, Marjorie Zucker, and William Duke.

Platelets circulate in close contact with the endothelium, continually monitoring its integrity. When the vessel wall is damaged, platelets bind to subendothelial proteins, initiating the process of primary hemostasis. At sites of blood loss, the platelets aggregate to form a vessel-sealing plug to halt bleeding. Activated platelets at sites of injury also provide a surface for assembly of coagulation reactions, resulting in the production of fibrin and consolidation of the thrombus. Both qualitative and quantitative deficiencies of the platelets cause bleeding. Platelets also have important functions in inflammation, tissue remodeling, and wound healing.[1]

Approximately $1 \times 10^{11}$ platelets are produced per day by an adult human, a number that can be increased 20-fold or more, if necessary.[2] One-third of the platelets are stored in the spleen, and the remaining two-thirds circulate in blood vessels.[3] Disorders that increase splenic volume cause more platelets to be trapped in the spleen, lowering the concentration of circulating platelets, although alone, this redistribution rarely causes a significant bleeding diathesis.

Under normal conditions, human platelets have a mean life span in the circulation of between 7 and 10 days.[4,5] Patients with thrombocytopenia secondary to platelet destruction have a markedly decreased platelet survival.[6,7] Patients with thrombocytopenia from marrow failure have mildly decreased platelet survival, mostly because the body's fixed daily consumption of platelets accounts for a progressively larger fraction of the reduced total daily production as the platelet count drops.[8] Platelet turnover is a measure of the net effect of platelet production and platelet destruction under steady-state conditions.[7] Several studies using $^{111}$In oxine–labeled platelets have established that, under normal conditions, platelet turnover in humans ranges from 40 to $50 \times 10^9$/L per day.[7] Although a high platelet turnover is expected in patients with immune thrombocytopenia (ITP), platelet production is not always increased in this disorder.[7] Low platelet production may result from binding of the antiplatelet antibodies to megakaryocytes, inhibiting their maturation or leading to their destruction and causing an inappropriately muted marrow response to the degree of thrombocytopenia.[9]

Every day approximately 10 to 12 percent of circulating platelets are removed by the mononuclear phagocyte system, primarily by macrophages in the spleen and liver. Although the precise mechanisms of platelet clearance are not completely understood, changes that occur as the platelets circulate are thought to lead them to be recognized by macrophages. One of these changes is the progressive loss of sialic acid from platelet surface proteins. Studies in animals and humans with anticancer drugs that inhibit apoptotic pathways have also identified a role for apoptotic proteins in platelet survival and clearance. According to these studies, a classical intrinsic apoptosis pathway regulates the life span of circulating platelets, and antiapoptotic proteins, especially Bcl-$_{XL}$, maintain platelet viability by restraining apoptosis.[10]

## THE PLATELET COUNT

The normal platelet count (defined as the values between percentiles 2.5 and 97.5 in normal individuals) is given as 150 to 400 × 10⁹/L; classically, thrombocytopenia is defined as a platelet count of less than 150 × 10⁹/L. However, a sustained lower platelet count (100 to 150 × 10⁹/L) can be seen in otherwise healthy individuals.[11,12] Long-term observation of individuals with platelet counts between 100 and 150 × 10⁹/L showed that 88 percent of these individuals had subsequently reached normal platelet counts or remained stable. In those individuals, the probability of developing ITP was 6.9 percent, an autoimmune disease other than ITP 12 percent, and myelodysplastic syndrome (MDS) 2 percent, after 64 months of follow-up. All patients with MDS in this cohort were found to be older than age 65 years.[13]

## THROMBOCYTOPENIA

Thrombocytopenia can be classified as severe (platelet count less than 20 × 10⁹/L), moderate (platelet count 20 to 70 × 10⁹/L), or mild (above 70 × 10⁹/L).[14] Although easy bruising occurs in patients with platelet counts less than 50 × 10⁹/L and spontaneous life-threatening bleeding can be expected in patients with platelet counts less than 15 × 10⁹/L, bleeding symptomatology is largely determined by comorbid conditions affecting platelets or the coagulation system, including liver cirrhosis, uremia, disseminated intravascular coagulation (DIC), or antiplatelet drug usage.

In clinical practice, platelet counting is automated and includes several different technologies: impedance, optical, two-dimensional laser, and optical-fluorescence methods. Although automated cell counter technology has progressed considerably during recent decades, the analytic performances of these machines for platelet counts and platelet indices is still not perfect, especially in patients with severe thrombocytopenia and macrothrombocytopenia.[15–17] Each step between the sampling of blood and its analysis is important: the blood sample should be obtained by a clean venipuncture without dilution with other IV solutions or drugs. Blood/anticoagulant ratio should be as recommended. The International Council for Standardization in Hematology (ICSH) recommends use of ethylenediaminetetraacetic acid (EDTA) as the anticoagulant. Adequate mixing of the blood sample with EDTA (the final EDTA concentration should be 1.5 to 2.2 mg/mL) is crucial to prevent clumping of the platelets. Blood samples should be kept at room temperature and analyzed within 6 hours of phlebotomy. If a sample is to be analyzed more than 6 hours after it is drawn, it can be kept at 4°C for 24 hours. The blood count analyzer should be cleaned according to laboratory standards.[17]

Although thrombocytopenia is variably attributed to single factors such as decreased platelet production, increased platelet destruction, or abnormal splenic pooling, combinations of factors are often involved in clinical settings. For instance, the thrombocytopenia seen in patients with viral infection can result from many factors, including platelet destruction (e.g., through an autoimmune mechanism or drug toxicity) or decreased platelet production because of direct megakaryocyte infection by the virus. Table 7–1 lists the multiple causes of thrombocytopenia and classifies them by pathogenesis.

## ● PSEUDO (SPURIOUS) THROMBOCYTOPENIA

Pseudothrombocytopenia (or spurious thrombocytopenia) is a relatively uncommon phenomenon with multiple causes, including *ex vivo* agglutination of platelets, the presence of abnormally large platelets (improper counting), or improper preparation of blood samples.

The incidence of pseudothrombocytopenia reported in different studies ranges from 0.09 to 0.21 percent, which accounts for 15 to 30 percent of all cases of isolated thrombocytopenia.[18–25] Pseudothrombocytopenia has been reported in association with the use of EDTA as an anticoagulant, with platelet cold agglutinins,[26] and with myeloma.[27] A very interesting report demonstrates pseudothrombocytopenia caused by platelet phagocytosis *ex vivo* in the presence of EDTA anticoagulant.[28]

**TABLE 7–1.** Classification of Thrombocytopenia

**I. Pseudo (spurious) thrombocytopenia**
A. Antibody-induced platelet aggregation
B. Platelet satellitism
C. Antiphospholipid antibodies
D. Glycoprotein IIb/IIIa antagonists
E. Miscellaneous

**II. Thrombocytopenia resulting from impaired platelet production**
A. Inherited platelet disorders
B. Acquired marrow disorders
 1. Nutritional deficiencies and alcohol-induced thrombocytopenia
 2. Clonal hematologic diseases (myelodysplastic syndrome, leukemias, myeloma, lymphoma, paroxysmal nocturnal hemoglobinuria)
 3. Aplastic anemia
 4. Marrow metastasis by solid tumors
 5. Marrow infiltration by infectious agents (HIV, tuberculosis, brucellosis, etc.)
 6. Hemophagocytosis
 7. Immune thrombocytopenia (ITP)
 8. Drug-induced thrombocytopenia
 9. Pregnancy-related thrombocytopenia

**III. Thrombocytopenia resulting from increased platelet destruction**
A. Immune thrombocytopenia
 1. Autoimmune thrombocytopenia (primary and secondary ITP)
 2. Alloimmune thrombocytopenia
B. Thrombotic microangiopathies (TTP, hemolytic uremic syndrome [HUS])
C. Disseminated intravascular coagulopathy (DIC)
D. Pregnancy-related thrombocytopenia
E. Hemangiomas (Kasabach-Merritt phenomenon)
F. Drug-induced immune thrombocytopenia (quinidine, heparin, abciximab)
G. Artificial surfaces (hemodialysis, cardiopulmonary bypass, extracorporeal membrane oxygenation)
H. Type 2B von Willebrand disease

**IV. Thrombocytopenia resulting from abnormal distribution of the platelets**
A. Hypersplenism
B. Hypothermia
C. Massive blood transfusions
D. Excessive fluid infusions

**V. Miscellaneous Causes**
A. Cyclic thrombocytopenia, acquired pure megakaryocytic thrombocytopenia

## ANTIBODY-INDUCED PLATELET AGGLUTINATION

Platelet agglutination *ex vivo* can be induced by antiplatelet antibodies or by activation of the platelets during collection. The responsible antibodies do not appear to be associated with a pathologic process, as they are found in normal individuals. One hypothesis put forth to explain their presence is that the antibodies are responsible for clearing aged and damaged platelets. Most antibodies implicated in pseudothrombocytopenia recognize platelet membrane glycoproteins that are modified to expose new epitopes when calcium is chelated. Typically, the artifact is most prominent in the presence of EDTA, but other anticoagulants can also cause platelet clumping, including sodium citrate, sodium oxalate, acid citrate dextrose, and heparin. The antibodies usually are of the immunoglobulin (Ig) G type; IgM and IgA antibodies also have been described.[29–31] Most antibodies react at room temperature; thus, the reaction can be prevented by keeping the blood sample at 37°C. In 20 percent of cases, however, the antibodies, usually of the IgM type, are reactive at both 22°C and 37°C.[30] Clumping usually is evident within 60 minutes after the blood is drawn, but may require incubations of 2 to 3 hours. Agglutination can be reproduced by incubating plasma from patients with pseudothrombocytopenia with blood from normal individuals in the presence of EDTA.

In most cases, the antibodies are directed against the integrin $\alpha_{IIb}\beta_3$ (also termed glycoprotein [GP] IIb/IIIa), a conclusion supported by the observation that platelets from patients with Glanzmann thrombasthenia, who lack the integrin $\alpha_{IIb}\beta_3$ complex, fail to agglutinate in the presence of patient sera.[32–35] Moreover, pretreatment of fresh blood with anti–integrin $\alpha_{IIb}\beta_3$ dramatically reduces EDTA-induced platelet agglutination.[36] The responsible epitope normally is cryptic and located in the integrin $\alpha_{IIb}$ subunit. Low temperature and calcium chelation combine to change the conformation of integrin $\alpha_{IIb}\beta_3$ and expose the epitope.[33]

## PLATELET SATELLITISM

Antibodies directed against integrin $\alpha_{IIb}\beta_3$ may react simultaneously with the leukocyte Fc$\gamma$ receptor III (Fc$\gamma$RIII) and attach the platelets to neutrophils and monocytes, inducing a phenomenon known as *platelet-leukocyte satellitism*,[32] another form of pseudothrombocytopenia (Fig. 7–1). These antibodies fail to produce satellitism in the presence of platelets from patients with type I Glanzmann thrombasthenia or in the presence of neutrophils from patients with congenital absence of Fc$\gamma$RIII.[32] Typically, the platelets form a rosette around the periphery of leukocytes. Neutrophils are most frequently involved, but the phenomenon also is occasionally observed with monocytes.[37,38] These antibodies also are naturally occurring, and their presence does not clearly correlate with any specific clinical situation, disease, or drug. As with the antibodies that induce only platelet clumping, exposure of a cryptic antigen on EDTA-treated platelets and leukocytes may trigger this phenomenon.

## ANTIPHOSPHOLIPID ANTIBODIES

Some antiplatelet antibodies from patients with pseudothrombocytopenia cross react with negatively charged phospholipids and may exhibit anticardiolipin activity.[30] The sera of these patients lose their ability to clump platelets when adsorbed onto either cardiolipin or activated normal platelets, supporting the hypothesis that antibody subpopulations directed against negatively charged phospholipids can bind to antigens modified by EDTA on the platelet membrane. Another possibility is that the antigens in this case are negatively charged phospholipids on the surface of platelets.

## INTEGRIN $\alpha_{IIb}\beta_3$ ANTAGONISTS

Thrombocytopenia has been described in patients suffering from acute coronary syndromes treated with the abciximab and other integrin $\alpha_{IIb}\beta_3$ antagonists.[39–41] Abciximab is associated with both pseudothrombocytopenia and true thrombocytopenia. The mechanism for platelet clumping with abciximab is unknown; the drug itself likely is not cross-linking the platelets because it is monovalent. More likely, other agglutinins bind integrin $\alpha_{IIb}\beta_3$ at new epitopes induced by the combination of abciximab binding and calcium chelation. True abciximab-induced thrombocytopenia occurs in approximately 0.3 to 1 percent of patients treated with the drug.[42] The mechanism is incompletely understood, but likely includes reaction of preformed antibodies with a neoepitope expressed after binding of abciximab to integrin $\alpha_{IIb}\beta_3$ (ligand-induced binding sites) or abciximab-induced platelet activation with subsequent platelet sequestration from the circulation. In some abciximab-treated patients, high antibody titers are detected in the plasma.

The incidence of pseudothrombocytopenia and thrombocytopenia related to abciximab was determined in four large placebo-controlled trials:[40] c7E3 Fab Antiplatelet Therapy in Unstable Refractory Angina (CAPTURE), Evaluation of 7E3 for the Prevention of Ischemic

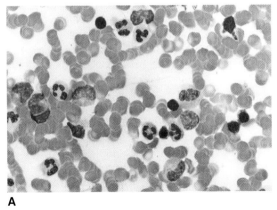
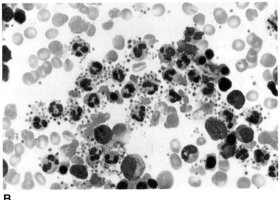

**A**    **B**

**Figure 7–1.** Platelet satellitism. **A.** Direct (non-anticoagulated) marrow film. No platelet satellitism. **B.** A concentrated marrow film anticoagulated with disodium ethylenediaminetetraacetic acid (Na$_2$EDTA) from same specimen as in **(A)**. Note platelets are adherent to the mature neutrophil surface (satellitism) in the presence of Na$_2$EDTA. The neutrophil precursors do not have surface features that interact with platelets, apparently a feature only present after the final steps in maturation. *(Reproduced with permission from Lichtman's Atlas of Hematology, www.accessmedicine.com.)*

Complications (EPIC), Evaluation of Percutaneous Transluminal Coronary Angioplasty to Improve Long-term Outcome of c7E3 GPIIb-IIIa Receptor Blockade (EPILOG), and Evaluation of Platelet IIb/IIIa Inhibitor for Stenting (EPISTENT). In these studies, pseudothrombocytopenia accounted for more than one-third of low platelet counts in patients undergoing coronary interventions and treated with abciximab. These studies demonstrated that pseudothrombocytopenia is a benign laboratory condition not associated with increased bleeding, stroke, transfusion requirements, or the need for repeat revascularization.

## MISCELLANEOUS ASSOCIATIONS

Some studies suggest that platelet agglutinins occur more frequently in hospitalized patients and in association with medical conditions such as autoimmune diseases, malignancy, liver disease, and sepsis.[25,43–46] However, others found no association with any particular pathology or with use of specific drugs.[30]

One study showed that antibodies from patients with pseudothrombocytopenia can induce agglutination of donor platelets in the presence of EDTA. This agglutination was prevented by warming the donor platelets to 37°C or by pretreating the platelets with aspirin, prostaglandin $E_1$, apyrase, and monoclonal antibodies against integrin $\alpha_{IIb}\beta_3$ that block the binding site for fibrinogen and von Willebrand factor (VWF), or arg-gly-asp (RGD) peptide, which binds the site on integrin $\alpha_{IIb}\beta_3$ that recognizes cytoadhesive proteins.[33] Whether the same reaction occurs *in vivo* is not known, but in that case, the antibodies should have a slow reactivity, or else bleeding would sometimes occur.

## MANAGEMENT OF PATIENTS WITH PSEUDOTHROMBOCYTOPENIA

An (unexpected) low platelet count reported by automated cell counters should be confirmed by microscopic examination of the blood film. Automated cell counters identify platelets merely based on their small volumes in comparison to those of other blood cells, generally defined as volumes between 2 and 20 fL. Because platelet clumps tend to exceed 20 fL, the clumps may be counted as leukocytes,[18] and even if counted as platelets, several platelets are counted as one. Thus, pseudothrombocytopenia may be accompanied by pseudoleukocytosis.[5,21,24,47] The greater the delay in processing of anticoagulated blood, the greater is the degree of platelet clumping and the greater the potential for artifact.[21] Platelet clumping can be prevented by collecting the sample in EDTA and maintaining its temperature at 37°C. Even with these measures, however, clumping will still occur in approximately 20 percent of cases.[30]

Another alternative is use of sodium citrate, which chelates calcium more weakly than does EDTA but still causes platelet clumping in approximately 10 to 20 percent of cases with EDTA-induced clumping. In some patients, an accurate platelet count can be obtained only by sampling blood directly into ammonium oxalate and manually counting the platelets using a Bruker chamber.[30] Flow cytometry may help for determining exact platelet number by immunostaining of the platelets.

Platelet agglutinins are not associated with bleeding or thrombosis, so they appear to have no clinical implications, except that they may lead to unnecessary therapy because of misdiagnosis. Transplacental transmission of agglutinins has been documented, but the pseudothrombocytopenia induced by these antibodies in the neonate resolves spontaneously.[48,49] No complications have been reported when platelet agglutinins are discovered during pregnancy.[48,50] Transfusion of blood products from patients with pseudothrombocytopenia produces an acceptable corrected count increment in the recipient, again supporting its benign nature.[23] Thus, the clinical importance of

pseudothrombocytopenia concerns conditions with which it is confused rather than any pathology associated with the condition. It is important that this syndrome be recognized promptly to avoid unnecessary diagnostic tests and treatment.

## ● INHERITED PLATELET DISORDERS

Megakaryopoiesis and thrombopoiesis are regulated by a number of hematopoietic growth factors and transcription factors (Chap. 3). Any genetic defect affecting platelet production, function, or morphology may cause inherited platelet disorders (IPDs; Chap. 11). In recent decades, knowledge of normal megakaryocyte and platelet physiology has grown enormously,[51] aided in part by the study of IPDs.[52,53]

IPDs are a very heterogeneous group of disorders. Some disorders, such as Bernard-Soulier syndrome, appear to be restricted to platelets,[54] whereas others appear as a part of a complex pathology, as seen in thrombocytopenia with absent radii (TAR) syndrome (Fig. 7–2). In some IPDs, the platelet count may be normal despite severely impaired platelet function, such as in Glanzmann thrombasthenia. Other disorders are accompanied by abnormal platelet numbers, usually thrombocytopenia. Table 7–2 summarizes the inherited thrombocytopenias.

Severe forms of IPDs that present as a bleeding tendency early in childhood are rare. IPD patients usually present with mucocutaneous bleeding, such as with purpura, epistaxis, and/or gingival bleeding. Menorrhagia and bleeding during pregnancy and labor are common problems in female patients. Spontaneous life-threatening bleeding is rare, including intracranial hemorrhage or massive gastrointestinal or genitourinary bleeding. Recent molecular investigations of IPD patients and their families with bleeding diathesis demonstrated that most IPDs cause mild bleeding tendencies, and IPDs may be more prevalent than previously thought.[55] In these milder cases, a bleeding diathesis may only be diagnosed after an episode of excessive bleeding, such as during surgery or following trauma.

Diagnosis of IPD presents a significant challenge because of the heterogeneity of clinical and laboratory findings of patients with the same disorder, even in the same family. IPD patients with isolated macrothrombocytopenia share common clinical and basic laboratory features with certain acquired platelet disorders and are sometimes misdiagnosed. It is very important to distinguish IPD patients from those with acquired platelet disorders, such as ITP, to avoid unnecessary or potentially harmful treatments. Helpful in this regard is information obtained during the history, including a family history of bleeding and consanguinity in the family, because the majority of IPDs are inherited as autosomal recessive traits. Because some IPDs are associated with increased risk of developing myeloid malignancies, the patient and family should be asked about a family history of myeloid malignancies. The presence of skeletal, facial, ocular, audiologic, neurologic, renal, cardiac, and immune problems associated with platelet disorders may also suggest IPD.[51,56]

Laboratory evaluation of a potential IPD should start with a careful blood film investigation, which could be helpful for patients with MYH9-related diseases (giant platelets and Döhle-like inclusion bodies within leukocytes; Fig. 7–3), Bernard-Soulier syndrome (macrothrombocytopenia), Gray platelet syndrome (pale platelets), and sitosterolemia (giant platelets surrounded by a circle of vacuoles, stomatocytosis). Platelet function analyzer (PFA-100) occlusion times are usually found to be prolonged. The skin bleeding time is not recommended for screening, because it is invasive and poorly reproducible. Although the PFA-100 test is very sensitive in detecting Bernard-Soulier syndrome and platelet-type von Willebrand disease (VWD), it may be normal in patients with variant forms of these disorders or patients with

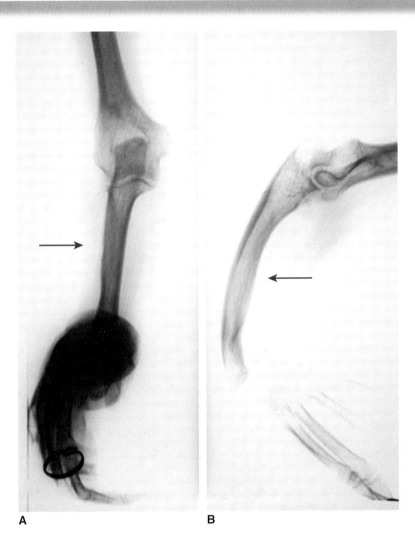

A          B

**Figure 7–2.** Thrombocytopenia with absent radii (TAR) syndrome. Radiograph of right forearm. A 48-year-old woman with repeated platelet counts in the range of 85 to 100 × 10⁹/L. Bleeding time was 11 minutes. No laboratory evidence of von Willebrand disease. Marrow examination was normal. Both forearms were short and bowed with angulated wrists and normal hands. No family history of forearm deformity. **A.** Anterior-posterior film of right arm. **B.** Lateral film of right arm. Absence of radius and bowed, hypertrophied ulna *(arrows)*. Angulation deformity at wrist. *(Reproduced with permission from Lichtman's Atlas of Hematology, www.accessmedicine.com. Kindly provided for the Atlas by Timothy J. Woodlock, Unity Health Systems, Rochester, NY.)*

storage pool deficiencies.⁵⁷ Light transmission aggregometry (LTA) using different concentrations of adenosine diphosphate (ADP), collagen, ristocetin, epinephrine, and arachidonic acid is accepted as a gold standard in diagnosing IPDs, but, again, may be normal in variant forms of IPDs and in some patients with storage pool diseases. Measurement of platelet nucleotide content and release is recommended in patients with platelet granule deficiencies. Flow cytometric analysis is very informative in patients with platelet surface GP deficiencies such as Bernard-Soulier syndrome. Marrow biopsy is needed in patients who have pancytopenia or severe thrombocytopenia, as in Fanconi anemia and congenital amegakaryocytic thrombocytopenia (CAMT), respectively. Unfortunately, these tests may help diagnose only a small portion of IPD patients. Further tests are only available in specialized centers and include electron microscopy, Western blotting, and others. Electron microscopy is able to define characteristic ultrastructural abnormalities; Western blotting, enzyme-linked immunosorbent assay (ELISA), or radioimmunoassay can be used for qualitative and quantitative analysis of specific platelet proteins.⁵¹,⁵⁶ Even with these expensive, complicated, and time-consuming tests, the results are inconclusive in nearly half of patients being evaluated for IPD.⁵⁶ Genetic analysis is often able to determine the underlying molecular pathology, but the very large number of candidate genes limits the traditional target gene approach. Within the past decade, next-generation sequencing techniques have not only improved the speed and cost of genetic investigations, but have also begun to generate very interesting data about the genetic causes of IPD.⁵²,⁵³

## ● NUTRITIONAL DEFICIENCIES AND ALCOHOL-INDUCED THROMBOCYTOPENIA

Iron, vitamin B₁₂, and folic acid deficiencies are the nutrient deficiencies most widely recognized to impair blood cell production. Severe nutritional deficiencies primarily cause anemia, rarely causing bicytopenia or pancytopenia. Isolated thrombocytopenia is rare in patients with nutritional deficiencies.

Iron is present in all human cells and mediates electron transfer reactions. Iron is a key component of hemoglobin, and iron deficiency causes a hypochromic and microcytic anemia. Iron-deficiency anemia (IDA) generally develops after acute or chronic bleeding and is usually accompanied by thrombocytosis rather than thrombocytopenia. Thrombocytopenia associated with IDA is relatively rare, reported in only 2.3 percent and 2.4 percent of pediatric and adult IDA patients, respectively.⁵⁸,⁵⁹

Cobalamin (vitamin B₁₂) and folate are both required for DNA synthesis and repair, but humans can synthesize neither vitamin. Dietary deficiencies, impaired absorption, or inhibition with drugs (as seen in methotrexate therapy) of these vitamins can cause megaloblastic anemia. Mild thrombocytopenia occurs in approximately 20 percent of patients with megaloblastic anemia resulting from vitamin B₁₂ deficiency in the United States.⁶⁰ The frequency may be higher in patients with folic acid

**TABLE 7–2.** Inherited Thrombocytopenia

**I. Congenital hypo-/amegakaryocytic thrombocytopenias**

A. Congenital amegakaryocytic thrombocytopenia (CAMT)

B. Congenital hypo-/amegakaryocytic thrombocytopenia with skeletal abnormalities

1. Thrombocytopenia with absent radii (TAR) syndrome

2. Amegakaryocytic thrombocytopenia with radioulnar synostosis (ATRUS)

3. Fanconi anemia

**II. MYH9-related diseases**

A. Macrothrombocytopenia, Döhle-like inclusion bodies in leukocytes; nephritis ± hearing loss ± cataracts

**III. Platelet granule deficiencies (storage pool disease)**

A. α-Granule defects

1. Gray platelet syndrome

2. Paris-Trousseau syndrome

3. Quebec platelet syndrome

4. Arthrogryposis–renal dysfunction–cholestasis (ARC) syndrome

B. Dense granule defects:

1. Hermansky-Pudlak syndrome

2. Chédiak-Higashi syndrome

3. Griscelli syndrome

C. α- and dense granule defects

**IV. Disorders of platelet surface receptors**

A. Glycoprotein (GP) Ib-IX-V defects

1. Bernard-Soulier syndrome

2. Platelet-type von Willebrand disease

3. Velocardiofacial syndrome

B. Integrin $\alpha_{IIb}\beta_{IIIa}$ defects: variant forms of Glanzmann thrombasthenia

**V. Wiskott-Aldrich syndrome (WAS) protein-related disorders**

A. Classical Wiskott-Aldrich syndrome

B. X-linked thrombocytopenia

C. X-linked neutropenia

**VI. GATA-1 mutations**

A. X-linked thrombocytopenia

B. X-linked thrombocytopenia and thalassemia-like phenotype

C. Congenital erythropoietic porphyria

**VII. Ankyrine repeat domain (ANKRD)-26 mutations**

A. Moderate thrombocytopenia with mild bleeding tendency, dysmegakaryopoiesis, increased risk of myeloid malignancies

**VIII. RUNX-1 mutations**

A. Familial platelet disorder with propensity to myeloid malignancy (FDP/AML)

**IX. Miscellaneous**

A. Sitosterolemia

B. Montreal platelet syndrome

C. Others

deficiency because of the high frequency of concomitant alcohol abuse. One large study of 139 patients examined the rates of cytopenias associated with megaloblastic anemia in India.[61] In this study, 76 percent had isolated vitamin $B_{12}$ deficiency, 7 percent had isolated folate deficiency, 9 percent had a combined deficiency, and 8 percent had normal vitamin levels. All were anemic by definition, and 80 percent had thrombocytopenia with mild to moderate depression of the platelet count. More than half of those with thrombocytopenia were also neutropenic. The authors of this study suggested that the cytopenias tended to progress from isolated anemia, to anemia plus thrombocytopenia, to pancytopenia, with the degree of cytopenia related to the severity of vitamin deficiency. Occasionally, thrombocytopenia is severe in patients with megaloblastic anemia and, when accompanied by fever, hepatomegaly, and splenomegaly, may suggest a diagnosis of acute leukemia. In these syndromes, the primary mechanism of thrombocytopenia is ineffective platelet production[62]; marrow megakaryocyte number usually is normal or increased. Abnormalities of megakaryocyte morphology are much less distinctive than the characteristic erythroid and myeloid defects, but often nuclear abnormalities are seen, with nuclei of larger size and dispersed nuclear segments, rather than single polyploid nuclei.[63] Thrombocytopenia may be seen in association with vitamin $B_{12}$ deficiency when the latter results from autoantibodies against parietal cells or intrinsic factor and is associated with ITP.[64,65] Various other autoimmune disorders can coexist with pernicious anemia, including autoimmune vitiligo and autoimmune thyroiditis.[66] Abnormalities of platelet function are sometimes seen associated with vitamin $B_{12}$ deficiency.[67,68] Diminished platelet aggregation and reduced release of ADP and ATP from granule stores in response to different agonists have been reported, and vitamin deficiency has been suggested to induce an acquired storage pool disease.[68]

Copper deficiency is usually seen in patients who have undergone gastric bypass surgery and may cause anemia, leukopenia, and thrombocytopenia associated with neurologic deficits resembling vitamin $B_{12}$ deficiency. Patients with copper deficiency also may be misdiagnosed as having MDS, because increased ring sideroblasts and dysplastic precursor cells can be seen on marrow smears.[69,70]

Acute and chronic alcohol (ethanol) consumption affects hematopoiesis and blood cell survival both directly and indirectly. Alcohol is one of the leading causes of thrombocytopenia in Western countries. Acute ethanol intoxication in healthy volunteers induces thrombocytopenia.[71] Platelet counts in these cases are usually mildly decreased (generally more than $100 \times 10^9$/L); severe thrombocytopenia is quite rare. Acute ethanol-induced thrombocytopenia usually resolves within 5 to 21 days with cessation of ethanol ingestion, sometimes with a transient rebound thrombocytosis that may reach up to $1,000,000 \times 10^9$/L.[72] Although the mechanism of acute alcohol-related thrombocytopenia is not clear, it has been suggested that metabolites of ethanol, especially acetaldehyde, impair the late stages of platelet production and increase platelet destruction.[73] Thus, thrombocytopenia associated with acute alcohol ingestion would be expected to be more frequent in those with poor nutrition (delayed oxidation of acetaldehyde) and those with partial acetaldehyde dehydrogenase defiance. Thrombocytopenia induced by alcohol ingestion is accompanied by a decreased number of marrow megakaryocytes. Vacuolated proerythroblasts and granulocyte precursors are sometimes seen, as are multinuclear erythroblasts and megaloblasts.[74] Vacuolization of the periphery of mature megakaryocytes has been reported.[75] Alcoholism (chronic ethanol consumption, which is defined as consumption of more than 80 g of ethanol per day), on the other hand, may cause thrombocytopenia by other mechanisms, such as alcoholic liver cirrhosis (both splenomegaly and thrombopoietin deficiency), folic acid deficiency, and alcohol-induced marrow suppression.[74–78]

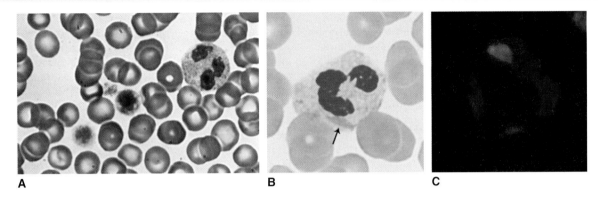

**Figure 7–3.** MYH9 abnormality. **A.** Blood film. May-Hegglin anomaly. Macrothrombocytes, thrombocytopenia, and light-blue cytoplasmic inclusions in neutrophils. Note two giant platelets approximately the diameter of red cells. The neutrophil has a large gray-blue inclusion in the cytoplasm at the 9 o'clock position. **B.** Blood film. Neutrophil of an individual with a mutation (E1841K) in exon 38 of the MYH9 gene. This mutation results in macrothrombocytopenia and Döhle-body–like inclusions in neutrophils (arrow). **C.** Blood film. Immunofluorescent analysis with antibodies to the A heavy chain of nonmuscle myosin in the neutrophils of the same patient as in **(B)**. The fluorescent body in the neutrophil indicates that the inclusion contains precipitated nonmuscle myosin heavy chains, characteristic of this family of disorders. (Reproduced with permission from Lichtman's Atlas of Hematology, www.accessmedicine.com. Images B and C kindly were provided for the Atlas by Dr. Shinji Kunishima, the Japanese Red Cross Aichi Blood Center, Nagoya, Japan.)

# ●ACQUIRED PURE AMEGAKARYOCYTIC THROMBOCYTOPENIA

Thrombocytopenia attributable to pure aplasia or hypoplasia of megakaryocytes is rare.[79] More common are instances in which amegakaryocytic thrombocytopenia anticipates the development of full-blown MDS or aplastic anemia and is associated with subtle abnormalities of other lineages, such as macrocytosis and dyserythropoiesis.[80-84] Most commonly, the disorder is caused by autoimmune suppression of megakaryocyte development, either idiopathic,[85] associated with autoimmune disorders such as systemic lupus erythematosus (SLE)[86] and eosinophilic fasciitis, or associated with infections such as hepatitis C.[87] Antibodies against thrombopoietin (TPO)[88] have been described to cause the disorder, as have antibodies against the TPO receptor.[89] Patients may achieve durable remission with therapies designed to blunt the autoimmune response, such as cyclosporine or antithymocyte globulin (ATG).[90]

## IMMUNE THROMBOCYTOPENIA

Table 7–3 summarizes the various types of ITP.

## PRIMARY IMMUNE THROMBOCYTOPENIA

ITP, formerly known as autoimmune thrombocytopenic purpura, is the most common cause of isolated thrombocytopenia in clinical practice. ITP is characterized by immune-mediated platelet destruction and impaired platelet production. ITP occurs in every age group. Childhood ITP typically is acute in onset, often developing after a viral infection or vaccination. Although thrombocytopenia may be severe, it usually resolves spontaneously, within a few weeks up to 6 months.[91] In contrast to childhood ITP, adult ITP generally is a chronic disease of insidious onset and rarely resolves spontaneously.

"Purpura" was recognized by Hippocrates (c. 460 to c. 370 BC) and Galen (AD 129 to c. 200/c. 216) as a sign associated with fever. Chronic purpura was first described in details by Ibn-i Sina (Avicenna, c. 980 to c. 1037) in his famous book "The Canon of Medicine." In 1705, Werlof suggested that purpura was related to infections and described it as "morbus maculosus haemorrhagicus." Patients with purpura were diagnosed as having "Werlof disease" for centuries. After the discovery of

platelets and their role in hemostasis, the relationship between purpura and low platelet count was understood.[92]

In 1915, Erich Frank renamed this disorder as "essential thrombocytopenia" and suggested that platelet production from megakaryocytes was impaired because of a toxic substance produced by the spleen.[93] Kaznelson, inspired by Frank's theory, proposed splenectomy for a patient with chronic thrombocytopenic purpura. The treatment was successful, and splenectomy was first-line therapy for ITP until the introduction of glucocorticoids in 1950s.

In the first issue of the journal *Blood* (in 1946), Damashek and Miller reviewed the megakaryocyte count and marrow morphology of patients with "idiopathic thrombocytopenic purpura."[94] They showed that most ITP patients had an increased number of megakaryocytes, but very few of them were producing platelets, so "actual platelet-producing tissue" might be decreased.[94]

---

**TABLE 7–3.** Immune-Mediated Thrombocytopenia

**I. Autoantibody-mediated thrombocytopenia**

  A. Primary immune thrombocytopenia

  B. Secondary immune thrombocytopenia

    1. Antiphospholipid syndrome, systemic lupus erythematosus, and other connective tissue disorders

    2. Infections: HIV, hepatitis C virus, hepatitis B virus, *Helicobacter pylori*, and others

    3. Vaccination

    4. Drugs and chemical substances

    5. Malignancies including lymphoproliferative disorders

    6. Transplantation

    7. Common variable immune deficiency

**II. Alloantibody-mediated thrombocytopenia/platelet destruction**

  A. Fetal/neonatal alloimmune thrombocytopenia

  B. Posttransfusion purpura

  C. Platelet alloimmunization after platelet transfusions

Although Marino first showed that antiplatelet antibodies might cause thrombocytopenia in animal studies in 1905, the Harrington-Hollingsworth experiment (1951) was an important milestone in the understanding of autoantibody-directed platelet destruction in the pathophysiology of ITP. In this pioneering work, normal volunteers (including Harrington himself, who received the highest dose) were infused with the plasma from patients with ITP, resulting in severe thrombocytopenia in the recipients, and they postulated that ITP could be caused by antiplatelet antibodies.[95,96] Subsequently, Shulman and coworkers[97] showed that the thrombocytopenic effect of ITP plasma was dose-dependent and associated with the globulin fraction. In the 1950s, glucocorticoids began to be used to treat ITP, and they became first-line therapy for adults. Shortly thereafter, other immunosuppressive agents were introduced for the treatment of chronic ITP.[92]

In the early 1970s, two groups showed that platelets from chronic ITP patients had elevated levels of platelet-associated immunoglobulin G (PAIgG).[98,99] In 1982, the first platelet target was identified: autoantibodies from patients with ITP failed to bind platelets deficient in the integrin $\alpha_{IIb}\beta_3$ complex (i.e., from patients with Glanzmann thrombasthenia).[100] In the late 1980s, two specific assays for the target antigens were described: the immunobead assay[101] and the monoclonal antibody-specific immobilization of platelet antigens (MAIPA) assay.[102] These assays showed that the majority of antiplatelet antibodies in patients with ITP are directed against integrin $\alpha_{IIb}\beta_{3(GPIIb-IIIa)}$ (approximately 80 percent), and the remainder are against the GPIb–IX–V complex and other platelet GPs such as GPIV and integrin $\alpha_2\beta_1$ (GPIa-IIa).[103,104] Some sera contain antibodies that recognize several antigens. Most antiplatelet autoantibodies are IgG; the remainder are IgM and IgA. Unfortunately, elevated levels of PAIgG later were found in patients with non-ITP. Therefore, PAIgG could not be used as a specific laboratory test for ITP in the same way that the direct antiglobulin test is used for the diagnosis of autoimmune hemolytic anemia.[105,106] To date, there is still no specific laboratory test for ITP, and the diagnosis of ITP is based on exclusion of other causes.

Antibody-coated platelets bind tissue macrophages through Fcγ receptors, leading to their destruction primarily in the spleen and, to a lesser extent, in the liver and marrow.[97,107,108] In 1981, Imbach reported successful treatment of pediatric ITP with intravenous immunoglobulin (IVIG) and suggested that the mechanism could involve blockade of macrophage Fc receptors. IVIG became first-line therapy in children and now is also used in adults when a prompt increase in the platelet count is desired.[109]

Early studies of PAIgG reported that the antibodies in ITP were polyclonal.[110] However, later studies showed that at least some ITP patients had clonal B-cell proliferation, as determined by DNA analysis for immunoglobulin heavy- and light-chain rearrangements and by flow cytometry of B cells from blood and spleen for surface Ig light chains.[111,112] This led to the use in ITP of the chimeric anti-CD20 monoclonal antibody, rituximab, which was designed for the treatment of CD20-positive B-cell lymphomas. The rapid elimination of B cells with rituximab encouraged the use of this agent in the treatment of ITP.

Numerous abnormalities in cell-mediated immunity have been described in patients with ITP, including abnormalities in antigen-presenting cells, T lymphocytes, and cytokine release. Under normal conditions, antigen-presenting cells recognize and process foreign antigens and express the antigens on their surface in association with major histocompatibility complex (MHC) molecules. MHC–antigen complexes activate resting (naïve) CD4+ T cells to differentiate into a variety of phenotypes such as T-helper 1 (Th1) and T-helper 2 (Th2), Th17, and T-regulatory (Treg) cells. Th1 cells are involved in cell-mediated immunity and host defense against intracellular bacteria and protozoa. Th2 cells are involved in humoral immunity and host defense

against extracellular parasites. Th17 cells are involved in host defense against extracellular bacteria and fungi. Treg cells (formerly known as suppressor T cells) play an important role in self-tolerance by inhibiting autoimmune responses. Abnormal T-cell responses drive the differentiation of autoreactive B-cell clones and autoantibody secretion. In patients with ITP, both Th1 and Th17 cells have been found to be upregulated, whereas the number and the suppressor functions of the Treg cells were found to be decreased.[113–115] This imbalance is believed to induce an autoimmune response against the platelets. It is unclear whether these abnormalities are causative or represent an epiphenomenon.[114,115] In addition, CD8+ cytotoxic T cells might be involved in the pathogenesis of ITP through cell-mediated destruction of platelets and megakaryocytes and through suppression of megakaryocytes, impairing platelet production.[115–117]

Antiplatelet autoantibodies may also activate platelet destruction by activating complement through the classical complement pathway. Increased platelet-associated C3, C4, and C9 have been demonstrated on the platelets from patients with ITP.[118,119] In vitro studies show that, in the presence of antiplatelet antibodies, C3 and C4 can bind platelets, increase the phagocytosis of the platelets by macrophages, and cause their lysis by stimulating assembly of the membrane attack complex.[120,121]

Early studies demonstrated that platelet survival is shortened in ITP patients and returns to normal after splenectomy-induced remission.[122] Platelet transfusion only transiently increases a patient's platelet count, and the transfused platelets also have a shortened survival, reflecting the fact that the major problem in ITP is platelet destruction. However, later studies showed that platelet life span was not short enough to account for the observed thrombocytopenia on the basis of destruction alone, again suggesting a concomitant defect in platelet production.[123] Potential mechanisms for this observation were provided by later studies that autoantibodies against platelet surface GPs might interfere with the maturation of megakaryocytes, resulting in reduced platelet production and contributing to the severity of thrombocytopenia in some ITP patients.[124] Antibodies that target the GPIb–IX–V complex may induce thrombocytopenia by decreasing platelet production, because GPIb autoantibodies inhibit megakaryopoiesis in vitro[124] and GPIb monoclonal antibodies inhibit proplatelet formation in vitro.[125]

In 1958, a hematopoietic growth factor regulating platelet production was proposed and named TPO by Kelemen.[126] Although interleukin (IL)-3, IL-6, IL-11, granulocyte-macrophage colony-stimulating factor, and c-KIT ligand increase megakaryocyte or platelet counts in vivo and in vitro, animal studies of these factors proved that they are not the main regulator of megakaryopoiesis.[127] In 1994, TPO was first characterized by five independent groups. TPO binds to its receptor MPL (formerly known as c-MPL); enhances megakaryocyte colony formation; increases the size, number, and ploidy of megakaryocytes; and increases platelet production (Chap. 3).[128–130] TPO is synthesized in greatest quantity in the liver but is found in other organs (kidney, muscle, and marrow stromal cells).[128] TPO is also required to maintain the viability of hematopoietic stem cells.[131] The regulation of TPO production is complex. Hepatic production of TPO is both constitutive (in the steady state) and inducible (by inflammation), and the concentration of TPO to which megakaryocytes are exposed is also determined by the platelet concentration. Platelets, bearing TPO receptors, remove the hormone from the circulation, at least partially accounting for the inverse relationship between TPO and platelet levels. TPO levels are markedly elevated in patients with thrombocytopenia associated with megakaryocytic hypoplasia, including disorders such as aplastic anemia or acute leukemia. In most reports, ITP patients have normal or slightly elevated TPO levels whether measured in plasma or serum, but the levels are always lower than the concentrations found in thrombocytopenias resulting from megakaryocytic hypoplasia.[128–130,132,133] Initial studies with recombinant and pegylated TPO molecules showed successful responses in patients with thrombocytopenia, but development of auto-antibodies against these molecules restricted their use in clinical settings. Based on the success of creating erythropoietin receptor agonist peptides, a number of screening efforts were undertaken to design small peptides or organic molecules that might bind to the TPO receptor and stimulate thrombopoiesis. One such molecule contains four copies of a 14-amino-acid peptide grafted onto an Ig Fc domain, forming a "peptibody" termed romiplostim. This agent, which binds to a region of the TPO receptor that overlaps that bound by authentic TPO, was shown to increase platelet counts in patients with ITP who had failed other modalities,[134] and was approved by the FDA for this indication in 2008. Another small organic thrombopoietic molecule, eltrombopag, was developed almost simultaneously[135] and approved in 2008 by FDA for the same indications.[127] This agent activates TPO receptor signaling by binding to the transmembrane domain of the receptor, a site quite distinct from the binding site for TPO and romiplostim. Both TPO-receptor agonists are currently being evaluated for additional clinical indications in clinical trials.[136]

Some patients with ITP appear to display a genetic predisposition. ITP has been documented in monozygotic twins[137] and shown to be highly prevalent in some families.[138] In addition to contributing to the development of ITP, like in other autoimmune disorders, heredity may also affect the response to ITP therapy. Human leukocyte antigen (HLA) class I and class II allele frequencies in patients with ITP have been studied by several investigators, with inconsistent results. Some investigators reported an increased frequency of HLA-Aw32, DRw2, and DRB1*0410.[108,139–141] Investigation has focused on genetic differences associated with dysregulation of immune tolerance and humoral immunity, but results have been inconclusive. For example, genetic polymorphisms of cytotoxic T-lymphocyte antigen (CTLA)-4, tumor necrosis factor, and Fcγ receptors IIA and IIIA have been suggested to influence the development of ITP and the response to therapy,[141–143] but as yet, no strong association has been found.

Accumulating data indicate that the pathophysiology of ITP is more complex than previously thought, with ITP comprising a heterogenous group of disorders with different etiologies and responding to different treatment modalities. The identification of the different subsets of ITP patients will help to better define treatment options.

## Definition and Classification

Although ITP has been recognized for centuries, there is as yet no consensus on either the definition or management of the disease. In 1996, the American Society of Hematology (ASH)[144] published practice guidelines for the diagnosis and management of ITP. In 2003, the British Committee for Standards in Haematology published its own guidelines.[145] Despite these guidelines, the heterogeneity of the definitions and clinical criteria used in different studies has made it difficult to interpret the data regarding the incidence, pathogenesis, and treatment of ITP. In 2008, the International Working Group (IWG) proposed a standardization of terminology, definitions, and outcome criteria for ITP patients.[146] In 2010, an international consensus report on the investigation and management of ITP was published.[147] Shortly thereafter, in 2011, ASH updated its 1996 ITP guidelines.[148]

The IWG definition proposed use of the term "immune thrombocytopenia" instead of "idiopathic thrombocytopenic purpura" as the basis for the ITP acronym, because the immune nature of ITP is clear but most ITP patients do not have purpura. A platelet count of 100 × $10^9$/L was proposed as the threshold level to entertain the diagnosis of ITP, because a sustained lower platelet count (100 to 150 × $10^9$/L) can be seen in otherwise healthy individuals,[11,12] and long-term observation of these individuals indicate that 88 percent reach normal platelet counts

or remain stable.[13] ITP is classified based on the absence or presence of other diseases as "primary" or "secondary." "Primary ITP" denotes the absence of any other identified pathology. All other autoimmune thrombocytopenias are classified as "secondary ITP" (see Table 7–3), and the associated primary disorder is indicated in parentheses, for example "secondary ITP (SLE-associated)" or "secondary ITP (drug-induced)." Heparin-induced thrombocytopenia (HIT) and alloimmune thrombocytopenias are not classified as ITP and maintain their standard classifications.[146]

The IWG described three phases of ITP: (1) newly diagnosed ITP (within 3 months of diagnosis); (2) persistent ITP (patients who do not achieve a stable remission between 3 and 12 months after diagnosis); and (3) chronic ITP (continuing for more than 12 months). ITP was formerly classified as mild, moderate, and severe depending on the platelet counts. However, the degree of thrombocytopenia does not always correlate with bleeding. The IWG proposed that the term "severe ITP" only be used for patients with clinically significant bleeding requiring additional therapy regardless of platelet count.[146]

One of the major problems with comparing ITP studies had been the definition of response to therapy. The IWG proposed the following terms and criteria for response to ITP treatment: "complete response, CR" (platelet count exceeding 100 × $10^9$/L and no bleeding symptoms), "response, R" (platelet count higher than 30 × $10^9$/L or at least a twofold increase from the baseline count and no bleeding symptoms), and "no response, NR" (platelet count below 30 × $10^9$/L or less than a twofold increase from the baseline count, or presence of bleeding symptoms). "Duration of response" is measured as the time between first measured CR or R and relapse. "Corticosteroid dependence" is defined as the need for ongoing or repeated glucocorticoid use for at least 2 months to maintain CR or R. Patients who relapse after splenectomy (failure to maintain CR or R) and require therapy are classified as having "refractory ITP." "On-demand therapy" is a term used for therapies employed to temporarily increase the platelet count in special situations such as trauma or surgery. "Adjunctive therapies" are treatments that are not designed to increase platelet counts, but that may decrease bleeding symptoms by other means, for example, treatment with oral contraceptives or anti-fibrinolytic drugs.[146]

## Incidence

ITP is relatively common, but demographic studies have yielded a wide range of incidence rates largely because of differences in the age and gender distribution of the populations studied and differences in cut-off platelet counts used to define the disease. ITP can affect males and females of any age. In one detailed study, the reported incidence of ITP was 3.9 per 100,000 per year. Although the overall incidence was higher in women than in men, a male predominance was seen in patients younger than 18 years of age and older than 65 years of age.[149]

## Clinical Features

ITP is of acute onset in children, often developing after vaccination or after a viral illness, and resolves spontaneously in 90 percent of cases. In adults, however, ITP usually is a chronic disease. Table 7–4 highlights the differences in ITP in children and adults. Approximately 25 percent of adult ITP patients are diagnosed incidentally on routine complete blood counts. Symptoms and signs of ITP depend not only on the platelet count, but also on the nature of coexisting conditions that can increase the tendency to bleed, such as uremia, trauma, and ingestion of drugs that affect platelet function (Table 7–5). Approximately one-third of patients have platelet counts greater than 30 × $10^9$/L at diagnosis and no significant bleeding.[150] Common bleeding signs include purpura (ecchymoses and petechiae), epistaxis, menorrhagia, and gingival bleeding. Hematuria, hemoptysis, and gastrointestinal bleeding

**TABLE 7–4.** Clinical Features of Idiopathic Thrombocytopenic Purpura in Children and Adults

|  | Children | Adults |
|---|---|---|
| **Occurrence** | | |
| Peak age (years) | 2–4 | 15–40 |
| Sex (female-to-male) | Equal | 1.2–1.7 |
| **Presentation** | | |
| Onset | Acute (most with symptoms lasting <1 week) | Insidious (most with symptoms lasting >2 months) |
| Symptoms | Purpura (<10% with severe bleeding) | Purpura (typically bleeding not severe) |
| Platelet count | Most cases <20,000/μL | Most cases <20,000/μL |
| **Course** | | |
| Spontaneous remission | 83% | 2% |
| Chronic disease | 24% | 43% |
| Response to splenectomy | 71% | 66% |
| Eventual complete recovery | 89% | 64% |
| **Morbidity and mortality** | | |
| Cerebral hemorrhage | <1% | 3% |
| Hemorrhagic death | <1% | 4% |
| Mortality of chronic refractory disease | 2% | 5% |

are less common. Intracerebral hemorrhage is rare and generally occurs in patients with platelet counts less than $10 \times 10^9$/L and usually is associated with trauma or vascular lesions. The incidence of life-threatening complications is highest in patients older than age 60 years.[150–154] The majority of ITP patients have a good prognosis, with the mortality rate being only slightly higher than that of the general population. However, ITP

**TABLE 7–5.** Situations That Increase the Bleeding Risk in Immune Thrombocytopenia Patients

Drugs: Anticoagulants, antiplatelet drugs, nonsteroidal antiinflammatory drugs, chemotherapy

Gastrointestinal pathologies that may cause bleeding (e.g., active peptic ulcer, inflammatory bowel disease)

Miscellaneous disorders that disturb hemostasis (e.g., congenital bleeding disorders, hepatic cirrhosis, uremia)

Older age (>60 years)

Nutritional factors such as herbal teas, kinin, and tonic water

Previous history of bleeding

Sport and occupational activities that increase bleeding risk

Trauma, surgery, and childbirth

Uncontrolled hypertension

patients who present with severe thrombocytopenia ($<30 \times 10^9$/L) and do not respond to any therapy within 2 years have a fourfold increased risk of death compared to the general population.[155]

The purpuric lesions seen in ITP are not palpable, do not blanch with pressure, and often develop on distal regions of the extremities and on skin areas exposed to pressure (e.g., around tight belts and stockings and at tourniquet sites). Hemorrhagic bullae, which may develop in the buccal mucosa, generally reflect acute, severe thrombocytopenia. Bleeding after surgery, trauma, or tooth extraction is common.

Besides the physical findings associated with platelet-type bleeding, the history and physical examination are usually unremarkable, except for the possibility of similar symptoms in other family members. Family history is especially important to discriminate familial thrombocytopenic syndromes from ITP. The spleen usually is not enlarged but may be palpable in some patients, a finding considered to occur with the same incidence as in normal adults.[156] Constitutional symptoms, such as fever, significant weight loss, marked splenomegaly, hepatomegaly, and lymphadenopathy, provide evidence that the thrombocytopenia has another cause. The presence of skeletal, cardiac, and renal abnormalities, hearing loss, albinism, or immune deficiencies in patients with thrombocytopenia should trigger suspicion of IPDs.

Fatigue is one of the common, but often neglected, complaints of patients with primary ITP. In a survey including United Kingdom (UK) and US ITP cohorts, the prevalence of fatigue was found to be significantly higher in adult primary ITP patients (39 percent and 22 percent for the UK and US cohorts, respectively) compared with healthy controls.[157] Fatigue has also been described in 20 percent of pediatric patients with ITP; fatigue resolved with the elevation of platelet counts.[158] Although glucocorticoids and immunosuppressive agents may induce fatigue, fatigue can occur in untreated ITP patients. The mechanism of fatigue in patients with ITP is unknown.

Patients with ITP are at slightly increased risk of venous and arterial thrombosis.[159] A recent retrospective study evaluating 986 patients with ITP showed the cumulative incidences of venous and arterial thrombosis to be 1.4 percent and 3.2 percent, respectively. This study found that increased thrombotic risk was associated with splenectomy, older age (>60 years), the presence of more than two thrombotic risk factors at the time of diagnosis, and glucocorticoid therapy.[160]

### Laboratory Features

In ITP patients, the blood film usually demonstrates isolated thrombocytopenia without erythrocyte or leukocyte abnormalities. Platelet anisocytosis is a common finding. Mean platelet volume and platelet distribution width are increased. Platelets may be abnormally large or abnormally small. The former reflect accelerated platelet production,[161] and the latter represent platelet fragments associated with platelet destruction.[162] The observation of giant platelets should trigger consideration of IPDs, which often are misdiagnosed as ITP.[163] The bleeding time correlates inversely with platelet count if the count is less than $50 \times 10^9$/L, but may be normal in patients with mild or moderate thrombocytopenia,[164] making it an unreliable test for use in such patients. The ultrastructure of ITP platelets viewed by electron microscopy is similar to that of normal platelets.[165]

Hemoglobin concentration and hematocrit are generally normal in patients with ITP. Anemia that is not easily explained (e.g., resulting from iron deficiency in bleeding patients or associated with thalassemia minor in endemic areas) must be investigated further. Autoimmune hemolytic anemia with a positive direct antiglobulin (Coombs) test and reticulocytosis may accompany ITP; this association is termed *Evans syndrome*.[166] Neither erythrocyte poikilocytosis nor schistocytes should be present. Total leukocyte counts and differential are generally normal.

Although atypical lymphocytes and eosinophilia may occur in children with ITP, leukocytosis and leukopenia with immature cells are not consistent with the diagnosis.

Marrow examination, which is not always required to make a diagnosis of ITP in adults, generally reveals a normal or increased number of megakaryocytes of normal morphology, although a decreased number of megakaryocytes does not rule out ITP. Erythropoiesis and myelopoiesis are normal. The international consensus report states that a marrow examination should usually be reserved for patients older than age 60 years, for those with systemic symptoms or other signs, and for those for whom splenectomy is contemplated. Biopsy for morphologic examination should be carried out, along with aspirate for flow cytometric and cytogenetic analysis.[147] The ASH 2011 guidelines, however, conclude that a marrow examination is unnecessary when the presentation is typical, even if the patients are older or being considered for splenectomy.[148]

In ITP patients, initial workup should be targeted to exclude secondary causes of thrombocytopenia (see Table 7–3). Testing for viral etiology (hepatitis C virus [HCV], HIV, and in endemic areas hepatitis B virus [HBV]) and *Helicobacter pylori* is also recommended.[147,148] Quantitative immunoglobulin assessment should be considered for pediatric cases to rule out common variable immunodeficiency (CVID).[147] Mild thrombocytopenia has been reported in patients with hypo- or hyperthyroidism, which returns to normal after appropriate therapy. Thyroid-stimulating hormone (TSH) and antithyroid antibodies may help to evaluate thyroid status in those patients.[147] Other tests to consider include blood group analysis and a pregnancy test for female patients of childbearing age, antiphospholipid antibodies, antinuclear antibody (ANA), viral polymerase chain reaction (PCR) for parvovirus, and cytomegalovirus (CMV). The results of these tests can change the treatment strategy.[147] On the other hand, the ASH 2011 guidelines do not recommend routine testing for antiphospholipid antibodies and ANAs in the initial workup of ITP,[148] unless signs or symptoms of an autoimmune disorder are present in the patient. Other tests, such as TPO levels, reticulated platelets, PAIgG, platelet survival studies, bleeding time, and serum complement levels are not recommended for the diagnosis and management of ITP patients in either of these guidelines.[147,148]

### Therapy and Course

What little is known of the natural course of moderate or severe ITP derives from before the glucocorticoid era and suggests that, left untreated, ITP in adults typically is a chronic disease, in contrast to ITP in children. In adults, the rate of spontaneous remission is reported as 9 percent,[167] and spontaneous remission can occur even after 3 years in patients who present with severe thrombocytopenia.[168] Although ITP is a benign disease, side effects of the therapies can cause serious morbidity and even mortality. Treatment for patients with ITP should be based on bleeding signs and symptoms and on the presence of factors that increase the bleeding risk (see Table 7–5). Possible side effects of the drugs and other treatments used in ITP should always be considered.

### Initial Management

**Observation** Because a significant portion of ITP patients are diagnosed incidentally in routine evaluation, signs and symptoms of bleeding are important in determining whether any treatment is required. The primary therapeutic goal is not simply to increase the platelet count, but to reach a safe platelet count where the risk of bleeding is minimal. Patients with no bleeding and consistent platelet counts in excess of $30 \times 10^9$/L do not require treatment and can be observed periodically. These patients are at low risk for clinically important bleeding. Simple observation is not recommended for patients with platelet

counts lower than $10 \times 10^9$/L, in those with platelet counts between 10 and $30 \times 10^9$/L and significant mucosal bleeding, or in those with risk factors for bleeding (see Table 7–5).[169] The presence of extensive purpura or hemorrhagic bullae in mucosal tissues (wet purpura) should be regarded as a harbinger of life-threatening bleeding and treated as such. Because ITP patients often have large platelets that may not be recognized by automated cell counters, a blood film should be evaluated before starting therapy in ITP patients with very low platelet counts who are not bleeding. Identification of secondary ITP cases is very important, and management of these patients should include treatment of the underlying pathology, if possible.

**Emergency Treatment of Acute Bleeding Resulting from Severe Thrombocytopenia** Bleeding symptoms generally are not severe in adult patients with ITP, even with very low platelet counts. However, life-threatening bleeding can occur, especially after trauma. Emergency treatment should be instituted in patients with intracranial or gastrointestinal bleeding, massive hematuria, or internal hematoma, and in those in need of emergency surgical intervention or about to go into labor. Patients who experience significant bleeding should be hospitalized and monitored closely. Recommended treatment includes IVIG and parenteral glucocorticoids in combination. IVIG is given as 1 g/kg per day for 2 days, and high-dose parenteral glucocorticoid therapy includes high-dose prednisone or methylprednisolone (1 g/d for 1 to 3 days). In most patients, IVIG increases the platelet count within 2 to 3 days.[147,148] Although platelet transfusions may not increase the platelet counts because the transfused platelets are destroyed rapidly, they nevertheless may contribute to the formation of platelet plugs at sites of bleeding and improve hemostasis. Platelet transfusion following IVIG infusion may increase the platelet count because IVIG may improve platelet survival.[147,148,170] Aminocaproic acid, which inhibits fibrinolysis, can be used to reduce bleeding[170] and is safe except in the presence of hematuria, in which case it can cause thrombi of the glomeruli, renal pelves, and ureters. This agent does not affect platelet count or function. Aminocaproic acid is usually administered intravenously (initial dose 0.1 g/kg over 30 minutes, then given either by continuous infusion at 0.5 to 1.0 g/h or as an equivalent intermittent dose every 2 to 4 hours). Aminocaproic acid also can be administered orally in a similar dose in emergency situations because it is absorbed very rapidly from the gastrointestinal tract.[147,148] Vincristine can be used in combination with glucocorticoids and IVIG in older patients.[108] Other hemostatic therapies, such as recombinant factor VIIa and fibrinogen infusions, have been reported to be effective in some ITP patients with life-threatening bleeding, but the risk-to-benefit ratio needs to be evaluated in controlled studies.[171,172] Emergency splenectomy has been reported to be successful in refractory ITP with bleeding, but reports of its use in this situation are rare.[173] Because of this, this therapy should only be considered in the most dire circumstances. Although there are some case reports describing successful results with plasmapheresis, this treatment is not recommended in current ITP guidelines.[147,148]

**Glucocorticoid Therapy** Glucocorticoids are accepted as the standard therapy for initial treatment in adult patients with ITP.[147,148] Glucocorticoids increase the platelet count in several ways, including by inhibiting phagocytosis of antibody-coated platelets by macrophages, decreasing autoantibody production, and improving marrow platelet production.[174,175] These agents also appear to reduce capillary leakage, thereby decreasing blood loss.[176] The major drawback of glucocorticoid therapy is that often the adverse effects of the treatment are worse than the disease itself. Important side effects, which can be severe, include facial swelling (chipmunk or moon facies), weight gain, folliculitis, hyperglycemia, hypertension, cataracts, osteoporosis, aseptic bone necrosis, opportunistic infections, and behavioral disturbances.[177,178]

Still under investigation is which glucocorticoid and dosing regimen are best for raising the platelet count. Prednisolone, dexamethasone, and methylprednisolone are all used. Generally, oral prednisone 1 to 2 mg/kg per day (or methylprednisolone at equivalent doses) is preferred as first-line therapy.[147,148] Patients usually respond to prednisone therapy within 3 weeks. In approximately two-thirds of patients, platelet counts increase to greater than $50 \times 10^9/L$ within 1 week, but decrease again when the prednisone dose is decreased.[152,177] Although no consensus exists regarding the duration of initial therapy, treatment should continue until platelet counts reach a safe range. In patients who respond, the recommendation is to continue glucocorticoid therapy 1 mg/kg per day for a total of 3 weeks before initiating a slow tapering of doses.[148] Sustained remission rates with glucocorticoid therapy are variable, with reported rates ranging from 5 to 50 percent.[108,155,177] If the patient does not respond to 3 weeks of prednisone therapy, other therapeutic options should be considered.

In addition to the standard 1 to 2 mg/kg per day dose of prednisone, lower[179,180] and higher doses[181–184] of prednisone, dexamethasone, and methylprednisolone have been investigated, with good results. The major aim of the high-dose glucocorticoid regimens is to reduce duration of therapy and therefore reduce the side effects of the glucocorticoids. Studies with dexamethasone 40 mg/d for 4 consecutive days for one course or with the same dose for four courses given every 2 weeks have reported responses in 50 percent and 89.2 percent of newly diagnosed ITP patients, respectively.[185,186] High-dose methylprednisolone therapy has also been shown to be effective, with an 80 percent response rate.[187] Despite the favorable results of these studies, high-dose glucocorticoid regimens as first-line therapy still have not been validated with randomized controlled trials. ASH 2011 guidelines recommend longer courses of standard doses of glucocorticoids (prednisone 1 to 2 mg/kg per day) as a first-line treatment of ITP.[148]

**Splenectomy** Splenectomy was demonstrated to be an effective treatment for patients with ITP a century ago,[188] and after the glucocorticoid era, it has been used for decades as a standard second-line therapy. The spleen is the major site both for synthesis of antiplatelet antibodies and for destruction of antibody-coated platelets. Splenectomy will decrease antibody production and platelet destruction and will be effective in patients in whom antibody-mediated platelet destruction rather than platelet production is the major cause of thrombocytopenia. Although splenectomy has been reported to be less preferred in recent ITP cohorts because of the emergence of new therapies such as TPO receptor agonists and rituximab,[189] splenectomy still produces the highest cure rates for ITP patients compared to all other therapies. Approximately 85 percent of patients with persistent or chronic ITP respond well to splenectomy, and 60 to 66 percent of the patients remain in remission after 5 years.[189–191] These high cure rates make splenectomy an important therapeutic option in the treatment of chronic ITP. The duration of the disease prior to splenectomy does not affect the outcome of the procedure, as it can be effective even years after ITP is diagnosed.[192,193] Splenectomy can be performed during pregnancy (preferably during the second trimester) and does not affect the response rates to other treatments except anti-D therapy in chronic ITP patients. Also, the cost of splenectomy is lower than that of newer treatments such as rituximab and TPO-receptor agonists.[191]

On the other hand, splenectomy is an invasive procedure, causes the permanent loss of an organ, and increases the risk of serious bacterial infection, bleeding, and thrombosis. Because ITP can remit spontaneously, splenectomy should be postponed at least 6 to 12 months after diagnosis if possible.[147,148] Splenectomy is not recommended in patients with CVID, with chronic infections such as chronic hepatitis and HIV, or with known thrombophilia.

No validated clinical or laboratory tests exist that can predict whether splenectomy will be effective in elevating platelet counts in ITP patients. Although it has been suggested that ITP patients with predominant splenic sequestration (as determined by radioisotope techniques) have better response rates than patients with predominantly nonsplenic sequestration, these data have not been validated in other studies[189] and the required radioisotope techniques are not widely available.

Over the past decade, minimally invasive laparoscopic splenectomy has gained preference over open splenectomy. Modern laparoscopic approaches reduce mortality rates (<1 percent), even in patients with severe thrombocytopenia.[194] The mortality rate increases in older patients, in patients with severe thrombocytopenia, and in the presence of coexisting illnesses.[177,195] Postsplenectomy sepsis is a major cause of morbidity and mortality in ITP. Extended steroid or other immunosuppressive therapy preceding splenectomy may increase the risk of perioperative infection. To minimize the risk of sepsis, patients should be immunized at least 2 weeks before splenectomy with polyvalent pneumococcal vaccine, *Haemophilus influenzae* type B vaccine, and quadrivalent meningococcal polysaccharide vaccine.[196] Interestingly, newer studies of ITP patients undergoing splenectomy show enteric organisms to be responsible for most of the cases of postsplenectomy sepsis, probably because of the widespread vaccination of ITP patients.[191] Splenectomized patients should be informed to be alert for the symptoms and signs of infection and be prepared for an emergency situation. Any fever should be carefully evaluated, and the patient treated with broad-spectrum antibiotics.

Splenectomy also increases the risk of thrombosis in ITP patients. In a large cohort of 9976 ITP patients, in whom 1762 underwent splenectomy, the cumulative incidences of abdominal venous thromboembolism and deep vein thrombosis/pulmonary embolism were increased in splenectomized patients compared to nonsplenectomized patients (1.6 percent vs. 1 percent for abdominal venous thrombosis, 4.3 percent vs. 1.7 percent for deep vein thrombosis–pulmonary embolism, respectively).[197] Several mechanisms may contribute to this enhanced risk for thrombosis, including postsplenectomy thrombocytosis and a failure to clear platelets, other cells, and microparticles that express the procoagulant lipid phosphatidylserine. Perioperative measures such as antiembolic stockings and anticoagulant prophylaxis should be considered in those cases.

Both the time required to reach a normal platelet count and the magnitude of platelet recovery are accepted as useful predictors of the long-term efficacy of splenectomy. In most cases, platelet counts recover within 10 days. Patients who attain a normal platelet count within 3 days of splenectomy generally have a good long-term response.[198] In patients refractory to splenectomy, the presence of accessory splenic tissue should be suspected, particularly if the blood film shows no evidence of splenectomy (i.e., pitting and Howell-Jolly bodies are absent in the erythrocytes). Such patients should be screened with sensitive radionuclide or magnetic resonance scans to identify residual or accessory splenic tissue.

**Intravenous Immunoglobulin** IVIG was first shown to be effective in childhood ITP in 1981,[109] then later in adult patients.[199] IVIG rapidly increases the platelet count in more than 75 percent of patients with chronic ITP and normalizes the platelet count in approximately 50 percent of the patients.[177,178] The effect of IVIG is similar whether or not the patient has undergone splenectomy and is transient, generally lasting only 3 to 4 weeks. Postulated mechanisms for the action of IVIG include blockade of macrophage Fc receptors, which slows clearance of antibody-coated platelets, antiidiotype neutralization of antiplatelet autoantibodies, cytokine modulation, immunomodulation (increased suppressor T-cell function and decreased autoantibody production), complement neutralization, and dendritic cell priming.[178,200,201] The recommended total dose of IVIG is 2 g/kg administered either as 0.4 g/kg per day on 5 consecutive days or as 1 g/kg per day on 2 consecutive days. If the need to increase the platelet count is urgent, the preferred dosing is 1 g/kg per day for 2 days combined with glucocorticoids.[148] For maintenance therapy, 0.5 to 1.0 g/kg as a single dose may be used, administered every 3 to 4 weeks or as needed. Although the annual total world consumption of IVIG exceeds 100 tons, the cost of IVIG is still high, and this also limits the use of IVIG in adults.[202] Adverse effects of IVIG therapy include headache, backache, nausea, fever, aseptic meningitis, alloimmune hemolysis, hepatitis, renal failure, pulmonary insufficiency, and thrombosis. Anaphylactic reactions may occur in patients with congenital IgA deficiency.[177] The patient may become refractory to the effect with repeated infusions of IVIG.[203] IVIG is used as a first-line therapy in childhood ITP, because the thrombocytopenia is usually transient. In adult ITP, however, IVIG is usually reserved for patients with life-threatening bleeding, when a prompt increase in platelet count is needed,[147,148] or as first-line therapy when glucocorticoids are contraindicated.[148]

**Anti-(Rh)D** Anti-(Rh)D is a polyclonal $\gamma$-globulin containing high titers of antibodies against the $Rh_o(D)$ antigen of erythrocytes. It is administered intravenously for treatment of ITP. Anti-(Rh)D binds Rh-positive erythrocytes and leads to their destruction in the spleen. Because splenic Fc receptors are blocked, more antibody-coated platelets survive in the circulation.[204,205] Anti-(Rh)D also can also modulate Fc$\gamma$ receptor expression and regulate the production of various cytokines, including IL-6, IL-10, and tumor necrosis factor-$\alpha$.[206] A positive direct antiglobulin test, a decrease in serum haptoglobin levels, and mild and transient hemolysis occur in all Rh-positive patients after anti-(Rh)D infusion, generally without requiring a blood transfusion.[205] The rate of serious hemolytic reactions has been estimated as one in 1115 patients; any reaction occurs within 4 hours of administration in almost all cases.[207] Anti-(Rh)D therapy is not effective in patients who have undergone splenectomy or in Rh-negative patients and is not recommended in patients with a positive direct antiglobulin test.[148]

It is recommended that anti-(Rh)D be given as a single dose of 50 to 100 mcg/kg by intravenous infusion over 3 to 5 minutes.[204,208,209] Adverse effects of anti-(Rh)D therapy resemble those observed with both $\gamma$-globulin infusion and autoimmune hemolytic anemia; symptoms include headache, asthenia, chills, fever, abdominal pain, diarrhea, vomiting, dizziness, and myalgia. Patients can experience immediate anaphylactic reactions and both type I (IgE-mediated) and type III (immune complex–mediated) hypersensitivity reactions.[204,205,208,210,211] Although anti-(Rh)D reportedly increases platelet counts within 1 week in more than 70 percent of patients who are Rh-positive and have their spleen,[212] and may obviate the need for splenectomy,[211] a randomized, controlled trial comparing anti-(Rh)D with conventional therapy showed no differences in the rates of spontaneous remission or the need for splenectomy.[209] Anti-(Rh)D is listed in current ASH ITP guidelines as a first-line agent when glucocorticoids are contraindicated.[148] Anti-(Rh)D is currently not available in Europe.

*Rituximab* B lymphocytes play many roles in the pathophysiology of ITP, including producing antibodies, presenting antigens, and regulating the functions of T cells and dendritic cells. B cells are targeted therapeutically with rituximab, a chimeric monoclonal antibody against CD20, which binds B cells and causes Fc-mediated lysis, thereby depleting these cells from blood, lymph nodes, and marrow. Rituximab rapidly depletes B cells in patients with autoimmune diseases, with the effect usually lasting 6 to 12 months.[114,213–217]

The optimal dosing regimen and duration of therapy have not been determined for patients with ITP. Usual rituximab doses are in the range of 100 to 375 mg/m². Most studies have used weekly infusion for 4 consecutive weeks at the dose used to treat B-cell lymphoma (375 mg/m²). Studies with low-dose rituximab (100 mg weekly for 4 weeks) showed similar activity to the standard dose.[218] Published studies with rituximab, however, have generally not been controlled and are extremely heterogeneous in terms of rituximab dosing and response criteria. Approximately 40 to 60 percent of the ITP patients demonstrate a response to rituximab at 1 year, and 20 to 25 percent of those have a long-term response (at 5 years).[215,219] Splenectomy does not affect response rates to rituximab therapy.[135,216] In ITP patients who have relapsed more than 1 year after rituximab therapy, retreatment with the drug will induce similar responses in 75 percent of patients who responded initially.[220] Despite the apparent benefit of rituximab, its use is still considered "off-label" for ITP.

Different patterns of response have been reported in ITP patients treated with rituximab. Although the majority of patients responded within 4 to 6 weeks (early responders), response was delayed for several months in some patients (late responders). In ITP patients who responded to rituximab, the increase in platelet count was associated with reduction in the quantity of platelet-associated autoantibodies. Rituximab also indirectly affects T cells, as depletion of autoreactive B cells prevents T-cell activation. Interestingly, despite the depletion of peripheral B cells, platelet-associated autoantibodies were still found in the plasma of ITP patients who do not respond to rituximab.[221] A study analyzing the spleens of ITP patients who did not respond to rituximab therapy demonstrated the presence in the spleen of long-lived plasma cells that produced antiplatelet antibodies for as long as 6 months after rituximab therapy ended. However, this class of cells was not found in the spleens of patients who had not received rituximab. The authors of this study suggested that depletion of peripheral B cells by rituximab promotes the differentiation of long-lived plasma cells in the spleen of ITP patients, which might be responsible for the persistence of antiplatelet antibodies.[222]

In a meta-analysis of 306 ITP patients treated with rituximab, adverse reactions were reported as mild to moderate in 66 patients (21.6 percent) and life-threatening in 10 patients (3.7 percent); nine patients (2.9 percent) died.[215] Although some of these deaths were attributed to ITP-related complications and not to rituximab itself, this mortality rate is higher than expected. Infusion-related reactions in rituximab therapy can be severe and, rarely, fatal. Premedication with methylprednisolone is recommend to avoid these reactions.[219] The risk of infection can increase as a result of depletion of B cells, decreased antibody production, and, rarely, neutropenia.[219] Treatment can also reactivate latent viruses, especially hepatitis B. Alteration of T- and B-cell populations and decreased antibody titers against HBV may stimulate HBV replication and, rarely, cause fatal fulminant hepatitis. All patients should be screened for HBV before rituximab therapy.[223] Although preventive lamivudine or entecavir can be used in HBV-positive ITP patients, it is instead recommended that alternative therapies be used.[219] Other viral reactivation syndromes are less common; progressive multifocal leukoencephalopathy (caused by reactivation of polyomavirus JC) is extremely rare.

**Thrombopoietin Receptor Agonists** The observation that platelet production in patients with ITP is impaired, the massive megakaryopoiesis seen in the marrow of mice and humans treated with recombinant TPO (far greater than seen in patients with ITP), and the unexpectedly normal or only modestly elevated TPO levels in patients with ITP suggested the potential benefit of megakaryocyte-stimulation therapy in patients with refractory ITP. Early use of an altered form of a recombinant TPO molecule to stimulate platelet production in normal platelet donors was halted because of its stimulation of autoantibodies that cleared endogenous TPO. Because of this untoward effect, the use of recombinant TPO was abandoned, and a search for molecules that might bind to and stimulate the TPO receptor ensued. Since then, the TPO receptor agonists romiplostim and eltrombopag have been clinically shown to stimulate platelet production.[224,225]

*Romiplostim* This drug is a peptibody that carries four copies of a 14-amino-acid TPO-receptor–binding peptide fused to an immunoglobulin scaffold, and binds to the TPO-binding site of the TPO receptor with high affinity. The TPO-receptor agonist induces megakaryocyte proliferation and differentiation by activating Janus-type tyrosine kinase (JAK)–signal transducer and activator of transcription (STAT) and mitogen-activated protein (MAP) kinase pathways.[224] The insertion of dimeric peptide into the IgG$_1$ heavy chain increases the half-life of the molecule.[225] Romiplostim has no homology with endogenous TPO; thus, the risk of the development of antibodies against TPO is very low. Romiplostim and TPO may also increase platelet responses to agonists. Weekly subcutaneous injection of romiplostim at doses of 1 to 3 mcg/kg produced a dose-dependent increase in the platelet count, starting from day 5, with peak platelet levels reached by days 12 to 15, and platelet counts returning to baseline by day 28.[131,135,224] Therapy for ITP is usually initiated at a dose of 1 mcg/kg per week, and the dose is then increased by 1 mcg/kg to a maximum of 10 mcg/kg until the patient reaches target platelet counts ($>50 \times 10^9$/L). Higher starting doses up to the maximum dose can be used in emergency situations. If the platelet count does not increase to safe levels after 4 weeks of romiplostim treatment at the maximum dose, the drug should be discontinued. Because platelet responses are highly variable, patients should be evaluated periodically, and the dose adjusted based on the platelet counts. Although discontinuation of romiplostim is recommended when the platelet count exceeds $400 \times 10^9$/L, it should be kept in mind that platelet counts can drop to extremely low levels. Close monitoring of the platelet counts is therefore crucial. Romiplostim can be used in patients with hepatic or renal insufficiency but is not recommended in pregnant patients because it can cross the placenta. Two parallel placebo-controlled trials examined response rates to romiplostim in both splenectomized and nonsplenectomized patients treated for 24 weeks.[134] Durable platelet responses and overall platelet responses were achieved by 38 percent and 79 percent of splenectomized patients, respectively, and by 61 percent and 88 percent of nonsplenectomized patients, respectively, who were given the drug. A newer study evaluating long-term (up to 5 years) results of romiplostim therapy showed that a platelet count of greater than $50 \times 10^9$/L was achieved at least once by 95 percent of treated ITP patients.[226]

*Eltrombopag* This agent is a small (442 Da) nonpeptide molecule that binds to the transmembrane domain of the TPO receptor and triggers megakaryocyte growth and differentiation, increasing platelet production. Eltrombopag has some distinctive features compared to recombinant human thrombopoietin (rhTPO) and romiplostim: eltrombopag does not compete with TPO binding, and although it induces the phosphorylation of STAT proteins, it does not affect the AKT pathway.[227] Eltrombopag has no effect on platelet activation in response to agonists.[225] In healthy volunteers, daily doses given for 10 days elevated platelet counts beginning at 8 days and peaking at 16 days. Eltrombopag is used orally at daily doses of 25 to 75 mg and should be given 2 hours before or after meals because food can affect its absorption. Ethnic differences in eltrombopag pharmacokinetics have been described. Lower initial doses and slower titration are preferred in East Asian patients.[228] Divalent cations such as calcium interfere with absorption of the drug, so it should not be taken with dairy products or antacids. Eltrombopag can also interfere with the uptake and metabolism of statins, increasing their plasma concentrations. Eltrombopag is metabolized in the liver and causes liver function abnormalities in approximately 13 percent of patients

administered the drug. Reduced initial doses are recommended in patients with liver disease.[225] Eltrombopag increases platelet counts ($50 \times 10^9$/L) in 80 percent of splenectomized and 88 percent of nonsplenectomized chronic ITP patients.[229] A newer study evaluated repeated short-term doses of eltrombopag (50 mg daily for up to 6 weeks followed by up to 4 weeks off therapy over three cycles) and suggested that eltrombopag can be used as on-demand therapy and repeated courses would be effective and safe.[230]

*Newer Thrombopoietin Receptor Agonists* Other congeners are currently being evaluated. An oral, nonpeptide TPO-receptor agonist, avatrombopag, binds to the transmembrane domain of TPO receptor and increases platelet counts. Lack of significant food interaction is an important feature of this new drug.[136] Its use is pending FDA approval.

Common side effects of TPO-receptor agonists include mild headache, arthralgia, nasopharyngitis, fatigue, diarrhea, and nausea. These side effects are generally mild and usually of insufficient severity to cause the discontinuation of the drugs. Abnormalities of liver function tests (elevated alanine aminotransferase [ALT], aspartate aminotransferase [AST], and bilirubin levels) occur in approximately 2 percent of ITP patients receiving eltrombopag therapy but not with romiplostim.[225] Autoantibodies against romiplostim may develop but rarely have neutralizing activity.

TPO-receptor agonists can induce extreme thrombocytosis, sometimes exceeding $1000 \times 10^9$/L. Careful dose titration is very important, because cessation of the TPO-receptor agonists causes rebound thrombocytopenia in approximately 10 percent of ITP patients.[225] Rates of thromboembolic events were reported as 6.5 percent and 4 percent with extended romiplostim and eltrombopag treatment, respectively.[225,230] The authors of these studies concluded that thromboembolic events are not associated with the dose of TPO receptor agonists or platelet counts, and at least one acquired and inherited thrombotic risk factor was present in most of the patients who experienced thrombosis while they were taking TPO-receptor agonists.[226,230] Nevertheless, the frequency of thrombosis in these studies was slightly higher than observed in other ITP studies.[160] Secondary myelofibrosis (increased marrow reticulin) is sometimes associated with therapy with TPO receptor agonists and is usually reversible. Concerns have also been expressed that these drugs might accelerate the progression of hematologic and solid malignancies. Under normal circumstances, expression of the TPO receptor (mpl) is highly restricted to hematologic tissues including marrow, spleen, placenta, brain, and fetal liver cells. TPO-receptor expression has been demonstrated on the leukemic cells of patients with acute myelogenous leukemia (AML) and MDS, but not in lymphoid malignancies, myeloproliferative neoplasms, or other nonhematologic malignancies.[231] Although romiplostim therapy was discontinued in a study of its use in patients with low-/intermediate-risk MDS and thrombocytopenia because of increased blast and AML rates (interim hazard ratio: 2.51), long-term analysis of the study showed similar survival and AML rates in the romiplostim and control groups.[232] The question of whether use of TPO-receptor agonists increase the risk of leukemia warrants further study.

*Azathioprine* This purine analogue is converted to 6-mercaptopurine following gastrointestinal absorption and works by suppressing the immune response. At least 4 months of azathioprine therapy at doses ranging from 50 to 250 mg/d are necessary to evaluate therapeutic efficacy. One study reported that azathioprine produced a sustained normalization of the platelet counts in up to 45 percent of patients with refractory ITP.[233] Azathioprine can be used in pregnancy if necessary (see "Thrombocytopenia During Pregnancy" below). As with other immunosuppressive drugs, major adverse effects are marrow suppression and possible increased risk of secondary malignancy.[177,234]

*Cyclophosphamide* This alkylating drug can be used orally (50 to 200 mg/d) or parenterally (1.0 to 1.5 g/m² IV every 4 weeks) in patients with refractory ITP.[235,236] It increases platelet counts in 60 to 80 percent of patients with ITP, and 20 to 40 percent of those patients will remain in remission for 2 to 3 years[177] after receiving 2 to 3 months of therapy. Its beneficial action is linked to its immunosuppression. The major complications of cyclophosphamide therapy are marrow suppression, hemorrhagic cystitis, infertility, alopecia, and secondary malignancy.

*Cyclosporine* Cyclosporine is an immunosuppressive drug inhibiting T-cell function and is primarily used to prevent rejection in patients with organ transplantation. Although cyclosporine may induce a durable remission in patients with ITP when used at relatively low doses (2.5 to 3.0 mg/kg per day),[237] experience with cyclosporine in ITP patients is usually based on small case series. Cyclosporine has several side effects, some potentially serious, including fever, increased risk of opportunistic infections, gingival hyperplasia, diarrhea, peptic ulcer, pancreatitis, renal dysfunction, elevated liver enzymes, hypertension, peripheral neuropathy, convulsions, hirsutism, and increased risk of secondary malignancy.

*Danazol* This synthetic androgen, with reduced virilizing effects compared to other androgens, has been used to treat patients with refractory ITP. Given at doses of 400 to 800 mg/d for at least 6 months, reported response rates range from 10 to 80 percent.[177,234] Danazol is postulated to decrease Fc receptor numbers on phagocytic cells by antagonizing the effects of estrogens.[153] Danazol should not be given to pregnant women or patients with liver disease. Common side effects of danazol therapy are weight gain, fluid retention, seborrhea, hirsutism, secondary amenorrhea, vocal changes, acne, hepatic toxicity, headache, lethargy, cholesterol spectrum abnormalities (i.e., reduced high-density lipoprotein [HDL] cholesterol), and myalgia. Because liver dysfunction is common with these doses of danazol therapy, liver function should be evaluated monthly.[153,177,234]

*Dapsone* Dapsone possesses antibacterial and antiinflammatory effects; it is primarily used for leprosy, malaria, and some types of dermatitis. When used at a dose of 75 to 100 mg/d, dapsone may increase platelet counts in patients with persistent, refractory, or chronic ITP.[147,238,239] The median time to response is long, up to 2 months. Partial response and CR rates are approximately 50 percent and 20 percent, respectively, but platelet counts return to baseline levels after discontinuation of the therapy.[238,239] The mechanism of dapsone action in ITP is not known. The most important side effects are nausea, headache, skin rashes, hepatitis, cholestasis, dose-dependent hemolysis, and methemoglobinemia. Dapsone should not be given to patients with glucose-6-phosphate dehydrogenase deficiency.

*Vinca Alkaloids* Both vincristine and vinblastine transiently increase the platelet count in approximately 70 percent of ITP patients within 5 to 21 days but produce sustained remissions in only 10 percent of treated patients.[108,153,177,234] The recommended dose of vincristine is 1 to 2 mg and of vinblastine is 0.1 mg/kg (maximum: 10 mg), both given by bolus injection at 1-week intervals for a minimum of three courses. It has been proposed that vinca alkaloids bind to platelet microtubules and thereby are transported to the spleen, where they subsequently inhibit the phagocytic functions of splenic macrophages. They may also stimulate megakaryopoiesis. Peripheral neuropathy, neutropenia, jaw pain, alopecia, and constipation are complications of treatment with vinca alkaloids.[234,240–242]

*Other Therapies* ITP patients with *H. pylori* infection should receive eradication therapy.[148] Many other therapies, including interferon-α,[243] immunoadsorption with staphylococcal protein A,[244] ascorbic acid,[245] colchicine,[246] and plasmapheresis,[247] have been studied for refractory ITP cases, but none has been clearly demonstrated to be effective.

## Accessory Therapies

Adjunctive therapies include agents designed to reduce bleeding without necessarily affecting the platelet count. Aminocaproic acid or tranexamic acid, both of which inhibit fibrinolysis, can be used for excessive mucosal bleeding. Local bleeding can be controlled by compression and use of gelatin sponges, fibrin sealants, or antifibrinolytic-embedded gauze. Avoiding the use of antiplatelet drugs, contact sports, and activities that increase bleeding risk and educating patients about maintaining dental hygiene are very important. Menorrhagia is a common problem in patients with chronic ITP; gynecologic evaluation of uterine problems is crucial. Oral contraceptives and hormonal intrauterine devices together with antifibrinolytic drugs may help to reduce excessive menstrual bleeding in these patients.

## SECONDARY IMMUNE THROMBOCYTOPENIA

Secondary ITP is defined as immune-mediated platelet destruction in the presence of other conditions, including infections, lymphoproliferative disorders, solid tumors, SLE, or the antiphospholipid syndrome (APS) (Fig. 7–4).[248] ITP can sometimes be the presenting sign of the illness or may develop during the course of the disease or with certain therapies. Thrombocytopenia in a patient with chronic disease may develop for other reasons, and the diagnosis of immune-mediated platelet destruction may require more detailed tests. Generally, thrombocytopenia is not severe in patients with secondary ITP, but bleeding risk may be enhanced at a particular platelet count because of the underlying disorder. The treatment strategy should be tailored to the individual patient.

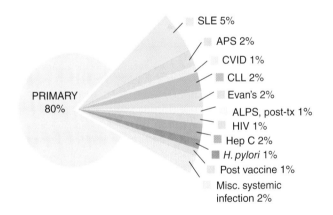

**Figure 7–4.** Estimated fraction of the various forms of secondary immune thrombocytopenia (ITP) based on clinical experience of the authors. The incidence of *Helicobacter pylori* (HP) ranges from approximately 1 percent in the United States to 60 percent in Italy and Japan. The incidence of the HIV and hepatitis C virus approximates 20 percent in some populations. Miscellaneous causes of immune thrombocytopenia, for example, posttransfusion purpura, myelodysplasia, drugs that lead to the production of autoantibodies, and other conditions, are not discussed further in this chapter. Post marrow or solid-organ transplantation autoimmune lymphoproliferative syndrome (ALPS) occurred in approximately 1 percent of the authors' patients. In the absence of a systematic analysis of the incidence of secondary ITP, the data shown represent the authors' assessment based on our experience and the findings reported in the literature. APS, antiphospholipid syndrome; CLL, chronic lymphocytic leukemia, CVID, common variable immune deficiency; SLE, systemic lupus erythematosus. *(Reproduced with permission from Cines DB, Bussel JB, Liebman HA, Luning Prak ET. The ITP syndrome: pathogenic and clinical diversity, Blood 2009 Jun 25;113(26):6511–6521.)*

# IMMUNE THROMBOCYTOPENIA IN PATIENTS WITH ANTIPHOSPHOLIPID SYNDROME, SYSTEMIC LUPUS ERYTHEMATOSUS, AND OTHER CONNECTIVE TISSUE DISORDERS

## Thrombocytopenia in the Antiphospholipid Syndrome

APS is characterized by recurrent arterial and/or venous thrombosis and well-defined morbidity during pregnancy in the presence of antiphospholipid antibodies (APLAs) (Chap. 22).[249] APS may affect any organ in the body, including the heart, brain, kidney, skin, lung, and placenta. This syndrome predominantly affects females (female-to-male ratio 5:1), especially during the childbearing years.[250] APLAs (lupus anticoagulant; anticardiolipin antibodies; anti–$\beta_2$-GPI antibodies) represent a heterogeneous family of antibodies that react with anionic phospholipids and phospholipid–protein complexes. Despite overwhelming evidence that APLAs are associated with thrombosis, the mechanisms remain uncertain. Many have been proposed, including endothelial cell damage and apoptosis, inhibition of prostacyclin release from endothelial cells, inhibition of the protein C–protein S anticoagulant system, induction of tissue factor, activation of platelets and the complement system, interference with antithrombin, impairment of fibrinolytic activity, and inhibition of annexin V binding to membrane phospholipids, eliminating the antithrombotic effect of annexin V.[251-254] APS is considered one of the most common causes of acquired thrombophilia.[255,256]

Thrombocytopenia is reported in approximately 20 to 40 percent of patients with APS, usually is mild (70 to $120 \times 10^9$/L), and does not require clinical intervention. Severe thrombocytopenia (platelet counts $<50 \times 10^9$/L) occurs in 5 to 10 percent of patients.[257-259] Although thrombocytopenia was a clinical criterion used to define the syndrome in the initial classification of APS,[260] it was not included in the most recently proposed classification.[261] Because ITP patients who present with APLAs are at increased risk for thrombosis,[262] measurement of APLA, especially lupus anticoagulant, in patients diagnosed with ITP may identify a subgroup at high risk for developing APS. The pathogenesis of thrombocytopenia in APS is not clear. Potential mechanisms explaining thrombocytopenia in APS patients include APLA-related direct platelet destruction, immune platelet destruction by antibodies against platelet GPs, complement-mediated platelet destruction, and platelet aggregation and consumption. Evidence indicates that APLAs bind platelet membranes and cause platelet destruction, but the link is not definitive. Some investigators suggest that antibodies against platelet GPs, rather than APLAs, are responsible for thrombocytopenia in patients with APS. Antibodies against the integrin $\alpha_{IIb}\beta_3$ or GPIb–IX–V complexes are found in approximately 40 percent of thrombocytopenic patients with APS.[263] Such antibodies do not cross react with antibodies against phospholipids or $\beta_2$-GPI.[264] Immunosuppressive treatment in these patients increases the platelet count and reduces the titers of anti-GP antibodies but not the titers of APLAs.[265] These data suggest that thrombocytopenia is a secondary immune phenomenon that develops concomitantly with APS. Against this conclusion, platelet antigens in thrombocytopenic patients with APS were found to be different from those in ITP and the antibodies to display virtually no reactivity with membrane GPs.[266] CD40 ligand on platelets is another possible antibody target. Anti-CD40 ligand antibodies have been found in patients with APS (13 percent) and ITP (12 percent) but not in healthy controls, and it was suggested that these antibodies cause thrombocytopenia.[267] Platelet activation, aggregation, and consumption (APS-associated thrombotic microangiopathy) may also contribute to thrombocytopenia.[259] Another issue of clinical importance in evaluating hemocytopenia associated with APS is the risk for future development of thrombosis. In one study in which APS patients were divided into three groups according to platelet

counts as normal, moderately thrombocytopenic (50 to $100 \times 10^9$/L), or severely thrombocytopenic ($<50 \times 10^9$/L), the rates of future thrombosis were 40 percent, 32 percent, and 9 percent, respectively.[268] These data show that moderate thrombocytopenia does not prevent thrombosis in patients with APS. Antithrombotic prophylaxis should be considered in these patients whenever it is possible.[257,268]

Although thrombocytopenia is a common finding in patients with APS, bleeding complications are rare, even with severe thrombocytopenia. Bleeding in an APS patient with moderate thrombocytopenia should trigger evaluation for the presence of antiprothrombin antibodies[269] and other disorders that may affect hemostasis, such as DIC, liver insufficiency, and uremia. Severe thrombocytopenia may require therapy, with treatment strategies similar to those used for patients with ITP. Glucocorticoids are effective in only 15 percent of patients.[257] IVIG and immunosuppressive drugs such as azathioprine and cyclophosphamide can be used in patients with severe bleeding and "catastrophic" APS. In general, splenectomy should be postponed as long as possible and is only preferred in patients with severe bleeding. Splenectomy may produce sustained remission in approximately two-thirds of patients as in patients with primary ITP.[167,270,271] Because of their increased risk of thrombosis, patients should be prophylactically anticoagulated in the immediate postoperative period. Rituximab has been used to treat refractory thrombocytopenia in patients with APS, with a wide range of results.[272-274] Although there is no consensus on dosing and schedule with rituximab therapy, it is generally administered as in patients with ITP (see ITP therapy in "Therapy and Course" above). TPO-receptor agonists may increase thrombosis risk in patients with APS and SLE, and these diagnoses in a patient with ITP were accepted as exclusion criteria in some randomized controlled studies of TPO-receptor agonists.[136] Two case reports described acute renal failure (one was a result of thrombotic microangiopathy) after use of eltrombopag.[275,276]

## Thrombocytopenia in Patients with Systemic Lupus Erythematosus and Other Connective Tissue Disorders

SLE is a complex autoimmune disease that primarily afflicts women of childbearing age. The autoimmune attack in SLE is not organ specific; it may affect any tissue in the body. The diagnostic criteria for SLE are based on a classification system proposed by the American College of Rheumatology.[277,278] The presence of hematologic findings (leukopenia, thrombocytopenia, or hemolytic anemia) is one of the criteria in the diagnosis and classification of SLE. Thrombocytopenia is common in patients with SLE, occurring in 20 to 40 percent of patients, and may be a presenting symptom.[279] Immunologic destruction of platelets is also seen in several other autoimmune conditions, including polyarteritis nodosa, rheumatoid arthritis, mixed connective tissue disease, and Sjögren syndrome, albeit at much lower rates than in SLE.

The causes of thrombocytopenia in SLE are many and include platelet destruction (ITP, DIC, thrombotic thrombocytopenic purpura [TTP] or hemolytic uremic syndrome [HUS], sepsis, drugs), ineffective hematopoiesis (megaloblastic anemia), abnormal platelet pooling (hypersplenism), marrow hypoplasia (from drugs and infections), and dilutional thrombocytopenia related to therapy. Severe thrombocytopenia is relatively rare, occurring in 5 percent of patients.[279] Although clinically significant bleeding is uncommon even in patients with severe thrombocytopenia, fatal gastrointestinal, cerebral, and pulmonary bleeding have been reported. Among the many potential contributors to thrombocytopenia in SLE patients, platelet destruction by autoantibodies is the major mechanism. Antiplatelet antibodies are present in up to 60 percent of SLE patients.[280,281] The presence of antiplatelet antibodies is correlated with low platelet counts and increased disease severity.[281] Besides the antiplatelet antibodies, APLAs (see "Thrombocytopenia in the Antiphospholipid Syndrome" above) and circulating immune complexes that bind platelets may nonspecifically accelerate platelet destruction.[282] Specific antiplatelet antibodies, especially those against integrin, have an important role in the pathogenesis of thrombocytopenia in SLE patients.[280,281,283] In general, marrow megakaryocytes are normal or increased, and platelet production is not affected in SLE patients with thrombocytopenia. However, decreased numbers of megakaryocytes and even amegakaryocytic thrombocytopenia have been reported.[86,284] High levels of TPO in the plasma, and both anti-TPO and anti-TPO receptor antibodies have been reported in SLE patients,[285,286] the latter associated with a decrease in marrow megakaryocytes and thrombocytopenia.[286] Thrombocytopenia in SLE is associated with serious organ pathology, leading to neuropsychiatric disease,[287] renal disease,[288,289] and APS,[290] and is an independent indicator of poor prognosis.[289,291,292] A study of selected SLE families in which at least one affected member was thrombocytopenic reported genetic linkage to loci at chromosomes 11p13 and 1q22–23.[293] A severe lupus phenotype was much more common in patients with thrombocytopenia and their affected family members than in patients from families with no thrombocytopenic patients. Therefore, thrombocytopenia in a family member may herald severe lupus in familial SLE.

There are no well-established treatment strategies for severe thrombocytopenia in patients with SLE. Because SLE ranges in severity from milder forms with easily controlled symptoms and signs to severe forms that can be fatal, the treatment of severe thrombocytopenia should be tailored to the individual patient. Patients with severe thrombocytopenia are generally treated with glucocorticoids as first-line therapy, but sustained remission is infrequent. Because most patients with severe thrombocytopenia also have nephritis and neurologic symptoms, they receive immunosuppressive therapy either alone or in combination with glucocorticoids.[294–297] IVIG is reserved for use in patients with severe bleeding.[298,299] It is well-known that B lymphocytes play an important role in the pathogenesis of SLE. Although lymphopenia is common in patients with active SLE, autoantibody-producing B cells have been shown to be expanded, and B cells were found to be more sensitive to inflammatory cytokines.[300] B-cell targeted therapy—rituximab—is effective in the treatment of refractory SLE patients, especially those with nephritis and severe thrombocytopenia.[300] A retrospective study evaluating the long-term effects of rituximab therapy in 65 patients with refractory ITP associated with SLE and mixed connective tissue disease reported an overall response rate of 80 percent.[301] Although case series indicate that splenectomy yields sustained remission in 61 percent of SLE patients with severe thrombocytopenia[295] and is relatively safe in terms of perioperative complications,[302] splenectomy may increase the risk of thrombotic complications in SLE patients[303] and may also increase the risk of infection if the patients require further immunosuppressive therapy.

## THROMBOCYTOPENIA IN INFECTIOUS DISEASES

The first recorded observation of purpura was made in patients with fever, and purpura was accepted as a sign of severe infections for centuries. Thrombocytopenia can be seen in patients with viral, bacterial, fungal, and parasitic infections. Infection can decrease platelet levels in several ways: by decreasing production in the marrow, by increased immune destruction, or by inducing microangiopathy, as seen in patients with infection-induced DIC or HUS. In addition, drugs used for the treatment of an infection can contribute to thrombocytopenia (see "Drug-Induced Thrombocytopenia" below).

Viral infections are an important cause of secondary ITP. ITP can be seen after a viral infection, especially in children, and usually resolves within 2 to 8 weeks. In patients with viral infections such as rubella, mumps, and infectious mononucleosis, thrombocytopenia can be present with other clinical signs and symptoms. Adult patients with isolated thrombocytopenia with no obvious causes should be screened for HIV, HCV and, in endemic areas, HBV. Because other clinical symptoms and signs associated with infection with these viruses may not be present initially, it may not be possible to distinguish these cases from primary ITP.

HIV is a leading cause of isolated thrombocytopenia in Western countries. Thrombocytopenia associated with HIV infection has numerous causes, many of which can be present simultaneously. These include accelerated platelet destruction primarily related to immune complexes, decreased platelet production, especially in advanced disease, splenic sequestration, and, rarely, platelet consumption associated with TTP. Medications, concurrent infections such as hepatitis C, and hematologic malignancies may contribute to the development of thrombocytopenia.[304–307]

HCV is another important cause of thrombocytopenia in adults. It is a hepatotrophic RNA virus of the Flaviviridae family. HCV infection is chronic in approximately 85 percent of infected individuals and progresses to cirrhosis in 20 percent of these individuals. The World Health Organization (WHO) estimates that approximately 3 percent of the world's population is infected with HCV, with the prevalence ranging from 0.5 to 2 percent in Western countries to 20 percent in some underdeveloped countries.[308] HCV causes thrombocytopenia through different mechanisms, including hypersplenism, decreased TPO level associated with liver insufficiency, the effect of drugs (pegylated interferon [IFN] and ribavirin), and immune-mediated platelet destruction.[309] Immune dysregulation in HCV is associated with several autoimmune disorders, including arthritis, Sjögren syndrome, cryoglobulinemia, and immune cytopenias.[310] As a potential mechanism of immune destruction, one study demonstrated binding of both free and IgG-complexed HCV to platelets.[311] In secondary ITP associated with HCV infection, antiviral therapy with pegylated IFN and ribavirin will decrease viral load and may also treat thrombocytopenia. However, platelet counts can be unaffected or even decrease after these therapies. Severe thrombocytopenia interferes with optimal HCV treatment and may increase bleeding risk. In this situation, the ASH 2011 guideline recommends IVIG as a first-line therapy, because glucocorticoids may increase viral load.[148] Glucocorticoids and splenectomy both appear to be effective treatments for thrombocytopenia, but their use should be balanced against other considerations after discussion with a hepatologist. TPO-receptor agonists may increase the risk of abdominal thrombosis in HCV patients with liver cirrhosis.[312]

The potential role of *H. pylori* in the pathogenesis of chronic ITP is controversial. Japanese and Italian studies showed that eradication of *H. pylori* with antibiotics resulted in marked platelet count increases in patients with ITP. However, this success was not reproduced in American and other European studies.[313] It appears that response rates are higher in countries where *H. pylori* infection is endemic. ITP patients treated for *H. pylori* had higher platelet counts than untreated ITP patients, even if the therapy was unsuccessful in eradicating the infection.[314] It has therefore been speculated that the antibiotic therapy, rather than eradication of *H. pylori*, may be the factor improving platelet counts. However, meta-analysis found that *H. pylori* eradication therapy was much more likely to increase platelet counts in patients with *H. pylori* infection than in uninfected patients,[315] strengthening the case for a causal relationship between infection and thrombocytopenia. On the other hand, eradication was shown to be less effective in patients with severe thrombocytopenia.[309] The recent ASH ITP guideline suggests that

ITP patients be screened for *H. pylori* and that eradication therapy should be used if testing is positive.[148]

# THROMBOCYTOPENIA DURING PREGNANCY

Thrombocytopenia is the second most common hematologic problem in pregnancy, after anemia. Table 7–6 lists the major causes of thrombocytopenia in pregnancy. Platelet counts tend to decrease during normal pregnancy, and mild thrombocytopenia (platelet counts ranging from 120 to $150 \times 10^9$/L) occurs with moderate frequency, especially during the third trimester.[316,317] Bleeding symptoms are generally mild, even in patients with severe thrombocytopenia, probably because of the procoagulant state of pregnancy. Nevertheless, it is important to investigate the cause of thrombocytopenia and exclude the disorders associated with significant morbidity such as eclampsia and hemolysis, elevated liver enzymes, low platelets (HELLP) syndrome (Table 7–6). A medical history should include previous blood counts, history of other diseases, nutritional status, and intake of drugs and herbal supplements. It is important to be alert to constitutional symptoms including fever and, especially, weight loss; neurologic abnormalities; arthritis; rash; and icterus. Key steps in the evaluation of thrombocytopenia in a pregnant woman include blood pressure measurement, evaluation of coagulation parameters, liver and kidney function tests, and examination of the blood film. Physical examination of the abdomen may be difficult in the third trimester, and abdominal ultrasound may be required to detect organomegaly. If there are no suspicious clinical or laboratory findings, marrow aspiration is considered unnecessary.[317,318]

## GESTATIONAL THROMBOCYTOPENIA

Gestational thrombocytopenia is detected in 5 to 7 percent of otherwise healthy pregnant women, accounting for 64 to 80 percent of patients with thrombocytopenia at term.[319–321] Gestational thrombocytopenia is a benign disorder and is not associated with an increased risk of bleeding. Platelet counts are greater than $70 \times 10^9$/L[316,317,319,320] and return to normal after delivery.

The pathogenesis of gestational thrombocytopenia is unknown. Several mechanisms have been proposed, including hemodilution, a compensated state of subclinical coagulopathy, endothelial cell injury, and immune destruction. Some authors have proposed platelet consumption by the placenta and hormonal depression of megakaryopoiesis as causes of gestational thrombocytopenia, as suggested by the rapid return of the platelet count to normal after delivery and by the transient normalization of the platelet count during pregnancy in some cases of essential thrombocythemia.[321–324] Discriminating gestational thrombocytopenia from ITP can be difficult because ITP is also common in young women and is often exacerbated by pregnancy. Neither condition can be definitively diagnosed by currently available tests. The diagnosis of ITP is favored if the patient had a previous episode of ITP unassociated with pregnancy or if the thrombocytopenia is severe and associated with bleeding that occurs in the first trimester. In healthy pregnant women, a platelet count greater than $70 \times 10^9$/L late in pregnancy does not require intensive investigation, because bleeding is not likely in the woman or her newborn child.[325]

# IMMUNE THROMBOCYTOPENIA IN PREGNANCY

ITP is responsible for 4 to 5 percent of all cases of pregnancy-associated thrombocytopenia.[319,321] Pregnancy itself may induce ITP, or exacerbate preexisting ITP, but generally, the platelet count returns to the prepregnancy level after delivery. Diagnosis of ITP in a pregnant woman requires the exclusion of other causes of thrombocytopenia as in a nonpregnant woman, but also requires the evaluation of other pregnancy-related causes (see Table 7–6). However, the management of ITP during pregnancy is different than in nonpregnant women. First, many of the drugs used to treat ITP may complicate pregnancy-related problems such as gestational diabetes, hypertension, and psychiatric disorders. Second, the fetus can also be affected by ITP and its treatment. Antiplatelet antibodies can cross the placenta, decrease the fetal platelet count, and sometimes cause bleeding.[320] ITP drugs can affect fetal development and growth, a fact to be considered in selecting therapy during pregnancy. And third, all pregnancies will end with delivery of the baby, a process that may happen unexpectedly. Preparation for delivery in a pregnant ITP patient requires close collaboration between the hematologist, the obstetrician, and the neonatologist.

In the management of pregnancy-related ITP, bleeding symptoms and platelet counts should be considered.[147,148] Although previous guidelines have defined threshold platelet levels for treatment during pregnancy and labor, these numbers are arbitrary and not based on randomized controlled studies. Generally, observation without therapy is appropriate if the platelet count is greater than $30 \times 10^9$/L and the patient has no bleeding symptoms. Therapy is required for a pregnant woman who is bleeding, has a platelet count less than $20 \times 10^9$/L in any trimester, or has a platelet count of 20 to $30 \times 10^9$/L in the third trimester.[147,318] Platelet counts should be increased to safe levels (generally $>30 \times 10^9$/L) if invasive procedures are planned. Glucocorticoids are the preferred initial therapy for these patients. Because of their side effects, glucocorticoids should be used at the minimal dose that will keep platelet counts in a safe range. The recommended starting dose of prednisone is 10 mg/d, which can be modified as appropriate.[147,318] Fetal side effects will be minimal with a low-dose glucocorticoid regimen, because approximately 90 percent of the glucocorticoid dose is metabolized in the placenta.[317] IVIG is indicated in pregnant patients who do not respond to or tolerate

**TABLE 7–6.** Causes of Thrombocytopenia During Pregnancy

Acute fatty liver of pregnancy

Antiphospholipid syndrome and systemic lupus erythematosus

Marrow disorders (e.g., aplastic anemia, acute leukemia)

Disseminated intravascular coagulation

Drugs (mostly heparins and antibiotics)

Gestational thrombocytopenia

Hemolysis, elevated liver function tests, low platelets (HELLP) syndrome

Hypersplenism

Immune thrombocytopenic purpura

Nutritional deficiencies including folate deficiency

Preeclampsia, eclampsia

Pseudothrombocytopenia

Thrombotic thrombocytopenic purpura–hemolytic uremic syndrome

Viral infections

glucocorticoid treatment, or when it is necessary to rapidly increase the platelet count. A dose of 1 g/kg per day for 2 days or 400 mg/kg per day for 5 days can be used alone or combined with low-dose prednisone. If the initial therapy with glucocorticoids and IVIG fails, all second-line therapies generate some concern. Anti-(Rh)D can cause severe hemolytic reactions in both the mother and the fetus and should be used only in patients refractory to glucocorticoids and IVIG.[148,318] Experience with azathioprine and cyclosporine in pregnancy is largely based on the case series from patients with rheumatologic disorders and solid-organ transplantation. These studies reported that exposure to these drugs during pregnancy was not associated with an increase in the risk of negative pregnancy outcomes and had no significant toxicity to the fetus.[326] Splenectomy can be used in pregnant ITP patients who are unresponsive or intolerant to available drugs and at significant risk of bleeding. If splenectomy is necessary, it is preferable that it be performed during the second trimester.[147,191]

Rituximab is not an optimal drug for use during pregnancy. It can cross the placenta, and transfer from mother to fetus increases with gestational age. The half-life of the drug is also very long; rituximab can be found in blood 6 months after an infusion. In a review evaluating 231 pregnancies with rituximab exposure reported in the literature, most of the patients had SLE, rheumatoid arthritis, and B-cell lymphoma, with rituximab being used in combination with other drugs. This retrospective study showed low risk of premature births, hematologic abnormalities, and birth defects. However, because of the lack of controlled studies, it is recommended that women avoid pregnancy for 1 year after rituximab infusion.[327]

TPO-receptor agonists were found to cause fetal loss and reduced fetal body weight in animal studies, and there are no data on humans.[328] Vinca alkaloids, cyclophosphamide, and danazol are not recommended during pregnancy.

The optimal mode of delivery in pregnant ITP patients has not been determined. Because earlier studies reported that thrombocytopenic neonates have an increased risk for intracranial hemorrhage, some physicians recommend delivering the baby by cesarean section in women with ITP to avoid injuries to the fetus during passage through the birth canal.[329] However, because of the rarity of intracerebral hemorrhage, there are no data proving the effectiveness of cesarean delivery in reducing the occurrence of intracerebral hemorrhage in the thrombocytopenic fetus.[322] Measurement of platelet counts in infants before delivery, such as by percutaneous umbilical cord blood sampling or fetal scalp vein sampling after cervical dilatation, is not recommended routinely because the risk of bleeding during these procedures is high.[330-332] The mother's platelet count at delivery does not correlate with the infant's platelet count. In ITP patients who gave birth more than once, however, the first infant's platelet count at birth may be a predictor of severe thrombocytopenia in subsequent pregnancies and may justify further obstetric management.[322,331,333] On the other hand, discordances in degree of thrombocytopenia between dichorionic twins in ITP indicate that fetal factors also are important.[334] In conclusion, there is as yet no definitive method to predict fetal platelet count in pregnant ITP patients, and the method of delivery should be determined by obstetrical evaluation. During vaginal delivery, the target maternal platelet count should be $50 \times 10^9$/L or higher. If cesarean section or epidural anesthesia is required, the platelet count should be maintained over 70 to $80 \times 10^9$/L.[147,148,318] Glucocorticoids, IVIG, and platelet transfusions may help to keep platelet counts in a safe range in these patients. Blood products should be available for possible severe bleeding during labor, although it is quite rare even in ITP patients with platelet counts lower than $20 \times 10^9$/L.

Severe neonatal thrombocytopenia (platelet counts <$20 \times 10^9$/L) occurs in 3 to 5 percent of ITP pregnancies, and moderate neonatal thrombocytopenia (platelet counts <$50 \times 10^9$/L) occurs in 9 percent.[330] Severe bleeding occurs in less than 1 percent of the babies. If the newborn is thrombocytopenic, the platelet count should be measured daily for 1 week. IVIG is preferred in neonates with severe thrombocytopenia. Platelet transfusions and glucocorticoids are added if bleeding is life-threatening.

If thrombocytopenia associated with SLE and APS has been complicated with prior pregnancy loss and thromboembolism, pregnant patients should receive antithrombotic prophylaxis with low-molecular-weight heparin and/or aspirin if possible. Although there is no defined threshold platelet level for these patients, platelet counts over $50 \times 10^9$/L are considered safe for both anticoagulant and antiplatelet therapy.[318]

## MICROANGIOPATHIC DISORDERS IN PREGNANCY: PREECLAMPSIA–ECLAMPSIA, HELLP, THROMBOTIC THROMBOCYTOPENIC PURPURA–HEMOLYTIC UREMIC SYNDROME, AND ACUTE FATTY LIVER OF PREGNANCY

### Preeclampsia

This condition is a systemic disorder characterized by new-onset hypertension after 20 weeks of gestation and primarily occurs near term. Although proteinuria occurs in the majority of these cases, the American College of Obstetricians and Gynecologists (ACOG) 2012 classification accepts the presence of one of the following in the absence of proteinuria: thrombocytopenia (<$100 \times 10^9$/L), abnormal liver function tests, renal insufficiency, pulmonary edema, or cerebral and visual symptoms. *Eclampsia* is defined by the occurrence of epileptic seizures in a preeclamptic woman during the peripartum period.[335-337] Preeclampsia complicates 5 to 8 percent of all pregnancies and is a major contributor to maternal and fetal morbidity and mortality.[335,338] Thrombocytopenia is seen in approximately 50 percent of women with preeclampsia, with the severity of thrombocytopenia correlating with the severity of the preeclampsia.[339]

Attempts to define the pathogenesis of preeclampsia have engendered numerous theories.[340] One clear aspect of the pathogenesis is the requirement for a placenta, given that the condition can be produced in abdominal pregnancies and molar pregnancies.[341] The disease appears to be initiated by defective invasion of the uterine spiral arteries by placental cytotrophoblasts. During normal implantation, these cells convert from epithelial to endothelial morphology, a process called *pseudovasculogenesis*.[342,343] In preeclampsia, this process is defective, resulting in diminished maternal blood flow to the placenta and placental hypoxia. Through unknown mechanisms, the production of membrane and soluble forms of the vascular endothelial growth factor (VEGF) receptor fms-like tyrosine kinase-1 (Flt1) is increased,[344] with resultant increases of soluble Flt1 (sFlt1) in the amniotic fluid[345] and maternal circulation.[346] sFlt1 is the product of an alternately spliced form of the Flt1 messenger RNA that lacks the transmembrane and cytoplasmic domains present in the full-length receptor. A large volume of evidence implicates sFlt1 as playing a key role in the pathogenesis of preeclampsia. By binding to VEGF and the related placental growth factor, sFlt1 blocks their favorable effects on vascular endothelium. Its expression in rats produces a syndrome akin to preeclampsia: hypertension and proteinuria associated with glomerular endotheliosis (occlusion of glomerular capillaries by swollen endothelial cells). Endoglin is another angiogenic receptor expressed on endothelial cells and placental syncytiotrophoblasts, functioning as a coreceptor for the potent angiogenic factor transforming growth factor-$\beta$.[347] Expression of its messenger RNA is increased in preeclamptic placenta.[347] The levels of the soluble extracellular domain, produced by proteolysis, are elevated in the blood of preeclamptic patients. In pregnant rats, soluble endoglin works synergistically with sFlt1 to produce vascular damage and a HELLP-like syndrome.[347] These findings strongly suggest that a tonic level of VEGF-like angiogenic factors is required to maintain the normal function of vascular endothelial cells and that this process is dysregulated during preeclampsia/eclampsia.

The connection between preeclampsia and thrombocytopenia is not clear, although many cases have evidence of activation of blood coagulation detected by elevated levels of fibrin-degradation products and thrombin–antithrombin complexes.[321] Low levels of the VWF-cleaving metalloprotease ADAMTS13 (a disintegrin and metalloprotease with a thrombospondin type 1 motif member 13) have also been described,[348] as have elevated levels of VWF, including the hyperadhesive ultralarge forms.[349]

### HELLP Syndrome

This syndrome occurs in the peripartum period and is defined by the presence of microangiopathic hemolytic anemia, elevated liver enzymes, and low platelets. In approximately 70 to 80 percent of patients, HELLP occurs in the setting of preeclampsia.[350] Microangiopathic hemolysis results from shearing of the erythrocytes as they pass through arterioles occluded by platelet–fibrin deposits. Adhesion and aggregation of platelets on damaged and activated endothelium presumably account for the low platelet count (Chap. 4). HELLP shares a number of features with TTP, including the presence of microangiopathic hemolysis and thrombocytopenia. Involvement of the central nervous system is a more prominent feature of TTP, whereas HELLP more commonly displays severe liver function abnormalities (Chap. 14).[351] Because the two syndromes can be confused with one other, one study attempted to distinguish the two by measuring the activity of ADAMTS13, which usually is absent or severely deficient in TTP.[348] The study found that essentially all 17 patients in a cohort with the HELLP syndrome had mild to moderate reductions in the activity of ADAMTS13 in the plasma, and none was severely deficient.

### Acute Fatty Liver of Pregnancy

This abnormality is a very severe, but fortunately very rare (1 in 20,000 to 100,000 pregnancies) condition that occurs during the third trimester of pregnancy or early postpartum period. Acute fatty liver of pregnancy (AFLP) is characterized by microvesicular fatty infiltration of liver resulting in hepatic failure and encephalopathy. The "Swansea Criteria" used for the diagnosis of AFLP include encephalopathy, vomiting, abdominal pain, polydipsia/polyuria, elevated transaminases, elevated ammonia, elevated uric acid, elevated bilirubin, leukocytosis, coagulopathy, renal impairment, hypoglycemia, ascites or bright liver on ultrasound evaluation, and microvesicular steatosis on liver biopsy. Six or more of these criteria should be present in a patient who has no obvious reason for hepatic failure. Both maternal and fetal mortality rates are high, ranging from 7 to 18 percent and 9 to 23 percent, respectively.[352]

Delivery of the fetus is the most effective treatment for preeclampsia, HELLP syndrome, and AFLP. The platelet count nadir and the peak of serum lactate dehydrogenase may occur postpartum, during the first postpartum day in most patients, but as late as 5 to 7 days in some. For patients with severe thrombocytopenia and microangiopathic hemolytic anemia, plasma exchange may be indicated if the fetus cannot be delivered or if improvement does not follow delivery. This treatment is empirically based on the similarity of the clinical picture to that of TTP. Postpartum day 3 often is considered the limit for supportive therapy in anticipation of a spontaneous recovery.[348] If thrombocytopenia and hemolysis (as assessed by serum lactate dehydrogenase levels) continue to worsen beyond this time, intervention with plasma exchange is

appropriate for the presumed diagnosis of TTP-HUS (Chap. 23). At this point, TTP-HUS cannot be distinguished from atypical preeclampsia/HELLP syndrome, for which plasma exchange treatment may be beneficial.[353] Earlier intervention with plasma exchange is indicated for more severe clinical problems, such as neurologic abnormalities or acute, anuric renal failure. In patients with AFLP, however, liver insufficiency, encephalopathy, and coagulopathy may not improve despite immediate delivery and intensive supportive care. These patients may require liver transplantation.[352]

## ● NEONATAL ALLOIMMUNE THROMBOCYTOPENIA

The platelet count in the fetus reaches normal adult levels ($>150 \times 10^9$/L) after the first trimester and is maintained throughout gestation. However, thrombocytopenia is more common in preterm infants, of several potential etiologies. Severe thrombocytopenia ($<50 \times 10^9$/L) is an important finding in neonates and should be carefully managed because of high bleeding risk.[354]

Fetal–neonatal alloimmune thrombocytopenia (NAIT) is a leading cause of severe thrombocytopenia and life-threatening bleeding in neonates. NAIT is caused by the transplacental transfer of maternal alloantibodies against fetal platelet antigens inherited from the father. NAIT resembles neonatal alloimmune hemolytic anemia (Rh hemolytic disease of the newborn) in many aspects. In both diseases, maternal alloantibodies against fetal blood cell antigens cross the placenta and destroy antigen-positive fetal cells, resulting in significant fetal/neonatal morbidity and mortality. However, unlike neonatal alloimmune hemolytic anemia, which tends to spare the first-born child, the first child is affected in 40 to 60 percent of NAIT cases.[317] Transplacental transfer of antiplatelet antibodies can also occur in babies born from mothers with ITP. Nevertheless, maternal ITP rarely causes serious thrombocytopenia or bleeding in the fetus, whereas thrombocytopenia tends to be more severe and the rate of intracranial hemorrhage is higher (10 to 20 percent) in NAIT.[106] In contrast to maternal ITP, in NAIT, the maternal platelet count is normal, a key differential diagnostic finding.

### PREVALENCE AND PATHOGENESIS

The estimated frequency of NAIT varies from 1 in 500 to 1 in 2000 livebirths.[355,356] Maternal alloantibodies against human platelet alloantigens (HPAs) are responsible for platelet destruction in NAIT. In populations of European ancestry, the most frequently implicated antigens are HPA-1a or Pl^A1 (78 percent of cases) and HPA-5b or Br^a (19 percent of cases).[357] These antigens are rare in Asian populations. HPA-4a (80 percent of cases) and HPA-3a (15 percent of cases) are responsible for platelet destruction in the majority of Asian NAIT cases. Besides targeting the HPA system, anti–HLA-2 antibodies have been reported, but whether they are responsible for NAIT is not clear.[355,358,359]

The frequency of NAIT in populations of European ancestry is lower than would be expected given that the prevalence of HPA-1a negativity is 2.5 percent. Only 10 percent of HPA-1a–negative mothers exposed to HPA-1a–positive platelets during pregnancy become immunized. HPA alloimmunization is strongly correlated with the presence of specific class II HLA antigens, with increased risk demonstrated in HPA-1a–negative mothers expressing HLA-B8, HLA-DR3, and HLA-DR52a antigens.[317,360,361] The presence of the HLA-DRB3*0101 allele in HPA-1a–negative women increases the NAIT risk as much as 140-fold.[361]

NAIT tends to be clinically more severe in cases with alloantibodies against HPA-1a.[106] HPA-1 (Pl[A]) antigens are expressed on platelet integrin $\beta_3$. Anti–HPA-1a antibodies possibly impair platelet aggregation, which may explain the severity of bleeding symptoms.[362]

## CLINICAL FEATURES

IgG alloantibodies can cross the placenta as early as week 14 of pregnancy, and placental passage increases with gestational age.[355] These antibodies bind to fetal platelets and lead to their destruction. In severe cases, intracranial hemorrhage and hydrocephalus may develop and cause fetal death or severe neurologic sequelae. The diagnosis can be difficult in the first affected fetus in a family. Ultrasonography is usually not helpful unless it detects bleeding or hydrocephalus. Unexplained fetal deaths in the maternal history or fetal hydrocephalus or bleeding in previous pregnancies may alert the physician to the possibility of NAIT. Usually the diagnosis of NAIT is possible after birth. NAIT should be suspected in a thrombocytopenic neonate with extensive purpura or visceral hemorrhage but no evidence of sepsis, skeletal anomalies, or other systemic diseases that may cause thrombocytopenia, including maternal ITP. Affected babies may have no signs or symptoms (13 to 59 percent of cases), or they may have signs of bleeding (18 to 65 percent of cases) or intracranial hemorrhage (22 to 23 percent of cases).[363] In a case series of 88 infants with NAIT resulting from anti–HPA-1a antibodies, 90 percent had purpura, 66 percent had hematomas, 30 percent had gastrointestinal bleeding, and 14 percent had intracerebral hemorrhage. Bleeding may be delayed, as the platelet count usually falls further during the first several days of life. Death or neurologic impairment occurs in up to 25 percent of infants. Platelet counts recover to normal in 1 to 2 weeks.[364]

The diagnosis of NAIT usually can be confirmed by tests for circulating maternal alloantibodies against fetal antigens (usually by MAIPA) or modified antigen capture enzyme-linked immunosorbent assay (MACE) or by platelet typing of the parents and neonate by either genotyping or ELISA. These tests may fail to yield the diagnosis because private HPA antigens may be responsible for NAIT.[317,322,357]

## MANAGEMENT

### Postnatal

In the clinical setting, the confirmation of a diagnosis of NAIT by platelet genotyping, MAIPA, or MACE will require days; thus, an infant born with severe thrombocytopenia with no obvious cause such as sepsis should be regarded as having NAIT. The alternatives in the management of affected neonates are IVIG, glucocorticoids (alone or combined with IVIG), and platelet transfusions. IVIG and/or glucocorticoid therapy may increase platelet counts rapidly, although a substantial increase of platelet counts usually occurs after 24 to 72 hours.[357] In cases with severe bleeding, platelets should be transfused. Transfused platelets should be ABO and (Rh)D compatible and HPA-1a–negative if possible.[365] If such platelet suspensions are not available, transfusion of washed and irradiated maternal platelets to the affected fetus is another alternative.[106] Repeated platelet transfusions may be required.[317] All affected infants should be screened with ultrasound for intracranial hemorrhage.[366]

### Prenatal

Pregnant women who had a previous thrombocytopenic infant attributable to NAIT should be carefully monitored in a center with experience with NAIT, because thrombocytopenia will be more severe in a second affected child. Current therapeutic alternatives for antenatal management of NAIT are unsatisfactory. Fetal platelet typing is important, but available tests usually require invasive procedures such as amniocentesis

or fetal blood sampling. Cell-free fetal DNA obtained from maternal blood has been studied for fetal platelet genotyping.[367] However, these tests need validation. The treatment options in high-risk NAIT are weekly IVIG administration to the mother, with or without glucocorticoids, serial *in utero* platelet transfusions, *in utero* IVIG administration, and early delivery (after 32 weeks of gestation). Maternal IVIG administration at a dose of 1 g/kg per week with or without glucocorticoids may increase fetal platelet counts,[368] although not all studies support this conclusion.[355,362] IVIG can be administered directly to severely thrombocytopenic fetuses, although this also may fail to raise fetal platelet counts.[369] In patients who do not respond to IVIG and glucocorticoid administration, serial transfusion of matched platelets should be considered. Matched platelet transfusions will only transiently increase the fetal platelet count because the transfused platelets also are targeted by the offending antibodies.[317] Serial platelet transfusions may increase the cumulative risk of hemorrhage and procedure-related hemorrhage and fetal loss.[362] In severely thrombocytopenic fetuses, early delivery by cesarean section may reduce the risk of intracranial hemorrhage.[362] New therapeutic strategies are under investigation, including vaccines and competitive molecules that competitively bind anti–HPA-1a antibodies.[365]

## ●ABNORMAL PLATELET DISTRIBUTION OR POOLING

### SPLENOMEGALY AND HYPERSPLENISM

Splenomegaly may lead to thrombocytopenia by inducing a reversible pooling of up to 90 percent of total body platelets.[370,371] This process can be thought of as an exaggeration of normal splenic pooling, in which approximately one-third of the platelet mass is contained within the spleen at any one time. The survival of platelets within the spleen can be normal or moderately reduced. Thus, the total blood platelet pool in a patient with splenomegaly could be normal even when the counts measured in venous blood are only 20 percent of normal. Platelet production is usually normal in patients with splenomegaly, as estimated by dividing the total body platelet mass by the platelet life span.[370] This finding provides further evidence that platelet production is more closely tied to total platelet mass than to circulating platelet count.

The most common disorder causing thrombocytopenia because of splenic pooling is chronic liver disease with portal hypertension and congestive splenomegaly. In patients with cirrhosis and portal hypertension, moderate thrombocytopenia is the rule. However, in such cases, the thrombocytopenia often results from both splenic pooling and reduced hepatic production of TPO.

Thrombocytopenia associated with splenomegaly is often of no clinical importance and generally does not require therapy. Signs and symptoms are related to the primary disorder, and bleeding manifestations result primarily from coagulation abnormalities caused by the underlying liver disease. This finding is consistent with the relatively moderate degree of thrombocytopenia, the near-normal total body content of platelets,[370] and the ability to mobilize platelets from the spleen to replenish losses.[372] When splenectomy is performed for another reason, however, the platelet count predictably returns to normal or thrombocytosis may even occur.[370] Platelet counts may also return to normal in patients following surgical correction of portal hypertension by portosystemic shunting.[373] Platelet transfusions usually are not needed for splenomegaly-associated thrombocytopenia and rarely produce significant increases in the platelet count because as much as 90 percent of the transfused platelets will be sequestered in the spleen.

## HYPERSPLENISM

Hypersplenism is distinguished from uncomplicated splenomegaly in that pooling is accompanied by increased destruction of platelets, leukocytes, and erythrocytes in association with increased marrow precursors of the deficient lines and correction of the cytopenia by splenectomy.[374–377] The clinical manifestations, laboratory findings, and specific treatment are aimed at the underlying disease.[378]

Imaging studies, such as computed tomographic scans, can be useful for defining the size of the spleen and identifying intrasplenic and extrasplenic disease. Magnetic resonance imaging defines the blood flow pattern, which is especially useful for detecting portal or splenic vein thromboses. Cell survival studies using radiolabeled platelets or red blood cells can be helpful for identifying hypersequestration when weighing the need for splenectomy. Most patients with splenomegaly require therapy for the underlying disease rather than for thrombocytopenia.

## THROMBOCYTOPENIA ASSOCIATED WITH MASSIVE TRANSFUSION

Several definitions are used for massive transfusion including transfusion of one blood volume or more than 10 units of packed red blood cells (RBCs) in 24 hours and transfusion of more than 4 units of packed RBC over 1 hour.[379] Massive transfusion is required in patients with uncontrolled and heavy bleeding. One study of patients requiring massive transfusion demonstrated that mild thrombocytopenia (47 to $100 \times 10^9$/L) occurred in all patients after transfusion of 15 red cell units, and more severe thrombocytopenia (25 to $61 \times 10^9$/L) developed after 20 red cell units.[380,381] Several factors contribute to thrombocytopenia in massive transfusion, including direct loss of platelets in the exsanguinated blood, dilution of platelets by the transfused RBCs, DIC triggered by the disease responsible for the blood loss or that develops after trauma, and hypothermia. Massively transfused patients should be treated with fresh-frozen plasma to replace coagulation factors and with platelets.[382] The precise ratio of platelets to red cells has not been determined, but studies show that massively transfused trauma patients demonstrated improved survival with increased transfusion of platelet concentrates.[383,384]

## THROMBOCYTOPENIA RESULTING FROM HYPOTHERMIA

Transient thrombocytopenia occurs during hypothermia, in both animals and humans, when the body temperature falls below 25°C.[385] The degree of thrombocytopenia correlates with the degree of the body temperature drop. Thus, thrombocytopenia is less severe in cardiac surgery patients supported by normothermic systemic perfusion (35°C to 37°C) than in those supported by moderately hypothermic systemic perfusion (25°C to 29°C).[386] In this case, the drop in platelet count likely results from splenic and hepatic pooling[387] and from cold activation and clearance of platelets. Cold induces clustering of the GPIb complex and rearrangement of its carbohydrate chains, which then serve as ligands for the macrophage integrin $\alpha_M\beta_2$, which mediates their clearance in hepatic macrophages.[388,389] In hypothermic dogs, radiolabeled platelets are sequestered in the spleen, liver, and other organs; the platelets return to the circulation when normal body temperature is restored.[385,390] The clinical relevance of these observations is illustrated by reports of patients, often elderly, who are hypothermic after periods of unconsciousness in inadequately heated rooms. In one report, a 69-year-old woman had 13 admissions over an 8-year period with repeated hypothermia, with her temperature ranging from 31°C to 34°C during the hospitalizations. On each admission, she was thrombocytopenic (platelet count 7 to $39 \times 10^9$/L). With no therapy other than rewarming, platelet counts returned to normal in 4 to 10 days.[391] However, a review of 75 patients admitted with hypothermia (body temperatures of 26°C to 35°C) demonstrated that only three patients were thrombocytopenic.[391]

## THROMBOCYTOPENIA RESULTING FROM PLATELET TRAPPING: KASABACH-MERRITT SYNDROME

Kasabach-Merritt syndrome is defined as profound thrombocytopenia related to platelet trapping within a vascular tumor, either a Kaposi-like hemangioendothelioma or a tufted angioma.[392–395] The syndrome presents predominantly during infancy, but several adult cases have been reported.[396] These vascular tumors should be differentiated from vascular malformations such as classic benign hemangiomas. Benign hemangiomas usually are superficial, multiple, and not associated with severe thrombocytopenia or DIC (Chap. 20), and usually disappear during childhood. On the other hand, Kaposi-like hemangioendothelioma and tufted angioma are low-grade malignant vascular tumors associated with high morbidity and mortality.

Vascular tumors usually are solitary, can reach 20 cm in diameter, and can be superficial or invade internal organs and the retroperitoneum.[397–399] Superficial tumors can be recognized by the local red to purple discoloration of the skin. The histologic types more frequently associated with Kasabach-Merritt syndrome are Kaposi-like hemangioendothelioma and tufted angiomas or angioblastomas.[392,393,400,401] Kaposi-like hemangioendothelioma is a locally aggressive, low-grade malignant tumor characterized by infiltrating sheets or lobules of poorly formed vascular channels and aberrant lymphatic vessels. These tumors are composed predominantly of plump, round, oval, and/or spindled endothelial cells with hemosiderin deposits.[392] A tufted angioma is a lesion characterized by the presence of vascular tufts and aggregates of round dilated capillaries, lymphangiomatosis, microthrombi, and hemosiderin deposits.[392,393,402,403] Electron microscopic examination shows abnormal endothelial cells with prominent cytoplasmic projections and wide intercellular gaps, fibrin deposition, and platelet aggregates within the vessels.[393] The histology of the tumor is useful for differentiating the vascular tumors associated with Kasabach-Merritt syndrome from benign capillary hemangiomas.[404]

Thrombocytopenia in Kasabach-Merritt syndrome usually is severe and associated with DIC.[405] Contributing factors include "platelet trapping" by abnormally proliferating endothelium within the hemangioma[406,407] and platelet consumption associated with DIC. Platelet trapping has been demonstrated by immunohistochemical staining of the tumors with anti-CD61 antibodies (a marker of platelets and megakaryocytes)[408] and by nuclear studies using $^{51}$Cr-labeled platelets[409] and $^{111}$In platelet scintigraphy to monitor response to therapy.[410,411] How platelets become trapped is not clear. Initial physical entrapment of the platelets within twisted abnormal vessels may favor their adhesion to abnormal endothelium, which can lead to platelet activation and aggregation followed by activation of the coagulation cascade, fibrin deposition, and formation of microthrombi. Excessive flow and shear rates generated by arteriovenous shunting within the tumor further increase the level of platelet activation. Continuous thrombus formation leads to platelet consumption and activation of the fibrinolytic cascade. Severe thrombocytopenia and DIC result.

The mainstay of treatment is eradication of the tumor. Several specific therapeutic modalities have been proposed, but none has been established as consistently effective.[412] Among the therapies are high-dose glucocorticoids,[412] IFN-$\alpha$,[412,413] vincristine,[414] cyclophosphamide,[415] combination chemotherapy,[416] and radiation.[417–419] For severe cases, interventions such as arterial embolization,[420,421] surgical resection,[422,423] and pneumatic compression can be attempted.

The mortality rate for advanced Kasabach-Merritt syndrome is approximately 12 percent; the rate is higher when associated with retroperitoneal or intraabdominal tumors. Patients die of complications resulting from DIC, low platelet count, and infections secondary to immunosuppression.

## ● CYCLIC THROMBOCYTOPENIA

Cyclic thrombocytopenia (CTP) is a very rare acquired disorder characterized by a periodic decrease in the platelet count, sometimes followed by rebound thrombocytosis without therapy ($>500 \times 10^9$/L).[424] Fluctuating levels of endogenous TPO, inversely related to the platelet count, were reported in one case.[425] Each thrombocytopenic cycle typically spans a period of 3 to 6 weeks, and women are more often affected than men. The platelet counts may fluctuate across a wide range. In reported cases, the median nadir and peak platelet counts were $10 \times 10^9$/L (range: 1 to 90 $\times 10^9$/L) and 330 $\times 10^9$/L (range: 72 to 2300 $\times 10^9$/L), respectively.[426] Rebound thrombocytosis is an important and distinctive feature of CTP. Although some cases are reported as associated with myeloproliferative neoplasms, most CTP cases are idiopathic.[427,428] The pathophysiology is unclear, and a number of potential mechanisms have been proposed, including autoimmune platelet destruction, megakaryocytic hypoplasia/aplasia, infections, and hormonal disturbances. Although most premenopausal female CTP patients studied have had low platelet counts during their menstrual periods, hysterectomy with bilateral salpingo-oophorectomy has not been shown to affect the course of the platelet fluctuations.[426]

The clinical presentation of CTP is similar to that of ITP. The bleeding tendency ranges from asymptomatic, to easy bruising, gingival bleeding, recurrent epistaxis, menorrhagia, and hematuria, to more serious bleeding, including gastrointestinal or central nervous system hemorrhage.[426] CTP is rarely considered in the differential diagnosis of thrombocytopenia, so patients are usually diagnosed and treated as having ITP. CTP is a rare disorder, but the diagnosis should be considered in patients with "ITP" who have not responded to therapies such as glucocorticoids, splenectomy, and IVIG and who have rebound thrombocytosis. Responses have been reported with hormone therapy and cyclosporine. In female patients, oral contraceptives may be useful to prolong the menstrual cycle and cover low-platelet-count days. Antifibrinolytic drugs such as aminocaproic acid or tranexamic acid may also be useful to decrease bleeding symptoms.

## ● DRUG-INDUCED THROMBOCYTOPENIA

Development of thrombocytopenia after quinine was first described by Vipan in 1865, and since then, a large number of drugs have been found to cause thrombocytopenia. Drugs should be considered as potentially causative in any thrombocytopenic patient on medication, taking herbal remedies, or using iodinated radiocontrast solutions.[429] Drug-induced thrombocytopenia generally affects only a small percentage of patients taking a particular drug and is usually not severe, although it can be fatal. Genetic and environmental factors both influence susceptibility to drugs. Discontinuation of the causative drug(s) is the main treatment strategy; glucocorticoids may help in some patients. Drugs may cause thrombocytopenia by different mechanisms. Dose-dependent myelosuppression and immune destruction of the platelets are two well-known causes. One of the most severe and life-threatening forms of drug-induced thrombocytopenia is HIT, an immune-mediated disorder caused by antibodies that recognize a neoepitope in platelet factor 4 that is exposed when platelet factor 4 binds heparin. The result is activation of platelets and the coagulation cascade and, ultimately, venous and arterial thrombosis. HIT affects up to 5 percent of patients exposed to therapeutic doses of unfractionated heparin (Chap. 23). This section discusses drugs, other than heparins, that cause isolated thrombocytopenia by immune platelet destruction.

### ETIOLOGY

Reviews of drug-induced thrombocytopenia often contain such extensive lists of implicated drugs, many of which are commonly used, that they are not helpful for decisions regarding which therapy to interrupt first. To address the issue of which drugs most likely cause thrombocytopenia, a systematic review of all published case reports defined levels of evidence to document the causal relation between the drug and thrombocytopenia.[430] This review distinguished drugs with definite or probable causal relationships from those for which the evidence was weaker.[430] Table 7–7 lists the drugs for which there is definite evidence of a causal role in producing thrombocytopenia (which includes recurrent thrombocytopenia with rechallenge in the same patient) and drugs for which the causal relation to thrombocytopenia has been validated by at least two reports with probable evidence (thus meeting all of the criteria for definite evidence except for the lack of rechallenge). Quinidine is by far the most commonly cited drug. Other commonly cited drugs are similar to drugs documented in a case-control study.[431] A remarkable observation from the systematic review was how many case reports did not provide sufficient clinical information to allow a determination of even a probable causal relation.[319]

### PATHOGENESIS

Thrombocytopenia is usually assumed to result from immune platelet destruction by drug-dependent antibodies.[429] Most of these antibodies bind the platelets only in the presence of the offending drugs. Drugs may trigger different immune mechanisms, as depicted in Table 7–8.

Drugs may bind covalently to membrane proteins and may induce hapten-dependent antibodies in patients receiving penicillin and cephalosporin. In quinine-induced thrombocytopenia, antibodies bind to membrane proteins only in the presence of soluble drug. In patients receiving tirofiban or eptifibatide, the drug binds to integrin $\alpha_{IIb}\beta_3$, creating a conformation-dependent neoepitope and inducing antibody production. Gold salts and procainamide, however, may induce true autoantibodies, with those induced by gold being unique in targeting platelet GPV.[432] These antibodies can bind and destroy platelets in the absence of the drug. In HIT, heparin–platelet factor 4 complexes induce autoantibodies.

Initial experimental observations suggested that drug–antibody complexes bind to platelets via the platelet Fc$\gamma$ receptor. This mechanism is confirmed for HIT (see below in this section), but for other drugs, the drug-dependent antibodies appear to bind to platelets via their Fab regions.[433]

The target antigens are the major platelet surface GPs (GPIb–IX–V and integrin $\alpha_{IIb}\beta_3$). Different drugs may provoke drug-dependent antibodies that preferentially react with one of these GPs, or drug-dependent antibodies from a single patient may react with multiple epitopes on both GPs. For example, a study of sera from 15 patients with quinine-induced thrombocytopenia demonstrated that, in the presence of quinine, the antibodies bound to two distinct domains on GPIb-IX, one on GPIb$\alpha$, and one on GPIX. Some patients had only one of the antibodies; some had both.[434] The same domains on GPIb-IX also appear

**TABLE 7–7.** Drugs Causing Thrombocytopenia

CASES: 1

| | | | |
|---|---|---|---|
| Adefovir dipivoxil (1, 0) | Diflunisal (0, 1) | Isotretinoin (0, 1) | Penicillin (0, 1) |
| Alatrofloxacin (0, 1) | Digitoxin (0, 1) | Itraconazole (0, 1) | Pentoxifylline (1, 0) |
| Albendazole (0, 1) | Diltiazem (0, 1) | Lithium (1, 0) | Piperazine (0, 1) |
| Alprenolol (1, 0) | Doxepin (0, 1) | Lopinavir/ritonavir (1, 0) | Primidone (0, 1) |
| Amlodipine (0, 1) | Eflornithine (1, 0) | Losartan (0, 1) | Pyrazinamide (0, 1) |
| Anakinra (0, 1) | Ezetimibe (0, 1) | Mebhydroline (0, 1) | Recombinant hepatitis B |
| Apalcillin (0, 1) | Famotidine (0, 1) | Meloxicam (0, 1) | vaccine (0, 1) |
| Aspirin (0, 1) | Felbamate (0, 1) | Meprobamate (0, 1) | Rifampicin (1, 0) |
| Atorvastatin (1, 0) | Fenoprofen (0, 1) | Mesalamine (1, 0) | Rituximab (1, 0) |
| Bismuth (0, 1) | Feprazone (0, 1) | Methazolamide (0, 1) | Rofecoxib (0, 1) |
| Butoconazole (0, 1) | Finasteride (0, 1) | Mexiletine (0, 1) | Rosiglitazone (0, 1) |
| Cefamandole (0, 1) | Formestane (0, 1) | Minoxidil (1, 0) | Sodium stibogluconate |
| Cephalothin (1, 0) | G-CSF (filgrastim) (0, 1) | Mirtazapine (0, 1) | (0, 1) |
| Chlorpheniramine (0, 1) | Haloperidol (1, 0) | Morphine (0, 1) | Sulfadiazine (0, 1) |
| Chlorpromazine (1, 0) | Inamrinone (1, 0) | Naphazoline (1, 0) | Sulfamethoxazole (0, 1) |
| Ciprofloxacin (0, 1) | Indomethacin (0, 1) | Nimesulide (0, 1) | Sulfathiazole (1, 0) |
| Clarithromycin (0, 1) | Infliximab (0, 1) | Nitroglycerin (1, 0) | Suramin (0, 1) |
| Clopidogrel (0, 1) | Influenza vaccine (0, 1) | Novobiocin (1, 0) | Teicoplanin (1, 0) |
| Deferoxamine (1, 0) | Interferon 2b (0, 1) | Octreotide (1, 0) | Thiothixene (1, 0) |
| Desipramine (0, 1) | Iocetamic acid (0, 1) | Oxcarbazepine (0, 1) | Tiagabine (0, 1) |
| Diazepam (1, 0) | Iopamidol (0, 1) | Oxytetracycline (0, 1) | Tolmetin (1, 0) |
| Diazoxide (1, 0) | Iron dextran (0, 1) | Penicillamine (0, 1) | Tranilast (0, 1) |
| Diethylstilbestrol (1, 0) | Isoniazid (1, 0) | | |

CASES: 2 TO 4

| | | | |
|---|---|---|---|
| Acetazolamide (1, 2) | Etretinate (0, 2) | Naproxen (0, 4) | Sulindac (0, 2) |
| Aminoglutethimide (2, 1) | Fluconazole (0, 2) | Oxaliplatin (0, 2) | Sulfamethoxypyridazine |
| Aminosalicylic acid (2, 1) | Glibenclamide (0, 2) | Oxprenolol (2, 1) | (0, 3) |
| Amphotericin b (2, 1) | Ibuprofen (0, 2) | Oxyphenbutazone (0, 2) | Sulfasalazine (1, 2) |
| Ampicillin (0, 2) | Indinavir (3, 0) | Phenytoin (0, 3) | Tamoxifen (2, 1) |
| Captopril (0, 2) | Interferon (0, 4) | Piperacillin (1, 1) | Terbinafine (0, 2) |
| Chlordiazepoxide (0, 2) | Iopanoic acid (1, 1) | Roxifiban (0, 2) | Ticlopidine (0, 3) |
| Chlorothiazide (1, 3) | Levamisole (2, 0) | Simvastatin (0, 2) | Trastuzumab (0, 2) |
| Digoxin (3, 0) | Meclofenamate (2, 0) | Sulfapyridine (0, 2) | Vancomycin (3, 0) |
| Ethambutol (1, 1) | Methicillin (2, 0) | | |

CASES: 5 TO 10

| | | | |
|---|---|---|---|
| Abciximab c7e3 Fab (1, 6) | Danazol (3, 4) | Hydrochlorothiazide (0, 5) | Procainamide (0, 7) |
| Amiodarone (2, 0) | Diatrizoate meglumine/ | Interferon-α (1, 6) | Ranitidine (0, 5) |
| Acetaminophen (3, 4) | diatrizoate sodium (3, 2) | Lotrafiban (0, 5) | Rifampin (5, 5) |
| Carbamazepine (0, 10) | Diclofenac (2, 3) | Methyldopa (3, 3) | Sulfisoxazole (1, 4) |
| Chlorpropamide (0, 5) | Efalizumab (Raptiva) (0, 6) | Nalidixic acid (1, 5) | Tirofiban (1, 6) |
| Cimetidine (1, 5) | Eptifibatide (0, 7) | | |

CASES: >10

| | | | |
|---|---|---|---|
| Gold (0, 11) | Quinidine (26, 32) | Quinine (14, 9) | Sulfamethoxazole (3, 12) |

G-CSF, granulocyte colony-stimulating factor.

Table of drugs that cause thrombocytopenia supported by one or more patient case reports with level I (definite) or level II (probable) clinical evidence. The table is broken down by the total number of single case reports with the individual number of level I cases and level II reports denoted in parentheses, respectively. The full list of articles reviewed, the methodology for establishing levels of evidence, and a complete updated database are available at www.ouhsc.edu/platelets/.

Data from www.ouhsc.edu/platelets/ditp.html.

**TABLE 7–8.** Mechanisms Underlying Drug-Induced Immune Thrombocytopenia

| Classification | Mechanism | Incidence | Example |
|---|---|---|---|
| Hapten-dependent antibody | Hapten links covalently to membrane protein and induces drug-specific immune response | Very rare | Penicillin, possibly some cephalosporin antibiotics |
| Quinine-type drug | Drug induces antibody that binds to membrane protein in presence of soluble drug | 26 cases per 1 million users of quinine per week; probably fewer cases with other drugs | Quinine, sulfonamide antibiotics, nonsteroidal antiinflammatory drugs |
| Fiban-type drug | Drug reacts with glycoprotein IIb/IIIa to induce a conformational change (neoepitope) recognized by antibody (not yet confirmed) | 0.2–0.5% | Tirofiban, eptifibatide |
| Drug-specific antibody | Antibody recognizes murine component of chimeric Fab fragment specific for platelet membrane glycoprotein IIIa | 0.5–1.0% after first exposure; 10–14% after second exposure | Abciximab |
| Autoantibody | Drug induces antibody that reacts with autologous platelets in absence of drug | 1% with gold; very rare with procainamide and other drugs | Gold salts, procainamide |
| Immune complex | Drug binds to platelet factor 4, producing immune complex for which antibody is specific; immune complex activates platelets through Fc receptors | 3–6% among patients treated with unfractionated heparin for 7 days; rare with low-molecular-weight heparin | Heparins |

Reproduced with permission from Aster RH, Bougie DW. Drug-induced immune thrombocytopenia, *N Engl J Med* 2007 Aug 9;357(6):580–587.

to be the antigenic targets for quinidine- and ranitidine-dependent antiplatelet antibodies.[434,435] Definition of the specific epitope involved in patient reactions with drug-dependent antibodies may not only elucidate the mechanism of drug-induced thrombocytopenia but also identify polymorphisms in GPIb-IX that cause sensitivity in producing drug-dependent antiplatelet antibodies. Sulfonamides, quinidine, and quinine are frequent causes of drug-induced thrombocytopenia. Studies of sera from 15 patients with thrombocytopenia caused by sulfamethoxazole or sulfisoxazole demonstrated that the antigenic epitope was part of integrin $\alpha_{IIb}\beta_3$.[436] Some antibodies from patients with quinidine- and quinine-dependent antiplatelet antibodies also react with integrin $\alpha_{IIb}\beta_3$.[437]

In addition to specificity for discrete epitopes on platelet surface GPs, drug-dependent antibodies are highly specific for the structure of the drug. For example, no cross-reactivity occurs between quinidine and quinine-dependent antibodies or between sulfamethoxazole and sulfisoxazole-dependent antibodies, even though both pairs of drugs have similar structures. Therefore, the neoantigens produced by drug binding to platelets create discrete epitopes that are sensitive to minor changes in drug structure.

The implications of this mechanism for platelet destruction are apparent. A patient with prior sensitivity to the drug has preformed antibodies that immediately react with the altered platelets upon repeat drug exposure, as demonstrated. An exception to this situation is the immediate acute thrombocytopenia that may occur with initial administration of antithrombotic agents that bind platelet integrin $\alpha_{IIb}\beta_3$,[42,438] especially abciximab. Abciximab is a humanized monoclonal antibody fragment that lacks the Fc domain, so thrombocytopenia is not caused by phagocytosis of the platelets by macrophages. Patients experiencing thrombocytopenia after receiving integrin $\alpha_{IIb}\beta_3$ inhibitors have been postulated to have preformed antibodies to epitopes exposed on the integrin by drug binding. These could be the same antibodies that cause *in vitro* EDTA-dependent platelet agglutination and pseudothrombocytopenia [see "Pseudo (Spurious) Thrombocytopenia" above].[33,439,440]

## DIAGNOSIS

The diagnosis of drug-induced thrombocytopenia can be made only by recovery from thrombocytopenia upon discontinuation of the drug and can be confirmed if thrombocytopenia recurs with rechallenge by

the drug. Prompt recovery within 5 to 7 days is usual.[430] Gold-induced thrombocytopenia is an exception because gold salts are retained for long periods of time within the body and thrombocytopenia can persist for months, becoming indistinguishable from ITP.[441] Rechallenge with a suspected drug is dangerous, because severe thrombocytopenia can develop rapidly with even very small drug doses. However, when multiple drugs are potentially involved and all are important for management, it may be appropriate to reintroduce them individually, followed by several days of close observation. In general, the smallest possible dose of the drug should be administered. The administration should be performed under direct supervision of the patient, with platelets available for bleeding should it occur. If rechallenge leads to thrombocytopenia, the patient should be advised to wear a Medic Alert bracelet. For common drugs, especially those that can be purchased without a prescription, it may be safer to supervise a rechallenge and unequivocally document risk rather than risk future unintentional use.

Laboratory assays can detect drug-dependent antibodies, and positive results can support a clinical diagnosis. However, the laboratory role remains largely investigational because results are not promptly available when a clinical decision must be made about discontinuing a drug. Furthermore, no laboratory test has been validated that supports continuing a suspected drug with no adverse effects following a negative laboratory test.

Drug-dependent antibodies can be detected by flow cytometric techniques,[436] MAIPA,[442] and solid-phase red cell adherence assays.[443] Strongly positive tests are apparent, but distinction of positive from negative tests is arbitrary and not yet clinically validated. Positive tests for heparin-dependent antibodies have been reported in patients without thrombocytopenia,[444-446] and patients with clinical evidence for drug-induced thrombocytopenia may have negative tests using multiple techniques.[436,447]

## CLINICAL AND LABORATORY FEATURES

In patients with newly discovered thrombocytopenia, all medications should be identified. Not only should the history explore use of prescription medications, but also use of nonprescription drugs should be queried, including products containing acetaminophen,[430] and drinks that may contain quinine ("tonic water").[448,449] Drug-induced thrombocytopenia is typically severe. Among the 247 case reports with evidence for a definite or probable causal relation of the drug to thrombocytopenia, 23 patients (9 percent) had major bleeding, including two patients who died of bleeding,[430] and 68 patients (28 percent) had overt but minor bleeding; 96 patients (39 percent) had only purpura or trivial bleeding, and the remainder had no bleeding.[430] The time from beginning the drug to the initial occurrence of thrombocytopenia varies from 1 day to 3 years, but the median time is 14 days. With rechallenge, acute thrombocytopenia may occur within minutes but almost always within 3 days.[430] Patients may have other signs and symptoms of drug sensitivity, such as nausea and vomiting, rash, fever, and abnormal liver function tests.[450] Laboratory data may demonstrate leukopenia, indicating that the drug-dependent antibodies target multiple cell types.[450] Patients who have systemic adverse reactions to drugs manifesting as TTP or HUS are described in Chap. 23.

## TREATMENT

Withdrawal of the offending drug is the most important therapeutic measure. Prednisone is commonly given because the distinction of drug-induced thrombocytopenia from ITP is almost never clear initially; however, glucocorticoids do not appear to speed recovery.[450] In patients with major bleeding, emergency treatment should be the same as for ITP: platelet transfusions, high doses of parenteral methylprednisolone, and possibly IVIG.[319]

## REFERENCES

1. Morrell CN, Aggrey AA, Chapman LM, Modjesks KL: Emerging roles for platelets as immune and inflammatory cells. *Blood* 123:2759–2767, 2014.
2. Kaushansky K: Historical review: Megakaryopoiesis and thrombopoiesis. *Blood* 111:981–986, 2008.
3. Brubaker DB, Marcus C, Holmes E: Intravascular and total body platelet equilibrium in healthy volunteers and in thrombocytopenic patients transfused with single donor platelets. *Am J Hematol* 58:165–176, 1998.
4. Hill-Zobel RL, McCandless B, Kang SA, et al: Organ distribution and fate of human platelets: Studies of asplenic and splenomegalic patients. *Am J Hematol* 23:231–238, 1986.
5. Heyns AD, Lotter MG, Badenhorst PN, et al: Kinetics, distribution and sites of destruction of 111indium-labelled human platelets. *Br J Haematol* 44:269–280, 1980.
6. Heyns AD, Lotter MG, Badenhorst PN, et al: Kinetics and sites of destruction of 111Indium-oxine-labeled platelets in idiopathic thrombocytopenic purpura: A quantitative study. *Am J Hematol* 12:167–177, 1982.
7. Leissinger CA: Platelet kinetics in immune thrombocytopenic purpura and human immunodeficiency virus thrombocytopenia. *Curr Opin Hematol* 8:299–305, 2001.
8. Hanson SR, Slichter SJ: Platelet kinetics in patients with bone marrow hypoplasia: Evidence for a fixed platelet requirement. *Blood* 66:1105–1109, 1985.
9. Pearse BM: Receptors compete for adaptors found in plasma membrane coated pits. *EMBO J* 7:3331–3336, 1988.
10. Kile BT: The role of apoptosis in megakaryocytes and platelets. *Br J Haematol* 165:217–226, 2015.
11. Bain BJ: Ethnic and sex differences in the total and differential white cell count and platelet count. *J Clin Pathol* 49:664–666, 1996.
12. Lozano M, Narvaez J, Faundez A: Platelet count and mean platelet volume in the Spanish population. *Med Clin (Barc)* 110:774–777, 1998.
13. Stasi R, Amadori S, Osborn J, et al: Long-term outcome of otherwise healthy individuals with incidentally discovered borderline thrombocytopenia. *PLoS Med* 3:e24, 2006.
14. Buckley MF, James JW, Brown DE: A novel approach to the assessment of variations in human platelet count. *Thromb Haemost* 83:480–484, 2000.
15. Buttarello M, Plebani M: Automated blood cell counts: State of the art. *Am J Clin Pathol* 130:104–116, 2008.
16. Segal HC, Briggs C, Kunka S: Accuracy of platelet counting haematology analysers in severe thrombocytopenia and potential impact on platelet transfusion. *Br J Haematol* 128:520–525, 2005.
17. Salignac S, Latger-Cannard V, Schlegel N, Lecompte TP: Platelet. *Methods Mol Biol* 992:193–205, 2013.
18. Yoneyama A, Nakahara K: [EDTA-dependent pseudothrombocytopenia—Differentiation from true thrombocytopenia] [in Japanese]. *Nihon Rinsho* 61:569–574, 2003.
19. García Suárez J, Merino JL, Rodriguez M, et al: [Pseudothrombocytopenia: Incidence, causes and methods of detection] [in Spanish]. *Sangre (Barc)* 36:197–200, 1991.
20. Payne BA, Pierre RV: Pseudothrombocytopenia: A laboratory artifact with potentially serious consequences. *Mayo Clin Proc* 59:123–125, 1984.
21. Savage RA: Pseudoleukocytosis due to EDTA-induced platelet clumping. *Am J Clin Pathol* 81:317–322, 1984.
22. Vicari A, Banfi G, Bonini PA: EDTA-dependent pseudothrombocytopaenia: A 12-month epidemiological study. *Scand J Clin Lab Invest* 48:537–542, 1988.
23. Sweeney JD, Holme S, Heaton WA, et al: Pseudothrombocytopenia in plateletpheresis donors. *Transfusion* 35:46–49, 1995.
24. Bartels PC, Schoorl M, Lombarts AJ: Screening for EDTA-dependent deviations in platelet counts and abnormalities in platelet distribution histograms in pseudothrombocytopenia. *Scand J Clin Lab Invest* 57:629–636, 1997.
25. Bragagni G, Bianconcini G, Brogna R, Zoli G: [Pseudothrombocytopenia: Clinical comment on 37 cases] [in Italian]. *Minerva Med* 92:13–17, 2001.
26. Kurata Y, Hayashi S, Jouzaki K, et al: [Four cases of pseudothrombocytopenia due to platelet cold agglutinins] [in Japanese]. *Rinsho Ketsueki* 47:781–786, 2006.
27. Reed BW, Go RS: Pseudothrombocytopenia associated with multiple myeloma. *Mayo Clin Proc* 81:869, 2006.
28. Campbell V, Fosbury E, Bain BJ: Platelet phagocytosis as a cause of pseudothrombocytopenia. *Am J Hematol* 84:362, 2009.
29. Onder O, Weinstein A, Hoyer LW: Pseudothrombocytopenia caused by platelet agglutinins that are reactive in blood anticoagulated with chelating agents. *Blood* 56:177–182, 1980.
30. Bizzaro N: EDTA-dependent pseudothrombocytopenia: A clinical and epidemiological study of 112 cases, with 10-year follow-up. *Am J Hematol* 50:103–109, 1995.
31. Hoyt RH, Durie BG: Pseudothrombocytopenia induced by a monoclonal IgM kappa platelet agglutinin. *Am J Hematol* 31:50–52, 1989.
32. Bizzaro N, Goldschmeding R, von dem Borne AE: Platelet satellitism is Fc gamma RIII (CD16) receptor-mediated. *Am J Clin Pathol* 103:740–744, 1995.
33. Casonato A, Bertomoro A, Pontara E, et al: EDTA dependent pseudothrombocytopenia caused by antibodies against the cytoadhesive receptor of platelet gpIIB-IIIA. *J Clin Pathol* 47:625–630, 1994.
34. Nomura S, Nagata H, Oda K, et al: Effects of EDTA on the membrane glycoproteins IIb-IIIa complex—Analysis using flow cytometry. *Thromb Res* 47:47–58, 1987.
35. Schrezenmeier H, Muller H, Gunsilius E, et al: Anticoagulant-induced pseudothrombocytopenia and pseudoleucocytosis. *Thromb Haemost* 73:506–513, 1995.
36. Ryo R, Sugano W, Goto M, et al: Platelet release reaction during EDTA-induced platelet agglutinations and inhibition of EDTA-induced platelet agglutination by anti-glycoprotein II b/III a complex monoclonal antibody. *Thromb Res* 74:265–272, 1994.
37. Cohen AM, Lewinski UH, Klein B, Djaldetti M: Satellitism of platelets to monocytes. *Acta Haematol* 64:61–64, 1980.
38. Djaldetti M, Fishman P: Satellitism of platelets to monocytes in a patient with hypogammaglobulinaemia. *Scand J Haematol* 21:305–308, 1978.
39. Schell DA, Ganti AK, Levitt R, Potti A: Thrombocytopenia associated with c7E3 Fab (abciximab). *Ann Hematol* 81:76–79, 2002.
40. Sane DC, Damaraju LV, Topol EJ, et al: Occurrence and clinical significance of pseudothrombocytopenia during abciximab therapy. *J Am Coll Cardiol* 36:75–83, 2000.
41. Peters MN, Press CD, Moscona JC: Acute profound thrombocytopenia secondary to local abciximab infusion. *Proc (Bayl Univ Med Cent)* 25:346–348, 2012.
42. Berkowitz SD, Sane DC, Sigmon KN, et al: Occurrence and clinical significance of thrombocytopenia in a population undergoing high-risk percutaneous coronary revascularization. Evaluation of c7E3 for the Prevention of Ischemic Complications (EPIC) Study Group. *J Am Coll Cardiol* 32:311–319, 1998.
43. Berkman N, Michaeli Y, Or R, Eldor A: EDTA-dependent pseudothrombocytopenia: A clinical study of 18 patients and a review of the literature. *Am J Hematol* 36:195–201, 1991.
44. Mori M, Kudo H, Yoshitake S, et al: Transient EDTA-dependent pseudothrombocytopenia in a patient with sepsis. *Intensive Care Med* 26:218–220, 2000.
45. Bizzaro N, Fiorin F: Coexistence of erythrocyte agglutination and EDTA-dependent platelet clumping in a patient with thymoma and plasmocytoma. *Arch Pathol Lab Med* 123:159–162, 1999.
46. Matarazzo M, Conturso V, Di MM, et al: EDTA-dependent pseudothrombocytopenia in a case of liver cirrhosis. *Panminerva Med* 42:155–157, 2000.
47. Recommended methods for radioisotope platelet survival studies: By the panel on Diagnostic Application of Radioisotopes in Hematology, International Committee for Standardization in Hematology. *Blood* 50:1137–1144, 1977.
48. Chiurazzi F, Villa MR, Rotoli B: Transplacental transmission of EDTA-dependent pseudothrombocytopenia. *Haematologica* 84:664, 1999.
49. Kortering JJ, Boersma B, Schoorl M, et al: Pseudothrombocytopenia in a neonate due to mother? *Eur J Pediatr* 172:987–989, 2013.
50. Solanki DL, Blackburn BC: Spurious thrombocytopenia during pregnancy. *Obstet Gynecol* 65:14S–17S, 1985.
51. Diz-Kucukkaya R: Inherited platelet disorders including Glanzmann thrombasthenia and Bernard-Soulier syndrome. *Hematology Am Soc Hematol Educ Program* 2013:275, 2013.
52. Bunimov N, Fuller N, Hayward CP: Genetic loci associated with platelet traits and platelet disorders. *Semin Thromb Hemost* 39:291–305, 2013.
53. Watson SP, Lowe GC, Lordkipanidze M, Morgan NY: Genotyping and phenotyping of platelet function disorders. *J Thromb Haemost* 2013:351–363, 2013.
54. Diz-Kucukkaya R, López JA: Inherited disorders of platelets: Membrane glycoprotein disorders. *Hematol Oncol Clin North Am* 27:613–627, 2013.
55. Gresele P: Diagnosis of inherited platelet function disorders: Guidance from the SSC of the ISTH. *J Thromb Haemost* 13:314–322, 2015.

56. Balduini CL, Pecci A, Noris P: Diagnosis and management of inherited thrombocy-topenias. *Semin Thromb Hemost* 39:161–171, 2015.

57. Harrison P, Mackie I, Mumford A, et al: Guidelines for the laboratory investigation of heritable disorders of platelet function. *Br J Haematol* 155:30–44, 2011.

58. Sandoval C, Berger E, Ozkaynak MF: Severe iron deficiency anemia in forty-two pediatric patients. *Pediatr Hematol Oncol* 19:157–161, 2002.

59. Kadikoylu G, Yavasoglu I, Bolaman Z, Senturk T: Platelet parameters in women with iron deficiency anemia. *J Natl Med Assoc* 98:398–402, 2006.

60. Stabler SP, Allen RH, Savage DG, Lindenbaum J: Clinical spectrum and diagnosis of cobalamin deficiency. *Blood* 76:871–881, 1990.

61. Sarode R, Garewal G, Marwaha N, et al: Pancytopenia in nutritional megaloblastic anaemia. A study from north-west India. *Trop Geogr Med* 41:331–336, 1989.

62. Slichter SJ, Harker LA: Thrombocytopenia: Mechanisms and management of defects in platelet production. *Clin Haematol* 7:523–539, 1978.

63. Epstein RD: Cells of the megakaryocyte series in pernicious anemia; in particular, the effect of specific therapy. *Am J Pathol* 25:239–251, 1949.

64. Rabinowitz AP, Sacks Y, Carmel R: Autoimmune cytopenias in pernicious anemia: A report of four cases and review of the literature. *Eur J Haematol* 44:18–23, 1990.

65. Junca J, Flores A, Granada ML, et al: The relationship between idiopathic thrombocy-topenic purpura and pernicious anaemia. *Br J Haematol* 111:513–516, 2000.

66. Dittmar M, Kahaly GJ: Polyglandular autoimmune syndromes: Immunogenetics and long-term follow-up. *J Clin Endocrinol Metab* 88:2983–2992, 2003.

67. Ingeberg S, Stoffersen E: Platelet dysfunction in patients with vitamin B$_{12}$ deficiency. *Acta Haematol* 61:75–79, 1979.

68. Terade H, Niikura H, Mori H, et al: [Megaloblastic anemia and platelet function—a qualitative platelet defect in pernicious anemia] [in Japanese]. *Rinsho Ketsueki* 31:254–255, 1990.

69. Green P: Anemias beyond B$_{12}$ and iron deficiency: The buzz about other B's elementary, and nonelementary problems. *Hematology Am Soc Hematol Educ Program* 2012:498, 2012.

70. Agnotti LB, Post GR, Robinson NS, et al: Pancytopenia with myelodysplasia due to copper deficiency. *Pediatr Blood Cancer* 51:693–695, 2008.

71. Ballard HS: The hematological complications of alcoholism. *Alcohol Health Res World* 21:45–52, 2015.

72. Haselager EM, Vreeken J: Rebound thrombocytosis after alcohol abuse: A possible factor in the pathogenesis of thromboembolic disease. *Lancet* 1:774–775, 1977.

73. Ballard HS: The hematological complications of alcoholism. *Alcohol Health Res World* 21:42–52, 2015.

74. Michot F, Gut J: Alcohol-induced bone marrow damage. A bone marrow study in alcohol-dependent individuals. *Acta Haematol* 78:252–257, 1987.

75. Latvala J, Parkkila S, Niemela O: Excess alcohol consumption is common in patients with cytopenia: Studies in blood and bone marrow cells. *Alcohol Clin Exp Res* 28:619–624, 2004.

76. Sullivan LW, Adams WH, Liu YK: Induction of thrombocytopenia by thrombopheresis in man: Patterns of recovery in normal subjects during ethanol ingestion and abstinence. *Blood* 49:197–207, 1977.

77. Smith CM, Tobin JD Jr, Burris SM, White JG: Alcohol consumption in the guinea pig is associated with reduced megakaryocyte deformability and platelet size. *J Lab Clin Med* 120:699–706, 1992.

78. Wolber EM, Jelkmann W: Thrombopoietin: The novel hepatic hormone. *News Physiol Sci* 17:6–10, 2002.

79. Hoffman R: Acquired pure amegakaryocytic thrombocytopenic purpura. *Semin Hematol* 28:303–312, 1991.

80. Antonijevic N, Terzic T, Jovanovic V, et al: [Acquired amegakaryocytic thrombocytopenia: Three case reports and a literature review] [in Serbian]. *Med Pregl* 57:292–297, 2004.

81. Dewulf G, Gouin I, Pautas E, et al: [Myelodisplasic syndromes diagnosed in a geriatric hospital: Morphological profile in 100 patients]. *Ann Biol Clin (Paris)* 62:197–202, 2004.

82. Rochant H: [Myelodysplastic syndromes: Unusual and mild forms] [in French]. *Pathol Biol (Paris)* 45:579–586, 1997.

83. Kini J, Khadilkar UN, Dayal JP: A study of the haematologic spectrum of myelodysplastic syndrome. *Indian J Pathol Microbiol* 44:9–12, 2001.

84. Nand S, Godwin JE: Hypoplastic myelodysplastic syndrome. *Cancer* 62:958–964, 1988.

85. Zafar T, Yasin F, Anwar M, Saleem M: Acquired amegakaryocytic thrombocytopenic purpura (AATP): A hospital based study. *J Pak Med Assoc* 49:114–117, 1999.

86. Nagasawa T, Sakurai T, Kashiwagi H, Abe T: Cell-mediated amegakaryocytic thrombo-cytopenia associated with systemic lupus erythematosus. *Blood* 67:479–483, 1986.

87. Slater LM, Katz J, Walter B, Armentrout SA: Aplastic anemia occurring as amegakaryo-cytic thrombocytopenia with and without an inhibitor of granulopoiesis. *Am J Hematol* 18:251–254, 1985.

88. Shiozaki H, Miyawaki S, Kuwaki T, et al: Autoantibodies neutralizing thrombopoietin in a patient with amegakaryocytic thrombocytopenic purpura. *Blood* 95:2187–2188, 2000.

89. Katsumata Y, Suzuki T, Kuwana M, et al: Anti-c-Mpl (thrombopoietin receptor) autoantibody-induced amegakaryocytic thrombocytopenia in a patient with systemic sclerosis. *Arthritis Rheum* 48:1647–1651, 2003.

90. Leach JW, Hussein KK, George JN: Acquired pure megakaryocytic aplasia report of two cases with long-term responses to antithymocyte globulin and cyclosporine. *Am J Hematol* 62:115–117, 1999.

91. Lusher JM, Iyer R: Idiopathic thrombocytopenic purpura in children. *Semin Thromb Hemost* 3:175–199, 1977.

92. Stasi R, Newland AC: ITP: A historical perspective. *Br J Haematol* 153:450, 2011.

93. Frank E: Die essentielle thrombopenie (konstitutionelle purpura-pseudoha mophilie). *Berl Klin Wochenschr* 52:454, 1915.

94. Dameshek W, Miller EB: The megakaryocytes in idiopathic thrombocytopenic purpura, a form of hypersplenism. *Blood* 1:27–50, 1946.

95. Harrington WJ, Minnich V, Hollingsworth JW, Moore CV: Demonstration of a throm-bocytopenic factor in the blood of patients with thrombocytopenic purpura. *J Lab Clin Med* 38:1–10, 1951.

96. Altman LK: Black and blue at the flick of a feather, in *Who Goes First?*, pp 273–282. Random House, New York, 1987.

97. Shulman NR, Weinrach RS, Libre EP, Andrews HL: The role of the reticuloendothelial system in the pathogenesis of idiopathic thrombocytopenic purpura. *Trans Assoc Am Physicians* 78:374–390, 1965.

98. McMillan R, Smith RS, Longmire RL, et al: Immunoglobulins associated with human platelets. *Blood* 37:316–322, 1971.

99. Dixon R, Rosse W, Ebbert L: Quantitative determination of antibody in idiopathic thrombocytopenic purpura. Correlation of serum and platelet-bound antibody with clinical response. *N Engl J Med* 292:230–236, 1975.

100. van Leeuwen EF, van der Ven JT, Engelfriet CP, von dem Borne AE: Specificity of auto-antibodies in autoimmune thrombocytopenia. *Blood* 59:23–26, 1982.

101. McMillan R, Tani P, Millard F, et al: Platelet-associated and plasma anti-glycoprotein autoantibodies in chronic ITP. *Blood* 70:1040–1045, 1987.

102. Kiefel V, Santoso S, Weisheit M, Mueller-Eckhardt C: Monoclonal antibody–specific immobilization of platelet antigens (MAIPA): A new tool for the identification of platelet-reactive antibodies. *Blood* 70:1722–1726, 1987.

103. Kiefel V, Santoso S, Kaufmann E, Mueller-Eckhardt C: Autoantibodies against platelet glycoprotein Ib/IX: A frequent finding in autoimmune thrombocytopenic purpura. *Br J Haematol* 79:256–262, 1991.

104. He R, Reid DM, Jones CE, Shulman NR: Spectrum of Ig classes, specificities, and titers of serum antiglycoproteins in chronic idiopathic thrombocytopenic purpura. *Blood* 83:1024–1032, 1994.

105. Mueller-Eckhardt C, Mueller-Eckhardt G, Kayser W, et al: Platelet associated IgG, platelet survival, and platelet sequestration in thrombocytopenic states. *Br J Haematol* 52:49–58, 1982.

106. Kelton JG, Powers PJ, Carter CJ: A prospective study of the usefulness of the mea-surement of platelet-associated IgG for the diagnosis of idiopathic thrombocytopenic purpura. *Blood* 60:1050–1053, 1982.

107. McMillan R: Autoantibodies and autoantigens in chronic immune thrombocytopenic purpura. *Semin Hematol* 37:239–248, 2000.

108. Cines DB, Blanchette VS: Immune thrombocytopenic purpura. *N Engl J Med* 346:995–1008, 2002.

109. Imbach P, Barandun S, d'Apuzzo V, et al: High-dose intravenous gammaglobulin for idiopathic thrombocytopenic purpura in childhood. *Lancet* 1:1228–1231, 1981.

110. Hymes K, Schur PH, Karpatkin S: Heavy-chain subclass of round antiplatelet IgG in autoimmune thrombocytopenic purpura. *Blood* 56:84–87, 1980.

111. van der HD, de Jong D, Limpens J, et al: Clonal B-cell populations in patients with idiopathic thrombocytopenic purpura. *Blood* 76:2321–2326, 1990.

112. Maguire RB, Stroncek DF, Campbell AC: Recurrent pancytopenia, coagulopathy, and renal failure associated with multiple quinine-dependent antibodies. *Ann Intern Med* 119:215–217, 1993.

113. Liu B, Zhao H, Poon MD: Abnormality of CD4(+)CD25(+) regulatory T cells in idiopathic thrombocytopenic purpura. *Eur J Haematol* 78:139–143, 2007.

114. Stasi R, Pagano A, Stipa E, Amadori S: Rituximab chimeric anti-CD20 monoclonal antibody treatment for adults with chronic idiopathic thrombocytopenic purpura. *Blood* 98:952–957, 2001.

115. McKenzie CG, Guo L, Freedman J, Semple JW: Cellular immune dysfunction in immune thrombocytopenia (ITP). *Br J Haematol* 163:10–23, 2013.

116. Zhang F, Chu X, Wang L, et al: Cell-mediated lysis of autologous platelets in chronic idiopathic thrombocytopenic purpura. *Eur J Haematol* 76:427–431, 2006.

117. Li S, Wang L, Zhao C, et al: CD8+ T cells suppress autologous megakaryocyte apoptosis in idiopathic thrombocytopenic purpura. *Br J Haematol* 139:605–611, 2007.

118. Hauch TW, Rosse WF: Platelet-bound complement (C3) in immune thrombocytopenia. *Blood* 50:1129–1136, 1977.

119. Kurata Y, Curd JG, Tamerius JD, McMillan R: Platelet-associated complement in chronic ITP. *Br J Haematol* 60:723–733, 1985.

120. Tsubakio T, Tani P, Curd JG, McMillan R: Complement activation in vitro by antiplatelet antibodies in chronic immune thrombocytopenic purpura. *Br J Haematol* 63:293–300, 1986.

121. Verschoor A, Langer HF: Crosstalk between platelets and the complement system in immune protection and disease. *Thromb Haemost* 110:910–919, 2013.

122. Aster RH, Keene WR: Sites of platelet destruction in idiopathic thrombocytopenic purpura. *Br J Haematol* 16:61–73, 1969.

123. Ballem PJ, Segal GM, Stratton JR, et al: Mechanisms of thrombocytopenia in chronic autoimmune thrombocytopenic purpura. Evidence of both impaired platelet production and increased platelet clearance. *J Clin Invest* 80:33–40, 1987.

124. Chang M, Nakagawa PA, Williams SA, et al: Immune thrombocytopenic purpura (ITP) plasma and purified ITP monoclonal autoantibodies inhibit megakaryocytopoiesis in vitro. *Blood* 102:887–895, 2003.

125. Takahashi R, Sekine N, Nakatake T: Influence of monoclonal antiplatelet glycoprotein antibodies on *in vitro* human megakaryocyte colony formation and proplatelet formation. *Blood* 93:1951–1958, 1999.

126. Kelemen E, Cserhati I, Tanos B: Demonstration and some properties of human thrombopoietin in thrombocythaemic sera. *Acta Haematol* 20:350–355, 1958.

127. Kuter DJ: Milestones in understanding platelet production: A historical overview. *Br J Haematol* 165:248–258, 2015.

128. Kaushansky K: Thrombopoietin: The primary regulator of megakaryocyte and platelet production. *Thromb Haemost* 74:521–525, 1995.

129. Chang M, Qian JX, Lee SM, et al: Tissue uptake of circulating thrombopoietin is increased in immune-mediated compared with irradiated thrombocytopenic mice. *Blood* 93:2515–2524, 1999.

130. Kosugi S, Kurata Y, Tomiyama Y, et al: Circulating thrombopoietin level in chronic immune thrombocytopenic purpura. *Br J Haematol* 93:704–706, 1996.

131. Kuter DJ: Thrombopoietin and thrombopoietin mimetics in the treatment of thrombocytopenia. *Annu Rev Med* 60:193–206, 2009.

132. Porcelijn L, Folman CC, Bossers B, et al: The diagnostic value of thrombopoietin level measurements in thrombocytopenia. *Thromb Haemost* 79:1101–1105, 1998.

133. Gouin-Thibault I, Cassinat B, Chomienne C, et al: Is the thrombopoietin assay useful for differential diagnosis of thrombocytopenia? Analysis of a cohort of 160 patients with thrombocytopenia and defined platelet life span. *Clin Chem* 47:1660–1665, 2001.

134. Kuter DJ, Bussel JB, Lyons RM, et al: Efficacy of romiplostim in patients with chronic immune thrombocytopenia: A double-blind randomised controlled trial. *Lancet* 371:395–403, 2008.

135. Psaila B, Bussel JB: Refractory immune thrombocytopenic purpura: Current strategies for investigation and management. *Br J Haematol* 143:16–26, 2008.

136. Bussel JB, Kuter DJ, Aledort LM: A randomized trial of avatrombopag, an investigational thrombopoietin-receptor agonist, in persistent and chronic immune thrombocytopenia. *Blood* 123:3887–3897, 2014.

137. Laster AJ, Conley CL, Kickler TS, et al: Chronic immune thrombocytopenic purpura in monozygotic twins: Genetic factors predisposing to ITP. *N Engl J Med* 307:1495–1498, 1982.

138. Bizzaro N: Familial association of autoimmune thrombocytopenia and hyperthyroidism. *Am J Hematol* 39:294–298, 1992.

139. Karpatkin S, Fotino M, Winchester R: Hereditary autoimmune thrombocytopenic purpura: An immunologic and genetic study. *Ann Intern Med* 94:781–782, 1981.

140. Stanworth SJ, Turner DM, Brown J, et al: Major histocompatibility complex susceptibility genes and immune thrombocytopenic purpura in Caucasian adults. *Hematology* 7:119–121, 2002.

141. Evers KG, Thouet R, Haase W, Kruger J: HLA frequencies and haplotypes in children with idiopathic thrombocytopenic purpura (ITP). *Eur J Pediatr* 129:267–272, 1978.

142. Pavkovic M, Georgievski B, Cevreska L, et al: CTLA-4 exon 1 polymorphism in patients with autoimmune blood disorders. *Am J Hematol* 72:147–149, 2003.

143. Foster CB, Zhu S, Erichsen HC, et al: Polymorphisms in inflammatory cytokines and Fcgamma receptors in childhood chronic immune thrombocytopenic purpura: A pilot study. *Br J Haematol* 113:596–599, 2001.

144. George JN, Woolf SH, Raskob GE, et al: Idiopathic thrombocytopenic purpura: A practice guideline developed by explicit methods for the American Society of Hematology. *Blood* 88:3–40, 1996.

145. Guidelines for the investigation and management of idiopathic thrombocytopenic purpura in adults, children and in pregnancy. *Br J Haematol* 120:574–596, 2003.

146. Rodeghiero F, Stasi R, Gernsheimer T, et al: Standardization of terminology, definitions and outcome criteria in immune thrombocytopenic purpura of adults and children: Report from an international working group. *Blood* 113:2386–2393, 2009.

147. Provan D, Stasi R, Newland AC, et al: International consensus report on the investigation and management of primary immune thrombocytopenia. *Blood* 115:168–186, 2010.

148. Neunert C, Lim W, Crowther M, et al: The American Society of Hematology 2011 evidence-based practice guideline for immune thrombocytopenia. *Blood* 117:4190–4207, 2011.

149. Schoonen WM, Kucera G, Coalson J, et al: Epidemiology of immune thrombocytopenic purpura in the General Practice Research Database. *Br J Haematol* 145:235–244, 2009.

150. Cortelazzo S, Finazzi G, Buelli M, et al: High risk of severe bleeding in aged patients with chronic idiopathic thrombocytopenic purpura. *Blood* 77:31–33, 1991.

151. Frederiksen H, Schmidt K: The incidence of idiopathic thrombocytopenic purpura in adults increases with age. *Blood* 94:909–913, 1999.

152. George JN, el-Harake MA, Raskob GE: Chronic idiopathic thrombocytopenic purpura. *N Engl J Med* 331:1207–1211, 1994.

153. McMillan R: Therapy for adults with refractory chronic immune thrombocytopenic purpura. *Ann Intern Med* 126:307–314, 1997.

154. Schattner E, Bussel J: Mortality in immune thrombocytopenic purpura: Report of seven cases and consideration of prognostic indicators. *Am J Hematol* 46:120–126, 1994.

155. Portielje JE, Ewstentdorp RG, Kluin-Nelemans HC: Morbidity and mortality in adults with idiopathic thrombocytopenic purpura. *Blood* 97:2549–2554, 2001.

156. McIntyre OR, Ebaugh FG Jr: Palpable spleens in college freshmen. *Ann Intern Med* 66:301–306, 1967.

157. Newton JL, Reese JA, Watson SI, et al: Fatigue in adult patients with primary immune thrombocytopenia. *Eur J Haematol* 86:420–429, 2011.

158. Blankenship JC, Tasissa G, O'Shea JC, et al: Effect of glycoprotein IIb/IIIa receptor inhibition on angiographic complications during percutaneous coronary intervention in the ESPRIT trial. *J Am Coll Cardiol* 38:653–658, 2001.

159. Sarpatwari A, Bennett D, Logie JW, et al: Thromboembolic events among adult patients with primary immune thrombocytopenia in the United Kingdom General Practice Research Database. *Haematologica* 95:1167–1175, 2010.

160. Ruggeri M, Tosetto A, Palandri F, et al: Thrombotic risk in patients with primary immune thrombocytopenia is only mildly increased and explained by personal and treatment-related risk factors. *J Thromb Haemost* 12:1266–1273, 2014.

161. Burstein SA, Downs T, Friese P, et al: Thrombocytopoiesis in normal and sublethally irradiated dogs: Response to human interleukin-6. *Blood* 80:420–428, 1992.

162. Khan I, Zucker-Franklin D, Karpatkin S: Microthrombocytosis and platelet fragmentation associated with idiopathic/autoimmune thrombocytopenic purpura. *Br J Haematol* 31:449–460, 1975.

163. Lopez JA, Andrews RK, Afshar-Kharghan V, Berndt MC: Bernard-Soulier syndrome. *Blood* 91:4397–4418, 1998.

164. Rodgers RP, Levin J: A critical reappraisal of the bleeding time. *Semin Thromb Hemost* 16:1–20, 1990.

165. Hughes M, Webert K, Kelton JG: The use of electron microscopy in the investigation of the ultrastructural morphology of immune thrombocytopenic purpura platelets. *Semin Hematol* 37:222–228, 2000.

166. Evans RS, Takahashi K, Duane RT, et al: Primary thrombocytopenic purpura and acquired hemolytic anemia; evidence for a common etiology. *Arch Intern Med* 87:48–65, 1951.

167. Stasi R, Stipa E, Masi M, et al: Long-term observation of 208 adults with chronic idiopathic thrombocytopenic purpura. *Am J Med* 98:436–442, 1995.

168. Sailer T, Lechner K, Panzer S, et al: The course of severe autoimmune thrombocytopenia in patients not undergoing splenectomy. *Haematologica* 91:1041–1045, 2006.

169. George JN, Raskob GE: Idiopathic thrombocytopenic purpura: Diagnosis and management. *Am J Med Sci* 316:87–93, 1998.

170. Baumann MA, Menitove JE, Aster RH, Anderson T: Urgent treatment of idiopathic thrombocytopenic purpura with single-dose gammaglobulin infusion followed by platelet transfusion. *Ann Intern Med* 104:808–809, 1986.

171. Larsen OH, Stentoft J, Radia D, et al: Combination of recombinant factor VIIa and fibrinogen corrects clot formation in primary immune thrombocytopenia at very low platelet counts. *Br J Haematol* 160:228–236, 2013.

172. Salama A, Rieke M, Kiesewetter H, von Depka H: Experiences with recombinant FVIIa in the emergency treatment of patients with autoimmune thrombocytopenia: A review of the literature. *Ann Hematol* 88:11–15, 2009.

173. Wanachiwanawin W, Piankijagum A, Sindhvananda K, et al: Emergency splenectomy in adult idiopathic thrombocytopenic purpura. A report of seven cases. *Arch Intern Med* 149:217–219, 1989.

174. Gernsheimer T, Stratton J, Ballem PJ, Slichter SJ: Mechanisms of response to treatment in autoimmune thrombocytopenic purpura. *N Engl J Med* 320:974–980, 1989.

175. Bussel JB: Fc receptor blockade and immune thrombocytopenic purpura. *Semin Hematol* 37:261–266, 2000.

176. Kitchens CS: Amelioration of endothelial abnormalities by prednisone in experimental thrombocytopenia in the rabbit. *J Clin Invest* 60:1129–1134, 1977.

177. George JN, Woolf SH, Raskob GE: Idiopathic thrombocytopenic purpura: A guideline for diagnosis and management of children and adults. American Society of Hematology. *Ann Med* 30:38–44, 1998.

178. George JN, Vesely SK: Immune thrombocytopenic purpura—Let the treatment fit the patient. *N Engl J Med* 349:903–905, 2003.

179. Mazzucconi MG, Francesconi M, Fidani P, et al: Treatment of idiopathic thrombocytopenic purpura (ITP): Results of a multicentric protocol. *Haematologica* 70:329–336, 1985.

180. Bellucci S, Charpak Y, Chastang C, Tobelem G: Low doses v conventional doses of corticoids in immune thrombocytopenic purpura (ITP): Results of a randomized clinical trial in 160 children, 223 adults. *Blood* 71:1165–1169, 1988.

181. Ozsoylu S, Irken G, Karabent A: High-dose intravenous methylprednisolone for acute childhood idiopathic thrombocytopenic purpura. *Eur J Haematol* 42:431–435, 1989.

182. Ozsoylu S, Sayli TR, Ozturk G: Oral megadose methylprednisolone versus intravenous immunoglobulin for acute childhood idiopathic thrombocytopenic purpura. *Pediatr Hematol Oncol* 10:317–321, 1993.

183. Albayrak D, Islek I, Kalayci AG, Gurses N: Acute immune thrombocytopenic purpura: A comparative study of very high oral doses of methylprednisolone and intravenously administered immune globulin. *J Pediatr* 125:1004–1007, 1994.

184. Cheng Y, Wong RS, Soo YO, et al: Initial treatment of immune thrombocytopenic purpura with high-dose dexamethasone. *N Engl J Med* 349:831–836, 2003.

185. Stasi R, Brunetti M, Pagano A: Pulsed intravenous high-dose dexamethasone in adults with chronic idiopathic thrombocytopenic purpura. *Blood Cells Mol Dis* 26:582–586, 2000.

186. Mazzucconi MG, Fazi P, Bernasconi S: Therapy with high dose dexamethasone (HD-DXM) in previously untreated patients affected by idiopathic thrombocytopenic purpura: A GIMEMA experience. *Blood* 109:1401–1407, 2007.

187. Alpdogan O, Budak-Alpdogan T, Ratip S: Efficacy of high-dose methylprednisolone as a first-line therapy in adult patients with idiopathic thrombocytopenic purpura. *Br J Haematol* 103:1061–1063, 1998.

188. Bell WR Jr: Long-term outcome of splenectomy for idiopathic thrombocytopenic purpura. *Semin Hematol* 37:22–25, 2000.

189. Kojouri K, Vesely SK, Terrell DR, George JN: Splenectomy for adult patients with idiopathic thrombocytopenic purpura: A systemic review to assess long-term platelet count responses, prediction of response, and surgical complications. *Blood* 104:2623–2635, 2004.

190. Mikhael J, Northridge K, Lindquist K, et al: Short-term and long-term failure of laparoscopic splenectomy in adult immune thrombocytopenic purpura patients: A systematic review. *Am J Hematol* 84:743–748, 2009.

191. Ghanima W, Godeau B, Cines DB, Bussel JB: How I treat immune thrombocytopenia: The choice between splenectomy or a medical therapy as a second-line treatment. *Blood* 120:960–969, 2012.

192. Najean Y, Rain JD, Billotey C: The site of destruction of autologous 111In-labelled platelets and the efficiency of splenectomy in children and adults with idiopathic thrombocytopenic purpura: A study of 578 patients with 268 splenectomies. *Br J Haematol* 97:547–550, 1997.

193. Pizzuto J, Ambriz R: Therapeutic experience on 934 adults with idiopathic thrombocytopenic purpura: Multicentric Trial of the Cooperative Latin American group on Hemostasis and Thrombosis. *Blood* 64:1179–1183, 1984.

194. Dolan JP, Sheppard BC, DeLoughery TG: Splenectomy for immune thrombocytopenic purpura: Surgery for the 21st century. *Am J Hematol* 83:93–96, 2007.

195. Lortan JE: Management of asplenic patients. *Br J Haematol* 84:566–569, 1993.

196. Atkinson WL, Pickering LK, Schwartz B, et al: General recommendations on immunization. Recommendations of the Advisory Committee on Immunization Practices (ACIP) and the American Academy of Family Physicians (AAFP). *MMWR Recomm Rep* 51:1–35, 2002.

197. Boyle S, White RH, Brunson A, Wun T: Splenectomy and the incidence of venous thromboembolism and sepsis in patients with immune thrombocytopenia. *Blood* 121:4782–4790, 2015.

198. Naouri A, Feghali B, Chabal J: Results for splenectomy for idiopathic thrombocytopenic purpura. *Acta Haematol* 89:200–203, 1993.

199. Newland AC, Treleaven JG, Minchinton RM, Waters AH: High-dose intravenous IgG in adults with autoimmune thrombocytopenia. *Lancet* 15:84–87, 1983.

200. Berchtold P, Dale GL, Tani P, McMillan R: Inhibition of autoantibody binding to platelet glycoprotein IIb/IIIa by anti-idiotypic antibodies in intravenous gammaglobulin. *Blood* 74:2414–2417, 1989.

201. Ramamurthi A, Lewis RS: Design of a novel apparatus to study nitric oxide (NO) inhibition of platelet adhesion. *Ann Biomed Eng* 26:1036–1043, 1998.

202. Imbach P: 30 Years of immunomodulation by intravenous immunoglobulin. *Immunotherapy* 4:651–654, 2015.

203. Bussel JB, Pham LC, Aledort L, Nachman R: Maintenance treatment of adults with chronic refractory immune thrombocytopenic purpura using repeated intravenous infusions of gammaglobulin. *Blood* 72:121–127, 1988.

204. Hong F, Ruiz R, Price H, et al: Safety profile of WinRho anti-D. *Semin Hematol* 35:9–13, 1998.

205. Ware RE, Zimmerman SA: Anti-D: Mechanisms of action. *Semin Hematol* 35:14–22, 1998.

206. Crow AR, Lazarus AH: The mechanisms of action of intravenous immunoglobulin and polyclonal anti-d immunoglobulin in the amelioration of immune thrombocytopenic purpura: What do we really know? *Transfus Med Rev* 22:103–116, 2008.

207. Despotovic J, Lambert MP, Herman J: RhIg for the treatment of immuno thrombocytopenia: Consensus and controversy. *Transfusion* 52:1126–1136, 2012.

208. Scaradavou A, Woo B, Woloski BM, et al: Intravenous anti-D treatment of immune thrombocytopenic purpura: Experience in 272 patients. *Blood* 89:2689–2700, 1997.

209. George JN, Raskob GE, Vesely SK, et al: Initial management of immune thrombocytopenic purpura in adults: A randomized controlled trial comparing intermittent anti-D with routine care. *Am J Hematol* 74:161–169, 2003.

210. Johnson GJ: Platelet thromboxane receptors: Biology and function, in *Handbook of Platelet Physiology and Pharmacology*, edited by G Rao, pp 38–79. Kluwer Academic, Boston, 1999.

211. Waintraub SE, Brody JI: Use of anti-D in immune thrombocytopenic purpura as a means to prevent splenectomy: Case reports from two University Hospital Medical Centers. *Semin Hematol* 37:45–49, 2000.

212. Marcus AJ: Transcellular metabolism of eicosanoids. *Prog Hemost Thromb* 8:127–142, 1986.

213. Narang M, Penner JA, Williams D: Refractory autoimmune thrombocytopenic purpura: Responses to treatment with a recombinant antibody to lymphocyte membrane antigen CD20 (rituximab). *Am J Hematol* 74:263–267, 2003.

214. Cooper N, Stasi R, Cunningham-Rundles S, et al: The efficacy and safety of B-cell depletion with anti-CD20 monoclonal antibody in adults with chronic immune thrombocytopenic purpura. *Br J Haematol* 125:232–239, 2004.

215. Arnold DM, Dentali F, Crowther MA, et al: Systematic review: Efficacy and safety of rituximab for adults with idiopathic thrombocytopenic purpura. *Ann Intern Med* 146:25–33, 2007.

216. Garvey B: Rituximab in the treatment of autoimmune haematological disorders. *Br J Haematol* 141:149–169, 2008.

217. Stasi R: Rituximab in autoimmune hematologic disease: Not just a matter of B cells. *Semin Hematol* 47:170–179, 2010.

218. Zaja F, Battista ML, Pirrotta MT: Lower dose rituximab is active in adult patients with idiopathic thrombocytopenic purpura. *Haematologica* 93:930–933, 2008.

219. Godeau B: B-cell depletion in immunothrombocytopenia. *Semin Hematol* 50:S75–S82, 2013.

220. Hasan A, Michel M, Patel V: Repeated courses of rituximab in chronic ITP: Three different regimens. *Am J Hematol* 84:661–665, 2010.

221. Cooper N, Stasi R, Cunningham-Rundles S: Platelet-associated antibodies, cellular immunity and FCGR3a genotype influence the response to rituximab in immune thrombocytopenia. *Br J Haematol* 158:539–547, 2012.

222. Mahevas M, Patin P, Huetz F: B cell deletion in immunothrombocytopenia reveals splenic long-lived plasma cells. *J Clin Invest* 123:432–442, 2013.

223. Tsutsumi Y, Yamamoto Y, Shimono J, et al: Hepatitis B virus reactivation with rituximab-containing regimen. *World J Hepatol* 5:612–620, 2013.

224. Siegal D, Crowther M, Cuker A: Thrombopoietin receptor agonists in primary ITP. *Semin Hematol* 50:S21, 2013.

225. Kuter DJ: The biology of thrombopoietin and thrombopoietin receptor agonists. *Int J Hematol* 98:10–23, 2013.

226. Kuter DJ, Bussel JB, Newland AC: Long-term treatment with romiplostim in patients with chronic immunothrombocytopenia: Safety and efficacy. *Br J Haematol* 161:411–423, 2013.

227. Erhardt JA, Erickson-Miller CL, Aivado M, et al: Comparative analyses of the small molecule thrombopoietin receptor agonist eltrombopag and thrombopoietin on in vitro platelet function. *Exp Hematol* 37:1030–1037, 2009.

228. Tomiyama Y, Miyakawa Y, Okamoto S: A lower dose of eltrombopag is efficacious in Japanese patients with previously treated chronic immune thrombocytopenia. *J Thromb Haemost* 10:799–806, 2012.

229. Saleh MN, Bussel JB, Cheng G: Safety and efficacy of eltrombopag for the treatment of chronic immunothrombocytopenia: Result of the long-term, open label EXTEND study. *Blood* 121:537–545, 2013.

230. Bussel JB, Saleh MN, Vasey SY, et al: Repeated short-term use of eltrombopag in patients with chronic immune thrombocytopenia (ITP). *Br J Haematol* 160:538–546, 2013.

231. Columbyova L, Loda M, Scadden DT: Thrombopoietin receptor expression in human cancer cell lines and primary tissues. *Cancer Res* 55:3509–3512, 1995.

232. Giagounidis A, Mufti GJ, Fenaux P: Results of a randomized, double-blind study of romiplostim versus placebo in patients with low/intermediate-1-risk myelodysplastic syndrome and thrombocytopenia. *Cancer* 120:1835–1846, 2014.

233. Quiquandon I, Fenaux P, Caulier MT, et al: Re-evaluation of the role of azathioprine in the treatment of adult chronic idiopathic thrombocytopenic purpura: A report on 53 cases. *Br J Haematol* 74:223–228, 1990.

234. Blanchette V, Freedman J, Garvey B: Management of chronic immune thrombocytopenic purpura in children and adults. *Semin Hematol* 35:36–51, 1998.

235. Verlin M, Laros RK Jr, Penner JA: Treatment of refractory thrombocytopenic purpura with cyclophosphamine. *Am J Hematol* 1:97–104, 1976.

236. Reiner A, Gernsheimer T, Slichter SJ: Pulse cyclophosphamide therapy for refractory autoimmune thrombocytopenic purpura. *Blood* 85:351–358, 1995.

237. Emillia G, Morselli M, Luppi M: Long-term salvage therapy with cyclosporine A in refractory idiopathic thrombocytopenic purpura. *Blood* 99:1482–1485, 2002.

238. Patel AP, Patil AS: Dapsone for immune thrombocytopenic purpura in children and adults. *Platelets* 26:164–167, 2015.

239. Zaja F, Marin L, Chiozzotto M, et al: Dapsone salvage therapy for adults with immune thrombocytopenia relapsed or refractory to steroid and rituximab. *Am J Hematol* 87:321–323, 2012.

240. Ahn YS, Byrnes JJ, Harrington WJ, et al: The treatment of idiopathic thrombocytopenia with vinblastine-loaded platelets. *N Engl J Med* 298:1101–1107, 1978.

241. Jackson CW, Edwards CC: Evidence that stimulation of megakaryocytopoiesis by low dose vincristine results from an effect on platelets. *Br J Haematol* 36:97–105, 1977.

242. Tangun Y, Atamer T: More on vincristine in treatment of ITP. *N Engl J Med* 297:894–895, 1977.

243. Sekreta CM, Baker DE: Interferon alfa therapy in adults with chronic idiopathic thrombocytopenic purpura. *Ann Pharmacother* 30:1176–1179, 1996.

244. Snyder HW Jr, Cochran SK, Balint JP Jr, et al: Experience with protein A-immunoadsorption in treatment-resistant adult immune thrombocytopenic purpura. *Blood* 79:2237–2245, 1992.

245. Emilia G, Messora C, Longo G, Bertesi M: Long-term salvage treatment by cyclosporin in refractory autoimmune haematological disorders. *Br J Haematol* 93:341–344, 1996.

246. Strother SV, Zuckerman KS, LoBuglio AF: Colchicine therapy for refractory idiopathic thrombocytopenic purpura. *Arch Intern Med* 144:2198–2200, 1984.

247. Bussel JB, Saal S, Gordon B: Combined plasma exchange and intravenous gammaglobulin in the treatment of patients with refractory immune thrombocytopenic purpura. *Transfusion* 28:38–41, 1988.

248. Cines DB, Bussel JB, Liebman HA, Luning Prak ET: The ITP syndrome: Pathogenic and clinical diversity. *Blood* 113:6511–6521, 2009.

249. Miyakis S, Lockshin MD, Atsumi T, et al: International consensus statement on an update of the classification criteria for definite antiphospholipid syndrome (APS). *J Thromb Haemost* 4:295–306, 2006.

250. Cervera R, Piette JC, Font J, et al: Antiphospholipid syndrome: Clinical and immunologic manifestations and patterns of disease expression in a cohort of 1,000 patients. *Arthritis Rheum* 46:1019–1027, 2002.

251. Oosting JD, Derksen RH, Bobbink IW, et al: Antiphospholipid antibodies directed against a combination of phospholipids with prothrombin, protein C, or protein S: An explanation for their pathogenic mechanism? *Blood* 81:2618–2625, 1993.

252. D'Cruz D, Hughes G: Antibodies, thrombosis and the endothelium. *Br J Rheumatol* 33:2–4, 1994.

253. Santoro SA: Antiphospholipid antibodies and thrombotic predisposition: Underlying pathogenetic mechanisms. *Blood* 83:2389–2391, 1994.

254. Rand JH, Wu XX: Antibody-mediated interference with annexins in the antiphospholipid syndrome. *Thromb Res* 114:383–389, 2004.

255. Asherson RA, Khamashta MA, Ordi-Ros J, et al: The "primary" antiphospholipid syndrome: Major clinical and serological features. *Medicine (Baltimore)* 68:366–374, 1989.

256. Alarcon-Segovia D, Deleze M, Oria CV, et al: Antiphospholipid antibodies and the anti-phospholipid syndrome in systemic lupus erythematosus. A prospective analysis of 500 consecutive patients. *Medicine (Baltimore)* 68:353–365, 1989.

257. Galli M, Finazzi G, Barbui T: Thrombocytopenia in the antiphospholipid syndrome. *Br J Haematol* 93:1–5, 1996.

258. Cuadrado MJ, Mujic F, Munoz E, et al: Thrombocytopenia in the antiphospholipid syndrome. *Ann Rheum Dis* 56:194–196, 1997.

259. Uthman I, Godeau B, Taher A, Khamashta M: The hematologic manifestations of the antiphospholipid syndrome. *Blood Rev* 22:187–194, 2008.

260. Harris EN: Antiphospholipid antibodies. *Br J Haematol* 74:1–9, 1990.

261. Wilson WA, Gharavi AE, Koike T, et al: International consensus statement on preliminary classification criteria for definite antiphospholipid syndrome: Report of an international workshop. *Arthritis Rheum* 42:1309–1311, 1999.

262. Diz-Kucukkaya R, Hacihanefioglu A, Yenerel M, et al: Antiphospholipid antibodies and antiphospholipid syndrome in patients presenting with immune thrombocytopenic purpura: A prospective cohort study. *Blood* 98:1760–1764, 2001.

263. Galli M, Daldossi M, Barbui T: Anti-glycoprotein Ib/IX and IIb/IIIa antibodies in patients with antiphospholipid antibodies. *Thromb Haemost* 71:571–575, 1994.

264. Lipp E, von Felten A, Sax H, et al: Antibodies against platelet glycoproteins and antiphospholipid antibodies in autoimmune thrombocytopenia. *Eur J Haematol* 60:283–288, 1998.

265. Stasi R, Stipa E, Masi M, et al: Prevalence and clinical significance of elevated anti-phospholipid antibodies in patients with idiopathic thrombocytopenic purpura. *Blood* 84:4203–4208, 1994.

266. Fabris F, Steffan A, Cordiano I, et al: Specific antiplatelet autoantibodies in patients with antiphospholipid antibodies and thrombocytopenia. *Eur J Haematol* 53:232–236, 1994.

267. Nakamura M, Tanaka Y, Satoh T, et al: Autoantibody to CD40 ligand in systemic lupus erythematosus: Association with thrombocytopenia but not thromboembolism. *Rheumatology (Oxford)* 45:150–156, 2006.

268. Thrombosis and thrombocytopenia in antiphospholipid syndrome (idiopathic and secondary to SLE): First report from the Italian Registry. Italian Registry of Antiphospholipid Antibodies (IR-APA). *Haematologica* 78:313–318, 1993.

269. Bernini JC, Buchanan GR, Ashcraft J: Hypoprothrombinemia and severe hemorrhage associated with a lupus anticoagulant. *J Pediatr* 123:937–939, 1993.

270. Font J, Jimenez S, Cervera R, et al: Splenectomy for refractory Evans' syndrome associated with antiphospholipid antibodies: Report of two cases. *Ann Rheum Dis* 59:920–923, 2000.

271. Hakim AJ, Machin SJ, Isenberg DA: Autoimmune thrombocytopenia in primary antiphospholipid syndrome and systemic lupus erythematosus: The response to splenectomy. *Semin Arthritis Rheum* 28:20–25, 1998.

272. Ames PR, Tommasino C, Fossati G, et al: Limited effect of rituximab on thrombocytopaenia and anticardiolipin antibodies in a patient with primary antiphospholipid syndrome. *Ann Hematol* 86:227–228, 2007.

273. Ahn ER, Lander G, Bidot CJ, et al: Long-term remission from life-threatening hypercoagulable state associated with lupus anticoagulant (LA) following rituximab therapy. *Am J Hematol* 78:127–129, 2005.

274. Kumar D, Roubey RA: Use of rituximab in the antiphospholipid syndrome. *Curr Rheumatol Rep* 12:40–44, 2010.

275. Sperati CL, Streiff MB: Acute renal failure in a patient with antiphospholipid syndrome and immune thrombocytopenic purpura treated with eltrombopag. *Am J Hematol* 85:724–726, 2010.

276. Jansen AJ, Swart RM, te Boekhorst PA: Thrombopoietin receptor agonists for immune thrombocytopenia. *N Engl J Med* 365:2240–2241, 2011.

277. Tan EM, Cohen AS, Fries JF, et al: The 1982 revised criteria for the classification of systemic lupus erythematosus. *Arthritis Rheum* 25:1271–1277, 1982.

278. Hochberg MC: Updating the American College of Rheumatology revised criteria for the classification of systemic lupus erythematosus. *Arthritis Rheum* 40:1725, 1997.

279. Rabinowitz Y, Dameshek W: Systemic lupus erythematosus after "idiopathic" thrombocytopenic purpura: A review. *Ann Intern Med* 52:1–28, 1960.

280. Michel M, Lee K, Piette JC, et al: Platelet autoantibodies and lupus-associated thrombocytopenia. *Br J Haematol* 119:354–358, 2002.

281. Pujol M, Ribera A, Vilardell M, et al: High prevalence of platelet autoantibodies in patients with systemic lupus erythematosus. *Br J Haematol* 89:137–141, 1995.

282. McMillan R: Immune thrombocytopenia. *Clin Haematol* 12:69–88, 1983.

283. Macchi L, Rispal P, Clofent-Sanchez G, et al: Anti-platelet antibodies in patients with systemic lupus erythematosus and the primary antiphospholipid antibody syndrome: Their relationship with the observed thrombocytopenia. *Br J Haematol* 98:336–341, 1997.

284. Griner PF, Hoyer LW: Amegakaryocytic thrombocytopenia in systemic lupus erythematosus. *Arch Intern Med* 125:328–332, 1970.

285. Fureder W, Firbas U, Nichol JL, et al: Serum thrombopoietin levels and anti-thrombopoietin antibodies in systemic lupus erythematosus. *Lupus* 11:221–226, 2002.

286. Kuwana M, Okazaki Y, Kajihara M, et al: Autoantibody to c-Mpl (thrombopoietin receptor) in systemic lupus erythematosus: Relationship to thrombocytopenia with megakaryocytic hypoplasia. *Arthritis Rheum* 46:2148–2159, 2002.

287. Feinglass EJ, Arnett FC, Dorsch CA, et al: Neuropsychiatric manifestations of systemic lupus erythematosus: Diagnosis, clinical spectrum, and relationship to other features of the disease. *Medicine (Baltimore)* 55:323–339, 1976.

288. Miller MH, Urowitz MB, Gladman DD: The significance of thrombocytopenia in systemic lupus erythematosus. *Arthritis Rheum* 26:1181–1186, 1983.

289. Mok CC, Lee KW, Ho CT, et al: A prospective study of survival and prognostic indicators of systemic lupus erythematosus in a southern Chinese population. *Rheumatology (Oxford)* 39:399–406, 2000.

290. Drenkard C, Villa AR, Alarcon-Segovia D, Perez-Vazquez ME: Influence of the antiphospholipid syndrome in the survival of patients with systemic lupus erythematosus. *J Rheumatol* 21:1067–1072, 1994.

291. Reveille JD, Bartolucci A, Alarcon GS: Prognosis in systemic lupus erythematosus. Negative impact of increasing age at onset, black race, and thrombocytopenia, as well as causes of death. *Arthritis Rheum* 33:37–48, 1990.

292. Abu-Shakra M, Urowitz MB, Gladman DD, Gough J: Mortality studies in systemic lupus erythematosus. Results from a single center. II. Predictor variables for mortality. *J Rheumatol* 22:1265–1270, 1995.

293. Scofield RH, Bruner GR, Kelly JA, et al: Thrombocytopenia identifies a severe familial phenotype of systemic lupus erythematosus and reveals genetic linkages at 1q22 and 11p13. *Blood* 101:992–997, 2003.

294. Boumpas DT, Austin HA, III, Fessler BJ, et al: Systemic lupus erythematosus: Emerging concepts. Part 1: Renal, neuropsychiatric, cardiovascular, pulmonary, and hematologic disease. *Ann Intern Med* 122:940–950, 1995.

295. Arnal C, Piette JC, Leone J, et al: Treatment of severe immune thrombocytopenia associated with systemic lupus erythematosus: 59 cases. *J Rheumatol* 29:75–83, 2002.

296. Boumpas DT, Barez S, Klippel JH, Balow JE: Intermittent cyclophosphamide for the treatment of autoimmune thrombocytopenia in systemic lupus erythematosus. *Ann Intern Med* 112:674–677, 1990.

297. Roach BA, Hutchinson GJ: Treatment of refractory, systemic lupus erythematosus-associated thrombocytopenia with intermittent low-dose intravenous cyclophosphamide. *Arthritis Rheum* 36:682–684, 1993.

298. Maier WP, Gordon DS, Howard RF, et al: Intravenous immunoglobulin therapy in systemic lupus erythematosus-associated thrombocytopenia. *Arthritis Rheum* 33:1233–1239, 1990.

299. Cohen MG, Li EK: Limited effects of intravenous IgG in treating systemic lupus erythematosus-associated thrombocytopenia. *Arthritis Rheum* 34:787–788, 1991.

300. Ding C, Foote S, Jones G: B-cell-targeted therapy for systemic lupus erythematosus: An update. *BioDrugs* 22:239–249, 2008.

301. Jovancevic B, Lindholm C, Pullerits R: Anti-B cell therapy against refractory thrombocytopenia in SLE and MCTD patients: Long-term follow up and review of the literature. *Lupus* 22:664–674, 2013.

302. Zhou J, Wu Z, Zhou Z, et al: Efficacy and safety of laparoscopic splenectomy in thrombocytopenia secondary to systemic lupus erythematosus. *Clin Rheumatol* 32:1131–1138, 2013.

303. Delgado AJ, Inanc M, Diz-Kucukkaya R, et al: Thrombocytopenic risk in patients submitted to splenectomy for systemic lupus erythematosus and antiphospholipid syndrome-related thrombocytopenia. *Eur J Intern Med* 15:162–167, 2004.

304. Ciernik IF, Cone RW, Fehr J, Weber R: Impaired liver function and retroviral activity are risk factors contributing to HIV-associated thrombocytopenia. Swiss HIV Cohort Study. *AIDS* 13:1913–1920, 1999.

305. Dominguez A, Gamallo G, Garcia R, et al: Pathophysiology of HIV related thrombocytopenia: An analysis of 41 patients. *J Clin Pathol* 47:999–1003, 1994.

306. Louache F, Vainchenker W: Thrombocytopenia in HIV infection. *Curr Opin Hematol* 1:369–372, 1994.

307. Brook MG, Ayles H, Harrison C, et al: Diagnostic utility of bone marrow sampling in HIV positive patients. *Genitourin Med* 73:117–121, 1997.

308. WHO Global Alert and Response. 2015. http://www.who.int/csr/disease/hepatitis/whocdscsrlyo2003/en/index1.html.

309. Stasi R: Therapeutic strategies for hepatitis- and other infection-related immune thrombocytopenias. *Semin Hematol* 46:S15–S25, 2001.

310. Calvaruso V, Craxi A: Immunological alterations in hepatitis C virus infection. *World J Gastroenterol* 19:8916–8923, 2013.

311. Hamaia S, Allain JP: The dynamics of hepatitis C virus binding to platelets and 2 mononuclear cell lines. *Blood* 98:2293–2300, 2001.

312. Cuker A: Toxicities of the thrombopoietic growth factors. *Semin Hematol* 47:289–298, 2010.

313. Jackson S, Beck PL, Pineo GF, Poon MC: *Helicobacter pylori* eradication: Novel therapy for immune thrombocytopenic purpura? A review of the literature. *Am J Hematol* 78:142–150, 2005.

314. Franchini M, Cruciani M, Mengoli C, et al: Effect of *Helicobacter pylori* eradication on platelet count in idiopathic thrombocytopenic purpura: A systematic review and meta-analysis. *J Antimicrob Chemother* 60:237–246, 2007.

315. Arnold DM, Bernotas A, Nazi I, et al: Platelet count response to *H. pylori* treatment in patients with immune thrombocytopenic purpura with and without *H. pylori* infection: A systematic review. *Haematologica* 94:850–856, 2009.

316. Burrows RF, Kelton JG: Incidentally detected thrombocytopenia in healthy mothers and their infants. *N Engl J Med* 319:142–145, 1988.

317. Letsky EA, Greaves M: Guidelines on the investigation and management of thrombocytopenia in pregnancy and neonatal alloimmune thrombocytopenia. Maternal and Neonatal Haemostasis Working Party of the Haemostasis and Thrombosis Task Force of the British Society for Haematology. *Br J Haematol* 95:21–26, 1996.

318. Gernsheimer T, James AH, Stasi R: How I treat thrombocytopenia in pregnancy. *Blood* 121:38–47, 2013.

319. George JN, Saucerman S: Platelet IgG, IgA, IgM, and albumin: Correlation of platelet and plasma concentrations in normal subjects and in patients with ITP or dysproteinemia. *Blood* 72:362–365, 1988.

320. Burrows RF, Kelton JG: Fetal thrombocytopenia and its relation to maternal thrombocytopenia. *N Engl J Med* 329:1463–1466, 1993.

321. McCrae KR, Samuels P, Schreiber AD: Pregnancy-associated thrombocytopenia: Pathogenesis and management. *Blood* 80:2697–2714, 1992.

322. Bussel JB: Immune thrombocytopenia in pregnancy: Autoimmune and alloimmune. *J Reprod Immunol* 37:35–61, 1997.

323. Shehata N, Burrows R, Kelton JG: Gestational thrombocytopenia. *Clin Obstet Gynecol* 42:327–334, 1999.

324. Kaplan C, Forestier F, Dreyfus M, et al: Maternal thrombocytopenia during pregnancy: Diagnosis and etiology. *Semin Thromb Hemost* 21:85–94, 1995.

325. Boehlen F, Hohlfeld P, Extermann P, et al: Platelet count at term pregnancy: A reappraisal of the threshold. *Obstet Gynecol* 95:29–33, 2000.

326. Ostensen M, Forger F: How safe are anti-rheumatic drugs during pregnancy. *Curr Opin Pharmacol* 13:470–475, 2015.

327. Chakravarty EF, Murray ER, Kelman A, Farmer P: Pregnancy outcomes after maternal exposure to rituximab. *Blood* 117:1499–1506, 2011.

328. Cheng G: Eltrombopag a thrombopoietin-receptor agonist in the treatment of adult chronic immune thrombocytopenia: A review of the efficacy and safety profile. *Ther Adv Hematol* 3:155–164, 2012.

329. al-Mofada SM, Osman ME, Kides E, et al: Risk of thrombocytopenia in the infants of mothers with idiopathic thrombocytopenia. *Am J Perinatol* 11:423–426, 1994.

330. Gill KK, Kelton JG: Management of idiopathic thrombocytopenic purpura in pregnancy. *Semin Hematol* 37:275–289, 2000.

331. Webert KE, Mittal R, Sigouin C, et al: A retrospective 11-year analysis of obstetric patients with idiopathic thrombocytopenic purpura. *Blood* 102:4306–4311, 2003.

332. Stamilio DM, Macones GA: Selection of delivery method in pregnancies complicated by autoimmune thrombocytopenia: A decision analysis. *Obstet Gynecol* 94:41–47, 1999.

333. Christiaens GC, Nieuwenhuis HK, Bussel JB: Comparison of platelet counts in first and second newborns of mothers with immune thrombocytopenic purpura. *Obstet Gynecol* 90:546–552, 1997.

334. Moise KJ Jr, Cotton DB: Discordant fetal platelet counts in a twin gestation complicated by idiopathic thrombocytopenic purpura. *Am J Obstet Gynecol* 156:1141–1142, 1987.

335. Mushambi MC, Halligan AW, Williamson K: Recent developments in the pathophysiology and management of pre-eclampsia. *Br J Anaesth* 76:133–148, 1996.

336. Leitch CR, Cameron AD, Walker JJ: The changing pattern of eclampsia over a 60-year period. *Br J Obstet Gynaecol* 104:917–922, 1997.

337. Thomas SV: Neurological aspects of eclampsia. *J Neurol Sci* 155:37–43, 1998.

338. Silver RM, Branch DW, Scott JR: Maternal thrombocytopenia in pregnancy: Time for a reassessment. *Am J Obstet Gynecol* 173:479–482, 1995.

339. McCrae KR: Thrombocytopenia in pregnancy: Differential diagnosis, pathogenesis, and management. *Blood Rev* 17:7–14, 2003.

340. Schlembach D: Pre-eclampsia—Still a disease of theories. *Fukushima J Med Sci* 49:69–115, 2003.

341. Brittain PC, Bayliss P: Partial hydatidiform molar pregnancy presenting with severe preeclampsia prior to twenty weeks gestation: A case report and review of the literature. *Mil Med* 160:42–44, 1995.

342. Luttun A, Carmeliet P: Soluble VEGF receptor Flt1: The elusive preeclampsia factor discovered? *J Clin Invest* 111:600–602, 2003.

343. Torry DS, Hinrichs M, Torry RJ: Determinants of placental vascularity. *Am J Reprod Immunol* 51:257–268, 2004.

344. Maynard SE, Min JY, Merchan J, et al: Excess placental soluble fms-like tyrosine kinase 1 (sFlt1) may contribute to endothelial dysfunction, hypertension, and proteinuria in preeclampsia. *J Clin Invest* 111:649–658, 2003.

345. Vuorela P, Helske S, Hornig C, et al: Amniotic fluid—Soluble vascular endothelial growth factor receptor-1 in preeclampsia. *Obstet Gynecol* 95:353–357, 2000.

346. Zhou Y, McMaster M, Woo K, et al: Vascular endothelial growth factor ligands and receptors that regulate human cytotrophoblast survival are dysregulated in severe preeclampsia and hemolysis, elevated liver enzymes, and low platelets syndrome. *Am J Pathol* 160:1405–1423, 2002.

347. Venkatesha S, Toporsian M, Lam C, et al: Soluble endoglin contributes to the pathogenesis of preeclampsia. *Nat Med* 12:642–649, 2006.

348. Lattuada A, Rossi E, Calzarossa C, et al: Mild to moderate reduction of a von Willebrand factor cleaving protease (ADAMTS-13) in pregnant women with HELLP microangiopathic syndrome. *Haematologica* 88:1029–1034, 2003.

349. Hulstein JJ, van Runnard Heimel PJ, Franx A, et al: Acute activation of the endothelium results in increased levels of active von Willebrand factor in hemolysis, elevated liver enzymes and low platelets (HELLP) syndrome. *J Thromb Haemost* 4:2569–2575, 2006.

350. Abildgaard U, Heimdal K: Pathogenesis of the syndrome of hemolysis, elevated liver enzymes, and low platelet count (HELLP): A review. *Eur J Obstet Gynecol Reprod Biol* 166:117–123, 2013.

351. Egerman RS, Sibai BM: HELLP syndrome. *Clin Obstet Gynecol* 42:381–389, 1999.

352. Hay JE: Liver disease in pregnancy. *Hepatology* 47:1067–1076, 2008.

353. Martin JN Jr, Files JC, Blake PG, et al: Postpartum plasma exchange for atypical preeclampsia-eclampsia as HELLP (hemolysis, elevated liver enzymes, and low platelets) syndrome. *Am J Obstet Gynecol* 172:1107–1125, 1995.

354. Chakravorty S, Roberts I: How I manage neonatal thrombocytopenia. *Br J Haematol* 156:155–162, 2011.

355. Kaplan C: Alloimmune thrombocytopenia of the fetus and the newborn. *Blood Rev* 16:69–72, 2002.

356. Peterson JA, McFarland JG, Curtis BR, Aster RH: Neonatal alloimmune thrombocytopenia: Pathogenesis, diagnosis and management. *Br J Haematol* 161:3–14, 2013.

357. Mueller-Eckhardt C, Kiefel V, Grubert A, et al: 348 Cases of suspected neonatal alloimmune thrombocytopenia. *Lancet* 1:363–366, 1989.

358. Grainger JD, Morrell G, Yates J, Deleacy D: Neonatal alloimmune thrombocytopenia with significant HLA antibodies. *Arch Dis Child Fetal Neonatal Ed* 86:F200–F201, 2002.

359. Chow MP, Sun KJ, Yung CH, et al: Neonatal alloimmune thrombocytopenia due to HLA-A2 antibody. *Acta Haematol* 87:153–155, 1992.

360. Davoren A, McParland P, Crowley J, et al: Antenatal screening for human platelet antigen-1a: Results of a prospective study at a large maternity hospital in Ireland. *BJOG* 110:492–496, 2003.

361. Williamson LM, Hackett G, Rennie J, et al: The natural history of fetomaternal alloimmunization to the platelet-specific antigen HPA-1a (PlA1, Zwa) as determined by antenatal screening. *Blood* 92:2280–2287, 1998.

362. Jolly MC, Letsky EA, Fisk NM: The management of fetal alloimmune thrombocytopenia. *Prenat Diagn* 22:96–98, 2002.

363. Murphy MF, Hambley H, Nicolaides K, Waters AH: Severe fetomaternal alloimmune thrombocytopenia presenting with fetal hydrocephalus. *Prenat Diagn* 16:1152–1155, 1996.

364. Kaplan C, Murphy MF, Kroll H, Waters AH: Feto-maternal alloimmune thrombocytopenia: Antenatal therapy with IvIgG and steroids—More questions than answers. European Working Group on FMAIT. *Br J Haematol* 100:62–65, 1998.

365. Ouwehand WH, Smith G, Ranasinghe E: Management of severe alloimmune thrombocytopenia in the newborn. *Arch Dis Child Fetal Neonatal Ed* 82:F173–F175, 2000.

366. Bertrand G, Kaplan C: How do we treat fetal and neonatal alloimmune thrombocytopenia? *Transfusion* 54:1698–1703, 2014.

367. Le Toriellec E, Chenet C, Kaplan C: Safe fetal platelet genotyping: New developments. *Transfusion* 53:1755–1762, 2013.

368. Porcelijn L, Kanhai HH: Fetal thrombocytopenia. *Curr Opin Obstet Gynecol* 10:117–122, 1998.

369. Weiner E, Zosmer N, Bajoria R, et al: Direct fetal administration of immunoglobulins: Another disappointing therapy in alloimmune thrombocytopenia. *Fetal Diagn Ther* 9:159–164, 1994.

370. Aster RH: Platelet sequestration studies in man. *Br J Haematol* 22:259–263, 1972.

371. Wadenvik H, Denfors I, Kutti J: Splenic blood flow and intrasplenic platelet kinetics in relation to spleen volume. *Br J Haematol* 67:181–185, 1987.

372. Heyns AD, Badenhorst PN, Lotter MG, et al: Kinetics and mobilization from the spleen of indium-111-labeled platelets during platelet apheresis. *Transfusion* 25:215–218, 1985.

373. Lawrence SP, Lezotte DC, Durham JD, et al: Course of thrombocytopenia of chronic liver disease after transjugular intrahepatic portosystemic shunts (TIPS). A retrospective analysis. *Dig Dis Sci* 40:1575–1580, 1995.

374. Peck-Radosavljevic M. Hypersplenism. *Eur J Gastroenterol Hepatol* 13:317–323, 2001.

375. Eichner ER: Splenic function: Normal, too much and too little. *Am J Med* 66:311–320, 1979.

376. Jacob HS: Hypersplenism: Mechanisms and management. *Br J Haematol* 27:1–5, 1974.

377. Cooney DP, Smith BA: The pathophysiology of hypersplenic thrombocytopenia. *Arch Intern Med* 121:332–337, 1968.

378. McCormick PA, Murphy KM: Splenomegaly, hypersplenism and coagulation abnormalities in liver disease. *Bailliers Best Pract Res Clin Gastroenterol* 14:1009–1031, 2000.

379. Sihler KC, Napolitano LM: Massive transfusion: New insights. *Chest* 136:1654–1667, 2009.

380. Hiippala ST, Myllyla GJ, Vahtera EM: Hemostatic factors and replacement of major blood loss with plasma-poor red cell concentrates. *Anesth Analg* 81:360–365, 1995.

381. Leslie SD, Toy PT: Laboratory hemostatic abnormalities in massively transfused patients given red blood cells and crystalloid. *Am J Clin Pathol* 96:770–773, 1991.

382. Hardy JF, de Moerloose P, Samama CM: The coagulopathy of massive transfusion. *Vox Sang* 89:123–127, 2005.

383. Cosgriff N, Moore EE, Sauaia A, et al: Predicting life-threatening coagulopathy in the massively transfused trauma patient: Hypothermia and acidoses revisited. *J Trauma* 42:857–861, 1997.

384. Cinat ME, Wallace WC, Nastanski F, et al: Improved survival following massive transfusion in patients who have undergone trauma. *Arch Surg* 134:964–968, 1999.

385. Villalobos TJ, Adelson E, Riley PA Jr, Crosby WH: A cause of the thrombocytopenia and leukopenia that occur in dogs during deep hypothermia. *J Clin Invest* 37:1–7, 1958.

386. Yau TM, Carson S, Weisel RD, et al: The effect of warm heart surgery on postoperative bleeding. *J Thorac Cardiovasc Surg* 103:1155–1162, 1992.

387. Pina-Cabral JM, Ribeiro-da-Silva A, Almeida-Dias A: Platelet sequestration during hypothermia in dogs treated with sulphinpyrazone and ticlopidine—Reversibility accelerated after intra-abdominal rewarming. *Thromb Haemost* 54:838–841, 1985.

388. Hoffmeister KM, Felbinger TW, Falet H, et al: The clearance mechanism of chilled blood platelets. *Cell* 112:87–97, 2003.

389. Hoffmeister KM, Josefsson EC, Isaac NA, et al: Glycosylation restores survival of chilled blood platelets. *Science* 301:1531–1534, 2003.

390. Reddick RL, Poole BL, Penick GD: Thrombocytopenia of hibernation. Mechanism of induction and recovery. *Lab Invest* 28:270–278, 1973.

391. Chan KM, Beard K: A patient with recurrent hypothermia associated with thrombocytopenia. *Postgrad Med* J 69:227–229, 1993.

392. Enjolras O, Wassef M, Mazoyer E, et al: Infants with Kasabach-Merritt syndrome do not have "true" hemangiomas. *J Pediatr* 130:631–640, 1997.

393. Sarkar M, Mulliken JB, Kozakewich HP, et al: Thrombocytopenic coagulopathy (Kasabach-Merritt phenomenon) is associated with Kaposiform hemangioendothelioma and not with common infantile hemangioma. *Plast Reconstr Surg* 100:1377–1386, 1997.

394. Vin-Christian K, McCalmont TH, Frieden IJ: Kaposiform hemangioendothelioma. An aggressive, locally invasive vascular tumor that can mimic hemangioma of infancy. *Arch Dermatol* 133:1573–1578, 1997.

395. Hall GW: Kasabach-Merritt syndrome: Pathogenesis and management. *Br J Haematol* 112:851–862, 2001.

396. Cooper JG, Edwards SL, Holmes JD: Kaposiform haemangioendothelioma: Case report and review of the literature. *Br J Plast Surg* 55:163–165, 2002.

397. Hoeger PH, Helmke K, Winkler K: Chronic consumption coagulopathy due to an occult splenic haemangioma: Kasabach-Merritt syndrome. *Eur J Pediatr* 154:365–368, 1995.

398. Brasanac D, Janic D, Boricic I, et al: Retroperitoneal kaposiform hemangioendothelioma with tufted angioma-like features in an infant with Kasabach-Merritt syndrome. *Pathol Int* 53:627–631, 2003.

399. Mukhtar IA, Letts M: Hemangioma of the radius associated with Kasabach-Merritt syndrome: Case report and literature review. *J Pediatr Orthop* 24:87–91, 2004.

400. Fukunaga M, Ushigome S, Ishikawa E: Kaposiform haemangioendothelioma associated with Kasabach-Merritt syndrome. *Histopathology* 28:281–284, 1996.

401. Alvarez-Mendoza A, Lourdes TS, Ridaura-Sanz C, Ruiz-Maldonado R: Histopathology of vascular lesions found in Kasabach-Merritt syndrome: Review based on 13 cases. *Pediatr Dev Pathol* 3:556–560, 2000.

402. Jones EW, Orkin M: Tufted angioma (angioblastoma). A benign progressive angioma, not to be confused with Kaposi's sarcoma or low-grade angiosarcoma. *J Am Acad Dermatol* 20:214–225, 1989.

403. Wong SN, Tay YK: Tufted angioma: A report of five cases. *Pediatr Dermatol* 19:388–393, 2002.

404. Mueller BU, Mulliken JB: The infant with a vascular tumor. *Semin Perinatol* 23:332–340, 1999.

405. Mazoyer E, Enjolras O, Laurian C, et al: Coagulation abnormalities associated with extensive venous malformations of the limbs: Differentiation from Kasabach-Merritt syndrome. *Clin Lab Haematol* 24:243–251, 2002.

406. Lyons LL, North PE, Mac-Moune LF, et al: Kaposiform hemangioendothelioma: A study of 33 cases emphasizing its pathologic, immunophenotypic, and biologic uniqueness from juvenile hemangioma. *Am J Surg Pathol* 28:559–568, 2004.

407. Gilon E, Ramot B, Sheba C: Multiple hemangiomata associated with thrombocytopenia: Remarks on the pathogenesis of the thrombocytopenia in this syndrome. *Blood* 14:74–79, 1959.

408. Seo SK, Suh JC, Na GY, et al: Kasabach-Merritt syndrome: Identification of platelet trapping in a tufted angioma by immunohistochemistry technique using monoclonal antibody to CD61. *Pediatr Dermatol* 16:392–394, 1999.

409. Brizel HE, Raccuglia G: Giant hemangioma with thrombocytopenia. Radioisotopic demonstration of platelet sequestration. *Blood* 26:751–764, 1965.

410. Shulkin BL, Argenta LC, Cho KJ, Castle VP: Kasabach-Merritt syndrome: Treatment with epsilon-aminocaproic acid and assessment by indium 111 platelet scintigraphy. *J Pediatr* 117:746–749, 1990.

411. Warrell RP Jr, Kempin SJ, Benua RS, et al: Intratumoral consumption of indium-111 labeled platelets in a patient with hemangiomatosis and intravascular coagulation (Kasabach-Merritt syndrome). *Cancer* 52:2256–2260, 1983.

412. Wananukul S, Nuchprayoon I, Seksarn P: Treatment of Kasabach-Merritt syndrome: A stepwise regimen of prednisolone, dipyridamole, and interferon. *Int J Dermatol* 42:741–748, 2003.

413. MacArthur CJ, Senders CW, Katz J: The use of interferon alfa-2a for life-threatening hemangiomas. *Arch Otolaryngol Head Neck Surg* 121:690–693, 1995.

414. Haisley-Royster C, Enjolras O, Frieden IJ, et al: Kasabach-Merritt phenomenon: A retrospective study of treatment with vincristine. *J Pediatr Hematol Oncol* 24:459–462, 2002.

415. Blei F, Karp N, Rofsky N, et al: Successful multimodal therapy for kaposiform hemangioendothelioma complicated by Kasabach-Merritt phenomenon: Case report and review of the literature. *Pediatr Hematol Oncol* 15:295–305, 1998.

416. Hu B, Lachman R, Phillips J, et al: Kasabach-Merritt syndrome-associated kaposiform hemangioendothelioma successfully treated with cyclophosphamide, vincristine, and actinomycin D. *J Pediatr Hematol Oncol* 20:567–569, 1998.

417. Frevel T, Rabe H, Uckert F, Harms E: Giant cavernous haemangioma with Kasabach-Merritt syndrome: A case report and review. *Eur J Pediatr* 161:243–246, 2002.

418. Atahan IL, Cengiz M, Ozyar E, Gurkaynak M: Radiotherapy in the management of Kasabach-Merritt syndrome: A case report. *Pediatr Hematol Oncol* 18:471–476, 2001.

419. Ogino I, Torikai K, Kobayasi S, et al: Radiation therapy for life- or function-threatening infant hemangioma. *Radiology* 218:834–839, 2001.

420. Billio A, Pescosta N, Rosanelli C, et al: Treatment of Kasabach-Merritt syndrome by embolisation of a giant liver hemangioma. *Am J Hematol* 66:140–141, 2001.

421. Hosono S, Ohno T, Kimoto H, et al: Successful transcutaneous arterial embolization of a giant hemangioma associated with high-output cardiac failure and Kasabach-Merritt syndrome in a neonate: A case report. *J Perinat Med* 27:399–403, 1999.

422. Zukerberg LR, Nickoloff BJ, Weiss SW: Kaposiform hemangioendothelioma of infancy and childhood. An aggressive neoplasm associated with Kasabach-Merritt syndrome and lymphangiomatosis. *Am J Surg Pathol* 17:321–328, 1993.

423. George M, Singhal V, Sharma V, Nopper AJ: Successful surgical excision of a complex vascular lesion in an infant with Kasabach-Merritt syndrome. *Pediatr Dermatol* 19:340–344, 2002.

424. Balduini CL, Stella CC, Rosti V, et al: Acquired cyclic thrombocytopenia-thrombocytosis with periodic defect of platelet function. *Br J Haematol* 85:718–722, 1993.

425. Yujiri T, Tanaka Y, Tanaka M, Tanizawa Y: Fluctuations in thrombopoietin, immature platelet fraction, and glycocalicin levels in a patient with cyclic thrombocytopenia. *Int J Hematol* 90:429–430, 2009.

426. Go RS: Idiopathic cyclic thrombocytopenia. *Blood Rev* 19:53–59, 2005.

427. Steensma DP, Harrison CN, Tefferi A: Hydroxyurea-associated platelet count oscillations in polycythemia vera: A report of four new cases and a review. *Leuk Lymphoma* 42:1243–1253, 2001.

428. Abe Y, Hirase N, Muta K, et al: Adult onset cyclic hematopoiesis in a patient with myelodysplastic syndrome. *Int J Hematol* 71:40–45, 2000.

429. Aster RH, Bougie DW: Drug-induced immune thrombocytopenia. *N Engl J Med* 357:580–587, 2007.

430. George JN, Raskob GE, Shah SR, et al: Drug-induced thrombocytopenia: A systematic review of published case reports. *Ann Intern Med* 129:886–890, 1998.

431. Kaufman DW, Kelly JP, Johannes CB, et al: Acute thrombocytopenic purpura in relation to the use of drugs. *Blood* 82:2714–2718, 1993.

432. Garner SF, Campbell K, Metcalfe P, et al: Glycoprotein V: The predominant target antigen in gold-induced autoimmune thrombocytopenia. *Blood* 100:344–346, 2002.

433. Christie DJ, Mullen PC, Aster RH: Fab-mediated binding of drug-dependent antibodies to platelets in quinidine- and quinine-induced thrombocytopenia. *J Clin Invest* 75:310–314, 1985.

434. Lopez JA, Li CQ, Weisman S, Chambers M: The glycoprotein Ib-IX complex-specific monoclonal antibody SZ1 binds to a conformation-sensitive epitope on glycoprotein IX: Implications for the target antigen of quinine/quinidine-dependent autoantibodies. *Blood* 85:1254–1258, 1995.

435. Chong BH, Du XP, Berndt MC, Horn S, Chesterman CN: Characterization of the binding domains on platelet glycoproteins Ib-IX and IIb/IIIa complexes for the quinine/quinidine-dependent antibodies. *Blood* 77:2190–2199, 1991.

436. Curtis BR, McFarland JG, Wu GG, Visentin GP, Aster RH: Antibodies in sulfonamide-induced immune thrombocytopenia recognize calcium-dependent epitopes on the glycoprotein IIb/IIIa complex. *Blood* 84:176–183, 1994.

437. Visentin GP, Newman PJ, Aster RH: Characteristics of quinine- and quinidine-induced antibodies specific for platelet glycoproteins IIb and IIIa. *Blood* 77:2668–2676, 1991.

438. Berkowitz SD, Harrington RA, Rund MM, Tcheng JE: Acute profound thrombocytopenia after C7E3 Fab (abciximab) therapy. *Circulation* 95:809–813, 1997.

439. Fiorin F, Steffan A, Pradella P, et al: IgG platelet antibodies in EDTA-dependent pseudothrombocytopenia bind to platelet membrane glycoprotein IIb. *Am J Clin Pathol* 110:178–183, 1998.

440. Cancio LC, Cohen DJ: Heparin-induced thrombocytopenia and thrombosis. *J Am Coll Surg* 186:76–91, 1998.

441. Coblyn JS, Weinblatt M, Holdsworth D, Glass D: Gold-induced thrombocytopenia. A clinical and immunogenetic study of twenty-three patients. *Ann Intern Med* 95:178–181, 1981.

442. Nieminen U, Kekomaki R: Quinidine-induced thrombocytopenic purpura: Clinical presentation in relation to drug-dependent and drug-independent platelet antibodies. *Br J Haematol* 80:77–82, 1992.

443. Leach MF, Cooper LK, AuBuchon JP: Detection of drug-dependent, platelet-reactive antibodies by solid-phase red cell adherence assays. *Br J Haematol* 97:755–761, 1997.

444. Visentin GP, Malik M, Cyganiak KA, Aster RH: Patients treated with unfractionated heparin during open heart surgery are at high risk to form antibodies reactive with heparin:platelet factor 4 complexes. *J Lab Clin Med* 128:376–383, 1996.

445. Boon DM, van Vliet HH, Zietse R, Kappers-Klunne MC: The presence of antibodies against a PF4-heparin complex in patients on haemodialysis. *Thromb Haemost* 76:480, 1996.

446. Bauer TL, Arepally G, Konkle BA, et al: Prevalence of heparin-associated antibodies without thrombosis in patients undergoing cardiopulmonary bypass surgery. *Circulation* 95:1242–1246, 1997.

447. Gentilini G, Curtis BR, Aster RH: An antibody from a patient with ranitidine-induced thrombocytopenia recognizes a site on glycoprotein IX that is a favored target for drug-induced antibodies. *Blood* 92:2359–2365, 1998.

448. Belkin GA: Cocktail purpura. An unusual case of quinine sensitivity. *Ann Intern Med* 66:583–586, 1967.

449. Siroty RR: Purpura on the rocks—With a twist. *JAMA* 235:2521–2522, 1976.

450. Pedersen-Bjergaard U, Andersen M, Hansen PB: Drug-induced thrombocytopenia: Clinical data on 309 cases and the effect of corticosteroid therapy. *Eur J Clin Pharmacol* 52:183–189, 1997.

# CHAPTER 8
# HEPARIN-INDUCED THROMBOCYTOPENIA

Adam Cuker and Mortimer Poncz

## SUMMARY

Heparin-induced thrombocytopenia (HIT) is a prothrombotic complication of treatment with heparin. It is associated with mild-to-moderate thrombocytopenia, although the main clinical concern is the high frequency of both arterial and venous thromboembolism, which may be limb- or life-threatening. HIT is an immune complex–based disorder involving platelet factor 4 complexed to negatively charged multimeric molecules, especially surface heparan side chains. It is initiated by exposure to heparin, particularly unfractionated heparin. There is growing understanding of the unusual nature of the underlying immune response in HIT, why certain individuals develop this disorder, and why HIT is prothrombotic. Diagnosis is based on an assessment of clinical probability and specialized laboratory testing. Management involves immediate cessation of heparin and initiation of inhibitors of thrombin or factor Xa.

## DEFINITION AND HISTORY

Heparin-induced thrombocytopenia (HIT) is a complication of heparin therapy in which there is a fall in platelet count and an unusually high incidence of arterial and/or venous thromboembolic complications in association with heparin therapy.

Although clinical usage of heparin as an anticoagulant began in the late 1950s, it was not until the early 1970s that a small percentage of treated patients were noted to develop a complication consisting of thrombocytopenia with paradoxical, life-threatening thromboemboli (for a historical review, see Ref. 1). In the 1980s, it became clear that HIT was caused by immunoglobulin (Ig) G antibodies that activate platelets. It was also recognized that HIT could be divided into two types, the classic immune-mediated prothrombotic disease that is the focus of this chapter (formerly called HIT type II) and a benign nonimmune condition associated with a mild, immediate, and transient drop in platelet count and no increased risk of thrombosis (formerly called HIT type I).[2] In this chapter, "HIT" means the immune-mediated form of the disease.

In the 1970s and 1980s, it became clear that HIT antibodies activated both platelets and endothelial cells.[3,4] Further analysis showed that blocking platelet FcγRIIA inhibited platelet activation by HIT sera in vitro,[5] suggesting that platelet activation involved an immune

complex. In the early 1990s, this complex was identified as heparin bound to the platelet-specific chemokine, platelet factor 4 (PF4).[6] Over the past 20 years, additional insights into the mechanism(s) underlying this immune complex disorder have emerged that have advanced our understanding of why this disorder is particularly prothrombotic and occurs in a only a small subset of patients. Additionally, advances have been made on the clinical side with respect to prevention, diagnosis, and treatment.

## EPIDEMIOLOGY

The frequency of HIT in heparin-treated patients ranges from less than 0.1 percent to 5.0 percent, depending on patient- and heparin-specific risk factors. These include the patient population, sex, nature of the heparin used, and duration of heparin exposure (Table 8–1).

The most important determinant of risk is the patient population. In a meta-analysis of seven prospective studies, the incidence of HIT was greater among surgical than medical patients (odds ratio [OR]: 3.25; 95 percent confidence interval [CI]: 1.98 to 5.35).[7] The incidence of HIT approaches 5 percent in patients who receive unfractionated heparin (UFH) after major orthopedic surgery.[8] Patients undergoing surgery with cardiopulmonary bypass have a very high frequency of anti-PF4/heparin antibody seroconversion (50 to 75 percent by postoperative day 10), but a lesser incidence of HIT (0.5 to 1.0 percent).[8–10] HIT occurs in 0.5 to 1.0 percent of medical patients[7] and in less than 0.1 percent of pregnant women[11,12] and children.[13] In a randomized trial of trauma patients, major trauma was associated with a significantly greater incidence of HIT than minor trauma (2.2 percent vs. 0.0 percent, p = 0.01) despite identical heparin exposure.[14]

Female sex is also a risk factor for HIT. A meta-analysis found an approximately twofold greater risk of HIT in women than men (OR: 2.37; 95 percent CI: 1.37 to 4.09). Analyses of a German database and a randomized trial of UFH versus low-molecular-weight heparin (LMWH) after orthopedic surgery yielded similar findings.[7]

HIT is more common with UFH than LMWH in surgical patients. In a meta-analysis of 15 studies, primarily involving orthopedic surgery patients, the incidence of HIT with UFH and LMWH was 2.6 percent and 0.2 percent, respectively.[15] Data are conflicting on whether the risk of HIT is reduced with LMWH in medical patients.[7,16,17] In a single-center study, institution-wide replacement of UFH with LMWH resulted in a 79 percent reduction in the incidence of HIT.[17a] Fondaparinux, a synthetic pentasaccharide anticoagulant, is associated with a nearly negligible risk of HIT, although several cases of fondaparinux-associated HIT have been reported.[18]

Duration of heparin exposure also influences the risk of HIT. In a meta-analysis of 3529 patients receiving UFH thromboprophylaxis for 6 or more days, the incidence of HIT was 2.6 percent.[15] Review of a hospital database indicated that briefer courses induce a substantially lower incidence of HIT (0.2 percent).[19]

High-quality data on the impact of dose and route of administration of heparin on the risk of HIT are lacking. Some studies suggest a lower rate of HIT with prophylactic dose subcutaneous UFH than therapeutic dose intravenous UFH,[19] but these analyses are confounded by differences in the patients who receive these treatments, including the clinical indication for heparin. Rarely, HIT has been reported with very low doses of heparin such as with use of heparin flushes or heparin-bonded catheters.[20,21]

## ETIOLOGY AND PATHOGENESIS

The development of HIT antibodies is nonclassical in that these antibodies typically begin as IgG and not IgM,[22] may disappear after a few months, and may not reappear with heparin reexposure.[23] It has been proposed

**TABLE 8–1.** Heparin-Induced Thrombocytopenia Risk Factors

| Patient-Specific Factors | Heparin-Specific Factors |
|---|---|
| Patient population (surgical > medical > obstetric > pediatric) | Type of heparin (unfractionated heparin > low-molecular-weight heparin) |
| Major trauma > minor trauma | Duration of heparin (~5 days >shorter courses) |
| Sex (female > male) | |

that the initial antigen exposure involves PF4 complexed with bacterial wall (Fig. 8–1) and that antibodies against this complex may be an important antimicrobial defensive mechanism.[24] These antigenic complexes, as well as circulating PF4–heparin complexes, are detected by splenic marginal B cells that subsequently produce pathogenic HIT antibodies.[25]

The nature of the antigenic heparin–PF4 complex has been partially defined. At the concentrations reached at sites of injury, PF4 exists as a tetramer. Crystal structure analysis shows that this tetramer is encircled by a ring of positive charge (Fig. 8–2),[26] and heparin is thought to bind to this region.[27] There are two closely spaced HIT antibody recognition domains (Fig. 8–2).[28] These domains are distinct from the heparin-binding domain. About half of patients have antibodies that react with one or the other HIT antigenic domain, and one-third of patients do not have antibodies that react to either domain, suggesting that there are other HIT antigenic sites on PF4. Studies of antihuman PF4 monoclonal antibodies suggest that unlike nonpathogenic anti-PF4 antibodies, HIT antibodies markedly increase their binding affinity for PF4 maintained in a tetrameric as opposed to dimeric state.[29] Moreover, tetrameric PF4 and UFH need to be at approximately 1:1 molar ratio for optimal HIT antigenicity.[30,31] At this ratio, ultralarge complexes (>670 kDa) of PF4 and heparin form that appear as visible colloidal complexes, and these are likely to be the antigenic source in HIT.[32,33] At higher or lower ratios, PF4 predominantly forms smaller and less antigenic PF4–heparin complexes. Ultralarge complexes are inefficiently

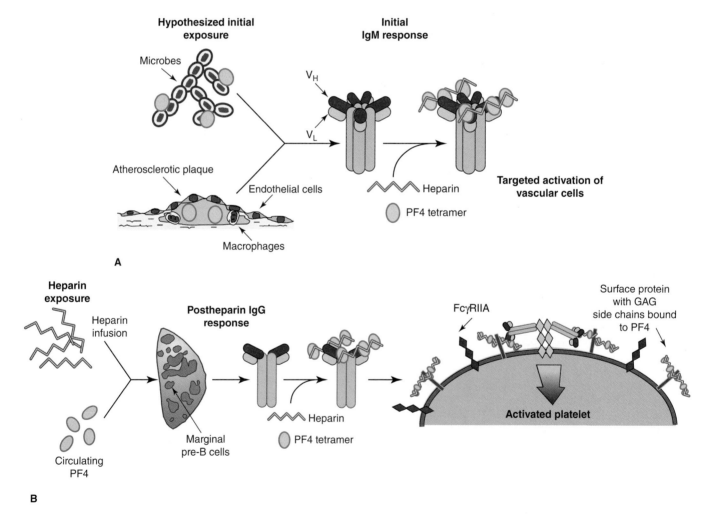

**Figure 8–1.** Proposed etiology of the immune response in heparin-induced thrombocytopenia (HIT). **A.** Proposed first exposure to HIT antigenic complex either during microbial invasion[24] or within growing atherosclerotic plaques, which are known to contain both platelet factor 4 (PF4) and immune-responsive cells.[49] In both cases, soluble PF4 and negatively charged molecules must be presented to B cells and result in an initial immunoglobulin M—perhaps low affinity—response. **B.** On exposure to heparin, especially unfractionated heparin, complexes form with free PF4 and are presented to splenic marginal B cells,[25] which subsequently produce pathogenic HIT antibodies that bind with high affinity to PF4 complexed to surface GAG complexes.[29] The concentrated binding of HIT antibodies to surface PF4–GAG complexes may enhance FcγRIIA aggregation and subsequent platelet activation.

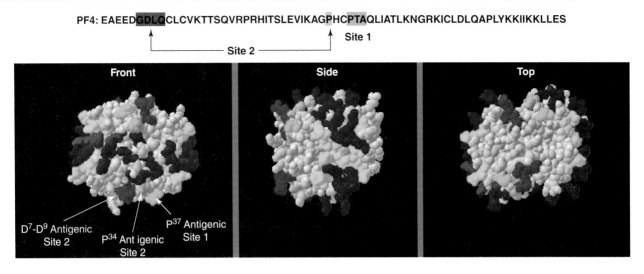

**Figure 8–2.** Platelet factor 4 (PF4) tetramer structure. At the top is the linear sequence of PF4. The regions that are known to contribute to heparin-induced thrombocytopenia (HIT) antigenicity when PF4 is complexed to heparin are boxed. Below are three views of the PF4 tetramer with the positively charged residues shown in both light and dark blue. Sites at which HIT neoepitopes are exposed on the PF4 tetramer are indicated. *(Adapted with permission from Li ZQ, Liu W, Park KS, et al: Defining a second epitope for heparin-induced thrombocytopenia antibodies using KKO, a murine HIT-like monoclonal antibody,* Blood *2002 Feb 15;99(4):1230–1236.)*

formed with LMWH, offering a potential explanation as to why this class of agents is associated with a lower incidence of HIT compared with UFH. Fondaparinux does not form large complexes with PF4, explaining the negligible incidence of HIT with this agent and supporting its potential utility in the prevention or treatment of HIT.

A passive immunization murine model of HIT has been used to demonstrate the following components are necessary to induce both thrombocytopenia and a prothrombotic state in HIT: the presence of human PF4 in platelets, FcγRIIA on the surface of platelets and possibly

other vascular cells, and the presence of a pathogenic HIT-like antibody.[34] Heparin has a more complex relationship to the pathogenesis of HIT (Fig. 8–3). In the passive immunization model of HIT, wherein a pathogenic HIT-like antibody is infused into mice expressing both human PF4 and FcγRIIA, heparin infusion is not needed to cause thrombocytopenia and a prothrombotic state.[35] The explanation for a lack of need to infuse heparin in this model is as follows: One important potential role of heparin in the pathogenesis of HIT is to form soluble, circulating PF4–heparin complexes that induce anti-PF4–heparin

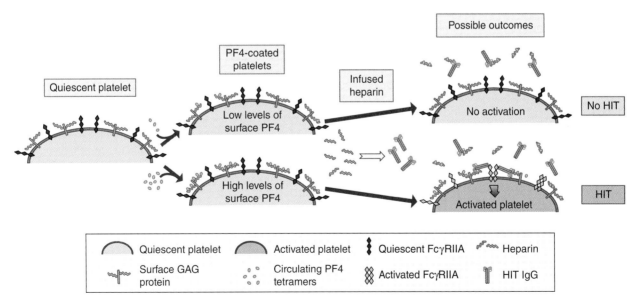

**Figure 8–3.** The role(s) of heparin in heparin-induced thrombocytopenia (HIT). On the *left* is depicted a quiescent platelet surface with GAG-expressing proteins as well as individual FcγRIIA receptors. Platelet factor 4 (PF4) is normally released by platelets in the steady-state, especially in individuals with underlying inflammation and/or atherosclerosis. Additionally, individuals have a wide range of platelet PF4 content, and this, too, contributes to having individuals with different levels of surface PF4 binding. Heparin infusions leads to HIT immunoglobulin G formation (see Fig. 8-1B) but also removes surface-bound PF4. If the individual has little initial surface-bound PF4, the surface of the platelets will be wiped clean of bound PF4 by the infused heparin and not be targeted by the HIT antibodies *(right, top)* so that HIT antibodies circulate but HIT does not develop. If there is significant residual surface-bound PF4 after heparin infusion, HIT antibodies will attach to the cell surface and activate the platelets *(right, bottom)*, potentially leading to HIT.

antibody production by presentation of the complex to splenic marginal B cells (see Figs. 8–1 and 8–3).[25] Passive immunization with HIT antibodies in these mice obviates the need for delivery of soluble antigenic complexes to the spleen. Another role for infused heparin is counterintuitive in that it may prevent HIT by partially or completely removing surface-bound PF4 (Fig. 8–3).[35] If the level of circulating, free human PF4 in the mice was initially low relative to the level of infused heparin, all surface-bound PF4 and detectable surface antigenicity would be removed and the circulating HIT antibodies would have no targets on platelets and other vascular cells (Fig. 8–3). HIT therefore would not develop despite the presence of heparin and circulating HIT antibody. On the other hand, if the level of circulating free human PF4 in the mice was initially high relative to the infused heparin, not all surface-bound PF4 would be removed. Circulating HIT antibodies could then target and activate platelets and other vascular cells, leading to thrombocytopenia and thrombosis (Fig. 8–3).

Most patients likely begin with little PF4 bound to surface glycosaminoglycans (GAGs). After therapeutic heparinization, the level of surface PF4 goes down markedly so that the platelets cannot be targeted by anti-PF4–heparin HIT antibodies. However, patients with high levels of surface PF4 and significant surface PF4 antigenic complexes remaining after heparinization may be at risk for binding of pathogenic anti-PF4–heparin HIT antibodies to platelets and other vascular cells. Bound pathogenic antibodies lead to thrombocytopenia by clearance of antibody-coated platelets by the reticuloendothelial system. Bound antibodies also lead to platelet activation through Fc$\gamma$RIIA and the formation of procoagulant platelet microparticles that contribute to thrombosis.[36]

As part of this activation, HIT antibodies also bind to endothelial cells likely via PF4–surface GAG complexes,[4,37] leading to local vascular activation and contributing to further local thrombosis. Additionally, HIT antibodies activate PF4-targeted monocytes[38,39] and neutrophils.[40] Monocyte activation may involve its surface Fc$\gamma$ receptors[41] with subsequent increased tissue factor expression and other changes consistent with a prothrombotic and inflammatory state. Monocyte and neutrophil GAGs are more complex than GAGs on the surface of platelets, which are mostly chondroitin sulfate[42] and have relatively low affinity for PF4.[43] Monocytes and neutrophils bind PF4 with greater avidity and are more resistant to removal of bound PF4 by circulating heparin than are platelets. In HIT, they may be preferentially targeted and activated relative to the platelets, contributing to the prothrombotic state of this immune thrombocytopenia.[44]

Are there any genetic polymorphisms that are associated with an increased risk of developing HIT or developing thrombosis after HIT begins? No clear linkage has been shown with known thrombophilic polymorphisms including factor V$^{Leiden}$, prothrombin$^{g20210a}$, MTHFR$^{C677T}$, $\alpha_{IIb}\beta_3$, and $\alpha_1\beta_2$.[45] Studies addressing a functional Fc$\gamma$RIIA$^{R/H131}$ polymorphism had varied outcome.[46,47] It is unclear whether patients with HIT have a higher density of Fc$\gamma$RIIA on their platelets.[48] High IgG affinity for the heparin–PF4 complex appears to affect the risk of developing HIT.

The model shown in Fig. 8–3 suggests that individuals with high PF4 content in their platelets and/or sustained platelet activation, as might be seen in patients with significant atherosclerosis, a postsurgery state, or trauma, would be most likely to develop HIT after heparinization and HIT antibody development. However, a relationship between formation of HIT antibodies and the degree of atherosclerosis in patients undergoing cardiopulmonary bypass surgery was not noted.[49] If levels of PF4 on the surface of circulating cells determine risk of developing HIT, this would offer a potential method for prescreening patients prior to heparinization and eliminate those at increased risk of HIT or be a useful tool in heparinized patients who develop thrombocytopenia to see whether they potentially can develop HIT. Theoretically, only those heparinized individuals with detectable surface PF4 would be potential candidates for developing HIT if they concurrently develop pathogenic antibodies.

# ● CLINICAL DIAGNOSIS

The clinical hallmark of HIT is development of thrombocytopenia in the setting of a proximate heparin exposure. The combination of thrombocytopenia and heparin exposure in hospitalized patients is common and has poor specificity for HIT.[50] Therefore, other clinical clues must be sought in estimating the clinical likelihood of HIT. These include timing, degree of platelet count fall, nadir platelet count, presence of thromboembolism or hemorrhage, and the likelihood of other causes of thrombocytopenia.

## TIMING

The platelet count in HIT characteristically begins to fall 5 to 10 days after initial heparin exposure.[23] There are three exceptions to this rule: (1) in rapid-onset HIT, patients with recent heparin exposure (within the previous 90 days) and preformed anti-PF4–heparin IgG experience a fall in platelet count immediately upon reexposure; (2) in delayed-onset HIT, clinical manifestations develop a median of 10 to 14 days after heparin is discontinued[51,52]; and (3) a small number of patients with spontaneous HIT have been reported. These patients present with a thrombotic thrombocytopenic disorder reminiscent of HIT in the absence of recognized heparin exposure.[53] Both delayed-onset HIT and spontaneous HIT occur in the absence of circulating heparin and may involve pathogenic HIT antibodies that recognize complexes of PF4 and endogenous GAGs on blood and vascular cells.

## DEGREE OF FALL IN PLATELET COUNT

The percentage fall in platelet count is measured from the peak platelet count after initiation of heparin to the nadir platelet count. Most patients with HIT experience a 50 percent or greater fall in platelet count; a more modest decline (30 to 50 percent) occurs in approximately 10 percent of patients.[54]

## NADIR PLATELET COUNT

As opposed to most other forms of drug-induced immune thrombocytopenia, thrombocytopenia associated with HIT is characteristically mild or moderate. The median nadir platelet count is approximately $60 \times 10^9$/L and rarely falls below $20 \times 10^9$/L in the absence of concomitant disseminated intravascular coagulation (DIC).[54] The nadir platelet count in HIT need not meet the traditional definition of thrombocytopenia ($<150 \times 10^9$/L). For example, patients with postoperative thrombocytosis may experience a subsequent greater than 50 percent decline in platelet count attributable to HIT that does not fall below this threshold.[55]

## THROMBOSIS

Thromboembolism is the presenting feature in up to 25 percent of patients with HIT and complicates approximately half of all cases.[56,57] Lower-extremity deep vein thrombosis and pulmonary embolism are the most common thrombotic manifestations, outnumbering arterial events by approximately 2:1.[56] Major venous obstruction can lead to limb gangrene. Catheter-associated upper extremity deep venous thrombosis is common.[58] Arterial thromboembolism most frequently involves the extremities but may also manifest as stroke or myocardial infarction.[56] Thrombosis of other vascular beds including cerebral sinuses, mesenteric vessels, and adrenal veins is well-documented, as is thrombotic occlusion of vascular grafts, fistulas, and extracorporeal circuitry.

## HEMORRHAGE

In contrast to most other forms of drug-induced immune thrombocytopenia, spontaneous hemorrhage is rare in HIT, even when thrombocytopenia is severe. In a prospective study, bleeding complications were not increased in HIT patients compared with nonthrombocytopenic controls.[59]

## UNUSUAL CLINICAL MANIFESTATIONS

Rare sequelae of HIT include anaphylactoid reactions after intravenous heparin bolus, transient global amnesia, and skin necrosis at subcutaneous heparin injection sites.[60,61] Curiously, these phenomena may occur in the absence of thrombocytopenia. Nonnecrotizing erythematous injection site lesions are generally caused by delayed type IV hypersensitivity rather than HIT.[62]

## OTHER CAUSES

The likelihood of other etiologies of thrombocytopenia must be carefully considered in patients with suspected HIT. Common causes of hospital-acquired thrombocytopenia include infection; drugs other than heparin; DIC; dilution; and intravascular devices and extracorporeal circuits such as intraaortic balloon pumps, cardiopulmonary bypass, and extracorporeal membrane oxygenation.[63]

Clinical scoring systems have been developed to permit estimation of the probability of HIT based on the aforementioned features. The most extensively studied of these systems, the 4T score,[64] classifies the probability of HIT as low, intermediate, or high on the basis of four criteria: thrombocytopenia, timing, thrombosis or other sequelae, and the likelihood of other causes of thrombocytopenia (Table 8–2). In a meta-analysis of 13 studies, the negative predictive value of a low-probability 4T score was 99.8 percent (95 percent CI: 97.0 to 100.0). The positive predictive values of an intermediate- and high-probability 4T score were 14 percent (95 percent CI: 9 to 22) and 64 percent (95 percent CI: 40 to 82), respectively.[65] The 4T score is limited by moderate interobserver agreement.[66] An alternative scoring system, the HIT Expert Probability (HEP) Score, exhibited improved reliability and favorable operating characteristics in a retrospective study but remains to be prospectively validated.[67]

# ●LABORATORY DIAGNOSIS

In light of the complexity and limited positive predictive value of clinical diagnosis,[65] clinicians rely heavily on laboratory testing to aid in diagnosis. Laboratory assays for HIT fall into two categories: immunoassays and functional assays.

## IMMUNOASSAYS

These assays detect the presence of circulating anti-PF4–heparin antibodies, irrespective of whether they are able to activate platelets and cause disease. The prototypical immunoassay is the solid-phase enzyme-linked immunosorbent assay (ELISA), in which dilute patient serum is added to microtiter wells coated with complexes of PF4–heparin (or PF4–polyvinylsulfonate).[6] The polyspecific ELISA detects circulating anti-PF4–heparin IgG, IgM, and IgA. In a systematic review and meta-analysis, the sensitivity and specificity of the polyspecific ELISA for HIT at the manufacturer-recommended cutoff were 96.7 percent (95 percent CI: 89.7 to 99.0) and 86.8 percent (95 percent CI: 82.0 to 90.5), respectively.[22,68–70a]

A key limitation of the polyspecific ELISA is its specificity. False-positive results are common and may result from detection of nonpathogenic anti-PF4–heparin antibodies[69] or antiphospholipid antibodies against either PF4[71] or PF4-bound $\beta_2$-glycoprotein I.[72] Specificity may be improved by raising the optical density (OD) cutoff. OD is directly associated with the 4T and HEP scores,[67] the risk of thrombosis,[73] and the likelihood of a positive functional assay.[74] In a Canadian study, only one of 37 patient samples exhibiting a weakly positive OD (0.40 to 0.99) demonstrated heparin-dependent platelet activation compared with 33 of 37 samples with a strongly positive OD (>2.0).[74] In a recent analysis of 1958 patients, increasing the cutoff from a manufacturer-recommended threshold of 0.4 to 0.8 OD units increased specificity from 85 percent to 93 percent with a slight reduction in sensitivity from 100 percent to 98 percent.[75]

Several modifications have been made to the PF4–heparin ELISA with the goal of improving specificity. Because pathogenic antibodies are primarily of the IgG class, detection systems specific for IgG have been developed. In a systematic review and meta-analysis of studies directly comparing the IgG-specific and polyspecific ELISA, the former showed greater specificity (87 percent [95 percent CI: 85 to 88] vs. 82 percent [95 percent CI: 80 to 84]) without sacrificing sensitivity (97 percent [95 percent CI: 95 to 99] for both assays).[76] Another modification involves the addition of a high heparin confirmatory step, in which reduction of the OD by 50 percent or more with the addition of excess heparin (100 U/mL) is considered to affirm the presence of heparin-dependent antibodies.[77] This method improves specificity, but false-positive results remain common and false-negative results may also occur, particularly at high OD values.[78,79]

Another limitation of the PF4–heparin ELISA is turnaround time. Although the analytical turnaround time of the ELISA is only approximately 2 hours, the assay is most cost-effective when multiple samples are run in batch. Consequently, many laboratories perform the ELISA only once or twice a week, leaving clinicians to make critical initial management decisions without the benefit of laboratory results.

**TABLE 8–2.** The 4T Score*

| Clinical Sign | Points Per Category | | |
|---|---|---|---|
| | **0** | **1** | **2** |
| **T**hrombocytopenia (acute) | Very low nadir (<10 × 10⁹/L) or <30% fall | Low nadir (10–20 × 10⁹/L) or 30–50% fall | Moderate nadir (20–100 × 10⁹/L) or >50% fall |
| **T**iming of first event (thrombocytopenia or thrombosis) | ≤4 Days (unless prior heparin exposure in last 3 months) | Within 5–10 days (but not well documented) or ≤1 day (with exposure in last 3 months) | Documented occurrence in 5–10 days or ≤1 day with recent prior exposure |
| **T**hrombotic-related event | None | Progressive, recurrent, or suspected (unconfirmed) thrombosis; erythematous nonnecrotic skin lesions | New thrombosis (confirmed) or skin necrosis or systemic reaction after heparin bolus |
| **T**hrombocytopenia (other causes) | Definite other cause is present | Possible other cause is present | No other strong explanation for thrombocytopenia |

*Scores of 0–3, 4–5, and 6–8 are classified as low, intermediate, and high probability, respectively.[64]

**TABLE 8–3.** Properties of Rapid Platelet Factor 4–Heparin Immunoassays

| Assay | Antibody Class Detection | Sensitivity (95% CI)* | Specificity (95% CI)* | Turnaround Time (Minutes) | Regulatory Approval |
|---|---|---|---|---|---|
| Particle gel immunoassay | IgG | 0.98 (0.94–1.00) | 0.88 (0.81–0.96) | 20 | Asia, Canada, Europe |
| Lateral flow immunoassay | IgG | 0.97 (0.92–1.00) | 0.91 (0.86–0.96) | 15 | Europe |
| Latex particle-enhanced immunoturbidimetric assay | IgG, IgA, IgM | 1.00 (0.66–1.00) | 0.91 (0.83–0.96) | 13 | Europe |
| Chemiluminescence assay | IgG, IgA, IgM | 0.97 (0.86–1.00) | 0.82 (0.77–0.87) | 30 | Europe |
| Chemiluminescence assay | IgG | 0.95 (0.90–1.00) | 0.94 (0.89–0.99) | 30 | Europe |

Ig, immunoglobulin.

*From [86a]

This drawback of the ELISA has spawned the development of several rapid immunoassays, which are designed to accommodate single samples and yield results in minutes. Table 8–3 summarizes the properties of these rapid assays.[68,80–86a] The latex particle-enhanced immunoturbidimetric assay and chemiluminescence assays are instrument-based and must be performed on proprietary analyzers. A rapid particle immunofiltration assay is approved in the Unites States, but published data suggest that it has unacceptable diagnostic accuracy.[87,88]

## FUNCTIONAL ASSAYS

Functional assays are more specific than commercial immunoassays because they detect only the subset of antibodies capable of inducing platelet activation in a heparin-dependent manner. The prototypical functional assays are the [14]C-serotonin release assay (SRA) and the heparin-induced platelet-activation assay (HIPA). In the SRA, various concentrations of heparin and heat-inactivated patient serum are added to washed donor platelets radiolabeled with [14]C. A positive test is signified by heparin-dependent release of [14]C-serotonin.[89] The HIPA is based on a similar principle but uses visual assessment of platelet aggregation as an end point.[90] The sensitivity and specificity of the SRA and HIPA are said to exceed 95 percent, but universally accepted reference standards against which to measure their performance do not exist.[63]

Washed platelet functional assays are technically demanding. Both the SRA and HIPA require reactive donor platelets, and the SRA requires radioisotope. Because these reagents are impracticable for most clinical laboratories, functional assays are performed at only a small number of reference laboratories around the world. Even among such laboratories, test methodology, result interpretation, and reporting are not well standardized.[91]

Novel immunoassays and functional assays for HIT designed to overcome the limitations of assays currently in use are in development.[92,93]

## ● MANAGEMENT

### NONHEPARIN ANTICOAGULANTS

Management of HIT requires immediate withdrawal of heparin, including cessation of heparin flushes and removal of heparin-coated catheters. However, discontinuation of heparin alone is insufficient to prevent thromboembolism. Historical studies of untreated patients document a 5 to 10 percent daily risk of thrombosis in the first 48 hours after heparin is stopped and a 30-day cumulative incidence of thrombosis of approximately 50 percent.[57,94] Discontinuation of heparin must therefore be accompanied by initiation of a rapid-acting, nonheparin anticoagulant.[95] Table 8–4 summarizes the properties of parenteral nonheparin anticoagulants used to treat HIT.

Argatroban and bivalirudin are direct thrombin inhibitors. Argatroban is the only FDA-approved drug for treatment of HIT available in the United States. Its approval was based on two open-label single-arm studies in which argatroban-treated subjects were compared with untreated historical controls.[96,97] In a pooled analysis of these two studies, argatroban reduced the relative risk of new thrombosis by two-thirds. The incidence of major bleeding was approximately 1 percent per day.[98] An important limitation of these studies was that serologic confirmation of HIT was not required for enrollment. Indeed, 36.4 percent of subjects were found to be anti-PF4–heparin antibody negative on *post hoc* testing,[99] suggesting that a sizable proportion of the study population did not have HIT.

Bivalirudin is a hirudin analogue. It is approved for patients with and without HIT undergoing percutaneous vascular procedures. It is not approved for treatment of HIT, although it has been used off-label for this indication, particularly in patients with critical illness and multiorgan failure[100] and those undergoing cardiac surgery.[101] Published evidence supporting its use is limited to retrospective single-center cohort studies.[100,102,103]

Two other direct thrombin inhibitors have been studied as treatments for HIT. Lepirudin, a recombinant hirudin, was shown to reduce the risk of thromboembolism compared with untreated historical controls but is no longer available.[94] A randomized clinical trial of desirudin closed because of poor accrual after only 16 subjects had been randomized.[104]

Danaparoid and fondaparinux are indirect factor Xa inhibitors. Danaparoid is approved for treatment of HIT in multiple jurisdictions but is no longer marketed in the United States, and drug shortages have limited its availability elsewhere. In an open-label randomized trial, 42 patients with HIT complicated by thrombosis were allocated to receive either danaparoid or dextran 70. Significantly more subjects in the danaparoid arm were judged to have complete recovery from thrombosis at hospital discharge (56 percent vs. 14 percent; p = 0.02).[105] *In vitro* cross-reactivity of HIT antibodies with danaparoid occurs in some patients, although the clinical relevance of this phenomenon has not been established.[106]

Fondaparinux in not approved for treatment of HIT. However, it is now widely used in this setting and appears to have similar efficacy and safety to approved agents.[63,107–110] A small number of cases of HIT induced or exacerbated by fondaparinux have been reported, although the attribution to fondaparinux in at least some of these cases remains uncertain.[111] Fondaparinux is more convenient to use than other agents given the ease of once-daily subcutaneous administration and a lack of need for laboratory monitoring (see Table 8–4).

Oral direct inhibitors of thrombin (e.g., dabigatran) and factor Xa (e.g., rivaroxaban, apixaban, edoxaban) do not induce platelet aggregation or PF4 release in the presence of HIT-positive sera *in vitro*[112] and constitute biologically rational approaches to the treatment of HIT. Clinical evidence is limited to a small number of case reports and case series.[113] A clinical trial of rivaroxaban in patients with suspected HIT

**TABLE 8–4.** Anticoagulants Used to Treat Heparin-Induced Thrombocytopenia

| Drug | Initial Dosing | Monitoring | Clearance (Half-Life) |
|---|---|---|---|
| **Direct Thrombin Inhibitors** | | | |
| Argatroban | Bolus: None<br>Continuous infusion:<br>Normal organ function → 2 mcg/kg/min<br>Liver dysfunction (total bilirubin >1.5 mg/dL), heart failure, postcardiac surgery, anasarca → 0.5–1.2 mcg/kg/min | Adjust dose to aPTT of 1.5–3.0 × patient baseline | Hepatobiliary (40–50 min) |
| Bivalirudin | Bolus: None<br>Continuous infusion:<br>Normal organ function → 0.15 mg/kg/h<br>Renal or hepatic insufficiency → consider dose reduction | Adjust dose to aPTT of 1.5–2.5 × patient baseline | Enzymatic and renal (25 min) |
| **Indirect Factor Xa Inhibitors** | | | |
| Danaparoid | Bolus:<br>  <60 kg → 1500 U<br>  60–75 kg → 2250 U<br>  75–90 kg → 3000 U<br>  >90 kg → 3750 U<br>Accelerated initial infusion:<br>  400 U/h × 4 h, then 300 U/h × 4 h<br>Maintenance infusion:<br>  Normal renal function → 200 U/h<br>  Renal insufficiency → 150 U/h | Adjust to anti–factor Xa of 0.5–0.8 U/mL | Renal (24 h) |
| Fondaparinux | <50 kg → 5 mg SC daily<br>50–100 kg → 7.5 mg SC daily<br>>100 kg → 10 mg SC daily<br>$Cl_{Cr}$ 30–50 mL/min → use caution<br>$Cl_{Cr}$ <30 mL/min → contraindicated | None | Renal (17–20 h) |

aPTT, activated partial thromboplastin time; $Cl_{Cr}$, creatinine clearance; SC, subcutaneous.

was closed after enrollment of only 22 patients because of slow accrual.[114] It is unlikely that other clinical trials will be conducted. Although current clinical practice guidelines do not recommend direct oral anticoagulants for the treatment of acute HIT,[95] it is likely that their use in this setting will continue to grow and evidence will continue to be accumulated through real-world clinical experience. An important toxicity of anticoagulants used for treatment of HIT is major bleeding, a risk compounded by the absence of effective reversal agents. Novel therapeutic approaches that target pathways proximal to activation of coagulation may provide effective antithrombotic therapy without the degree of bleeding risk associated with anticoagulants. Candidate strategies include a desulfated form of heparin with minimal anticoagulant activity[112] and small-molecule PF4 antagonists,[115] which interfere with formation of PF4–heparin complexes; inhibitors of FcγRIIA-mediated platelet activation by HIT immune complexes; and inhibitors of splenic tyrosine kinase and $Ca^{2+}$[116] and diacylglycerol-regulated guanine nucleotide exchange factor I,[117] which disrupt intracellular transduction triggered by immune complex binding.

## WHO TO TREAT

Because of the frequency of heparin use and thrombocytopenia among hospitalized patients, the modest specificity of immunologic assays, and clinicians' fears of missing a case of HIT, overdiagnosis and unnecessary treatment with nonheparin anticoagulants of patients without HIT are common.[118] Inappropriate use of these agents is associated with increased costs and bleeding risk.[119] In light of the very high negative predictive value (99.8 percent) of a low-probability 4T score,[65] a reasonable first step toward reducing unnecessary treatment is to avoid use of nonheparin anticoagulants in patients with a low-probability 4T score. Heparin should be discontinued and a nonheparin anticoagulant initiated in patients with an intermediate- or high-probability 4T score until the results of HIT laboratory testing become available.[65,95,120]

## TRANSITIONING TO A VITAMIN K ANTAGONIST

Warfarin and other vitamin K antagonists should not be prescribed as the initial anticoagulant in patients with acute HIT because their use increases the risk of venous limb gangrene as a result of rapid lowering of protein C activity.[121] For patients receiving a vitamin K antagonist at the time HIT is diagnosed, the vitamin K antagonist should be discontinued and its effects reversed with vitamin K. A vitamin K antagonist may be initiated once the platelet count has recovered to a stable plateau. Large loading doses (e.g., warfarin >5 mg/d) should be avoided. The vitamin K antagonist should be overlapped with a parenteral nonheparin anticoagulant for at least 5 days and until the international normalized ratio (INR) has reached its intended target.[63,95] If the patient is being transitioned from argatroban to warfarin, guidelines regarding the appropriate INR target should be followed,[122] because both argatroban and warfarin increase the INR. This target will vary according to the sensitivity of the prothrombin time reagent to argatroban used in each institution.

## DURATION OF ANTICOAGULATION

Patients with HIT-associated thromboembolism are typically treated with therapeutic anticoagulation for 3 to 6 months. The optimal duration of anticoagulation in patients with HIT without thrombosis (i.e., isolated HIT) is unknown. In a historical series of untreated patients with isolated HIT, the cumulative incidence of thromboembolism at 30 days was 53 percent.[57] Most events occurred within 10 days of heparin cessation, corresponding to the platelet recovery phase. It is therefore generally accepted that anticoagulation be continued in patients with isolated HIT until platelet count recovery. Some authorities recommend longer courses (e.g., 4 weeks).[120]

## PLATELET TRANSFUSION

There is a long-held concern that platelet transfusion may precipitate thrombosis in HIT by "adding fuel to the fire." Two case series challenge this dogma. Collectively, these series included 41 patients with suspected HIT who underwent platelet transfusion. None developed thrombosis during extended follow-up.[123,124] Nevertheless, because HIT is characteristically prothrombotic rather than prohemorrhagic, prophylactic platelet transfusion is rarely indicated. Transfusion may be considered in the setting of clinically significant bleeding, high bleeding risk, or diagnostic uncertainty.

## HEPARIN REEXPOSURE IN PATIENTS WITH A HISTORY OF HEPARIN-INDUCED THROMBOCYTOPENIA

In general, heparin reexposure should be avoided in patients with a history of HIT because of the risk of reoccurrence.[125] An exception to this rule is the use of intraoperative heparin in patients with a history of HIT who are undergoing cardiovascular surgery. The HIT immune response wanes over time. Functional assays become negative at a median of 50 days after heparin cessation, whereas anti-PF4–heparin antibody titers decline more slowly and are no longer detectable in 60 percent of patients by day 100.[23] HIT laboratory testing can be used to determine the safety of heparin reexposure during cardiovascular surgery. Patients with a negative immunologic and functional assay may safely receive UFH during surgery. This was first demonstrated in 10 patients with a history of HIT undergoing cardiac surgery, none of whom developed clinical reoccurrence.[126] In a newer report, 11 of 17 such patients developed recrudescence of anti-PF4–heparin antibodies, but only one developed HIT.[127] Heparin should be strictly avoided in patients with a positive functional assay. If possible, surgery should be delayed in these individuals until functional and immunologic assays become negative. If surgery cannot be delayed, a nonheparin anticoagulant (e.g., bivalirudin) should be used.[101] Appropriate intraoperative anticoagulation of patients with a functional assay that has become negative but an immunologic assay that remains positive is uncertain. The 2012 American College of Chest Physicians Guidelines recommend a nonheparin anticoagulant in this setting.[95] However, intraoperative heparin was used uneventfully in three such patients undergoing urgent heart transplantation.[128] Similar findings were observed in a recently published series of 10 patients.[129] When heparin is administered to patients with a history of HIT, it should be limited to the intraoperative setting. Pre- and postoperative exposure should be scrupulously avoided, although patients with a history of HIT who are (inadvertently) reexposed to longer courses of heparin do not always develop recurrent HIT.[127]

In light of its documented efficacy and safety in large coronary angiography trials, bivalirudin is recommended over heparin in patients with a history of HIT who require percutaneous vascular procedures, irrespective of the results of HIT laboratory testing.[95]

## HEMODIALYSIS

Although approximately 10 percent of patients on chronic hemodialysis develop circulating anti-PF4–heparin antibodies,[130] the incidence of HIT in this population is less than 1 percent.[131] Ongoing heparin exposure during dialysis in patients with a history of HIT is contraindicated. Alternative strategies including regional citrate, saline flushing, danaparoid, argatroban, and vitamin K antagonists have been reported.[95]

## PREGNANCY

HIT is rare (<0.1 percent) in pregnant women exposed to heparin.[11,12] When it does occur, initiation of a nonheparin anticoagulant is warranted. The largest published experience is with danaparoid. A retrospective cohort of 30 women with acute HIT received danaparoid during pregnancy.[132] Five patients developed thrombosis and three developed major bleeding. Danaparoid does not cross the placenta, and there was no measurable anti-Xa activity in the cord blood of six neonates who were tested after delivery. If danaparoid is unavailable, fondaparinux may be considered, although evidence supporting its use in pregnant women with HIT is limited to case reports[133,134] and partial transplacental passage has been demonstrated.[135]

## REFERENCES

1. Kelton JG, Warkentin TE: Heparin-induced thrombocytopenia: A historical perspective. *Blood* 112:2607, 2008.
2. Chong BH, Berndt MC: Heparin-induced thrombocytopenia. *Blut* 58:53, 1989.
3. Fratantoni JC, Pollet R, Gralnick HR: Heparin-induced thrombocytopenia: Confirmation of diagnosis with in vitro methods. *Blood* 45:395, 1975.
4. Cines DB, Tomaski A, Tannenbaum S: Immune endothelial-cell injury in heparin-associated thrombocytopenia. *N Engl J Med* 316:581, 1987.
5. Kelton JG, Sheridan D, Santos A, et al: Heparin-induced thrombocytopenia: Laboratory studies. *Blood* 72:925, 1988.
6. Amiral J, Bridey F, Dreyfus M, et al: Platelet factor 4 complexed to heparin is the target for antibodies generated in heparin-induced thrombocytopenia. *Thromb Haemost* 68:95, 1992.
7. Warkentin TE, Sheppard JA, Sigouin CS, et al: Gender imbalance and risk factor interactions in heparin-induced thrombocytopenia. *Blood* 108:2937, 2006.
8. Warkentin TE, Shepard JA, Horsewood P, et al: Impact of the patient population on the risk for heparin-induced thrombocytopenia. *Blood* 96:1703, 2000.
9. Pouplard C, May MA, Regina S, et al: Changes in platelet count after cardiac surgery can effectively predict the development of pathogenic heparin-dependent antibodies. *Br J Haematol* 128:837, 2005.
10. Selleng S, Malowsky B, Strobel U, et al: Early-onset and persisting thrombocytopenia in post-cardiac surgery patients is rarely due to heparin-induced thrombocytopenia, even when antibody tests are positive. *J Thromb Haemost* 8:30, 2010.
11. Sanson BJ, Lensing AW, Prins MH, et al: Safety of low-molecular-weight heparin in pregnancy: As systematic review. *Thromb Haemost* 81:668, 1999.
12. Fausett MB, Vogtlander M, Lee RM, et al: Heparin-induced thrombocytopenia is rare in pregnancy. *Am J Obstet Gynecol* 185:148, 2001.
13. Avila ML, Shah V, Brandão LR: Systematic review on heparin-induced thrombocytopenia in children: A call to action. *J Thromb Haemost* 11:660, 2013.
14. Lubenow N, Hinz P, Thomaschewski S, et al: The severity of trauma determines the immune response to PF4/heparin and the frequency of heparin-induced thrombocytopenia. *Blood* 115:1797, 2010.
15. Martel N, Lee J, Wells PS: Risk for heparin-induced thrombocytopenia with unfractionated and low-molecular-weight heparin thromboprophylaxis: A meta-analysis. *Blood* 106:2710, 2005.
16. Morris TA, Castrejon S, Devendra G, Gamst AC: No difference in risk for thrombocytopenia during treatment of pulmonary embolism and deep venous thrombosis with either low-molecular-weight heparin or unfractionated heparin: A metaanalysis. *Chest* 132:1131, 2007.
17. Pohl C, Kredteck A, Bastians B, et al: Heparin-induced thrombocytopenia in neurologic patients treated with low-molecular-weight heparin. *Neurology* 64:1285, 2005.
17a. McGowan KE, Makari J, Diamantouros A, et al: Reducing the hospital burden of heparin-induced thrombocytopenia: Impact of an avoid-heparin program. *Blood* 127:1954, 2016.

18. Warkentin TE: Fondaparinux: Does it cause HIT? Can it treat HIT? *Expert Rev Hematol* 3:567, 2010.

19. Smythe M, Koerber JM, Mattson JC: The incidence of recognized heparin-induced thrombocytopenia in a large, tertiary care teaching hospital. *Chest* 131:1644, 2007.

20. Muslimani AA, Ricaurte B, Daw HA: Immune heparin-induced thrombocytopenia resulting from preceding exposure to heparin catheter flushes. *Am J Hematol* 82:652, 2007.

21. Laster J, Silver D: Heparin-coated catheters and heparin-induced thrombocytopenia. *J Vasc Surg* 7:667, 1988.

22. Juhl D, Eichler P, Lubenow N, et al: Incidence and clinical significance of anti-PF4/heparin antibodies of the IgG, IgM, and IgA class in 755 consecutive patient samples referred for diagnostic testing for heparin-induced thrombocytopenia. *Eur J Haematol* 76:420, 2006.

23. Warkentin TE, Kelton JG: Temporal aspects of heparin-induced thrombocytopenia. *N Engl J Med* 344:1286, 2001.

24. Krauel K, Pötschke C, Weber C, et al: Platelet factor 4 binds to bacteria, [corrected] inducing antibodies cross-reacting with the major antigen in heparin-induced thrombocytopenia. *Blood* 117:1370, 2011.

25. Zheng Y, Yu M, Podd A, et al: Critical role for mouse marginal zone B cells in PF4/heparin antibody production. *Blood* 121:3484, 2013.

26. Zhang X, Chen L, Bancroft DP, et al: Crystal structure of recombinant human platelet factor 4. *Biochemistry* 33:8361, 1994.

27. Stuckey JA, St Charles R, Edwards BF: A model of the platelet factor 4 complex with heparin. *Proteins* 14:277, 1992.

28. Li ZQ, Liu W, Park KS, et al: Defining a second epitope for heparin-induced thrombocytopenia antibodies using KKO, a murine HIT-like monoclonal antibody. *Blood* 99:1230, 2002.

29. Litvinov RI, Yarovoi SV, Rauova L, et al: Distinct specificity and single-molecule kinetics characterize the interaction of pathogenic and non-pathogenic antibodies against platelet factor 4-heparin complexes with platelet factor 4. *J Biol Chem* 288:33060, 2013.

30. Greinacher A, Pötzsch B, Amiral J, et al: Heparin-associated thrombocytopenia: Isolation of the antibody and characterization of a multimolecular PF4-heparin complex as the major antigen. *Thromb Haemost* 71:247, 1994.

31. Horne MK 3rd, Alkins BR: Platelet binding of IgG from patients with heparin-induced thrombocytopenia. *J Lab Clin Med* 127:435, 1996.

32. Rauova L, Poncz M, McKenzie SE, et al: Ultralarge complexes of PF4 and heparin are central to the pathogenesis of heparin-induced thrombocytopenia. *Blood* 105:131, 2005.

33. Suvarna S, Espinasse B, Qi R, et al: Determinants of PF4/heparin immunogenicity. *Blood* 110:4253, 2007.

34. Reilly MP, Taylor SM, Hartman NK, et al: Heparin-induced thrombocytopenia/thrombosis in a transgenic mouse model requires human platelet factor 4 and platelet activation through FcγRIIA. *Blood* 98:2442, 2001.

35. Rauova L, Zhai L, Kowalska MA, et al: Role of platelet surface PF4 antigenic complexes in heparin-induced thrombocytopenia pathogenesis: Diagnostic and therapeutic implications. *Blood* 107:2346, 2006.

36. Warkentin TE, Hayward CP, Boshkov LK, et al: Sera from patients with heparin-induced thrombocytopenia generate platelet-derived microparticles with procoagulant activity: An explanation for the thrombotic complications of heparin-induced thrombocytopenia. *Blood* 84:3691, 1994.

37. Visentin GP, Malik M, Cyganiak KA, Aster RH: Patients treated with unfractionated heparin during open heart surgery are at high risk to form antibodies reactive with heparin:platelet factor 4 complexes. *J Lab Clin Med* 128:376, 1996.

38. Pouplard C, Iochmann S, Renard B, et al: Induction of monocyte tissue factor expression by antibodies to heparin-platelet factor 4 complexes developed in heparin-induced thrombocytopenia. *Blood* 97:3300, 2001.

39. Arepally GM, Mayer IM: Antibodies from patients with heparin-induced thrombocytopenia stimulate monocytic cells to express tissue factor and secret interleukin-8. *Blood* 98:1252, 2001.

40. Xiao Z, Visentin GP, Dayananda KM, Neelagaham S: Immune complexes formed following the binding of anti-platelet factor 4 (CXCL4) antibodies to CXCL4 stimulate human neutrophil activation and cell adhesion. *Blood* 112:1091, 2008.

41. Kasthuri RS, Glover SL, Jonas W, et al: PF4/heparin-antibody complex induces monocyte tissue factor expression and release of tissue factor positive microparticles by activation of FcγRI. *Blood* 119:5285, 2012.

42. Ward JV, Packham MA: Characterization of the sulfated glycosaminoglycans on the surface and in the storage granules of rabbit platelets. *Biochim Biophys Acta* 583:196, 1979.

43. Handin RI, Cohen HJ: Purification and binding properties of human platelet factor four. *J Biol Chem* 251:4273, 1976.

44. Rauova L, Hirsch JD, Greene TK, et al: Monocyte-bound PF4 in the pathogenesis of heparin-induced thrombocytopenia. *Blood* 116:5021, 2010.

45. Carlsson LE, Lubenow N, Blumentritt C, et al: Platelet receptor and clotting factor polymorphisms as genetic risk factors for thromboembolic complications in heparin-induced thrombocytopenia. *Pharmacogenetics* 13:253, 2003.

46. Arepally G, McKenzie SE, Jiang XM, et al: Fc gamma RIIA H/R 131 polymorphism, subclass-specific IgG anti-heparin/platelet factor 4 antibodies and clinical course in patients with heparin-induced thrombocytopenia and thrombosis. *Blood* 89:370, 1997.

47. Carlsson LE, Santoso S, Baurichter G, et al: Heparin-induced thrombocytopenia: New insights into the impact of the FcgammaRIIa-R-H131 polymorphism. *Blood* 92:1526, 1998.

48. Chong BH, Pilgrim RL, Cooley MA, Chesterman CN: Increased expression of platelet IgG Fc receptors in immune heparin-induced thrombocytopenia. *Blood* 81:988, 1993.

49. Cuker A, Rauova L, Bolgiano D, et al: Atherosclerosis is not a risk factor for anti-platelet factor 4/heparin antibody formation after cardiopulmonary bypass surgery. *Thromb Haemost* 111:1191, 2014.

50. Oliveira GB, Crespo EM, Becker RC, et al: Complications After Thrombocytopenia Caused by Heparin (CATCH) Registry Investigators: Incidence and prognostic significance of thrombocytopenia in patients treated with prolonged heparin therapy. *Arch Intern Med* 168:94, 2008.

51. Warkentin TE, Kelton JG: Delayed-onset heparin-induced thrombocytopenia and thrombosis. *Ann Intern Med* 135:502, 2001.

52. Rice L, Attisha WK, Drexler A, Francis JL: Delayed-onset heparin-induced thrombocytopenia. *Ann Intern Med* 136:210, 2002.

53. Warkentin TE, Basciano PA, Knopman J, Bernstein RA: Spontaneous heparin-induced thrombocytopenia syndrome: 2 new cases and a proposal for defining this disorder. *Blood* 123:3651, 2014.

54. Warkentin TE: Clinical presentation of heparin-induced thrombocytopenia. *Semin Hematol* 35:9, 1998.

55. Warkentin TE, Roberts RS, Hirsh J, Kelton JG: An improved definition of immune heparin-induced thrombocytopenia in postoperative orthopedic patients. *Arch Intern Med* 163:2518, 2003.

56. Greinacher A, Farner B, Kroll H, et al: Clinical features of heparin-induced thrombocytopenia including risk factors for thrombosis. A retrospective analysis of 408 patients. *Thromb Haemost* 94:132, 2005.

57. Warkentin TE, Kelton JG: A 14-year study of heparin-induced thrombocytopenia. *Am J Med* 101:502, 1996.

58. Hong AP, Cook DJ, Sigouin CS, Warkentin TE: Central venous catheters and upper-extremity deep-vein thrombosis complicating immune heparin-induced thrombocytopenia. *Blood* 101:3049, 2003.

59. Warkentin TE, Levine MN, Hirsh J, et al: Heparin-induced thrombocytopenia in patients treated with low-molecular-weight heparin or unfractionated heparin. *N Engl J Med* 332:1330, 1995.

60. Warkentin TE, Roberts RS, Hirsh J, Kelton JG: Heparin-induced skin lesions and other unusual sequelae of the heparin-induced thrombocytopenia syndrome: A nested cohort study. *Chest* 127:1857, 2005.

61. Warkentin TE, Greinacher A: Heparin-induced anaphylactic and anaphylactoid reactions: Two distinct but overlapping syndromes. *Expert Opin Drug Saf* 8:129, 2009.

62. Schindewolf M, Kroll H, Ackermann H, et al: Heparin-induced non-necrotizing skin lesions: Rarely associated with heparin-induced thrombocytopenia. *J Thromb Haemost* 8:1486, 2010.

63. Cuker A, Cines DB: How I treat heparin-induced thrombocytopenia. *Blood* 119:2209, 2012.

64. Lo GK, Juhl D, Warkentin TE, et al: Evaluation of pretest clinical score (4 T's) for the diagnosis of heparin-induced thrombocytopenia in two clinical settings. *J Thromb Haemost* 4:759, 2006.

65. Cuker A, Gimotty PA, Crowther MA, Warkentin TE: Predictive value of the 4Ts scoring system for heparin-induced thrombocytopenia: A systematic review and meta-analysis. *Blood* 120:4160, 2012.

66. Nagler M, Fabbro T, Wuillemin WA: Prospective evaluation of the interobserver reliability of the 4Ts score in patients with suspected heparin-induced thrombocytopenia. *J Thromb Haemost* 10:151, 2012.

67. Cuker A, Arepally G, Crowther MA, et al: The HIT Expert Probability (HEP) Score: A novel pre-test probability model for heparin-induced thrombocytopenia based on broad expert opinion. *J Thromb Haemost* 8:2642, 2010.

68. Bakchoul T, Giptner A, Najaoui A, et al: Prospective evaluation of PF4/heparin immunoassays for the diagnosis of heparin-induced thrombocytopenia. *J Thromb Haemost* 7:1260, 2009.

69. Lo GK, Sigouin CS, Warkentin TE: What is the potential for overdiagnosis of heparin-induced thrombocytopenia? *Am J Hematol* 82:1037, 2007.

70. Greinacher A, Juhl D, Strobel U, et al: Heparin-induced thrombocytopenia: A prospective study on the incidence, platelet-activating capacity and clinical significance of anti-platelet factor 4/heparin antibodies of the IgG, IgM, and IgA classes. *J Thromb Haemost* 5:1666, 2007.

70a. Nagler M, Bachmann LM, ten Cate H, ten Cate-Hoek A: Diagnostic value of immunoassays for heparin-induced thrombocytopenia: A systematic review and meta-analysis. *Blood* 127:546, 2016.

71. Pauzner R, Greinacher A, Selleng K, et al: False-positive tests for heparin-induced thrombocytopenia in patients with antiphospholipid syndrome and systemic lupus erythematosus. *J Thromb Haemost* 7:1070, 2009.

72. Sikara MP, Routsias JG, Samiotaki M, et al: β2 Glycoprotein I (β2GPI) binds platelet factor 4 (PF4): Implications for the pathogenesis of antiphospholipid syndrome. *Blood* 115:713, 2010.

73. Zwicker JI, Uhl L, Huang WY, et al: Thrombosis and ELISA optical density values in hospitalized patients with heparin-induced thrombocytopenia. *J Thromb Haemost* 2:2133, 2004.

74. Warkentin TE, Sheppard JI, Moore JC, et al: Quantitative interpretation of optical density measurements using PF4-dependent enzyme-immunoassays. *J Thromb Haemost* 6:1304, 2008.

75. Raschke RA, Curry SC, Warkentin TE, Gerkin RD: Improving clinical interpretation of the anti-platelet factor 4/heparin enzyme-linked immunosorbent assay for the diagnosis of heparin-induced thrombocytopenia through the use of receiver operating characteristic analysis, stratum-specific likelihood ratios, and Bayes theorem. *Chest* 144:1269, 2013.

76. Husseinzadeh HD, Gimotty PA, Pishko AM, et al: Diagnostic accuracy of IgG-specific versus polyspecific enzyme-linked immunoassays in heparin-induced thrombocytopenia: a systematic review and meta-analysis. *J Thromb Haemost* 15:1203, 2017.

77. Whitlatch NL, Kong DF, Metjian AD, et al: Validation of the high-dose heparin confirmatory step for the diagnosis of heparin-induced thrombocytopenia. *Blood* 116:1761, 2010.

78. Warkentin TE, Sheppard JI: No significant improvement in diagnostic specificity of an anti-PF4/polyanion immunoassay with use of high heparin confirmatory procedure. *J Thromb Haemost* 4:281, 2006.

79. Selleng S, Schreier N, Wollert HG, Greinacher A: The diagnostic value of the anti-PF4/heparin immunoassay high-dose heparin confirmatory test in cardiac surgery patients. *Anesth Analg* 112:774, 2011.

80. Sachs UJ, von Hesberg J, Santoso S, et al: Evaluation of a new nanoparticle-based lateral-flow immunoassay for the exclusion of heparin-induced thrombocytopenia (HIT). *Thromb Haemost* 106:1197, 2011.

81. Meyer O, Salama A, Pittet N, Schwind P: Rapid detection of heparin-induced platelet antibodies with particle gel immunoassay (ID-HPF4). *Lancet* 354:1525, 1999.

82. Leroux D, Hezard N, Lebreton A, et al: Prospective evaluation of a rapid nano-particle-based lateral flow immunoassay (STic Expert HIT) for the diagnosis of heparin-induced thrombocytopenia. *Br J Haematol* 166:774, 2014.

83. Davidson SJ, Ortel TL, Smith LJ: Performance of a new, rapid, automated immunoassay for the detection of anti-platelet factor 4/heparin complex antibodies. *Blood Coagul Fibrinolysis* 22:340, 2011.

84. Althaus K, Hron G, Strobel U, et al: Evaluation of automated immunoassays in the diagnosis of heparin induced thrombocytopenia. *Thromb Res* 131:e85, 2013.

85. Legnani C, Cini M, Pili C, et al: Evaluation of a new automated panel of assays for the detection of anti-PF4/heparin antibodies in patients suspected of having heparin-induced thrombocytopenia. *Thromb Haemost* 104:402, 2010.

86. Van Hoecke F, Devreese K: Evaluation of two new automated chemiluminescent assays (HemosIL AcuStar HIT-IgG and HemosIL AcuStar HIT-Ab) for the detection of heparin-induced antibodies in the diagnosis of heparin-induced thrombocytopenia. *Int J Lab Hematol* 34:410, 2012.

86a. Sun L, Gimotty PA, Lakshmanan S, Cuker A: Diagnostic accuracy of rapid immunoassays for heparin-induced thrombocytopenia: a systematic review and meta-analysis. *Thromb Haemost* 115:1044, 2016.

87. Warkentin TE, Sheppard JI, Raschke R, Greinacher A: Performance characteristics of a rapid assay for anti-PF4/heparin antibodies: The particle immunofiltration assay. *J Thromb Haemost* 5:2308, 2007.

88. Andrews DM, Cubillos GF, Paulino SK, et al: Prospective evaluation of the particle immunofiltration anti-platelet factor 4 rapid assay in MICU patients with thrombocytopenia. *Crit Care* 17:R143, 2013.

89. Sheridan D, Carter C, Kelton JG: A diagnostic test for heparin-induced thrombocytopenia. *Blood* 67:27, 1986.

90. Greinacher A, Michels I, Kiefel V, Mueller-Eckhardt C: A rapid and sensitive test for diagnosing heparin-associated thrombocytopenia. *Thromb Haemost* 66:734, 1991.

91. Price EA, Hayward CP, Moffat KA, et al: Laboratory testing for heparin-induced thrombocytopenia is inconsistent in North America: A survey of North American specialized coagulation laboratories. *Thromb Haemost* 98:1357, 2007.

92. Cuker A, Rux AH, Hinds JL, et al: Novel diagnostic assays for heparin-induced thrombocytopenia. *Blood* 121:3727, 2013.

93. Nazi I, Arnold DM, Smith JW, et al: FcγRIIa proteolysis as a diagnostic biomarker for heparin-induced thrombocytopenia. *J Thromb Haemost* 11:1146, 2013.

94. Greinacher A, Eichler P, Lubenow N, et al: Heparin-induced thrombocytopenia with thromboembolic complications: Meta-analysis of 2 prospective trials to assess the value of parenteral treatment with lepirudin and its therapeutic aPTT range. *Blood* 96:846, 2000.

95. Linkins LA, Dans AL, Moores LK, et al: American College of Chest Physicians: Treatment and prevention of heparin-induced thrombocytopenia: Antithrombotic Therapy and Prevention of Thrombosis, 9th ed: American College of Chest Physicians Evidence-Based Clinical Practice Guidelines. *Chest* 141:e495S, 2012.

96. Lewis BE, Wallis DE, Berkowitz SD, et al: ARG-911 Study Investigators: Argatroban anticoagulant therapy in patients with heparin-induced thrombocytopenia. *Circulation* 103:1838, 2001.

97. Lewis BE, Wallis DE, Leya F, et al: Argatroban-915 Investigators: Argatroban anticoagulation in patients with heparin-induced thrombocytopenia. *Arch Intern Med* 163:1849, 2003.

98. Lewis BE, Wallis DE, Hursting MJ, et al: Effects of argatroban therapy, demographic variables, and platelet count on thrombotic risks in heparin-induced thrombocytopenia. *Chest* 129:1407, 2006.

99. Walenga JM, Fasanella AR, Iqbal OH, et al: Coagulation laboratory testing in patients treated with argatroban. *Semin Thromb Hemost* 25:61, 1999.

100. Kiser TH, Fish DN: Evaluation of bivalirudin treatment for heparin-induced thrombocytopenia in critically ill patients with hepatic and/or renal dysfunction. *Pharmacotherapy* 26:452, 2006.

101. Koster A, Dyke CM, Aldea G, et al: Bivalirudin during cardiopulmonary bypass in patients with previous or acute heparin-induced thrombocytopenia and heparin antibodies: Results of the CHOOSE-ON trial. *Ann Thorac Surg* 83:572, 2007.

102. Skrupky LP, Smith JR, Deal EN, et al: Comparison of bivalirudin and argatroban for the management of heparin-induced thrombocytopenia. *Pharmacotherapy* 30:1229, 2010.

103. Joseph L, Casanegra AI, Dhariwal M, et al: Bivalirudin for the treatment of patients with confirmed or suspected heparin-induced thrombocytopenia. *J Thromb Haemost* 12:1044, 2014.

104. Boyce SW, Bandyk DF, Bartholomew JR, et al: A randomized, open-label pilot study comparing desirudin and argatroban in patients with suspected heparin-induced thrombocytopenia with or without thrombosis: PREVENT-HIT Study. *Am J Ther* 18:14, 2011.

105. Chong BH, Gallus AS, Cade JF, et al; Australian HIT Study Group: Prospective randomised open-label comparison of danaparoid with dextran 70 in the treatment of heparin-induced thrombocytopaenia with thrombosis: A clinical outcome study. *Thromb Haemost* 86:1170, 2001.

106. Magnani HN, Gallus A: Heparin-induced thrombocytopenia (HIT). A report of 1,478 clinical outcomes of patients treated with danaparoid (Orgaran) from 1982 to mid-2004. *Thromb Haemost* 95:967, 2006.

107. Schindewolf M, Steindl J, Beyer-Westendorf J, et al: Frequent off-label use of fondaparinux in patients with suspected acute heparin-induced thrombocytopenia (HIT): Findings from the GerHIT multi-centre registry study. *Thromb Res* 134:29, 2014.

108. Kang M, Alahmadi M, Sawh S, et al: Fondaparinux for the treatment of suspected heparin-induced thrombocytopenia: A propensity score-matched study. *Blood* 125:924, 2015.

109. Warkentin TE, Pai M, Sheppard JI, et al: Fondaparinux treatment of acute heparin-induced thrombocytopenia confirmed by the serotonin-release assay: A 30-month, 16-patient case series. *J Thromb Haemost* 9:2389, 2011.

110. Goldfarb MJ, Blostein MD: Fondaparinux in acute heparin-induced thrombocytopenia: A case series. *J Thromb Haemost* 9:2501, 2011.

111. Warkentin TE: Fondaparinux: Does it cause HIT? Can it treat HIT? *Expert Rev Hematol* 3:567, 2010.

112. Krauel K, Hackbarth C, Furll B, Greinacher A: Heparin-induced thrombocytopenia: In vivo studies on the interaction of dabigatran, rivaroxaban, and low-sulfated heparin, with platelet factor 4 and anti-PF4/heparin antibodies. *Blood* 119:1248, 2012.

113. Tran PN, Tran MH: Emerging role of direct oral anticoagulants in the management of heparin-induced thrombocytopenia. *Clin Appl Thromb Hemost* 1:1076029617696582, 2017.

114. Linkins LA, Warkentin TE, Pai M, et al: Rivaroxaban for treatment of suspected or confirmed heparin-induced thrombocytopenia study. *J Thromb Haemost* 14:1206, 2016.

115. Sachias BS, Rux AH, Cines DB, et al: Rational design and characterization of platelet factor 4 antagonists for the study of heparin-induced thrombocytopenia. *Blood* 119:5955, 2012.

116. Reilly MP, Sinha U, André P, et al: PRT-060318, a novel Syk inhibitor, prevents heparin-induced thrombocytopenia and thrombosis in a transgenic mouse model. *Blood* 117:2241, 2011.

117. Stolla M, Stefanini L, André P, et al: CalDAG-GEFI deficiency protects mice in a novel model of Fcγ RIIA-mediated thrombosis and thrombocytopenia. *Blood* 118:1113, 2011.

118. Cuker A: Heparin-induced thrombocytopenia (HIT) in 2011: An epidemic of overdiagnosis. *Thromb Haemost* 106:993, 2011.

119. Smythe MA, Koerber JM, Mehta TP, et al: Assessing the impact of a heparin-induced thrombocytopenia protocol on patient management, outcomes, and costs. *Thromb Haemost* 108:992, 2012.

120. Watson H, Davidson S, Keeling D: Haemostasis and Thrombosis Task Force of the British Committee for Standards in Haematology: Guidelines on the diagnosis and management of heparin-induced thrombocytopenia: Second edition. *Br J Haematol* 159:528, 2012.

121. Warkentin TE, Elavathil LJ, Hayward CP, et al: The pathogenesis of venous limb gangrene associated with heparin-induced thrombocytopenia. *Ann Intern Med* 127:804, 1997.

122. Sheth SB, DiCicco RA, Hursting MJ, et al: Interpreting the international normalized ratio (INR) in individuals receiving argatroban and warfarin. *Thromb Haemost* 85:453, 2001.

123. Hopkins CK, Goldfinger D: Platelet transfusions in heparin-induced thrombocytopenia: A report of four cases and review of the literature. *Transfusion* 48:2128, 2008.

124. Refaai MA, Chuang C, Menegus M, et al: Outcomes after platelet transfusion in patients with heparin-induced thrombocytopenia. *J Thromb Haemost* 8:1419, 2010.

125. Gruel Y, Lang M, Darnige L, et al: Fatal effect of re-exposure to heparin after previous heparin-associated thrombocytopenia and thrombosis. *Lancet* 336:1077, 1990.

126. Pötzsch B, Klövekorn WP, Madlener K: Use of heparin during cardiopulmonary bypass in patients with a history of heparin-induced thrombocytopenia. *N Engl J Med* 343:515, 2000.

127. Warkentin TE, Sheppard JA: Serological investigation of patients with a previous history of heparin-induced thrombocytopenia who are reexposed to heparin. *Blood* 123:2485, 2014.

128. Selleng S, Haneya A, Hirt S, et al: Management of anticoagulation in patients with subacute heparin-induced thrombocytopenia scheduled for heart transplantation. *Blood* 112:4024, 2008.

129. Warkentin TE, Anderson JA: How I treat patients with a history of heparin-induced thrombocytopenia. *Blood* 128:348, 2016.

130. Carrier M, Knoll GA, Kovacs MJ, et al: The prevalence of antibodies to the platelet factor 4–heparin complex and associated with access thrombosis in patients on chronic hemodialysis. *Thromb Res* 120:215, 2007.

131. Hutchison CA, Dasgupta I: National survey of heparin-induced thrombocytopenia in the haemodialysis population of the UK population. *Nephrol Dial Transplant* 22:1680, 2007.

132. Magnani HN: An analysis of clinical outcomes of 91 pregnancies in 83 women treated with danaparoid (Orgaran). *Thromb Res* 125:297, 2010.

133. Hajj-Chahine J, Jayle C, Tomasi J, Corbi P: Successful surgical management of massive pulmonary embolism during the second trimester in a parturient with heparin-induced thrombocytopenia. *Interact Cardiovasc Thorac Surg* 11:679, 2010.

134. Ciurzyński M, Jankowski K, Pietrzak B, et al: Use of fondaparinux in a pregnant woman with pulmonary embolism and heparin-induced thrombocytopenia. *Med Sci Monit* 17:CS56, 2011.

135. Dempfle CE: Minor transplacental passage of fondaparinux in vivo. *N Engl J Med* 350:1914, 2004.

# CHAPTER 9
# REACTIVE THROMBOCYTOSIS

Kenneth Kaushansky

## SUMMARY

The three major pathophysiologic causes of thrombocytosis are (1) clonal, including essential (or primary) thrombocythemia and other myeloproliferative neoplasms; (2) familial, including rare cases of nonclonal myeloproliferation resulting from thrombopoietin and thrombopoietin receptor mutations; and (3) reactive, in which thrombocytosis occurs secondary to a variety of acute and chronic clinical conditions. This chapter deals with the latter causes of thrombocytosis.

The upper limit of the normal platelet count in most clinical laboratories is between 350,000/$\mu$L (350 × 10$^9$/L) and 450,000/$\mu$L (450 × 10$^9$/L). In a sample of 10,000 healthy individuals 18 to 65 years of age, 1 percent had platelet counts greater than 400,000/$\mu$L. Only in eight of these 99 individuals was thrombocytosis confirmed 6 months to 1 year later.[1] Nevertheless, it is clear that thrombocytosis is a feature of several important disorders, including cancer, and that even a high normal platelet count is associated with morbidity and mortality. In a longitudinal study of healthy Norwegian men, a platelet count in the top quartile of the normal range (from 275 × 10$^9$/L to 350 × 10$^9$/L) was associated with a twofold increase in cardiovascular mortality over a 12-year follow-up.[2] Whether the platelet count per se or an underlying inflammatory condition resulting in both thrombocytosis and accelerated atherogenesis is responsible for these observations is not certain. The causes of thrombocytosis in which the platelet count exceeds the upper limit can be broadly categorized as (1) clonal, including essential thrombocythemia and other myeloproliferative neoplasms, (2) familial, and (3) reactive, or secondary. This chapter focuses on the causes and molecular mechanisms that underlie reactive, or secondary, thrombocytosis.

## ● NORMAL THROMBOPOIESIS

The regulation of platelet production is discussed extensively in Chap. 1, but a brief discussion here provides the appropriate background for discussion of reactive thrombocytosis. Thrombopoietin (TPO), the ligand for the megakaryocytic growth factor receptor c-Mpl,

Acronyms and Abbreviations: EPO, erythropoietin; ESA, erythropoiesis-stimulating agent; FGF, fibroblast growth factor; GM-CSF, granulocyte-macrophage colony-stimulating factor; IFN, interferon; IL, interleukin; JAK, Janus kinase; LIF, leukemia inhibitory factor; MHC, major histocompatibility complex; NF, nuclear factor; SDF, stromal cell-derived factor; STAT, signal transducer and activator of transcription; TPO, thrombopoietin.

is the major humoral regulator of megakaryocyte survival, growth, and development, although, curiously, it does not stimulate the final step in thrombopoiesis: platelet release from megakaryocyte proplatelet processes. Although TPO supports the entire continuum of megakaryocyte development from stem cell to mature megakaryocyte,[3] other cytokines including interleukin (IL)-6,[4] IL-3,[5,6] IL-11,[7] leukemia inhibitory factor (LIF),[8,9] fibroblast growth factor (FGF)-4,[10] stromal cell-derived factor (SDF)-1,[10,11] interferon (IFN)-$\gamma$,[12] and granulocyte-macrophage colony-stimulating factor (GM-CSF)[13] also affect thrombopoiesis, both in vitro and in vivo. Many of these cytokines act in synergy with other cytokines, including TPO.[11,12,14]

The regulation of thrombopoiesis occurs primarily by humoral mechanisms, with the levels of TPO inversely related to platelet counts.[15,16] In contrast, other cytokines shown to affect megakaryopoiesis in vitro do not vary with platelet levels.[17] Despite these important insights, the regulation of TPO blood levels is complex and incompletely understood. The liver produces approximately half of all the hormone that circulates, based on platelet production in liver-specific knockout mice.[18] However, platelet levels do not affect hepatic TPO production; instead, platelets themselves have an important role in regulating plasma levels, as their receptors for TPO (c-mpl) remove it from plasma.[19] Thus, as the platelet count drops, increased free plasma TPO levels stimulate megakaryopoiesis; conversely, as the platelet count rises, depletion of free plasma TPO decreases platelet production. This modulatory mechanism results in the steady-state level of platelet production. However, marrow stromal cells also produce TPO[20] and are responsive to platelet products, which serve to down-modulate expression of the hormone.[21] A third mechanism by which platelets regulate TPO levels occurs through the Ashwell-Morell hepatocyte receptor, whereby their binding of senescent platelets leads to stimulation of hepatocyte signaling pathways and subsequent expression of TPO.[22]

## ● ENHANCED THROMBOPOIESIS IN PATHOLOGIC STATES

### THROMBOCYTOSIS IN INFLAMMATORY CONDITIONS

Inflammation is the most common cause of secondary thrombocytosis. In one survey, thrombocytosis was believed secondary to one or more inflammatory conditions in nearly 80 percent of all patients with an elevated platelet count. Table 9–1 lists the clinical conditions associated with reactive thrombocytosis. The most common diagnoses in such patients are inflammatory bowel disease and rheumatoid arthritis,[23] although most conditions in which the erythrocyte sedimentation rate or C-reactive protein is elevated have been reported to cause secondary thrombocytosis. Although several cytokines and lymphokines are elevated in the blood of such patients, the most compelling evidence suggests that IL-6 and IFN-$\gamma$ are responsible for the thrombocytosis seen in patients with inflammation.

### Interleukin-6
IL-6 was cloned by several groups of investigators using a number of distinct assays, including antiviral activity, myeloma cell growth, hepatocyte growth, and immunoglobulin secretion.[24] The recombinant protein was later found to affect megakaryocyte growth and differentiation, both in vitro and in vivo.[4,25,26] The IL-6 gene is present on the short arm of human chromosome 7; encodes a 26-kDa polypeptide produced in almost all tissues from T cells, fibroblasts, macrophages, and stromal cells; and is a key regulator of the inflammatory response.[27,28]

---

**TABLE 9–1.** Major Causes of Thrombocytosis

A. Reactive (secondary) thrombocytosis
  1. Transient reactive processes
  2. Acute blood loss
  3. Recovery ("rebound") from thrombocytopenia
  4. Acute infection, inflammation
  5. Response to exercise
B. Sustained processes
  1. Iron deficiency
  2. Postsplenectomy, asplenic states
  3. Malignancies
  4. Chronic inflammatory and infectious diseases (inflammatory bowel disease, rheumatoid arteritis, tuberculosis, chronic pneumonitis)
  5. Response to drugs (vincristine, epinephrine, all-*trans*-retinoic acid, some antibiotics, cytokines, and growth factors)
  6. Hemolytic anemia

---

IL-6 production is dependent on the presence of IL-1 and tumor necrosis factor (TNF)-α, cytokines produced by lymphocytes and monocytes in response to phagocytosis of microorganisms, the binding of immune complexes, and several other innate immune stimuli. IL-6 production is regulated primarily by transcriptional enhancement; regulatory elements responsible for IL-6 promoter activation include nuclear factor-κB (NFκB), adapter protein (AP)-1, CCAAT/enhancer binding protein (C/EBP) α, and C/EBPβ.

Although not critical for steady-state thrombopoiesis, as the combined genetic elimination of *c-mpl* and the signaling component of the IL-6 receptor (gp130) produces no more severe thrombocytopenia than elimination of *c-mpl* alone,[29] IL-6 contributes to inflammatory thrombopoiesis, primarily by stimulating the hepatic production of TPO.[30] Most studies report that patients with inflammation display an increased level of TPO,[31,32] but TPO is not the only cytokine responsible for this effect,[33] especially when corrected for the thrombocytosis, which would normally act to reduce levels of the hormone. Stimulation of hepatocytes with IL-6 results in enhanced production of TPO mRNA and protein.[34,35]

## INTERFERON-γ

A second inflammatory cytokine that contributes to inflammatory thrombopoiesis is IFN-γ. The interferons are proteins first defined by their ability to induce an antiviral state in mammalian cells. Biochemical fractionation revealed three classes of interferons: IFN-α, a family of 17 distinct but highly homologous molecules; IFN-β, a single molecule more distantly related to the various isoforms of IFN-α; and IFN-γ, a unique molecule that shares functional properties but not structure with the others. IFN-γ exerts the most profound hematologic effects of the three classes of protein, including direct suppression of erythroid colony-forming cell growth and the activation of macrophages to secrete a number of inflammatory cytokines; several comprehensive reviews on IFN-γ have been published.[36,37]

IFN-γ is produced by activated T lymphocytes and natural killer (NK) cells in response to T-cell antigen crosslinking and in response to stimulation by the inflammatory mediators TNF-α, IL-12, and IL-15.[38] Prominent hematologic effects include activation of macrophages to assume an inflammatory phenotype (e.g., secretion of TNF-α and enhanced tumor cell killing), upregulation of major histocompatibility

complex (MHC) class I and class II molecules enhancing antigen recognition responses,[37] and inhibition of proliferative responses in stem cells and erythroid progenitors.[39,40] These latter effects account for the association of IFN-γ and aplastic anemia.[41] However, in stark contrast to the inhibitory effects of IFN-γ on erythropoiesis, the cytokine stimulates megakaryocyte growth and differentiation.[42] This is likely related to its stimulation of signal transducer and activator of transcription (STAT)-1 in megakaryocytes, as transgenic expression of the transcription factor mimics the effect of the cytokine and corrects the thrombocytopenia seen in a genetic model system.[43] These findings argue that IFN-γ also contributes to the thrombocytosis seen in inflammatory states in humans.

Notwithstanding the above two mechanisms, patients with inflammatory conditions and thrombocytosis might have an additional cause of the elevated platelet count. The evaluation of iron deficiency is often difficult in patients with inflammation, as the most reliable indicator of tissue iron stores, serum ferritin, is an acute-phase reactant, possibly obscuring a diagnosis of iron deficiency in patients with an inflammatory condition. In a recent study of patients with inflammatory bowel disease, thrombocytosis was eliminated in half of the subjects by the administration or iron.[44]

## THROMBOCYTOSIS CAUSED BY IRON DEFICIENCY

Although most patients with inflammation-related thrombocytosis display increased production of the hormone, TPO levels in patients with iron deficiency and thrombocytosis are not elevated.[45] In contrast, erythropoietin (EPO) levels are elevated in patients with iron-deficiency anemia and are thought by some to be responsible for the thrombocytosis seen in iron deficiency, at least in part. Consistent with this hypothesis, administration of EPO to animals and humans leads to a modest increase in the platelet count.[46] Although some have suggested that this is a result of cross-reactivity of EPO on the TPO receptor,[47] direct EPO- and TPO-receptor binding studies refute this hypothesis.[48] Rather, megakaryocytic progenitors display EPO receptors, and their binding of the hormone leads to many of the same intracellular biochemical signals as induced by TPO.

However, several lines of evidence indicate that pathophysiologic mechanisms other than anemia must be responsible, at least in part, for the thrombocytosis seen in patients with iron deficiency. For example, many patients with iron-deficiency anemia do not have thrombocytosis.[45] Moreover, EPO levels are elevated in nearly all types of anemia, but iron deficiency is the only type of anemia that is regularly associated with thrombocytosis, other than the anemia of chronic inflammation, in which the inflammatory state that causes the anemia by modulation of hepcidin levels also causes thrombocytosis (as discussed in "Thrombocytosis in Inflammatory Conditions" above). Thus, although several lines of evidence suggest that enhanced levels of EPO as a consequence of the anemia associated with iron deficiency contribute to this form of reactive thrombocytosis, elevated EPO levels cannot completely account for it.

## THERAPEUTIC ERYTHROPOIETIN AND ENHANCED CARDIOVASCULAR MORTALITY

Several reports have linked the use of large doses of EPO or other erythropoiesis-stimulating agents (ESAs) to enhanced cardiovascular mortality[49] and to progression to dialysis in patients with renal insufficiency,[50] although not all studies concur with these landmark results.[51] Evidence is accumulating that the rapid expansion of erythropoiesis caused by pharmacologic levels of EPO often induces functional iron deficiency. If so, because iron deficiency leads to thrombocytosis, the excessive cardiovascular morbidity and mortality associated with the administration of EPO and ESAs to patients are hypothesized to be secondary to the thrombocytosis. Consistent with this view is that even a high-normal platelet count was found to be associated with enhanced cardiovascular morbidity and mortality in a longitudinal study of healthy Norwegian men.[2] In support of this hypothesis (that the excessive cardiovascular morbidity and mortality are secondary to the thrombocytosis) is the finding that patients with renal insufficiency on high therapeutic doses of EPO (>20,000 U/week) and hemoglobin (Hgb) values in excess of 13 g/dL are more likely to develop functional iron deficiency and thrombocytosis and that those individuals in whom the platelet count exceeds $300,000/\mu L$ display a statistically significantly higher 3-year mortality rate.[52] An alternate explanation is that EPO directly increases thrombopoiesis independently of iron deficiency and/or enhances the vascular reactivity of platelets. This hypothesis is based on the finding that megakaryocytes and platelets bear EPO receptors[53] and that TPO, which stimulates very similar signaling pathways as EPO in receptor-bearing cells, primes platelets to enhanced aggregation responses to classic platelet agonists.[54] Still other researchers have hypothesized that an alternate form of the EPO receptor, made up of the classic EPO receptor and the $\beta$ subunit of the GM-CSF, IL-3, and IL-5 receptors, is displayed on vascular endothelial cells,[55] and in that site could mediate enhanced vascular events. Thus, given the widespread use of ESAs in patients with anemia caused by cancer, kidney failure, myelodysplastic syndromes, and many other conditions, verifying these hypotheses or disproving them and establishing new ones appears to be important and a field ripe for new discovery.

# ● CLINICAL FEATURES OF REACTIVE THROMBOCYTOSIS

The clinical features of secondary thrombocytosis are almost always a result of the underlying disorder provoking the reaction, usually an inflammatory condition or iron-deficiency anemia. It is also highly unusual for the thrombocytosis per se to provoke any untoward symptoms. Although pathologic thrombosis is a major feature of primary thrombocythemia, it is virtually absent in reactive thrombocytosis, unless provoked by other features of the underlying condition (e.g., vasculitis) or completely unrelated conditions in the patient (e.g., atherosclerotic disease). Whether this is because patients with reactive thrombocytosis do not have as high platelet counts, on average, as patients with primary thrombocythemia[56]; or because they have smaller mean platelet volumes[56]; or because of the activated signaling characteristic of the platelets or other blood cells in patients with myeloproliferative diseases; or because of the presence of a mutant Janus kinase (JAK) 2[57] or a constitutively active TPO receptor[58] is uncertain at this time. Nevertheless, because vascular complications of reactive thrombocytosis are so unlikely to be a consequence of the elevated platelet count, treatment of the thrombocytosis *per se* is not recommended in reactive thrombocytosis except in very unusual circumstances.

# REFERENCES

1. Ruggeri M, Tosetto A, Frezzato M, Rodeghiero F: The rate of progression to polycythemia vera or essential thrombocythemia in patients with erythrocytosis or thrombocytosis. *Ann Intern Med* 139:470, 2003.
2. Thaulow E, Erikssen J, Sandvik L, et al: Blood platelet count and function are related to total and cardiovascular death in apparently healthy men. *Circulation* 84:613, 1991.
3. Kaushansky K: The molecular mechanisms that control thrombopoiesis. *J Clin Invest* 115:3339, 2005.
4. Williams N, De Giorgio T, Banu N, et al: Recombinant interleukin 6 stimulates immature megakaryocytes. *Exp Hematol* 18:69, 1990.
5. Yonemura Y, Kawakita M, Masuda T, et al: Synergistic effects of interleukin 3 and interleukin 11 on murine megakaryopoiesis in serum-free culture. *Exp Hematol* 20:1011, 1992.
6. Carrington PA, Hill RJ, Stenberg PE, et al: Multiple *in vivo* effects of interleukin 3 and interleukin 6 on mouse megakaryocytopoiesis. *Blood* 77:34, 1991.
7. Schlerman FJ, Bree AG, Kaviani MD, et al: Thrombopoietic activity of recombinant human interleukin 11 in normal and myelosuppressed nonhuman primates. *Stem Cells* 14:517, 1996.
8. Debili N, Massé J-M, Katz A, et al: Effects of the recombinant hematopoietic growth factors interleukin-3, interleukin-6, stem cell factor, and leukemia inhibitory factor on the megakaryocytic differentiation of CD34+ cells. *Blood* 82:84, 1993.
9. Farese A, Myers LA, MacVittie TJ: Therapeutic efficacy of recombinant leukemia inhibitory factor in a primate model of radiation-induced marrow aplasia. *Blood* 84: 3675, 1994.
10. Avecilla ST, Hattori K, Heissig B, et al: Chemokine-mediated interaction of hematopoietic progenitors with the bone marrow vascular niche is required for thrombopoiesis. *Nat Med* 10:64, 2004.
11. Hodohara K, Fujii N, Yamamoto N, Kaushansky K: Stromal cell derived factor 1 acts synergistically with thrombopoietin to enhance the development of megakaryocytic progenitor cells. *Blood* 95:769, 2000.
12. Tsuji-Takayama K, Tahata H, Izumi N, et al: IFN-gamma in combination with IL-3 accelerates platelet recovery in mice with 5-fluorouracil-induced marrow aplasia. *J Interferon Cytokine Res* 16:447, 1996.
13. Kaushansky K, O'Hara PJ, Berkner K, et al: Genomic cloning, characterization, and multilineage expression of human granulocyte-macrophage colony-stimulating factor. *Proc Natl Acad Sci U S A* 83:3101, 1986.
14. Broudy VC, Lin NL, Kaushansky K: Thrombopoietin (c-mpl ligand) acts synergistically with erythropoietin, stem cell factor, and IL-11 to enhance murine megakaryocyte colony growth and increases megakaryocyte ploidy *in vitro. Blood* 85:1719, 1995.
15. Kuter DJ, Rosenberg RD: The reciprocal relationship of thrombopoietin (c-Mpl Ligand) to changes in the platelet mass during busulfan-induced thrombocytopenia in the rabbit. *Blood* 85:2720, 1995.
16. Kuter DJ: The physiology of platelet production. *Stem Cells* 14(Suppl 1):88, 1996.
17. Cockrell EM, Gorman J, Hord JD, et al: Endogenous interleukin-11 (IL-11) levels in newly diagnosed children with acquired severe aplastic anemia (SAA). *Cytokine* 28:55, 2004.
18. Qian S, Fu F, Li W, et al: Primary role of the liver in thrombopoietin production shown by tissue-specific knockout. *Blood* 92:2189, 1998.
19. Fielder PJ, Hass P, Nagel M, et al: Human platelets as a model for the binding and degradation of thrombopoietin. *Blood* 89:2782, 1997.
20. Sungaran R, Markovic B, Chong BH: Localization and regulation of thrombopoietin mRNA expression in human kidney, liver, bone marrow and spleen using in situ hybridization. *Blood* 89:101, 1997.
21. McIntosh B, Kaushansky K: Marrow stromal production of thrombopoietin is regulated by transcriptional mechanisms in response to platelet products. *Exp Hematol* 36:799, 2008.
22. Grozovsky R, Begonja AJ, Liu K, et al: The Ashwell-Morell receptor regulates hepatic thrombopoietin production via JAK2-STAT3 signaling. *Nat Med* 21:47, 2015.
23. Griesshammer M, Bangerter M, Sauer T, et al: Aetiology and clinical significance of thrombocytosis: Analysis of 732 patients with an elevated platelet count. *J Intern Med* 245:295, 1999.
24. Kishimoto T: The biology of interleukin-6. *Blood* 74:1, 1989.
25. Asano S, Okano A, Ozawa K, et al: In vivo effects of recombinant human interleukin 6 in primates: Stimulated production of platelets. *Blood* 75:1602, 1990.
26. Ishibashi T, Kimura H, Shikama Y, et al: Interleukin-6 is a potent thrombopoietic factor *in vivo* in mice. *Blood* 74:1241, 1989.
27. Naka T, Nishimoto N, Kishimoto T: The paradigm of IL-6: From basic science to medicine. *Arthritis Res* 4(Suppl 3):S233, 2002.
28. Sehgal PB: Regulation of IL6 gene expression. *Res Immunol* 143:724, 1992.
29. Gainsford T, Nandurkar H, Metcalf D, et al: The residual megakaryocyte and platelet production in c-Mpl-deficient mice is not dependent on the actions of interleukin-6, interleukin-11, or leukemia inhibitory factor. *Blood* 95:528, 2000.
30. Wolber EM, Fandrey J, Frackowski U, Jelkmann W: Hepatic thrombopoietin mRNA is increased in acute inflammation. *Thromb Haemost* 86:1421, 2001.
31. Heits F, Stahl M, Ludwig D, et al: Elevated serum thrombopoietin and interleukin-6 concentrations in thrombocytosis associated with inflammatory bowel disease. *J Interferon Cytokine Res* 19:757, 1999.
32. Ishiguro A, Suzuki Y, Mito M, et al: Elevation of serum thrombopoietin precedes thrombocytosis in acute infections. *Br J Haematol* 116:612, 2002.
33. Ceresa IF, Noris P, Ambaglio C, et al: Thrombopoietin is not uniquely responsible for thrombocytosis in inflammatory disorders. *Platelets* 18:579, 2007.
34. Wolber EM, Jelkmann W: Interleukin-6 increases thrombopoietin production in human hepatoma cells HepG2 and Hep3B. *J Interferon Cytokine Res* 20:499, 2000.
35. Kaser A, Brandacher G, Steurer W, et al: Interleukin-6 stimulates thrombopoiesis through thrombopoietin: Role in inflammatory thrombocytosis. *Blood* 98:2720, 2001.
36. Theofilopoulos AN, Baccala R, Beutler B, Kono DH: Type I interferons (alpha/beta) in immunity and autoimmunity. *Annu Rev Immunol* 23:307, 2005.
37. Young HA, Bream JH: IFN-gamma: Recent advances in understanding regulation of expression, biological functions, and clinical applications. *Curr Top Microbiol Immunol* 316:97, 2007.
38. Schoenborn JR, Wilson CB: Regulation of interferon-gamma during innate and adaptive immune responses. *Adv Immunol* 96:41, 2007.
39. Choi I, Muta K, Wickrema A, et al: Interferon gamma delays apoptosis of mature erythroid progenitor cells in the absence of erythropoietin. *Blood* 95:3742, 2000.

40. Yu JM, Emmons RV, Hanazono Y, et al: Expression of interferon-gamma by stromal cells inhibits murine long-term repopulating hematopoietic stem cell activity. *Exp Hematol* 27:895, 1999.

41. Young NS, Scheinberg P, Calado RT: Aplastic anemia. *Curr Opin Hematol* 15:162, 2008.

42. Tsuji-Takayama K, Tahata H, Harashima A, et al: Interferon-gamma enhances megakaryocyte colony-stimulating activity in murine bone marrow cells. *J Interferon Cytokine Res* 16:701, 1996.

43. Huang Z, Richmond TD, Muntean AG, et al: STAT1 promotes megakaryopoiesis downstream of GATA-1 in mice. *J Clin Invest* 117:3890, 2007.

44. Kulnigg-Dabsch S, Schmid W, Howaldt S, et al: Iron deficiency generates secondary thrombocytosis and platelet activation in IBD: The randomized, controlled thrombo-VIT trial. *Inflamm Bowel Dis* 19:1609, 2013.

45. Akan H, Güven N, Aydogdu I, et al: Thrombopoietic cytokines in patients with iron deficiency anemia with or without thrombocytosis. *Acta Haematol* 103:152, 2000.

46. Loo M, Beguin Y: The effect of recombinant human erythropoietin on platelet counts is strongly modulated by the adequacy of iron supply. *Blood* 93:3286, 1999.

47. Bilic E, Bilic E: Amino acid sequence homology of thrombopoietin and erythropoietin may explain thrombocytosis in children with iron deficiency anemia. *J Pediatr Hematol Oncol* 25:675, 2003.

48. Geddis AE, Kaushansky K: Cross reactivity between erythropoietin and thrombopoietin at the level of Mpl does not account for the thrombocytosis seen in iron deficiency. *J Pediatr Hematol Oncol* 25:919, 2003.

49. Singh AK, Szczech L, Tang KL, et al: Correction of anemia with epoetin alfa in chronic kidney disease. *N Engl J Med* 355:2085, 2006.

50. Drüeke TB, Locatelli F, Clyne N, et al: Normalization of hemoglobin level in patients with chronic kidney disease and anemia. *N Engl J Med* 355:2071, 2006.

51. Rossert J, Levin A, Roger SD, et al: Effect of early correction of anemia on the progression of CKD. *Am J Kidney Dis* 47:738, 2006.

52. Streja E, Kovesdy CP, Greenland S, et al: Erythropoietin, iron depletion, and relative thrombocytosis: A possible explanation for hemoglobin-survival paradox in hemodialysis. *Am J Kidney Dis* 52:727, 2008.

53. Geddis AE, Fox NE, Hitchcock, I: Erythropoietin stimulates thrombopoiesis in the absence of c-Mpl signaling. *Blood* 112(Suppl 1):2451, 2008.

54. Rodríguez-Liñares B, Watson SP: Thrombopoietin potentiates activation of human platelets in association with JAK2 and TYK2 phosphorylation. *Biochem J* 316:93, 1996.

55. Brines M, Grasso G, Fiordaliso F, et al: Erythropoietin mediates tissue protection through an erythropoietin and common beta-subunit heteroreceptor. *Proc Natl Acad Sci U S A* 101:14907, 2004.

56. Osselaer JC, Jamart J, Scheiff JM: Platelet distribution width for differential diagnosis of thrombocytosis. *Clin Chem* 43:1072, 1997.

57. Kaushansky K: On the molecular origins of the chronic myeloproliferative disorders: It all makes sense. *Blood* 105:4187, 2005.

58. Pikman Y, Lee BH, Mercher T, et al: MPLW515L is a novel somatic activating mutation in myelofibrosis with myeloid metaplasia. *PLoS Med* 3:e270, 2006.

# CHAPTER 10
# HEREDITARY QUALITATIVE PLATELET DISORDERS

A. Koneti Rao and Barry S. Coller

## SUMMARY

Abnormalities of platelet function manifest themselves primarily as excessive hemorrhage at mucocutaneous sites, with ecchymoses, petechiae, epistaxis, gingival hemorrhage, and menorrhagia most common. Both quantitative and qualitative platelet abnormalities can produce these symptoms, so it is necessary to exclude thrombocytopenia (Chap. 7) by performing a platelet count. Chapter 11 discusses acquired qualitative platelet abnormalities, and this chapter discusses the hereditary qualitative platelet abnormalities.

The hereditary qualitative platelet disorders can be classified according to the major locus of the defect (see Table 10–1 and Fig. 10–1). Thus, abnormalities of platelet glycoproteins, platelet granules, and signal transduction and secretion can all result in hemorrhagic diatheses and prolonged bleeding times. Glanzmann thrombasthenia results from abnormalities in one of two integrin subunits, either $\alpha_{IIb}$ (glycoprotein [GP] IIb) or $\beta_3$ (GPIIIa), resulting in loss or dysfunction of the $\alpha_{IIb}\beta_3$ (GPIIb/IIIa) receptor. This results in a profound defect in platelet aggregation and secondary defects in platelet adhesion, secretion, and platelet coagulant activity. Heterozygous gain-of-function mutations in $\alpha_{IIb}\beta_3$ can result in a syndrome of macrothrombocytopenia. Loss of the platelet GPIb–IX–V complex because of abnormalities in GPIb$\alpha$, GPIb$\beta$, or GPIX results in the Bernard-Soulier syndrome, which is characterized by giant platelets and modest thrombocytopenia. The major defect is in platelet adhesion because of a decrease in platelet interactions with von Willebrand factor, but abnormalities in $\alpha_{IIb}\beta_3$ activation and thrombin-induced aggregation are also present. A gain-of-function defect in GPIb$\alpha$ (platelet-type [pseudo-] von Willebrand disease) can produce a hemorrhagic disorder via depletion of high-molecular-weight von Willebrand multimers. Inherited defects in platelet dense or $\alpha$ granules, agonist receptors, or proteins and mechanisms involved in signal transduction and secretion also lead to platelet dysfunction and produce hemorrhagic symptoms.

Abnormalities of platelet coagulant activity, that is, the ability of platelets to facilitate thrombin generation (Chap. 2), can lead to a hemorrhagic diathesis. Impaired platelet function may occur in association with mutations in transcription factors RUNX1, GATA-1, FLI-1, and GFI1B, and these patients have thrombocytopenia as well.

## ● PLATELET FUNCTION IN HEMOSTASIS

Abnormalities of platelet function manifest themselves primarily as excessive hemorrhage at mucocutaneous sites, with ecchymoses, petechiae, epistaxis, gingival hemorrhage, and menorrhagia being most common. Mild platelet function abnormalities will not cause spontaneous bleeding but may cause (excessive) hemorrhage after trauma or medical interventions. Both quantitative and qualitative platelet abnormalities can produce these symptoms, so it is necessary to exclude thrombocytopenia (Chap. 7) by performing a platelet count. Although no longer performed widely, a prolonged bleeding time in a patient with a normal platelet count is suggestive of a qualitative platelet abnormality. Some patients may have abnormalities in both platelet number and function. Chapter 11 discusses acquired qualitative platelet abnormalities, and this chapter discusses hereditary qualitative platelet abnormalities.

Following injury to the blood vessel, platelets adhere to exposed subendothelium by a process that involves, among other events, the interaction of a plasma protein, von Willebrand factor (VWF), and a specific glycoprotein complex on the platelet surface, the glycoprotein (GP) Ib–IX–V complex. Adhesion is followed by recruitment of additional platelets that form clumps (aggregation), which involves binding of fibrinogen to specific platelet surface receptors, a complex comprised of integrin $\alpha_{IIb}\beta_3$ (GPIIb/IIIa). Platelet activation is required for fibrinogen binding; resting platelets do not bind fibrinogen. Activated platelets release the contents of their granules (secretion), including adenosine diphosphate (ADP) and serotonin from the dense granules, which causes the recruitment of additional platelets. Moreover, platelets play a major role in coagulation mechanisms; several key enzymatic reactions occur on the platelet membrane phospholipid surface. A number of physiologic agonists interact with platelet surface receptors to induce responses, including a change in platelet shape from discoid to spherical (shape change), aggregation, secretion, and thromboxane $A_2$ (TXA$_2$) production. The binding of agonists to their platelet receptors initiates numerous intracellular events (Chap. 2) including the production or release of several messenger molecules. One pathway leads to the hydrolysis of phosphoinositide (PI) by phospholipase C, leading to the formation of diacylglycerol and inositol 1,4,5-triphosphate [IP$_3$]). These and other mediators induce or modulate the various platelet responses of Ca$^{2+}$ mobilization, protein phosphorylation, aggregation, secretion, and thromboxane production. Numerous other mechanisms, such as activation of tyrosine kinases and phosphatases, are also triggered by platelet activation (Chap. 2). Inherited or acquired defects in the above and other platelet mechanisms may lead to impaired platelet function and a bleeding diathesis.

**Acronyms and Abbreviations:** ADP, adenosine diphosphate; BLOC, biogenesis of lysosome-related organelles complex; BSS, Bernard-Soulier syndrome; βTG, β-thromboglobulin; cAMP, cyclic adenosine monophosphate; EDTA, ethylenediaminetetraacetic acid; GFI1b, growth factor independent 1B; GPS, gray platelet syndrome; GT, Glanzmann thrombasthenia; HLA, human leukocyte antigen; HPS, Hermansky-Pudlak syndrome; Ig, immunoglobulin; LAD, leukocyte adhesion deficiency; MIDAS, metal ion-dependent adhesion site; PAR, protease-activated receptor; PF4, platelet factor 4; PKC; protein kinase C; PLC, phospholipase C; rFVIIa, recombinant factor VIIa; TGF, transforming growth factor; TXA$_2$, thromboxane A$_2$; VWD, von Willebrand disease; VWF, von Willebrand factor.

## ● CLASSIFICATION OF HEREDITARY QUALITATIVE PLATELET DISORDERS

The hereditary qualitative platelet disorders can be classified according to the major locus of the defect (Table 10–1 and Fig. 10–1). Glanzmann thrombasthenia (GT) is caused by abnormalities in either integrin $\alpha_{IIb}$ (GPIIb)

**TABLE 10–1.** Inherited Disorders of Platelet Function

I. Abnormalities of glycoprotein adhesion receptors

  A. Integrin $\alpha_{IIb}\beta_3$ (glycoprotein IIb/IIIa; CD41/CD61): Glanzmann thrombasthenia

  B. Glycoproteins Ib (CD42b,c)/IX (CD42a)/V: Bernard-Soulier syndrome

  C. Glycoprotein Ibα (CD42b,c): Platelet-type (pseudo-) von Willebrand disease

  D. Integrin $\alpha_2\beta_1$ (glycoprotein Ia/IIa; VLA-2; CD49b/CD29)

  E. CD36 (glycoprotein IV)

  F. Glycoprotein VI

II. Abnormalities of platelet granules

  A. δ-Storage pool deficiency

  B. Gray platelet syndrome (α-storage pool deficiency)

  C. α,δ-Storage pool deficiency

  D. Quebec platelet disorder

III. Abnormalities of platelet signaling and secretion

  A. Defects in platelet agonist receptors or agonist-specific signal transduction (thromboxane A$_2$ receptor defect, adenosine diphosphate [ADP] receptor defects [P2Y$_{12}$, P2X$_1$], epinephrine receptor defect, platelet activating factor receptor defect)

  B. Defects in guanosine triphosphate (GTP)–binding proteins (Gαq deficiency, Gαs hyperfunction and genetic variation in extra-large Gαs, Gαi1 deficiency, CaLDAG-GEFI deficiency)

  C. Phospholipase C (PLC)-$\beta_2$ deficiency and defects in PLC activation

  D. Defects in protein phosphorylation protein kinase C (PKC)-θ deficiency

  E. Defects in arachidonic acid metabolism and thromboxane production (phospholipase A$_2$ deficiency cyclooxygenase [prostaglandin H$_2$ sythase-1 deficiency], thromboxane sythase deficiency)

IV. Abnormalities of platelet coagulant activity (Scott syndrome)

V. Abnormalities of a cytoskeletal structural protein: $\beta_1$ tubulin, filamin A

VI. Abnormalities in cytoskeletal linking proteins

  A. Wiskott-Aldrich syndrome protein (WASP)

  B. Kindlin-3: Leukocyte adhesion defect (LAD)-III; LAD-1 variant; integrin activation deficiency disease defect (IADD)

VII. Abnormalities of transcription factors leading to functional defects

  A. RUNX1 (familial platelet dysfunction with predisposition to acute myelogenous leukemia)

  B. GATA-1

  C. FLI1 (dimorphic dysmorphic platelets with giant α granules and thrombocytopenia; Paris-Trousseau/Jacobsen syndrome)

  D. GFI1B

platelet adhesion owing to a decrease in platelet interactions with VWF. A gain-of-function defect in GPIbα (platelet-type [pseudo-] von Willebrand disease [VWD]) can also produce a hemorrhagic disorder via depletion of high-molecular-weight VWF multimers. Defects in secretion of granule contents because of deficiencies in the granules or in the mechanisms that mediate secretion results in impaired platelet function. Inherited defects in agonist receptors or proteins or mediators involved in signal transduction or thromboxane synthesis may also produce hemorrhagic symptoms. Abnormalities of platelet coagulant activity, that is, the ability of platelets to facilitate thrombin generation (Chap. 3), and in cytoskeletal-linking proteins can also lead to a hemorrhagic diathesis. Lastly, it is becoming clear that some patients may have abnormalities in multiple aspects of platelet function and number related to a mutation in a hematopoietic transcription factor that regulates gene expression in megakaryocytes and platelets.

## CLINICAL MANIFESTATIONS

Disorders of platelet function are characterized by highly variable mucocutaneous bleeding manifestations and excessive hemorrhage following surgical procedures or trauma. These include ecchymoses, petechiae, epistaxis, gingival bleeding, and menorrhagia. Spontaneous hemarthrosis are distinctly rare, distinguishing them from the hemophilias, and deep hematomas and spontaneous central nervous system bleeding are highly unusual in these patients. Postpartum hemorrhage and postsurgical bleeding may be severe in some patients. In general, most patients with platelet function defects have mild to moderate bleeding manifestations, but bleeding manifestations may be severe in some entities, such as GT and BSS. Individual patients with the same functional defect or even the same genetic defect may also vary in the intensity of bleeding manifestations, suggesting one or more disease-modifying genes exist. Moreover, the severity of bleeding symptoms may vary over the lifetime of the same individual, implying that factors in addition to the platelet defect may be contributing to the bleeding risk. Sometimes, a mild platelet function defect becomes clinically manifest when the patient uses medication interfering with primary hemostasis (e.g., nonsteroidal antiinflammatory drugs [NSAIDs]).

Although normal in many of the inherited platelet function defects, the platelet count may be decreased in some entities, such as BSS and the gray platelet syndrome (GPS), and in association with mutations in hematopoietic transcription factors. Most patients with platelet function defects, but not all, have a prolonged bleeding time, a test no longer available in most centers because of its inherent inaccuracies. *In vitro* platelet aggregation and secretion studies provide evidence for the dysfunction but are not generally predictive of the severity of clinical manifestations. In some patients, such as those with abnormal platelet coagulant activities, these studies may be normal. Some patients with platelet dysfunction are initially detected through abnormalities on testing with the platelet function analyzer (PFA-100).

## GENERAL APPROACH TO PATIENTS WITH MUCOCUTANEOUS BLEEDING SYMPTOMS FOR ABNORMALITIES IN PLATELET NUMBER OR FUNCTION

Platelet disorders are characterized by alterations in platelet number or function or both. A general approach is shown in Fig. 10-1. A reduced platelet count can occur as an isolated platelet disorder (inherited or acquired) or with evidence of a concomitant defect in platelet function. Platelet size and examination of the blood film may provide insights

or $\beta_3$ (GPIIIa), resulting in loss or dysfunction of the integrin $\alpha_{IIb}\beta_3$ receptor. This results in a profound defect in platelet aggregation and secondary defects in platelet adhesion, secretion, and coagulant activity. Loss of the platelet GPIb–IX–V complex because of abnormalities in GPIbα, GPIbβ, or GPIX results in the Bernard-Soulier syndrome (BSS), which is characterized by giant platelets and thrombocytopenia. The major defect is in

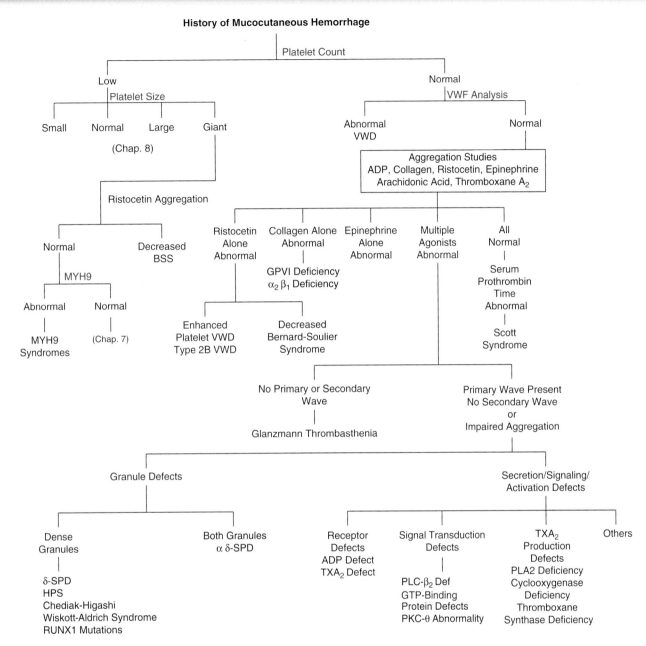

**Figure 10–1.** Evaluation of patients for inherited abnormalities in platelet number or function. The major and well-recognized entities are shown here. A reduced platelet count occurs in patients with purely quantitative platelet disorders (inherited or acquired) as well as in patients who have inherited qualitative platelet disorders. Chapter 7 discusses inherited thrombocytopenias. Notable among patients with thrombocytopenia and inherited platelet dysfunction is the Bernard-Soulier syndrome (BSS), which is characterized by giant platelets. Patients with the gray platelet syndrome are characterized by thrombocytopenia and gray appearance of platelets on the blood smear due to paucity of granules. Platelet aggregation studies can provide clues regarding the nature of the underlying platelet abnormality. Decreased response to ristocetin alone with normal responses to other agonists is found in BSS and von Willebrand disease (VWD; type I and type III). The response to ristocetin is enhanced in VWD type IIB and the platelet-type VWD. Impaired response to collagen or epinephrine alone may suggest a defect in their respective receptors. Patients with adenosine diphosphate (ADP) and thromboxane receptor defects have impaired responses to multiple agonists because of the feedback amplification provided by ADP and thromboxane $A_2$ (TXA$_2$) when activated by different agonists. Absence of both primary and secondary waves of aggregation in response to all physiologic agonists occurs in Glanzmann thrombasthenia (GT). A heterogeneous group of platelet defects is characterized by a decreased secondary wave of platelet aggregation in response to ADP and epinephrine and diminished responses to low doses of collagen, TXA$_2$, and thrombin. They can be broadly separated into granule defects (involving dense [$\delta$] or both dense and $\alpha$ granules) and defects in the platelet secretion or release reaction associated with normal dense granule stores. The granule defects may occur in isolation or in association with other syndromes. Secretion abnormalities arise from defects in mechanisms that regulate the release of granule contents and include defects at the level of platelet receptors (ADP, TXA$_2$), signaling events involving guanosine triphosphate (GTP)-binding proteins that link surface receptors to intracellular enzymes, phospholipase C activation, and protein phosphorylation (protein kinase C [PKC]-$\theta$). They may also arise from defects in TXA$_2$ synthesis because of deficiencies of phospholipase A$_2$ (PLA$_2$), cyclooxygenase, or thromboxane synthase. Patients with Scott syndrome are characterized by a normal bleeding time, normal responses in aggregation studies, and a shortened prothrombin time, which reflects the defect in the platelet–coagulant protein interactions. Additional details on the various entities are described in the section "General Approach to Patients with Mucocutaneous Bleeding Symptoms for Abnormalities in Platelet Number or Function." GP, glycoprotein; PLA2, phospholipase A2; PLC, phospholipase C; SPD, storage pool deficiency; u-PA, urokinase plasminogen activator; VWF, von Willebrand factor.

into the underlying mechanism or cause. Platelet size provides clues in some entities (Chap. 7).[1,2] Decreased platelet size is characteristic of the Wiskott-Aldrich syndrome. In the Paris-Trousseau/Jacobsen syndrome, thrombocytopenia is associated with giant $\alpha$ granules in a subpopulation of platelets in association with mutations in the transcription factor *FLI1*. Transcription factor *RUNX1* mutations are associated with familial thrombocytopenia, abnormal platelet function, and predisposition to leukemia. Large platelets that lack the purple granules on the peripheral smear are observed in GPS ($\alpha$-storage pool disease). The diagnosis is obtained with biochemical analysis of $\alpha$-granule contents. Patients with platelet-type (pseudo-) VWD and type 2b VWD have moderate thrombocytopenia and large platelets. Studies of GPIb function and biochemistry establish the diagnosis. Patients who are hemizygous for GPIb$\beta$ because of deletion of 22q11.2, those with mutations in transcription factor *GATA-1* or $\beta_1$ tubulin (R318W), and some patients who are heterozygous for defects in GPIb/IX have variable thrombocytopenia and large platelets. Mutations that activate $\alpha_{IIb}\beta_3$ are also associated with large platelets and thrombocytopenia. The platelets in BSS are truly giant; the diagnosis is confirmed with biochemical and functional analyses of the GPIb–IX–V complex.

A variety of methods have been developed to assess platelet function, and new instrumentation continues to be developed.[3–8] Platelet aggregation studies performed using platelet-rich plasma can loosely separate patients into those with defects in the primary wave of platelet aggregation (dependent on fibrinogen, VWF, their respective receptors, or agonist receptors for collagen, ADP, or TXA$_2$) and those with defects in the secondary wave of aggregation. Enhanced ristocetin-induced platelet aggregation at low doses of ristocetin is characteristic of patients with platelet-type VWD (who have a defect in the GPIb receptor) and patients with type 2b VWD (who have gain-of-function defect in VWF) (Chap. 16). These two diseases differ in the binding of the patient's VWF to normal platelets or the ability of purified VWF, cryoprecipitate, or asialo-VWF to aggregate patient platelets; the diagnosis of platelet-type VWD or its confirmation requires genetic analysis of GPIb.

Neither ristocetin nor the snake venom botrocetin induces platelet aggregation if the plasma lacks functional VWF, as in VWD (Chap. 16), or if the platelets lack functional GPIb–IX complexes, as in BSS. The defect in VWD, but not BSS, can be corrected by adding normal plasma or purified VWF. Direct analysis of VWF and the platelet GPIb–IX complex is used to confirm the diagnosis.

Patients whose plasma lacks fibrinogen (afibrinogenemia; Chap. 15) or whose platelets cannot bind fibrinogen because of abnormal $\alpha_{IIb}\beta_3$ receptors (GT) or inability to activate integrin $\alpha_{IIb}\beta_3$ (leukocyte adhesion deficiency [LAD]-3) as the result of a kindlin-3 abnormality will have no primary wave of platelet aggregation in response to all physiologic agonists, including ADP, epinephrine, collagen, TXA$_2$, and thrombin. Simple coagulation tests (prothrombin time, partial thromboplastin time, and measurement of plasma fibrinogen) and analysis of platelet integrin $\alpha_{IIb}\beta_3$ receptors and kindlin-3 can differentiate between these two groups. Isolated defects in the primary response to collagen have been observed in patients with abnormalities in platelet integrin $\alpha_2\beta_1$ (GPIa/IIa) or GPVI. Platelet glycoprotein analysis can separate these from each other. Because antibodies to GPVI can result in receptor depletion from circulating platelets, a search for anti-GPVI should be undertaken in patients with reduced platelet GPVI. Defects in ADP, epinephrine, or TXA$_2$ receptors will result in decreased platelet aggregation in response to the specific agonist. However, patients with isolated ADP and TXA$_2$ receptor abnormalities have impaired aggregation in response to other agonists as well because of the feedback potentiation provided by ADP and TXA$_2$.

A very heterogeneous group of platelet defects can result in a decreased secondary wave of platelet aggregation in response to ADP and epinephrine and diminished responses to low doses of collagen

and thrombin. They can be separated into granule defects and defects in platelet secretion or the release reaction. Operationally, these two groups can be separated on the basis of their release of dense granule contents in response to high doses of thrombin. High-dose thrombin activation can overcome most or all of the release reaction (secretion) abnormalities, so platelets from patients with these disorders will release normal amounts of granule contents; in contrast, patients with reduced granule contents have abnormal granule release responses even when using high doses of thrombin. $\alpha$-Granule contents and dense-body contents can be measured immunologically and biochemically; electron microscopy can establish granule defects. Specific analysis of the genes or proteins implicated in the different granule biogenesis abnormalities (Wiskott-Aldrich syndrome [*WASP*], Hermansky-Pudlak syndrome [*HPS1–9*], Chédiak-Higashi syndrome [*LYST*], Paris-Trousseau/Jacobson syndrome [*FLI1*], and inherited platelet disorder with predisposition to leukemia [*RUNX1*]) can establish the diagnosis. The Quebec platelet disorder is characterized by increased urokinase plasminogen activator (u-PA) in $\alpha$ granules and degradation of several $\alpha$-granule proteins. The diagnosis can be established by immunoblot analysis or analysis of u-PA activity and confirmed by genetic analysis of *u-PA*. Secretion abnormalities arise as a result of defects in mechanisms that regulate the secretion of granule contents and may include abnormalities at various levels, including surface receptors, guanosine triphosphate (GTP)-binding proteins that link surface receptors to intracellular enzymes, phospholipase C (PLC) activation, and protein phosphorylation (protein kinase C [PKC]-$\theta$). They also arise from defects in TXA$_2$ synthesis caused by deficiencies of phospholipase A$_2$ (PLA$_2$), cyclooxygenase, or thromboxane synthase. Specific studies on signal transduction mechanisms, PI metabolism, Ca$^{2+}$ mobilization, protein phosphorylation, and thromboxane production are needed to define these defects. Because transcription factor abnormalities can affect the expression of multiple proteins involved in megakaryopoiesis and platelet function, they can simultaneously produce alterations in platelet count, structure, and function.

In the disorder of platelet coagulant activity (Scott syndrome), platelet aggregation studies are normal and the serum prothrombin time is the preferred screening assay. Other tests of platelet coagulant activity, microvesiculation, and phospholipid transfer are used to establish the diagnosis.

The introduction of microfluidic multiparameter assessments of platelet function[7,8] and advances in proteomics, RNA expression profiling, and DNA sequencing are shifting the diagnosis of platelet function disorders from a target gene approach to one in which unbiased comprehensive functional and genetic analyses are employed. These methods have identified mutations in *RUNX1* and *FLI-1*[9] in patients with platelet function disorders, in *NBEAL2* in GPS,[10–12] in *TMEM16* in Scott syndrome,[13] and in *RBM8A* in thrombocytopenia with absent radii (TAR) syndrome.[14,15] Many additional genetic alterations, including ones that affect multiple systems, are likely to be identified in the near future as these techniques are employed more broadly.

# ● ABNORMALITIES OF ADHESION RECEPTORS

## INTEGRIN $\alpha_{IIb}\beta_3$ (GLYCOPROTEIN IIB/IIIA; CD41/CD61)–GLANZMANN THROMBASTHENIA

### Definition and History

GT is an inherited hemorrhagic disorder characterized by a severe reduction in, or absence of, platelet aggregation in response to multiple physiologic agonists as a result of qualitative or quantitative abnormalities of platelet integrin $\alpha_{IIb}$ (GPIIb; CD41) and/or integrin $\beta_3$ (GPIIIa; CD61).[16]

In 1918, Eduard Glanzmann, a Swiss pediatrician, described a group of patients with hemorrhagic symptoms and a defect in platelet function, namely the ability to retract clots ("weak" platelets or thrombasthenia).[17] Subsequent studies demonstrated that thrombasthenic patients have prolonged bleeding times and that their platelets fail to aggregate in response to physiologic agonists[18-21] and have markedly reduced[18,20-22] platelet fibrinogen. In the mid-1970s, Nurden and Caen[23] and Phillips and colleagues[24] discovered that thrombasthenic platelets are deficient in both integrin $\alpha_{IIb}$ and $\beta_3$. Later studies demonstrated that integrin $\alpha_{IIb}$ and $\beta_3$ form a calcium-dependent complex in the platelet membrane that functions as a receptor for fibrinogen and other adhesive glycoproteins.[25-28] Cloning and sequencing of the complementary DNAs for integrin $\alpha_{IIb}$[29] and $\beta_3$[30] identified them as separate protein subunits that are members of the integrin receptor superfamily[31] and permitted the molecular biological characterization of patients with the disorder (see database of Glanzmann patients at https://glanzmann.mcw.edu/).

### Etiology and Pathogenesis

GT is a rare disorder characterized by autosomal recessive inheritance with a worldwide distribution. In regions where consanguineous matings are common, groups of patients with the disorder have been identified, and in several populations, founder mutations have been identified by analyzing polymorphisms in the DNA surrounding the affected mutation. These include 42 patients from South India; 39 patients from the Iraqi-Jewish population in Israel; 46 Arab patients from Israel,

Jordan, and Saudi Arabia; 30 patients from Italy; a smaller number of patients from three Gypsy families; and 43 patients from Pakistan.[22,32-40] Perhaps the highest frequency of a GT mutation is found in the Iraqi-Jewish population where the most common mutation causing GT was found in six of 700 individuals.[39]

The platelet integrin $\alpha_{IIb}\beta_3$ receptor is required for platelet aggregation induced by all physiologic agonists (ADP, epinephrine, thrombin, collagen, TXA$_2$) (Chap. 2).[41] Consequently, abnormalities in the receptor result in a failure of platelet plug formation at sites of vascular injury and excessive bleeding.

The integrin $\alpha_{IIb}\beta_3$ receptor is also responsible for the uptake of fibrinogen from plasma into $\alpha$ granules[42]; hence, patients with GT have markedly reduced platelet fibrinogen.[18,20,21,43,44] Clot retraction requires platelets with intact integrin $\alpha_{IIb}\beta_3$ receptors[45,46] and is, therefore, usually abnormal in GT.[18]

Defects in either integrin $\alpha_{IIb}$ or $\beta_3$ result in the same functional defect because both subunits are required for receptor function (Chap. 2). Biosynthetic studies indicate that integrin $\alpha_{IIb}$ and $\beta_3$ form a complex soon after protein synthesis in the rough endoplasmic reticulum[47-49]; subsequent posttranslational processing[50] and transport to the platelet membrane require that the complex be intact (Fig. 10-2).[51,52] Complex formation protects each of the glycoproteins from proteolytic digestion,[47-50] so if either integrin $\alpha_{IIb}$ or $\beta_3$ is absent or unable to form a normal complex, the other subunit will be rapidly degraded, most likely through a proteasomal mechanism. Thus, a deficiency in either glycoprotein produces a deficiency in both. Because complex formation and vesicular transport are also required for proteolytic processing of pro-$\alpha_{IIb}$ into its constituent $\alpha_{IIb}\alpha$ and $\alpha_{IIb}\beta$ subunits,[50] if these processes

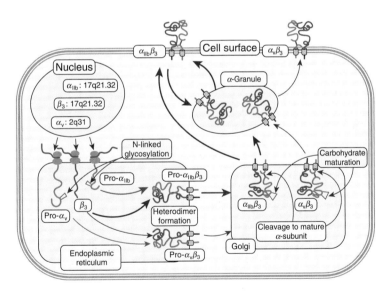

**Figure 10-2.** Biogenesis of integrin $\alpha_{IIb}\beta_3$ and integrin $\alpha_V\beta_3$ receptors. The nuclear genes for integrins $\alpha_{IIb}$ (chromosome localization 17q21.32; gene designation *ITGA2B*; 30 exons), $\alpha_V$ (2q31; *ITGAV*; 30 exons), and $\beta_3$ (17q21.32; *ITGB3*; 14 exons) are transcribed into messenger RNA and translated by ribosomes attached to the membranes of the endoplasmic reticulum (ER). The proteins undergo initial glycosylation and form the integrins $\alpha_{IIb}\beta_3$ and $\alpha_V\beta_3$ heterodimers in the ER. It is presumed that many more integrin $\alpha_{IIb}\beta_3$ complexes form than $\alpha_V\beta_3$ complexes because the final copy number of platelet integrin $\alpha_{IIb}\beta_3$ receptors is approximately 100,000, whereas it is only 50 to 100 for $\alpha_V\beta_3$. This is shown schematically by the differences in the width of the arrows depicting integrin $\alpha_{IIb}\beta_3$ versus $\alpha_V\beta_3$ complex formation. The heteroduplexes are transported to the Golgi where the carbohydrate chains undergo modification to their mature structures and both $\alpha_{IIb}$ and $\alpha_V$ subunits undergo proteolytic cleavage within a disulfide-bonded loop, resulting in two-chain forms of the receptor subunits. Mature integrin $\alpha_{IIb}\beta_3$ receptors are transported to $\alpha$-granule membranes, where they undergo cycling to and from the plasma membrane. This process results in the internalization of fibrinogen and perhaps other plasma proteins. Integrin $\alpha_{IIb}\beta_3$ may be transported directly to the plasma membrane and is transported to $\alpha$-granule membranes. Of the total of approximately 100,000 integrin $\alpha_{IIb}\beta_3$ receptors, approximately two-thirds are on the surface at any given time and the remaining one-third can be brought to the surface by platelet activation. The distribution of integrin $\alpha_V\beta_3$ between the plasma membrane and $\alpha$ granules and the potential cycling of the receptors between $\alpha$ granules and the plasma membrane have not be defined. *(Used with permission from Dr. W. Beau Mitchell, New York Blood Center, New York, NY.)*

do not occur normally, the very small amount of residual integrin $\alpha_{IIb}$ will be pro-$\alpha_{IIb}$, not mature $\alpha_{IIb}$.[53] Pro-$\alpha_{IIb}$ has been reported to bind to the membrane-bound endoplasmic reticulum chaperone calnexin, providing a potential mechanism for assessing whether the protein has undergone proper folding (calnexin cycle) and perhaps explaining how the receptor adopts a bent configuration.[54,55]

Integrin $\beta_3$ (GPIIIa) can also combine with the integrin $\alpha_V$ (CD51) subunit to form the integrin $\alpha_V\beta_3$ "vitronectin" receptor[30,56,57] (see Fig. 10–2; Chap. 2). This receptor can bind many of the same adhesive glycoproteins as integrin $\alpha_{IIb}\beta_3$, although there are some differences in ligand preference and binding sequences.[57–61] A small number of integrin $\alpha_V\beta_3$ receptors are present on platelets (50 to 100 per platelet)[60,62,63]; osteoclasts, endothelial cells, macrophages, vascular smooth muscle, and uterine cells, among others, also have integrin $\alpha_V\beta_3$ receptors.[64,65] In general, GT patients with defects in integrin $\beta_3$ also are deficient in integrin $\alpha_V\beta_3$, whereas patients with defects in integrin $\alpha_{IIb}$ have either normal or increased numbers of platelet integrin $\alpha_V\beta_3$ receptors.[60,63,64,66–68] One exception to this rule is a patient with a defect in $\beta_3$ (H280P) that interferes with integrin $\alpha_{IIb}\beta_3$ biogenesis to a much greater extent than integrin $\alpha_V\beta_3$ biogenesis.[69] At present, there is no evidence that patients who lack integrin $\alpha_V\beta_3$ receptors in addition to lacking integrin $\alpha_{IIb}\beta_3$ receptors have a more severe hemorrhagic diathesis or suffer from any other abnormalities, perhaps because alternative receptors containing integrin $\alpha_V$ associated with other $\beta$ subunits can substitute for integrin $\alpha_V\beta_3$.[63] Upregulation of integrin $\alpha_2\beta_1$ on osteoclasts of Iraqi-Jewish patients with GT has been reported as a potential compensatory mechanism to explain the lack of bone changes despite the deficiency in osteoclast integrin $\alpha_V\beta_3$.[70]

The molecular biologic abnormalities in more than 100 patients with GT have been identified, and they are listed in an Internet database that is updated continuously[71] (https://glanzmann.mcw.edu/). Figure 10–3 contains information on mutations of particular interest.

Of note, many of the patients with identified mutations are compound heterozygotes rather than homozygotes, indicating that a sizable number of silent carriers are present in the population. Where consanguinity is common, the disorder is more likely to be caused by a homozygous mutation arising in a founder, but even under these circumstances, more than one mutation may be present. Thus, in the Iraqi-Jewish population, in which consanguinity has been present from 586 BCE to the present, two separate mutations have been identified in more than one family.[39] Most of the missense mutations result in decreased expression of integrin $\alpha_{IIb}\beta_3$ on the surface of platelets. This probably reflects the stringent structural requirements for proper folding and complex formation.

**Mutations in Integrin $\alpha_{IIb}\beta_3$ Within the Metal Ion-Dependent Adhesion Site of Integrin $\beta_3$ and the Interface with the Integrin $\alpha_{IIb}$ $\beta$-Propeller** A metal coordination site or MIDAS domain, which is highly conserved in six integrin receptor $\alpha$-chain subunits and required for ligand binding, is also present in the $\beta$-A (or I-like) domain of the integrin $\beta_3$ subunit.[72] Mutagenesis and molecular modeling experiments suggested that a highly conserved D$x$S$x$S amino acid sequence[73] motif plus additional coordinating residues are brought together in the three-dimensional structure of the $\beta_3$ subunit to form a cation-binding sphere of the MIDAS domain,[74] and this was confirmed by the crystal structures of integrin $\alpha_V\beta_3$ and later integrin $\alpha_{IIb}\beta_3$ (see Chap. 2, Fig. 2–11, and Fig. 10–3).[75,76] Thus, the $\beta_3$ MIDAS is composed of Asp[119], Ser[121], Ser[123], Glu[220], and Asp[251]. A region originally termed the ligand-associated metal binding site (LIMBS) in integrin $\alpha_V\beta_3$,[77] but now termed the synergy metal binding site (SyMBS) in integrin $\alpha_{IIb}\beta_3$,[78] binds a $Ca^{2+}$ ion and is required for binding of ligands to the MIDAS. It is composed of atoms from D158, N215, D217, P219, and E220. Integrin $\beta_3$ residues 214 and 216 are in close proximity with both the SyMBS residues and the interface with the $\alpha_{IIb}$ subunit. Adjacent to the MIDAS domain is a metal ion site termed the ADMIDAS (adjacent to metal ion-dependent adhesion site), in which calcium is coordinated by

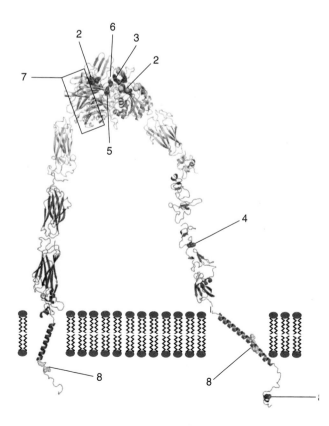

**Figure 10–3.** Diagram of $\alpha_{IIb}\beta_3$ structure and identification of select mutations causing Glanzmann thrombasthenia. The website https://glanzmann.mcw.edu/ contains a full listing of reported Glanzmann thrombasthenia mutations. The $\alpha_{IIb}\beta_3$ structure depicted is a composite of data from crystal and NMR structures, as well as molecular modeling of missing regions. Among the missense mutations identified are ones that (1) interfere with inside-out and outside-in signaling ($\beta_3$ S752P); (2) interfere with ligand binding to either the metal ion-dependent adhesion site (MIDAS) in $\beta_3$ ($\beta_3$ D119Y and D119N) or the $\alpha_{IIb}$ component of the ligand binding site (Y143H, P145L/A, insert R160/T161); (3) result in receptors that are sensitive to dissociation by divalent cation chelation ($\beta_3$ R214W, R214Q, R216Q); (4) result in a constitutively active receptor ($\beta_3$ C560R); (5) alter the interface between $\alpha_{IIb}$ and $\beta_3$ and disrupt ligand binding ($\beta_3$ L262Y); (6) result in a $\beta_3$ protein that can complex more effectively with $\alpha V$ than $\alpha_{IIb}$ (S162L, R216Q, H280P); or (7) alter the $\alpha_{IIb}$ propeller structure and prevent normal $\alpha_{IIb}\beta_3$ complex formation, processing, and/or transport. The mutations identified by number 8 in $\alpha_{IIb}$ (G991C and R995Q/W) and $\beta_3$ (L718P and D723H) are gain-of-function mutations associated with macro-/anisothrombocytopenia. (Reproduced with permission from Dr. Ana Negri based on PDBids 3FCS, 3G9W, 2K9J, 2KNC, and 2KV9 and molecular modeling of the missing segments of the $\alpha_{IIb}$ calf domain, the $\beta$3 hybrid domain, and the link between the $\beta$3 EGF-1 and EGF-2 domains.)

Ser[123], Asp[126], Asp[127], and Met[335] in unliganded integrin $\alpha_V\beta_3$ and integrin $\alpha_{IIb}\beta_3$, but Asp[251] substitutes for Met[335] in the ligand-bound structures of both integrin $\alpha_V\beta_3$ and integrin $\alpha_{IIb}\beta_3$. The crystal structures also demonstrated that peptide ligands containing the Arg-Gly-Asp (RGD) cell adhesion sequence interact with integrin $\alpha_{IIb}\beta_3$ and integrin $\alpha_V\beta_3$ in part by coordination of the metal ion in the MIDAS by the aspartic acid in the RGD peptide.[77,79] The low-molecular-weight drugs eptifibatide and tirofiban, which block ligand binding to the $\alpha_{IIb}$ subunit, have negatively charged regions that also interact with the MIDAS cation.[76] The fibrinogen $\gamma$-chain C-terminal dodecapeptide mediates binding to integrin $\alpha_{IIb}\beta_3$, and a crystal structure of the complex demonstrates that an aspartic acid carboxyl oxygen coordinates the MIDAS cation, whereas the carboxy terminal valine interacts with the nearby cation in the ADMIDAS.[76,79] A number of mutations in patients with GT have been identified within the cation-binding sphere of the MIDAS domain (see Fig. 10–3, and Chap. 2, Fig. 2–11). Two mutations, D119Y (Cam variant)[80] and D119N (patient NR),[81] are located within the conserved D$x$S$x$S amino acid motif and produce severe abnormalities of ligand binding to integrin $\alpha_{IIb}\beta_3$ but do not affect its surface expression. Mutations at residues R214 and R216 result in abnormal integrin $\alpha_{IIb}\beta_3$ receptors that cannot bind ligand and are very sensitive to dissociation by calcium chelation, perhaps because they are at the integrin $\alpha_{IIb}$–$\beta_3$ interface.[32,82–84] Disrupting the SyMBS with a D217V mutation also leads to GT despite the expression of normal amounts of the integrin protein.[85] Further support for the importance of the MIDAS domain, SyMBS, and adjacent residues comes from studies in which the mutations D119N, R214W, D217N, E220Q, and E220K were introduced into Chinese hamster ovary CHO cells *in vitro* and shown to result in functional abnormalities.[86]

The interface between the $\alpha_{IIb}$ $\beta$-propeller and the $\beta_3$ subunit also involves, in part, the interaction between $\beta_3$ R261, contained in a four-amino-acid $3_{10}$ helix, with a number of hydrophobic residues in the $\alpha_{IIb}$ $\beta$-propeller arranged as inner and outer rings, making up a cage.[75] A $\beta_3$ subunit L262Y mutation, adjacent to R261 results in disruption of the helix and an unstable integrin $\alpha_{IIb}\beta_3$ complex that is expressed on the surface of platelets but is unable to bind fibrinogen.[87] The platelets of the patient with this mutation were able to bind fibrin and support clot retraction, suggesting different requirements for fibrinogen and fibrin binding.

**Mutations in Integrin $\alpha_{IIb}\beta_3$ Within the $\alpha_{IIb}$ $\beta$-Propeller Sequence** Based on their homology to another integrin $\alpha$ subunit, the aminoterminal 450 amino acids of integrin $\alpha_{IIb}$ and the homologous region in integrin $\alpha_V$, which contain the minimal ligand-binding sequence,[88] were predicted to fold into seven repeat (blade) $\beta$-propellers, containing four cation-binding sites,[89] and this prediction was confirmed by the crystal structures of both $\alpha_V$ and $\alpha_{IIb}$ integrin subunits.[75,76] The upper surface of the propeller interacts with the $\beta_3$ subunit $\beta$-A (or I-like) domain to form the head of the integrin $\alpha_{IIb}\beta_3$ complex, which is the site of ligand binding. Each repeat (blade) contains four $\beta$ strands that are connected by loops. The four calcium-binding sites in the $\alpha_{IIb}$ subunit, which are in $\beta$-hairpin structures, are located in loops on the undersurface of the propeller. Ligand binding in integrin $\alpha_{IIb}$ has been localized to a hydrophobic (F160, Y190, F231) and negatively charged (D224) pocket that lies adjacent to the MIDAS domain in the $\beta_3$ subunit and is composed of contributions from the loops that link blade 2 to blade 3 (residues 144 to 171), $\beta$ strand 2 to $\beta$ strand 3 in blade 3 (residues 186 to 193), and blade 3 to blade 4 (residues 223 to 236). Integrin $\alpha_{IIb}$ contains a unique "cap" subdomain made up of four insertions in $\beta$-propeller loops (residues 72 to 88, 111 to 126, 147 to 166, and 200 to 217) that also plays a role in ligand binding.[76]

GT missense mutations located within the integrin $\alpha_{IIb}$ $\beta$-propeller (see Fig. 10–3) primarily affect transport of the integrin $\alpha_{IIb}\beta_3$ complex

to the cell surface,[68,90–93] but several missense mutations and an insertion result in functionally defective receptors. Thus, Y143H affects soluble ligand binding but not adhesion or clot retraction,[94] and P145A, which has been identified in several kindreds,[32,95] and P145L prevent ligand binding. A two-amino-acid insertion at residues 161 and 162 and a T176I missense mutation also affect ligand binding.[96–98] An L183P mutation, which is near to but not in the loop containing Y190, affects both receptor expression and function.[99]

**Mutations in Integrin $\alpha_{IIb}\beta_3$ That Affect Receptor Activation** Several $\beta_3$ subunit missense mutations (C560R, V193M) result in the receptor adopting a high-affinity ligand-binding state, which is paradoxical because it results in a bleeding diathesis.[100,101] A $\beta_3$ subunit S527F mutation in the third I-EGF domain was also associated with a constitutively active receptor, presumably because it prevents the receptor from assuming a bent, inactive conformation.[102] The cytoplasmic domain of the $\beta_3$ subunit plays a functional role in integrin activation and the regulation of ligand binding.[103,104] Two GT mutations have been identified in this region. One is an R724X nonsense mutation (patient RM)[105] that results in the deletion of the carboxyterminal 39 residues of integrin $\beta_3$, and the other is a $\beta_3$ subunit S752P missense mutation (patient P or Paris I).[106–108] This latter patient is unusual in that he had a generally mild history of excessive hemorrhage, but he did have a prolonged bleeding time and his platelets did not aggregate in response to ADP. These mutations do not severely affect surface expression of platelet integrin $\alpha_{IIb}\beta_3$ complexes, but both mutant receptors are unresponsive to agonist stimulation. Mammalian cell expression studies of these mutations show normal adhesion to immobilized fibrinogen but abnormal cell spreading. Cells expressing the S752P mutant receptors have reduced focal adhesion plaque formation, and cells expressing the R724X mutant receptors have undetectable tyrosine phosphorylation of focal adhesion kinase, pp125[FAK]. These mutations provide evidence for the role of the $\beta_3$ subunit cytoplasmic tail in inside-out signaling (i.e., platelet signals that lead to integrin $\alpha_{IIb}\beta_3$ adopting a high-affinity ligand-binding conformation) and outside-in signaling (i.e., signaling to the interior of the platelet as a result of integrin $\alpha_{IIb}\beta_3$ binding ligand; see Chap. 2, Figs. 2–3, 2–4, and 2–12).

**Variants of Integrin $\alpha_{IIb}\beta_3$ in the Population** The application of missense variant whole-exome and whole-genome sequencing to large numbers of individuals has provided valuable information on the frequency of missense variants in the general population and the frequency of the genetic alterations leading to GT. For the most part, the frequency of a variant in a population is a reflection of its impact on reproductive fitness and when it entered the population, with lower frequencies for variants that entered the population more recently. Thus, variants with minor allele frequencies (MAFs) of approximately 0.5 percent or less probably entered the population less than 2500 years ago, when the recent explosive growth in human populations began.[109] Data from a study[109A] involving approximately 33,000 alleles from approximately 16,500 people demonstrated the presence of 114 novel missense variants affecting approximately 10 percent of the integrin $\alpha_{IIb}$ amino acids and approximately 9 percent of the $\beta_3$ subunit amino acids. Thus, approximately 1.1 percent of the population studied carried at least one missense variant. None of the known GT mutations was observed in any of the alleles studied, indicating that they have MAFs of less than 0.01 percent and thus entered the population very recently. In fact, studies of two GT populations with high intragroup marriages, Palestinian Arabs and French Manouche gypsies, estimated that the GT mutations entered the population approximately 300 to 600 and approximately 300 to 400 years ago, respectively.[110,111] Several novel missense variants identified in this study affected one of the amino acids mutated in patients with GT, and in two cases, these variants were shown to profoundly affect expression of the receptor.

In one case, a missense variant reduced expression by approximately 50 percent but did not alter function. A series of prediction tools indicated that somewhere between 45 and 74 percent of the 114 novel missense mutations may be deleterious. Thus, perhaps approximately 0.6 percent of individuals in the general population are silent carriers for a GT variant that profoundly affects structure and/or function. In addition, some of the rare individuals in the healthy population with levels of integrin $\alpha_{IIb}\beta_3$ receptor expression intermediate between those of obligate GT carriers and normal individuals may reflect heterozygosity for "hypomorphic" variants that partially affect receptor expression but not function.[112]

## Clinical Features

Table 10–2 summarizes the clinical manifestations of 177 patients with GT obtained from two reviews.[22,33] Menorrhagia occurs in nearly all female patients. Purpura can be present immediately after birth but often is not dramatic. Petechiae of the face and subconjunctival hemorrhage associated with crying may be the first symptoms in neonates and babies. Spontaneous hemarthroses and central nervous system bleeding are very rare. The hemorrhagic diathesis in patients with GT is notable for its variability and the lack of correlation between the biochemical platelet abnormalities and clinical severity.[22] Even within groups of patients such as the Iraqi Jews, most of whom share the same genetic $\alpha_{IIb}$ or $\beta_3$ subunit abnormalities, there is a wide spectrum of clinical severity.[33,39] Moreover, the severity of bleeding symptoms can vary significantly during the lifetime of individual patients. GT does not appear to protect against the development of atherosclerosis as judged by the carotid artery intima-to-media ratio.[113] Carriers of GT are usually asymptomatic or only mildly symptomatic and generally have normal results in platelet function tests.[22,33,112,114,115]

## Laboratory Features

Table 10–3 provides characteristic laboratory findings in GT. Patients have normal platelet counts and morphology, prolonged bleeding times, decreased or absent clot retraction, and abnormal platelet aggregation responses to physiologic stimuli. The initial slope of high-dose ristocetin-induced aggregation is normal (or near normal), reflecting the normal plasma VWF and the normal platelet GPIb/IX content; at lower doses of ristocetin, however, where GPIb/IX–mediated activation of integrin $\alpha_{IIb}\beta_3$ (Chap. 2) normally contributes to the aggregation response, patients have decreased second wave aggregation.[116] GT platelets undergo normal shape change in response to ADP and thrombin, demonstrating their ability to undergo metabolic and cytoskeletal changes in response to these agents. Similarly, high doses of thrombin and collagen produce normal release of dense body and $\alpha$-granule contents[18,20,117]; the decreased secretion observed with lower doses of these agents reflects the lack of augmentation of the release reaction normally produced by platelet aggregation.[18,116,118–120]

Platelets in whole blood or platelet-rich plasma adhere to glass because fibrinogen first becomes deposited on the glass and the platelets then adhere to the immobilized fibrinogen.[121,122] Platelets from

**TABLE 10–2.** Bleeding in Patients with Glanzmann Thrombasthenia

| | No. of Affected Patients | Frequency (%) |
|---|---|---|
| **Symptoms** | | |
| Menorrhagia | 54/55 | 98 |
| Easy bruising, purpura | 152/177 | 86 |
| Epistaxis | 129/177 | 73 |
| Gingival bleeding | 97/177 | 55 |
| Gastrointestinal hemorrhage | 22/177 | 12 |
| Hematuria | 10/177 | 6 |
| Hemarthrosis | 5/177 | 3 |
| Intracranial hemorrhage | 3/177 | 2 |
| Visceral hematoma | 1/177 | 1 |
| **Severity** | | |
| Requirement for red cell transfusions | | |
| Patients from literature* | 32/48 | 67 |
| Paris patients | 54/64 | 84 |

*Data are from 177 patients reviewed by George and colleagues,[22] of whom 113 were from the literature and 64 were studied in Paris.

Reproduced with permission from Bloom AL: *Hemostasis and Thrombosis.* UK: Churchill Livingstone, 1992.

**TABLE 10–3.** Laboratory Features of Glanzmann Thrombasthenia

I. Platelet count: Normal

II. Bleeding time: Markedly prolonged

III. Tests of platelet function

   A. Platelet aggregation

      1. Epinephrine—no observable response

      2. ADP and thrombin—shape change, but no aggregation

      3. Collagen—shape change followed by variable increase in light transmission most likely from progressive adhesion to collagen fibers (pseudoaggregation)

      4. Ristocetin—normal initial slope of aggregation; at low doses, inhibition of second wave; at high doses, cyclical aggregation–disaggregation

   B. Aperture closure time (PFA-100): Prolonged

   C. Clot retraction: Absent or reduced

   D. Platelet release reaction: Decreased with epinephrine and low-dose adenosine diphosphate (ADP), thrombin, and collagen; normal with high-dose thrombin and collagen

   E. Interaction with glass (platelet retention test): Absent or reduced

   F. Platelet coagulant activity: Variably abnormal

   G. Microparticle formation: Variably abnormal

   H. *Ex vivo* interaction with deendothelialized blood vessels in flow chambers: Marked abnormality in platelet thrombus formation and defective platelet spreading; decreased platelet adhesion at high shear rates

IV. Tests of $\alpha_{IIb}\beta_3$ and $\alpha_V\beta_3$ receptors: Number and functional integrity

   A. $\alpha_{IIb}\beta_3$ content: Reduced or absent, except in variants

   B. $\alpha_V\beta_3$ content: Reduced or absent in patients with $\beta_3$ defects; normal or increased in patients with $\alpha_{IIb}$ defects

   C. Platelet binding of fibrinogen and other adhesive glycoproteins to $\alpha_{IIb}\beta_3$: Reduced or absent

   D. Platelet fibrinogen content: Markedly reduced, except in some variants

patients with GT fail to adhere to glass,[18,20,121] and this forms the basis of their abnormality in the glass bead retention assay.[123] Platelet coagulant activity has been variably reported as normal or abnormal.[18–21,124–126] A defect in platelet microparticle formation and support of thrombin generation has been identified in some patients,[125–128] but not in all patients.[129] Integrins $\alpha_{IIb}\beta_3$ and $\alpha_V\beta_3$ bind prothrombin, probably accounting for some of the abnormalities identified.[130,131]

In flow-chamber studies, thrombasthenic platelets adhere normally to deendothelialized blood vessels at low and intermediate shear rates but do not spread normally or form platelet thrombi.[132–134] A defect in adhesion occurs at higher shear rates. A paradoxical increase in fibrin formation on these surfaces has been observed with thrombasthenic platelets, but the explanation for this phenomenon remains unknown.[135] In contrast to normal blood, blood from nearly all patients with GT fails to occlude a 150-$\mu$m PFA-100 aperture in collagen-coated membranes under high sheer, either in the presence of ADP or epinephrine.[136,137]

Platelet integrins $\alpha_{IIb}\beta_3$ and $\alpha_V\beta_3$ can be quantitated by several techniques, including monoclonal antibody binding (using flow cytometry or radiolabeled binding), immunoblotting, and surface labeling followed by sodium dodecylsulfate polyacrylamide gel electrophoresis (SDS-PAGE). Based on such studies, GT patients are subcategorized by integrin $\alpha_{IIb}\beta_3$ content into those with less than 5 percent of normal (type I), 5 to 20 percent (type II), or 50 percent or more (variants).[22,138] In one review of 64 patients, 78 percent were type I, 14 percent were type II, and 8 percent were variants.[22] This subtyping predated the identification of integrin $\alpha_{IIb}\beta_3$ abnormalities as the cause of GT and was based on functional data; this categorization provides only limited information.

Measuring integrin $\alpha_V\beta_3$ content is technically more demanding than measuring that of integrin $\alpha_{IIb}\beta_3$ because there are only approximately 50 to 100 integrin $\alpha_V\beta_3$ receptors per platelet.[63] The integrin $\alpha_V\beta_3$ level is very useful, however, in making a preliminary assessment of whether the patient has a defect in the $\alpha_{IIb}$ or $\beta_3$ subunits, because, in general, patients who lack integrin $\alpha_V\beta_3$ receptors have a defect in the $\beta_3$ rather than $\alpha_{IIb}$ subunit.[139] A $\beta_3$ subunit missense mutation (H280P) that differentially affected integrin $\alpha_{IIb}\beta_3$ more than $\alpha_V\beta_3$ has, however, been described.[69]

Fibrinogen-binding studies assess the function of the integrin $\alpha_{IIb}\beta_3$ complex.[25] Early studies used radiolabeled fibrinogen to the binding of fibrinogen when the platelets are stimulated with ADP[25] or a similar agonist. Fibrinogen can also be labeled with a fluorescent molecule, and then flow cytometry can be used to measure fibrinogen binding. These techniques are most useful in detecting qualitative abnormalities of integrin $\alpha_{IIb}\beta_3$ in patients with variant GT. The binding of a monoclonal antibody (PAC1) to platelets gives similar information because the antibody only binds to the activated form of the integrin.[140]

Carriers of GT have essentially normal platelet function.[34] Their platelets, however, only contain approximately 60 percent of the normal number of integrin $\alpha_{IIb}\beta_3$ receptors; the overlap in values between normal individuals and carriers, however, does not permit for unequivocal diagnosis of carriers by this technique.[112] Carrier detection is most accurately performed by DNA analysis.

Platelet fibrinogen is reduced to approximately 10 percent of normal in patients with marked reductions in integrin $\alpha_{IIb}\beta_3$[18,21,43,44] but is variably reduced in patients with significant amounts of integrin $\alpha_{IIb}\beta_3$.[138,141,142]

### Therapy and Prognosis

Therapy of GT patients is discussed in the section entitled "Management of Inherited Platelet Function Disorders." Although GT is a severe disease, the prognosis for survival is generally good. In one series, two of 64 patients died of hemorrhage, and in another series, three of 43 patients died of hemorrhage.[22,33] A nationwide survey in Japan identified 98 GT patients in 1976 and 192 in 1991.[143] The mortality rate decreased substantially during this time interval.

$\alpha_{IIb}\beta_3$: **Select Macrothrombocytopenias** Five heterozygous missense mutations in four different amino acids in integrin $\alpha_{IIb}\beta_3$ ($\alpha_{IIb}$ G991C, R995Q, and R995W, and $\beta_3$ L718P and D723H), as well as several different deletions, lead to variably mild reductions in both integrin $\alpha_{IIb}\beta_3$ expression and platelet aggregation, as well as constitutively active receptors, in patients with inherited aniso- and macrothrombocytopenia.[144–150] The defects cluster on both sides of the transmembrane domains and include both members of the $\alpha_{IIb}$ R995-$\beta_3$ D723 salt bridge proposed to maintain the receptor in a low-affinity state.[151] Proplatelet formation has been reported to be abnormal in several reported cases.

## GLYCOPROTEIN IB (CD42b,c)–IX (CD42a)–V: BERNARD-SOULIER SYNDROME

### Definition and History

BSS is an inherited disorder of the platelet GPIb–IX–V complex characterized by thrombocytopenia, giant platelets, and a failure of the platelets to bind GPIb ligands, most importantly, VWF and thrombin.[152–155]

In 1948, Bernard and Soulier described two children from a consanguineous family who had a severe bleeding disorder characterized by mucocutaneous hemorrhage, variable thrombocytopenia, and giant platelets.[156,157] Beginning in the early 1970s, BSS platelets were shown to have a functional defect in VWF-dependent platelet adhesion and agglutination.[158–160] In 1975, Nurden and Caen identified an abnormality in platelet GPIb as the cause of the functional defect.[161] Later studies confirmed the defect in VWF–GPIb interactions[162–164] and identified additional defects in platelet GPV and GPIX.[165,166] Subsequent studies have identified additional ligands for the GPIb–IX complex, including thrombin,[167] P-selectin,[168] leukocyte integrin $\alpha_M\beta_2$,[169] high-molecular-weight kininogen,[170] thrombospondin-1,[171] and coagulation factors XI[172] and XII[173] (Chap. 2), but the precise contributions of these interactions to the disorder are not well defined. Molecular defects in the genes for GPIb$\alpha$, GPIb$\beta$, and GPIX, but not GPV, have been identified in BSS. Mouse models of BSS have been produced by gene targeting of *GPIb$\alpha$*[174] and *GPIb$\beta$*,[175] and like humans, mice deficient in *GPV* do not demonstrate the typical features of human BSS.[176,177]

### Etiology and Pathogenesis

This rare disease, with a prevalence estimated as less than one in 1,000,000, has been reported from countries around the world.[152,154,157,165] Both autosomal recessive ("biallelic") and autosomal dominant ("monoallelic") forms of the disorder have been described, with the biallelic producing the most severe symptoms and the monoallelic causing macrothrombocytopenia and a mild or no bleeding syndrome. Consanguinity is common in the biallelic form, with 85 percent of the reported cases being homozygous for the causative mutation.[154]

Six different features of BSS may contribute to the hemorrhagic diathesis: thrombocytopenia, abnormal platelet adhesive interactions with VWF, abnormal platelet interactions with thrombin, abnormal platelet coagulant activity, abnormal platelet interactions with P-selectin, and abnormal platelet interactions with leukocyte integrin $\alpha_M\beta_2$.

The pathophysiology of the thrombocytopenia is uncertain. Early studies suggested a marked shortening of platelet survival, presumably from the decrease in platelet surface charge resulting from the GPIb defect.[178,179] Later studies using [111]In-oxine to label platelets reported more modest or no shortening of platelet survival, indicating that ineffective thrombopoiesis and/or decreased thrombopoiesis may contribute to the thrombocytopenia.[180,181] Morphologic abnormalities have been identified in BSS megakaryocytes, and these may contribute to abnormal platelet production.[182] Based on observations in other giant platelet syndromes (Chap. 7), the large size of Bernard-Soulier platelets would tend to diminish the adverse hemostatic effects of the thrombocytopenia because the platelet mass is better preserved. With only rare exceptions,[183] however, the bleeding diathesis with BSS is more severe than expected from the thrombocytopenia, reinforcing the conclusion that a qualitative platelet defect is the predominant problem.[157,184]

The platelet GPIb–IX complex functions as a receptor for VWF (Chaps. 2 and 16).[152,185,186] This interaction is crucial in the adhesion of platelets to subendothelial surfaces, especially under high shear conditions, where VWF acts as a bridge between the subendothelial matrix and the platelet.[133,134] The relative roles of subendothelial VWF, plasma VWF, and platelet VWF have not been completely defined, but they probably all contribute to platelet adhesion.[187] The interaction of VWF with GPIb/IX initiates activation of integrin $\alpha_{IIb}\beta_3$,[188,189] which can also bind to VWF, but at a different site on the molecule.[190] The interaction of GPIb/IX with VWF also directly contributes to platelet–platelet interactions.[191-193]

GPIb/IX–VWF interactions can also occur in platelet suspensions at high shear rates; this can lead to platelet activation, with subsequent aggregation mediated by integrin $\alpha_{IIb}\beta_3$.[187,194-196] Whether sustained shear rates *in vivo* ever reach the levels required to initiate VWF binding, however, is not established.

Abnormalities of the GPIb–IX complex can be a result of genetic defects in *GPIbα*, *GPIbβ*, or *GPIX*, all of which are required for surface expression. BSS is the most severe form of the disease and is caused by defects in both alleles of one of the proteins as a result of a homozygous mutation, compound heterozygosity, or a combination of hemizygosity of *GPIbβ* because of a microdeletion and a mutation affecting the other *GPIbβ* allele. These abnormalities have been termed the *biallelic forms*.[154] A macrothrombocytopenic syndrome associated with a mild bleeding syndrome has been reported with heterozygous defects in *GPIbα* and *GPIbβ*.[154] Because obligate heterozygotes for the biallelic BSS mutations do not commonly demonstrate macrothrombocytopenia, the heterozygous defects associated with macrothrombocytopenia may exert a dominant negative effect.[154]

The platelets of patients with BSS have a decreased response to platelet activation by thrombin, especially at limiting concentrations of thrombin.[197-199] BSS platelets are deficient in two different proteins that interact with thrombin, namely GPIbα, which binds thrombin,[167] and GPV, which is a thrombin substrate (Chap. 2). The precise nature of the interactions of thrombin with GPIbα and its biologic consequences are still unclear, but binding of thrombin to GPIbα can initiate signaling within the platelet, perhaps directly through GPIbα crosslinking or indirectly by augmenting activation of other thrombin receptors (protease-activated receptors [PARs] 1 and 4) or other thrombin-dependent events at the platelet surface.[167] Paradoxically, mice deficient in GPV actually have increased sensitivity to thrombin activation and variably increased thrombus formation, perhaps because GPV limits access of thrombin to GPIb.[200,201] Because thrombin is one of the major physiologic activators of platelets, the loss of thrombin binding to GPIbα may contribute to the hemorrhagic diathesis.

Platelets from patients with BSS are defective in supporting thrombin generation as judged by the serum prothrombin time (PT),[202] a test performed with whole blood, but in other tests of platelet coagulant activity, BSS platelets support coagulation as well as, or better than, normal platelets.[124,203] Defects in collagen-induced coagulant activity and the association of factors V, VIII, and XI with BSS platelets have been described,[203] but their significance is unclear. Similarly, GPIb/IX has been identified as a binding site for other proteins involved in coagulation, including high-molecular-weight kininogen

and factor XII, but the contributions of these interactions to the coagulant abnormality are also uncertain.[170,172,173] Binding of VWF to GPIb/IX has been implicated in fibrin-dependent, but not fibrin-independent, augmentation of platelet coagulant activity, and thus, fibrin-dependent coagulant activity is likely to be abnormal in BSS.[126] This finding may partially explain the variability in findings between the serum PT and some of the other assays as fibrin only forms in the serum PT. Abnormal membrane lipids have also been reported.[204]

The mechanism(s) producing the giant platelets in BSS has not been identified, but since giant platelets are found in BSS variants in which GPIb/IX is present, but unable to bind ligand, it has been postulated that the abnormality is a result of the inability of GPIb/IX to bind an unknown marrow ligand.[152] It cannot be because of an inability to bind VWF as, with only rare exceptions,[205] patients lacking VWF do not have large platelets. Moreover, in a mouse model of BSS, restoring a receptor with the GPIb transmembrane and cytoplasmic domains, but not the ligand-binding domain, partially corrected both the thrombocytopenia and large platelet size.[206] A defect in GPIb/IX–mediated signaling has also been proposed to cause the large platelets as a deficiency of PLC has also been described in BSS.[152,207] A mechanical alteration in the plasma membrane of BSS platelets has been identified by micropipette experiments, showing the plasma membrane to be more deformable than normal.[208] Megakaryocytes in BSS have increased ploidy and volume, as well as alterations in the membrane demarcation system, granules, and microtubules.[181,182] Both the increased size and deformability may reflect the loss of the normal interaction of GPIb/IX with the cytoskeleton via actin-binding protein (filamin-1; Chap. 2).

Platelets from patients with BSS are deficient not only in GPIbα, GPIbβ, and GPIX, which are known to be associated as a complex, but also in GPV (Chap. 2).[152,166] All of these proteins share highly conserved leucine-rich regions.[152,187] One possible explanation for the loss of surface expression of all the proteins is that they need to form a complex during biosynthesis in order to be transported to the surface[187]; evidence supports the need for GPIbα, GPIbβ, and GPIX to all be present for optimal surface expression,[209] but data from mice deficient in GPV indicate that this glycoprotein is not required for surface expression of the GPIb–IX complex.[200] GPV may, however, improve the efficiency of expression of the other members of the complex.[210] Moreover, data from the BSS mouse expressing a chimeric GPIbα molecule in which the leucine-rich repeat domain was replaced with the external domain of another receptor indicate that complex formation does not require the GPIbα leucine-rich domain.[206]

At the molecular level, the platelets from different patients with BSS are heterogeneous, with many having no detectable GPIb and others having variable amounts, up to 50 percent of normal.[152,207,211-214] There also is variability in the degree of concordance in the reduction of GPIb and the other deficient proteins.[215,216]

**Molecular Defects** The molecular biologic basis of BSS has been determined in 161 patients from 132 unrelated families,[154] and an online registry of defects is available at http://www.bernardsoulier.org/.[217] An international consortium reported on 211 families with the recessive form of BSS, which they termed "biallelic."[154] In total, 45 different mutations have been reported in *GPIbα*, 52 in *GPIbβ*, and 28 in *GPIX*. No defects in *GPV* have been identified in patients with BSS. The association with consanguineous matings was reinforced as 85 percent of the families had homozygous mutations and 13 percent were compound heterozygotes for defects in one of the genes. None of the variants were identified in several gene variant databases,[154] suggesting that they are all rare and likely entered the population relatively recently. A number of likely founder mutations have been identified in each of the three genes in different populations.[154,218] The ancestry of seven apparently unrelated families with a *GPIbβ* W89D mutation was traced to a common ancestor in 1671 in India.[218] Five mutations in *GPIX* account for 137 of the 184 affected *GPIX* alleles, and *GPIX* N61S is found in 64 European families. A number of mutations have been identified to cause the heterozygous monoallelic form, including the *GPIbα* A172V mutation, which has been associated with biallelic and monoallelic forms of the disorder in 42 apparently unrelated families with macrothrombocytopenia in Italy.[154] Many of the defects affect the leucine-rich repeats or the conserved flanking sequences, supporting the importance of these structural elements in the biogenesis and surface expression of the GPIb–IX–V complex (see Chap. 2, Fig. 2–14, and Fig. 10–4). Three patients have been described who are homozygous for a deletion in the last two bases of codon 492 of GPIbα, resulting in a frameshift that alters the membrane-spanning region and results in premature termination, and another patient has been described who is heterozygous for this deletion and a missense mutation of GPIbα.[219–222] These defects appear to result in a poorly anchored GPIbα with GPIbα antigen present in plasma. *GPIbβ* mutations have affected the promoter region, at a binding site for the GATA-1 transcription factor,[223] the signal peptide,[224] and the transmembrane and intracellular domains.[225] A homozygous Y88C defect in GPIbβ has been reported to cause BSS in two Japanese families, and heterozygotes with this mutation have a giant platelet syndrome.[221,226] Similarly, a patient heterozygous for a GPIbβ R17C mutation also had a giant platelet syndrome.[227] An N45S mutation in GPIX, affecting leucine-rich repeat 1, has been reported in at least 12 different white patients, including four patients from a large Swiss family with variable clinical manifestations[228–230] and one Turkish patient.[231]

BSS has been reported in seven patients in association with hemizygous deletion of GPIbβ and several neighboring genes on chromosome 22q11.2, leading to variable manifestations of the DiGeorge syndrome,

including cardiac defects, dysmorphic facial features, thymic hypoplasia, and velopharyngeal insufficiency.[154,232–239] Hemizygous mutations in the remaining *GPIbβ* allele have included P96S and P29L.[236,237] In other studies of patients with the 22q11.2 deletion syndrome, modest reductions in platelet count and increases in platelet volume, as well as reduced platelet agglutination to ristocetin and decreased platelet GPIb/IX expression, have been variably reported, consistent with hemizygosity for *GPIbβ*.[240–244]

A number of monoallelic, heterozygous mutations in the genes of the GPIb–IX complex have been described as causing macrothrombocytopenia, some, but not all, of which have also been implicated in causing the biallelic form either because of homozygosity or compound heterozygosity.[154] These include a heterozygous mutation in the second leucine-rich repeat (L57F)[245] in which the affected patients have moderate bleeding symptoms, moderate thrombocytopenia, and giant platelets. Additional monoallelic mutations of *GPIbα* that appear to produce dominant effects are N41H[246] and Y54D.[247]

The "Bolzano" defect, which involves a mutation in the sixth leucine-rich repeat of GPIbα (A156V), results in a GPIbα molecule that has reduced ability to bind VWF but can bind thrombin. It has been described in both biallelic and monoallelic forms. Two patients with biallelic forms have been described. In one patient, the Bolzano defect was homozygous, and the patient had a lifelong history of mucocutaneous hemorrhage in association with an approximately 50 percent reduction in GPIb surface expression and total loss of ability to bind VWF.[248] In the other, the Bolzano mutation coexisted with a 12-amino-acid deletion and an amino acid substitution (Q181K).[249] The monoallelic form of the Bolzano defect has been reported in more than 100 patients from 48 pedigrees, primarily from southern Italy.[250] Most patients have no bleeding symptoms, but some have mild to moderate bleeding symptoms. Mild thrombocytopenia, increased mean platelet volume, reduced expression of GPIb/IX/V, and normal or borderline abnormal values for ristocetin-induced platelet aggregation are characteristic of this disorder.

### Clinical Features

Epistaxis is the most common symptom of BSS (70 percent); also common are ecchymoses (58 percent), menometrorrhagia (44 percent), gingival hemorrhage (42 percent), and gastrointestinal bleeding (22 percent).[157] The combination of BSS with angiodysplasia can result in particularly severe recurrent hemorrhage.[251–253] Hemorrhagic symptoms that occur with lower frequency include posttraumatic bleeding (13 percent), hematuria (7 percent), cerebral hemorrhage (4 percent), and retinal hemorrhage (2 percent). There is considerable variability in symptoms among patients, even among patients within a single family.[152,254] A review that includes brief descriptions of the clinical features of 55 patients, reported through 1998, has been published.[152]

### Laboratory Features

Thrombocytopenia is present in nearly all patients but is variable in its severity, ranging from approximately $20 \times 10^9$ platelets/L to near-normal levels. Platelets are large on smear, with more than one-third usually having diameters greater than 3.5 $\mu$m and some being as large or larger than lymphocytes. By electron microscopy, platelets display only minor variations in vesicular structures and the open canalicular system,[157] but megakaryocytes have more notable abnormalities in their demarcation membranes.[182] The cell membranes of platelets from patients with BSS appear to be more deformable than normal,[208] perhaps because GPIb ordinarily interacts with the platelet cytoskeleton[255] (Chap. 2).

Closure times of the apertures of collagen-coated membranes are markedly prolonged in the presence of ADP or epinephrine (PFA-100).[136] The hallmark findings in the BSS are the failure of platelets to aggregate

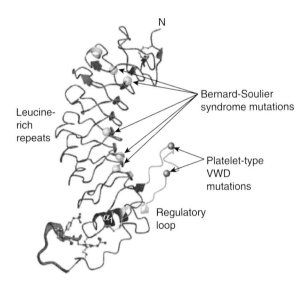

**Figure 10–4.** Localization of select missense mutations causing platelet-type von Willebrand disease (VWD) and Bernard-Soulier syndrome (BSS) in the GPIbα N-terminal domain. Ribbon diagram of the topology of GPIbα N-terminal domain viewed from the side. The regulatory loop is colored *blue* with activating platelet-type VWD mutations G233V and M239V indicated as open *black balls*. Five BSS mutations, which cause loss of von Willebrand factor binding, are shown as *blue balls*. L57F and C65R localize to leucine-rich repeat (LRR) 2 with L129P, A156V, and L179del localized to the LRR5, LRR6, and LRR7 β-strands, respectively. The molecular structure of the sulfated tyrosine residues 276, 278, and 279 are shown. (*Adapted with permission from Uff S, Clemetson JM, Harrison T, Clemetson KJ, et al. Crystal structure of the platelet glycoprotein Ib(alpha) N-terminal domain reveals an unmasking mechanism for receptor activation, J BiolChem 2002 Sep 20;277(38):35657–35663.*)

in response to ristocetin[159] or botrocetin,[162,256] agents that require VWF–GPIb interactions. In VWD, but not BSS, this defect can be corrected by adding normal plasma (or VWF).

Although, the large size of the platelets in BSS and the thrombocytopenia make it technically difficult to perform platelet aggregation studies, in general, aggregation induced by ADP, epinephrine, or collagen is either normal or enhanced.[160,257,258] The aggregation response to thrombin is usually dose dependent, being essentially normal in response to high doses of thrombin but characterized by a prolonged lag phase and diminished aggregation in response to low doses of thrombin.[197,259]

**Platelet Coagulant Activity** The coagulant activity of platelets from patients with BSS has been variably reported as reduced, normal, or increased.[124,202,203] The variable presence of fibrin in the different assays used to assess platelet coagulant activity may account for these inconsistent results as GPIb–VWF interactions enhance platelet coagulant activity when fibrin is present, but not when it is absent.[126]

**Platelet–Thrombin Interactions** Both GPIb and the seven-transmembrane domains PAR-1 and PAR-4 receptors are required for maximal response to thrombin.[167,259] Two different crystal structures of the interactions between thrombin and GPIbα have been reported; in one, two molecules of thrombin bind to each GPIbα molecule, raising the possibility that free thrombin or thrombin adherent to fibrinogen can cluster GPIb–IX–V complexes.[167,260,261] GPV, which is missing from the platelet surface in BSS, is cleaved by thrombin, but the cleavage is neither necessary nor sufficient for thrombin-induced platelet activation.[262,263] In fact, platelets of mice lacking GPV have increased responsiveness to thrombin, perhaps because GPV ordinarily limits access of thrombin to GPIbα or inhibits GPIbα crosslinking.[200,201]

***Ex Vivo* Interaction with Subendothelial Surfaces** Platelets from patients with BSS demonstrate defective adhesion to subendothelial surfaces, especially at shear rates greater than 650 s$^{-1}$.[133,134,158,264] The results are similar to those in patients with VWD.

**Shear-Induced Platelet Aggregation** Unlike normal platelets, platelets from patients with BSS are not aggregated by high shear rates.[194,195] The initial interaction in this process appears to be binding of VWF to GPIb,[187] with subsequent activation of integrin $\alpha_{IIb}\beta_3$, perhaps through signaling via the protein 14-3-3ζ associated with the cytoplasmic domain of GPIbα,[196,265] Fcγ receptor IIA, GPVI, and/or the Fc receptor γ chain (Chap. 2).[266–268] Pathologic shear stress has been reported to increase binding of α-actin to GPIb/IX as part of the signaling process.[268–270]

### Therapy

The therapy of BSS is described in the section "Management of Inherited Platelet Function Disorders" below. Splenectomy has been performed when the diagnosis of immune thrombocytopenia was mistakenly made, but this usually does not normalize the platelet count or improve the bleeding diathesis.[249]

## GPIBα (CD42b,c): PLATELET-TYPE (PSEUDO-) VON WILLEBRAND DISEASE

### Definition and History

A heterogeneous group of patients has been described with mild to moderate bleeding symptoms, variably enlarged platelets, variable thrombocytopenia, and diminished plasma high-molecular-weight VWF multimers.[271] The fundamental defect in these patients is thought to be an enhanced interaction between an abnormal platelet GPIb/IX receptor and normal plasma VWF.[272–281] Because these patients have some of the hallmarks of VWD, but the defect is in platelet GPIb/IX, the condition has been termed both *pseudo-VWD* and *platelet-type VWD*. At present, 55 patients are listed in the database of patients with this disorder (www.pt-vwd.org).[282,283]

### Etiology and Pathogenesis

A qualitative abnormality in GPIb is responsible for this disorder, with ongoing *in vivo* binding of high-molecular-weight VWF multimers to platelets causing depletion of the plasma high-molecular-weight multimers. In addition, the binding of the VWF to platelets may lead to shortened platelet survival, perhaps accounting for the variable thrombocytopenia. Inheritance is autosomal dominant.

Abnormalities in the Mr of GPIb were identified in two families,[277] but these may have resulted from a now-recognized polymorphism in GPIb (Chap. 2) rather than being related to the functional disorder. Heterozygous point mutations in the *GPIbα* gene causing a variety of missense alterations (G233V, G233S, M239V, D235Y, W230L) have been found in several different families.[271,278,284–289] The G238V mutation is the most common among the patients in the database, affecting 31 of 35 patients. All of these mutations are in the R-loop (also termed β-switch) in the carboxyterminal flanking sequence of the leucine-rich repeats, a region implicated in ligand binding (see Fig. 10–4).[152,187,290–293] Molecular modeling suggests that the M239V substitution produces a significant conformational change in the molecule,[294] and this was confirmed by crystallographic analysis.[295] It has been proposed that the platelet-type VWD mutations either destabilize the compact triangular structure of the R-loop by interfering with the D235-K237 salt bridge or stabilizing the extended β-hairpin form of the R-loop, which is better able to engage the VWF A1 domain.[282] A mouse model of the GPIbα G233V mutation recapitulated many of the human manifestations and had an unexpected increase in bone mass.[296] Recombinant GPIbα fragments containing the G233V and M239V mutations demonstrated enhanced interactions with VWF in several different systems, including ones under shear stress.[297,298] An increase in platelet GPIb/IX expression has also been reported.[278,281] An in-frame 27-base-pair (bp) deletion in the macroglycopeptide region of GPIbα has also been reported to cause platelet-type VWD.[279] Because the deletion may lead to the loss of up to four glycosylation sites, it has been proposed that the glycans play a negative regulatory role in ligand binding.[282]

### Clinical Features

Patients have variable thrombocytopenia and mild to moderate mucocutaneous hemorrhage. A study of 13 patients with six different mutations using a standardized bleeding assessment tool found a wide range of clinical severity, with approximately 40 percent having a normal bleeding score and the remainder having a wide range of abnormal scores.[271] Bleeding scores did not correlate with age or sex, but did correlate with reductions in both platelet count and ristocetin cofactor activity. All patients had macrothrombocytopenia. Of note, pregnancy may exacerbate the thrombocytopenia and bleeding symptoms.[278]

### Laboratory Features and Differential Diagnosis

Mild thrombocytopenia and somewhat enlarged platelets are present in some, but not all, patients. Plasma VWF levels are variably reduced, with a disproportionate reduction in plasma high-molecular-weight multimers. Platelet VWF multimers are normal.

The most characteristic laboratory finding in platelet-type VWD is enhanced platelet aggregation in response to low concentrations of ristocetin[272–276,278,288] or botrocetin.[299] This same abnormality is present in patients with type 2b VWD, as is selective depletion of plasma high-molecular-weight VWF multimers (Chap. 16). In platelet-type VWD, however, the defect is in platelet GPIbα, whereas in type 2b VWD, the defect is in the VWF. In one study comparing platelet-type and type 2b

VWD, patients with type 2b VWD had more severe bleeding, especially menorrhagia, and lower platelet counts.[271] Several assays can help differentiate between these abnormalities[274,300-302]: (1) normal VWF (purified or in cryoprecipitate) will aggregate platelets from patients with platelet-type VWD, but not platelets from patients with type 2b VWD; (2) isolated platelets from patients with platelet-type VWD will bind normal VWF at lower concentrations of ristocetin than will normal platelets or platelets from patients with type 2b VWD; (3) plasma VWF from patients with type 2b VWD will bind to normal platelets at lower-than-normal concentrations of ristocetin, whereas higher-than-normal concentrations of ristocetin are required to promote the plasma VWF from patients with platelet-type VWF to bind to normal platelets[301]; and (4) VWF lacking sialic acid residues (asialo-VWF) will agglutinate platelets from patients with platelet-type VWD in the presence of ethylenediaminetetraacetic acid (EDTA).[303] A number of patients with platelet-type VWD were originally diagnosed as having type 2b VWD, leading to the conclusion that platelet-type VWD may be underdiagnosed, and an international registry–based study supports this contention.[278,280,304]

### Therapy

Because normal VWF (especially the high-molecular-weight forms) can bind excessively to the platelets of patients with platelet-type VWD and potentially lead to rapid platelet clearance from the circulation, increasing the VWF level by any means (desmopressin infusion or VWF replacement with cryoprecipitate or VWF concentrates) poses a potential risk of inducing thrombocytopenia.[300,305] It may be possible to estimate this risk by assessing whether the patient's platelets aggregate *ex vivo* in response to VWF (as in cryoprecipitate).[273] Low-dose cryoprecipitate has successfully supported hemostasis, without inducing thrombocytopenia.[275,305,306] Currently, cryoprecipitate is generally less favored for VWF replacement therapy than plasma-derived factor VIII concentrates such as Humate-P, which is approved in the United States for the therapy of VWD, because the plasma-derived factor VIII concentrates have a reduced risk of viral infection. Consideration should also be given to platelet transfusion in appropriate circumstances. Recombinant factor VIIa infusion may be beneficial and is licensed for this indication in Europe, but this therapy is not yet approved by the FDA; it has the theoretical advantage of avoiding excessive interactions between VWF and the abnormal GPIbα receptor.[307,308]

## INTEGRIN $\alpha_2\beta_1$ DEFICIENCY (GLYCOPROTEIN IA/IIA; VLA-2; CD49B/CD29)

Integrin $\alpha_2\beta_1$ (GPIa/IIa) can mediate platelet adhesion to collagen and platelet activation under certain conditions (Chap. 2). A female patient with excessive posttraumatic bruising and menorrhagia but no epistaxis, gum bleeding, or excessive bleeding after tonsillectomy or appendectomy was described whose platelets selectively failed to aggregate or undergo shape change in response to collagen.[309,310] The bleeding time was markedly prolonged, and the patient's platelets failed to adhere and spread normally on subendothelial surfaces. The patient's platelets only contained approximately 15 to 25 percent of the normal amount of integrin $\alpha_2$[309,311] and a reduction in the $\beta_1$ subunit was also apparent.[309] It is difficult to draw conclusions about the physiologic role of integrin $\alpha_2\beta_1$ in platelet function from this patient because her $\alpha_2\beta_1$ deficiency was incomplete, her bleeding symptoms were mild and variable, and some of the platelet function abnormalities (e.g., abnormal platelet–collagen interactions in the presence of the divalent chelating agent EDTA) are difficult to ascribe to the deficiency in $\alpha_2\beta_1$.[309,312]

Another patient with integrin $\alpha_2$ deficiency has been described.[313] She had a history of mucocutaneous and postoperative bleeding. Her bleeding time was prolonged and platelet aggregation in response to collagen was selectively reduced, but not absent. In addition to her $\alpha_2$ subunit defect, she also had little or no intact thrombospondin, and exogenous thrombospondin corrected the defect in platelet aggregation. The patient's hemorrhagic symptoms and platelet defects disappeared when she entered menopause.

The variation in platelet integrin $\alpha_2\beta_1$ expression in healthy individuals is very wide (10-fold), and platelet levels have been correlated with allelic variants.[314] Reduced $\alpha_2\beta_1$ expression has been associated with alterations in megakaryocyte production and decreased mean platelet volume.[315]

Mice with targeted deletion of integrin $\alpha_2\beta_1$ do not have a hemorrhagic phenotype or prolonged tail bleeding times, but they do have reduced platelet adhesion to collagen and reduced thrombus formation after vascular injury[316]; mice with a conditional loss of integrin $\alpha_2\beta_1$ in megakaryocytes and platelets have a decreased mean platelet volume.[315]

## CD36 (GPIV; FATTY ACYL TRANSLOCASE [FAT]; SCAVENGER RECEPTOR CLASS B, MEMBER 3 [SCARB3])

CD36 (GPIV) is a highly but variably expressed platelet glycoprotein that is present on many cell types and documented to participate in long-chain fatty acid transport (Chap. 2). Approximately 3 percent of Japanese, 2 percent of African Americans, and 0.3 percent of whites in the United States have platelets that lack CD36 (GPIV).[317,318] Although CD36 (GPIV) has been implicated in platelet interactions with collagen, thrombospondin, advanced glycation products,[319] and myeloid-related protein (MRP)-14,[320-323] as well as in platelet–monocyte interactions,[324] individuals lacking CD36 (GPIV) do not have a hemorrhagic diathesis. Platelets from these patients can bind thrombospondin via alternative receptors,[325] and there are differing data on its role in adhesion to collagen.[326-328] A multiparameter analysis of platelet thrombus formation to different matrix proteins at differing shear rates identified a role for CD36 at low, but not high, shear rates.[8] CD36 (GPIV) has also been implicated as a receptor for oxidized low-density lipoprotein (LDL), and the binding of very-low-density lipoprotein (VLDL) to CD36 (GPIV) has been reported to enhance collagen-induced platelet aggregation and thromboxane production.[329] CD36 (GPIV) platelet expression varies widely among healthy individuals (200 to 14,000 molecules per platelet) and correlates with activation by oxidized LDL and genetic single-nucleotide variants.[330]

Two forms of CD36 (GPIV) deficiency have been described in Japan: type I, in which both platelets and monocytes are deficient, and type II, in which only platelets are deficient.[331-333] A P90S substitution that also leads to abnormal posttranslational modification is a common abnormality contributing to both type I and type II deficiencies. In the type I form, patients are homozygous for the abnormality, whereas in type II deficiency, patients are doubly heterozygous for the P90S abnormality and an unidentified platelet-specific expression defect.[331,334,335] Other abnormalities that have been associated with type I deficiency include a dinucleotide deletion (539–540) in exon 5, a 161-bp deletion (331–491) corresponding to loss of exon 4, a nucleotide insertion at position 1159 in codon 317 leading to a frameshift and premature stop, and splice-site mutations.[336-338] Other mutations have been identified in other populations.

CD36 (GPIV) deficiency can result in refractoriness to platelet transfusions because of isoimmunization and has been implicated in posttransfusion purpura (Chap. 7),[339] as well as thrombocytopenia caused by the passive transfer of anti-CD36 antibodies.[340]

## GLYCOPROTEIN VI DEFICIENCY

GPVI can mediate platelet adhesion to collagen and is important in collagen-induced signal transduction (Chap. 2). Twelve patients with mild to moderate bleeding disorders and variable deficiencies of platelet GPVI or signaling have been described; one had concomitant GPS (α-granule deficiency).[341–350] The others had selective abnormalities in platelet–collagen interactions. Platelet GPVI deficiency associated with an autoantibody to GPVI has been described in several patients, one of whom also had systemic lupus erythematosus and another of whom had coexisting antibodies to integrin $\alpha_{IIb}\beta_3$.[351–353] Antibody to GPVI may be detectable in eluates prepared from patient platelets even when it is not detectable in patient plasma.[354] Acquired forms of GPVI-specific signal transduction have also been described in patients with myelodysplastic syndromes and chronic lymphocytic leukemia.[347] Studies in mice and primates demonstrated that antibodies to GPVI can result in loss of GPVI from the platelet surface through either proteolytic shedding or a cyclic adenosine monophosphate (cAMP)-mediated internalization mechanism, even though the platelets continue to circulate.[346,355] Thus, it is likely that the deficiency of GPVI most commonly results from the autoantibodies.[353] It is unclear whether the patients reported earlier as having GPVI deficiency might also have had an immune basis for their GPVI deficiency.

Three different inherited forms of GPVI deficiency have been described. One patient with a lifelong history of "mild" mucocutaneous, posttraumatic, and postsurgery bleeding had a marked deficiency of platelet membrane GPVI resulting from both a 16-base out-of-frame deletion and a S175N missense mutation.[350] The patient's platelets failed to respond to collagen, convulxin, or collagen-related peptide. Of note, FcRγ expression was normal. Another patient with easy bruising, a prolonged bleeding time, abnormal PFA-100 closure time to collagen/epinephrine, and no platelet aggregation in response to collagen had a combination of an R38C mutation in one allele and a five-nucleotide duplication insertion in the other, leading to a nonsense codon.[356] The R38C mutation led to misfolding of the protein, reduced surface expression, and a qualitative defect in collagen binding. Five subjects from four apparently unrelated families in Chile with variable histories of easy bruising, epistaxis, excessive bleeding after minor trauma, and gingival bleeding were found to have no platelet aggregation in response to collagen, convulxin, or collagen-related peptide.[357] DNA analysis showed a homozygous adenine insertion between bases 711 and 712. Heterozygotes were asymptomatic and had nearly normal platelet function.

## ● ABNORMALITIES OF PLATELET GRANULES

Platelets contain at least three types of granules: dense or δ granules containing ADP, ATP, calcium, serotonin, and pyrophosphate; α granules containing a variety of proteins, some derived from plasma and others synthesized by the megakaryocyte; and lysosomes containing acid hydrolases. Following platelet activation, the contents of the α and dense granules are secreted. Inability to release these granule contents by virtue of a deficiency of the granules or their contents or in the cellular mechanisms governing the secretory process is associated with impaired platelet function. A heterogeneous group of disorders involving platelet granules has been described. They are broadly categorized into defects affecting dense granules (δ-storage pool deficiency [SPD]), α granules (α-SPD, or GPS), or both dense bodies and α granules (αδ-SPD). Another disorder affecting granules is the Quebec platelet disorder, which affects the α granules.

## δ-STORAGE POOL DEFICIENCY

### Definition and History

In 1969, a family with impaired platelet aggregation was described whose platelets displayed decreased levels of ADP.[358] Holmsen and Weiss subsequently established that the defect was a deficiency in the nonmetabolic pool or "storage pool" of ADP present in the dense granules.[359] δ-SPD is a heterogeneous disorder characterized by a bleeding tendency, abnormalities in the second wave of platelet aggregation, and variable deficiencies of platelet dense granule contents.

### Etiology and Pathogenesis

Normal platelets contain two pools of adenine nucleotides that exchange very slowly.[360] One pool is a metabolic nongranule pool in which the ratio of ATP to ADP content is 8 to 10:1. The second pool is the "storage pool" present in the dense granules and contains 65 percent of the platelet adenine nucleotides with an ATP-to-ADP ratio of 2:3. It is this storage pool that is deficient in δ-SPD. Dense granules also contain serotonin, which is taken up from plasma at a ratio of approximately 1000:1 via a pH-dependent amine-trapping mechanism. Platelet serotonin levels are also decreased in δ-SPD.

δ-SPD can be a primary, inherited platelet disorder or a component of a multisystem (syndromic) disorder, such as the Hermansky-Pudlak syndrome (HPS)[361–365] (variable oculocutaneous albinism, hemorrhagic disorder, and neurologic manifestations), the Chédiak-Higashi syndrome[361,365,366] (partial oculocutaneous albinism, giant lysosomal granules, and frequent pyogenic infections), and the Wiskott-Aldrich syndrome[361,367,368] (see below). Other diseases associated with δ-SPD are Ehlers-Danlos syndrome,[369] osteogenesis imperfecta,[370] and TAR syndrome.[361,371] The mode of inheritance in δ-SPD is not well defined, but an autosomal dominant pattern for the primary form has been identified in some patients.[372] The inheritance pattern of the syndromic forms follows the autosomal recessive and X-linked patterns characteristic of those disorders. Essential criteria for the diagnosis of HPS are the tyrosinase-positive oculocutaneous albinism and the δ-SPD in platelets.[373] The hallmarks of albinism are diffuse hypopigmentation of skin, iris, hair and retina, although there is phenotypic heterogeneity.

Studies from animal models and, particularly, in patients with the syndromic variants indicate that defects in biogenesis of lysosome-related organelles form the basis of the disorders.[361,374] These organelles share features with lysosomes but have distinct morphology, composition, and functions, and include melanosomes in melanocytes, platelet δ granules, and Weibel-Palade bodies in endothelial cells.[361,374] In δ-SPD associated with HPS, there may be a total failure of δ-granule formation as judged by electron microscopy of platelets and megakaryocytes[375] and the absence of CD63 (granulophysin; ME491; LIMP-1; LAMP-3), a lysosomal and dense granule membrane protein of Mr 40,000 that is also found in melanosomes.[361,363,376,377] The defect in melanosomes accounts for the oculocutaneous albinism. The defect in lysosomes results in accumulation of ceroid lipofuscin, a lipid–protein complex leading to granulomatous colitis and pulmonary fibrosis, which are variably manifest in these patients. Abnormalities of nine genes have been implicated in causing HPS (Fig. 10–5). Ultrastructural studies in patients with a variety of types of HPS indicate that α granules and other organelles are unaffected.[378] Mutations in HPS-associated genes result in defects in intracellular protein trafficking and in the biogenesis of lysosomes and lysosomes-related organelles.[361] The HPS gene products operate in distinct complexes termed *biogenesis of lysosome-related organelles complexes* (BLOCs), which consist of multiple proteins.[361] HPS is unusually common in patients from northwest Puerto Rico (frequency: 1:1800), and linkage analysis of these patients led to the identification of the abnormality in the HPS gene (*HPS1*). The gene encodes a 700-amino-acid

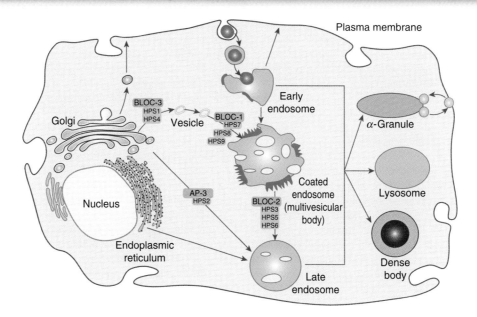

**Figure 10–5.** Hypothetical model of platelet granule formation and location of defects resulting in Hermansky-Pudlak syndrome (HPS). Early endosomes derive from invaginations from the plasma membrane, whereas membrane-bound structures from the Golgi and endoplasmic reticulum contribute to the production of coated endosomes and late endosomes. Three multiprotein complexes termed *biogenesis of lysosome-related organelles complexes* (BLOCS) are involved in the transport and interconversion of the different endosomal species. The gene products of HPS1 and HPS4 are involved in BLOC-3, whereas those of HPS3, HPS5, and HPS6 are involved in BLOC-2, and those of HPS7, HPS8, and HPS9 contribute to BLOC-1. HPS2 is a result of mutations in adaptor complex-3 (AP-3). It has not yet been determined which endosomal species contribute to *a* granules, lysosomes, and dense bodies, but all three organelles are affected in HPS. *a* Granules are in dynamic exchange with the plasma membrane, selectively taking up fibrinogen via integrin $a_{IIb}\beta_3$ receptors. *(Used with permission of Dr. Marjan Huizing and Dr. William Gahl, National Human Genome Research Institute, National Institutes of Health.)*

protein that participates in the complex of proteins called BLOC-3.[361,363] The mutation in the Puerto Rican kindreds is a 16-bp duplication in HPS1 exon 15; other mutations of the same gene have been identified in patients from this region and in other ethnic groups.[363,379,380] HPS2 is caused by mutations in the gene *AP3B1 (HPS2)*, which codes for the $\beta_3A$ subunit of the heterotetrameric adaptor complex-3 (AP-3), which, in turn, facilitates the formation of vesicles of lysosomal lineage from membranes of the *trans*-Golgi network or late endosomes. Patients with mutations in this protein tend to also have neutropenia and childhood infections.[373,381]

Defects in the *HPS3* gene cause a relatively mild form of HPS, and pulmonary involvement is usually minimal.[382] *HPS4* encodes a protein that interacts with the *HPS1* protein in the BLOC-3 complex.[383] Patients with mutations in this gene tend to have severe disease, and like patients with defects in *HPS1*, pulmonary involvement is common. The gene products of HPS5 and HPS6 interact with the *HPS3* gene product to form BLOC-2.[384,385] Proteins implicated in HPS7 (encoded by *DTNBP1*) and HPS8 (encoded by *BLOC1S3*) are components of BLOC-1.[386,387] Improper trafficking of melanocyte-specific proteins, including tyrosinase, has been found in the melanosomes of patients with *HPS5*.[388] HPS is also associated with mutations in pallidin (*BLOC1S6/PLDN*), a protein of BLOC-1 and labeled as HPS9.[389]

Not all patients with δ-SPD have HPS. Some of the patients described to have δ-SPD have been subsequently shown to have mutations in RUNX1.[358,372,390,391]

In other forms of δ-SPD, data obtained with uranaffin, a dye that specifically stains amine-containing granules, indicate that dense granule membranes are formed but are not properly filled.[392–394] The defects in the different substances contained in dense granules are also heterogeneous, with some patients able to secrete significant amounts of calcium and pyrophosphate even when adenine nucleotide secretion is nearly absent.[392]

Chédiak-Higashi syndrome results from mutation of the *LYST* gene, which encodes a protein of estimated molecular mass of 429 kDa, predicted from domain analysis to participate in vesicle transport and to interact with microtubules; an *HPS1*-like region is also present.[361,366]

Numerous animal models of human δ-SPD and HPS have been reported, and several represent specific counterparts of the human disease. Thus, more than 20 separate inherited mouse defects have been reported to include dense granule deficiencies; of these, pale ear *(ep)* is linked to the mouse equivalent of the *HPS1* gene; pearl *(pe)* to the mouse equivalent of *HSP2* (β₃A subunit of AP-3 complex); cocoa to *HPS3*; light ear *(le)* to *HPS4*; ruby-eye-2 *(ru2)* to *HPS5*; ruby-eye *(ru)* to *HPS6*; sandy *(sdy)* to *HPS7*; and pallid to HPS9 *(PLDN)*.[361,395] The beige mouse and rat serve as models for Chédiak-Higashi syndrome.[361]

### Clinical Features

Patients with δ-SPD as part of the HPS may have severe, or even lethal, hemorrhage.[363] For all other forms of the disorder, the bleeding tendency is variable and mild to moderate.

### Laboratory Features

When tested with the PFA-100 instrument, both prolonged and normal closure times have been reported, akin to prior findings with bleeding times.[396–399] Interestingly, flow-dependent thrombus formation, assessed using a multisurface and multiparameter flow assay, is reported to be decreased.[8] In platelet aggregation studies, ADP and epinephrine induce a normal primary wave of aggregation, but the secondary wave is variably abnormal. The abnormal platelet response is more easily discernible at low collagen doses than high doses. Secretion of ATP from platelets can be measured by luminescence simultaneously with platelet aggregation using a specially designed instrument.[400] ATP release in response to activation is absent or decreased in δ-SPD patients. Thrombin at high doses causes maximal release of platelet dense body contents, even in patients with secretion abnormalities unrelated to granule deficiency, and therefore, this reagent may distinguish between δ-SPD (diminished release) and abnormalities of platelet secretory mechanisms, wherein the release may be normal or near-normal.

Measurement of platelet granule contents can establish further the platelet abnormality. The total platelet content of adenine nucleotides is reduced in δ-SPD, and the ratio of total platelet ATP to ADP is increased because it more closely reflects the ratio in the cytoplasmic, "metabolic" pool of adenine nucleotides (approximately 8:1) than in the "storage" pool in dense granules (approximately 2:3).[360,401] Platelet serotonin is variably reduced.[402] Serotonin is taken up by platelets of patients with δ-SPD, but because it cannot be stored in dense granules, it is rapidly catabolized.[402] Abnormalities in platelet secretion and arachidonic acid metabolism have been identified but are quite variable.[403] Reduced plasma and platelet VWF activity in association with a decrease in plasma high-molecular-weight multimers has been reported in HPS[404,405] and may reflect abnormalities involving the endothelial Weibel-Palade bodies.

The decrease or absence of platelet dense bodies can be confirmed by electron microscopy, using either whole mounts or thin sections of platelets fixed in the presence of calcium, although it requires expertise to interpret the results.[5,406] Some patients have abnormal granules. Uranaffin and osmium may help to identify dense granules. The fluorescent amine mepacrine can be used to quantify dense bodies by fluorescent microscopy or by flow cytometry.[407,408] Immunoblot analysis of skin fibroblasts in HPS may facilitate identification of the protein responsible for the defect.[409]

### Therapy, Course, and Prognosis

The general principles of patient management are similar to those described for all patients with platelet function defects. Patients with HPS suffer from a number of specific problems related to their albinism, colitis, and pulmonary fibrosis.[373] In particular, they should avoid sun exposure. An antifibrotic agent, pirfenidone, demonstrated modest benefit in the initial study.[410] A second study[411] failed to confirm this and was terminated because of futility.

## GRAY PLATELET SYNDROME (α-STORAGE POOL DEFICIENCY)

### Definition and History

GPS is a markedly heterogeneous bleeding disorder characterized by selective deficiency of platelet α granules and their contents, in combination with thrombocytopenia and large platelet size.[412,413] The name derives from the initial observation by Raccuglia, in 1971,[414] of the gray appearance of platelets with paucity of granules on peripheral blood films from a patient with a lifelong bleeding disorder.

### Etiology and Pathogenesis

Normal platelets contain approximately 50 spherical or elongated α granules that contain a large number of proteins, some relatively specific for platelets (platelet factor 4 [PF4], β-thromboglobulin [βTG]), others that are also found in plasma, and yet others whose role in platelets is poorly understood.[412,415,416] Plasma proteins present in α granules include fibrinogen, VWF, albumin, coagulation factor V, immunoglobulin (Ig) G, fibronectin, and several protease inhibitors. Some of these proteins, such as VWF, are synthesized by megakaryocytes, whereas others, such as albumin and IgG, are incorporated into platelets by endocytosis. The α-granule membrane contains several proteins present in the platelet plasma membrane (integrin $\alpha_{IIb}\beta_3$, GPIb–IX–V) and some specific for α granules (P-selectin and osteonectin).

The molecular mechanisms leading to α-granule deficiency in GPS and the combined αδ-SPD are also heterogeneous; thus, they have been attributed to failure of α-granule maturation during MK differentiation, transport or targeting of proteins to α granules, and/or synthesis of granule membranes.[412,415] Proteomic studies in a GPS patient suggested a failure to incorporate endogenously synthesized MK proteins into α granules.[415] Some GPS patients have elevated plasma PF4,[412] suggesting that PF4 synthesis was normal and the primary defect was impaired granule biogenesis with leakage of PF4. Some patients with decreased α-granule contents have a mutation in the gene for the transcription factor RUNX1,[372,390] and PF4 is a transcriptional target of RUNX1.[417] This suggests that decreased platelet PF4 levels in these patients represents a defect in transcriptional regulation and synthesis of PF4. GPS has been reported in association with an X-linked thrombocytopenia, thalassemia, and an R216N mutation in GATA-1, a major regulator of megakaryopoiesis.[418] Autosomal dominant GPS resulting from mutations in transcription factor gene GFI1B has been reported in two kindreds.[419,420]

Three groups[10–12] have reported mutations in NBEAL2 in patients with GPS, a gene that encodes for a protein linked to vesicle transport in neuronal cells. These studies implicate defective vesicle transport as a major mechanism in many forms of GPS. Studies in Nbeal2-deficient mice provide evidence[421,422] that Nbeal2 is required for α-granule biogenesis, platelet function, and MK survival, development, and platelet production—key evidence linking GPS and Nbeal2. These mice were also found to have abnormalities in arterial thrombosis, inflammation, and wound repair. A mutation in the gene encoding the VPS33B protein (a member of the Sec1/Munc18 protein family) involved in vesicle trafficking has also been associated with human α-granule deficiency in the arthrogryposis multiplex congenital, renal dysfunction, and cholestasis (ARC) syndrome.[423] A mutation in the VPS16B gene has also been linked to α-granule deficiency in the ARC syndrome, and it appears that VPS16B and VPS33B interact with each other.[424] Thus, multiple mechanisms can lead to GPS. The inheritance of α-granule deficiency has been autosomal recessive in most reports, but autosomal dominant and sex-linked cases have also been described.[372,390,412,418]

### Clinical Features

GPS patients have a lifelong mild to moderate bleeding diathesis, which is variable in its manifestations.[412]

### Laboratory Features

Platelets appear as larger-than-normal, pale, ghost-like, oval forms on blood films and are often difficult to identify (Fig. 10–6). Thrombocytopenia is variable but can be moderately severe, with counts below 50,000/μL. Platelet aggregation abnormalities vary considerably.[343,412,413,425–427] ADP- and epinephrine-induced aggregation is normal or nearly normal. Collagen- and thrombin-induced aggregation tends to be more abnormal, but this is not a consistent finding. Concomitant GPVI deficiency was reported in one patient, and if the association is more widespread, it may explain the variable abnormalities in collagen-induced aggregation.[343] Studies in one patient showed flow-dependent thrombus formation to be decreased.[8] Additional abnormalities in PI metabolism, protein phosphorylation, calcium mobilization, platelet factor Va, and platelet secretion have been described[428–430] and may contribute to the platelet aggregation abnormalities and clinical symptoms. The failure of exogenous α-granule proteins to fully correct the aggregation defects suggests that these abnormalities may be important in the overall platelet dysfunction in GPS.[425]

Under the electron microscope, platelets and megakaryocytes from GPS patients reveal absent or markedly decreased α granules

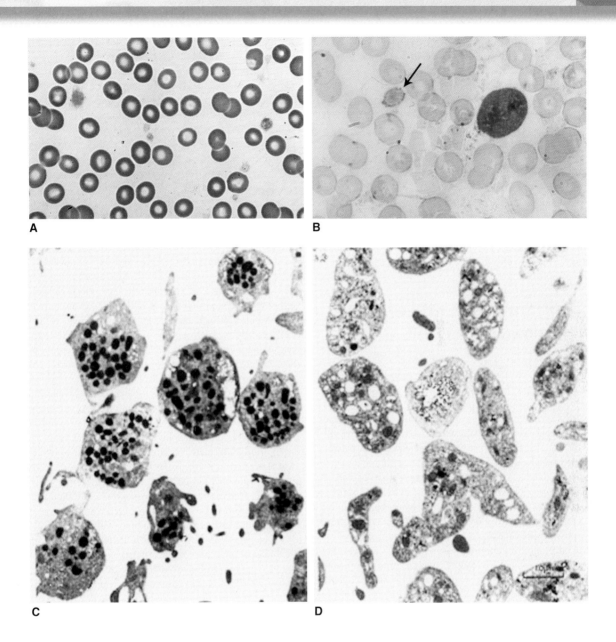

**Figure 10–6.** Gray platelet syndrome (*a*-granule deficiency). **A.** Blood film. Note gray staining of many, but not all, platelets with loss of internal granular structure. Two are megathrombocytes, with one platelet being very large, almost the size of a red cell (giant platelet). **B.** Blood film. Treated with periodic acid–Schiff (PAS) stain for carbohydrate. Note large "gray platelet" stained with PAS *(arrow)* and typical PAS staining of neutrophil cytoplasm. **C.** Transmission electron microscopy of normal human platelets with abundant electron-dense *a* granules. **D.** Transmission electron microscopy of platelets from a patient with gray platelet syndrome. Note profound reduction in electron-dense *a* granules. *(Reproduced with permission from Lichtman's Atlas of Hematology, www.accessmedicine.com.)*

(see Fig. 10-6).[412] The platelets are deficient in *α*-granule proteins: PF4, *β*TG, VWF, thrombospondin, fibronectin, factor V, high-molecular-weight kininogen, transforming growth factor (TGF)-*β*₁, and platelet-derived growth factor (PDGF); albumin and IgG may also be decreased. There is increased reticulin in the marrow of some patients with GPS,[431–433] which may be associated with splenomegaly and evidence of extramedullary hematopoiesis.[431,434] The marrow fibrosis has been attributed to elevated marrow levels of PDGF and TGF-*β*₁ leaked from megakaryocytes.[412] Megakaryocytes show emperipolesis and the capture of neutrophils. P-selectin is a protein present in the *α*-granule membranes and translocates to platelet surface on platelet activation. The content and surface expression of P-selectin has been reported as normal[412,435] or decreased,[436] which underscores the heterogeneity of the GPS.

## *α,δ*-STORAGE POOL DEFICIENCY

This disorder is characterized by moderate to severe defects in both *α* and *δ* granules, with heterogeneous expression in the few patients in whom it has been reported.[372] Clinical and laboratory features are similar to those of *δ*-SPD. In general, the functional consequences of the defect in dense granules are more severe than the defect in *α* granules.

## QUEBEC PLATELET DISORDER

Quebec platelet disorder (QPD) is an autosomal dominant bleeding disorder associated with reduced platelet counts and decreased *α*-granule proteins as a result of increased plasmin-mediated degradation of the *α*-granule proteins.[437,438] Originally described as factor V

Quebec, the early description of this disorder included severe bleeding after trauma, mild thrombocytopenia, decreased functional platelet factor V, and normal plasma factor V.[437,439] The bleeding time is normal to mildly prolonged, and epinephrine-induced platelet aggregation is selectively decreased. Aggregation response to other agonists is variable. Platelets from patients with QPD display reduced levels of several $\alpha$-granule proteins (factor V, fibrinogen, VWF, fibronectin, thrombospondin, multimerin, and osteonectin) as a consequence of enhanced proteolysis.[437,440] The excessive plasmin generation inducing the degradation of $\alpha$-granule proteins results from increased megakaryocyte expression of u-PA because of a tandem duplication mutation of the cis regulatory elements of the u-PA gene (PLAU).[441,442] Plasma tests of systemic fibrinolysis (fibrinogen, D-dimer, plasminogen, plasmin-$\alpha_2$ antiplasmin complexes, and u-PA) are normal in these patients. Genetic testing for the PLAU mutation provides a definitive diagnosis. Treatment with fibrinolytic inhibitors appears to be effective in controlling bleeding.[437]

# ● ABNORMALITIES OF PLATELET SIGNALING AND SECRETION

A sizable percentage of patients with variably severe mucocutaneous bleeding manifestations, mostly mild, have defects in platelet aggregation and secretion. In most of these patients, the underlying platelet molecular mechanisms are unknown. The most common pattern on laboratory studies is blunted platelet aggregation and absence of the second wave of aggregation on exposure to ADP, epinephrine, collagen, or U46619, and decreased dense granule secretion. Such patients have been lumped together, more out of convenience than because of an understanding of the mechanisms, categorized as primary secretion defects, activation defects, or signal transduction defects.[443–446] Simplistically, platelet activation is a complex process involving agonist binding to surface receptors; signal transduction through G-protein–coupled receptors and other types of receptors; phosphoinositol metabolism resulting in calcium mobilization and phosphorylation of target proteins; arachidonic acid metabolism leading to TXA$_2$ production; activation of the integrin $\alpha_{IIb}\beta_3$ receptor; and release of granule contents (Chap. 2). Defects involving these and other processes can result in impaired platelet function.

## DEFECTS IN PLATELET AGONIST RECEPTORS OR AGONIST-SPECIFIC SIGNAL TRANSDUCTION

### Thromboxane A$_2$ Receptor Defect
Platelets contain two different isoforms of the TXA$_2$ receptor. Both forms activate PLC, but they differ in their effects on adenylyl cyclase, with one stimulating and the other inhibiting this enzyme.[447] A mutation in the first cytoplasmic loop of the TXA$_2$ receptor (R601L) has been described as causing an inherited bleeding disorder in several families from Japan.[448,449] The platelets of these patients do not aggregate in response to TXA$_2$ mimetics. The aggregation defect also extends to other agonists, such as ADP, in which TXA$_2$ made by activated platelets and released into the surrounding medium, augments the response. The defect appears to be in signal initiation rather than ligand binding. TXA$_2$-induced activation of PLC (measured as Ca$^{2+}$ mobilization, inositol trisphosphate, and phosphatidic acid formation) is impaired, whereas PLA$_2$ activation and TXA$_2$ production are normal. Of note, the mutation appears to inhibit PLC activation by both receptor isoforms and impairs adenylyl cyclase stimulation by one of the isoforms; it does

not, however, affect the inhibition of adenylyl cyclase produced by the other isoform. Both dominant and recessive inheritance patterns have been reported. The abnormal aggregation responses in heterozygous family members suggests a dominant negative effect of the mutation.[449] Another report[450] describes a heterozygous D304N substitution in the seventh transmembrane region of the TXA$_2$ receptor associated with a bleeding history, a 50 percent reduction in ligand binding, and loss of receptor function. A heterozygous TXA$_2$R mutation (V2416) in the third intracellular loop has been reported[7] in a subject without any bleeding symptoms. This subject had impaired aggregation and Ca$^{2+}$ mobilization in response to U46619, normal platelet receptor levels, and aspirin resistance in microfluidic experiments assessing platelet deposition under flow.

### Adenosine Diphosphate Receptor Defects (P2Y$_{12}$ and P2X$_1$)
Multiple receptors (P2Y$_{12}$, P2Y$_1$, and P2X$_1$) mediate ADP interactions with platelets (Chap. 2).[451] P2Y$_1$ receptors induce PLC activation, intracellular Ca$^{2+}$ mobilization, and shape change, while P2Y$_{12}$ receptors mediate inhibition of cAMP formation by adenylyl cyclase. ADP-induced platelet aggregation requires activation of both P2Y$_1$ and P2Y$_{12}$ receptors. P2X$_1$ receptors function as an ATP- and ADP-gated cation channel (Chap. 2). Patients with P2Y$_{12}$ receptor abnormalities have blunted ADP-induced platelet aggregation responses, impaired suppression of prostaglandin E$_1$ (PGE$_1$)-induced elevations in cAMP, and normal ADP-stimulated shape change.[452–456] Bleeding symptoms have been variable, with some demonstrating moderately severe hemorrhage in association with surgery and trauma. Because ADP released from platelets potentiates the responses to other agonists, such as collagen and TXA$_2$, platelet aggregation in response to these agonists is also abnormal in these patients. Platelet binding of ADP or the ADP analogue 2-methylthio-ADP[452–454,456] was decreased in all but one patient studied.[457] Decreased platelet 2-methylthio-ADP binding has also been reported in other patients with impaired aggregation and secretion in response to several agonists, including ADP.[458,459]

The genetic defects have been defined in some of these patients. In three patients, homozygous deletions have been demonstrated in the P2Y$_{12}$ gene, resulting in premature termination and a lack of P2Y$_{12}$ protein.[445,452,456] A homozygous missense mutation in the translation initiation codon was described in another patient,[454] and another patient was reported to have a two-nucleotide deletion (at amino acid 240) in one P2Y$_{12}$ gene allele, resulting in a frameshift and a premature stop codon.[453,460] Although this last patient had one P2Y$_{12}$ allele with a normal coding region, the patient's platelets lacked P2Y$_{12}$ receptors, suggesting repression of the normal allele or an unrelated abnormality in its transcriptional regulation. In contrast, platelets from the patient's daughter had an intermediate number of ADP-binding sites, a normal platelet response to ADP, and one frame-shifted allele and one normal allele, suggesting that the mutant allele does not act in a dominant negative manner.[453] Studies in yet another patient with abnormal ADP-induced aggregation revealed a compound heterozygous state with one allele containing an R256N substitution in the sixth transmembrane domain, and the other allele containing an R265W substitution in the third extracellular loop of the receptor.[457] Platelet binding of $^{33}$P-2MeS ADP was normal; neither mutation affected the translocation of the P2Y$_{12}$ receptor to the cell surface, but ADP-induced inhibition of adenylyl cyclase was partially reduced, indicating a functionally abnormal receptor. A heterozygous mutation (K174E) in the second extracellular loop of P2Y$_{12}$ was identified in one patient[455]; this was associated with decreased 2-methylthio-ADP binding. Another heterozygous mutation, P258T, in the third extracellular loop has been described in association with a bleeding diathesis.[461] Interestingly, a heterozygous mutation in P2Y$_{12}$ (P341A) has been shown to induce altered interaction with Rab guanosine triphosphatases (GTPases) and endosomal trafficking of the receptor leading to its decreased surface expression.[462]

A defect in the $P2X_1$ purinergic receptor has been described in a 6-year-old patient with bleeding manifestations.[463] The patient had isolated impairment of ADP-induced platelet aggregation and was heterozygous for a deletion of a single leucine in a stretch of four leucine residues[351-354] in the second transmembrane domain of $P2X_1$. The mutant protein apparently caused a dominant negative effect on $P2X_1$-mediated calcium channel activity.

### Epinephrine Receptor Defects

Abnormalities of $\alpha$-adrenergic receptors and $\alpha$-adrenergic–specific signal transduction have been described in several patients,[464-466] but the relationship to bleeding manifestations remains unclear, particularly because responses to epinephrine are blunted even in some otherwise normal individuals. Responses to epinephrine are blunted in QPD.[437]

### Platelet-Activating Factor Receptor Defect

A defect in the platelet-activating factor receptor or platelet-activating factor–specific signal transduction has been reported.[467]

## GUANOSINE TRIPHOSPHATE–BINDING PROTEIN DEFECTS

GTP-binding proteins are a heterotrimeric class of proteins (consisting of $\alpha$, $\beta$, and $\gamma$ subunits) that link surface receptors and intracellular enzymes (Chap. 2). Abnormalities involving $G\alpha q$, $G\alpha i_1$, and $G\alpha s$ proteins have been described.

### Gαq Deficiency

$G\alpha q$ plays a major role in mediating platelet responses to activation of G-protein–coupled receptors. One patient has been described with a selective platelet $G\alpha q$ deficiency in association with a mild bleeding disorder, abnormal platelet aggregation and secretion in response to a number of agonists, and diminished GTPase activity (a reflection of $G\alpha$-subunit dysfunction) in response to platelet activation.[468,469] The downstream events from $G\alpha q$, including $Ca^{2+}$ mobilization, release of arachidonic acid from phospholipids, and activation of integrin $\alpha_{IIb}\beta_3$ receptors, were impaired. The $G\alpha q$ coding sequence in this patient was normal, but $G\alpha q$ mRNA levels were decreased in platelets, suggesting a potential defect in transcriptional regulation of the gene. This abnormality appeared to be selective for platelets as the patient's neutrophils had normal $G\alpha q$ protein.[470]

### Gαs Hyperfunction and Genetic Variation in Extra Large Gαs

Two unrelated families have been described with inducible hyperactivity of $G\alpha s$.[471] These patients had a bleeding diathesis, prolonged bleeding times, variable mental retardation, and mild skeletal malformations. Platelet aggregation responses to physiologic agonists were normal, but the platelets showed increased sensitivity to inhibition by agents ($PGE_1$, prostacyclin [$PGI_2$]) that elevate cAMP. Platelet $G\alpha s$, which when activated increases platelet cAMP levels and inhibits platelet aggregation and secretion, was increased in these patients. The $G\alpha s$ gene (GNAS1) has multiple alternative promoters and isoforms as a result of alternative splicing, including extralarge $G\alpha s$ (XL$\alpha s$). XL$\alpha s$ is imprinted and thus normally only expressed from the paternal allele. A heterozygous 36-bp insertion and a 2-bp substitution were identified in exon 1 of the paternal XL$\alpha s$ gene in these patients. Because XL$\alpha s$ is not activated by the usual platelet $G\alpha s$-coupled receptors, the mechanisms leading to increased cAMP levels and enhanced expression of $G\alpha s$ protein is unclear. Of note, 2.2 percent of control subjects also had

the same polymorphism, but only those individuals inheriting it from their father had inducible $G\alpha s$ hyperfunction and increased platelet $G\alpha s$ protein.

Platelet $G\alpha s$ deficiency has also been described in a patient with pseudohypoparathyroidism Ib in association with disturbed imprinting and altered methylation in the GNAS1 gene cluster that encompasses the four GNAS1 splice variants, including the $G\alpha s$ subunit.[472] The $G\alpha s$ coding sequence was normal. As expected from the deficiency in $G\alpha s$ protein, there was decreased platelet cAMP formation upon activation of receptors linked to $G\alpha s$. The authors did not indicate whether the patient had a bleeding diathesis.

### Gαi1 Deficiency

Platelet $G\alpha i1$ deficiency has been reported in association with a bleeding disorder and abnormalities in integrin $\alpha_{IIb}\beta_3$ activation, platelet aggregation, and dense granule secretion upon activation with one or more agonists.[473] In keeping with the known function of $G\alpha i$ in inhibiting the activation of adenylyl cyclase and the subsequent increases in cAMP levels, the patient's platelets failed to inhibit forskolin-stimulated cAMP levels on activation. Platelet $G\alpha i1$ protein was decreased by 75 percent, whereas other members of the $G\alpha i$ family ($G\alpha i2$, $G\alpha i3$, $G\alpha iz$) and $G\alpha q$ were normal. Although a large subset of patients has been considered as having a defect in Gi signaling,[474] this is based on abnormal responses on platelet aggregation and secretion studies to ADP and epinephrine, and direct evidence at the molecular level to support this conclusion has not been provided.

### CalDAG-GEFI Deficiency

Three siblings from first-cousin parents with severe mucocutaneous bleeding manifestations had prolonged bleeding times and reduced platelet aggregation in response to ADP or epinephrine and to low doses, but not high doses, of a thrombin receptor–activating peptide and collagen.[475] Clot retraction was normal. Whole-exome analysis revealed a homozygous G248W mutation in RAS guanyl-releasing protein-2 (RASGRP2), the gene for the protein calcium- and diacylglycerol (DAG)-regulated guanine exchange factor-1 (CalDAG-GEFI), affecting the CDC25 catalytic domain critical for interacting with GTPases. The platelets demonstrated decreased Rap1 activation and fibrinogen binding and abnormal adhesion and spreading on immobilized fibrinogen and collagen. These results support a model of platelet activation in which CalDAG-GEFI stimulates GTP loading of Rap1 and Rac1 in response to an increase in intracellular $Ca^{2+}$ and the activated Rap1 leads to integrin $\alpha_{IIb}\beta_3$ activation and the activated Rac1 enhances platelet spreading. The heterozygotes were asymptomatic, but their platelets had a defective spreading.[475]

## PHOSPHOLIPASE C–$\beta_2$ DEFICIENCY AND DEFECTS IN PHOSPHOLIPASE C ACTIVATION

Several investigators have described patients with relatively mild bleeding diatheses and impaired platelet aggregation and dense granule secretion, despite normal granule stores and the ability to synthesize $TXA_2$.[445,446,476-478] An early event after stimulating several platelet G-protein–coupled receptors is activation of PLC-$\beta$, leading to formation of the intracellular mediators $IP_3$ and DAG (Chap. 2); the former mediates $Ca^{2+}$ mobilization, and the latter mediates PKC-induced protein phosphorylation. Defects in one or more of these responses has been documented in several patients. In one study of eight patients with abnormal platelet aggregation and secretion in response to several different receptor-mediated agonists, $Ca^{2+}$ mobilization and/or pleckstrin phosphorylation was abnormal in seven patients, suggesting that the impaired secretion and aggregation resulted from upstream abnormalities in early signaling events.[478] Specific defects at the level of PLC-$\beta_2$,[479,480]

$G\alpha q$,[468] and PKC-$\theta$[481] were identified in these eight patients. In another study, eight patients were described who had decreased initial rates and extents of platelet aggregation in response to ADP, epinephrine, and the TXA$_2$ mimetic U44069[476]; subsequent studies in one patient demonstrated impaired phosphatidylinositol hydrolysis, phosphatidic acid formation, and pleckstrin phosphorylation.[482,483]

In two related patients described with PLC-$\beta_2$ deficiency, platelet aggregation and secretion were impaired in association with impaired IP$_3$ and DAG formation, calcium mobilization, and pleckstrin phosphorylation following activation with ADP, collagen, platelet-activating factor, or thrombin, indicating a defect in PLC activation.[479] These patients had a mild bleeding disorder. Human platelets contain at least seven PLC isozymes, and a selective decrease was observed in only the PLC-$\beta_2$ isozyme.[480] The decreased platelet PLC-$\beta_2$ protein levels were associated with a normal gene coding sequence but with diminished PLC-$\beta_2$ mRNA levels in platelets, but not neutrophils, suggesting a hematopoietic lineage-specific defect in PLC-$\beta_2$ gene regulation.[484] Defects in phosphatidylinositol metabolism and protein phosphorylation have been described in other such patients, although the primary protein abnormalities were not defined.[482,483,485–488]

## DEFECTS IN PROTEIN PHOSPHORYLATION: PROTEIN KINASE C-$\theta$ DEFICIENCY

PKC isozymes, a family of serine- and threonine-specific protein kinases, phosphorylate a wide array of proteins involved in signal transduction. PKC enzymes regulate several aspects of platelet function, including activation of integrin $\alpha_{IIb}\beta_3$ receptors, platelet aggregation and secretion, and platelet production (Chap. 2). Deficiency of a human platelet PKC isozyme (PKC-$\theta$) has been described in a patient with lifelong mucocutaneous bleeding manifestations, mild thrombocytopenia, and markedly abnormal platelet aggregation (including primary wave) and dense granule secretion in response to multiple agonists.[481,489] Agonist-induced phosphorylation of pleckstrin and myosin light chain were diminished in the patient's platelets. This subject was subsequently shown to have a heterozygous mutation in a transcription factor, RUNX1 (also termed core-binding factor A2, CBFA2, or *AML1*), which has been linked to a familial platelet function defect, associated with thrombocytopenia and predisposition to acute leukemia[481,490] (see "Transcription Factor Mutations and Associated Platelet Dysfunction" below). Platelet expression of myosin light chain *(MYL9)* was also decreased in this patient.[491]

## DEFECTS IN ARACHIDONIC ACID METABOLISM AND THROMBOXANE PRODUCTION

### Defects in Arachidonic Acid Release from Phospholipids

Release of free arachidonic acid from phospholipids, mediated by cytosolic PLA$_2$, is the initial and rate-limiting step in thromboxane synthesis upon platelet activation. Several patients have been described with abnormalities in the release of arachidonic acid.[469,485,492–494] In general, their platelets aggregated normally in response to arachidonic acid but not to ADP, epinephrine, and/or collagen. In one of these patients, this defect was related to an upstream abnormality in $G\alpha q$ (see "$G\alpha q$ Deficiency" above).[468] Another patient had HPS with $\delta$-SPD and abnormal PLA$_2$ activity.[492] An inherited deficiency in cytosolic PLA$_2$ has been reported in a patient with recurrent small intestinal ulceration, markedly decreased eicosanoid synthesis (including in thromboxane, 12-hydroxyeicosatetraenoic acid [12-HETE], and leukotriene B$_4$), and impaired aggregation with ADP and collagen but normal with arachidonic acid.[493] This patient had two heterozygous single-base-pair

mutations in the PLA$_2$ coding region, leading to S111P and R485H substitutions. Another report documents twins with a history of gastrointestinal ulcers, associated with similarly impaired platelet function associated with a homozygous D575H mutation in PLA$_2$ *(PLA2G4A)*.[494] These patients had mildly decreased plasma factor XI as well.

### Cyclooxygenase (Prostaglandin H$_2$ Synthase-1) Deficiency

Deficient platelet cyclooxygenase (prostaglandin H$_2$ synthase-1) activity leading to impaired platelet function and a mild bleeding disorder has been identified in a number of patients.[495–502] Platelets from such patients cannot make thromboxane from arachidonic acid but can make it from cyclic endoperoxides (prostaglandin G$_2$ and prostaglandin H$_2$). While some patients have had decreased platelet cyclooxygenase protein, others have had evidence of a dysfunctional molecule.[501,502]

### Thromboxane Synthase Deficiency

Presumed platelet thromboxane synthase deficiencies have been identified in two families based on the failure of cyclic endoperoxides to be converted into TXA$_2$.[503,504]

## ● ABNORMALITIES OF PLATELET COAGULANT ACTIVITY (SCOTT SYNDROME)

### DEFINITION AND HISTORY

Activated platelets play an essential role in providing the membrane surface on which specific blood coagulation reactions occur, leading to thrombin generation.[505,506] Patients whose platelets fail to facilitate thrombin generation are defined as having defects in platelet coagulant activity (PCA) (Chap. 2). Only a few patients have been described with isolated defects in PCA and normal aggregation and secretion responses.[505,507–513] Defects in PCA may also be secondary to abnormalities in platelet aggregation, such as in patients with SPD and thrombasthenia.[505] Patients with isolated abnormalities in PCA are referred to as having the Scott syndrome after the first patient described in 1979 by Weiss and colleagues.[505,507–510]

### ETIOLOGY AND PATHOGENESIS

The main functional abnormality in Scott syndrome is the impaired ability of activated platelets to promote coagulation reactions; a second abnormality in these patients is a defect in release of microvesicles on cell activation.[514,515] In resting platelets, membrane phospholipids are asymmetrically distributed, with the aminophospholipids phosphatidylserine (PS) and phosphatidylethanolamine (PE) concentrated in the inner membrane leaflet, and phosphatidylcholine (PC) and sphingomyelin concentrated in the outer leaflet. Cell activation induces phospholipid translocation, with PS moving to the outer leaflet. This process is regulated by several proteins that are descriptively identified by their functions. They include a "flippase" (i.e., an aminophospholipid translocase identified as a P4 adenosine triphosphatase [ATPase]) that promotes inward transport of lipids; a "floppase" that regulates outward phospholipid transport (encoded by gene *ABCC1*); and one or more "scramblases" that promote bidirectional movement of lipids between the two layers.[506] Surface expression of PS is essential for platelets to accelerate coagulation reactions, in particular, activation of the tenase complex leading to the activation of factors X to Xa and of the prothrombinase complex that converts prothrombin to thrombin (Chaps. 3 and 4). Scott syndrome platelets have a defect in PS translocation resulting in decreased binding of factors Va-Xa and VIIIa-IXa,[505,506] thus leading to impaired blood coagulation. Erythrocytes and lymphocytes also demonstrate similar defects in both microvesicle formation and coagulant activity.[505,512] In a French family with Scott syndrome,[508] the propositus's platelets were found to have a defect in protein tyrosine phosphorylation, suggesting an additional defect in signal transduction.[510]

Apart from the above patients with Scott syndrome, four patients from three unrelated families have been reported to have abnormal PCA, a bleeding disorder, impaired serum prothrombin consumption, and reduced microparticle formation.[516] However, in contrast to the Scott syndrome, the prothrombinase activity was normal.

The inheritance pattern in Scott syndrome appears to be autosomal recessive.[505,508] A heterozygous missense mutation has been reported in one patient in the gene *ABCA1*, which encodes the ATP-binding cassette transporter protein implicated in PS translocation; the significance of this remains unclear.[517] Mutations in TMEM16F have been identified in two patients with Scott syndrome. The patient Scott was found to have a homozygous mutation at the splice acceptor site for intron 12 of *TMEM16F*, resulting in a frameshift and premature termination of protein translation.[518] A second patient had compound heterozygosity for a mutation at the donor splice site of intron 6 and a single nucleotide insertion in exon 12, causing a frameshift and premature termination of translation.[13] Although these findings constitute strong evidence linking *TMEM16F* mutations to Scott syndrome, they leave open whether TMEM16F is itself the membrane scramblase or a protein that regulates the scramblase.

## CLINICAL AND LABORATORY FEATURES

The bleeding symptoms in patients with Scott syndrome are similar to those in patients with other platelet defects. In contrast to other qualitative platelet abnormalities, the bleeding time in Scott syndrome patients is normal.[508,509,514] The serum PT, which reflects the completeness of clotting of whole blood and consumption of prothrombin, is abnormal, indicating incomplete coagulation.[507-509] More specific assays of "platelet factor 3," the phenomenologic designation of the platelet contribution to accelerating clot formation, are also abnormal.[519]

Patients with the Scott syndrome have normal platelet aggregation and secretion in response to the usually used agonists.[505] The patient Scott[505] also had normal platelet phospholipid content, normal to enhanced platelet adhesion to subendothelium with diminished thrombus formation, diminished factor Va binding to platelets and platelet microparticles, and diminished platelet acceleration of both factor X activation and prothrombin activation. Abnormalities in exposure of negatively charged phospholipids and shedding of microparticles have been consistent findings in all patients described.[506,508-512]

## TREATMENT

Platelet or whole blood transfusions have been effective as prophylaxis and as therapy for bleeding episodes.[505,507-509] Prothrombin complex concentrates were effective in the patient Scott,[392] but these preparations may be associated with thrombotic complications.

## ⬤ ABNORMALITIES OF A CYTOSKELETAL STRUCTURAL PROTEIN: $\beta_1$-TUBULIN AND FILAMIN A

Megakaryocytes and platelets express primarily and selectively the $\beta_1$ isoform of tubulin. A heterozygous $\beta_1$-tubulin Q43P polymorphism was identified in a group of patients with a recessive form of

macrothrombocytopenia; the polymorphism could not account fully for the macrothrombocytopenia because of the difference in inheritance and its presence in approximately 11 percent of the normal population.[520] Individuals heterozygous for the polymorphism had normal platelet counts, relatively high mean platelet volume values, abnormally rounded platelets with abnormal marginal bands of microtubules, and mild abnormalities of platelet aggregation, secretion, and adhesion to collagen. One study found the polymorphism was associated with decreased collagen-induced platelet aggregation and increased risk of intracerebral hemorrhage in men.[521]

Subsequently, two patients with macrothrombocytopenia from a single kindred were reported to be heterozygous for a R318W $\beta_1$ tubulin mutation.[522] The mutation is strategically located at the $\alpha$–$\beta$ tubulin interface. Of note, the Q43P polymorphism and an R207H substitution were also found in this family, but neither was judged to be responsible for the macrothrombocytopenia.

Filamins are large dimeric actin-binding proteins that stabilize actin filament networks. Filamin A is the predominant platelet filamin. Several patients have been reported with dominant mutations of the X-linked *Filamin A (FLNA)* gene associated with thrombocytopenia and abnormalities in platelet aggregation, secretion, GPVI signaling, and thrombus growth on collagen.[522A]

## ⬤ ABNORMALITIES OF CYTOSKELETAL LINKING PROTEINS

### WISKOTT-ALDRICH SYNDROME PROTEIN

The Wiskott-Aldrich syndrome (WAS) is an X chromosome–linked inherited disorder characterized by small platelets, thrombocytopenia, recurrent infections, eczema, and an increased incidence of autoimmunity and malignancies.[523,524] In addition, a variety of immunologic abnormalities affecting T-lymphocyte function, Ig levels, cellular immunity, and responsiveness to polysaccharide antigens are commonly present. Death from infection, hemorrhage, or malignancy is common before adulthood. Some patients with WAS mutations may have only thrombocytopenia (X-linked thrombocytopenia [XLT]) without other features. WAS is caused by mutations in the WAS gene, which encodes the WAS protein (WASP), a multidomain protein that relays signals from the cell surface to the actin skeleton and modulates the latter's reorganization. In platelets, WASP is localized to the cytoskeleton.[524,525] It is phosphorylated on platelet activation by several different protein kinases, including Btk, Grb2, PLC-$\gamma_2$, PKC-$\theta$, and SGK1.[524]

Microthrombocytopenia is a consistent feature of WAS and XLT and the major contributor to the bleeding diathesis, which may be life-threatening in some patients because of gastrointestinal hemorrhage or intracranial hemorrhage. Marrow megakaryocytes are normal in number, but platelet formation is abnormal and platelet survival is decreased.[523,524]

Abnormalities in platelet surface glycoprotein sialophorin (CD43, gp115, leukosialin), GPIb, platelet integrin $\alpha_2$, integrin $\alpha_{IIb}\beta_3$, and GPIV have been reported in some WAS patients.[526,527] Platelets from patients with WAS also have qualitative defects, including SPD[367,368,528] and impaired energy metabolism.[528,529]

Platelet aggregation in WAS has been reported to be reduced, normal, or enhanced.[524,530-533] Interpreting these studies is confounded by the low platelet count, methodologic differences, and timing in relation to splenectomy.[524] Despite the role of WASP in cytoskeletal reorganization, shape change and actin polymerization are normal in WAS platelets.[531,534,535]

WASP has been implicated in regulating responses dependent on integrin $\alpha_{IIb}\beta_3$ outside-in signaling.[536] Although Pac-1 binding is normal in WAS platelets, there is decreased spreading on fibrinogen and decreased clot retraction associated with enhanced PS exposure.[536]

Splenectomy usually improves the thrombocytopenia.[523,524] Hematopoietic stem cell transplantation is the accepted curative approach for WAS and can correct all aspects of the disease provided reconstitution is achieved.[523,524] Autologous gene-modified hematopoietic stem cell transplantation is an emerging therapy for WAS patients.[523,524]

# ● KINDLIN-3 (LEUKOCYTE ADHESION DEFECT-3; LEUKOCYTE ADHESION DEFECT—1 VARIANT; INTEGRIN ACTIVATION DEFICIENCY DISEASE)

## DEFINITION AND HISTORY/ETIOLOGY AND PATHOGENESIS

A syndrome with the features of both mild LAD-1 and GT was first described in 1997[537] and termed LAD-1 variant or LAD-3. Since then more than 10 families have been reported, with several from Turkey.[538–541] The etiology is a deficiency or defect in the cytoskeletal linking protein kindlin-3 (FERMTS3). Kindlin-3 is a protein expressed exclusively in hematopoietic cells with homology to talin that also binds to the cytoplasmic domain of the $\beta_3$ subunit of integrin $\alpha_{IIb}\beta_3$ (Chap. 2). It has been implicated in the inside-out activation of integrin $\alpha_{IIb}\beta_3$ in mice.[542] It also participates in the activation of leukocyte integrins, which accounts for the defects in immune function. It may also affect red blood cell structure. Defects in CALDAGGEF1, the gene for another exchange factor, also cause abnormalities in platelet function and are discussed in the section "Guanosine Triphosphate–Binding Protein Defects."[538,543]

The disorder is characterized by a hemorrhagic diathesis in combination with a variable predisposition to infections and inflammation without pus formation, poor wound healing, delayed umbilical cord stump detachment, and variable osteopetrosis. Intracerebral hemorrhage at birth or soon thereafter has been reported in several of the patients, as well as relatively severe mucosal and gastrointestinal bleeding. Thus, the bleeding diathesis is more severe than is found in patients with GT, perhaps because of additional abnormalities in blood vessels. The need for red blood cell transfusions in infancy has been reported in several patients as a result of blood loss from mucosal surfaces and perhaps red blood cell abnormalities. Leukocytosis, as is found in other LAD syndromes, is a constant finding. Normal platelet counts are the usual finding, but thrombocytopenia has been reported. Platelet aggregation studies demonstrate defects similar to those observed in GT.[541–543] Hematopoietic stem cell transplantation has been successful in restoring normal hematopoietic function in patients with life-threatening hemorrhagic and infectious complications of the disease.[541]

# ● TRANSCRIPTION FACTOR MUTATIONS AND ASSOCIATED PLATELET DYSFUNCTION

Transcription factors, and the cis-regulatory sequences to which they bind, regulate lineage-specific gene expression. Transcription factors RUNX1, FLI1 (a member of the ETS [E-twenty-six] family), GATA-1, and GFI1B (growth factor independent 1B) are important regulators of hematopoietic lineage differentiation, megakaryopoiesis, and platelet

production.[419,420,544] They interact in a combinatorial manner in regulating megakaryocytic genes.[544] A single transcription factor mutation may alter expression of numerous genes, affect diverse cellular mechanisms, and lead to defects in both platelet number and function. Until recently, the pursuit of the molecular mechanisms in patients with platelet dysfunction has focused on delineating mutations in the genes encoding postulated candidate proteins. Therefore, the increasing spotlight on transcription factor mutations to explain platelet dysfunction is a paradigm shift.[9,545,545A]

## RUNX1 (FAMILIAL PLATELET DISORDER WITH PREDISPOSITION TO ACUTE MYELOGENOUS LEUKEMIA)

An association between inherited platelet dysfunction, thrombocytopenia, and a predisposition to acute myeloid leukemia has been reported in several families in which the platelet abnormalities antedated the leukemia.[390,490,546–551] Inherited mutations in RUNX1 (AML1, CBFA2) are the basis for this constellation, which is inherited as an autosomal dominant trait, because of haploinsufficiency.[490] Patients generally display mild thrombocytopenia from birth and a bleeding disorder disproportionate to the thrombocytopenia. Approximately one-third of patients develop leukemia, with a median age of onset of 33 years.[552]

Platelet abnormalities reported in patients with RUNX1 mutations include decreased aggregation, secretion, protein phosphorylation (myosin light chain and pleckstrin), and production of 12-hydroxyeicosapentaenoic acid; decreased integrin $\alpha_{IIb}\beta_3$ activation upon platelet activation; $\delta$- and/or $\alpha$-granule SPD; and a selective decrease in one PKC isoform (PKC-$\theta$).[372,390,553–555] Of note, several patients described earlier as having SPD ($\delta$ or $\alpha$ granules) have been subsequently shown to harbor RUNX1 mutations.[358,372,390,391] In one patient, platelet albumin and IgG were diminished, suggesting a defect in the uptake and packaging of these proteins into $\alpha$ granules.[481,489]

Most mutations of RUNX1 have been in the conserved Runt domain,[390] although a mutation in the transactivating domain (Y260X) has been reported.[390] Platelet transcript expression profiling in a patient with RUNX1 haploinsufficiency revealed downregulation of numerous genes involved in platelet structure and function, including MYL9 (myosin light chain), ALOX12 (12-lipoxygenase), PF4, and PRKCQ (PKC-$\theta$).[491,554–556] ALOX12, PRKCQ, PF4, and MYL9[554–556] are direct transcriptional targets of RUNX1. Patients with RUNX1 haploinsufficiency also have impaired megakaryopoiesis[490] and decreased platelet thrombopoietin receptors (Mpl).[551] Targeted correction of RUNX1 mutation in induced pluripotent stem cells (iPSCs) developed from skin fibroblasts from two patients resulted in normalization of the defect in megakaryopoiesis.[391] These studies raise the potential for targeted gene therapy for this disorder. Using next-generation sequencing, Stockley and colleagues[9] identified mutations in RUNX1 and FLI1, in six of 13 patients with excessive bleeding, and impaired aggregation and platelet dense granule secretion in response to multiple agonists. Thus, transcription factor mutations are an important mechanism for inherited platelet dysfunction.[545,545A]

## GATA-1

GATA-1 is a critical regulator of both megakaryocyte and erythroid development. GATA-1 mutations have been associated with an X-linked syndrome consisting of dyserythropoiesis, anemia, thrombocytopenia, and large platelets[2]; selectively impaired responses to collagen and ristocetin related to abnormalities in GPIb$\beta$[557,558]; diminished platelet G$\alpha$s protein and mRNA[557]; and a form of GPS (with R216N mutation).[418]

## FLI-1 (DIMORPHIC DYSMORPHIC PLATELETS WITH GIANT *A*-GRANULES AND THROMBOCYTOPENIA [PARIS-TROUSSEAU/ JACOBSEN SYNDROME])

The Paris-Trousseau syndrome, a variant of Jacobsen syndrome, is a rare autosomal dominant disorder[559-562] characterized by mental retardation, congenital macrothrombocytopenia, giant α granules (1 to 2 $\mu$m in diameter) in a subpopulation (1 to 5 percent) of circulating platelets, and marrow dysmegakaryopoiesis in association with deletion of the distal part of either the maternally or paternally derived chromosome 11 (11q23.3–24). Among the genes deleted is the transcription factor FLI-1, which is important in megakaryocyte development via its effects on expression of several genes, including *ITGA2, GPIX, GPIbα*, and *c-MPL*.[2] Although platelet survival is normal, there is dramatic expansion of marrow megakaryocytes resulting from arrested megakaryocyte development. Thrombin-induced platelet release of α-granule contents is impaired.[559] Both the inheritance pattern and the dimorphic population of normal and dysmorphic giant α granules are explained by the observation that during a period in early megakaryocyte development, only one of the two FLI-1 alleles appears to be expressed in any single megakaryocyte precursor.[561,562]

## GFI1B

Two studies[419,420] implicate autosomal dominant mutations in GFI1B with a bleeding disorder, multiple alterations in platelet number and function, and red cell anisopoikilocytosis. In one study,[420] the affected family members had a single nucleotide insertion in exon 7 of GFI1B, leading to a frameshift mutation associated with macrothrombocytopenia, impaired platelet aggregation responses, α-granule deficiency, and decreased platelet P-selectin, fibrinogen, GPIbα, and integrin $\beta_3$. The second study identified[419] a dominant negative truncating mutation (c.859C to T) in the zinc finger 5 region of GFI1B in a family originally reported in 1968 with macrothrombocytopenia and platelet dysfunction.[563] The family members had decreased platelet α granules, PF4, $\beta$TG, and GP1bα, and deficiency of platelet factor 3. There was myelofibrosis and emperipolesis in the marrow.

## ● MISCELLANEOUS INHERITED DISORDERS ASSOCIATED WITH PLATELET FUNCTION DEFECTS

The TAR syndrome is characterized by a reduction in platelet counts, absence of the radius bone in the forearm, skeletal abnormalities, and decreased marrow megakaryocytes. Dense granule SPD and impaired platelet aggregation and secretion have also been reported in TAR syndrome.[371] Early studies reported that the majority of these patients have a deletion on chromosome 1q21.1,[15] and later studies showed that these patients have both a rare null allele of *RBM8A* along with one of two low-frequency single nucleotide polymorphisms (SNPs) in the gene's regulatory regions.[14] *RBM8A* encodes for the Y14 subunit of the exon-junction complex (EJC), which plays an essential role in RNA processing.

Platelet function abnormalities have also been reported in inherited connective tissue disorders such as osteogenesis imperfecta, the Ehlers-Danlos syndrome, and the Marfan syndrome[369,370,564,565]; bleeding manifestations are more likely caused by the underlying connective tissue defect than by the platelet dysfunction. Abnormalities in platelet responses and/or granules have been reported in patients with

hexokinase deficiency,[566] glucose-6 phosphatase deficiency (glycogen storage disease, type I),[567,568] and Down syndrome.[569-573] In glucose-6 phosphatase deficiency, the platelet abnormalities were reversed following total parenteral nutrition for 10 to 12 days,[567,568] indicating that the platelets may be intrinsically normal. The *MYH9*-related disorders (May-Hegglin anomaly) are characterized by giant platelets, thrombocytopenia, and basophilic granulocyte inclusions; some patients with this anomaly have platelet function and ultrastructural abnormalities.[8,574,575] Despite the large platelet size, the surface membrane glycoproteins appear to be normal.[576] Markedly impaired platelet responses to multiple agonists have been reported with partial trisomy 18p associated with three copies of the *PACAP* (pituitary adenylate cyclase–activating polypeptide) gene and elevated plasma levels of *PACAP*, which induces increased platelet cAMP levels via stimulation of Gαs.[577]

Familial hemophagocytic lymphohistiocytosis (FHLH) is a genetic disorder of lymphocyte cytotoxicity associated with mutations in the gene encoding perforin or proteins important for vesicular trafficking and exocytosis. Flow cytometric analyses of the platelets of FHLH type 5 patients, who have MUNC18–2 *(STXBP2)* mutations, revealed that thrombin-induced secretion from both α and δ granules is impaired.[578,579] Platelets from an FHLH type 4 patient with a mutation in syntaxin-11 *(STX11)* also had a defect in agonist-induced secretion associated with normal cargo levels.[580]

## ● MANAGEMENT OF INHERITED PLATELET FUNCTION DISORDERS

Management of patients with inherited platelet function disorders needs to be individualized because of the wide variation in clinical manifestations, even in patients with the same defect. A general approach is described here; additional features specific to some individual entities are provided in their respective descriptions. Management of these patients involves preventive measures and treatment of specific bleeding episodes.[581-583] Dental hygiene is important in minimizing gingival hemorrhage. Antiplatelet agents should be avoided as they increase the bleeding manifestations. Iron and folate supplementation may be needed in patients with chronic hemorrhage. Hepatitis B vaccine should be administered early in life.

### PLATELET TRANSFUSIONS AND GENERAL APPROACHES

Transfusion of platelets is a time-tested therapy for serious bleeding and as prophylaxis prior to surgery or invasive procedures. In addition to the usual risks associated with transfusions (transmission of infections, allergic reactions, Rh-immunization in Rh-negative individuals, and rarely hemolytic reactions) patients with GT and BSS may develop specific antibodies against the missing glycoproteins, which may seriously compromise efficacy of future platelet transfusions.[581,582] This occurs particularly in patients whose platelets have no detectable integrin $\alpha_{IIb}\beta_3$.[584] Therefore, platelet transfusions should be kept to a minimum. Transfusions of both platelets and red blood cells should be given with leukocyte depletion filters to decrease the risk of alloimmunization and cytomegalovirus transmission. It is reasonable to use human leukocyte antigen (HLA)-matched and ABO-matched platelets to minimize the risk of alloimmunization and side effects.[581-583]

Treatment with 1-deamino-8-D-arginine vasopressin (DDAVP; desmopressin) may shorten the bleeding time and/or improve hemostasis in some, but not all, patients with platelet function defects.[585-588] Responses to DDAVP appear dependent on the cause of the platelet dysfunction.[585,587,588] Most patients with thrombasthenia do not respond to DDAVP with a shortening of the bleeding time[585,587–589] with exceptions,[590] but it is unknown whether DDAVP improves hemostasis in these patients despite a lack of shortening of the bleeding time. Responses to DDAVP in SPD patients have been variable, with a shortening of the bleeding time in some patients[588,591] but not others.[585,587] In uncontrolled studies, it has been feasible to manage selected patients with inherited platelet defects undergoing surgical procedures with DDAVP alone.[585,587] However, this approach needs to be individualized based on the nature and location of the surgery and the intensity of the patient's bleeding symptoms, and platelets need to be readily available for transfusion in the event of excess hemorrhage. The abnormal *in vitro* platelet aggregation or secretion responses in patients with platelet defects are usually not corrected by DDAVP.[587,592] It has been proposed that one mechanism by which DDAVP improves platelet function is via increased formation of procoagulant "COAT" platelets induced by combined activation by collagen and thrombin.[592]

Investigators have reported the successful use of recombinant factor VIIa (rFVIIa) in the management of bleeding events in patients with inherited platelet defects, including GT (including patients with antibodies to integrin $\alpha_{IIb}\beta_3$), BSS, and SPD.[581,583,593–596] rFVIIa is thought to increase thrombin generation through both tissue factor–dependent and –independent mechanisms.

The antifibrinolytic agents epsilon-aminocaproic acid (EACA) and tranexamic acid,[581–583] which may be given orally, intravenously, or topically, have been successfully used in patients with coagulation disorders and platelet function abnormalities.[586,597] Antifibrinolytic agents are useful in patients with gingival bleeding, epistaxis, and menorrhagia and those undergoing dental extractions. A tranexamic acid mouthwash (10 mL of a 5 percent solution used four times daily) has been found effective in controlling gum bleeding and bleeding after tooth extractions.[582] A short 3- to 4-day course of prednisone (20 to 50 mg)[598] has also been used.

Topical agents can also help arrest bleeding and have been used in GT patients. Gelfoam (a form of resolvable, oxidized, regenerated cellulose) soaked in either tranexamic acid or topical thrombin may be effective.[599] Fibrin sealants prepared from a source of fibrinogen and a source of thrombin (exogenous or from the patient's own plasma), with or without antifibrinolytic agents or other components,[599] have been used successfully in patients with GT.[600] Some preparations of bovine thrombin induced antibody formation to itself and contaminated factor V and factor XI and have been associated with serious hemorrhage; recombinant human thrombin is now available and appears to have low immunogenicity.[601]

Allogeneic marrow transplantation has successfully treated patients with GT, BSS,[581] LAD-3,[541] and WAS.[523,524] Progress has been made in gene therapy approaches to correcting the genetic defect in GT in megakaryocytes.[602–604] Several GT animal models are available, including the integrin subunits $\alpha_{IIb}$ and $\beta_3$-null mouse models[605] and dog models involving mutations in the $\alpha_{IIb}$ subunit.[604,606,607] With respect to BSS, in mouse models, lentiviral transduction of hematopoietic stem cells with human GPIbα under the control of the integrin $\alpha_{IIb}$ promoter has been effective in improving hemostasis when transplanted into animals.[289] Thus, as methods of marrow transplantation and gene transfer therapy improve, it will be important to reassess the risk-to-benefit ratios of these therapies for individual patients with GT.

## BLEEDING AT SPECIFIC SITES

Control of epistaxis can be particularly difficult in some patients.[608] When topical measures fail, platelet transfusions or factor VIIa should be considered. Nosebleeds occur primarily along the anterior nasal septum at the Kiesselbach area[608]; posterior nosebleeds can occur either along the septum or the lateral nasal wall. Self-administered home therapy for anterior hemorrhage consists of pinching the outer aspect of the nose against the septum for 15 minutes to tamponade the septal vessels.[608] If this fails, topical application by medical personnel of an anesthetic such as lidocaine in combination with a vasoconstrictor such as phenylephrine or oxymetazoline is commonly effective. Electrical cautery sometimes is effective when chemical cauterization fails. In many cases, anterior or posterior packing may be needed for persistent severe epistaxis.

Menarche may be associated with severe bleeding manifestations and require transfusions in some patients. Antifibrinolytics have been used for menorrhagia; hormonal therapy with progesterone alone or combined progesterone-estrogen is effective in those with persistent hemorrhage.[581,583]

## PREGNANCY

Management during pregnancy and delivery requires close interaction between the hematologist and the obstetrician. Most patients with severe bleeding symptoms, particularly those with GT and BSS, will need platelet transfusions during childbirth, and this need may continue for several days after delivery.[581–583] Postpartum bleeding may occur 2 to 4 weeks after delivery in some patients. rFVIIa has been used successfully in women with GT with persistent bleeding despite platelet transfusions and those with integrin $\alpha_{IIb}\beta_3$ antibodies.[581–583,609,610] Of note, fetal thrombocytopenia and intracranial hemorrhage may occur because of transplacental passage of the antibodies.

## SURGERY

Management during surgical procedures needs to be individualized and depends on the bleeding history of the patient, the nature of the surgery, and information such as alloimmunization and refractoriness to prior transfusions. Therapeutic options include DDAVP, platelet transfusions, rFVIIa, and ancillary measures, such as antifibrinolytics, which may be continued for several days after surgery.[581–583]

## REFERENCES

1. Noris P, Biino G, Pecci A, et al: Platelet diameters in inherited thrombocytopenias: Analysis of 376 patients with all known disorders. *Blood* 124:e4–e10, 2014.
2. Kumar R, Kahr WHA: Congenital thrombocytopenia: Clinical manifestations, laboratory abnormalities, and molecular defects of a heterogeneous group of conditions. *Hematol Oncol Clin N Am* 27:465–494, 2013.
3. Harrison P, Lordkipanidze M: Clinical tests of platelet function in AD, in *Platelets,* 3rd ed, edited by AD Michelson, pp 519–545. Elsevier, San Diego, CA, 2013.
4. Cattaneo M, Hayward CP, Moffat KA, et al: Results of a worldwide survey on the assessment of platelet function by light transmission aggregometry: A report from the platelet physiology subcommittee of the SSC of the ISTH. *J Thromb Haemost* 7:1029, 2009.
5. Hayward CP, Moffat KA, Spitzer E, et al: Results of an external proficiency testing exercise on platelet dense-granule deficiency testing by whole mount electron microscopy. *Am J Clin Pathol* 131:671–675, 2009.
6. Hayward CP, Pai M, Liu Y, et al: Diagnostic utility of light transmission platelet aggregometry: Results from a prospective study of individuals referred for bleeding disorder assessments. *J Thromb Haemost* 7:676–684, 2009.
7. Flamm MH, Colace TV, Chatterjee MS, et al: Multiscale prediction of patient-specific platelet function under flow. *Blood* 120:190–198, 2012.
8. de Witt SM, Swieringa F, Cavill R, et al: Identification of platelet function defects by multi-parameter assessment of thrombus formation. *Nat Commun* 5:4257, 2014.
9. Stockley J, Morgan NV, Bem D, et al: Enrichment of FLI1 and RUNX1 mutations in families with excessive bleeding and platelet dense granule secretion defects. *Blood* 122:4090–4093, 2013.
10. Albers CA, Cvejic A, Favier R, et al: Exome sequencing identifies NBEAL2 as the causative gene for gray platelet syndrome. *Nat Genet* 43:735–737, 2011.
11. Kahr WH, Hinckley J, Li L, et al: Mutations in NBEAL2, encoding a BEACH protein, cause gray platelet syndrome. *Nat Genet* 43:738–740, 2011.
12. Gunay-Aygun M, Falik-Zaccai TC, Vilboux T, et al: NBEAL2 is mutated in gray platelet syndrome and is required for biogenesis of platelet alpha-granules. *Nat Genet* 43:732–734, 2011.

13. Castoldi E, Collins PW, Williamson PL, Bevers EM: Compound heterozygosity for 2 novel TMEM16F mutations in a patient with Scott syndrome. *Blood* 117:4399–4400, 2011.

14. Albers CA, Paul DS, Schulze H, et al: Compound inheritance of a low-frequency regulatory SNP and a rare null mutation in exon-junction complex subunit RBM8A causes TAR syndrome. *Nat Genet* 44:435–439, S1–S2, 2012.

15. Klopocki E, Schulze H, Strauss G, et al: Complex inheritance pattern resembling autosomal recessive inheritance involving a microdeletion in thrombocytopenia-absent radius syndrome. *Am J Hum Genet* 80:232–240, 2007.

16. Nurden P, Nurden AT: Congenital disorders associated with platelet dysfunctions. *Thromb Haemost* 99:253–263, 2008.

17. Glanzmann E: Hereditäre hämmorhagische Thrombasthenie. *Ein Beitrag zur Pathologie der Blutplättchen Jahrbuch fur Kinderheilkunde und physische Erziehung* 88:113–141, 1918.

18. Caen JP, Castaldi PA, Leclerc JC, et al: Congenital bleeding disorders with long bleeding time and normal platelet count. I. Glanzmann's thrombasthenia. *Am J Med* 41:4, 1966.

19. Hardisty RM, Dormandy KM, Hutton RA: Thrombasthenia: Studies on three cases. *Br J Haematol* 10:371, 1964.

20. Zucker MB, Pert JH, Hilgartner MW: Platelet function in a patient with thrombasthenia. *Blood* 28:524, 1966.

21. Weiss HJ, Kochwa S: Studies of platelet function and proteins in 3 patients with Glanzmann's thrombasthenia. *J Lab Clin Med* 71:153–165, 1968.

22. George JN, Caen JP, Nurden AT: Glanzmann's thrombasthenia: The spectrum of clinical disease. *Blood* 75:1383–1395, 1990.

23. Nurden AT, Caen JP: An abnormal platelet glycoprotein pattern in three cases of Glanzmann's thrombasthenia. *Br J Haematol* 28:253–260, 1974.

24. Phillips DR, Jenkins CS, Luscher EF, Larrieu M: Molecular differences of exposed surface proteins on thrombasthenic platelet plasma membranes. *Nature* 257:599–600, 1975.

25. Peerschke EI: The platelet fibrinogen receptor. *Semin Hematol* 22:241–259, 1985.

26. Bennett JS: The platelet-fibrinogen interaction, in *Platelet Membrane Glycoproteins*, edited by JN George, AT Nurden, DR Phillips, p 193. Plenum, New York, 1985.

27. Phillips DR, Charo IF, Parise LV, Fitzgerald LA: The platelet membrane glycoprotein IIb-IIIa complex. *Blood* 71:831–843, 1988.

28. Plow EF, Ginsberg MH: Cellular adhesion: GPIIb-IIIa as a prototypic adhesion receptor. *Prog Hemost Thromb* 9:117–156, 1989.

29. Poncz M, Eisman R, Heidenreich R, et al: Structure of the platelet membrane glycoprotein IIb. Homology to the alpha subunits of the vitronectin and fibronectin membrane receptors. *J Biol Chem* 262:8476–8482, 1987.

30. Fitzgerald LA, Steiner B, Rall SC, et al: Protein sequence of endothelial glycoprotein IIIa derived from a cDNA clone. Identity with platelet glycoprotein IIIa and similarity to "integrin." *J Biol Chem* 262:3936–3939, 1987.

31. Hynes RO: Integrins: Bidirectional, allosteric signaling machines. *Cell* 110:673–687, 2002.

32. D'Andrea G, Colaizzo D, Vecchione G, et al: Glanzmann's thrombasthenia: Identification of 19 new mutations in 30 patients. *Thromb Haemost* 87:1034–1042, 2002.

33. Seligsohn U, Peretz H, Newman PJ, Coller BS: Glanzmann thrombasthenia in Israel: Clinical, biochemical and molecular genetic characterization, in *Genetic Diversity Among Jews*, edited by B Bonne-Tamir, A Adam, pp 275–282. Oxford University Press, Oxford, 1992.

34. Reichert N, Seligsohn U, Ramot B: Clinical and genetic studies of Glanzmann's thrombasthenia in Israel. *Thromb Diath Haemorrh* 34:806, 1975.

35. Awidi AS: Increased incidence of Glanzmann's thrombasthenia in Jordan as compared with Scandinavia. *Scand J Haematol* 30:218–222, 1983.

36. Khanduri U, Pulimood R, Sudarsanam A, et al: Glanzmann's thrombasthenia. A review and report of 42 cases from South India. *Thromb Haemost* 46:717–721, 1981.

37. Ahmed MA, Al Sohaibani MO, Al Mohaya SA, et al: Inherited bleeding disorders in the Eastern Province of Saudi Arabia. *Acta Haemat* 79:202–206, 1988.

38. Awidi AS: Rare inherited bleeding disorders secondary to coagulation factors in Jordan: A nine-year study. *Acta Haemat* 88:11–13, 1992.

39. Rosenberg N, Yatuv R, Orion Y, et al: Glanzmann thrombasthenia caused by an 11.2-kb deletion in the glycoprotein IIIa (beta3) is a second mutation in Iraqi Jews that stemmed from a distinct founder. *Blood* 89:3654–3662, 1997.

40. Borhany M, Fatima H, Naz A, et al: Pattern of bleeding and response to therapy in Glanzmann thrombasthenia. *Haemophilia* 18:e423–e425, 2012.

41. Coller BS, Shattil SJ: The GPIIb/IIIa (integrin alphaIIbbeta3) odyssey: A technology-driven saga of a receptor with twists, turns, and even a bend. *Blood* 112:3011–3025, 2008.

42. Harrison P: Platelet α-granular fibrinogen. *Platelets* 3:1–10, 1992.

43. Coller BS, Seligsohn U, West SM, et al: Platelet fibrinogen and vitronectin in Glanzmann thrombasthenia: Evidence consistent with specific roles for glycoprotein IIb/IIIA and αVβ3 integrins in platelet protein trafficking. *Blood* 78:2603–2610, 1991.

44. Disdier M, Legrand C, Bouillot C, et al: Quantitation of platelet fibrinogen and thrombospondin in Glanzmann's thrombasthenia by electroimmunoassay. *Thromb Res* 53:521–533, 1989.

45. Cohen I, Gerrard JM, White JG: Ultrastructure of clots during isometric contraction. *J Cell Biol* 91:775, 1982.

46. Gartner TK, Ogilvie ML: Peptides and monoclonal antibodies which bind to platelet glycoproteins IIb and/or IIIa inhibit clot retraction. *Thromb Res* 49:43–53, 1988.

47. Duperray A, Troesch A, Berthier R, et al: Biosynthesis and assembly of platelet GPIIb-IIIa in human megakaryocytes: Evidence that assembly between pro-GPIIb and GPIIIa is a prerequisite for expression of the complex on the cell surface. *Blood* 74:1603–1611, 1989.

48. Bodary SC, Napier MA, McLean JW: Expression of recombinant platelet glycoprotein IIbIIIa results in a functional fibrinogen-binding complex. *J Biol Chem* 264:18859–18862, 1989.

49. O'Toole TE, Loftus JC, Plow EF, et al: Efficient surface expression of platelet GPIIb-IIIa requires both subunits. *Blood* 74:14–18, 1989.

50. Kolodziej MA, Vilaire G, Gonder D, et al: Study of the endoproteolytic cleavage of platelet glycoprotein IIb using oligonucleotide-mediated mutagenesis. *J Biol Chem* 266:23499–23504, 1991.

51. Bennett JS: The molecular biology of platelet membrane proteins. *Semin Hematol* 27:186–204, 1990.

52. Kieffer N, Phillips DR: Platelet membrane glycoproteins: Functions in cellular interactions. *Annu Rev Cell Biol* 6:329–357, 1990.

53. Seligsohn U, Coller BS, Zivelin A, et al: Immunoblot analysis of platelet GPIIb in patients with Glanzmann thrombasthenia in Israel. *Br J Haematol* 72:415–423, 1989.

54. Mitchell WB, Li J, French DL, Coller BS: AlphaIIbbeta3 biogenesis is controlled by engagement of alphaIIb in the calnexin cycle via the N15-linked glycan. *Blood* 107:2713–2719, 2006.

55. Mitchell WB, Li J, Murcia M, et al: Mapping early conformational changes in alphaIIb and beta3 during biogenesis reveals a potential mechanism for alphaIIbbeta3 adopting its bent conformation. *Blood* 109:3725–3732, 2007.

56. Zimrin AB, Eisman R, Vilaire G, et al: Structure of platelet glycoprotein IIIa. A common subunit for two different membrane receptors. *J Clin Invest* 81:1470–1475, 1988.

57. Cheresh DA: Human endothelial cells synthesize and express an Arg-Gly-Asp-directed adhesion receptor involved in attachment to fibrinogen and von Willebrand factor. *Proc Natl Acad Sci U S A* 84:6471–6475, 1987.

58. Smith JW, Cheresh DA: The Arg-Gly-Asp binding domain of the vitronectin receptor. *J Biol Chem* 263:18726–18731, 1988.

59. Cheresh DA, Berliner SA, Vicente V, Ruggeri ZM: Recognition of distinct adhesive sites on fibrinogen by related integrins on platelets and endothelial cells. *Cell* 58:945–953, 1989.

60. Lawler J, Hynes RO: An integrin receptor on normal and thrombasthenic platelets which binds thrombospondin. *Blood* 74:2022–2027, 1989.

61. Yokoyama K, Zhang XP, Medved L, Takada Y: Specific binding of integrin alpha v beta 3 to the fibrinogen gamma and alpha E chain C-terminal domains. *Biochemistry* 38:5872–5877, 1999.

62. Lam SC, Plow EF, D'Souza SE, et al: Isolation and characterization of a platelet membrane protein related to the vitronectin receptor. *J Biol Chem* 264:3742–3749, 1989.

63. Coller BS, Cheresh DA, Asch E, Seligsohn U: Platelet vitronectin receptor expression differentiates Iraqi-Jewish from Arab Patients with Glanzmann thrombasthenia in Israel. *Blood* 77:75–83, 1991.

64. Krissansen GW, Elliott MJ, Lucas CM, et al: Identification of a novel integrin beta subunit expressed on cultured monocytes (macrophages). *J Biol Chem* 265:823, 1990.

65. Byzova TV, Rabbani R, D'Souza SE, Plow EF: Role of integrin alpha(v)beta3 in vascular biology. *Thromb Haemost* 80:726–734, 1998.

66. Newman PJ, Seligsohn U, Lyman S, Coller BS: The molecular genetic basis of Glanzmann thrombasthenia in the Iraqi-Jewish and Arab populations in Israel. *Proc Natl Acad Sci U S A* 88:3160–3164, 1991.

67. Burk CD, Newman PJ, Lyman S, et al: A deletion in the gene for glycoprotein IIb associated with Glanzmann's thrombasthenia. *J Clin Invest* 87:270–276, 1991.

68. Poncz M, Rifat S, Coller BS, et al: Glanzmann thrombasthenia secondary to a Gly273Asp mutation adjacent to the first calcium-binding domain of platelet glycoprotein IIb. *J Clin Invest* 93:172–179, 1994.

69. Tadokoro S, Tomiyama Y, Honda S, et al: Missense mutations in the beta(3) subunit have a different impact on the expression and function between alpha(IIb)beta(3) and alpha(v)beta(3). *Blood* 99:931–938, 2002.

70. Horton MA, Massey HM, Rosenberg N, et al: Upregulation of osteoclast alpha2beta1 integrin compensates for lack of alphavbeta3 vitronectin receptor in Iraqi-Jewish-type Glanzmann thrombasthenia. *Br J Haematol* 122:950–957, 2003.

71. French DL, Coller BS: Hematologically important mutations: Glanzmann thrombasthenia. *Blood Cells Mol Dis* 23:39–51, 1997.

72. Coller BS: αIIbB3: Structure and function. *Thrombos Haemostas* 13(Suppl 1):S17–S25, 2015.

73. Bajt ML, Loftus JC: Mutation of a ligand binding domain of beta 3 integrin. Integral role of oxygenated residues in alpha IIb beta 3 (GPIIb-IIIa) receptor function. *J Biol Chem* 269:20913–20919, 1994.

74. Lee JO, Rieu P, Arnaout MA, Liddington R: Crystal structure of the A domain from the alpha subunit of integrin CR3 (CD11b/CD18). *Cell* 80:631–638, 1995.

75. Xiong JP, Stehle T, Diefenbach B, et al: Crystal structure of the extracellular segment of integrin alphaVbeta3. *Science* 294:339–345, 2001.

76. Xiao T, Takagi J, Coller BS, et al: Structural basis for allostery in integrins and binding to fibrinogen-mimetic therapeutics. *Nature* 432:59–67, 2004.

77. Xiong JP, Stehle T, Zhang R, et al: Crystal structure of the extracellular segment of integrin alpha Vbeta3 in complex with an Arg-Gly-Asp ligand. *Science* 296:151–155, 2002.

78. Zhu J, Luo BH, Xiao T, et al: Structure of a complete integrin ectodomain in a physiologic resting state and activation and deactivation by applied forces. *Mol Cell* 32:849–861, 2008.

79. Springer TA, Zhu J, Xiao T: Structural basis for distinctive recognition of fibrinogen gammaC peptide by the platelet integrin alphaIIbbeta3. *J Cell Biol* 182:791–800, 2008.

80. Loftus JC, O'Toole TE, Plow EF, et al: A β3 integrin mutation abolishes ligand binding and alters divalent cation-dependent conformation. *Science* 249:915–918, 1990.

81. Ward CM, Chao YL, Kato GJ, et al: Substitution of Asn, but not Tyr, for ASP119 of the β3 integrin subunit preserves fibrin binding and clot retraction. *Blood* 90:26a, 1997.
82. Fournier DJ, Kabral A, Castaldi PA, Berndt MC: A variant of Glanzmann's thrombasthenia characterized by abnormal glycoprotein IIb/IIIa complex formation. *Thromb Haemost* 62:977–983, 1989.
83. Newman PJ, Weyerbusch-Bottum S, Visentin GP, et al: Type II Glanzmann thrombasthenia due to a destabilizing amino acid substitution in platelet membrane glycoprotein IIIa. *Thromb Haemost* 69:1017, 1993.
84. Lanza F, Stierle A, Fournier D, et al: A new variant of Glanzmann's thrombasthenia (Strasbourg I). Platelets with functionally defective glycoprotein IIb-IIIa complexes and a glycoprotein IIIa Arg214Trp mutation. *J Clin Invest* 89:1995–2004, 1992.
85. D'Andrea G, Bafunno V, Del VL, et al: A beta3 Asp217—>Val substitution in a patient with variant Glanzmann thrombasthenia severely affects integrin alphaIIBbeta3 functions. *Blood Coagul Fibrinolysis* 19:657–662, 2008.
86. Baker EK, Tozer EC, Pfaff M, et al: A genetic analysis of integrin function: Glanzmann thrombasthenia in vitro. *Proc Natl Acad Sci U S A* 94:1973–1978, 1997.
87. Ward CM, Kestin AS, Newman PJ: A Leu262Pro mutation in the integrin beta(3) subunit results in an alpha(IIb)-beta(3) complex that binds fibrin but not fibrinogen. *Blood* 96:161–169, 2000.
88. Loftus JC, Halloran CE, Ginsberg MH, et al: The amino-terminal one-third of alpha IIb defines the ligand recognition specificity of integrin alpha IIb beta 3. *J Biol Chem* 271:2033–2039, 1996.
89. Springer TA: Folding of the N-terminal, ligand-binding region of integrin α-subunits into a β-propeller domain. *Proc Natl Acad Sci U S A* 94:65–72, 1997.
90. Ruan J, Peyruchaud O, Alberio L, et al: Double heterozygosity of the GPIIb gene in a Swiss patient with Glanzmann's thrombasthenia. *Br J Haematol* 102:918–925, 1998.
91. Wilcox DA, Paddock CM, Lyman S, et al: Glanzmann thrombasthenia resulting from a single amino acid substitution between the second and third calcium-binding domains of GPIIb. Role of the GPIIb amino terminus in integrin subunit association. *J Clin Invest* 95:1553–1560, 1995.
92. Wilcox DA, Wautier JL, Pidard D, Newman PJ: A single amino acid substitution flanking the fourth calcium binding domain of alpha IIb prevents maturation of the alpha IIb beta 3 integrin complex. *J Biol Chem* 269:4450–4457, 1994.
93. Basani RB, Vilaire G, Shattil SJ, et al: Glanzmann thrombasthenia due to a two amino acid deletion in the fourth calcium-binding domain of alpha IIb: Demonstration of the importance of calcium-binding domains in the conformation of alpha IIb beta 3. *Blood* 88:167–173, 1996.
94. Kiyoi T, Tomiyama Y, Honda S, et al: A naturally occurring Tyr143His alpha IIb mutation abolishes alpha IIb beta 3 function for soluble ligands but retains its ability for mediating cell adhesion and clot retraction: Comparison with other mutations causing ligand-binding defects. *Blood* 101:3485–3491, 2003.
95. Basani RB, French DL, Vilaire G, et al: A naturally-occurring mutation near the amino terminus of $\alpha_{IIb}$ defines a new region involved in ligand binding to $\alpha_{IIb}\beta_3$. *Blood* 95:180–188, 2000.
96. Westrup D, Santoso S, Becker-Hagendorff K, et al: Transfection of GPIIbIIe176/IIIa (Frankfurt I) in mammalian cells. *Thromb Haemost* 77:671, 1997.
97. Honda S, Tomiyama Y, Shiraga M, et al: A two-amino acid insertion in the Cys146-Cys167 loop of the $\alpha_{IIb}$ subunit is associated with a variant of Glanzmann thrombasthenia. *J Clin Invest* 102:1183–1192, 1998.
98. Kirchmaier CM, Westrup D, Becker-Hagendorff K, et al: A new variant of Glanzmann thrombasthenia (Frankfurt I). *Thromb Haemost* 73:1058, 1995.
99. Grimaldi CM, Chen F, Wu C, et al: Glycoprotein IIb Leu214Pro mutation produces Glanzmann thrombasthenia with both quantitative and qualitative abnormalities in GPIIb/IIIa. *Blood* 91:1562–1568, 1998.
100. Fullard J, Murphy R, O'Neill S, et al: A Val193Met mutation in GPIIIa results in a GPIIb/IIIa receptor with a constitutively high affinity for a small ligand. *Br J Haematol* 115:131–139, 2001.
101. Ruiz C, Liu CY, Sun QH, et al: A point mutation in the cysteine-rich domain of glycoprotein (GP) IIIa results in the expression of a GPIIb-IIIa (alphaIIbbeta3) integrin receptor locked in a high-affinity state and a Glanzmann thrombasthenia-like phenotype. *Blood* 98:2432–2441, 2001.
102. Vanhoorelbeke K, De Meyer SF, Pareyn I, et al: The novel S527F mutation in the integrin beta3 chain induces a high affinity alphaIIbbeta3 receptor by hindering adoption of the bent conformation. *J Biol Chem* 284:14914–14920, 2009.
103. Chen YP, Djaffar I, Pidard D, et al: Ser-752—>Pro mutation in the cytoplasmic domain of integrin $\beta$ 3 subunit and defective activation of platelet integrin $\alpha$ IIb $\beta$ 3 (glycoprotein IIb-IIIa) in a variant of Glanzmann thrombasthenia. *Proc Natl Acad Sci U S A* 89:10169–10173, 1992.
104. Ylanne J, Chen Y, O'Toole TE, et al: Distinct functions of integrin $\alpha$ and $\beta$ subunit cytoplasmic domains in cell spreading and formation of focal adhesions. *J Cell Biol* 122:223–233, 1993.
105. Wang R, Shattil SJ, Ambruso DR, Newman PJ: Truncation of the cytoplasmic domain of β3 in a variant form of Glanzmann thrombasthenia abrogates signaling through the integrin $\alpha_{IIb}\beta3$ complex. *J Clin Invest* 100:2393–2403, 1997.
106. Chen YP, Djaffar I, Pidard E: Ser752Pro mutation in the cytoplasmic domain of integrin $\beta_3$ subunit and defective activation of platelet integrin $\alpha_{IIb}\beta_3$ (glycoprotein IIb-IIIa) in a variant of Glanzmann thrombasthenia. *Proc Natl Acad Sci U S A* 89:10169–10173, 1992.
107. Ylanne J, Huuskonen J, O'Toole TE, et al: Mutation of the cytoplasmic domain of the integrin beta 3 subunit. Differential effects on cell spreading, recruitment to adhesion plaques, endocytosis, and phagocytosis. *J Biol Chem* 270:9550–9557, 1995.
108. Chen YP, O'Toole TE, Ylanne J, et al: A point mutation in the integrin beta 3 cytoplasmic domain (S752—>P) impairs bidirectional signaling through alpha IIb beta 3 (platelet glycoprotein IIb-IIIa). *Blood* 84:1857–1865, 1994.
109. Coventry A, Bull-Otterson LM, Liu X, et al: Deep resequencing reveals excess rare recent variants consistent with explosive population growth. *Nat Commun* 1:131, 2010.
109A. Buitrago L, Rendon A, Liang Y, et al: αIIbβ3 variants defined by next-generation sequencing: Predicting variants likely to cause Glanzmann thrombasthenia. *Proc Natl Acad Sci U S A* E1898–E1907, 2015.
110. Rosenberg N, Hauschner H, Peretz H, et al: A 13-bp deletion in alpha(IIb) gene is a founder mutation that predominates in Palestinian-Arab patients with Glanzmann thrombasthenia. *J Thromb Haemost* 3:2764–2772, 2005.
111. Fiore M, Pillois X, Nurden P, et al: Founder effect and estimation of the age of the French Gypsy mutation associated with Glanzmann thrombasthenia in Manouche families. *Eur J Hum Genet* 19:981–987, 2011.
112. Coller BS, Seligsohn U, Zivelin A, et al: Immunologic and biochemical characterization of homozygous and heterozygous Glanzmann's thrombasthenia in Iraqi-Jewish and Arab populations of Israel: Comparison of techniques for carrier detection. *Br J Haematol* 62:723–735, 1986.
113. Shpilberg O, Rabi I, Schiller K, et al: Patients with Glanzmann thrombasthenia lacking platelet glycoprotein alpha(IIb)beta(3) (GPIIb/IIIa) and alpha(v)beta(3) receptors are not protected from atherosclerosis. *Circulation* 105:1044–1048, 2002.
114. Cronberg S, Nilsson IM, Zetterqvist E: Investigation of a family with members with both severe and mild degree of thrombasthenia. *Acta Paediatr Scand* 56:189–197, 1967.
115. Stormorken H, Gogstad GO, Solum NO, Pande H: Diagnosis of heterozygotes in Glanzmann's thrombasthenia. *Thromb Haemost* 48:217–221, 1982.
116. Coller BS, Peerschke EI, Scudder LE, Sullivan CA: A murine monoclonal antibody that completely blocks the binding of fibrinogen to platelets produces a thrombasthenic-like state in normal platelets and binds to glycoproteins IIb and/or IIIa. *J Clin Invest* 72:325–338, 1983.
117. Malmsten C, Kindahl H, Samuelsson B, et al: Thromboxane synthesis and the platelet release reaction in Bernard-Soulier syndrome, thrombasthenia Glanzmann and Hermansky-Pudlak syndrome. *Br J Haematol* 35:511–520, 1977.
118. Charo IF, Feinman RD, Detwiler TC: Interrelations of platelet aggregation and secretion. *J Clin Invest* 60:866–873, 1977.
119. Heptinstall S, Taylor PM: The effects of citrate and extracellular calcium ions on the platelet release reaction induced by adenosine diphosphate and collagen. *Thromb Haemost* 42:778–793, 1979.
120. Caen JP, Cronberg S, Levy-Toledano S, et al: New data on Glanzmann's thrombasthenia. *Proc Soc Exp Biol Med* 136:1082–1086, 1971.
121. Zucker MB, Vroman L: Platelet adhesion induced by fibrinogen adsorbed onto glass. *Proc Soc Exp Biol Med* 131:318–320, 1969.
122. Stanford MF, Munoz PC, Vroman L: Platelets adhere where flow has left fibrinogen on glass. *Ann N Y Acad Sci* 416:504–512, 1983.
123. Zucker MB, McPherson J: Reactions of platelets near surfaces in vitro: Lessons from the platelet retention test. *Ann N Y Acad Sci* 283:128, 1977.
124. Bevers EM, Comfurius P, Nieuwenhuis HK, et al: Platelet prothrombin converting activity in hereditary disorders of platelet function. *Br J Haematol* 63:335–345, 1986.
125. Reverter JC, Beguin S, Kessels H, et al: Inhibition of platelet-mediated, tissue factor-induced thrombin generation by the mouse/human chimeric 7E3 antibody. Potential implications for the effect of c7E3 Fab treatment on acute thrombosis and "clinical restenosis." *J Clin Invest* 98:863–874, 1996.
126. Beguin S, Kumar R, Keularts I, et al: Fibrin-dependent platelet procoagulant activity requires GPIb receptors and von Willebrand factor. *Blood* 93:564–570, 1999.
127. Gemmell CH, Sefton MV, Yeo EL: Platelet-derived microparticle formation involves glycoprotein IIb-IIIa. Inhibition by RGDS and a Glanzmann's thrombasthenia defect. *J Biol Chem* 268:14586–14589, 1993.
128. Nomura S, Komiyama Y, Matsuura E, et al: Participation of $\alpha$ IIb $\beta$ 3 in platelet microparticle generation by collagen plus thrombin. *Haemostasis* 26:31–37, 1996.
129. Nomura S, Komiyama Y, Murakami T, et al: Flow cytometric analysis of surface membrane proteins on activated platelets and platelet-derived microparticles from healthy and thrombasthenic individuals. *Int J Hematol* 58:203–212, 1993.
130. Byzova TV, Plow EF: Networking in the hemostatic system. Integrin alphaiibbeta3 binds prothrombin and influences its activation. *J Biol Chem* 272:27183–27188, 1997.
131. Byzova TV, Plow EF: Activation of alphaVbeta3 on vascular cells controls recognition of prothrombin. *J Cell Biol* 143:2081–2092, 1998.
132. Tschopp TB, Weiss HJ, Baumgartner HR: Interaction of thrombasthenic platelets with subendothelium: Normal adhesion, absent aggregation. *Experientia* 31:113–116, 1975.
133. Sakariassen KS, Nievelstein PFEM, Coller BS, Sixma JJ: The role of platelet membrane glycoproteins Ib and IIb-IIIa in platelet adherence to human artery subendothelium. *Br J Haematol* 63:681–691, 1986.
134. Weiss HJ, Turitto VT, Baumgartner HR: Platelet adhesion and thrombus formation on subendothelium in platelets deficient in glycoproteins IIb-IIIa, Ib, and storage granules. *Blood* 67:322, 1986.
135. Weiss HJ, Turitto VT, Baumgartner HR: The role of shear rate and platelets in promoting fibrin formation on rabbit subendothelium: Studies utilizing patients with quantitative and qualitative platelet defects. *J Clin Invest* 78:1072–1082, 1986.
136. Harrison P, Robinson M, Liesner R, et al: The PFA-100: A potential rapid screening tool for the assessment of platelet dysfunction. *Clin Lab Haematol* 24:225–232, 2002.
137. Buyukasik Y, Karakus S, Goker H, et al: Rational use of the PFA-100 device for screening of platelet function disorders and von Willebrand disease. *Blood Coagul Fibrinolysis* 13:349–353, 2002.

138. Lee H, Nurden AT, Thomaidis A, Caen JP: Relationship between fibrinogen binding and platelet glycoprotein deficiencies in Glanzmann's thrombasthenia type I and type II. *Br J Haematol* 48:47, 1981.

139. Coller BS, Seligsohn U, Peretz H, Newman PJ: Glanzmann thrombasthenia: New insights from an historical perspective. *Semin Hematol* 31:301–311, 1994.

140. Shattil SJ, Hoxie JA, Cunningham M, Brass LF: Changes in the platelet membrane glycoprotein IIb.IIIa complex during platelet activation. *J Biol Chem* 260:11107–11114, 1985.

141. Karpatkin M, Howard L, Karpatkin S: Studies of the origin of platelet-associated fibrinogen. *J Lab Clin Med* 104:223–237, 1984.

142. Grimaldi CM, Chen F, Scudder LE, et al: A Cys374Tyr homozygous mutation of platelet glycoprotein IIIa (beta 3) in a Chinese patient with Glanzmann's thrombasthenia. *Blood* 88:1666–1675, 1996.

143. Yasunaga K, Nomura S: Statistical analysis of Glanzmann's thrombasthenia in Japan. *Acta Haematol* 89:165–166, 1993.

144. Kashiwagi H, Kunishima S, Kiyomizu K, et al: Demonstration of novel gain-of-function mutations of alphaIIbbeta3: Association with macrothrombocytopenia and Glanzmann thrombasthenia-like phenotype. *Mol Genet Genomic Med* 1:77–86, 2013.

145. Kunishima S, Kashiwagi H, Otsu M, et al: Heterozygous ITGA2B R995W mutation inducing constitutive activation of the alphaIIbbeta3 receptor affects proplatelet formation and causes congenital macrothrombocytopenia. *Blood* 117:5479–5484, 2011.

146. Ghevaert C, Salsmann A, Watkins NA, et al: A nonsynonymous SNP in the ITGB3 gene disrupts the conserved membrane-proximal cytoplasmic salt bridge in the alphaIIb-beta3 integrin and cosegregates dominantly with abnormal proplatelet formation and macrothrombocytopenia. *Blood* 111:3407–3414, 2008.

147. Nurden AT, Pillois X, Fiore M, et al: Glanzmann thrombasthenia-like syndromes associated with macrothrombocytopenias and mutations in the genes encoding the alphaIIbbeta3 integrin. *Semin Thromb Hemost* 37:698–706, 2011.

148. Schaffner-Reckinger E, Salsmann A, Debili N, et al: Overexpression of the partially activated alpha(IIb)beta3D723H integrin salt bridge mutant downregulates RhoA activity and induces microtubule-dependent proplatelet-like extensions in Chinese hamster ovary cells. *J Thromb Haemost* 7:1207–1217, 2009.

149. Jayo A, Conde I, Lastres P, et al: L718P mutation in the membrane-proximal cytoplasmic tail of beta 3 promotes abnormal alpha IIb beta 3 clustering and lipid microdomain coalescence, and associates with a thrombasthenia-like phenotype. *Haematologica* 95:1158–1166, 2010.

150. Peyruchaud O, Nurden AT, Milet S, et al: R to Q amino acid substitution in the GFFKR sequence of the cytoplasmic domain of the integrin IIb subunit in a patient with a Glanzmann's thrombasthenia-like syndrome. *Blood* 92:4178–4187, 1998.

151. Hughes PE, Diaz-Gonzalez F, Leong L, et al: Breaking the integrin hinge. A defined structural constraint regulates integrin signaling. *J Biol Chem* 271:6571–6574, 1996.

152. Lopez JA, Andrews RK, Afshar-Kharghan V, Berndt MC: Bernard-Soulier syndrome. *Blood* 91:4397–4418, 1998.

153. Lopez JA, Berndt MC: The GPIb-IX-V complex, in *Platelets*, edited by AD Michelson, p 85. Academic Press, San Diego, 2002.

154. Savoia A, Kunishima S, De Rocco D, et al: Spectrum of the mutations in Bernard-Soulier syndrome. *Hum Mutat* 35:1033–1045, 2014.

155. Andrews RK, Berndt MC: Bernard-Soulier syndrome: An update. *Semin Thromb Hemost* 39:656–662, 2013.

156. Bernard J, Soulier JP: Sur une nouvelle variete de dystrophie thrombocytaire-hemorragipare congenitale. *Semin Hop Paris* 24:3217, 1948.

157. Bernard J: History of congenital hemorrhagic thrombocytopathic dystrophy. *Blood Cells* 9:179, 1983.

158. Weiss HJ, Tschopp TB, Baumgartner HR, et al: Decreased adhesion of giant (Bernard-Soulier) platelets to subendothelium. Further implications on the role of the von Willebrand factor in hemostasis. *Am J Med* 57:920–925, 1974.

159. Howard MA, Hutton RA, Hardisty RM: Hereditary giant platelet syndrome: A disorder of a new aspect of platelet function. *Br Med J* 2:586–588, 1973.

160. Bithell TC, Parekh SJ, Strong RR: Platelet-function studies in the Bernard-Soulier syndrome. *Ann N Y Acad Sci* 201:145–160, 1972.

161. Nurden AT, Caen JP: Specific roles for platelet surface glycoproteins in platelet function. *Nature* 255:720–722, 1975.

162. Howard MA, Perkin J, Salem HH, Firkin BG: The agglutination of human platelets by botrocetin: Evidence that botrocetin and ristocetin act at different sites on the factor VIII molecule and platelet membrane. *Br J Haematol* 57:25–35, 1984.

163. Moake JL, Olson JD, Troll JH, et al: Binding of radioiodinated human von Willebrand factor to Bernard-Soulier, thrombasthenic and von Willebrand's disease platelets. *Thromb Res* 19:21–27, 1980.

164. Zucker MB, Kim SJ, McPherson J, Grant RA: Binding of factor VIII to platelets in the presence of ristocetin. *Br J Haematol* 35:535–549, 1977.

165. Berndt MC, Gregory C, Chong BH, et al: Additional glycoprotein defects in Bernard-Soulier's syndrome: Confirmation of genetic basis by parental analysis. *Blood* 62:800–807, 1983.

166. Clemetson KJ, McGregor JL, James E, et al: Characterization of the platelet membrane glycoprotein abnormalities in Bernard-Soulier syndrome and comparison with normal by surface-labeling techniques and high-resolution two-dimensional gel electrophoresis. *J Clin Invest* 70:304–311, 1982.

167. Vanhoorelbeke K, Ulrichts H, Romijn RA, et al: The GPIbalpha-thrombin interaction: Far from crystal clear. *Trends Mol Med* 10:33–39, 2004.

168. Romo GM, Dong JF, Schade AJ, et al: The glycoprotein Ib-IX-V complex is a platelet counterreceptor for P-selectin. *J Exp Med* 190:803–814, 1999.

169. Simon DI, Chen Z, Xu H, et al: Platelet glycoprotein Ibα is a counterreceptor for the leukocyte integrin Mac-1 (CD11b/CD18). *J Exp Med* 192:193–204, 2000.

170. Bradford HN, Dela Cadena RA, Kunapuli SP, et al: Human kininogens regulate thrombin binding to platelets through the glycoprotein Ib-IX-V complex. *Blood* 90:1508–1515, 1997.

171. Jurk K, Clemetson KJ, de Groot PG, et al: Thrombospondin-1 mediates platelet adhesion at high shear via glycoprotein Ib (GPIb): An alternative/backup mechanism to von Willebrand factor. *FASEB J* 17:1490–1492, 2003.

172. Baglia FA, Badellino KO, Li CQ, et al: Factor XI binding to the platelet glycoprotein Ib-IX-V complex promotes factor XI activation by thrombin. *J Biol Chem* 277: 1662–1668, 2002.

173. Bradford HN, Pixley RA, Colman RW: Human factor XII binding to the glycoprotein Ib-IX-V complex inhibits thrombin-induced platelet aggregation. *J Biol Chem* 275: 22756–22763, 2000.

174. Ware J, Russell S, Ruggeri ZM: Generation and rescue of a murine model of platelet dysfunction: The Bernard-Soulier syndrome. *Proc Natl Acad Sci U S A* 97:2803–2808, 2000.

175. Kato K, Martinez C, Russell S, et al: Genetic deletion of mouse platelet glycoprotein Ibbeta produces a Bernard-Soulier phenotype with increased alpha-granule size. *Blood* 104:2339–2344, 2004.

176. Ramakrishnan V, Reeves PS, DeGuzman F, et al: Increased thrombin responsiveness in platelets from mice lacking glycoprotein V. *Proc Natl Acad Sci U S A* 96:13336–13341, 1999.

177. Nonne C, Hechler B, Cazenave JP, et al: Reassessment of in vivo thrombus formation in glycoprotein V deficient mice backcrossed on a C57Bl/6 strain. *J Thromb Haemost* 6:210–212, 2008.

178. Grottum KA, Solum NO: Congenital thrombocytopenia with giant platelets: A defect in the platelet membrane. *Br J Haematol* 16:277–290, 1969.

179. Greenberg JP, Packham MA, Guccione MA, et al: Survival of rabbit-platelets treated in vitro with chymotrypsin, plasmin, trypsin, and neuraminidase. *Blood* 53:916–927, 1979.

180. Heyns Ad, Badenhorst PN, Wessels P, et al: Kinetics, *in vivo* redistribution and sites of sequestration of indium-111-labelled platelets in giant platelet syndromes. *Br J Haematol* 60:323–330, 1985.

181. Tomer A, Scharf RE, McMillan R, et al: Bernard-Soulier syndrome: Quantitative characterization of megakaryocytes and platelets by flow cytometric and platelet kinetic measurements. *Eur J Haematol* 52:193–200, 1994.

182. Nurden P, Nurden A: Giant platelets, megakaryocytes and the expression of glycoprotein Ib-IX complexes. *C R Acad Sci III* 319:717–726, 1996.

183. Vettore S, Scandellari R, Scapin M, et al: A case of Bernard-Soulier Syndrome due to a homozygous four bases deletion (TGAG) of GPIbalpha gene: Lack of GPIbalpha but absence of bleeding. *Platelets* 19:388–391, 2008.

184. George JN, Nurden AT: Inherited disorders of the platelet membrane: Glanzmann's thrombasthenia and Bernard-Soulier syndrome, in *Hemostasis and Thrombosis: Basic Principles and Clinical Practice*, edited by RW Colman, J Hirsh, VJ Marder, EW Salzman, p 726. Lippincott, Philadelphia, 1987.

185. Ruggeri Z: The platelet glycoprotein Ib-IX complex. *Prog Hemost Thromb* 10:35–68, 1991.

186. Andrews RK, Lopez JA, Berndt MC: The GPIb-IX-V complex, in *Platelets*, 3rd ed, edited by AD Michelson. Academic Press, San Diego, 2013.

187. Roth GJ: Developing relationships: Arterial platelet adhesion, glycoprotein Ib, and leucine-rich glycoproteins. *Blood* 77:5–19, 1991.

188. Yap CL, Hughan SC, Cranmer SL, et al: Synergistic adhesive interactions and signaling mechanisms operating between platelet glycoprotein Ib/IX and integrin alpha IIbbeta 3. Studies in human platelets and transfected Chinese hamster ovary cells. *J Biol Chem* 275:41377–41388, 2000.

189. Gardiner EE, Arthur JF, Shen Y, et al: GPIbalpha-selective activation of platelets induces platelet signaling events comparable to GPVI activation events. *Platelets* 21:244–252, 2010.

190. Zhou YF, Eng ET, Zhu J, et al: Sequence and structure relationships within von Willebrand factor. *Blood* 120:449–458, 2012.

191. Wu YP, Vink T, Schiphorst M, et al: Platelet thrombus formation on collagen at high shear rates is mediated by von Willebrand factor-glycoprotein Ib interaction and inhibited by von Willebrand factor-glycoprotein IIb/IIIa interaction. *Arterioscler Thromb Vasc Biol* 20:1661–1667, 2000.

192. Kulkarni S, Dopheide SM, Yap CL, et al: A revised model of platelet aggregation. *J Clin Invest* 105:783–791, 2000.

193. Matsui H, Sugimoto M, Mizuno T, et al: Distinct and concerted functions of von Willebrand factor and fibrinogen in mural thrombus growth under high shear flow. *Blood* 100:3604–3610, 2002.

194. Ikeda Y, Handa M, Kawano K, et al: The role of von Willebrand factor and fibrinogen in platelet aggregation under varying shear stress. *J Clin Invest* 87:1234–1240, 1991.

195. Peterson DM, Stathopoulos NA, Giorgio TD, et al: Shear-induced platelet aggregation requires von Willebrand factor and platelet membrane glycoproteins Ib and IIb-IIIa. *Blood* 69:625–628, 1987.

196. Ruggeri ZM: Mechanisms of shear-induced platelet adhesion and aggregation. *Thromb Haemost* 70:119, 1993.

197. Jamieson GA, Okumura T: Reduced thrombin binding and aggregation in Bernard-Soulier platelets. *J Clin Invest* 61:861–864, 1978.

198. Jandrot-Perrus M, Rendu F, Caen JP, et al: The common pathway for alpha- and gamma-thrombin-induced platelet activation is independent of GPIb: A study of Bernard-Soulier platelets. *Br J Haematol* 75:385–392, 1990.

199. Smith PT, Landry ML, Carey H, et al: Papular-purpuric gloves and socks syndrome associated with acute parvovirus B19 infection: Case report and review. *Clin Infect Dis* 27:164–168, 1998.

200. Ramakrishnan V, Reeves PS, DeGuzman F, et al: Increased thrombin responsiveness in platelets from mice lacking glycoprotein V. *Proc Natl Acad Sci U S A* 96:13336–13341, 1999.

201. Ni H, Ramakrishnan V, Ruggeri ZM, et al: Increased thrombogenesis and embolus formation in mice lacking glycoprotein V. *Blood* 98:368–373, 2001.

202. Caen J, Bellucci S: The defective prothrombin consumption in Bernard-Soulier syndrome. Hypotheses from 1948 to 1982. *Blood Cells* 9:389–399, 1983.

203. Walsh PN, Mills DC, Pareti FI, et al: Hereditary giant platelet syndrome. Absence of collagen-induced coagulant activity and deficiency of factor-XI binding to platelets. *Br J Haematol* 29:639–655, 1975.

204. Perret B, Levy-Toledano S, Platavid M: Abnormal phospholipid organization in Bernard-Soulier platelets. *Thromb Res* 31:529, 1983.

205. Nurden P, Nurden AT, La Marca S, et al: Platelet morphological changes in 2 patients with von Willebrand disease type 3 caused by large homozygous deletions of the von Willebrand factor gene. *Haematologica* 94:1627–1629, 2009.

206. Kanaji T, Russell S, Ware J: Amelioration of the macrothrombocytopenia associated with the murine Bernard-Soulier syndrome. *Blood* 100:2102–2107, 2002.

207. McNicol A, Drouin J, Clemetson KJ, Gerrard JM: Phospholipase C activity in platelets from Bernard-Soulier syndrome patients. *Arterioscler Thromb.* 13:1567–1571, 1993.

208. White JG, Burris SM, Hasegawa D, Johnson M: Micropipette aspiration of human blood platelets: A defect in Bernard-Soulier's syndrome. *Blood* 63:1249–1252, 1984.

209. Lopez JA, Leung B, Reynolds CC, et al: Efficient plasma membrane expression of a functional platelet glycoprotein Ib-IX complex requires the presence of its three subunits. *J Biol Chem* 267:12851–12859, 1992.

210. Li CQ, Dong JF, Lanza F, et al: Expression of platelet glycoprotein (GP) V in heterologous cells and evidence for its association with GP Ib alpha in forming a GP Ib-IX-V complex on the cell surface. *J Biol Chem* 270:16302–16307, 1995.

211. Drouin J, McGregor JL, Parmentier S, et al: Residual amounts of glycoprotein Ib concomitant with near-absence of glycoprotein IX in platelets of Bernard-Soulier patients. *Blood* 72:1086–1088, 1988.

212. Stevens MC, Blanchette VS, Freedman MH, et al: A variant form of Bernard-Soulier syndrome: Mild haemostatic defect associated with partial platelet GPIb deficiency. *Clin Lab Haematol* 10:443–451, 1988.

213. Finch CN, Miller JL, Lyle VA, Handin RI: Evidence that an abnormality in the glycoprotein Ib alpha gene is not the cause of abnormal platelet function in a family with classic Bernard-Soulier disease. *Blood* 75:2357–2362, 1990.

214. Poulsen LO, Taaning E: Variation in surface platelet glycoprotein Ib expression in Bernard-Soulier syndrome. *Haemostasis* 20:155–161, 1990.

215. Wright SD, Michaelides K, Johnson DJ, et al: Double heterozygosity for mutations in the platelet glycoprotein IX gene in three siblings with Bernard-Soulier syndrome. *Blood* 81:2339–2347, 1993.

216. Nurden AT, Jallu V, Hourdille P: GP Ib and Bernard-Soulier platelets. *Blood* 73:2225–2227, 1989.

217. Nurden AT, Nurden P: Inherited disorders of platelet function, in *Platelets*, edited by AD Michelson. Academic Press, San Diego, 2007.

218. Lanza F, Baas MJ, Dupuis A, et al: Founder effect for a novel GPIBB mutations in Bernard-Soulier patients from La Reunion island. *J Thromb Haemost* 11:1322 (abstract), 2013.

219. Kenny D, Newman PJ, Morateck PA, Montgomery RR: A dinucleotide deletion results in defective membrane anchoring and circulating soluble glycoprotein Ibalpha in a novel form of Bernard-Soulier syndrome. *Blood* 90:2626–2633, 1997.

220. Holmberg L, Karpman D, Nilsson I, Olofsson T: Bernard-Soulier syndrome Karlstad: Trp 498-Stop mutation resulting in a truncated glycoprotein Ibalpha that contains part of the transmembrane domain. *Br J Haematol* 98:57, 1997.

221. Kunishima S, Lopez JA, Kobayashi S, et al: Missense mutations of the glycoprotein (GP) Ib beta gene impairing the GPIb alpha/beta disulfide linkage in a family with giant platelet disorder. *Blood* 89:2404–2412, 1997.

222. Koskela S, Partanen J, Salmi TT, Kekomaki R: Molecular characterization of two mutations in platelet glycoprotein (GP) Ibalpha in two Finnish Bernard-Soulier syndrome families. *Eur J Haematol* 62:160–168, 1999.

223. Ludlow LB, Schick BP, Budarf ML, et al: Identification of a mutation in a GATA binding site of the platelet glycoprotein Ibbeta promoter resulting in the Bernard-Soulier syndrome. *J Biol Chem* 271:22076–22080, 1996.

224. Strassel C, Alessi MC, Juhan-Vague I, et al: A 13 base pair deletion in the GPIbbeta gene in a second unrelated Bernard-Soulier family due to slipped mispairing between direct repeats. *J Thromb Haemost* 2:1663–1665, 2004.

225. Strassel C, David T, Eckly A, et al: Synthesis of GPIb beta with novel transmembrane and cytoplasmic sequences in a Bernard-Soulier patient resulting in GPIb-defective signaling in CHO cells. *J Thromb Haemost* 4:217–228, 2006.

226. Kurokawa Y, Ishida F, Kamijo T, et al: A missense mutation (Tyr88 to Cys) in the platelet membrane glycoprotein Ibbeta gene affects GPIb/IX complex expression—Bernard-Soulier syndrome in the homozygous form and giant platelets in the heterozygous form. *Thromb Haemost* 86:1249–1256, 2001.

227. Kunishima S, Naoe T, Kamiya T, Saito H: Novel heterozygous missense mutation in the platelet glycoprotein Ib beta gene associated with isolated giant platelet disorder. *Am J Hematol* 68:249–255, 2001.

228. Koskela S, Javela K, Jouppila J, et al: Variant Bernard-Soulier syndrome due to homozygous Asn45Ser mutation in the platelet glycoprotein (GP) IX in seven patients of five unrelated Finnish families. *Eur J Haematol* 62:256–264, 1999.

229. Vanhoorelbeke K, Schlammadinger A, Delville JP, et al: Occurrence of the Asn45Ser mutation in the GPIX gene in a Belgian patient with Bernard-Soulier syndrome. *Platelets* 12:114–120, 2001.

230. Zieger B, Jenny A, Tsakiris DA, et al: A large Swiss family with Bernard-Soulier syndrome-Correlation phenotype and genotype. *Hamostaseologie* 29:161–167, 2009.

231. Dagistan N, Kunishima S: First Turkish case of Bernard-Soulier syndrome associated with GPIX N45S. *Acta Haematol* 118:146–148, 2007.

232. Bartsch I, Sandrock K, Lanza F, et al: Deletion of human GP1BB and SEPT5 is associated with Bernard-Soulier syndrome, platelet secretion defect, polymicrogyria, and developmental delay. *Thromb Haemost* 106:475–483, 2011.

233. Kunishima S, Imai T, Kobayashi R, et al: Bernard-Soulier syndrome caused by a hemizygous GPIbbeta mutation and 22q11.2 deletion. *Pediatr Int* 55:434–437, 2013.

234. Budarf ML, Konkle BA, Ludlow LB, et al: Identification of a patient with Bernard-Soulier syndrome and a deletion in the DiGeorge/velo-cardio-facial chromosomal region in 22q11.2. *Hum Mol Genet* 4:763, 1995.

235. Lascone MR, Sacchelli M, Vittorini S, Giusti S: Complex conotruncal heart defect, severe bleeding disorder and 22q11 deletion: A new case of Bernard-Soulier syndrome and of 22q11 deletion syndrome? *Ital Heart J* 2:475–477, 2001.

236. Tang J, Stern-Nezer S, Liu PC, et al: Mutation in the leucine-rich repeat C-flanking region of platelet glycoprotein Ibbeta impairs assembly of von Willebrand factor receptor. *Thromb Haemost* 92:75–88, 2004.

237. Hillmann A, Nurden A, Nurden P, et al: A novel hemizygous Bernard-Soulier syndrome (BSS) mutation in the amino terminal domain of glycoprotein (GP)Ibbeta—Platelet characterization and transfection studies. *Thromb Haemost* 88:1026–1032, 2002.

238. Nakagawa M, Okuno M, Okamoto N, et al: Bernard-Soulier syndrome associated with 22q11.2 microdeletion. *Am J Med Genet* 99:286–288, 2001.

239. Liang HP, Morel-Kopp MC, Curtin J, et al: Heterozygous loss of platelet glycoprotein (GP) Ib-V-IX variably affects platelet function in velocardiofacial syndrome (VCFS) patients. *Thromb Haemost* 98:1298–1308, 2007.

240. Van Geet C, Devriendt K, Eyskens B, et al: Velocardiofacial syndrome patients with a heterozygous chromosome 22q11 deletion have giant platelets. *Pediatr Res* 44:607–611, 1998.

241. Lawrence S, McDonald-McGinn DM, Zackai E, Sullivan KE: Thrombocytopenia in patients with chromosome 22q11.2 deletion syndrome. *J Pediatr* 143:277–278, 2003.

242. Kato T, Kosaka K, Kimura M, et al: Thrombocytopenia in patients with 22q11.2 deletion syndrome and its association with glycoprotein Ib-beta. *Genet Med* 5:113–119, 2003.

243. Latger-Cannard V, Bensoussan D, Gregoire MJ, et al: Frequency of thrombocytopenia and large platelets correlates neither with conotruncal cardiac anomalies nor immunological features in the chromosome 22q11.2 deletion syndrome. *Eur J Pediatr* 163:327–328, 2004.

244. Ryan AK, Goodship JA, Wilson DI, et al: Spectrum of clinical features associated with interstitial chromosome 22q11 deletions: A European collaborative study. *J Med Genet* 34:798–804, 1997.

245. Miller JL, Lyle VA, Cunningham D: Mutation of leucine-57 to phenylalanine in a platelet glycoprotein Ib alpha leucine tandem repeat occurring in patients with an autosomal dominant variant of Bernard-Soulier disease. *Blood* 79:439–446, 1992.

246. Vettore S, Scandellari R, Moro S, et al: Novel point mutation in a leucine-rich repeat of the GPIbalpha chain of the platelet von Willebrand factor receptor, GPIb/IX/V, resulting in an inherited dominant form of Bernard-Soulier syndrome affecting two unrelated families: The N41H variant. *Haematologica* 93:1743–1747, 2008.

247. Kunishima S, Imai T, Hamaguchi M, Saito H: Novel heterozygous missense mutation in the second leucine rich repeat of GPIbalpha affects GPIb/IX/V expression and results in macrothrombocytopenia in a patient initially misdiagnosed with idiopathic thrombocytopenic purpura. *Eur J Haematol* 76:348–355, 2006.

248. De Marco L, Mazzucato M, Fabris F, et al: Variant Bernard-Soulier syndrome type Bolzano. A congenital bleeding disorder due to a structural and functional abnormality of the platelet glycoprotein Ib-IX complex. *J Clin Invest* 86:25–31, 1990.

249. Margaglione M, D'Andrea G, Grandone E, et al: Compound heterozygosity (554–589 del, C515-T transition) in the platelet glycoprotein Ib alpha gene in a patient with a severe bleeding tendency. *Thromb Haemost* 81:486–492, 1999.

250. Noris P, Perrotta S, Bottega R, et al: Clinical and laboratory features of 103 patients from 42 Italian families with inherited thrombocytopenia derived from the monoallelic Ala156Val mutation of GPIbalpha (Bolzano mutation). *Haematologica* 97:82–88, 2012.

251. Yuksel O, Koklu S, Ucar E, et al: Severe recurrent gastrointestinal bleeding due to angiodysplasia in a Bernard-Soulier patient: An onerous medical concomitance. *Dig Dis Sci* 49:885–887, 2004.

252. Okita R, Hihara J, Konishi K, et al: Intractable gastrointestinal bleeding from angiodysplasia in a patient of Bernard-Soulier syndrome—Report of a case. *Hiroshima J Med Sci* 54:113–115, 2005.

253. Kaya Z, Gursel T, Dalgic B, Aslan D: Gastric angiodysplasia in a child with Bernard-Soulier syndrome: Efficacy of octreotide in long-term management. *Pediatr Hematol Oncol* 22:223–227, 2005.

254. George JN, Reimann TA, Moake JL, et al: Bernard-Soulier disease: A study of four patients and their parents. *Br J Haematol* 48:459, 1981.

255. Fox JE: Linkage of a membrane skeleton to integral membrane glycoproteins in human platelets. Identification of one of the glycoproteins as glycoprotein Ib. *J Clin Invest* 76:1673–1683, 1985.

256. Eaton LA Jr, Read MS, Brinkhous KM: Glycoprotein Ib bioassays. Activity levels in Bernard-Soulier syndrome and in stored blood bank platelets. *Arch Pathol Lab Med* 115:488–493, 1991.

257. Waldenstrom E, Holmberg L, Axelsson U, et al: Bernard-Soulier syndrome in two Swedish families: Effect of DDAVP on bleeding time. *Eur J Haematol* 46:182–187, 1991.

258. Evensen SA, Solum NO, Grottum KA, Hovig T: Familial bleeding disorder with a moderate thrombocytopenia and giant blood platelets. *Scand J Haematol* 13:203–214, 1974.

259. Greco NJ, Tandon NN, Jones GD, et al: Contributions of glycoprotein Ib and the seven transmembrane domain receptor to increases in platelet cytoplasmic [Ca 2+] induced by α-thrombin. *Biochemistry* 35:906–914, 1996.

260. Celikel R, McClintock RA, Roberts JR, et al: Modulation of alpha-thrombin function by distinct interactions with platelet glycoprotein Ibalpha. *Science* 301:218–221, 2003.

261. Dumas JJ, Kumar R, Seehra J, et al: Crystal structure of the GpIbalpha-thrombin complex essential for platelet aggregation. *Science* 301:222–226, 2003.

262. McGowan EB, Ding A, Detwiler TC: Correlation of thrombin-induced glycoprotein V hydrolysis and platelet activation. *J Biol Chem* 258:11243, 1983.

263. Bienz D, Schnippering W, Clemetson KJ: Glycoprotein V is not the thrombin activation receptor on human blood platelets. *Blood* 68:720–725, 1986.

264. Caen JP, Nurden AT, Jeanneau C, et al: Bernard-Soulier syndrome: A new platelet glycoprotein abnormality. Its relationship with platelet adhesion to subendothelium and with the factor VIII von Willebrand protein. *J Lab Clin Med* 87:586–596, 1976.

265. Andrews RK, Harris SJ, McNally T, Berndt MC: Binding of purified 14-3-3 zeta signaling protein to discrete amino acid sequences within the cytoplasmic domain of the platelet membrane glycoprotein Ib-IX-V complex. *Biochemistry* 37:638–647, 1998.

266. Sullam PM, Hyun WC, Szollosi J, et al: Physical proximity and functional interplay of the glycoprotein Ib-IX-V complex and the Fc receptor FcgammaRIIA on the platelet plasma membrane. *J Biol Chem* 273:5331–5336, 1998.

267. Falati S, Edmead CE, Poole AW: Glycoprotein Ib-V-IX, a receptor for von Willebrand factor, couples physically and functionally to the Fc receptor g chain, Fyn, and Lyn to activate human platelets. *Blood* 94:1648–1656, 1999.

268. Arthur JF, Gardiner EE, Matzaris M, et al: Glycoprotein VI is associated with GPIb-IX-V on the membrane of resting and activated platelets. *Thromb Haemost* 93:716–723, 2005.

269. Feng S, Resendiz JC, Christodoulides N, et al: Pathological shear stress stimulates the tyrosine phosphorylation of alpha-actinin associated with the glycoprotein Ib-IX complex. *Biochemistry* 41:1100–1108, 2002.

270. Aziz KA: An acquired form of Bernard Soulier syndrome associated with acute myeloid leukemia. *Saudi Med J* 26:1095–1098, 2005.

271. Kaur H, Ozelo M, Scovil S, et al: Systematic analysis of bleeding phenotype in PT-VWD compared to type 2B VWD using an electronic bleeding questionnaire. *Clin Appl Thromb Hemost* 20:765–771, 2014.

272. Takahashi H: Studies on the pathophysiology and treatment of von Willebrand's disease. IV. Mechanism of increased ristocetin-induced platelet aggregation in von Willebrand's disease. *Thromb Res* 19:857–867, 1980.

273. Krizek DM, Rick ME, Williams SB, Gralnick HR: Cryoprecipitate transfusion in variant von Willebrand's disease and thrombocytopenia. *Ann Intern Med* 98:484–486, 1983.

274. Weiss HJ, Meyer D, Rabinowitz R, et al: Pseudo-von Willebrand's disease. An intrinsic platelet defect with aggregation by unmodified human factor VIII/von Willebrand factor and enhanced adsorption of its high-molecular-weight multimers. *N Engl J Med* 306:326–333, 1982.

275. Miller JL, Castella A: Platelet-type von Willebrand's disease: Characterization of a new bleeding disorder. *Blood* 60:790–794, 1982.

276. Gralnick HR, Williams SB, Shafer BC, Corash L: Factor VIII/von Willebrand factor binding to von Willebrand's disease platelets. *Blood* 60:328–332, 1982.

277. Takahashi H, Handa M, Watanabe K, et al: Further characterization of platelet-type von Willebrand's disease in Japan. *Blood* 64:1254–1262, 1984.

278. Nurden P, Lanza F, Bonnafous-Faurie C, Nurden A: A second report of platelet-type von Willebrand disease with a Gly233Ser mutation in the GPIBA gene. *Thromb Haemost* 97:319–321, 2007.

279. Othman M, Notley C, Lavender FL, et al: Identification and functional characterization of a novel 27-bp deletion in the macroglycopeptide-coding region of the GPIBA gene resulting in platelet-type von Willebrand disease. *Blood* 105:4330–4336, 2005.

280. Enayat MS, Guilliatt AM, Lester W, et al: Distinguishing between type 2B and pseudo-von Willebrand disease and its clinical importance. *Br J Haematol* 133:664–666, 2006.

281. Bryckaert MC, Pietu G, Ruan C, et al: Abnormality of glycoprotein Ib in two cases of "pseudo"-von Willebrand's disease. *J Lab Clin Med* 106:393–400, 1985.

282. Othman M, Kaur H, Emsley J: Platelet-type von Willebrand disease: New insights into the molecular pathophysiology of a unique platelet defect. *Semin Thromb Hemost* 39:663–673, 2013.

283. Othman M, Emsley J: Platelet-type von Willebrand disease: Toward an improved understanding of the "sticky situation." *Semin Thromb Hemost* 40:146–150, 2014.

284. Miller JL, Cunningham D, Lyle VA, Finch CN: Mutation in the gene encoding the alpha chain of platelet glycoprotein Ib in platelet-type von Willebrand disease. *Proc Natl Acad Sci U S A* 88:4761–4765, 1991.

285. Russell SD, Roth GJ: Pseudo-von Willebrand disease: A mutation in the platelet glycoprotein Ib alpha gene associated with a hyperactive surface receptor. *Blood* 81:1787–1791, 1993.

286. Takahashi H, Murata M, Moriki T, et al: Substitution of Val for Met at residue 239 of platelet glycoprotein Ib alpha in Japanese patients with platelet-type von Willebrand disease. *Blood* 85:727–733, 1995.

287. Kunishima S, Heaton DC, Naoe T, et al: De novo mutation of the platelet glycoprotein Ib alpha gene in a patient with pseudo-von Willebrand disease. *Blood Coagul Fibrinolysis* 8:311–315, 1997.

288. Matsubara Y, Murata M, Sugita K, Ikeda Y: Identification of a novel point mutation in platelet glycoprotein Ibalpha, Gly to Ser at residue 233, in a Japanese family with platelet-type von Willebrand disease. *J Thromb Haemost* 1:2198–2205, 2003.

289. Kanaji S, Fahs SA, Ware J, et al: Non-myeloablative conditioning with busulfan before hematopoietic stem cell transplantation leads to phenotypic correction of murine Bernard-Soulier syndrome. *J Thromb Haemost* 12:1726–1732, 2014.

290. Uff S, Clemetson JM, Harrison T, et al: Crystal structure of the platelet glycoprotein Ib(alpha) N-terminal domain reveals an unmasking mechanism for receptor activation. *J Biol Chem* 277:35657–35663, 2002.

291. Huizinga EG, Tsuji S, Romijn RA, et al: Structures of glycoprotein Ibalpha and its complex with von Willebrand factor A1 domain. *Science* 297:1176–1179, 2002.

292. Enayat S, Ravanbod S, Rassoulzadegan M, et al: A novel D235Y mutation in the GP1BA gene enhances platelet interaction with von Willebrand factor in an Iranian family with platelet-type von Willebrand disease. *Thromb Haemost* 108:946–954, 2012.

293. Woods AI, Sanchez-Luceros A, Bermejo E, et al: Identification of p.W246L as a novel mutation in the GP1BA gene responsible for platelet-type von Willebrand disease. *Semin Thromb Hemost* 40:151–160, 2014.

294. Pincus MR, Carty RP, Miller JL: Structural implications of the substitution of Val for Met at residue 239 in the alpha chain of human platelet glycoprotein Ib. *J Protein Chem* 13:629–633, 1994.

295. Dumas JJ, Kumar R, McDonagh T, et al: Crystal structure of the wild-type von Willebrand factor A1-glycoprotein Ibalpha complex reveals conformation differences with a complex bearing von Willebrand disease mutations. *J Biol Chem* 279:23327–23334, 2004.

296. Suva LJ, Hartman E, Dilley JD, et al: Platelet dysfunction and a high bone mass phenotype in a murine model of platelet-type von Willebrand disease. *Am J Pathol* 172:430–439, 2008.

297. Doggett TA, Girdhar G, Lawshe A, et al: Alterations in the intrinsic properties of the GPIbalpha-VWF tether bond define the kinetics of the platelet-type von Willebrand disease mutation, Gly233Val. *Blood* 102:152–160, 2003.

298. Tait AS, Cranmer SL, Jackson SP, et al: Phenotype changes resulting in high-affinity binding of von Willebrand factor to recombinant glycoprotein Ib-IX: Analysis of the platelet-type von Willebrand disease mutations. *Blood* 98:1812–1818, 2001.

299. Takahashi H, Nagayama R, Hattori A, Shibata A: Botrocetin- and polybrene-induced platelet aggregation in platelet-type von Willebrand disease. *Am J Hematol* 18:179–189, 1985.

300. Miller JL, Kupinski JM, Castella A, Ruggeri ZM: Von Willebrand factor binds to platelets and induces aggregation in platelet-type but not type IIB von Willebrand disease. *J Clin Invest* 72:1532–1542, 1983.

301. Scott JP, Montgomery RR: The rapid differentiation of type IIb von Willebrand's disease from platelet-type (pseudo-) von Willebrand's disease by the "neutral" monoclonal antibody binding assay. *Am J Clin Pathol* 96:723–728, 1991.

302. Miller JL: Sorting out heightened interactions between platelets and von Willebrand factor. "IIB or not IIB?" is becoming an increasingly answerable question in the molecular era. *Am J Clin Pathol* 96:681–683, 1991.

303. Miller JL, Ruggeri ZM, Lyle VA: Unique interactions of asialo von Willebrand factor with platelets in platelet-type von Willebrand disease. *Blood* 70:1804–1809, 1987.

304. Hamilton A, Ozelo M, Leggo J, et al: Frequency of platelet type versus type 2B von Willebrand disease. An international registry-based study. *Thromb Haemost* 105:501–508, 2011.

305. Takahashi H: Replacement therapy in platelet-type von Willebrand disease. *Am J Hematol* 18:351–362, 1985.

306. Miller JL: Platelet-type von Willebrand's disease. *Clin Lab Med* 4:319–331, 1984.

307. Poon MC: Factor VIIa, in *Platelets*, 2nd ed, edited by AD Michelson, p 867. Academic Press, San Diego, 2007.

308. Fressinaud E, Signaud-Fiks M, Le Boterff C, Piot B: Use of recombinant factor VIIa (NovoSevenr) for dental extraction in a patient affected by platelet-type (pseudo-) von Willebrand disease. *Haemophilia* 4:299, 1998.

309. Nieuwenhuis HK, Akkerman JW, Houdijk WP, Sixma JJ: Human blood platelets showing no response to collagen fail to express surface glycoprotein Ia. *Nature* 318:470–472, 1985.

310. Nieuwenhuis HK, Sakariassen KS, Houdijk WP, et al: Deficiency of platelet membrane glycoprotein Ia associated with a decreased platelet adhesion to subendothelium: A defect in platelet spreading. *Blood* 68:692–695, 1986.

311. Beer JH, Nieuwenhuis HK, Sixma JJ, Coller BS: Deficiency of antibody 6F1 binding to the platelets of a patient with an isolated defect in platelet-collagen interaction. *Circulation* 78(Suppl):II-308, 1988.

312. Coller BS, Beer JH, Scudder LE, Steinberg MH: Collagen-platelet interactions: Evidence for a direct interaction of collagen with platelet GPIa/IIa and an indirect interaction with platelet GPIIb/IIa mediated by adhesive proteins. *Blood* 74:182–192, 1989.

313. Kehrel B, Balleisen L, Kokott R, et al: Deficiency of intact thrombospondin and membrane glycoprotein Ia in platelets with defective collagen-induced aggregation and spontaneous loss of disorder. *Blood* 71:1074–1078, 1988.

314. Kunicki TJ, Williams SA, Nugent DJ: Genetic variants that affect platelet function. *Curr Opin Hematol* 19:371–379, 2012.

315. Habart D, Cheli Y, Nugent DJ, et al: Conditional knockout of integrin alpha2beta1 in murine megakaryocytes leads to reduced mean platelet volume. *PLoS One* 8:e55094, 2013.

316. McCall-Culbreath KD, Zutter MM: Collagen receptor integrins: Rising to the challenge. *Curr Drug Targets* 9:139–149, 2008.

317. Yamamoto N, Ikeda H, Tandon NN, et al: A platelet membrane glycoprotein (GP) deficiency in healthy blood donors: Naka-platelets lack detectable GPIV (CD36). *Blood* 76:1698–1703, 1990.

318. Curtis BR, Aster RH: Incidence of the Nak(a)-negative platelet phenotype in African Americans is similar to that of Asians. *Transfusion* 36:331–334, 1996.

319. Zhu W, Li W, Silverstein RL: Advanced glycation end products induce a prothrombotic phenotype in mice via interaction with platelet CD36. *Blood* 119:6136–6144, 2012.

320. Asch AS, Barnwell J, Silverstein RL, Nachman RL: Isolation of the thrombospondin membrane receptor. *J Clin Invest* 79:1054–1061, 1987.

321. Tandon NN, Kralisz U, Jamieson GA: Identification of glycoprotein IV (CD36) as a primary receptor for platelet-collagen adhesion. *J Biol Chem* 264:7576–7583, 1989.

322. Wang Y, Fang C, Gao H, et al: Platelet-derived S100 family member myeloid-related protein-14 regulates thrombosis. *J Clin Invest* 124:2160–2171, 2014.

323. Matsuno K, Diaz-Ricart M, Montgomery RR, et al: Inhibition of platelet adhesion to collagen by monoclonal anti-CD36 antibodies. *Br J Haematol* 92:960–967, 1996.

324. Silverstein RL, Asch AS, Nachman RL: Glycoprotein IV mediates thrombospondin-dependent platelet-monocyte and platelet-U937 cell adhesion. *J Clin Invest* 84:546–552, 1989.

325. Kehrel B, Kronenberg A, Schwippert B, et al: Thrombospondin binds normally to glycoprotein IIIb deficient platelets. *Biochem Biophys Res Commun* 179:985–991, 1991.

326. Tandon NN, Ockenhouse CF, Greco NJ, Jamieson GA: Adhesive functions of platelets lacking glycoprotein IV (CD36). *Blood* 78:2809–2813, 1991.

327. Saelman EU, Kehrel B, Hese KM, et al: Platelet adhesion to collagen and endothelial cell matrix under flow conditions is not dependent on platelet glycoprotein IV. *Blood* 83:3240–3244, 1994.

328. Kuijpers MJ, de Witt S, Nergiz-Unal R, et al: Supporting roles of platelet thrombospondin-1 and CD36 in thrombus formation on collagen. *Arterioscler Thromb Vasc Biol* 34:1187–1192, 2014.

329. Englyst NA, Taube JM, Aitman TJ, et al: A novel role for CD36 in VLDL-enhanced platelet activation. *Diabetes* 52:1248–1255, 2003.

330. Ghosh A, Murugesan G, Chen K, et al: Platelet CD36 surface expression levels affect functional responses to oxidized LDL and are associated with inheritance of specific genetic polymorphisms. *Blood* 117:6355–6366, 2011.

331. Kashiwagi H, Tomiyama Y, Honda S, et al: Molecular basis of CD36 deficiency. Evidence that a 478C—>T substitution (proline90—>serine) in CD36 cDNA accounts for CD36 deficiency. *J Clin Invest* 95:1040–1046, 1995.

332. Hirano K, Kuwasako T, Nakagawa-Toyama Y, et al: Pathophysiology of human genetic CD36 deficiency. *Trends Cardiovasc Med* 13:136–141, 2003.

333. Febbraio M, Silverstein RL: CD36: Implications in cardiovascular disease. *Int J Biochem Cell Biol* 39:2012–2030, 2007.

334. Kashiwagi H, Tomiyama Y, Kosugi S, et al: Family studies of type II CD36 deficient subjects: Linkage of a CD36 allele to a platelet-specific mRNA expression defect(s) causing type II CD36 deficiency. *Thromb Haemost* 74:758–763, 1995.

335. Ikeda H: Platelet membrane protein CD36. *Hokkaido Igaku Zasshi* 74:99–104, 1999.

336. Kashiwagi H, Tomiyama Y, Kosugi S, et al: Identification of molecular defects in a subject with type I CD36 deficiency. *Blood* 83:3545–3552, 1994.

337. Kashiwagi H, Tomiyama Y, Nozaki S, et al: A single nucleotide insertion in codon 317 of the CD36 gene leads to CD36 deficiency. *Arterioscler Thromb Vasc Biol* 16:1026–1032, 1996.

338. Hanawa H, Watanabe K, Nakamura T, et al: Identification of cryptic splice site, exon skipping, and novel point mutations in type I CD36 deficiency. *J Med Genet* 39:286–291, 2002.

339. Bierling P, Godeau B, Fromont P, et al: Posttransfusion purpura-like syndrome associated with CD36 (Naka) isoimmunization. *Transfusion* 35:777–782, 1995.

340. Morishita K, Wakamoto S, Miyazaki T, et al: Life-threatening adverse reaction followed by thrombocytopenia after passive transfusion of fresh frozen plasma containing anti-CD36 (Nak) isoantibody. *Transfusion (Paris)* 45:803–806, 2005.

341. Moroi M, Jung SM, Okuma M, Shinmyozu K: A patient with platelets deficient in glycoprotein VI that lack both collagen-induced aggregation and adhesion. *J Clin Invest* 84:1440–1445, 1989.

342. Ryo R, Yoshida A, Sugano W, et al: Deficiency of P62, a putative collagen receptor, in platelets from a patient with defective collagen-induced platelet aggregation. *Am J Hematol* 39:25–31, 1992.

343. Nurden P, Jandrot-Perrus M, Combrie R, et al: Severe deficiency of glycoprotein VI in a patient with gray platelet syndrome. *Blood* 104:107–114, 2004.

344. Arai M, Yamamoto N, Moroi M, et al: Platelets with 10% of the normal amount of glycoprotein VI have an impaired response to collagen that results in a mild bleeding tendency. *Br J Haematol* 89:124–130, 1995.

345. Arthur JF, Dunkley S, Andrews RK: Platelet glycoprotein VI-related clinical defects. *Br J Haematol* 139:363–372, 2007.

346. Chu XX, Hou M: [Advances in the studies of platelet glycoprotein VI (GPVI): Review] [in Chinese]. *Zhongguo Shi Yan Xue Ye Xue Za Zhi* 14:1040–1044, 2006.

347. Bellucci S, Huisse MG, Boval B, et al: Defective collagen-induced platelet activation in two patients with malignant haemopathies is related to a defect in the GPVI-coupled signalling pathway. *Thromb Haemost* 93:130–138, 2005.

348. Kojima H, Moroi M, Jung SM, et al: Characterization of a patient with glycoprotein (GP) VI deficiency possessing neither anti-GPVI autoantibody nor genetic aberration. *J Thromb Haemost* 4:2433–2442, 2006.

349. Dunkley S, Arthur JF, Evans S, et al: A familial platelet function disorder associated with abnormal signalling through the glycoprotein VI pathway. *Br J Haematol* 137:569–577, 2007.

350. Hermans C, Wittevrongel C, Thys C, et al: A compound heterozygous mutation in glycoprotein VI in a patient with a bleeding disorder. *J Thromb Haemost* 7:1356–1363, 2009.

351. Sugiyama T, Okuma M, Ushikubi F, et al: A novel platelet aggregating factor found in a patient with defective collagen-induced platelet aggregation and autoimmune thrombocytopenia. *Blood* 69:1712–1720, 1987.

352. Takahashi H, Moroi M: Antibody against platelet membrane glycoprotein VI in a patient with systemic lupus erythematosus. *Am J Hematol* 67:262–267, 2001.

353. Boylan B, Chen H, Rathore V, et al: Anti-GPVI-associated ITP: An acquired platelet disorder caused by autoantibody-mediated clearance of the GPVI/FcRγ-chain complex from the human platelet surface. *Blood* 104:1350–1355, 2004.

354. Akiyama M, Kashiwagi H, Todo K, et al: Presence of platelet-associated anti-GPVI autoantibodies and restoration of GPVI expression in patients with GPVI deficiency. *J Thromb Haemost* 7:1373-1383, 2009.

355. Nieswandt B, Schulte V, Bergmeier W, et al: Long-term antithrombotic protection by in vivo depletion of platelet glycoprotein VI in mice. *J Exp Med* 193:459–469, 2001.

356. Dumont B, Lasne D, Rothschild C, et al: Absence of collagen-induced platelet activation caused by compound heterozygous GPVI mutations. *Blood* 114:1900–1903, 2009.

357. Matus V, Valenzuela G, Saez CG, et al: An adenine insertion in exon 6 of human GP6 generates a truncated protein associated with a bleeding disorder in four Chilean families. *J Thromb Haemost* 11:1751–1759, 2013.

358. Weiss HJ, Chervenick PA, Zalusky R, Factor A: A familial defect in platelet function associated with impaired release of adenosine diphosphate. *N Engl J Med* 281:1264–1270, 1969.

359. Holmsen H, Weiss HJ: Hereditary defect in the platelet release reaction caused by a deficiency in the storage pool of platelet adenine nucleotides. *Br J Haematol* 19:643–649, 1970.

360. Holmsen H: Secretable storage pools in platelets. *Annu Rev Med* 30:119–134, 1979.

361. Huizing M, Helip-Wooley A, Westbroek W, et al: Disorders of lysosome-related organelle biogenesis: Clinical and molecular genetics. *Annu Rev Genomics Hum Genet* 9:359–386, 2008.

362. Hermansky F, Pudlak P: Albinism associated with hemorrhagic diathesis and unusual pigmented reticular cells in the bone marrow: Report of two cases with histochemical studies. *Blood* 14:162, 1959.

363. Gahl WA, Brantly M, Kaiser-Kupfer MI, et al: Genetic defects and clinical characteristics of patients with a form of oculocutaneous albinism (Hermansky-Pudlak syndrome). *N Engl J Med* 338:1258–1264, 1998.

364. Wei ML: Hermansky-Pudlak syndrome: A disease of protein trafficking and organelle function. *Pigment Cell Res* 19:19–42, 2006.

365. Gunay-Aygun M, Huizing M, Gahl WA: Molecular defects that affect platelet dense granules. *Semin Thromb Hemost* 30:537–547, 2004.

366. Shiflett SL, Kaplan J, Ward DM: Chédiak-Higashi syndrome: A rare disorder of lysosomes and lysosome related organelles. *Pigment Cell Res* 15:251–257, 2002.

367. Grottum KA, Hovig T, Holmsen H, et al: Wiskott-Aldrich syndrome: Qualitative platelet defects and short platelet survival. *Br J Haematol* 17:373–388, 1969.

368. Stormorken H, Hellum B, Egeland T, et al: X-linked thrombocytopenia and thrombocytopathia: Attenuated Wiskott- Aldrich syndrome. Functional and morphological studies of platelets and lymphocytes. *Thromb Haemost* 65:300–305, 1991.

369. Onel D, Ulutin SB, Ulutin ON: Platelet defect in a case of Ehlers-Danlos syndrome. *Acta Haematol* 50:238–244, 1973.

370. Hathaway WE, Solomons CC, Ott JE: Platelet function and pyrophosphates in osteogenesis imperfecta. *Blood* 39:500–509, 1972.

371. Day HJ, Holmsen H: Platelet adenine nucleotide "storage pool deficiency" in thrombocytopenia absent radii syndrome. *JAMA* 221:1053, 1972.

372. Weiss HJ, Witte LD, Kaplan KL, et al: Heterogeneity in storage pool deficiency: Studies on granule-bound substances in 18 patients including variants deficient in alpha-granules, platelet factor 4, beta-thromboglobulin, and platelet-derived growth factor. *Blood* 54:1296–1319, 1979.

373. Seward SL Jr, Gahl WA: Hermansky-Pudlak syndrome: Health care throughout life. *Pediatrics* 132:153–160, 2013.

374. Bonifacino JS: Insights into the biogenesis of lysosome-related organelles from the study of the Hermansky-Pudlak syndrome. *Ann N Y Acad Sci* 1038:103–114, 2004.

375. White JG: Inherited abnormalities of the platelet membrane and secretory granules. *Hum Pathol* 18:123–139, 1987.

376. Nishibori M, Cham B, McNicol A, et al: The protein CD63 is in platelet dense granules, is deficient in a patient with Hermansky-Pudlak syndrome, and appears identical to granulophysin. *J Clin Invest* 91:1775–1782, 1993.

377. Huizing M, Boissy RE, Gahl WA: Hermansky-Pudlak syndrome: Vesicle formation from yeast to man. *Pigment Cell Res* 15:405–419, 2002.

378. Huizing M, Parkes JM, Helip-Wooley A, et al: Platelet alpha granules in BLOC-2 and BLOC-3 subtypes of Hermansky-Pudlak syndrome. *Platelets* 18:150–157, 2007.

379. Hermos CR, Huizing M, Kaiser-Kupfer MI, Gahl WA: Hermansky-Pudlak syndrome type 1: Gene organization, novel mutations, and clinical-molecular review of non-Puerto Rican cases. *Hum Mutat* 20:482, 2002.

380. Carmona-Rivera C, Hess RA, O'Brien K, et al: Novel mutations in the HPS1 gene among Puerto Rican patients. *Clin Genet* 79:561–567, 2011.

381. Dell'Angelica EC, Shotelersuk V, Aguilar RC, et al: Altered trafficking of lysosomal proteins in Hermansky-Pudlak syndrome due to mutations in the beta 3A subunit of the AP-3 adaptor. *Mol Cell* 3:11–21, 1999.

382. Huizing M, Anikster Y, Fitzpatrick DL, et al: Hermansky-Pudlak syndrome type 3 in Ashkenazi Jews and other non-Puerto Rican patients with hypopigmentation and platelet storage-pool deficiency. *Am J Hum Genet* 69:1022–1032, 2001.

383. Anderson PD, Huizing M, Claassen DA, et al: Hermansky-Pudlak syndrome type 4 (HPS-4): Clinical and molecular characteristics. *Hum Genet* 113:10–17, 2003.

384. Huizing M, Helip-Wooley A, Dorward H, et al: Hermansky-Pudlak syndrome: A model for abnormal vesicle formation and trafficking. *Pigment Cell Res* 16:584, 2003.

385. Zhang Q, Zhao B, Li W, et al: Ru2 and Ru encode mouse orthologs of the genes mutated in human Hermansky-Pudlak syndrome types 5 and 6. *Nat Genet* 33:145–153, 2003.

386. Li W, Zhang Q, Oiso N, et al: Hermansky-Pudlak syndrome type 7 (HPS-7) results from mutant dysbindin, a member of the biogenesis of lysosome-related organelles complex 1 (BLOC-1). *Nat Genet* 35:84–89, 2003.

387. Morgan NV, Pasha S, Johnson CA, et al: A germline mutation in BLOC1S3/reduced pigmentation causes a novel variant of Hermansky-Pudlak syndrome (HPS8). *Am J Hum Genet* 78:160–166, 2006.

388. Helip-Wooley A, Westbroek W, Dorward HM, et al: Improper trafficking of melanocyte-specific proteins in Hermansky-Pudlak syndrome type-5. *J Invest Dermatol* 127:1471–1478, 2007.

389. Cullinane AR, Curry JA, Carmona-Rivera C, et al: A BLOC-1 mutation screen reveals that PLDN is mutated in Hermansky-Pudlak Syndrome type 9. *Am J Hum Genet* 88: 778–787, 2011.

390. Michaud J, Wu F, Osato M, et al: In vitro analyses of known and novel RUNX1/AML1 mutations in dominant familial platelet disorder with predisposition to acute myelogenous leukemia: Implications for mechanisms of pathogenesis. *Blood* 99:1364–1372, 2002.

391. Connelly JP, Kwon EM, Gao Y, et al: Targeted correction of RUNX1 mutation in FPD patient-specific induced pluripotent stem cells rescues megakaryopoietic defects. *Blood* 124:1926–1930, 2014.

392. Weiss HJ: Inherited disorders of platelet granules and signal transduction, in *Hemostasis and Thrombosis: Basic Principles and Clinical Practice*, 3rd ed, edited by RW Colman, J Hirsh, VJ Marder, M Samama, pp 673–684. Lippincott, Philadelphia, 1993.

393. Payne CM: A qualitative ultrastructural evaluation of the cell organelle specificity of the uranaffin reaction to normal human platelets. *Am J Clin Pathol* 31:62, 1984.

394. Weiss HJ, Lages B, Vicic W, et al: Heterogeneous abnormalities of platelet dense granule ultrastructure in 20 patients with congenital storage pool deficiency. *Br J Haematol* 83:282–295, 1993.

395. Masliah-Planchon J, Darnige L, Bellucci S: Molecular determinants of platelet delta storage pool deficiencies: An update. *Br J Haematol* 160:5–11, 2013.

396. Akkerman JW, Nieuwenhuis HK, Mommersteeg-Leautaud ME, et al: ATP-ADP compartmentation in storage pool deficient platelets: Correlation between granule-bound ADP and the bleeding time. *Br J Haematol* 55:135–143, 1983.

397. Cattaneo M, Lecchi A, Agati B, et al: Evaluation of platelet function with the PFA-100 system in patients with congenital defects of platelet secretion. *Thromb Res* 96:213–217, 1999.

398. Harrison C, Khair K, Baxter B, et al: Hermansky-Pudlak syndrome: Infrequent bleeding and first report of Turkish and Pakistani kindreds. *Arch Dis Child* 86:297–301, 2002.

399. Hayward CP, Harrison P, Cattaneo M, et al: Platelet function analyzer (PFA)-100 closure time in the evaluation of platelet disorders and platelet function. *J Thromb Haemost* 4:312–319, 2006.

400. Cattaneo M: Light transmission aggregometry and ATP release for the diagnostic assessment of platelet function. *Semin Thromb Hemost* 35:158–167, 2009.

401. Akkerman JWN, Nieuwenhuis HK, Mommersteeg-Leautaud ME, et al: ATP-ADP compartmentation in storage pool deficient platelets: Correlation between granule-bound ADP and the bleeding time. *Br J Haematol* 55:135–143, 1983.

402. Weiss HJ, Tschopp TB, Rogers J, Brand H: Studies of platelet 5-hydroxytryptamine (serotonin) in storage pool disease and albinism. *J Clin Invest* 54:421–433, 1974.

403. Weiss HJ, Lages B: Platelet malondialdehyde production and aggregation responses induced by arachidonate, prostaglandin-G2, collagen, and epinephrine in 12 patients with storage pool deficiency. *Blood* 58:27–33, 1981.

404. Witkop CJ Jr, Bowie EJ, Krumwiede MD, et al: Synergistic effect of storage pool deficient platelets and low plasma von Willebrand factor on the severity of the hemorrhagic diathesis in Hermansky-Pudlak syndrome. *Am J Hematol* 44:256–259, 1993.

405. McKeown LP, Hansmann KE, Wilson O, et al: Platelet von Willebrand factor in Hermansky-Pudlak syndrome. *Am J Hematol* 59:115–120, 1998.

406. White JG: Electron opaque structures in human platelets: Which are or are not dense bodies? *Platelets* 19:455–466, 2008.

407. Lorez HP, Richards JG, Da Prada M, et al: Storage pool disease: Comparative fluorescence microscopical, cytochemical and biochemical studies on amine-storing organelles of human blood platelets. *Br J Haematol* 43:297–305, 1979.

408. Gordon N, Thom J, Cole C, Baker R: Rapid detection of hereditary and acquired platelet storage pool deficiency by flow cytometry. *Br J Haematol* 89:117–123, 1995.

409. Nazarian R, Huizing M, Helip-Wooley A, et al: An immunoblotting assay to facilitate the molecular diagnosis of Hermansky-Pudlak syndrome. *Mol Genet Metab* 93:134–144, 2008.

410. Gahl WA, Brantly M, Troendle J, et al: Effect of pirfenidone on the pulmonary fibrosis of Hermansky-Pudlak syndrome. *Mol Genet Metab* 76:234–242, 2002.

411. O'Brien K, Troendle J, Gochuico BR, et al: Pirfenidone for the treatment of Hermansky-Pudlak syndrome pulmonary fibrosis. *Mol Genet Metab* 103:128–134, 2011.

412. Nurden AT, Nurden P: The gray platelet syndrome: Clinical spectrum of the disease. *Blood Rev* 21:21–36, 2007.

413. Nurden AT, Nurden P, Bermejo E, et al: Phenotypic heterogeneity in the Gray platelet syndrome extends to the expression of TREM family member, TLT-1. *Thromb Haemost* 100:45–51, 2008.

414. Raccuglia G: Gray platelet syndrome: A variety of qualitative platelet disorder. *Am J Med* 51:818, 1971.

415. Maynard DM, Heijnen HF, Gahl WA, Gunay-Aygun M: The alpha granule proteome: Novel proteins in normal and ghost granules in gray platelet syndrome. *J Thromb Haemost* 8:1786–1796, 2010.

416. Zufferey A, Schvartz D, Nolli S, et al: Characterization of the platelet granule proteome: Evidence of the presence of MHC1 in alpha-granules. *J Proteomics* 101:130–140, 2014.

417. Aneja K, Jalagadugula G, Mao G, et al: Mechanism of platelet factor 4 (PF4) deficiency with RUNX1 haplodeficiency: RUNX1 is a transcriptional regulator of *PF4. J Thromb Haemost* 9:383–391, 2011.

418. Tubman VN, Levine JE, Campagna DR, et al: X-linked gray platelet syndrome due to a GATA1 Arg216Gln mutation. *Blood* 109:3297–3299, 2007.

419. Monteferrario D, Bolar NA, Marneth AE, et al: A dominant-negative GFI1B mutation in the gray platelet syndrome. *N Engl J Med* 370:245–253, 2014.

420. Stevenson WS, Morel-Kopp MC, Chen Q, et al: GFI1B mutation causes a bleeding disorder with abnormal platelet function. *J Thromb Haemost* 11:2039–2047, 2013.

421. Deppermann C, Cherpokova D, Nurden P, et al: Gray platelet syndrome and defective thrombo-inflammation in Nbeal2-deficient mice. *J Clin Invest* 123:3331–3342, 2013.

422. Kahr WH, Lo RW, Li L, et al: Abnormal megakaryocyte development and platelet function in Nbeal2(-/-) mice. *Blood* 122:3349–3358, 2013.

423. Lo B, Li L, Gissen P, et al: Requirement of VPS33B, a member of the Sec1/Munc18 protein family, in megakaryocyte and platelet alpha-granule biogenesis. *Blood* 106:4159–4166, 2005.

424. Urban D, Li L, Christensen H, et al: The VPS33B binding protein VPS16B is required in megakaryocyte and platelet alpha-granule biogenesis. *Blood* 120:5032–5040, 2012.

425. Srivastava PC, Powling MJ, Nokes TJ, et al: Grey platelet syndrome: Studies on platelet alpha-granules, lysosomes and defective response to thrombin. *Br J Haematol* 65:441–446, 1987.

426. Greenberg-Sepersky SM, Simons ER, White JG: Studies of platelets from patients with the grey platelet syndrome. *Br J Haematol* 59:603–609, 1985.

427. Lages B, Sussman II, Levine SP, et al: Platelet alpha granule deficiency associated with decreased P-selectin and selective impairment of thrombin-induced activation in a new patient with gray platelet syndrome (alpha-storage pool deficiency). *J Lab Clin Med* 129:364–375, 1997.

428. Rendu F, Marche P, Hovig T, et al: Abnormal phosphoinositide metabolism and protein phosphorylation in platelets from a patient with the grey platelet syndrome. *Br J Haematol* 67:199–206, 1987.

429. Baruch D, Lindhout T, Dupuy E, Caen JP: Thrombin-induced platelet factor Va formation in patients with a gray platelet syndrome. *Thromb Haemost* 58:768–771, 1987.

430. Enouf J, Lebret M, Bredoux R, et al: Abnormal calcium transport into microsomes of grey platelet syndrome. *Br J Haematol* 65:437–440, 1987.

431. Jantunen E, Hanninen A, Naukkarinen A, et al: Gray platelet syndrome with splenomegaly and signs of extramedullary hematopoiesis: A case report with review of the literature. *Am J Hematol* 46:218–224, 1994.

432. Caen JP, Deschamps JF, Bodevin E, et al: Megakaryocytes and myelofibrosis in gray platelet syndrome. *Nouv Rev Fr Hematol* 29:109–114, 1987.

433. Coller BS, Hultin MB, Nurden AT: Isolated alpha-granule deficiency (gray platelet syndrome) with slight increase in bone marrow reticulin and possible glycoprotein and/or protease defect. *Thromb Haemost* 50:211, 1983.

434. Falik-Zaccai TC, Anikster Y, Rivera CE, et al: A new genetic isolate of gray platelet syndrome (GPS): Clinical, cellular, and hematologic characteristics. *Mol Genet Metab* 74:303–313, 2001.

435. Lages B, Shattil SJ, Bainton DF, Weiss HJ: Decreased content and surface expression of alpha-granule membrane protein GMP-140 in one of two types of platelet alpha delta storage pool deficiency. *J Clin Invest* 87:919–929, 1991.

436. Lages B, Sussman II, Levine SP, et al: Platelet alpha granule deficiency associated with decreased P-selectin and selective impairment of thrombin-induced activation in a new patient with gray platelet syndrome (alpha-storage pool deficiency). *J Lab Clin Med* 129:364–375, 1997.

437. Blavignac J, Bunimov N, Rivard GE, Hayward CP: Quebec platelet disorder: Update on pathogenesis, diagnosis, and treatment. *Semin Thromb Hemost* 37:713–720, 2011.

438. Hayward CPM, Rivard GE, Kane WH: An autosomal dominant, qualitative platelet disorder associated with multimerin deficiency, abnormalities in platelet factor V, thrombospondin, von Willebrand factor, and fibrinogen, and an epinephrine aggregation defect. *Blood* 87:4967–4978, 1996.

439. Tracy PB, Giles AR, Mann KG, et al: Factor V (Quebec): A bleeding diathesis associated with a qualitative platelet factor V deficiency. *J Clin Invest* 74:1221–1228, 1984.

440. Hayward CP, Rivard GE, Kane WH, et al: An autosomal dominant, qualitative platelet disorder associated with multimerin deficiency, abnormalities in platelet factor V, thrombospondin, von Willebrand factor, and fibrinogen and an epinephrine aggregation defect. *Blood* 87:4967–4978, 1996.

441. Veljkovic DK, Rivard GE, Diamandis M, et al: Increased expression of urokinase plasminogen activator in Quebec platelet disorder is linked to megakaryocyte differentiation. *Blood* 113:1535–1542, 2009.

442. Diamandis M, Paterson AD, Rommens JM, et al: Quebec platelet disorder is linked to the urokinase plasminogen activator gene (PLAU) and increases expression of the linked allele in megakaryocytes. *Blood* 113:1543–1546, 2009.

443. Rao AK: Hereditary disorders of platelet secretion and signal transduction, in *Hemostasis and Thrombosis: Basic Principles and Clinical Practice*, 5th ed, edited by RW Colman, VJ Marder, AW Clowes, JN George, SZ Goldhaber, pp 961–974. Lippincott Williams & Wilkins, Philadelphia, 2006.

444. Rao AK, Jalagadugula G, Sun L: Inherited defects in platelet signaling mechanisms. *Semin Thromb Hemost* 30:525–535, 2004.

445. Cattaneo M: Inherited platelet-based bleeding disorders. *J Thromb Haemost* 1:1628–1636, 2003.

446. Rao AK: Inherited platelet function disorders: Overview and disorders of granules, secretion, and signal transduction. *Hematol Oncol Clin North Am* 27:585–611, 2013.

447. Hirata T, Ushikubi F, Kakizuka A, et al: Two thromboxane A2 receptor isoforms in human platelets. Opposite coupling to adenylyl cyclase with different sensitivity to Arg60 to Leu mutation. *J Clin Invest* 97:949–956, 1996.

448. Hirata T, Kakizuka A, Ushikubi F, et al: Arg60 to Leu mutation of the human thromboxane A2 receptor in a dominantly inherited bleeding disorder. *J Clin Invest* 94:1662–1667, 1994.

449. Higuchi W, Fuse I, Hattori A, Aizawa Y: Mutations of the platelet thromboxane A2 (TXA2) receptor in patients characterized by the absence of TXA2-induced platelet aggregation despite normal TXA2 binding activity. *Thromb Haemost* 82:1528–1531, 1999.

450. Mumford AD, Dawood BB, Daly ME, et al: A novel thromboxane A2 receptor D304N variant that abrogates ligand binding in a patient with a bleeding diathesis. *Blood* 115:363–369, 2010.

451. Gachet C: P2 receptors, platelet function and pharmacological implications. *Thromb Haemost* 99:466–472, 2008.

452. Cattaneo M, Lecchi A, Randi AM, et al: Identification of a new congenital defect of platelet function characterized by severe impairment of platelet responses to adenosine diphosphate. *Blood* 80:2787–2796, 1992.

453. Nurden P, Savi P, Heilmann E, et al: An inherited bleeding disorder linked to a defective interaction between ADP and its receptor on platelets. Its influence on glycoprotein IIb-IIIa complex function. *J Clin Invest* 95:1612–1622, 1995.

454. Shiraga M, Miyata S, Kato H, et al: Impaired platelet function in a patient with P2Y12 deficiency caused by a mutation in the translation initiation codon. *J Thromb Haemost* 3:2315–2323, 2005.

455. Daly ME, Dawood BB, Lester WA, et al: Identification and characterization of a novel P2Y 12 variant in a patient diagnosed with type 1 von Willebrand disease in the European MCMDM-1VWD study. *Blood* 113:4110–4113, 2009.

456. Cattaneo M: The platelet P2Y12 receptor for adenosine diphosphate: Congenital and drug-induced defects. *Blood* 117:2102–2012, 2011.

457. Cattaneo M, Zighetti ML, Lombardi R, et al: Molecular bases of defective signal transduction in the platelet P2Y12 receptor of a patient with congenital bleeding. *Proc Natl Acad Sci U S A* 100:1978–1983, 2003.

458. Cattaneo M, Lombardi R, Zighetti ML, et al: Deficiency of (33)P-2MeS-ADP binding sites on platelets with secretion defect, normal granule stores and normal thromboxane A2 production. *Thromb Haemost* 77:986–990, 1997.

459. Cattaneo M, Lecchi A, Lombardi R, et al: Platelets from a patient heterozygous for the defect of P2(CYC) receptors for ADP have a secretion defect despite normal thromboxane A(2) production and normal granule stores: Further evidence that some cases of platelet "primary secretion defect" are heterozygous for a defect of P2(CYC) receptors. *Arterioscler Thromb Vasc Biol* 20:E101–E106, 2000.

460. Hollopeter G, Jantzen HM, Vincent D, et al: Identification of the platelet ADP receptor targeted by antithrombotic drugs. *Nature* 409:202–207, 2001.

461. Remijn JA, Ijsseldijk MJ, Strunk AL, et al: Novel molecular defect in the platelet ADP receptor P2Y12 of a patient with haemorrhagic diathesis. *Clin Chem Lab Med* 45:187–189, 2007.

462. Cunningham MR, Nisar SP, Cooke AE, et al: Differential endosomal sorting of a novel P2Y12 purinoreceptor mutant. *Traffic* 14:585–598, 2013.

463. Oury C, Toth-Zsamboki E, Van Geet C, et al: A natural dominant negative P2X1 receptor due to deletion of a single amino acid residue. *J Biol Chem* 275:22611–22614, 2000.

464. Scrutton MC, Clare KA, Hutton RA, Bruckdorfer KR: Depressed responsiveness to adrenaline in platelets from apparently normal human donors: A familial trait. *Br J Haematol* 49:303–314, 1981.

465. Rao AK, Willis J, Kowalska MA, et al: Differential requirements for platelet aggregation and inhibition of adenylate cyclase by epinephrine. Studies of a familial platelet alpha 2-adrenergic receptor defect. *Blood* 71:494–501, 1988.

466. Tamponi G, Pannocchia A, Arduino C, et al: Congenital deficiency of alpha-2-adrenoceptors on human platelets: Description of two cases. *Thromb Haemost* 58:1012–1016, 1987.

467. Pelczar-Wissner CJ, McDonald EG, Sussman II: Absence of platelet activating factor (PAF) mediated platelet aggregation: A new platelet defect. *Am J Hematol* 16:419–422, 1984.

468. Gabbeta J, Yang X, Kowalska MA, et al: Platelet signal transduction defect with Galpha subunit dysfunction and diminished Galphaq in a patient with abnormal platelet responses. *Proc Natl Acad Sci U S A* 94:8750–8755, 1997.

469. Rao AK, Koike K, Willis J, et al: Platelet secretion defect associated with impaired liberation of arachidonic acid and normal myosin light chain phosphorylation. *Blood* 64:914–921, 1984.

470. Gabbeta J, Vaidyula VR, Dhanasekaran DN, Rao AK: Human platelet Gaq deficiency is associated with decreased Gaq gene expression in platelets but not neutrophils. *Thromb Haemost* 87:129–133, 2002.

471. Freson K, Hoylaerts MF, Jaeken J, et al: Genetic variation of the extra-large stimulatory G protein alpha-subunit leads to Gs hyperfunction in platelets and is a risk factor for bleeding. *Thromb Haemost* 86:733–738, 2001.

472. Freson K, Thys C, Wittevrongel C, et al: Pseudohypoparathyroidism type Ib with disturbed imprinting in the GNAS1 cluster and Gsalpha deficiency in platelets. *Hum Mol Genet* 11:2741–2750, 2002.

473. Patel YM, Patel K, Rahman S, et al: Evidence for a role for Galphai1 in mediating weak agonist-induced platelet aggregation in human platelets: Reduced Galphai1 expression and defective Gi signaling in the platelets of a patient with a chronic bleeding disorder. *Blood* 101:4828–4835, 2003.

474. Dawood BB, Lowe GC, Lordkipanidze M, et al: Evaluation of participants with suspected heritable platelet function disorders including recommendation and validation of a streamlined agonist panel. *Blood* 120:5041–5049, 2012.

475. Canault M, Ghalloussi D, Grosdidier C, et al: Human CalDAG-GEFI gene (RASGRP2) mutation affects platelet function and causes severe bleeding. *J Exp Med* 211:1349–1362, 2014.

476. Lages B, Weiss HJ: Heterogeneous defects of platelet secretion and responses to weak agonists in patients with bleeding disorders. *Br J Haematol* 68:53–62, 1988.

477. Koike K, Rao AK, Holmsen H, Mueller PS: Platelet secretion defect in patients with the attention deficit disorder and easy bruising. *Blood* 63:427–433, 1984.

478. Yang X, Sun L, Gabbeta J, Rao AK: Platelet activation with combination of ionophore A23187 and a direct protein kinase C activator induces normal secretion in patients with impaired receptor mediated secretion and abnormal signal transduction. *Thromb Res* 88:317–328, 1997.

479. Yang X, Sun L, Ghosh S, Rao AK: Human platelet signaling defect characterized by impaired production of inositol-1,4,5-triphosphate and phosphatidic acid and diminished Pleckstrin phosphorylation: Evidence for defective phospholipase C activation. *Blood* 88:1676–1683, 1996.

480. Lee SB, Rao AK, Lee KH, et al: Decreased expression of phospholipase C-beta 2 isozyme in human platelets with impaired function. *Blood* 88:1684–1691, 1996.

481. Sun L, Mao G, Rao AK: Association of CBFA2 mutation with decreased platelet PKC-theta and impaired receptor-mediated activation of GPIIb-IIIa and pleckstrin phosphorylation: Proteins regulated by CBFA2 play a role in GPIIb-IIIa activation. *Blood* 103:948–954, 2004.

482. Lages B, Weiss HJ: Impairment of phosphatidylinositol metabolism in a patient with a bleeding disorder associated with defects of initial platelet responses. *Thromb Haemost* 59:175–179, 1988.

483. Speiser-Ellerton S, Weiss HJ: Studies on platelet protein phosphorylation in patients with impaired responses to platelet agonists. *J Lab Clin Med* 115:104–111, 1990.

484. Mao GF, Vaidyula VR, Kunapuli SP, Rao AK: Lineage-specific defect in gene expression in human platelet phospholipase C-beta2 deficiency. *Blood* 99:905–911, 2002.

485. Holmsen H, Walsh PN, Koike K, et al: Familial bleeding disorder associated with deficiencies in platelet signal processing and glycoproteins. *Br J Haematol* 67:335–344, 1987.

486. Cartwright J, Hampton KK, Macneil S, et al: A haemorrhagic platelet disorder associated with altered stimulus-response coupling and abnormal membrane phospholipid composition. *Br J Haematol* 88:129–136, 1994.

487. Fuse I, Mito M, Hattori A, et al: Defective signal transduction induced by thromboxane A2 in a patient with a mild bleeding disorder: Impaired phospholipase C activation despite normal phospholipase A2 activation. *Blood* 81:994–1000, 1993.

488. Mitsui T: Defective signal transduction through the thromboxane A2 receptor in a patient with a mild bleeding disorder. Deficiency of the inositol 1,4,5-triphosphate formation despite normal G-protein activation. *Thromb Haemost* 77:991–995, 1997.

489. Gabbeta J, Yang X, Sun L, et al: Abnormal inside-out signal transduction-dependent activation of glycoprotein IIb-IIIa in a patient with impaired pleckstrin phosphorylation. *Blood* 87:1368–1376, 1996.

490. Song WJ, Sullivan MG, Legare RD, et al: Haploinsufficiency of CBFA2 causes familial thrombocytopenia with propensity to develop acute myelogenous leukaemia. *Nat Genet* 23:166–175, 1999.

491. Sun L, Gorospe JR, Hoffman EP, Rao AK: Decreased platelet expression of myosin regulatory light chain polypeptide (MYL9) and other genes with platelet dysfunction and CBFA2/RUNX1 mutation: Insights from platelet expression profiling. *J Thromb Haemost* 5:146–154, 2007.

492. Rendu F, Breton-Gorius J, Trugnan G, et al: Studies on a new variant of the Hermansky-Pudlak syndrome: Qualitative, ultrastructural, and functional abnormalities of the platelet-dense bodies associated with a phospholipase A defect. *Am J Hematol* 4:387–399, 1978.

493. Adler DH, Cogan JD, Phillips JA, et al: Inherited human cPLA(2alpha) deficiency is associated with impaired eicosanoid biosynthesis, small intestinal ulceration, and platelet dysfunction. *J Clin Invest* 118:2121–2131, 2008.

494. Faioni EM, Razzari C, Zulueta A, et al: Bleeding diathesis and gastro-duodenal ulcers in inherited cytosolic phospholipase-A2 alpha deficiency. *Thromb Haemost* 112:1182–1189, 2014.

495. Malmsten C, Hamberg M, Svensson J, Samuelsson B: Physiological role of an endoperoxide in human platelets: Hemostatic defect due to platelet cyclo-oxygenase deficiency. *Proc Natl Acad Sci U S A* 72:1446–1450, 1975.

496. Lagarde M, Byron PA, Vargaftig BB, Dechavanne M: Impairment of platelet thromboxane A2 generation and of the platelet release reaction in two patients with congenital deficiency of platelet cyclo-oxygenase. *Br J Haematol* 38:251–266, 1978.

497. Pareti FI, Mannucci PM, D'Angelo A, et al: Congenital deficiency of thromboxane and prostacyclin. *Lancet* 1:898–901, 1980.

498. Rak K, Boda Z: Haemostatic balance in congenital deficiency of platelet cyclo-oxygenase. *Lancet* 2:44, 1980.

499. Horellou MH, Lecompte T, Lecrubier C, et al: Familial and constitutional bleeding disorder due to platelet cyclo-oxygenase deficiency. *Am J Hematol* 14:1–9, 1983.

500. Rao AK, Koike K, Day HJ, et al: Bleeding disorder associated with albumin-dependent partial deficiency in platelet thromboxane production. Effect of albumin on arachidonate metabolism in platelets. *Am J Clin Pathol* 83:687–696, 1985.

501. Roth GJ, Machuga R: Radioimmune assay of human platelet prostaglandin synthetase. *J Lab Clin Med* 99:187–196, 1982.

502. Matijevic-Aleksic N, McPhedran P, Wu KK: Bleeding disorder due to platelet prostaglandin H synthase-1 (PGHS-1) deficiency. *Br J Haematol* 92:212–217, 1996.

503. Defreyn G, Machin SJ, Carreras LO, et al: Familial bleeding tendency with partial platelet thromboxane synthetase deficiency: Reorientation of cyclic endoperoxide metabolism. *Br J Haematol* 49:29–41, 1981.

504. Mestel F, Oetliker O, Beck E, et al: Severe bleeding associated with defective thromboxane synthetase. *Lancet* 1:157, 1980.

505. Weiss HJ: Impaired platelet procoagulant mechanisms in patients with bleeding disorders. *Semin Thromb Hemost* 35:233–241, 2009.

506. Lhermusier T, Chap H, Payrastre B: Platelet membrane phospholipid asymmetry: From the characterization of a scramblase activity to the identification of an essential protein mutated in Scott syndrome. *J Thromb Haemost* 9:1883–1891, 2011.

507. Weiss HJ, Vicic WJ, Lages BA, Rogers J: Isolated deficiency of platelet procoagulant activity. *Am J Med* 67:206–213, 1979.

508. Toti F, Satta N, Fressinaud E, et al: Scott syndrome, characterized by impaired transmembrane migration of procoagulant phosphatidylserine and hemorrhagic complications, is an inherited disorder. *Blood* 87:1409–1415, 1996.

509. Weiss HJ, Lages B: Platelet prothrombinase activity and intracellular calcium responses in patients with storage pool deficiency, glycoprotein IIb-IIIa deficiency, or impaired platelet coagulant activity—A comparison with Scott syndrome. *Blood* 89:1599–1611, 1997.

510. Dachary-Prigent J, Pasquet JM, Fressinaud E, et al: Aminophospholipid exposure, microvesiculation and abnormal protein tyrosine phosphorylation in the platelets of a patient with Scott syndrome: A study using physiologic agonists and local anaesthetics. *Br J Haematol* 99:959–967, 1997.

511. Zwaal RF, Comfurius P, Bevers EM: Scott syndrome, a bleeding disorder caused by defective scrambling of membrane phospholipids. *Biochim Biophys Acta* 1636:119–128, 2004.

512. Munnix IC, Harmsma M, Giddings JC, et al: Store-mediated calcium entry in the regulation of phosphatidylserine exposure in blood cells from Scott patients. *Thromb Haemost* 89:687–695, 2003.

513. Solum NO: Procoagulant expression in platelets and defects leading to clinical disorders. *Arterioscler Thromb Vasc Biol* 19:2841–2846, 1999.

514. Weiss HJ: Scott syndrome: A disorder of platelet coagulant activity. *Semin Hematol* 31:312–319, 1994.

515. Sims PJ, Wiedmer T, Esmon CT, et.al: Assembly of the platelet prothrombinase complex is linked to vesiculation on the platelet plasma membrane. Studies in Scott syndrome: An isolated defect in platelet procoagulant activity. *J Biol Chem* 264:137–148, 1989.

516. Castaman G, Yu-Feng L, Battistin E, Rodeghiero F: Characterization of a novel bleeding disorder with isolated prolonged bleeding time and deficiency of platelet microvesicle generation. *Br J Haematol* 96:458–463, 1997.

517. Albrecht C, McVey JH, Elliott JI, et al: A novel missense mutation in ABCA1 results in altered protein trafficking and reduced phosphatidylserine translocation in a patient with Scott syndrome. *Blood* 106:542–549, 2005.

518. Suzuki J, Umeda M, Sims PJ, Nagata S: Calcium-dependent phospholipid scrambling by TMEM16F. *Nature* 468:834–838, 2010.

519. Weiss HJ: Platelet aggregation, adhesion and adenosine diphosphate release in thrombopathia (platelet factor 3 deficiency). A comparison with Glanzmann's thrombasthenia and von Willebrand's disease. *Am J Med* 43:570–578, 1967.

520. Freson K, De Vos R, Wittevrognel C, et al: The $\beta_1$-tubulin Q43P functional polymorphism reduces the risk of cardiovascular disease in men by modulating platelet function and structure. *Blood* 106:2356–2362, 2005.

521. Navarro-Nunez L, Lozano ML, Rivera J, et al: The association of the beta1-tubulin Q43P polymorphism with intracerebral hemorrhage in men. *Haematologica* 92:513–518, 2007.

522. Kunishima S, Kobayashi R, Itoh TJ, et al: Mutation of the beta1-tubulin gene associated with congenital macrothrombocytopenia affecting microtubule assembly. *Blood* 113:458–461, 2009.

522A. Berrou, E, Adam, F, Lebret, M et al: Heterogeneity of platelet functional alterations in patients with filamin A mutations. *Arterioscler Thromb Vasc Biol* 33:e11–18, 2013.

523. Buchbinder D, Nugent DJ, Fillipovich AH: Wiskott-Aldrich syndrome: Diagnosis, current management, and emerging treatments. *Appl Clin Genet* 7:55–66, 2014.

524. Massaad MJ, Ramesh N, Geha RS: Wiskott-Aldrich syndrome: A comprehensive review. *Ann N Y Acad Sci* 1285:26–43, 2013.

525. Lutskiy MI, Shcherbina A, Bachli ET, et al: WASP localizes to the membrane skeleton of platelets. *Br J Haematol* 139:98–105, 2007.

526. Parkman R, Remold-O'Donnell E, Kenney DM, et al: Surface protein abnormalities in lymphocytes and platelets from patients with Wiskott-Aldrich syndrome. *Lancet* 2:1387–1389, 1981.

527. Semple JW, Siminovitch KA, Mody M, et al: Flow cytometric analysis of platelets from children with the Wiskott-Aldrich syndrome reveals defects in platelet development, activation and structure. *Br J Haematol* 97:747–754, 1997.

528. Baldini MG: Nature of the platelet defect in the Wiskott-Aldrich syndrome. *Ann N Y Acad Sci* 201:437–444, 1972.

529. Verhoeven AJ, van Oostrum IE, van Haarlem H, Akkerman JW: Impaired energy metabolism in platelets from patients with Wiskott-Aldrich syndrome. *Thromb Haemost* 61:10–14, 1989.

530. Marone G, Albini F, di Martino L, et al: The Wiskott-Aldrich syndrome: Studies of platelets, basophils and polymorphonuclear leucocytes. *Br J Haematol* 62:737–745, 1986.

531. Gross BS, Wilde JI, Quek L, et al: Regulation and function of WASp in platelets by the collagen receptor, glycoprotein VI. *Blood* 94:4166–4176, 1999.

532. Shcherbina A, Rosen FS, Remold-O'Donnell E: Pathological events in platelets of Wiskott-Aldrich syndrome patients. *Br J Haematol* 106:875–883, 1999.

533. Tsuboi S, Nonoyama S, Ochs HD: Wiskott-Aldrich syndrome protein is involved in alphaIIb beta3-mediated cell adhesion. *EMBO Rep* 7:506–511, 2006.

534. Rengan R, Ochs HD, Sweet LI, et al: Actin cytoskeletal function is spared, but apoptosis is increased, in WAS patient hematopoietic cells. *Blood* 95:1283–1292, 2000.

535. Falet H, Hoffmeister KM, Neujahr R, Hartwig JH: Normal Arp2/3 complex activation in platelets lacking WASp. *Blood* 100:2113–2122, 2002.

536. Shcherbina A, Cooley J, Lutskiy MI, et al: WASP plays a novel role in regulating platelet responses dependent on alphaIIbbeta3 integrin outside-in signalling. *Br J Haematol* 148:416–427, 2010.

537. Kuijpers TW, van de Vijver E, Weterman MA, et al: LAD-1/variant syndrome is caused by mutations in FERMT3. *Blood* 113:4740–4746, 2009.

538. Harris ES, Smith TL, Springett GM, et al: A. Leukocyte adhesion deficiency-I variant syndrome (LAD-Iv, LAD-III): Molecular characterization of the defect in an index family. *Am J Hematol* 87:311–313, 2012.

539. Mory A, Feigelson SW, Yarali N, et al: Kindlin-3: A new gene involved in the pathogenesis of LAD-III. *Blood* 112:2591, 2008.

540. Svensson L, Howarth K, McDowall A, et al: Leukocyte adhesion deficiency-III is caused by mutations in KINDLIN3 affecting integrin activation. *Nat Med* 15:306–312, 2009.

541. Malinin NL, Zhang L, Choi J, et al: A point mutation in KINDLIN3 ablates activation of three integrin subfamilies in humans. *Nat Med* 15:313–318, 2009.

542. Moser M, Nieswandt B, Ussar S, et al: Kindlin-3 is essential for integrin activation and platelet aggregation. *Nat Med* 14:325–330, 2008.

543. Pasvolsky R, Feigelson SW, Kilic SS, et al: A LAD-III syndrome is associated with defective expression of the Rap-1 activator CalDAG-GEFI in lymphocytes, neutrophils, and platelets. *J Exp Med* 204:1571–1582, 2007.

544. Tijssen MR, Cvejic A, Joshi A, et al: Genome-wide analysis of simultaneous GATA1/2, RUNX1, FLI1, and SCL binding in megakaryocytes identifies hematopoietic regulators. *Dev Cell* 20:597–609, 2011.

545. Rao AK: Spotlight on *FLI1, RUNX1* and platelet dysfunction. *Blood* 122:4004–4006, 2013.

545A. Songdej N, Rao AK: Hematopoietic transcription factor mutations and inherited platelet dysfunction. *F1000Prime Reports* 7:66, 2015.

546. Gerrard JM, Israels ED, Biship AJ, et al: Inherited platelet-storage pool deficiency associated with a high incidence of acute myeloid leukaemia. *Br J Haematol* 79:246–255, 1991.

547. Ganly P, Walker LC, Morris CM: Familial mutations of the transcription factor RUNX1 (AML1, CBFA2) predispose to acute myeloid leukemia. *Leuk Lymphoma* 45:1–10, 2004.

548. Dowton SB, Beardsley D, Jamison D, et al: Studies of a familial platelet disorder. *Blood* 65:557, 1985.

549. Ho CY, Otterud B, Legare RD, et al: Linkage of a familial platelet disorder with a propensity to develop myeloid malignancies to human chromosome 21q22.1–22.2. *Blood* 87:5218–5224, 1996.

550. Arepally G, Rebbeck TR, Song W, et al: Evidence for genetic homogeneity in a familial platelet disorder with predisposition to acute myelogenous leukemia (FPD/AML). *Blood* 92:2600–2602, 1998.

551. Walker LC, Stevens J, Campbell H, et al: A novel inherited mutation of the transcription factor RUNX1 causes thrombocytopenia and may predispose to acute myeloid leukaemia. *Br J Haematol* 117:878–881, 2002.

552. Owen CJ, Toze CL, Koochin A, et al: Five new pedigrees with inherited RUNX1 mutations causing familial platelet disorder with propensity to myeloid malignancy. *Blood* 112:4639–4645, 2008.

553. Sun L, Mao G, Rao AK: Association of CBFA2 mutation with decreased platelet PKC-$\theta$ and impaired receptor-mediated activation of GPIIb-IIIa and pleckstrin phosphorylation: Proteins regulated by CBFA2 play a role in GPIIb-IIIa activation. *Blood* 103:948–954, 2004.

554. Rao AK: Inherited platelet function disorders: Overview and disorders of granules, secretion, and signal transduction. *Hematol Oncol Clin North Am* 27:585–611, 2013.

555. Kaur G, Jalagadugula G, Mao G, Rao AK: RUNX1/core binding factor A2 regulates platelet 12-lipoxygenase gene (ALOX12): Studies in human RUNX1 haplodeficiency. *Blood* 115:3128–3135, 2010.

556. Jalagadugula G, Mao G, Kaur G, et al: Regulation of platelet myosin light chain (*MYL9*) by RUNX1: Implications for thrombocytopenia and platelet dysfunction in *RUNX1* haplodeficiency. *Blood* 116:6037–6045, 2010.

557. Freson K, Devriendt K, Matthijs G, et al: Platelet characteristics in patients with X-linked macrothrombocytopenia because of a novel GATA1 mutation. *Blood* 98:85–92, 2001.

558. Hughan SC, Senis Y, Best D, et al: Selective impairment of platelet activation to collagen in the absence of GATA1. *Blood* 105:4369–4376, 2005.

559. Breton-Gorius J, Favier R, Guichard J, et al: A new congenital dysmegakaryopoietic thrombocytopenia (Paris-Trousseau) associated with giant platelet alpha-granules and chromosome 11 deletion at 11q23. *Blood* 85:1805–1814, 1995.

560. Favier R, Jondeau K, Boutard P, et al: Paris-Trousseau syndrome: Clinical, hematological, molecular data of ten new cases. *Thromb Haemost* 90:893–897, 2003.

561. Raslova H, Komura E, Le Couedic JP, et al: FLI1 monoallelic expression combined with its hemizygous loss underlies Paris-Trousseau/Jacobsen thrombopenia. *J Clin Invest* 114:77–84, 2004.

562. Shivdasani RA: Lonely in Paris: When one gene copy isn't enough. *J Clin Invest* 114:17–19, 2004.

563. Kurstjens R, Bolt C, Vossen M, Haanen C: Familial thrombopathic thrombocytopenia. *Br J Haematol* 15:305–317, 1968.

564. Estes JW: Platelet abnormalities in heritable disorders of connective tissue. *Ann N Y Acad Sci* 201:445–450, 1972.

565. Evensen SA, Myhre L, Stormorken H: Haemostatic studies in osteogenesis imperfecta. *Scand J Haematol* 33:177–179, 1984.

566. Akkerman JWN, Rijksen G, Gorter G, et al: Platelet functions and energy metabolism in a patient with hexokinase deficiency. *Blood* 63:147–153, 1984.

567. Corby DG, Putnam CW, Greene HL: Impaired platelet function in glucose-6-phosphatase deficiency. *J Pediatr* 85:71–76, 1974.

568. Czapek EE, Deykin D, Salzman EW: Platelet dysfunction in glycogen storage disease type I. *Blood* 41:235–247, 1973.

569. Boullin DJ, O'Brien RA: Abnormalities of 5-hydroxytryptamine uptake and binding by blood platelets from children with Down's syndrome. *J Physiol* 212:287–297, 1971.

570. Lott IT, Chase TN, Murphy DL: Down's syndrome: Transport, storage, and metabolism of serotonin in blood platelets. *Pediatr Res* 6:730–735, 1972.

571. McCoy EE, Sneddon JM: Decreased calcium content and 45Ca2+ uptake in Down's syndrome blood platelets. *Pediatr Res* 18:914–916, 1984.

572. More R, Amir N, Meyer S, et al: Platelet abnormalities in Down's syndrome. *Clin Genet* 22:128–136, 1982.

573. Sheppard JR, Schumacher W, White JG, et al: The alpha adrenergic response of Down's syndrome platelets. *J Pharmacol Exp Ther* 225:584–588, 1983.

574. Hamilton RW, Shaikh BS, Ottie JN, et al: Platelet function, ultrastructure, and survival in the May-Hegglin anomaly. *Am J Clin Pathol* 74:663–668, 1980.

575. Lusher JM, Schneider J, Mizukami I, et al: The May-Hegglin anomaly: Platelet function, ultrastructure and chromosome studies. *Blood* 32:950–961, 1968.

576. Coller BS, Zarrabi MH: Platelet membrane studies in the May-Hegglin anomaly. *Blood* 58:279–284, 1981.

577. Freson K, Hashimoto H, Thys C, et al: The pituitary adenylate cyclase-activating polypeptide is a physiological inhibitor of platelet activation. *J Clin Invest* 113:905–912, 2004.

578. Sandrock K, Nakamura L, Vraetz T, et al: Platelet secretion defect in patients with familial hemophagocytic lymphohistiocytosis type 5 (FHL-5). *Blood* 116:6148–6150, 2010.

579. Al Hawas R, Ren Q, Ye S, et al: Munc18b/STXBP2 is required for platelet secretion. *Blood* 120:2493–2500, 2012.

580. Ye S, Karim ZA, Al Hawas R, et al: Syntaxin-11, but not syntaxin-2 or syntaxin-4, is required for platelet secretion. *Blood* 120:2484–2492, 2012.

581. Alamelu J, Liesner R: Modern management of severe platelet function disorders. *Br J Haematol* 149:813–823, 2010.

582. Seligsohn U: Treatment of inherited platelet disorders. *Haemophilia* 18(Suppl 4):161–165, 2012.

583. Bolton-Maggs PH, Chalmers EA, Collins PW, et al: A review of inherited platelet disorders with guidelines for their management on behalf of the UKHCDO. *Br J Haematol* 135:603–633, 2006.

584. Fiore M, Firah N, Pillois X, et al: Natural history of platelet antibody formation against alphaIIbbeta3 in a French cohort of Glanzmann thrombasthenia patients. *Haemophilia* 18:e201–209, 2012.

585. Mannucci PM: Desmopressin (DDAVP) in the treatment of bleeding disorders: The first 20 years. *Blood* 90:2515–2521, 1997.

586. Mannucci PM: Hemostatic drugs. *N Engl J Med* 339:245–253, 1998.

587. Rao AK, Ghosh S, Sun L, et al: Effect of mechanism of platelet dysfunction on response to DDAVP in patients with congenital platelet function defects. A double-blind placebo-controlled trial. *Thromb Haemost* 74:1071–1078, 1995.

588. Kobrinsky NL, Israels ED, Gerrard JM, et al: Shortening of bleeding time by 1-deamino-8-D-arginine vasopressin in various bleeding disorders. *Lancet* 1:1145–1148, 1984.

589. Schulman S, Johnson H, Egberg N, Blombäck M: DDAVP-induced correction of prolonged bleeding time in patients with congenital platelet function defects. *Thromb Res* 45:165–174, 1987.

590. DiMichele DM, Hathaway WE: Use of DDAVP in inherited and acquired platelet dysfunction. *Am J Hematol* 33:39–45, 1990.

591. Nieuwenhuis HK, Sixma JJ: 1-Desamino-8-D-arginine vasopressin (desmopressin) shortens the bleeding time in storage pool deficiency. *Ann Intern Med* 108:65–67, 1988.

592. Colucci G, Stutz M, Rochat S, et al: The effect of desmopressin on platelet function: A selective enhancement of procoagulant COAT platelets in patients with primary platelet function defects. *Blood* 123:1905–1916, 2014.

593. Almeida AM, Khair K, Hann I, Liesner R: The use of recombinant factor VIIa in children with inherited platelet function disorders. *Br J Haematol* 121:477–481, 2003.

594. Poon MC, d'Oiron R: Recombinant activated factor VII (NovoSeven) treatment of platelet-related bleeding disorders. International Registry on Recombinant Factor VIIa and Congenital Platelet Disorders Group. *Blood Coagul Fibrinolysis* 11(Suppl 1):S55–S68, 2000.

595. Poon MC, Demers C, Jobin F, Wu JW: Recombinant factor VIIa is effective for bleeding and surgery in patients with Glanzmann thrombasthenia. *Blood* 94:3951–3953, 1999.

596. del Pozo Pozo AI, Jimenez-Yuste V, Villar A, et al: Successful thyroidectomy in a patient with Hermansky-Pudlak syndrome treated with recombinant activated factor VII and platelet concentrates. *Blood Coagul Fibrinolysis* 13:551–553, 2002.

597. Sindet-Pedersen S, Ramstrom G, Bernvil S, Blomback M: Hemostatic effect of tranexamic acid mouthwash in anticoagulant-treated patients undergoing oral surgery. *N Engl J Med* 320:840–843, 1989.

598. Mielke CH Jr, Levine PH, Zucker S: Preoperative prednisone therapy in platelet function disorders. *Thromb Res* 21:655–662, 1981.

599. Spotnitz WD, Burks S: Hemostats, sealants, and adhesives: Components of the surgical toolbox. *Transfusion* 48:1502–1516, 2008.

600. Chuansumrit A, Suwannuraks M, Sri-Udomporn N, et al: Recombinant activated factor VII combined with local measures in preventing bleeding from invasive dental procedures in patients with Glanzmann thrombasthenia. *Blood Coagul Fibrinolysis* 14:187–190, 2003.

601. Singla NK, Foster KN, Alexander WA, Pribble JP: Safety and immunogenicity of recombinant human thrombin: A pooled analysis of results from 10 clinical trials. *Pharmacotherapy* 32:998–1005, 2012.

602. Wilcox DA, Olsen JC, Ishizawa L, et al: Integrin alphaIIb promoter-targeted expression of gene products in megakaryocytes derived from retrovirus-transduced human hematopoietic cells. *Proc Natl Acad Sci U S A* 96:9654–9659, 1999.

603. Wilcox DA, White GC 2nd: Gene therapy for platelet disorders: Studies with Glanzmann's thrombasthenia. *J Thromb Haemost* 1:2300–2311, 2003.

604. Fang J, Jensen ES, Boudreaux MK, et al: Platelet gene therapy improves hemostatic function for integrin alphaIIbbeta3-deficient dogs. *Proc Natl Acad Sci U S A* 108:9583–9588, 2011.

605. Hodivala-Dilke KM, Tsakiris DA, Rayburn H, et al: Beta3-integrin-deficient mice are a model for Glanzmann thrombasthenia showing placental defects and reduced survival. *J Clin Invest* 103:229–238, 1999.

606. Boudreaux MK, Lipscomb DL: Clinical, biochemical, and molecular aspects of Glanzmann's thrombasthenia in humans and dogs. *Vet Pathol* 38:249–260, 2001.

607. Niemeyer GP, Boudreaux MK, Goodman-Martin SA, et al: Correction of a large animal model of type I Glanzmann's thrombasthenia by nonmyeloablative bone marrow transplantation. *Exp Hematol* 31:1357–1362, 2003.

608. Schlosser RJ: Clinical practice. Epistaxis. *N Engl J Med* 360:784–789, 2009.

609. Siddiq S, Clark A, Mumford A: A systematic review of the management and outcomes of pregnancy in Glanzmann thrombasthenia. *Haemophilia* 17:e858–e869, 2011.

610. Peitsidis P, Datta T, Pafilis I, et al: Bernard Soulier syndrome in pregnancy: A systematic review. *Haemophilia* 16:584–591, 2010.

# CHAPTER 11
# ACQUIRED QUALITATIVE PLATELET DISORDERS

Charles S. Abrams, Sanford J. Shattil, and Joel S. Bennett

## SUMMARY

Acquired qualitative platelet disorders are frequent causes of abnormal platelet function measured *in vitro*, although by themselves, they are usually associated with little or no clinical bleeding. However, there are important exceptions. Nevertheless, their major clinical impact becomes apparent in the additional presence of thrombocytopenia or additional acquired or congenital disorders of hemostasis. Acquired disorders of platelet function can be conveniently classified into those that result from drugs, hematologic diseases, and systemic disorders. Drugs are the most frequent cause of acquired qualitative platelet dysfunction. Aspirin is the most notable drug in this regard because of its frequent use, its irreversible effect on platelet prostaglandin synthesis, and its documented effect on hemostatic competency, although this effect is minimal in normal individuals. Other nonsteroidal antiinflammatory drugs reversibly inhibit platelet prostaglandin synthesis and usually have little effect on hemostasis. The antiplatelet effects of a number of drugs have proven useful in preventing arterial thrombosis, but as would be anticipated, excessive bleeding can be a complication of their use. In addition to aspirin, these drugs include the $P2Y_{12}$ adenosine diphosphate receptor antagonists, clopidogrel, prasugrel and ticagrelor, vorapaxar, an inhibitor of the PAR1 thrombin receptor, and drugs that specifically inhibit adhesive ligand binding to platelet integrin $\alpha_{IIb}\beta_3$ (GPIIb/IIIa). Other drugs used to treat thrombosis, such as heparin and fibrinolytic agents, may also impair platelet function *in vitro* and *ex vivo*, but the clinical significance of these observations is uncertain. High doses of the $\beta$-lactam antibiotics can impair platelet function *in vitro*, whereas clinically significant bleeding is unusual in the absence of a coexisting hemostatic defect. Similarly, a number of miscellaneous drugs, including a variety of psychotropic, chemotherapeutic, and anesthetic agents, as well as a number of foods and food additives, can affect platelet function *in vitro* but do not appear to be of clinical significance by themselves. Hematologic diseases associated with abnormal platelet function include marrow processes in which platelets may be intrinsically abnormal such as the myeloproliferative neoplasms, leukemias, and myelodysplastic syndromes; dysproteinemias in which monoclonal immunoglobulins can impair platelet function; and acquired forms of von Willebrand disease. Of the systemic diseases, renal failure is most prominently associated with abnormal platelet function because of the retention in the circulation of platelet inhibitory compounds. Platelet function may also be abnormal in the presence of antiplatelet antibodies, following cardiopulmonary bypass, and in association with liver disease or disseminated intravascular coagulation.

Platelet function may be adversely affected by drugs and by hematologic and nonhematologic diseases. Because the use of aspirin and other nonsteroidal antiinflammatory agents is pervasive, acquired platelet dysfunction is much more frequent than inherited platelet dysfunction. Acquired disorders of platelet function can be classified according to the underlying clinical conditions with which they are associated (Table 11–1).

It is important to have a balanced view of the clinical significance of acquired disorders of platelet function. On the one hand, their severity is usually mild. On the other hand, there are important exceptions to this rule, particularly when platelet dysfunction is associated with other hemostatic defects. If a patient does not present with a history of bleeding, it may be difficult to predict the risk of future bleeding. This is not surprising since even patients with thrombocytopenia may experience little or no spontaneous bleeding until their platelet count is less than $10 \times 10^9$/L. Furthermore, clinical assessment of these disorders is made problematic by difficulties in standardization and interpretation of laboratory tests of platelet function, including platelet aggregometry. These tests are more useful in diagnosing platelet dysfunction than in predicting the risk of bleeding.[1,2]

## ● DRUGS THAT AFFECT PLATELET FUNCTION

Drugs are the most common cause of platelet dysfunction (Table 11–2). For example, in an analysis of 72 hospitalized patients with a prolonged bleeding time (a test no longer considered reliable), 54 percent were receiving large doses of antibiotics known to prolong the bleeding time and 10 percent were taking aspirin or other nonsteroidal antiinflammatory drugs.[3] Some drugs can prolong the bleeding time and either cause or exacerbate a bleeding diathesis. Other drugs may prolong the bleeding time but not cause bleeding, while many only affect platelet function *ex vivo* or when added to platelets *in vitro*. It is important for the hematologist to understand the clinical significance of these distinctions.

## ASPIRIN AND OTHER NONSTEROIDAL ANTIINFLAMMATORY DRUGS

### Aspirin

Aspirin irreversibly inactivates the enzyme cyclooxygenase (COX), also known as prostaglandin endoperoxide H synthase, by acetylating a serine residue at position 529.[4] Two isoforms of COX have been identified (COX-1 and COX-2),[5] as well as a splice variant of COX-1, COX-1b (COX-3), whose functional significance is uncertain.[6] COX-1 is constitutively expressed by many tissues, including platelets, the gastric mucosa, and endothelial cells (Chap. 24 discusses the use of aspirin as an antithrombotic agent).[5] COX-2 is undetectable in most tissues, but its synthesis is rapidly induced in cells such as endothelial cells,

**Acronyms and Abbreviations:** ADP, adenosine diphosphate; BCNU, *bis*-chloroethylnitrosourea; BTK, Bruton tyrosine kinase; cAMP, cyclic adenosine monophosphate; cGMP, cyclic guanosine monophosphate; COX, cyclooxygenase; coxibs, COX inhibitors; CYP, cytochrome P; DDAVP, desmopressin or 1-desamino-8-D-arginine vasopressin; DIC, disseminated intravascular coagulation; EPO, erythropoietin; GP, glycoprotein; Ig, immunoglobulin; ITP, immune thrombocytopenia; KGD, lysine-glycine-aspartic acid tripeptide; NO, nitric oxide; NSAID, nonsteroidal antiinflammatory drug; PAR, protease-activated receptor; PCI, percutaneous coronary intervention; PG, prostaglandin; $PGI_2$, prostacyclin; PKC, protein kinase C; RGD, arginine-glycine-aspartic acid tripeptide; SLE, systemic lupus erythematosus; t-PA, tissue plasminogen activator; TTP, thrombotic thrombocytopenic purpura; $TXA_2$, thromboxane $A_2$; VWF, von Willebrand factor.

**TABLE 11–1.** Acquired Qualitative Platelet Disorders

Drugs that affect platelet function

    Aspirin and other nonsteroidal antiinflammatory drugs

    P2Y$_{12}$ antagonists (clopidogrel, prasugrel, ticagrelor)

    PAR1 thrombin receptor antagonist (vorapaxar)

    Integrin $\alpha_{IIb}\beta_3$ receptor antagonists (abciximab, eptifibatide, tirofiban)

    Drugs that increase platelet cyclic adenosine monophosphate

    Antibiotics

    Anticoagulants and fibrinolytic agents

    Cardiovascular drugs

    Volume expanders

    Psychotropic agents and anesthetics

    Oncologic drugs

    Foods and food additives

Hematologic disorders associated with abnormal platelet function

    Chronic myeloproliferative neoplasms

    Leukemias and myelodysplastic syndromes

    Dysproteinemias

    Acquired von Willebrand syndrome

Systemic disorders associated with abnormal platelet function

    Uremia

    Antiplatelet antibodies

    Cardiopulmonary bypass

    Liver disease

    Disseminated intravascular coagulation

    Infection with HIV

---

**TABLE 11–2.** Drugs That Affect Platelet Function

Nonsteroidal antiinflammatory drugs

    Aspirin, ibuprofen, sulindac, naproxen, meclofenamic acid, mefenamic acid, diflunisal, piroxicam, tolmetin, zomepirac, sulfinpyrazone, indomethacin, phenylbutazone, celecoxib

P2Y$_{12}$ antagonists

    Clopidogrel, prasugrel, ticagrelor

PAR1 receptor antagonist

    Vorapaxar

Integrin $\alpha_{IIb}\beta_3$ antagonists

    Abciximab, eptifibatide, tirofiban

Drugs that affect platelet cyclic adenosine monophosphate levels or function

    Prostacyclin, iloprost, dipyridamole, cilostazol

Antibiotics

    Penicillins

        Penicillin G, carbenicillin, ticarcillin, methicillin, ampicillin, piperacillin, azlocillin, mezlocillin, sulbenicillin, temocillin

    Cephalosporins

        Cephalothin, moxalactam, cefoxitin, cefotaxime, cefazolin

    Nitrofurantoin

    Miconazole

Anticoagulants, fibrinolytic agents, and antifibrinolytic agents

    Heparin

    Streptokinase, tissue plasminogen activator, urokinase

    $\varepsilon$-Aminocaproic acid

Cardiovascular drugs

    Nitroglycerin, isosorbide dinitrate, propranolol, nitroprusside, nifedipine, verapamil, diltiazem, quinidine

Volume expanders

    Dextran, hydroxyethyl starch

Psychotropic drugs and anesthetics

    Psychotropic drugs

        Imipramine, amitriptyline, nortriptyline, chlorpromazine, promethazine, fluphenazine, trifluoperazine, haloperidol

    Anesthetics

        Local

            Dibucaine, tetracaine, Cyclaine, butacaine, nupercaine, procaine, cocaine

    General

        Halothane

Oncologic drugs

    Mithramycin, daunorubicin, carmustine, ibrutinib

Miscellaneous drugs

    Ketanserin

Antihistamines

    Diphenhydramine, chlorpheniramine, mepyramine

Radiographic contrast agent

    Iopamidol, iothalamate, ioxaglate, meglumine diatrizoate, sodium diatrizoate

Foods and food additives

    $\omega$-3 Fatty acids, ethanol, Chinese black tree fungus, onion extract, ajoene, cumin, turmeric

---

fibroblasts, and monocytes by growth factors, cytokines, endotoxin, and hormones.[5] Platelets express only COX-1, whereas endothelial cells can express both COX-1 and COX-2.[7,8] In the cardiovascular system, COX products regulate complex interactions between platelets and the vessel wall. The platelet product of COX-1–mediated prostaglandin synthesis, thromboxane A$_2$ (TXA$_2$), produces vasoconstriction and is a receptor-mediated agonist for platelet aggregation and secretion.[4] Thus, inactivation of COX-1 by aspirin prevents platelet synthesis of TXA$_2$, thereby inhibiting platelet responses that depend on this substance. Accordingly, platelet responses to adenosine diphosphate (ADP), epinephrine, low doses of collagen and thrombin, and arachidonic acid are affected (arachidonic acid completely), but there is almost no effect on the responses to higher doses of collagen or thrombin.[9,10] On the other hand, the endothelial cell prostaglandin (PG) product, prostacyclin (PGI$_2$), produces smooth muscle cell relaxation and vasodilation and increases the platelet content of cyclic adenosine monophosphate (AMP), thereby decreasing overall platelet reactivity.[11]

Platelet PG synthesis in an adult is nearly completely inhibited by a single 100-mg dose of aspirin or by 30 mg taken daily for 7 to 10 days.[4] Although single doses of aspirin irreversibly inhibit platelet and endothelial cell COX,[12] they have no lasting effect on PG synthesis by endothelial cells because of the ability of these cells to synthesize additional COX unaffected by aspirin.[13] In vitro studies also suggest that the presence of erythrocytes contributes to agonist-stimulated platelet reactivity,[14] an effect that can be inhibited by aspirin at doses greater than those required to inhibit platelet COX-1.[15] A meta-analysis of clinical trials indicates that aspirin doses varying from 50 to 1500 mg daily are equally efficacious in preventing adverse cardiovascular and cerebrovascular events.[16] This has led many to suggest that the lowest effective doses should be prescribed to minimize gastrointestinal toxicity. Nonetheless, even low doses of aspirin can be associated with significant gastrointestinal hemorrhage.[17–19]

Aspirin is one of the relatively few drugs that prolongs the bleeding time in humans and appears to do so by blocking aggregation rather than adhesion. In normal individuals, the effect on the bleeding time is slight (generally no more than 1.2 to 2.0 times the preaspirin bleeding time),[20,21] is observed in both males and females, and requires that almost all the COX in the circulating platelets be inhibited.[11] The sensitivity of the bleeding time to aspirin is dependent on such technical variables as the direction of the incision on the forearm and the degree of hydrostatic pressure applied to the arm,[22] and hence the current view that the test is unreliable. The bleeding time may remain prolonged for 1 to 4 days after aspirin has been discontinued, and platelet aggregation tests may remain abnormal for up to a week until platelets affected by aspirin are replaced as the result of thrombopoiesis.[23]

The significance of aspirin ingestion on the hemostatic competency of normal individuals appears to be minimal. Nevertheless, patients taking aspirin chronically report significant increases in bruising, epistaxis, and gastrointestinal blood loss.[17–19] Gastrointestinal blood loss appears to be the result of a direct effect of aspirin on the gastric mucosa.[24,25] Furthermore, there is an increase in the incidence of hemorrhagic stroke when aspirin is used in the primary and secondary prevention of vascular disease, as well as an increase in major gastrointestinal and other extracranial bleeding.[26] Aspirin may also increase bleeding in the mother and the neonate during parturition.[27] In addition, some studies show that aspirin taken preoperatively increases the amount of blood loss following cardiothoracic surgery.[28,29] In contrast, a retrospective analysis has documented the safety of performing epidural and spinal anesthesia in patients who had ingested aspirin.[30] Aspirin may increase the amount of blood loss following general surgery.[31] The significance of aspirin ingestion in this setting was tested in the POISE-2 study[32] in which patients at risk for vascular complications were randomized to aspirin or placebo prior to their noncardiac surgery. Although taking aspirin did not reduce the incidence of cardiovascular events, there was a small increase in hemorrhagic complications. This suggests that discontinuing aspirin prior to surgery is a useful practice, particularly prior to plastic or neurosurgical procedures in which the limits of tolerable bleeding are narrow.[33] On the other hand, patients taking aspirin and other antiplatelet agents for severe cardiovascular disease may be at risk for thrombosis if these medications are discontinued. Thus, the clinician must thoroughly weigh the potential risks and benefits of discontinuing aspirin prior to noncardiac surgery. This is especially true in patients with other hemostatic disorders; for example, aspirin precipitates hemorrhage in individuals with von Willebrand disease, hemophilia A, warfarin ingestion, uremia, and disorders of platelet function.[34–36] Infusion of desmopressin (DDAVP) has been effective in correcting a prolonged bleeding time caused by aspirin.[37,38]

Resistance to the antiplatelet effects of aspirin ("aspirin resistance") is a controversial topic, and whether it exists depends to large extent on whether resistance is considered from a biochemical or clinical perspective.[39] Biochemical resistance to the platelet-inhibitory effects of aspirin, that is, the failure to achieve pharmacologic inhibition of $TXA_2$ production, is uncommon.[39] For example, when healthy subjects were given either standard or enteric-coated aspirin, 49 percent given a single dose of enteric-coated aspirin failed to inhibit $TXA_2$ synthesis, whereas the failure to inhibit $TXA_2$ synthesis was never seen in subjects given standard aspirin.[40] Nevertheless, subjects given enteric-coated aspirin eventually responded when taking it daily, implying that although some patients absorb enteric-coated aspirin preparations poorly, they will ultimately absorb sufficient amounts of aspirin to prevent platelet $TXA_2$ synthesis. Most commonly, aspirin resistance occurs because patients are nonadherent with aspirin therapy, often because of gastrointestinal toxicity.[41] Clinically, the term aspirin resistance has been applied to patients who develop cardiovascular events despite taking aspirin. Given that aspirin treatment selectively inhibits platelet synthesis of only one endogenous platelet agonist, $TXA_2$, it is not surprising that aspirin does not completely abolish platelet-mediated vascular events.

### Traditional Nonsteroidal Antiinflammatory Drugs

Unlike aspirin, nonsteroidal antiinflammatory drugs (NSAIDs), such as ibuprofen, naproxen, diclofenac, sulindac, piroxicam, indomethacin, and sulfinpyrazone, *reversibly* inhibit COX enzymes.[42] Although these drugs can cause a transient prolongation of the bleeding time when given in therapeutic doses, this is usually not clinically significant.[43] Population studies have suggested that concurrent treatment with NSAIDs and anticoagulants increases the risk of bleeding complication, but many bleeding events were limited to the gastrointestinal tract where NSAIDs are known to induce gastritis and peptic ulcerations.[44] As evidence of the modest effect of NSAIDs on platelet function, ibuprofen has been given safely to patients with hemophilia A.[45,46] Nonetheless, care must be taken when ibuprofen is given to patients with hemophilia and HIV infection receiving zidovudine because increased bleeding has been reported in this circumstance.[47] Because ibuprofen, and probably other NSAIDs, binds to COX-1, blocking its acetylation by aspirin,[42] coadministration of NSAIDs and aspirin may impair the irreversible, antithrombotic effects of aspirin on platelets.[48] For this reason, patients who require both medications should ingest aspirin at least 2 hours prior to the ingestion of traditional NSAIDs.

### Coxibs (COX-2 Inhibitors)

COX-1 is present in the gastric mucosa where its products protect the integrity of the gastric lining cells. In inflammatory cells, COX-2 products such as $PGE_2$ and $PGI_2$ elicit an increased sense of pain and perpetuate the inflammatory process.[40] Thus, the coxibs (COX inhibitors), designed to be relatively more specific for COX-2 versus COX-1, were intended to reduce pain and inflammation with fewer gastric side effects than traditional NSAIDs.[40,42] However, clinical trials revealed that coxib administration was associated with cardiovascular toxicity (myocardial infarction, stroke, edema, exacerbation of hypertension), partly because of inhibiting $PGI_2$ synthesis.[11,49–52] On the basis of these results, rofecoxib and valdecoxib were withdrawn from the market (valdecoxib was also associated with cases of Stevens-Johnson syndrome), and a black box warning regarding serious cardiovascular events was added to prescribing information for celecoxib, the only coxib now available in the United States.[50] Nonetheless, clinical evidence suggests there is no excess cardiovascular risk from daily doses of celecoxib of 200 mg or less.[51] Traditional NSAIDs also inhibit COX-2 to a variable extent, and several observational trials have revealed excess cardiovascular events associated with use of these drugs.[50,53–55] Thus, a warning has also been added to their prescribing information. If indicated, analgesics such as acetaminophen, sodium or choline salicylate, and narcotics may be substituted for aspirin and NSAIDs for treating musculoskeletal pain.[50] One report suggests that acetaminophen can selectively inhibit COX-2,[56] but the clinical significance of this observation is not clear.

## THIENOPYRIDINES

Ticlopidine, clopidogrel, and prasugrel are thienopyridines that are used as antiplatelet agents in arterial diseases (Chap. 24) with results at least comparable to aspirin in the secondary prevention of cerebrovascular and cardiovascular events.[16,57]

Thienopyridines differ from aspirin in their mechanism of anti-platelet activity and their toxicity profile. All three thienopyridines are prodrugs that depend on oxidation by cytochrome P450 (CYP) enzymes in the liver (ticlopidine and clopidogrel) or in liver and intestine (prasugrel) to form the active metabolites that irreversibly inhibit the platelet $P2Y_{12}$ ADP receptor.[58-61] Ticlopidine at 250 mg twice a day, clopidogrel at 75 mg once per day, and prasugrel at 10 mg once a day inhibit platelet aggregation *ex vivo* in humans. The extent of this effect is equivalent to or greater than that of aspirin, and the effect of thienopyridines and aspirin appears additive.[62,63] When given at their usual oral doses, the effect of thienopyridines on platelet aggregation and the bleeding time can be seen within hours of the first dose, but are not maximal for 4 to 6 days. A 300-mg loading dose of clopidogrel or 60 mg of prasugrel, followed by their usual daily doses, shortens the time required for their maximal antiplatelet effect to a few hours.[64,65] The common CYP polymorphism CYP2C19 results in lower levels of active clopidogrel and ticlopidine metabolites and has been reported to be associated with decreased platelet inhibition and an elevated risk for major adverse cardiovascular events.[55,66,67] Because the enzyme CYP3A is present in the intestine and can oxidize prasugrel to its pharmacologically active metabolite, intestinal metabolism may account for the rapid appearance and higher levels of the active metabolite in plasma after an oral dose.[61,68-70] Furthermore, prasugrel metabolism and inhibition of platelet function are not affected by CYP2C19 polymorphisms.[61,68-70]

The clinical efficacy of prasugrel has been compared to clopidogrel in patients with acute coronary syndrome scheduled for percutaneous coronary intervention in the Triton-TIMI 38 trial. Patients who received prasugrel had a significantly decreased incidence of ischemic events compared to patients who received clopidogrel (9.9 percent vs. 12.1 percent, p <0.001).[69] However, major bleeding was also significantly increased in patients receiving prasugrel compared to clopidogrel (2.4 percent vs. 1.8 percent, p <0.03). Thus, although prasugrel appeared to be more efficacious than clopidogrel, this benefit was partially offset by a higher rate of hemorrhage.[69]

The platelet-inhibitory effects of thienopyridines persist for 4 to 10 days after the drugs have been discontinued, either because of their extended half-life after multiple dosing or their irreversible effect on platelets.[58] Ticlopidine administration is associated with potentially serious hematologic complications, including neutropenia (neutrophils <1200 × $10^9$/L in 2.4 percent of individuals)[58,71,72] and, less commonly, aplastic anemia and thrombocytopenia.[73,74] In addition, at least one in 5000 patients develops a thrombotic thrombocytopenic purpura (TTP)-like syndrome.[75-77] Results from a large clinical trial suggest that hematologic complications may be less common with clopidogrel or prasugrel.[57] Clopidogrel may also be rarely associated with a TTP-like syndrome (one in 270,000),[78] although this rate is close to the TTP incidence in the general population. Because of its toxicity profile, ticlopidine has been replaced by the other thienopyridines in the United States.

Because aspirin and the thienopyridines inhibit platelet function by different mechanisms, their antithrombotic effects may be additive. In theory, this would be beneficial in the treatment of diseases associated with platelet activation such as ischemic heart disease, peripheral vascular disease, and ischemic strokes.[62,79,80] This hypothesis was tested in the CURE trial of patients with acute coronary syndromes.[62] Although clopidogrel plus aspirin decreased the combined incidence of cardiovascular deaths, myocardial infarctions, and strokes from 11.4 percent to 9.3 percent, the benefit was partially offset by an increase in severe bleeding from 2.7 to 3.7 percent. Similarly, in the CHARISMA trial of a broad population of patients at risk for cardiovascular events, there were 94 fewer ischemic events in patients treated with both clopidogrel and aspirin, but this occurred at the expense of 93 more

moderate or severe bleeding events.[81] Furthermore, a meta-analysis of seven randomized controlled trials involving more than 39,000 patients confirmed that intracranial hemorrhage was more frequent in patients who received both clopidogrel plus aspirin compared to clopidogrel alone.[82] Thus, except for special circumstances such as coronary artery stenting, it appears that the added benefit of dual antiplatelet therapy is small and has the added risk of increased bleeding.[83]

## OTHER ADENOSINE DIPHOSPHATE RECEPTOR ANTAGONISTS

Ticagrelor, cangrelor, and elinogrel are oral, reversible, nonthienopyridine $P2Y_{12}$ receptor antagonists. Because they are not prodrugs and do not require metabolic activation, the onset of their inhibitory activity is more rapid than that of the thienopyridines. A novel, and as yet unexplained, side effect of treatment with this class of the $P2Y_{12}$ antagonists is the occurrence of dyspnea, which can complicate the management of patients with coronary artery disease.[84]

Ticagrelor, the first drug of the class, has been approved for use in acute coronary syndromes. Its efficacy versus clopidogrel was tested in the PLATO trial in which patients with an acute coronary syndrome were randomized to treatment with either ticagrelor or clopidogrel.[85-87] At 1 year, the combined end point of death, myocardial infarction, and stroke was 9.8 percent in patients treated with ticagrelor compared to 11.7 percent in patients treated with clopidogrel.[88] Although stent thrombosis was also decreased in the ticagrelor-treated group, major bleeding not associated with coronary artery bypass surgery was increased in this group. The incidence of fatal intracranial hemorrhage was also greater in the ticagrelor-treated patients, but it was a rare event (0.1 percent of treated patients). In the ATLANTIC trial, patients suffering from an ST-segment elevation myocardial infarction were randomized to receive ticagrelor in the ambulance or in the catheterization laboratory.[89] Although initiating therapy before hospitalization was safe and lowered the incidence of stent thrombosis, there was no overall improvement in preventing major cardiovascular adverse events. Thus, ticagrelor, like prasugrel, appears to be more efficacious than clopidogrel at preventing adverse cardiovascular events but with more hemorrhagic complications.

## THROMBIN RECEPTOR ANTAGONISTS

Thrombin is the most potent physiologic platelet agonist. Three G-protein–coupled thrombin receptors have been identified in humans (protease-activated receptors [PARs] 1, 3, and 4).[90] Although human platelets express both PAR-1 and PAR-4, the major platelet thrombin receptor is PAR-1 and can be activated by nanomolar concentrations of thrombin. PAR-4 signaling appears to be unnecessary for platelet activation if PAR-1 signaling is intact.[90] Vorapaxar is a potent, selective, long-acting, oral PAR-1 inhibitor generated from the naturally occurring muscarinic receptor antagonist himbacine.[91] A high-resolution crystal structure of vorapaxar bound to PAR-1 revealed that the binding pocket for the drug is unusual for a peptide-activated G-protein–coupled receptor in that it consists of a superficial tunnel with little of the bound drug surface exposed to aqueous solvent, perhaps accounting for the very slow dissociation rate of vorapaxar from PAR-1.[92]

The efficacy of vorapaxar for the secondary prevention of arterial thrombosis was examined in the phase III TRA 2P–TIMI 50 trial in which patients with a history of myocardial infarction, stroke, or peripheral arterial disease were randomized between vorapaxar and placebo.[93] Most patients were also taking either aspirin or a thienopyridine. Because of a high incidence of intracranial bleeding in the first years of the study, entry criteria were modified to eliminate patients with a history of a stroke. At 3 years, the incidence of the primary end point (cardiovascular death, myocardial infarction, and stroke) was significantly reduced in vorapaxar-treated patients (9.3 percent vs. 11.2 percent, p <0.001). However, moderate to severe bleeding, including intracranial bleeding, was significantly increased in the vorapaxar-treated patients (4.2 percent vs. 2.5 percent, p <0.001). Nonetheless, based on efficacy, vorapaxar received FDA approval in 2014. Atopaxar, a second PAR-1 antagonist, is currently being evaluated in clinical trials.[94] Atopaxar has a shorter half-life than vorapaxar, suggesting that potential bleeding complications might be easier to manage.

## INTEGRIN $\alpha_{IIb}\beta_3$ RECEPTOR ANTAGONISTS

Drugs that specifically impair the function of the major platelet integrin $\alpha_{IIb}\beta_3$ (GPIIb/IIIa) have been developed for short-term use as antithrombotic agents in the setting of ischemic coronary artery disease.[95,96] Integrin $\alpha_{IIb}\beta_3$ mediates platelet–platelet cohesion by binding the divalent ligand fibrinogen, thereby crosslinking the integrin on adjacent platelets, causing the formation of platelet aggregates.[97] Thus, integrin $\alpha_{IIb}\beta_3$ is a viable therapeutic target to prevent arterial thrombosis. Abciximab, eptifibatide, and tirofiban are three FDA-approved structurally dissimilar integrin $\alpha_{IIb}\beta_3$ inhibitors that rapidly impair platelet aggregation. Abciximab is a human-murine chimeric Fab fragment, eptifibatide is a cyclic heptapeptide based on the sequence Lys-Gly-Asp (KGD), and tirofiban is an Arg-Gly-Asp (RGD)-based peptidomimetic. All three drugs have demonstrated efficacy in the management of patients with acute coronary syndromes, particularly in the setting of percutaneous coronary interventions (PCI) where iatrogenic artery wall injury occurs.[97]

Inherited integrin $\alpha_{IIb}\beta_3$ abnormalities cause the bleeding disorder Glanzmann thrombasthenia (Chap. 10).[98,99] Thus, it is not surprising that integrin $\alpha_{IIb}\beta_3$ antagonists can predispose to bleeding. In EPIC, a clinical trial of abciximab in patients undergoing PCI, 14 percent of patients given abciximab experienced major bleeding compared to 7 percent of patients given placebo.[100] However, patients were also given aspirin and heparin. When the heparin dose was decreased in the subsequent EPILOG trial, the incidence of major bleeding in patients receiving abciximab decreased to 2.0 percent compared to 3.1 percent in the control group receiving heparin and aspirin alone.[101] Nonetheless, in both EPIC and EPILOG, minor bleeding was significantly more frequent in patients given abciximab and standard-dose heparin compared to patients given standard-dose heparin alone, attesting to the ability of an integrin $\alpha_{IIb}\beta_3$ antagonist to impair normal hemostasis. In the PRISM-PLUS trial of tirofiban and the PURSUIT trial of eptifibatide, major and minor bleeding were slightly more frequent in patients receiving the study drug compared to controls.[102,103] Similarly, patients receiving the oral integrin $\alpha_{IIb}\beta_3$ inhibitors xemilofiban and sibrafiban for 30 and 28 days, respectively, frequently experienced mucocutaneous bleeding similar to that experienced by patients with congenital thrombasthenia.[104,105] Although short-term use of the parenteral integrin $\alpha_{IIb}\beta_3$ antagonists is often beneficial in patients with acute coronary syndrome or following PCI, paradoxically, the long-term use of oral integrin $\alpha_{IIb}\beta_3$ inhibitors was associated with an increase in mortality.[106] The cause of this paradoxical effect is not clear but has been attributed by some to an antagonist-induced conformational change in integrin $\alpha_{IIb}\beta_3$ simulating the effect of physiologic platelet agonists.[107]

The risk of bleeding in patients undergoing PCI in the presence of integrin $\alpha_{IIb}\beta_3$ antagonists can be minimized by using heparin on a weight basis,[101] by avoiding treatment of patients who are receiving warfarin at therapeutic doses, by early vascular sheath removal, and by meticulous care of vascular puncture sites.[108] Platelet transfusions can

rapidly reverse the platelet function defect in patients receiving abciximab, presumably by decreasing the overall extent of integrin blockade. The ability of platelet transfusion to reverse the effects of the other integrin $\alpha_{IIb}\beta_3$ antagonists is less clear, but these drugs have very short half-lives if renal and hepatic function are normal.

Thrombocytopenia occurring within 24 hours of initiating therapy has been observed in small numbers of patients following the administration of all integrin $\alpha_{IIb}\beta_3$ antagonists.[102,105,108,109] In EPIC, the incidence of platelet counts of less than $100 \times 10^9$/L and of less than $50 \times 10^9$/L in patients receiving abciximab for the first time was 3.9 percent and 0.9 percent, respectively.[109] Thrombocytopenia has also been reported in patients receiving eptifibatide, tirofiban, and a variety of small-molecule RGD- and non–RGD-based integrin $\alpha_{IIb}\beta_3$ inhibitors with an incidence of up to 13 percent.[102,105,109–113]

The mechanism responsible for thrombocytopenia following the administration of these drugs is uncertain but may be related to the presence of preexisting antiintegrin $\alpha_{IIb}\beta_3$ antibodies that recognize epitopes exposed by the antagonist or, in the case of abciximab, to murine sequences incorporated into the abciximab Fab fragment.[114] The thrombocytopenia usually reverses readily when the drug is stopped, but it may also be reversed by platelet transfusion if clinically indicated.[108] Thrombocytopenia in patients receiving integrin $\alpha_{IIb}\beta_3$ antagonists must be differentiated from pseudothrombocytopenia as a result of drug-induced platelet clumping, from heparin-induced thrombocytopenia in patients receiving heparin concurrently, and from other causes of thrombocytopenia, depending on the clinical circumstances.[115,116] It is important to identify thrombocytopenia early because integrin $\alpha_{IIb}\beta_3$ antagonists are administered as long infusions, and the drug should be stopped as soon as true thrombocytopenia has been confirmed. In most cases of profound thrombocytopenia, a platelet count obtained 2 to 4 hours after initiating therapy will provide evidence of a significant decrease in platelet count, although cases of delayed thrombocytopenia have been observed after treatment with abciximab.[114]

## DRUGS THAT AFFECT PLATELET CYCLIC NUCLEOTIDE LEVELS OR FUNCTION

The pyrimidopyrimidine derivative, dipyridamole, inhibits platelet cyclic nucleotide phosphodiesterase, resulting in the intraplatelet accumulation of the inhibitory cyclic nucleotide cyclic AMP (cAMP). Dipyridamole may also inhibit the breakdown of cyclic guanosine monophosphate (cGMP), resulting in potentiation of the platelet-inhibitory effect of nitric oxide.[117] Although the platelet-inhibitory effects of dipyridamole are seen *in vitro*, the clinical utility of dipyridamole has been controversial.[118,119] A meta-analysis failed to demonstrate the clinical benefit of adding dipyridamole to aspirin.[16] However, many older dipyridamole trials used formulations with limited dipyridamole bioavailability.[120] In the European Stroke Prevention Study 2 (ESPS 2), dipyridamole was beneficial in preventing stroke and transient ischemic attack, but there was no difference in mortality between patients taking dipyridamole and placebo or among patients taking dipyridamole plus aspirin compared to either dipyridamole or aspirin alone.[121] The basis for the benefit of dipyridamole in the ESPS 2 trial is unclear but could be from a higher dipyridamole dosage or a result of the sustained-release dipyridamole preparation used in the trial.

Intravenous infusions of $PGE_1$, $PGI_2$, or stable $PGI_2$ analogues stimulate platelet adenylyl cyclase, causing an increase in platelet cAMP and a decrease in platelet responsiveness.[122] These agents cause a transient inhibition of platelet shape change, aggregation, and secretion. However, their clinical utility is limited by their short half-life and side effects that include peripheral vasodilation.[123] Cilostazol, a phosphodiesterase III inhibitor, has been approved in the United States for the treatment of peripheral vascular disease[124] and may have utility in the prevention of cardiac stent occlusion.[125] Nitric oxide (NO) and organic nitrates such as nitroglycerin inhibit platelet function *in vitro*, probably by activating guanylyl cyclase, thereby increasing cGMP.[126] Their effect on *in vivo* platelet function is uncertain. High concentrations of caffeine and theophylline also inhibit platelet phosphodiesterases *in vitro*.

## ANTIBIOTICS

Penicillins contain a $\beta$-lactam ring and a unique side chain. Most cause a dose-dependent prolongation of the bleeding time in normal volunteers.[127] Because they reduce platelet aggregation and secretion, as well as ristocetin-induced platelet agglutination, they may affect both platelet adhesion and platelet activation. Tests of platelet aggregation are abnormal in 50 to 75 percent of individuals receiving large doses (at least several grams per day) of carbenicillin, penicillin G, ticarcillin, ampicillin, nafcillin, and azlocillin and in 25 to 50 percent of patients taking piperacillin, azlocillin, or mezlocillin.[127-129] Differences in the antiplatelet effects of these antibiotics probably relate to differences in blood levels and drug potency. Their effect on platelets is maximal after 1 to 3 days of administration and may remain for several days after the antibiotic has been stopped, suggesting that the effect of these antibiotics on platelets *in vivo* is irreversible.

Penicillins can impair the interaction of agonists and von Willebrand factor (VWF) with the platelet membrane.[130] Indeed, when many penicillins are incubated with washed platelets, albeit at concentrations higher than those attained *in vivo*, they inhibit the interaction of VWF and agonists, such as ADP and epinephrine, with their platelet receptors.[131] The relative *in vitro* antiplatelet potency of the penicillins correlates well with their lipid solubility and with the inhibitory potency of the isolated side chains.[132] Moreover, the inhibitory effect of penicillin G on platelet function *in vitro* is potentiated by the presence of probenecid.[133] When platelet function was tested after intravenous administration of penicillin, oxacillin, or mezlocillin for 3 to 17 days to patients or normal volunteers, irreversible inhibition of agonist-induced aggregation was noted, along with a 40 percent reduction in low-affinity TXA$_2$ receptors.[134] Thus, penicillins probably inhibit platelet function by binding to one or more membrane components necessary for adhesive interactions with the vessel wall or for stimulus-response coupling.

Although clinically significant bleeding is associated with the use of carbenicillin, penicillin G, ticarcillin, and nafcillin, it is far less common than prolongation of the bleeding time.[127,135] Patients with coexisting hemostatic defects (e.g., thrombocytopenia, vitamin K deficiency, uremia) may be particularly prone to this complication. On the other hand, high doses of penicillin G did not increase gastrointestinal blood loss in a thrombocytopenic rabbit model.[136] In our experience, bleeding attributable to antibiotic-induced platelet dysfunction is uncommon and unpredictable. Because $\beta$-lactam–induced platelet dysfunction resolves with time following cessation of the drug, this class of drugs should only be considered as a cause of bleeding in the appropriate clinical setting. A similar pattern of platelet dysfunction has been reported with some cephalosporins or related antibiotics, but not with others.[127,137,138] Broad-spectrum antibiotics can also cause a bleeding diathesis attributable to killing of gut flora, resulting in vitamin K deficiency. Nitrofurantoin, a structurally unrelated antibiotic, may cause a mild prolongation of the bleeding time and impair platelet aggregation when blood levels of the drug are higher than 20 $\mu$M, as may occur in patients with renal insufficiency.[139] Miconazole, an antifungal agent, inhibits human and rabbit platelet COX *in vitro* and rabbit platelet COX after intravenous infusion.[140]

## ANTICOAGULANTS, FIBRINOLYTIC AGENTS, AND ANTIFIBRINOLYTIC AGENTS

Heparin predisposes to bleeding primarily through its anticoagulant effect, but it may also impair platelet function. For example, a bolus injection of heparin (100 U/kg) can cause a significant prolongation of the bleeding time in normal subjects and in patients prior to cardiopulmonary bypass, suggesting that therapeutic doses of heparin may impair platelet function.[126] Heparin likely impairs platelet function by inhibiting the generation and action of the potent platelet agonist thrombin. On the other hand, *in vitro* studies suggest that heparin can enhance platelet aggregation induced by other platelet agonists.[141] Heparin binds to a single class of high-affinity binding sites on resting platelets and to an additional class of lower-affinity binding sites on fully activated platelets.[142] High heparin doses also impair VWF-dependent platelet function, possibly by binding to the heparin-binding domain of VWF.[143] The contributions of these effects on platelet function to the bleeding complications of heparin therapy are uncertain.

Bleeding during fibrinolytic therapy is predominantly a result of the combined effects of structural lesions in blood vessels and the fibrin(ogen)olytic activity of the agent used. However, pharmacologic doses of streptokinase, urokinase, and tissue plasminogen activator (t-PA) can affect platelet function.[144] High concentrations of plasmin *ex vivo* cause platelet aggregation.[145] Moreover, marked increases in the urinary excretion of the TXA$_2$ metabolite 2,3-dinor-TXB$_2$ have been detected in patients receiving streptokinase or t-PA for coronary thrombolysis, suggesting that *in vivo* platelet activation had occurred during infusion of the drug.[146,147] Nevertheless, several *in vitro* studies indicate that plasmin generation has an inhibitory effect on platelet function. First, very high levels of fibrin(ogen) degradation products, coupled with very low levels of fibrinogen, may impair platelet aggregation.[148] Second, plasminogen can bind to platelets[149] and, after its conversion to plasmin, enzymatically degrade platelet glycoprotein (GP) Ib, impairing the interaction of platelets with VWF.[150,151] Third, plasmin can inhibit platelet arachidonic acid metabolism.[152] Fourth, t-PA promotes the disaggregation of platelet aggregates, presumably by inducing lysis of the fibrinogen that mediates aggregate formation.[153] Finally, after initial activation, platelets incubated with plasmin and recombinant t-PA *in vitro* become refractory to activation by other agonists.[154] Whether any of these *in vitro* and *ex vivo* observations apply to the *in vivo* situation and are clinically significant remains uncertain.[155] The antifibrinolytic drug $\varepsilon$-aminocaproic acid can increase the bleeding time when administered for several days at doses of 24 g/d or greater.[150]

## CARDIOVASCULAR DRUGS

Administration of nitroprusside, which increases platelet cGMP,[156-160] nitroglycerine,[161] and propranolol,[162,163] can decrease platelet aggregation and secretion *ex vivo*. Nitroprusside can increase the bleeding time twofold when administered at infusion rates of 6 to 8 mcg/kg/min.[156,164] Inhalation of NO advocated for the treatment of pulmonary hypertension and the adult respiratory distress syndrome, can impair agonist-induced platelet aggregation *ex vivo*, although the clinical significance of these observations is unclear.[165-167] Calcium channel blockers such as verapamil, nifedipine, and diltiazem inhibit platelet aggregation when added at very high concentrations to washed platelets.[123] This effect is seen primarily with epinephrine-induced aggregation and does not appear to be related to calcium channel blockade.[168] At therapeutic doses, calcium channel blockers do not prolong the bleeding time, although one agent, nisoldipine, has been reported to inhibit agonist-induced calcium transients and platelet aggregation after 10 days of oral administration.[169] At high concentrations, the antiarrhythmic drug quinidine has been reported to cause a mild prolongation of the bleeding time and to potentiate the effect of aspirin.[170]

## VOLUME EXPANDERS

Dextran is a neutral polysaccharide that is heterogeneous in molecular size. Two preparations with average molecular weights of 40,000 and 70,000 are in clinical use. Although dextran infusions may prolong the bleeding time of normal subjects and patients with von Willebrand disease, this phenomenon has not been observed in most normal subjects.[9,171,172] Infused dextran adsorbs to the platelet surface and can impair platelet aggregation, secretion, and procoagulant activity. The maximal effect of dextran may require several hours, suggesting that larger molecules with a slower rate of clearance are responsible.[9] Curiously, the drug has no effect when added to platelet-rich plasma.[9] Dextran infusion produces a modest reduction in plasma VWF antigen levels and ristocetin cofactor activity.[171] Despite these effects on primary hemostasis, prospective studies indicate that dextran is not associated with significant postoperative bleeding, unless it is administered together with low-dose heparin.[173,174] Hydroxyethyl starch, another volume expander, while generally safe, may prolong the bleeding time and predispose to hemorrhage, particularly if it is administered in doses exceeding 20 mL/kg of a 6 percent solution. Lower doses of hydroxyethyl starch may contribute to bleeding if administered simultaneously with low-dose heparin or if given to patients with preexistent hemostatic defects or after major cardiothoracic surgery.[175–178] Different hydroxyethyl starch preparations vary in the average number of hydroxymethyl groups per glucose unit, and this may affect both intravascular survival and effects on hemostasis.[179,180]

## PSYCHOTROPIC DRUGS, ANESTHETICS, AND COCAINE

Platelets from patients taking antidepressants or phenothiazines may exhibit impaired aggregation, but this is not associated with bleeding.[181,182] The effect on aggregation has been attributed to inhibition of intracellular signaling molecules such as protein kinase C (PKC).[183] Selective serotonin reuptake inhibitors, such as paroxetine, have been shown to decrease platelet serotonin storage.[184] Fluoxetine does not appear to impair platelet aggregation *in vitro* and has only rarely been associated with clinical bleeding.[185,186] General anesthesia with halothane or propofol may cause a slight prolongation of the bleeding time, most likely the result of an effect on calcium signaling, but this has no adverse effect on surgical hemostasis.[187,188] In addition to an association with thrombocytopenia, cocaine has been reported to either inhibit[189,190] or stimulate platelet activation.[191] It has been suggested that heroin decreases platelet NO production.[192] The clinical relevance of these observations is unknown.

## ONCOLOGIC DRUGS

Administering mithramycin to a total dose of 6 to 21 mg decreases platelet aggregation and is associated with mucocutaneous bleeding.[193] An *ex vivo* defect in platelet secretion and secondary aggregation has been reported in patients with solid tumors within 48 hours of receiving infusions of autologous marrow and high-dose chemotherapy consisting of cisplatin, cyclophosphamide, and either *bis*-chloroethylnitrosourea (BCNU; carmustine) or melphelan.[194] Both daunorubicin and BCNU can inhibit platelet aggregation and secretion when added to platelet-rich plasma, but they have not been shown to cause clinically significant platelet dysfunction.[195–197] Administration of recombinant forms of thrombopoietin to thrombocytopenic patients with cancer results in the production

of normally functioning platelets.[198,199] Dasatinib, the broad-spectrum protein tyrosine kinase inhibitor, impairs collagen-induced platelet activation *in vitro* and increases tail bleeding times in mice, perhaps explaining some bleeding episodes in patients with chronic myelogenous leukemia who have been treated with the drug.[200] Ibrutinib, a Bruton tyrosine kinase (BTK) inhibitor efficacious in a wide variety of lymphoid malignanies,[201,202] is associated with hemorrhagic complications in up to half of patients, with significant hemorrhagic toxicity in 5 percent.[201–203] Exposing platelets to ibrutinib *ex vivo* can produce defective platelet adhesion.[204] Furthermore, humans or mice lacking BTK have impaired *ex vivo* platelet function, although the impairment is quite mild.[205,206] Whether the hemorrhagic toxicity of ibrutinib is caused by platelet BTK inhibition or by an off-target effect remains to be determined.

## MISCELLANEOUS AGENTS

The immunosuppressive drug cyclosporine has been reported to enhance ADP-stimulated platelet aggregation *in vitro*.[207] It is unclear whether this contributes to the TTP-like syndrome associated with this drug. Antihistamines,[208] the serotonin antagonist ketanserin,[209] and certain radiographic contrast agents[210,211] can impair platelet aggregation responses *ex vivo* by unknown mechanisms.

## FOODS AND FOOD ADDITIVES

Certain foods and food additives affect platelet function *in vitro*, and it is conceivable that some may affect hemostasis, particularly in association with other hemostatic defects. For example, diets rich in fish oils containing $\omega$-3 fatty acids (eicosapentaenoic acid, docosahexaenoic acid) cause a slight prolongation of the bleeding time.[212] These fatty acids act by reducing the platelet content of arachidonic acid and by competing with arachidonic acid for COX.[213,214] Easy bruising noted after eating Chinese food has been attributed to an antiplatelet effect of the black tree fungus.[215] A component of extract of onion can inhibit platelet arachidonic acid metabolism.[216] Ajoene, a component of garlic, is an inhibitor of fibrinogen binding and platelet aggregation.[217] Extracts of two commonly used spices, cumin and turmeric, also inhibit platelet aggregation and eicosanoid biosynthesis.[218]

## ● HEMATOLOGIC DISORDERS ASSOCIATED WITH ABNORMAL PLATELET FUNCTION

### CHRONIC MYELOPROLIFERATIVE NEOPLASMS

#### *Definition and History*

Bleeding and thrombosis are significant causes of morbidity and mortality in the chronic myeloproliferative neoplasms, particularly in essential thrombocythemia, polycythemia vera, and primary myelofibrosis.[219–221] Thrombocytosis is a constant finding in essential thrombocythemia, but the differential diagnosis includes these other myeloproliferative neoplasms, including chronic myelogenous leukemia, as well as other diseases associated with reactive thrombosis (Chap. 9).[222,223] Most of the information about platelets, bleeding, and thrombosis in the myeloproliferative neoplasms comes from studies of essential thrombocythemia and polycythemia vera.

#### *Etiology and Pathogenesis*

Several factors contribute to the hemostatic abnormalities in the myeloproliferative neoplasms: (1) Increased whole-blood viscosity in polycythemia vera: The engorgement of blood vessels associated with polycythemia is a risk factor for thrombosis and bleeding, particularly in postoperative situations.[224-226] (2) Intrinsic defects in platelet function: Many intrinsic platelet function defects have been reported in the myeloproliferative neoplasms, although their precise relationships to clinical bleeding are generally unclear.[227,228] (3) Elevated platelet counts: The contribution of an elevated platelet count, *per se*, to the risk of hemorrhage and thrombosis in myeloproliferative neoplasms is controversial, as the risk does not extend to patients with reactive thrombocytosis.[229,230] A number of retrospective studies indicate that the risk of abnormal hemostasis cannot be confidently predicted from the degree of thrombocytosis.[227] On the other hand, acquired von Willebrand syndrome, which represents a potential major cause of bleeding in the chronic myeloproliferative neoplasms, is most frequently associated with extreme elevations of the platelet count (e.g., $\geq 1000$ to $1500 \times 10^9$/L)[231-233]; in some, the VWF abnormality can be corrected, albeit transiently, by infusion of DDAVP or factor VIII/VWF concentrates, while in others, it can be partially or completely corrected by cytoreductive therapy.[234] (4) Leukocytosis may represent a risk factor for thrombosis in the myeloproliferative neoplasms.[221,235] In this context, leukocyte and/or endothelial dysfunction may contribute to the thrombotic phenotype in some individuals with polycythemia vera[236,237] or essential thrombocythemia[232] through leukocyte–platelet and leukocyte–endothelial cell interactions.[232,238,239]

Under the light or electron microscope, platelets in these disorders may be larger or smaller than normal, may be abnormally shaped, and may exhibit a reduction in the number of storage granules.[240] In essential thrombocythemia, platelet survival may be modestly reduced.[241] A number of functional and biochemical abnormalities have been described in platelets from patients with myeloproliferative neoplasms. The most frequently encountered functional abnormality is a decrease in platelet aggregation and granule secretion in response to epinephrine, ADP, or collagen.[227] The defect in epinephrine-induced aggregation often includes absence of the primary wave of aggregation, which is unusual in other conditions. This is not simply the result of an elevated platelet count because it is not encountered in reactive thrombocytosis.[222,242] Thus, loss of platelet responsiveness to epinephrine may help to support the presence of a myeloproliferative neoplasm in otherwise ambiguous cases, although the discovery of genetic abnormalities (e.g., JAK2, thrombopoietin receptor [MPL], calreticulin) is beginning to eliminate all ambiguity in the diagnosis of a myeloproliferative neoplasm.

Reduced platelet aggregation and secretion in the myeloproliferative neoplasms is associated with one or more of the following: decreased agonist-induced release of arachidonic acid from membrane phospholipids[243,244]; reduced conversion of arachidonic acid to PG endoperoxides or lipoxygenase products[245]; reduced platelet responsiveness to $TXA_2$[246]; decreased numbers of $\alpha_2$-adrenergic receptors associated with reduced or absent platelet responses to epinephrine[247,248]; deficiency of integrin $\alpha_2\beta_1$, resulting in variable changes in platelet responsiveness to collagen[249]; diminished stimulus–response coupling downstream of several agonists associated with reduced activation of phosphatidylinositide 3′-kinase, Rap1, and integrin $\alpha_{IIb}\beta_3$[250]; and deficiency of dense or $\alpha$ granules.[251,252] Reduction in platelet procoagulant activity has been reported in some patients with myeloproliferative neoplasms and thrombocytosis,[253] as have specific platelet membrane abnormalities, including decreased expression and activation of integrin $\alpha_{IIb}\beta_3$,[254] decreased amounts of the GPIb–V–IX complex, resulting in an acquired form of Bernard-Soulier syndrome[255]; decreased numbers of receptors for $PGD_2$[256]; increased numbers of Fc$\gamma$RIIa receptors[257]; an increase in GPIV (CD36) with[258,259] or without[260] a corresponding decrease in GPIb; and impaired expression of MPL in polycythemia vera[261] and essential thrombocythemia.[111]

On the other hand, evidence for *in vitro* platelet or coagulation hyperactivity has been reported in the myeloproliferative neoplasms. This includes spontaneous platelet aggregation in a patient with essential thrombocythemia and thrombosis,[262] increased thromboxane biosynthesis by platelets in patients with essential thrombocythemia[263] or polycythemia vera,[264] and increased "procoagulant imbalance" in patients manifested by increased endogenous thrombin potential[265] and increased procoagulant activity in circulating microparticles.[266]

Several features of these protean *in vitro* platelet functional defects require emphasis relative to the clinical setting. First, none are unique to a particular myeloproliferative neoplasm. Second, their relative frequencies have varied widely in reported series. Third, none has been prospectively shown to be predictive of bleeding or thrombosis. Fourth, although the chronic myeloproliferative neoplasms comprise several distinct clinicopathologic entities, they represent clonal abnormalities of hematopoiesis.[267] Consequently, megakaryocytes and their platelet progeny may acquire genetic, biochemical, and structural abnormalities as they develop from clones of abnormal progenitors. Examples of clonal defects in the chronic myeloproliferative neoplasms are acquisition of activating mutations in JAK2 (e.g., V617F in polycythemia vera, essential thrombocythemia, and myelofibrosis; or in exon 12 in polycythemia vera)[268-272] or MPL (W515L/K in essential thrombocythemia and myelofibrosis).[273,274] Mutations in the calreticulin gene have been found in most of the essential thrombocythemia and myelofibrosis patients who lack activating mutations in JAK2 or MPL.[275,276] It is biologically plausible that mutations in these or other leukocyte and platelet proteins might influence hemostatic mechanisms, including the activation state of platelets.[277-279] However, the precise impact of their presence or allele burden on human platelet function and on thrombotic risk is only now beginning to be understood.[232,280] For example, most,[232,268] but not all,[237,281] studies have concluded that the presence of the JAK2 (V617F) mutation or a high JAK2 (V617F) allele burden confers increased thrombotic risk in essential thrombocythemia, the latter in part a result of higher hemoglobin values. On the other hand, essential thrombocythemia or myelofibrosis patients with calreticulin mutations tend to have higher platelet counts, lower hemoglobin and leukocyte values, and fewer thromboses compared to patients with JAK2 mutations.[275,282-285] The same may hold true for rare patients with familial essential thrombocythemia or myelofibrosis and somatically acquired calreticulin mutations.[282]

### Clinical and Laboratory Features

Pathologic bleeding occurs in approximately one-third of patients with myeloproliferative neoplasms and contributes to mortality in 10 percent of those affected patients. Thrombosis also occurs in one-third of patients with myeloproliferative disorders, contributing to mortality in 15 to 40 percent of affected patients.[228,232] Most symptomatic patients experience either bleeding or thrombosis; however, some develop both complications during the course of their disease. Bleeding usually involves the skin or mucous membranes but may also occur after surgery or trauma. Thrombosis can involve arteries or veins and may occur in unusual locations such as abdominal wall vessels or the hepatic, portal, and mesenteric circulations.[286-291] Indeed, full-blown or latent chronic myeloproliferative neoplasms account for a substantial proportion of patients with splanchnic vein thrombosis.[286,291-294] Individuals with essential thrombocythemia may experience ischemia and necrosis of the fingers and toes from digital artery thrombosis, microvascular occlusion in the coronary circulation, or transient neurologic symptoms, including headaches,[295] because of cerebrovascular occlusion.[296] A syndrome of redness and burning pain in the extremities, termed *erythromelalgia*, is strongly associated with essential thrombocythemia and polycythemia vera and is thought to be partly caused by arteriolar platelet thrombi, although it may also have vasculopathic and neuropathic components.[297,298] It has been difficult to predict the risk of bleeding or thrombosis in an asymptomatic patient,[229] but an increase in leukocyte count[221,232,235] or the number of reticulated platelets in patients with thrombocytosis, thought to reflect an increase in platelet turnover, has been associated with an increased risk for thrombosis.[299] Vascular complications are also more likely to occur in patients older than 60 years of age and, most importantly, in patients with other cardiovascular risk factors, such as diabetes, hypertension, hyperlipidemia, and obesity.[221,300–303]

### Therapy

Therapy should be risk-adapted and considered for symptomatic patients, for patients with a history of thrombosis or bleeding, for those with standard cardiovascular risk factors, for patients older than 60 years of age, and for individuals about to undergo surgery. Readers are referred to expert recommendations for a summary of the treatment of essential thrombocythemia and polycythemia vera, with particular relevance to risk factors for hemostasis and thrombosis.[221,232,301,303–306] Treatment includes phlebotomy to correct the polycythemia and maintenance of a normal red cell mass, with the goal to achieve a hematocrit of less than 45 percent,[235,307,308] as well as therapy of the underlying disorder.[228,232,309,310] Platelet count reduction to less than $400 \times 10^9$/L in patients with thrombocytosis, either by plateletpheresis or cytoreductive agents, has been considered to be a target value associated with clinical improvement in patients with essential thrombocythemia.[228,302,311]

Effective cytoreductive agents include the ribonuclease reductase inhibitor hydroxyurea,[312] interferon-α (most recently the pegylated form of interferon alfa-2a), and anagrelide.[301,311,313,314] In a prospective, randomized trial of 114 "high-risk" individuals with essential thrombocythemia who were either older than 60 years of age or had a previous history of thrombosis, hydroxyurea significantly reduced the incidence of new thrombosis from 24.0 to 3.6 percent.[312] Anagrelide, an imidazoquinazoline derivative, is thought to decrease platelet counts by impairing megakaryocyte maturation.[315] Anagrelide has essentially no effect on red and white cell counts and is not known to be leukemogenic. Nevertheless, 10 to 20 percent of patients experience neurologic, gastrointestinal, and cardiac side effects, in particular fluid retention, often necessitating discontinuation of the drug.[314,316,317] When hydroxyurea and anagrelide were compared head-to-head in a randomized trial of 809 patients with essential thrombocythemia (all of whom were taking aspirin), subjects in the anagrelide group showed an increased rate of arterial thrombosis, major bleeding, and transformation to myelofibrosis relative to the group treated with hydroxyurea; however, the anagrelide group showed a relative decreased rate of venous thrombosis.[318] Progression to myelofibrosis despite treatment with anagrelide has also been observed in a phase II study.[319] However, in a newer, although relatively small, randomized, phase III study of 259 previously untreated high-risk patients with essential thrombocythemia, anagrelide was found to be noninferior to hydroxyurea in the prevention of arterial or venous thrombotic complications.[320] It should be noted that this study used a long-lasting anagrelide drug that is not currently available in the United States. During an episode of acute bleeding in the chronic myeloproliferative neoplasms, DDAVP infusion may temporarily improve hemostasis if the patient has an acquired storage pool defect or acquired von Willebrand syndrome.[252,321] In the case of acquired von Willebrand syndrome, cytoreduction to reduce the platelet count may also ameliorate the process, although this may take time and require more temporizing interventions including DDAVP or factor VIII/VWF concentrates.[234]

Low-dose aspirin (~80 to 100 mg/d) may be useful in patients with essential thrombocythemia and thrombosis, particularly those with erythromelalgia or with digital or cerebrovascular ischemia.[231,232,298,322] However, the evidence to date remains largely anecdotal, and aspirin can exacerbate a bleeding tendency in patients with myeloproliferative neoplasms, particularly in individuals with acquired von Willebrand syndrome or with World Health Organization (WHO)-defined prefibrotic myelofibrosis masquerading as essential thrombocythemia.[221,301,303,323] Consequently, even though a single, daily, low-dose aspirin is recommended for thromboprophylaxis in essential thrombocythemia, a risk-adapted approach is advised.[221,305] In addition, because platelet volume and turnover may be enhanced in essential thrombocythemia and polycythemia vera, the platelets of some individuals may not achieve total COX-1 inhibition with a single daily dose of aspirin. In such circumstances, 12-hour dosing may be considered, although this protocol has not been formally evaluated in a prospective clinical trial.[324,325]

In a double-blind, placebo-controlled study of 518 patients with polycythemia vera who were judged to have no contraindications to daily low-dose (100 mg) aspirin, subjects in the aspirin arm exhibited a reduced risk of nonfatal arterial and venous cardiovascular end points. Although aspirin was well tolerated, there was no effect of aspirin on overall and cardiovascular mortality.[326] As has been noted,[307] this study population was heavily pretreated to normalize the platelet count, although some individuals may have had residual elevations in red cell mass. Consequently, the safety and efficacy of aspirin as observed in this study may not be relevant to all patients with polycythemia vera.

Pregnant women with essential thrombocythemia or polycythemia vera pose special challenges because of an apparent increased risk of unsuccessful pregnancy, thrombotic or bleeding complications, and potential teratogenicity of hydroxyurea.[305,327] In essential thrombocythemia, the risk of first-trimester miscarriages may be higher among women with the JAK2 (V617F) mutation.[328] Although evidence-based recommendations are not available, Barbui and Finazzi recommend a risk-adapted approach to management in pregnancy. High-risk women are defined as those with previous major bleeding or thrombotic episodes, previous pregnancy complications, or a platelet count greater than $1500 \times 10^9$/L.[329] Low-risk individuals are recommended to be maintained at a hematocrit of less than 45 percent and to receive aspirin, 100 mg/d, during pregnancy and low-molecular-weight heparin, 4000 U/d, for 6 weeks after delivery. Interferon-α, rather than aspirin, is considered if there has been previous major bleeding or if platelets are greater than $1500 \times 10^9$/L. High-risk patients are recommended to receive low-molecular-weight heparin throughout pregnancy.

## LEUKEMIAS AND MYELODYSPLASTIC SYNDROMES

### Clinical and Laboratory Features

The most frequent cause of bleeding in patients with leukemia or a myelodysplastic syndrome is thrombocytopenia. However, abnormal platelet function *in vitro* has been described in acute myelogenous leukemia, and in some patients, this may be clinically significant. In acute myelogenous leukemia and its variants, platelets may be larger than normal, abnormally shaped, and exhibit a marked variation in the number of granules. There may be decreased aggregation and serotonin release in response to ADP, epinephrine, or collagen, decreased surface P-selectin expression in response to platelet activation via the PAR-1 thrombin receptor, and decreased platelet procoagulant activity. These functional abnormalities may be caused by either acquired storage pool deficiency or a defect in the process of platelet activation through one or more signaling pathways.[330–334] These defects are intrinsic to the platelet and probably relate to the fact that the megakaryocytes from which platelets were derived originated from a leukemic stem cell. Indeed, in a familial platelet disorder with a predisposition to acute leukemia, platelet dysfunction prior to the development of leukemia occurs, at least in part, because of downregulation of genes such as *NF-E2* or *ALOX12*, themselves target genes of *RUNX1*, a transcription factor that is germline-mutated in these individuals.[335,336]

As discussed in the section on oncology drugs, drugs used to treat acute leukemias may affect platelet function, at least *in vitro*.[200,337,338] Bleeding in the acute leukemias usually responds to platelet transfusions and to treatment of the underlying disease. Similar *in vitro* platelet abnormalities may be seen in the myelodysplastic syndromes, sometimes accompanied by clinical bleeding disproportionate to that expected for the degree of thrombocytopenia.[330,339–344] In these syndromes, platelets may be less uniformly affected, perhaps because there is a residual population of normal platelets admixed with those from the malignant clone.

Reduced platelet aggregation has been reported in children with acute lymphocytic leukemia.[331] Unless the leukemia is biphenotypic, it is difficult to ascribe the platelet defect to the leukemic process itself. Platelets are normal in children with acute lymphoblastic leukemia in complete remission.[345] Single cases have been reported of patients with acute B-lymphoblastic leukemia[346] or Hodgkin lymphoma[347] whose severe bleeding was attributed, in part, to acquired Glanzmann thrombasthenia associated with antiintegrin $\alpha_{IIb}\beta_3$ antibodies. Hairy cell leukemia is a lymphoproliferative disease in which platelet dysfunction may rarely complicate the clinical picture; bleeding is usually due to thrombocytopenia rather than platelet dysfunction.[348] Some patients may exhibit storage pool deficiency or a defect in the process of platelet activation. These abnormalities have been reported to disappear following splenectomy,[349] which usually corrects the thrombocytopenia as well. Acquired von Willebrand syndrome has been reported in association with hairy cell leukemia.[350]

## DYSPROTEINEMIAS

### Definition and History

Platelet dysfunction is observed in approximately one-third of patients with immunoglobulin (Ig) A multiple myeloma or Waldenström macroglobulinemia, 15 percent of patients with IgG myeloma, and in occasional patients with monoclonal gammopathy of undetermined significance.[351,352] In addition to platelet dysfunction, other causes of bleeding should be considered in these patients, including the hyperviscosity syndrome,[353] thrombocytopenia, complications of amyloidosis such as amyloid angiopathy[354] or acquired factor X deficiency,[355,356] and, rarely, a circulating heparin-like anticoagulant[357–359] or systemic fibrino(gen)lysis.[360,361] The monoclonal immunoglobulin may also affect *in vitro* coagulation tests by interfering with fibrin polymerization and with the function of other coagulation proteins. On occasion, paraproteins can impair *in vivo* hemostasis as well.

### Etiology and Pathogenesis

The bleeding time may be prolonged in patients with dysproteinemias, even in the absence of clinical bleeding. The platelet defect is caused by the monoclonal protein. It has been suggested that some monoclonal immunoglobulins interact with the platelet surface to interfere nonspecifically with platelet adhesion or stimulus–response coupling. This concept is supported by the observations that platelet dysfunction is more common when the concentration of the paraprotein in plasma or on the platelet membrane is very high[362]; that platelet aggregation, secretion, clot retraction, and platelet procoagulant activity may all be affected; and that normal platelets can acquire these defects when incubated with the purified monoclonal immunoglobulin.[363]

In some cases, specific interactions of the monoclonal protein with platelets or with components of the extracellular matrix have been described. One reported IgA myeloma protein inhibited the ability of a suspension of aortic connective tissue to aggregate normal platelets.[364] The bleeding time and bleeding diathesis of the patient from whom this myeloma protein was obtained were corrected by removal of the protein by plasmapheresis. In another patient with IgD$\lambda$ myeloma, $\lambda$ dimers were found to bind to the A1 domain of VWF, inhibiting shear-induced platelet aggregation.[365] In still another patient, an IgG myeloma protein bound specifically to the platelet integrin $\beta_3$ subunit. Both the intact immunoglobulin and its F(ab')2 fragment inhibited the binding of fibrinogen to activated integrin $\alpha_{IIb}\beta_3$, thus inducing a thrombasthenic-like state.[366] A number of patients with myeloma, monoclonal gammopathy of undetermined significance, lymphoma, or chronic lymphocytic leukemia have been reported to have an acquired form of von Willebrand disease in which the level of plasma VWF is reduced or the high-molecular-weight multimers of VWF are selectively reduced.[321,352,367–374]

### Therapy

When clinically significant platelet dysfunction occurs in a patient with a dysproteinemia, cytoreductive therapy should be considered as a means to reduce the production and plasma level of the monoclonal immunoglobulin.[351,352] Plasmapheresis can also control bleeding by reducing the level of the abnormal protein and can be lifesaving during acute bleeds.[352,375,376] Cryoprecipitate, DDAVP, and/or plasmapheresis may be transiently effective in patients with acquired von Willebrand syndrome.[321,368,377,378] However, high-dose intravenous gamma-globulin (IVIG) appears to be particularly effective in individuals with acquired von Willebrand syndrome associated with an IgG monoclonal gammopathy of undetermined significance, although intermittent infusions may be required at approximately 3-week intervals (Chap. 16).[352,369–371,379–381] The reported experience with rituximab for the latter condition is extremely limited, but so far disappointing.[382]

## ACQUIRED VON WILLEBRAND SYNDROME

Acquired von Willebrand syndrome is a relatively rare disorder that typically occurs in the setting of an autoimmune or clonal hematologic disease.[231,381,383–385] It is being increasingly recognized in conditions associated with high shear and turbulence in the circulation, such as severe aortic stenosis, hypertrophic obstructive cardiomyopathy, and circulatory assist devices.[381,386–390] It also can occur in association with a number of other unrelated medical conditions,[381] including Gaucher disease,[391] hypothyroidism[392,393] and Noonan syndrome.[394] As discussed above, it can represent one cause of bleeding in multiple myeloma,[321,377] Waldenström macroglobulinemia,[395] monoclonal gammopathy of undetermined significance,[370] low-grade non-Hodgkin lymphoma,[396,397] chronic lymphocytic leukemia,[398] and chronic myeloproliferative neoplasms, the latter particularly in association with very high platelet counts.[233]

The pathophysiology of acquired von Willebrand syndrome involves a reduction in circulating VWF (and its associated factor VIII molecule), generally because of rapid VWF turnover in the circulation.[381] VWF levels and multimer patterns may simulate type I, II, or III von Willebrand disease. In lymphoproliferative disorders, a specific, often nonneutralizing anti-VWF antibody is present,[321,352,377,399] whereas in autoimmune disorders, anti-VWF antibodies are part of a generalized autoimmune response.[400] In other situations, the syndrome may result from increased adsorption of VWF by tumor cells (e.g., Wilms tumor, osteosarcoma[401]) or platelets (myeloproliferative neoplasms),[315,350,402–404] increased VWF proteolysis (e.g., aortic stenosis, ventricular assist devices), or decreased VWF production (hypothyroidism).[381,405,406]

Mucocutaneous bleeding should raise the suspicion of acquired von Willebrand syndrome in patients without a prior personal or family history of bleeding. This is especially important in patients with a known autoimmune, lymphoproliferative, or myeloproliferative disorder.[315,381] Diagnostic evaluation includes measurements of factor VIII activity, VWF antigen, ristocetin cofactor activity, and VWF multimer analysis.[407] The presence of an *in vitro* inhibitor may or may not be detected depending on whether the antibody binds to VWF and neutralizes its function or merely leads to accelerated VWF clearance by the reticuloendothelial system.[315] An abnormally high ratio of VWF propeptide to von Willebrand antigen may be present as a result of the rapid clearance of von Willebrand antigen but not VWF.[44]

Given the uncommon prevalence of this syndrome, reports of patient management have been retrospective and largely anecdotal. Treatment should be reserved for patients with active bleeding or those who are likely to bleed if left untreated.[352,381] Infusions of DDAVP[321,398,400] or factor VIII/VWF concentrates[408,409] may be useful, although the rapid clearance of VWF may limit efficacy. Treatment has included glucocorticoids or rituximab in patients with lupus[231,385,410] and recombinant factor VIIa[411] or high-dose IVIG.[190,384,412] High-dose IVIG is particularly effective when acquired von Willebrand syndrome is associated with a lymphoproliferative disorder or, as discussed in the section "Dysproteinemias," with an IgG monoclonal gammopathy of undetermined significance. IVIG likely acts by delaying VWF clearance via reticuloendothelial cell blockade, although other mechanisms have been postulated.[297,369,370,379,380,397,413] Treatment of the underlying disease can be effective in some situations[381,414,415] (e.g., hypothyroidism with thyroid replacement,[416,417] Gaucher disease with enzyme replacement therapy,[391] and extreme thrombocytosis with cytoreduction[233,315,323,418]). As with inherited von Willebrand disease, longstanding acquired von Willebrand syndrome can be associated with and complicated by gastrointestinal tract arteriovenous malformations, resulting in severe bleeding.[419] An example of such gastrointestinal bleeding is found in patients with severe aortic stenosis and is referred to as Heyde syndrome. In this situation, valve replacement can correct the hemostatic defect.[387,420]

# ● SYSTEMIC DISORDERS ASSOCIATED WITH ABNORMAL PLATELET FUNCTION

## UREMIA

### Definition and History
In the predialysis era, hemorrhage occurred in approximately 50 percent of uremic patients and was a cause of death in approximately 30 perccent.[421,422] With the advent of dialysis, the frequency of spontaneous hemorrhage in patients with renal failure has decreased.[422] Experience with percutaneous renal biopsy in several thousand patients with renal disease supports the notion that the hemostatic defect in patients with renal disease is usually mild. Although the incidence of small perirenal hematomas following biopsy may be as high as 85 percent when patients are examined by computed tomography, gross hematuria is observed in only 5 to 10 percent of cases and is usually transient.[423,424] Severe bleeding following biopsy requiring surgical intervention is even less common and usually can be attributed to factors other than a uremic hemostatic defect, such as needle lacerations of the kidney or spleen, anomalous vessels, heparin anticoagulation, or the presence of amyloid in the kidney.

### Etiology and Pathogenesis
The hemostatic defect in uremia has been attributed to defects in platelet function and appears to be multifactorial.[425] One prominent factor is renal failure–associated anemia.[426] A lowered hematocrit *ex vivo*

induces a defect in platelet adhesion that can be corrected by increasing the hematocrit to 30 percent or more.[427] In uremic patients, successful treatment of anemia with red blood cell transfusion or recombinant human erythropoietin (EPO) results in partial or complete correction of prolonged bleeding times when the hematocrit is increased to 27 to 32 percent.[428–431] The effect of anemia on primary hemostasis is not unique to uremia. In normal individuals, the bleeding time correlates with the hematocrit, and bleeding times can be prolonged in patients with severe anemia of any etiology.[426] Red cells may have a beneficial effect on hemostasis both because they displace platelets toward the periphery of the column of circulating blood[432] and they may enhance platelet reactivity.[14]

Because correction of anemia does not always return the bleeding time to normal, other factors present in renal failure may perturb platelet function.[427] Ristocetin-induced platelet aggregation, a surrogate for VWF binding to the platelet GPIb–IX–V complex, may be decreased in uremia. However, plasma VWF concentrations are normal or elevated in renal failure,[433] and qualitative VWF abnormalities have not been uniformly observed.[434,435] Mixing studies using uremic platelets and normal plasma, and vice versa, do not demonstrate consistent quantitative or qualitative abnormalities in GPIb–IX–V.[434–436] Nonetheless, uremic plasma can inhibit the adhesion of normal platelets to deendothelialized human umbilical artery segments, whereas uremic platelets adhere normally in the presence of normal plasma.[434] Because the defective adhesion appears independent of VWF, an unidentified component of uremic plasma may be responsible for the adhesion defect.[434] Uremic platelets also exhibit markedly reduced spreading on the subendothelium of rabbit vessels, a defect attributed to impaired VWF binding to platelet integrin $\alpha_{IIb}\beta_3$.[437] Because VWF binding to integrin $\alpha_{IIb}\beta_3$ requires platelet stimulation, this observation suggests a uremia-induced defect in platelet signal transduction.

There are a number of reports describing defective agonist-induced platelet activation in uremic patients, including reduced fibrinogen binding, aggregation, and secretion. These abnormalities may be retained after platelets are separated from uremic plasma, and in some cases, uremic plasma imparts the defect to normal platelets.[438] Furthermore, the ability of activated platelets to express procoagulant activity is reduced in uremia.[439] These functional defects likely result from uremia-induced abnormalities in platelet biochemistry, including reduced agonist-induced increases in cytoplasmic free calcium,[440] reduced release of arachidonic acid from platelet phospholipids,[421] and reduced conversion of released arachidonic acid to PG endoperoxides and $TXA_2$.[138,441,442]

A number of dialyzable and nondialyzable substances have been reported to be responsible for the platelet function defects in uremia,[443] but urea itself is not responsible. *Ex vivo* platelet aggregation can be inhibited by small dialyzable substances, such as guanidinosuccinic acid and phenolic acids, as well as by poorly characterized "middle molecules" at concentrations found in uremic plasma.[444,445] Venous and arterial segments from uremic patients have been reported to produce more $PGI_2$ than segments from normal individuals, an abnormality not corrected by dialysis.[446] Altered NO metabolism has been observed in uremia.[447,448] In a uremic rat model, defective platelet adhesion was normalized by an inhibitor of NO formation,[449] suggesting that increased NO synthesis by endothelial cells or platelets is at least partially responsible for the defective platelet function.[450] Why renal failure increases NO synthesis is not entirely clear, although exposing endothelial cells to guanidinosuccinic acid can mimic the effects of NO, suggesting that retained guanidinosuccinic acid may be the relevant substrate.[451] Uremia has been reported to upregulate the y+L system for L-arginine transport into platelets, enabling platelets to maintain or enhance NO synthesis, even in the face of low circulating L-arginine concentrations.[452,453]

By contrast, some substances found in high concentrations in uremic plasma, such as urea and parathyroid hormone, appear to play no role in platelet dysfunction.[454]

Concurrent medications and thrombocytopenia must always be considered when a patient with renal failure exhibits a bleeding tendency. Aspirin can prolong the bleeding time inordinately in uremia. Unlike aspirin's effect on COX, this effect is transient and correlates with blood levels of aspirin.[34,35] Bleeding may be potentiated by the administration of heparin during hemodialysis; in this situation, the use of an ethylene-vinyl alcohol copolymer hollow fiber dialyzer or intermittent saline infusion and high blood flow rates may eliminate the need for heparin.[455] β-Lactam antibiotics that prolong the bleeding time may have a greater effect in uremic patients and increase the occurrence of bleeding.[456]

Mild thrombocytopenia has been reported in chronic renal failure, particularly in patients on dialysis,[457] as a result of diminished marrow production and decreased platelet survival.[458] Serum thrombopoietin levels in hemodialysis patients are increased,[457,459] perhaps reflecting increased platelet turnover or a decrease in megakaryocyte mass. But when platelet counts are greater than $100 \times 10^9/L$, it is necessary to consider whether a systemic disease or medication, such as multiple myeloma, systemic vasculitis, hemolytic uremic syndrome, eclampsia, renal allograft rejection, or heparin, could be responsible for bleeding in a uremic patient.

### Clinical and Laboratory Features

Despite dialysis, abnormal platelet function in uremia remains a clinical issue because it may contribute to bleeding following surgery or trauma or in conjunction with anatomic lesions of the gastrointestinal tract.[441,455] The bleeding time has often been used as an indication of hemorrhagic risk in uremia, but critical reviews of the literature indicate that it is not appropriate to use for this purpose.[460,461]

### Therapy

Abnormal platelet aggregation is common in uremic patients, but by itself is not an indication for therapeutic intervention.[425] The frequency of excessive bleeding after biopsies or other surgical procedures in uremic patients who have not received specific treatment is not known, but it may be uncommon. Thus, if bleeding does complicate a procedure, a thorough search for causes of bleeding other than uremia should be initiated without assuming that uremia is the etiology. However, when therapy for a uremic bleeding diathesis is necessary, the uremic platelet defect can usually be successfully treated.

There are several therapeutic maneuvers that can either partially or completely correct an abnormal bleeding time in uremic patients, and anecdotal observations indicate that they may also improve hemostasis. Because prospective studies comparing various treatment regimens have not been performed, the choice of therapy should be based on the severity of the bleeding, the anticipated severity of the hemostatic stress imposed by surgery or trauma, the predicted duration of the therapeutic effect, and the risks of therapy.

The mainstay of therapy is *dialysis*. Intensive dialysis can correct the bleeding diathesis in many patients but is only partially effective in others.[462] Peritoneal dialysis and hemodialysis are equally effective.[462,463] If a patient undergoing dialysis bleeds, it may be worthwhile to increase the intensity of the dialysis.

In uremic individuals, increasing the hematocrit by transfusion or treatment with recombinant human EPO to 27 to 32 percent is often associated with diminished clinical bleeding.[428–430,464,465] A number of reports suggest that EPO has an effect on platelets independent of an increase in hematocrit,[431] perhaps the result of an increase in the number of young platelets in the circulation.[466]

DDAVP, a vasopressin analogue whose pressor effects are substantially less than its antidiuretic effects, causes the release of VWF from tissue stores and has been reported to shorten the bleeding time in 50 to 75 percent of patients with uremia. In many cases, surgery has been carried out safely after administration of this drug, although no controlled trials have been performed.[467] DDAVP is usually administered intravenously in a dose of 0.3 mcg/kg over 15 to 30 minutes (maximum dose: 20 mcg), but it is also effective at this dose when given subcutaneously.[467] Alternatively, the drug can be given intranasally.[468] Improvement in the bleeding time is seen within 30 to 60 minutes of administration, lasts for approximately 4 hours, and roughly correlates with the rise in the plasma levels of VWF and the appearance in the circulation of high-molecular-weight VWF multimers.[467] In some patients, the drug has been given repeatedly at 12- to 24-hour intervals, although tachyphylaxis can occur.[469]

Side effects of DDAVP have been mild and uncommon and have included a 10 to 15 percent decrease in mean arterial pressure, a 20 to 30 percent increase in pulse rate, facial flushing, water retention, and hyponatremia leading to seizures; the latter is more common after repeated administration and when fluids are given freely.[467] Water retention and hyponatremia have not been observed in patients whose kidneys cannot respond to the hormone. Several uremic and nonuremic individuals with atherosclerosis have been reported to develop stroke or myocardial infarction after DDAVP administration, although such complications appear to be rare.[470,471] If dialysis is not effective, DDAVP is the treatment of choice for uremic bleeding, particularly if only a short-term effect is required.[467]

*Conjugated estrogens* at a dose of 0.6 mg/kg intravenously for 5 days have also been reported to shorten the bleeding time in most, but not all, uremic individuals, both in uncontrolled studies and in randomized, double-blind studies.[34,472–474] They may also be useful in some patients with uremia who bleed from gastrointestinal telangiectasia.[475] No changes in the plasma levels or multimer distribution of VWF have been noted with this treatment, and it has been postulated that the active component in conjugated estrogens, 17β-estradiol, acts through an estrogen receptor mechanism.[476]

Lastly, uncontrolled studies suggest that infusions of cryoprecipitate can shorten the bleeding time in uremic patients and ameliorate bleeding.[243] However, others have reported inconsistent results,[477] and because of concerns of viral contamination, cryoprecipitate is very rarely used for this indication.

## ANTIPLATELET ANTIBODIES

### Definition and History

Antibody binding to platelets in several pathologic conditions, including immune thrombocytopenia (ITP), systemic lupus erythematosus (SLE), and platelet alloimmunization, can cause thrombocytopenia as a result of decreased platelet survival. Less commonly, bleeding times may be shorter than expected for the degree of thrombocytopenia, suggesting enhanced platelet function.[478] On occasion, platelet function is impaired in ITP.[479–483]

### Etiology and Pathogenesis

The mechanism by which autoantibodies or alloantibodies impair platelet function is likely antibody binding to specific platelet GPs. Most antiplatelet antibodies are directed against integrin $\alpha_{IIb}\beta_3$,[479–482] but antibodies directed against GPIb–IX–V, integrin $\alpha_2\beta_1$, and GPIV have been detected as well.[484,485] In most instances, the functional consequences of antibody binding are obscured by the presence of thrombocytopenia. However, patients have been reported with normal platelet counts, absent platelet aggregation, autoantibodies against integrin $\alpha_{IIb}\beta_3$, and a bleeding diathesis reminiscent of Glanzmann thrombasthenia.[479–482,486–489] Similarly, autoantibodies against GPIb and integrin $\alpha_2\beta_1$ have been detected that selectively inhibit ristocetin-induced platelet aggregation[490,491] and collagen-induced platelet aggregation,[492,493] respectively. A patient with ITP has also been identified whose anti-GPVI autoantibody produced GPVI shedding from the platelet surface and platelets unresponsive to stimulation by collagen.[494]

Besides interfering with platelet function, some autoantibodies can activate platelets and induce aggregation and secretion *in vitro*. Such antibodies can activate platelets through immune complex binding to platelet Fc receptors, by depositing sublytic quantities of the membrane attack complex of complement (C5b-9) on the cell surface,[495] or by binding to a specific membrane antigen.[246] The prototypic example of this phenomenon is heparin-induced thrombocytopenia in which antibodies bound to neoepitopes exposed on the platelet factor 4 molecule by heparin activate platelets after binding to platelet Fc receptors (Chap. 8).[496]

### Clinical Laboratory Features and Therapy

Platelet dysfunction should be suspected in any patient with ITP or SLE who has mucocutaneous bleeding with a platelet count that is not ordinarily associated with bleeding (e.g., equal to or greater than approximately $30 \times 10^9$/L). Likewise, this scenario has been described occasionally in patients with Hodgkin disease,[347,480] non-Hodgkin lymphoma and myeloma,[497,498] and hairy cell leukemia.[499] The clinical spectrum of autoimmune platelet dysfunction may also include some individuals with "easy bruising" and a normal platelet count. These patients may have ITP with "compensated thrombocytolysis," as a substantial proportion have circulating antiplatelet antibodies and large platelets.[500]

Patients with antiplatelet antibodies may exhibit defective platelet function *in vitro*, even if they do not manifest a prolonged bleeding time or excessive bleeding. These deficits include impaired platelet aggregation to ADP, epinephrine, and collagen,[501–504] as well as impaired adhesion to the subendothelial matrix.[20] The most frequently reported abnormalities are absence of platelet aggregation in response to low concentrations of collagen and absence of the second wave of aggregation in response to ADP or epinephrine. This pattern is identical to that seen in individuals with inherited storage pool disease. In fact, both ITP and SLE may be associated with an acquired form of storage pool disease manifested by a reduced platelet content of dense- and $\alpha$-granule components.[432,505] In one report, platelets in ITP also exhibited an activation defect manifested by impaired conversion of arachidonic acid to $TXA_2$.[506]

Because antibody-mediated platelet dysfunction and bleeding almost always occur in the setting of ITP, therapeutic efforts should be directed to the treatment of these disorders.

## CARDIOPULMONARY BYPASS

### Definition and History

Circulating blood through an extracorporeal bypass circuit during cardiac surgery induces a variety of hemostatic defects. The most significant of these are thrombocytopenia, platelet dysfunction, and hyperfibrinolysis.[507–509] At their extreme, these defects can result in substantial postoperative bleeding that may last hours to days after bypass. Approximately 5 percent of patients experience excessive postoperative bleeding after extracorporeal bypass; roughly half of the bleeding is from surgical causes; much of the remainder is caused by qualitative platelet defects and hyperfibrinolysis.

### Etiology and Pathogenesis

Thrombocytopenia is a consistent feature of bypass surgery.[126,508] Typically, platelet counts begin to decrease to approximately 50 percent of presurgical levels within the first half hour after the initiation of bypass, but thrombocytopenia can occur within 5 minutes and often does not nadir for the first few days.[507,509,510] The major factor responsible for thrombocytopenia is hemodilution from priming the pump with colloid or crystalloid solutions, but it is often more profound than can be accounted for by hemodilution alone.[509–511] Platelet adhesion to artificial surfaces in the circuit has been demonstrated by scanning electron microscopy.[512] The mechanism of this interaction is uncertain, but it may be a result of the deposition of fibrinogen on the bypass circuit and platelet adhesion mediated by integrin $\alpha_{IIb}\beta_3$.[513] Less common causes of thrombocytopenia during bypass are disseminated intravascular coagulation, sequestration of damaged platelets in the liver, and heparin-induced thrombocytopenia.[514] Like antibodies against the complex of platelet factor 4 and heparin that are commonly detected after bypass surgery and can be responsible for heparin-induced thrombocytopenia,[496] antibodies against protamine and protamine–heparin complexes are commonly detected as well.[82,515,516] Such antibodies may contribute to the thrombocytopenia and possibly to thromboembolic events following cardiopulmonary bypass.[517]

Qualitative platelet defects are the primary nonstructural hemostatic defects induced by the bypass circuit[508,518] and are manifest as abnormal *ex vivo* platelet aggregation, decreased ristocetin-induced platelet agglutination, deficiency of platelet $\alpha$ and $\delta$ granules, release of soluble CD40 ligand, and the generation of platelet microparticles.[507,509,510,519–522] The severity of these abnormalities correlates with the duration of extracorporeal bypass,[523] and they generally resolve within 2 to 24 hours.[508]

Bypass-induced defects in platelet function are likely caused by platelet activation and fragmentation,[521,524] hypothermia, contact with fibrinogen-coated synthetic surfaces, contact with the blood–air interface, cardiotomy suction and retransfusion of cardiotomy suction blood, and platelet exposure thrombin, plasmin, ADP, or complement.[513,519,525–528] Drugs such as heparin, protamine, integrin $\alpha_{IIb}\beta_3$ antagonists, and aspirin, as well as the production of fibrin degradation products, can also impair platelet function.[126,529–531] Controversy exists about the significance of these defects *in vivo*. Some investigators suggest that the entire qualitative platelet defect is a result of the use of heparin during bypass and its inhibitory effect on thrombin activity[529]; however, this would not account for the bleeding diathesis that can exist hours after heparin reversal.

Hyperfibrinolysis may also contribute to the bleeding diathesis associated with cardiopulmonary bypass.[532,533] This is likely from thrombus formation in the pericardial cavity followed by local, and subsequently systemic, fibrinolysis.[532] The relevance of hyperfibrinolysis to postbypass bleeding is bolstered by the efficacy of antifibrinolytic therapy in minimizing cardiopulmonary bypass surgery blood loss.

### Therapy

A preoperative evaluation of cardiac surgical candidates should include a history of bleeding in either the patient or family member. Some authors recommend a screening prothrombin time, partial prothrombin time, and bleeding time even in individuals with no history of bleeding.[534] However, the validity of this approach is controversial.[535] Regardless, prophylactic transfusion of allogeneic blood components is not indicated.[508,536,537] Preoperative administration of recombinant human EPO has been reported to reduce the need for allogeneic blood transfusion in undergoing elective open-heart surgery.[538–541] Cell savers are now often used during bypass surgery and the collected washed autologous red blood cells are reinfused after completion of cardiopulmonary bypass. In addition, blood collected from chest tube drainage has been reinfused to minimize allogeneic transfusions.[541] The safety of transfusing large quantities of blood by this technique has not fully been established.[528,542]

A number of maneuvers have been taken to reduce the hemostatic abnormalities associated with cardiac surgery. These include coating the artificial surfaces of cardiopulmonary bypass devices with heparin,[543-547] using centrifugal rather than roller pumps,[548] use of a number of pharmacologic agents,[549] and performing coronary artery surgery without bypass.[301,550] Off-pump coronary artery bypass surgery appears to preserve platelet function, but concerns have been raised about adverse thromboembolic events after surgery because of the concurrence of normal platelet function, late thrombin generation, and reduced fibrinolysis.[551-553] Several pharmacologic maneuvers have been tried to assist in the management of postoperative bleeding. Postoperative patients with a prolonged bleeding time and excessive blood loss may respond to DDAVP, as evidenced by a shortening of the bleeding time. However, results of trials using this agent have been contradictory, with some studies showing a reduced blood loss and most showing no benefit.[554-556] Based on the assumption that platelet activation during bypass could be a major cause of postoperative platelet dysfunction, infusion of platelet activation inhibitors such as $PGE_1$, $PGI_2$, or stable $PGI_2$ analogues has been carried out in animal models and in humans. By increasing platelet cAMP and reducing platelet responsiveness, these agents prevent bypass-induced thrombocytopenia and platelet dysfunction. However, randomized trials using $PGI_2$ and its analogue, iloprost, have not shown a clear overall benefit, in part because of significant toxicity, including hypotension.[123,557] Recombinant factor VIIa has been recommended to treat uncontrolled postoperative bleeding that has not responded to routine hemostatic therapy.[558] However, the off-label use of recombinant factor VIIa is associated with an increased risk for arterial and venous thromboembolism,[559] and a retrospective case-matched review of patients who had received recombinant factor VIIa perioperatively during major cardiac surgery indicated that it was associated with worse survival.[223] Nonetheless, it remains a potentially useful therapeutic consideration in view of the prognosis of uncontrolled postoperative hemorrhage.[560] Based primarily on the cardiovascular complications encountered by patients in two randomized studies of the use of parecoxib/valdecoxib to treat pain after cardiac surgery, the use of coxibs and traditional NSAIDs appears contraindicated in this setting.[561,562]

Inhibiting fibrinolysis using $\varepsilon$-aminocaproic acid or tranexamic acid during cardiopulmonary bypass can reduce mediastinal blood loss and transfusion requirements.[549] Aprotinin (Trasylol), a broad-spectrum protease inhibitor, was also used for this purpose, but observational studies,[563-565] as well as a blinded clinical trial,[566] revealed that its use is associated with serious end-organ damage and a higher mortality than the use of $\varepsilon$-aminocaproic acid or no antifibrinolytic agent.

The most important determinant of blood loss following cardiopulmonary surgery is the surgical procedure itself. If excessive nonsurgical postoperative bleeding occurs, one should verify that the patient is no longer hypothermic and that heparin has been fully reversed. At this point, the administration of pharmacologic agents, along with judicious transfusions of platelets, cryoprecipitate, fresh frozen plasma, and red blood cells, is appropriate.

## MISCELLANEOUS DISORDERS

Measurements of hemostatic function are frequently abnormal in patients with end-stage and fulminant liver disease and result from decreased coagulation factor production, fibrinolysis, dysfibrinogenemia, thrombocytopenia as a result of hypersplenism and thrombopoietin deficiency, and disseminated intravascular coagulation (DIC).[425,567] However, the clinical consequences of these laboratory abnormalities have been reassessed because they do not take into account that both anti- and prohemostatic pathways are perturbed in liver disease.[568,569] Thus, hemostasis in liver disease is considered to be "rebalanced,"

although it remains unstable, with patients prone to both bleeding and thrombosis. Chronic liver disease can be associated with a prolonged bleeding time and reduced platelet aggregation and procoagulant activity,[567,570,571] but there is no evidence for a platelet function defect specific to liver disease.[572] Rather, they are the result of multiple factors, including thrombocytopenia, hypofibrinogenemia, and anemia, none of which imply an intrinsic defect in platelet function.[573] Regardless, the prolonged bleeding in these patients may respond to infusion of DDAVP,[574] but clinical relevance of this observation is uncertain.[575]

Patients with DIC may exhibit reduced platelet aggregation and acquired storage pool deficiency.[576,577] These result from platelet activation in vivo by thrombin or other agonists. Alternatively, elevated levels of fibrin(ogen) degradation products and the low fibrinogen levels that accompany DIC may contribute to the platelet defect. Although purified low-molecular-weight fibrinogen degradation products can impair platelet aggregation, this effect requires concentrations of degradation products unlikely to occur in vivo.[578] Moreover, it is difficult to assess the significance of platelet dysfunction in most patients with DIC because of the simultaneous presence of thrombocytopenia and other hemostatic defects.

Decreased platelet aggregation and secretion in response to ADP and epinephrine has been reported in Bartter syndrome, a group of rare inherited disorders characterized by severe restrictions of salt reabsorption by the thick ascending limb of Henle, perhaps caused by excessive $PGE_2$ synthesis.[579-582] However, reviews of series of patients with Bartter syndrome make no mention of hemostatic problems,[580] so the clinical significance of the platelet aggregation abnormalities is doubtful.

In addition to thrombocytopenia, platelet dysfunction has been observed in some patients with hemorrhagic fevers caused by Dengue, Hanta, Lassa, Junín, and Ebola viruses.[583] There are also isolated reports of a slight prolongation of the bleeding time and/or ex vivo platelet function defects in a number of other clinical conditions. These include nonthrombocytopenic purpura with eosinophilia,[584-586] atopic asthma and hay fever,[587] acute respiratory failure,[588] and Wilms tumor elaborating hyaluronic acid.[589] The clinical significance of these associations is not clear.

## REFERENCES

1. Hayward CP: Diagnostic evaluation of platelet function disorders. *Blood Rev* 25(4):169–173, 2011.
2. Nurden P, Nurden A, Jandrot-Perrus M: Diagnostic assessment of platelet function, in *Quality in Laboratory Hemostasis and Thrombosis*, edited by S Kitchen, JD Olson, FE Preston, pp 159–173. Blackwell Publishing, London, 2013.
3. Wisloff F, Godal H: Prolonged bleeding time with adequate platelet count in hospital patients. *Scand J Haematol* 27(1):45–50, 1981.
4. Patrono C: Aspirin as an antiplatelet drug. *N Engl J Med* 330(18):1287–1294, 1981.
5. Smith WL, DeWitt DL, Garavito RM: Cyclooxygenases: Structural, cellular, and molecular biology. *Annu Rev Biochem* 69:145–182, 2000.
6. Kis B, Snipes JA, Busija DW: Acetaminophen and the cyclooxygenase-3 puzzle: Sorting out facts, fictions, and uncertainties. *J Pharmacol Exp Ther* 315(1):1–7, 2005.
7. Smith W, Garavito R, DeWitt D: Prostaglandin endoperoxide H synthases (cyclooxygenases)-1 and 2. *Biol Chem* 271:33157, 1996.
8. Chandrasekharan NV, Dai H, Roos KL, et al: COX-3, a cyclooxygenase-1 variant inhibited by acetaminophen and other analgesic/antipyretic drugs: Cloning, structure, and expression. *Proc Natl Acad Sci U S A* 99(21):13926–13931, 2002.
9. Weiss H, Aledort L: Impaired platelet/connective tissue reaction in man after aspirin ingestion. *Lancet* 2:495, 1967.
10. O'Brien JR: Effect of salicylates on human platelets. *Lancet* 1(7557):1431, 1968.
11. Grosser T, Fries S, FitzGerald GA: Biological basis for the cardiovascular consequences of COX-2 inhibition: Therapeutic challenges and opportunities. *J Clin Invest* 116(1): 4–15, 2006.
12. Kyrle PA, Eichler HG, Jager U, Lechner K: Inhibition of prostacyclin and thromboxane A2 generation by low-dose aspirin at the site of plug formation in man *in vivo. Circulation* 75(5):1025–1029, 1987.
13. Jaffe EA, Weksler BB: Recovery of endothelial cell prostacyclin production after inhibition by low doses of aspirin. *J Clin Invest* 63(3):532–535, 1979.
14. Marcus AJ, Safier LB: Thromboregulation: Multicellular modulation of platelet reactivity in hemostasis and thrombosis. *FASEB J* 7(6):516–522, 1993.

15. Rich JB: The efficacy and safety of aprotinin use in cardiac surgery. *Ann Thorac Surg* 66(5 Suppl):S6–S11, 1998.

16. Antithrombotic Trialists Collaboration: Collaborative meta-analysis of randomised trials of antiplatelet therapy for prevention of death, myocardial infarction, and stroke in high risk patients. *BMJ* 324(7329):71–86, 2002.

17. Seshasai SR, Wijesuriya S, Sivakumaran R, et al: Effect of aspirin on vascular and non-vascular outcomes: Meta-analysis of randomized controlled trials. *Arch Intern Med* 172(3):209–216, 2012.

18. Raju N, Sobieraj-Teague M, Hirsh J, et al: Effect of aspirin on mortality in the primary prevention of cardiovascular disease. *Am J Med* 124(7):621–629, 2011.

19. Bartolucci AA, Tendera M, Howard G: Meta-analysis of multiple primary prevention trials of cardiovascular events using aspirin. *Am J Cardiol* 107(12):1796–1801, 2011.

20. Kallmann R, Nieuwenhuis HK, de Groot PG, et al: Effects of low doses of aspirin, 10 mg and 30 mg daily, on bleeding time, thromboxane production and 6-keto-PGF1 alpha excretion in healthy subjects. *Thromb Res* 45:355, 1987.

21. Nakajima H, Takami H, Yamagata K, Kariya K, Tamai Y, Nara H: Aspirin effects on colonic mucosal bleeding. *Dis Colon Rectum* 40:1484, 1997.

22. Mielke CH Jr: Aspirin prolongation of the template bleeding time: Influence of venostasis and direction of incision. *Blood* 60(5):1139–1142, 1982.

23. Hirsh J, Salzman EW, Harker L, et al: Aspirin and other platelet active drugs. Relationship among dose, effectiveness, and side effects. *Chest* 95(2 Suppl):12S–18S, 1989.

24. Page IH: Salicylate damage to the gastric mucosal barrier. *N Engl J Med* 276:1307, 1967.

25. Leonards JR, Levy G: The role of dosage form in aspirin-induced gastrointestinal bleeding. *Clin Pharmacol* 8:400, 1969.

26. Baigent C, Blackwell L, Collins R, et al: Aspirin in the primary and secondary prevention of vascular disease: Collaborative meta-analysis of individual participant data from randomised trials. *Lancet* 373(9678):1849–1860, 2009.

27. Stuart MJ, Gross SJ, Elrad H, Graeber JE: Effects of acetylsalicylic-acid ingestion on maternal and neonatal hemostasis. *N Engl J Med* 307(15):909–912, 1982.

28. Ferraris VA, Ferraris SP, Lough FC, Berry WR: Preoperative aspirin ingestion increases operative blood loss after coronary artery bypass grafting. *Ann Thorac Surg* 45(1):71–74, 1988.

29. Sethi GK, Copeland JG, Goldman S, et al: Implications of preoperative administration of aspirin in patients undergoing coronary artery bypass grafting. Department of Veterans Affairs Cooperative Study on Antiplatelet Therapy. *J Am Coll Cardiol* 15(1):15–20, 1990.

30. Horlocker TT, Wedel DJ, Offord KP: Does preoperative antiplatelet therapy increase the risk of hemorrhagic complications associated with regional anesthesia? *Anesth Analg* 70(6):631–634, 1990.

31. Kitchen L, Erichson RB, Sideropoulos H: Effect of drug-induced platelet dysfunction on surgical bleeding. *Am J Surg* 143(2):215–217, 1982.

32. Devereaux PJ, Mrkobrada M, Sessler DI, et al; POISE-2 Investigators: Aspirin in patients undergoing noncardiac surgery. *N Engl J Med* 370(16):1494–1503, 2014.

33. Kennedy BM: Aspirin and surgery—A review. *Ir Med J* 77(11):363–369, 1984.

34. Livio M, Benigni A, Vigano G, et al: Moderate doses of aspirin and risk of bleeding in renal failure. *Lancet* 1(8478):414–416, 1986.

35. Gaspari F, Vigano G, Orisio S, et al: Aspirin prolongs bleeding time in uremia by a mechanism distinct from platelet cyclooxygenase inhibition. *J Clin Invest* 79(6):1788–1797, 1987.

36. Chesebro JH, Fuster V, Elveback LR, et al: Trial of combined warfarin plus dipyridamole or aspirin therapy in prosthetic heart valve replacement: Danger of aspirin compared with dipyridamole. *Am J Cardiol* 51(9):1537–1541, 1983.

37. Kobrinsky NL, Israels ED, Gerrard JM, et al: Shortening of bleeding time by 1-deamino-8-D-arginine vasopressin in various bleeding disorders. *Lancet* 1(8387):1145–1148, 1984.

38. Lethagen S, Rugarn P: The effect of DDAVP and placebo on platelet function and prolonged bleeding time induced by oral acetyl salicylic acid intake in healthy volunteers. *Thromb Haemost* 67(1):185–186, 1992.

39. Kasmeridis C, Apostolakis S, Lip GY: Aspirin and aspirin resistance in coronary artery disease. *Curr Opin Pharmacol* 13(2):242–250, 2013.

40. Grosser T, Fries S, Lawson JA, et al: Drug resistance and pseudoresistance: An unintended consequence of enteric coating aspirin. *Circulation* 127(3):377–385, 2013.

41. Floyd CN, Ferro A: Mechanisms of aspirin resistance. *Pharmacol Ther* 141(1):69–78, 2014.

42. Catella-Lawson F, Reilly MP, Kapoor SC, et al: Cyclooxygenase inhibitors and the antiplatelet effects of aspirin. *N Engl J Med* 345(25):1809–1817, 2001.

43. Mielke CH Jr, Kahn SB, Muschek LD, et al: Effects of zomepirac on hemostasis in healthy adults and on platelet function *in vitro*. *J Clin Pharmacol* 20(5–6 Pt 2):409–417, 1980.

44. Lamberts M, Lip GY, Hansen ML, et al: Relation of nonsteroidal anti-inflammatory drugs to serious bleeding and thromboembolism risk in patients with atrial fibrillation receiving antithrombotic therapy: A nationwide cohort study. *Ann Intern Med* 161(10):690–698, 2014.

45. Thomas P, Hepburn B, Kim HC, Saidi P: Nonsteroidal anti-inflammatory drugs in the treatment of hemophilic arthropathy. *Am J Hematol* 12(2):131–137, 1982.

46. McIntyre BA, Philp RB, Inwood MJ: Effect of ibuprofen on platelet function in normal subjects and hemophiliac patients. *Clin Pharmacol Ther* 24(5):616–621, 1978.

47. Ragni MV, Miller BJ, Whalen R, Ptachcinski R: Bleeding tendency, platelet function, and pharmacokinetics of ibuprofen and zidovudine in HIV(+) hemophilic men. *Am J Hematol* 40(3):176–182, 1992.

48. Li X, Fries S, Li R, et al: Differential impairment of aspirin-dependent platelet cyclo-oxygenase acetylation by nonsteroidal antiinflammatory drugs. *Proc Natl Acad Sci U S A* 111(47):16830–16835, 2014.

49. Kearney PM, Baigent C, Godwin J, et al: Do selective cyclo-oxygenase-2 inhibitors and traditional non-steroidal anti-inflammatory drugs increase the risk of atherothrombosis? Meta-analysis of randomised trials. *BMJ* 332(7553):1302–1308, 2006.

50. Antman EM, Bennett JS, Daugherty A, et al: Use of nonsteroidal antiinflammatory drugs: An update for clinicians: A scientific statement from the American Heart Association. *Circulation* 115(12):1634–1642, 2007.

51. Solomon SD, Wittes J, Finn PV, et al: Cardiovascular risk of celecoxib in 6 randomized placebo-controlled trials: The cross trial safety analysis. *Circulation* 117(16):2104–2113, 2008.

52. Trelle S, Reichenbach S, Wandel S, et al: Cardiovascular safety of non-steroidal anti-inflammatory drugs: Network meta-analysis. *BMJ* 342:c7086, 2011.

53. McGettigan P, Henry D: Cardiovascular risk and inhibition of cyclooxygenase: A systematic review of the observational studies of selective and nonselective inhibitors of cyclooxygenase 2. *JAMA* 296(13):1633–1644, 2006.

54. Coxib and Traditional NSAID Trialists' (CNT) Collaboration, Bhala N, Emberson J, Merhi A, et al: Vascular and upper gastrointestinal effects of non-steroidal anti-inflammatory drugs: Meta-analyses of individual participant data from randomised trials. *Lancet* 382(9894):769–779, 2013.

55. Schmidt M, Christiansen CF, Mehnert F, et al: Non-steroidal anti-inflammatory drug use and risk of atrial fibrillation or flutter: Population based case-control study. *BMJ* 343:d3450, 2011.

56. Hinz B, Cheremina O, Brune K: Acetaminophen (paracetamol) is a selective cyclooxygenase-2 inhibitor in man. *FASEB J* 22(2):383–390, 2008.

57. CAPRIE Steering Committee: A randomised, blinded, trial of clopidogrel versus aspirin in patients at risk of ischaemic events (CAPRIE). CAPRIE Steering Committee. *Lancet* 348(9038):1329–1339, 1996.

58. McTavish D, Faulds D, Goa KL: Ticlopidine. An updated review of its pharmacology and therapeutic use in platelet-dependent disorders. *Drugs* 40(2):238–259, 1990.

59. Geiger J, Brich J, Honig-Liedl P, et al: Specific impairment of human platelet P2Y(AC) ADP receptor-mediated signaling by the antiplatelet drug clopidogrel. *Arterioscler Thromb Vasc Biol* 19(8):2007–2011, 1999.

60. Daniel JL, Dangelmaier C, Jin J, et al: Molecular basis for ADP-induced platelet activation. I. Evidence for three distinct ADP receptors on human platelets. *J Biol Chem* 273(4):2024–2029, 1998.

61. Farid NA, Kurihara A, Wrighton SA: Metabolism and disposition of the thienopyridine antiplatelet drugs ticlopidine, clopidogrel, and prasugrel in humans. *J Clin Pharmacol* 50(2):126–142, 2010.

62. Yusuf S, Zhao F, Mehta SR, et al: Effects of clopidogrel in addition to aspirin in patients with acute coronary syndromes without ST-segment elevation. *N Engl J Med* 345(7):494–502, 2001.

63. De Caterina R, Sicari R, Bernini W, et al: Benefit/risk profile of combined antiplatelet therapy with ticlopidine and aspirin. *Thromb Haemost* 65(5):504–510, 1991.

64. Helft G, Osende JI, Worthley SG, et al: Acute antithrombotic effect of a front-loaded regimen of clopidogrel in patients with atherosclerosis on aspirin. *Arterioscler Thromb Vasc Biol* 20(10):2316–2321, 2000.

65. Parodi G, Valenti R, Bellandi B, et al: Comparison of prasugrel and ticagrelor loading doses in ST-segment elevation myocardial infarction patients: RAPID (Rapid Activity of Platelet Inhibitor Drugs) primary PCI study. *J Am Coll Cardiol* 61(15):1601–1606, 2013.

66. Collet JP, Hulot JS, Pena A, et al: Cytochrome P450 2C19 polymorphism in young patients treated with clopidogrel after myocardial infarction: A cohort study. *Lancet* 373(9660):309–317, 2009.

67. Mega JL, Close SL, Wiviott SD, et al: Cytochrome p-450 polymorphisms and response to clopidogrel. *N Engl J Med* 360(4):354–362, 2009.

68. Jernberg T, Payne CD, Winters KJ, et al: Prasugrel achieves greater inhibition of platelet aggregation and a lower rate of non-responders compared with clopidogrel in aspirin-treated patients with stable coronary artery disease. *Eur Heart J* 27(10):1166–1173, 2006.

69. Brandt JT, Payne CD, Wiviott SD, et al: A comparison of prasugrel and clopidogrel loading doses on platelet function: Magnitude of platelet inhibition is related to active metabolite formation. *Am Heart J* 153(1):66 e9–e16, 2007.

70. Wiviott SD, Braunwald E, McCabe CH; TRITON-TIMI 38 Investigators: Prasugrel versus clopidogrel in patients with acute coronary syndromes. *N Engl J Med* 357(20):2001–2015, 2007.

71. Hass WK, Easton JD, Adams HP Jr, et al: A randomized trial comparing ticlopidine hydrochloride with aspirin for the prevention of stroke in high-risk patients. Ticlopidine Aspirin Stroke Study Group. *N Engl J Med* 321(8):501–507, 1989.

72. Gent M, Blakely JA, Easton JD, et al: The Canadian American Ticlopidine Study (CATS) in thromboembolic stroke. *Lancet* 1(8649):1215–1220, 1989.

73. Mataix R, Ojeda E, Perez MC, Jimenez S: Ticlopidine and severe aplastic anaemia. *Br J Haematol* 80(1):125–126, 1992.

74. Garnier G, Taillan B, Pesce A, et al: Ticlopidine and severe aplastic anaemia. *Br J Haematol* 81(3):459–460, 1992.

75. Bennett CL, Weinberg PD, Rozenberg-Ben-Dror K, et al: Thrombotic thrombocytopenic purpura associated with ticlopidine. A review of 60 cases. *Ann Intern Med* 128(7):541–544, 1998.

76. Steinhubl SR, Tan WA, Foody JM, Topol EJ: Incidence and clinical course of thrombotic thrombocytopenic purpura due to ticlopidine following coronary stenting. EPISTENT Investigators. Evaluation of Platelet IIb/IIIa Inhibitor for Stenting. *JAMA* 281(9):806–810, 1999.

77. Chen DK, Kim JS, Sutton DM: Thrombotic thrombocytopenic purpura associated with ticlopidine use: A report of 3 cases and review of the literature. *Arch Intern Med* 159(3):311–314, 1999.

78. Bennett CL, Connors JM, Carwile JM, et al: Thrombotic thrombocytopenic purpura associated with clopidogrel. *N Engl J Med* 342(24):1773–1777, 2000.

79. Leon MB, Baim DS, Popma JJ, et al: A clinical trial comparing three antithrombotic-drug regimens after coronary-artery stenting. Stent Anticoagulation Restenosis Study Investigators. *N Engl J Med* 339(23):1665–1671, 1998.

80. Steinhubl SR, Berger PB, Mann JT 3rd, et al: Early and sustained dual oral antiplatelet therapy following percutaneous coronary intervention: A randomized controlled trial. *JAMA* 288(19):2411–2420, 2002.

81. Bhatt DL, Fox KA, Hacke W, et al: Clopidogrel and aspirin versus aspirin alone for the prevention of atherothrombotic events. *N Engl J Med* 354(16):1706–1717, 2006.

82. Lee GM, Welsby IJ, Phillips-Bute B, et al: High incidence of antibodies to protamine and protamine/heparin complexes in patients undergoing cardiopulmonary bypass. *Blood* 121(15):2828–2835, 2013.

83. Bellemain-Appaix A, O'Connor SA, Silvain J, et al; ACTION Group: Association of clopidogrel pretreatment with mortality, cardiovascular events, and major bleeding among patients undergoing percutaneous coronary intervention: A systematic review and meta-analysis. *JAMA* 308(23):2507–2516, 2012.

84. Parodi G, Storey RF: Dyspnoea management in acute coronary syndrome patients treated with ticagrelor. *Eur Heart J Acute Cardiovasc Care* 4(6):555-560, 2015.

85. Alexopoulos D, Xanthopoulou I, Gkizas V, et al: Randomized assessment of ticagrelor versus prasugrel antiplatelet effects in patients with ST-segment-elevation myocardial infarction. *Circ Cardiovasc Interv* 5(6):797–804, 2012.

86. Franchi F, Rollini F, Muniz-Lozano A, et al: Cangrelor: A review on pharmacology and clinical trial development. *Expert Rev Cardiovasc Ther* 11(10):1279–1291, 2013.

87. Bhatt DL, Stone GW, Mahaffey KW, et al; CHAMPION PHOENIX Investigators: Effect of platelet inhibition with cangrelor during PCI on ischemic events. *N Engl J Med* 368(14):1303–1313, 2013.

88. Wallentin L, Becker RC, Budaj A, et al: Ticagrelor versus clopidogrel in patients with acute coronary syndromes. *N Engl J Med* 361(11):1045–1057, 2009.

89. Montalescot G, van't Hof AW, Lapostolle F, et al; ATLANTIC Investigators: Prehospital ticagrelor in ST-segment elevation myocardial infarction. *N Engl J Med* 371(11):1016–1027, 2014.

90. Kahn ML, Nakanishi-Matsui M, Shapiro MJ, et al: Protease-activated receptors 1 and 4 mediate activation of human platelets by thrombin. *J Clin Invest* 103(6):879–887, 1999.

91. Chackalamannil S, Xia Y, Greenlee WJ, et al: Discovery of potent orally active thrombin receptor (protease activated receptor 1) antagonists as novel antithrombotic agents. *J Med Chem* 48(19):5884–5887, 2005.

92. Zhang C, Srinivasan Y, Arlow DH, et al: High-resolution crystal structure of human protease-activated receptor 1. *Nature* 492(7429):387–392, 2012.

93. Morrow DA, Braunwald E, Bonaca MP, et al; TRA 2P–TIMI 50 Steering Committee and Investigators: Vorapaxar in the secondary prevention of atherothrombotic events. *N Engl J Med* 366(15):1404–1413, 2012.

94. Goto S, Ogawa H, Takeuchi M, et al; J-LANCELOT (Japanese-Lesson from Antagonizing the Cellular Effect of Thrombin) Investigators: Double-blind, placebo-controlled phase II studies of the protease-activated receptor 1 antagonist E5555 (atopaxar) in Japanese patients with acute coronary syndrome or high-risk coronary artery disease. *Eur Heart J* 31(21):2601–2613, 2010.

95. Lefkovits J, Plow EF, Topol EJ: Platelet glycoprotein IIb/IIIa receptors in cardiovascular medicine. *N Engl J Med* 332(23):1553–1559, 1995.

96. Bennett JS, Mousa S: Platelet function inhibitors in the Year 2000. *Thromb Haemost* 85(3):395–400, 2001.

97. Hook KM, Bennett JS: Glycoprotein IIb/IIIa antagonists. *Handb Exp Pharmacol* 2012(210):199–223, 1994.

98. French DL, Seligsohn U: Platelet glycoprotein IIb/IIIa receptors and Glanzmann's thrombasthenia. *Arterioscler Thromb Vasc Biol* 20(3):607–610, 2000.

99. Nurden AT: Inherited abnormalities of platelets. *Thromb Haemost* 82(2):468–480, 1999.

100. Use of a monoclonal antibody directed against the platelet glycoprotein IIb/IIIa receptor in high-risk coronary angioplasty. The EPIC Investigation. *N Engl J Med* 330(14):956–961, 1994.

101. EPILOG Investigators: Platelet glycoprotein IIb/IIIa receptor blockade and low-dose heparin during percutaneous coronary revascularization. *N Engl J Med* 336(24):1689–1696, 1997.

102. Inhibition of the platelet glycoprotein IIb/IIIa receptor with tirofiban in unstable angina and non-Q-wave myocardial infarction. Platelet Receptor Inhibition in Ischemic Syndrome Management in Patients Limited by Unstable Signs and Symptoms (PRISM-PLUS) Study Investigators. *N Engl J Med* 338(21):1488–1497, 1998.

103. Inhibition of platelet glycoprotein IIb/IIIa with eptifibatide in patients with acute coronary syndromes. The PURSUIT Trial Investigators. Platelet Glycoprotein IIb/IIIa in Unstable Angina: Receptor Suppression Using Integrilin Therapy. *N Engl J Med* 339(7):436–443, 1998.

104. Simpfendorfer C, Kottke-Marchant K, Lowrie M, et al: First chronic platelet glycoprotein IIb/IIIa integrin blockade. A randomized, placebo-controlled pilot study of xemilofiban in unstable angina with percutaneous coronary interventions. *Circulation* 96(1):76–81, 1997.

105. Cannon CP, McCabe CH, Borzak S, et al: Randomized trial of an oral platelet glycoprotein IIb/IIIa antagonist, sibrafiban, in patients after an acute coronary syndrome: Results of the TIMI 12 trial. Thrombolysis in Myocardial Infarction. *Circulation* 97(4):340–349, 1998.

106. Bhatt DL, Chew DP, Hirsch AT, et al: Superiority of clopidogrel versus aspirin in patients with prior cardiac surgery. *Circulation* 103(3):363–368, 2001.

107. Bassler N, Loeffler C, Mangin P, et al: A mechanistic model for paradoxical platelet activation by ligand-mimetic alphaIIb beta3 (GPIIb/IIIa) antagonists. *Arterioscler Thromb Vasc Biol* 27(3):e9–e15, 2007.

108. Ferguson JJ, Kereiakes DJ, Adgey AA, et al: Safe use of platelet GP IIb/IIIa inhibitors. *Eur Heart J* 19(Suppl D):D40–D51, 1998.

109. Berkowitz SD, Sane DC, Sigmon KN, et al: Occurrence and clinical significance of thrombocytopenia in a population undergoing high-risk percutaneous coronary revascularization. Evaluation of c7E3 for the Prevention of Ischemic Complications (EPIC) Study Group. *J Am Coll Cardiol* 32(2):311–319, 1998.

110. Giugliano RP, McCabe CH, Sequeira RF, et al: First report of an intravenous and oral glycoprotein IIb/IIIa inhibitor (RPR 109891) in patients with recent acute coronary syndromes: Results of the TIMI 15A and 15B trials. *Am Heart J* 140(1):81–93, 2000.

111. Comparison of sibrafiban with aspirin for prevention of cardiovascular events after acute coronary syndromes: A randomised trial. The SYMPHONY Investigators. Sibrafiban versus Aspirin to Yield Maximum Protection from Ischemic Heart Events Post-acute Coronary Syndromes. *Lancet* 355(9201):337–345, 2000.

112. Hongo RH, Brent BN: Association of eptifibatide and acute profound thrombocytopenia. *Am J Cardiol* 88(4):428–431, 2001.

113. McClure MW, Berkowitz SD, Sparapani R, et al: Clinical significance of thrombocytopenia during a non-ST-elevation acute coronary syndrome. The platelet glycoprotein IIb/IIIa in unstable angina: Receptor suppression using Integrilin therapy (PURSUIT) trial experience. *Circulation* 99(22):2892–2900, 1999.

114. Abrams CS, Cines DB: Platelet glycoprotein IIb/IIIa inhibitors and thrombocytopenia: Possible link between platelet activation, autoimmunity and thrombosis. *Thromb Haemost* 88(6):888–889, 2002.

115. Christopoulos CG, Machin SJ: A new type of pseudothrombocytopenia: EDTA-mediated agglutination of platelets bearing Fab fragments of a chimaeric antibody. *Br J Haematol* 87(3):650–652, 1994.

116. Sane DC, Damaraju LV, Topol EJ, et al: Occurrence and clinical significance of pseudothrombocytopenia during abciximab therapy. *J Am Coll Cardiol* 36(1):75–83, 2000.

117. Ivy DD, Kinsella JP, Ziegler JW, Abman SH: Dipyridamole attenuates rebound pulmonary hypertension after inhaled nitric oxide withdrawal in postoperative congenital heart disease. *J Thorac Cardiovasc Surg* 115(4):875–882, 1998.

118. Gresele P, Arnout J, Deckmyn H, Vermylen J: Mechanism of the antiplatelet action of dipyridamole in whole blood: Modulation of adenosine concentration and activity. *Thromb Haemost* 55(1):12–18, 1986.

119. FitzGerald GA: Dipyridamole. *N Engl J Med* 316:1247, 1987.

120. Reilly M, FitzGerald GA: Gathering intelligence on antiplatelet drugs: The view from 30 000 feet. When combined with other information overviews lead to conviction. *BMJ* 324(7329):59–60, 2002.

121. Diener HC, Cunha L, Forbes C, et al: European Stroke Prevention Study. 2. Dipyridamole and acetylsalicylic acid in the secondary prevention of stroke. *J Neurol Sci* 143(1–2):1–13, 1996.

122. Fisher CA, Kappa JR, Sinha AK, et al: Comparison of equimolar concentrations of iloprost, prostacyclin, and prostaglandin E1 on human platelet function. *J Lab Clin Med* 109(2):184–190, 1987.

123. Fish KJ, Sarnquist FH, van Steennis C, et al: A prospective, randomized study of the effects of prostacyclin on platelets and blood loss during coronary bypass operations. *J Thorac Cardiovasc Surg* 91(3):436–442, 1986.

124. Sorkin EM, Markham A: Cilostazol. *Drugs Aging* 14(1):63–71; discussion 72–73, 1999.

125. Biondi-Zoccai GG, Lotrionte M, Anselmino M, et al: Systematic review and meta-analysis of randomized clinical trials appraising the impact of cilostazol after percutaneous coronary intervention. *Am Heart J* 155(6):1081–1089, 2008.

126. Khuri SF, Valeri CR, Loscalzo J, et al: Heparin causes platelet dysfunction and induces fibrinolysis before cardiopulmonary bypass [see comments]. *Ann Thorac Surg* 60(4):1008–1014, 1995.

127. Sattler FR, Weitekamp MR, Ballard JO: Potential for bleeding with the new beta-lactam antibiotics. *Ann Intern Med* 105(6):924–931, 1986.

128. Pillgram-Larsen J, Wisloff F, Jorgensen JJ, et al: Effect of high-dose ampicillin and cloxacillin on bleeding time and bleeding in open-heart surgery. *Scand J Thorac Cardiovasc Surg* 19(1):45–48, 1985.

129. Fass RJ, Copelan EA, Brandt JT, et al: Platelet-mediated bleeding caused by broad-spectrum penicillins. *J Infect Dis* 155(6):1242–1248, 1987.

130. Cazenave JP, Packham MA, Guccione MA, Mustard JF: Effects of penicillin G on platelet aggregation, release, and adherence to collagen. *Proc Soc Exp Biol Med* 142(1):159–166, 1973.

131. Shattil SJ, Bennett JS, McDonough M, Turnbull J: Carbenicillin and penicillin G inhibit platelet function in vitro by impairing the interaction of agonists with the platelet surface. *J Clin Invest* 65(2):329–337, 1980.

132. Fletcher C, Pearson C, Choi SC, et al: *In vitro* comparison of antiplatelet effects of beta-lactam penicillins. *J Lab Clin Med* 108(3):217–223, 1986.

133. Packham MA, Rand ML, Perry DW, et al: Probenecid inhibits platelet responses to aggregating agents in vitro and has a synergistic inhibitory effect with penicillin G. *Thromb Haemost* 76(2):239–244, 1996.

134. Burroughs SF, Johnson GJ: Beta-lactam antibiotic-induced platelet dysfunction: Evidence for irreversible inhibition of platelet activation in vitro and in vivo after prolonged exposure to penicillin. *Blood* 75(7):1473–1480, 1990.

135. Sattler FR, Weitekamp MR, Sayegh A, Ballard JO: Impaired hemostasis caused by beta-lactam antibiotics. *Am J Surg* 155(5A):30–39, 1988.

136. Giles AR, Greenwood P, Tinlin S: A platelet release defect induced by aspirin or penicillin G does not increase gastrointestinal blood loss in thrombocytopenic rabbits. *Br J Haematol* 57(1):17–23, 1984.

137. Andrassy K, Koderisch J, Trenk D, et al: Hemostasis in patients with normal and impaired renal function under treatment with cefodizime. *Infection* 15(5):348–350, 1987.

138. Bloom A, Greaves M, Preston FE, Brown CB: Evidence against a platelet cyclooxygenase defect in uraemic subjects on chronic haemodialysis. *Br J Haematol* 62:143, 1986.

139. Rossi EC, Levin NW: Inhibition of primary ADP-induced platelet aggregation in normal subjects after administration of nitrofurantoin (furadantin). *J Clin Invest* 52(10):2457–2467, 1973.

140. Ishikawa S, Manabe S, Wada O: Miconazole inhibition of platelet aggregation by inhibiting cyclooxygenase. *Biochem Pharmacol* 35(11):1787–1792, 1986.

141. Salzman EW, Rosenberg RD, Smith MH, et al: Effect of heparin and heparin fractions on platelet aggregation. *J Clin Invest* 65(1):64–73, 1980.

142. Horne MK 3rd, Chao ES: Heparin binding to resting and activated platelets. *Blood* 74(1):238–243, 1989.

143. Sobel M, McNeill PM, Carlson PL, et al: Heparin inhibition of von Willebrand factor-dependent platelet function in vitro and in vivo. *J Clin Invest* 87(5):1787–1793, 1991.

144. Coller BS: Platelets and thrombolytic therapy. *N Engl J Med* 322(1):33–42, 1990.

145. Niewiarowski S, Senyi AF, Gillies P: Plasmin-induced platelet aggregation and platelet release reaction. Effects on hemostasis. *J Clin Invest* 52(7):1647–1659, 1973.

146. Fitzgerald DJ, Catella F, Roy L, FitzGerald GA: Marked platelet activation in vivo after intravenous streptokinase in patients with acute myocardial infarction. *Circulation* 77(1):142–150, 1988.

147. Kerins DM, Roy L, FitzGerald GA, Fitzgerald DJ: Platelet and vascular function during coronary thrombolysis with tissue-type plasminogen activator. *Circulation* 80(6):1718–1725, 1989.

148. Thorsen LI, Brosstad F, Gogstad G, et al: Competitions between fibrinogen with its degradation products for interactions with the platelet-fibrinogen receptor. *Thromb Res* 44(5):611–623, 1986.

149. Miles LA, Ginsberg MH, White JG, Plow EF: Plasminogen interacts with human platelets through two distinct mechanisms. *J Clin Invest* 77(6):2001–2009, 1986.

150. Adelman B, Michelson AD, Loscalzo J, et al: Plasmin effect on platelet glycoprotein Ib-von Willebrand factor interactions. *Blood* 65(1):32–40, 1985.

151. Stricker RB, Wong D, Shiu DT, et al: Activation of plasminogen by tissue plasminogen activator on normal and thrombasthenic platelets: Effects on surface proteins and platelet aggregation. *Blood* 68(1):275–280, 1986.

152. Schafer AI, Adelman B: Plasmin inhibition of platelet function and of arachidonic acid metabolism. *J Clin Invest* 75(2):456–461, 1985.

153. Loscalzo J, Vaughan DE: Tissue plasminogen activator promotes platelet disaggregation in plasma. *J Clin Invest* 79(6):1749–1755, 1987.

154. Penny WF, Ware JA: Platelet activation and subsequent inhibition by plasmin and recombinant tissue-type plasminogen activator. *Blood* 79(1):91–98, 1992.

155. Winters KJ, Eisenberg PR, Jaffe AS, Santoro SA: Dependence of plasmin-mediated degradation of platelet adhesive receptors on temperature and Ca2+. *Blood* 76(8):1546–1557, 1990.

156. Hines R, Barash PG: Infusion of sodium nitroprusside induces platelet dysfunction in vitro. *Anesthesiology* 70(4):611–615, 1989.

157. Kroll MH, Schafer AI: Biochemical mechanisms of platelet activation. *Blood* 74:1181–1195, 1989.

158. Anfossi G, Russo I, Massucco P, et al: Studies on inhibition of human platelet function by sodium nitroprusside. Kinetic evaluation of the effect on aggregation and cyclic nucleotide content. *Thromb Res* 102(4):319–330, 2001.

159. Bozzo J, Hernandez MR, Galan AM, et al: Antiplatelet effects of sodium nitroprusside in flowing human blood: Studies under normoxic and hypoxic conditions. *Thromb Res* 97(4):217–225, 2000.

160. Jang EK, Azzam JE, Dickinson NT, et al: Roles for both cyclic GMP and cyclic AMP in the inhibition of collagen-induced platelet aggregation by nitroprusside. *Br J Haematol* 117(3):664–675, 2002.

161. Schafer AI, Alexander RW, Handin RI: Inhibition of platelet function by organic nitrate vasodilators. *Blood* 55(4):649–654, 1980.

162. Weksler BB, Gillick M, Pink J: Effect of propranolol on platelet function. *Blood* 49(2):185–196, 1977.

163. Leon R, Tiarks CY, Pechet L: Some observations on the *in vivo* effect of propranolol on platelet aggregation and release. *Am J Hematol* 5(2):117–121, 1978.

164. Hines R: Preservation of platelet function during trimethaphan infusion. *Anesthesiology* 72(5):834–837, 1990.

165. Hogman M, Frostell C, Arnberg H, Hedenstierna G: Bleeding time prolongation and NO inhalation. *Lancet* 341(8861):1664–1665, 1993.

166. Samama CM, Diaby M, Fellahi JL, et al: Inhibition of platelet aggregation by inhaled nitric oxide in patients with acute respiratory distress syndrome. *Anesthesiology* 83(1):56–65, 1995.

167. Gries A, Bode C, Peter K, et al: Inhaled nitric oxide inhibits human platelet aggregation, P-selectin expression, and fibrinogen binding *in vitro* and *in vivo*. *Circulation* 97(15):1481–1487, 1998.

168. Barnathan ES, Addonizio VP, Shattil SJ: Interaction of verapamil with human platelet alpha-adrenergic receptors. *Am J Physiol* 242(1):H19–H23, 1982.

169. Fujinishi A, Takahara K, Ohba C, et al: Effects of nisoldipine on cytosolic calcium, platelet aggregation, and coagulation/fibrinolysis in patients with coronary artery disease. *Angiology* 48(6):515–521, 1997.

170. Lawson D, Mehta J, Mehta P, et al: Cumulative effects of quinidine and aspirin on bleeding time and platelet a₂-adrenoceptors: Potential mechanism of bleeding diathesis in patients receiving this combination. *J Lab Clin Med* 108:581, 1986.

171. Aberg M, Hedner U, Bergentz SE: Effect of dextran 70 on factor VIII and platelet function in von Willebrand's disease. *Thromb Res* 12(5):629–634, 1978.

172. Mishler JM 4th: Synthetic plasma volume expanders—Their pharmacology, safety and clinical efficacy. *Clin Haematol* 13(1):75–92, 1984.

173. Kelton JG, Hirsh J: Bleeding associated with antithrombotic therapy. *Semin Hematol* 17(4):259–291, 1980.

174. Korttila K, Lauritsalo K, Sarmo A, et al: Suitability of plasma expanders in patients receiving low-dose heparin for prevention of venous thrombosis after surgery. *Acta Anaesthesiol Scand* 27(2):104–107, 1983.

175. Cope JT, Banks D, Mauney MC, et al: Intraoperative hetastarch infusion impairs hemostasis after cardiac operations. *Ann Thorac Surg* 63(1):78–82; discussion 82–83, 1997.

176. Ruttmann TG, James MF, Aronson I: *In vivo* investigation into the effects of haemodilution with hydroxyethyl starch (200/0.5) and normal saline on coagulation. *Br J Anaesth* 80(5):612–616, 1998.

177. Roberts JS, Bratton SL: Colloid volume expanders. Problems, pitfalls and possibilities. *Drugs* 55(5):621–630, 1998.

178. Avorn J, Patel M, Levin R, Winkelmayer WC: Hetastarch and bleeding complications after coronary artery surgery. *Chest* 124(4):1437–1442, 2003.

179. Treib J, Haass A, Pindur G: Coagulation disorders caused by hydroxyethyl starch. *Thromb Haemost* 78(3):974–983, 1997.

180. Scharbert G, Deusch E, Kress HG, et al: Inhibition of platelet function by hydroxyethyl starch solutions in chronic pain patients undergoing peridural anesthesia. *Anesth Analg* 99(3):823–827, 2004.

181. Svehla C, Spankova H, Mlejnkova M: The effect of tricyclic antidepressive drugs on adrenaline and adenosine diphosphate induced platelet aggregation. *J Pharm Pharmacol* 18(9):616–617, 1966.

182. Warlow C, Ogston D, Douglas AS: Platelet function after the administration of chlorpromazine to human subjects. *Haemostasis* 5(1):21–26, 1976.

183. Morishita S, Aoki S, Watanabe S: Different effect of desipramine on protein kinase C in platelets between bipolar and major depressive disorders. *Psychiatry Clin Neurosci* 53(1):11–15, 1999.

184. Hergovich N, Aigner M, Eichler HG, et al: Paroxetine decreases platelet serotonin storage and platelet function in human beings. *Clin Pharmacol Ther* 68(4):435–442, 2000.

185. Alderman CP, Seshadri P, Ben-Tovim DI: Effects of serotonin reuptake inhibitors on hemostasis. *Ann Pharmacother* 30(11):1232–1234, 1996.

186. Pai VB, Kelly MW: Bruising associated with the use of fluoxetine. *Ann Pharmacother* 30(7–8):786–788, 1996.

187. Corbin F, Blaise G, Sauve R: Differential effect of halothane and forskolin on platelet cytosolic Ca2+ mobilization and aggregation. *Anesthesiology* 89(2):401–410, 1998.

188. Aoki H, Mizobe T, Nozuchi S, Hiramatsu N: *In vivo* and *in vitro* studies of the inhibitory effect of propofol on human platelet aggregation. *Anesthesiology* 88(2):362–370, 1998.

189. Heesch CM, Negus BH, Steiner M, et al: Effects of *in vivo* cocaine administration on human platelet aggregation. *Am J Cardiol* 78(2):237–239, 1996.

190. Jennings LK, White MM, Sauer CM, et al: Cocaine-induced platelet defects. *Stroke* 24(9):1352–1359, 1993.

191. Togna G, Graziani M, Sorrentino C, Caprino L: Prostanoid production in the presence of platelet activation in hypoxic cocaine-treated rats. *Haemostasis* 26(6):311–318, 1996.

192. Batista A, Macedo T, Tavares P, et al: Nitric oxide production and nitric oxide synthase expression in platelets from heroin abusers before and after ultrarapid detoxification. *Ann N Y Acad Sci* 965:479–486, 2002.

193. Ahr DJ, Scialla SJ, Kimball DB Jr: Acquired platelet dysfunction following mithramycin therapy. *Cancer* 41(2):448–454, 1978.

194. Panella TJ, Peters W, White JG, et al: Platelets acquire a secretion defect after high-dose chemotherapy. *Cancer* 65(8):1711–1716, 1990.

195. Pogliani EM, Fantasia R, Lambertenghi-Deliliers G, Cofrancesco E: Daunorubicin and platelet function. *Thromb Haemost* 45(1):38–42, 1981.

196. McKenna R, Ahmad T, Ts'ao CH, Frischer H: Glutathione reductase deficiency and platelet dysfunction induced by 1,3-bis(2-chloroethyl)-1-nitrosourea. *J Lab Clin Med* 102(1):102–115, 1983.

197. Karolak L, Chandra A, Khan W, et al: High-dose chemotherapy-induced platelet defect: Inhibition of platelet signal transduction pathways. *Mol Pharmacol* 43(1):37–44, 1993.

198. O'Malley CJ, Rasko JE, Basser RL, et al: Administration of pegylated recombinant human megakaryocyte growth and development factor to humans stimulates the production of functional platelets that show no evidence of *in vivo* activation. *Blood* 88(9):3288–3298, 1996.

199. Vadhan-Raj S, Murray LJ, Bueso-Ramos C, et al: Stimulation of megakaryocyte and platelet production by a single dose of recombinant human thrombopoietin in patients with cancer. *Ann Intern Med* 126(9):673–681, 1997.

200. Gratacap MP, Martin V, Valera MC, et al: The new tyrosine-kinase inhibitor and anti-cancer drug dasatinib reversibly affects platelet activation *in vitro* and *in vivo*. *Blood* 114(9):1884–1892, 2009.

201. Byrd JC, Furman RR, Coutre SE, et al: Targeting BTK with ibrutinib in relapsed chronic lymphocytic leukemia. *N Engl J Med* 369(1):32–42, 2013.

202. Wang ML, Rule S, Martin P, et al: Targeting BTK with ibrutinib in relapsed or refractory mantle-cell lymphoma. *N Engl J Med* 369(6):507–516, 2013.

203. Advani RH, Buggy JJ, Sharman JP, et al: Bruton tyrosine kinase inhibitor ibrutinib (PCI-32765) has significant activity in patients with relapsed/refractory B-cell malignancies. *J Clin Oncol* 31(1):88–94, 2013.

204. Levade M, David E, Garcia C, et al: Ibrutinib treatment affects collagen and von Willebrand Factor-dependent platelet functions. *Blood* 124(26):3991–3995, 2014.

205. Quek LS, Bolen J, Watson SP: A role for Bruton's tyrosine kinase (Btk) in platelet activation by collagen. *Curr Biol* 8(20):1137–1140, 1998.

206. Atkinson BT, Ellmeier W, Watson SP: Tec regulates platelet activation by GPVI in the absence of Btk. *Blood* 102(10):3592–3599, 2003.

207. Cohen H, Neild GH, Patel R, et al: Evidence for chronic platelet hyperaggregability and in vivo activation in cyclosporin-treated renal allograft recipients. *Thromb Res* 49(1):91–101, 1988.

208. Thomson C, Forbes CD, Prentice CR: A comparison of the effects of antihistamines on platelet function. *Thromb Diath Haemorrh* 30(3):547–556, 1973.

209. Platelet function during long-term treatment with ketanserin of claudicating patients with peripheral atherosclerosis. A multi-center, double-blind, placebo-controlled trial. The PACK Trial Group. *Thromb Res* 55(1):13–23, 1989.

210. Parvez Z, Moncada R, Fareed J, Messmore HL: Antiplatelet action of intravascular contrast media. Implications in diagnostic procedures. *Invest Radiol* 19(3):208–211, 1984.

211. Rao AK, Rao VM, Willis J, et al: Inhibition of platelet function by contrast media: Iopamidol and ioxaglate versus iothalamate. Work in progress. *Radiology* 156(2):311–313, 1985.

212. Goodnight SH Jr, Harris WS, Connor WE: The effects of dietary omega 3 fatty acids on platelet composition and function in man: A prospective, controlled study. *Blood* 58(5):880–885, 1981.

213. Moncada S, Higgs EA: Arachidonate metabolism in blood cells and the vessel wall. *Clin Haematol* 15(2):273–292, 1986.

214. Leaf A, Weber PC: Cardiovascular effects of n-3 fatty acids. *N Engl J Med* 318(9):549–557, 1988.

215. Hammerschmidt DE: Szechwan purpura. *N Engl J Med* 302(21):1191–1193, 1980.

216. Srivastava KC: Onion exerts antiaggregatory effects by altering arachidonic acid metabolism in platelets. *Prostaglandins Leukot Med* 24(1):43–50, 1986.

217. Apitz-Castro R, Escalante J, Vargas R, Jain MK: Ajoene, the antiplatelet principle of garlic, synergistically potentiates the antiaggregatory action of prostacyclin, forskolin, indomethacin and dipyridamole on human platelets. *Thromb Res* 42(3):303–311, 1986.

218. Srivastava KC: Extracts from two frequently consumed spices—cumin (*Cuminum cyminum*) and turmeric (*Curcuma longa*)—inhibit platelet aggregation and alter eicosanoid biosynthesis in human blood platelets. *Prostaglandins Leukot Essent Fatty Acids* 37(1):57–64, 1989.

219. Pearson TC: The risk of thrombosis in essential thrombocythemia and polycythemia vera. *Semin Oncol* 29(3 Suppl 10):16–21, 2002.

220. Kessler CM: Propensity for hemorrhage and thrombosis in chronic myeloproliferative disorders. *Semin Hematol* 41(2 Suppl 3):10–14, 2004.

221. Tefferi A: Polycythemia vera and essential thrombocythemia: 2013 update on diagnosis, risk-stratification, and management. *Am J Hematol* 88(6):507–516, 2013.

222. Schafer AI: Thrombocytosis. *N Engl J Med* 350(12):1211–1219, 2004.

223. Alfirevic A, Duncan A, You J, et al: Recombinant factor VII is associated with worse survival in complex cardiac surgical patients. *Ann Thorac Surg* 98(2):618–624, 2014.

224. Wasserman LR, Gilbert HS: The treatment of polycythemia vera. *Med Clin North Am* 50(6):1501–1518, 1966.

225. Murphy S: Polycythemia vera. *Dis Mon* 38(3):153–212, 1992.

226. Carobbio A, Finazzi G, Antonioli E, et al: Thrombocytosis and leukocytosis interaction in vascular complications of essential thrombocythemia. *Blood* 112(8):3135–3137, 2008.

227. Schafer AI: Essential thrombocythemia. *Prog Hemost Thromb* 10:69–96, 1990.

228. Elliott MA, Tefferi A: Pathogenesis and management of bleeding in essential thrombocythemia and polycythemia vera. *Curr Hematol Rep* 3(5):344–351, 2004.

229. Kessler CM, Klein HG, Havlik RJ: Uncontrolled thrombocytosis in chronic myeloproliferative disorders. *Br J Haematol* 50(1):157–167, 1982.

230. McIntyre KJ, Hoagland HC, Silverstein MN, Petitt RM: Essential thrombocythemia in young adults. *Mayo Clin Proc* 66(2):149–154, 1991.

231. Michiels JJ, Berneman Z, Gadisseur A, et al: Immune-mediated etiology of acquired von Willebrand syndrome in systemic lupus erythematosus and in benign monoclonal gammopathy: Therapeutic implications. *Semin Thromb Hemost* 32(6):577–588, 2006.

232. Carobbio A, Antonioli E, Guglielmelli P, et al: Leukocytosis and risk stratification assessment in essential thrombocythemia. *J Clin Oncol* 26(16):2732–2736, 2008.

233. Budde U, Schaefer G, Mueller N, et al: Acquired von Willebrand's disease in the myeloproliferative syndrome. *Blood* 64(5):981–985, 1984.

234. Tiede A, Rand JH, Budde U, et al: How I treat the acquired von Willebrand syndrome. *Blood* 117(25):6777–6785, 2011.

235. Hernandez-Boluda JC, Gomez M: Target hematologic values in the management of essential thrombocythemia and polycythemia vera. *Eur J Haematol* 94(1):4–11, 2015.

236. Landolfi R, Di Gennaro L, Barbui T, et al: Leukocytosis as a major thrombotic risk factor in patients with polycythemia vera. *Blood* 109(6):2446–2452, 2007.

237. Gangat N, Strand J, Li CY, et al: Leucocytosis in polycythaemia vera predicts both inferior survival and leukaemic transformation. *Br J Haematol* 138(3):354–358, 2007.

238. Villmow T, Kemkes-Matthes B, Matzdorff AC: Markers of platelet activation and platelet-leukocyte interaction in patients with myeloproliferative syndromes. *Thromb Res* 108(2–3):139–145, 2002.

239. Falanga A, Marchetti M, Vignoli A, et al: Leukocyte-platelet interaction in patients with essential thrombocythemia and polycythemia vera. *Exp Hematol* 33(5):523–530, 2005.

240. Maldonado JE, Pintado T, Pierre RV: Dysplastic platelets and circulating megakaryocytes in chronic myeloproliferative diseases. I. The platelets: Ultrastructure and peroxidase reaction. *Blood* 43(6):797–809, 1974.

241. Bautista AP, Buckler PW, Towler HM, et al: Measurement of platelet life-span in normal subjects and patients with myeloproliferative disease with indium oxine labelled platelets. *Br J Haematol* 58(4):679–687, 1984.

242. Ginsberg AD: Platelet function in patients with high platelet counts. *Ann Intern Med* 82:506–511, 1975.

243. Janson PA, Jubelirer SJ, Weinstein MS, Deykin D: Treatment of bleeding tendency in uremia with cryoprecipitate. *N Engl J Med* 303:1318, 1980.

244. Pareti FI, Gugliotta L, Mannucci L, et al: Biochemical and metabolic aspects of platelet dysfunction in chronic myeloproliferative disorders. *Thromb Haemost* 47(2):84–89, 1982.

245. Schafer AI: Deficiency of platelet lipoxygenase activity in myeloproliferative disorders. *N Engl J Med* 306(7):381–386, 1982.

246. Sugiyama T, Okuma M, Ushikubi F, et al: A novel platelet aggregating factor found in a patient with defective collagen-induced platelet aggregation and autoimmune thrombocytopenia. *Blood* 69:1712–1720, 1987.

247. Kaywin P, McDonough M, Insel PA, Shattil SJ: Platelet function in essential thrombocythemia: Decreased epinephrine responsiveness associated with a deficiency of platelet alpha-adrenergic receptors. *N Engl J Med* 299:505–509, 1978.

248. Swart SS, Pearson D, Wood JK, Barnett DB: Functional significance of the platelet alpha2-adrenoceptor: Studies in patients with myeloproliferative disorders. *Thromb Res* 33(5):531–541, 1984.

249. Handa M, Watanabe K, Kawai Y, et al: Platelet unresponsiveness to collagen: Involvement of glycoprotein Ia-IIa (alpha 2 beta 1 integrin) deficiency associated with a myeloproliferative disorder. *Thromb Haemost* 73(3):521–528, 1995.

250. Moore SF, Hunter RW, Harper MT, et al: Dysfunction of the PI3 kinase/Rap1/integrin alpha(IIb)beta(3) pathway underlies ex vivo platelet hypoactivity in essential thrombocythemia. *Blood* 121(7):1209–1219, 2013.

251. Malpass TW, Savage B, Hanson SR, et al: Correlation between prolonged bleeding time and depletion of platelet dense granule ADP in patients with myelodysplastic and myeloproliferative disorders. *J Lab Clin Med* 103(6):894–904, 1984.

252. Mohri H: Acquired von Willebrand disease and storage pool disease in chronic myelocytic leukemia. *Am J Hematol* 22(4):391–401, 1986.

253. Walsh PN, Murphy S, Barry WE: The role of platelets in the pathogenesis of thrombosis and hemorrhage in patients with thrombocytosis. *Thromb Haemost* 38(4):1085–1096, 1977.

254. Kaplan R, Gabbeta J, Sun L, et al: Combined defect in membrane expression and activation of platelet GPIIb–IIIa complex without primary sequence abnormalities in myeloproliferative disease. *Br J Haematol* 111(3):954–964, 2000.

255. Berndt MC, Kabral A, Grimsley P, et al: An acquired Bernard-Soulier-like platelet defect associated with juvenile myelodysplastic syndrome. *Br J Haematol* 68(1):97–101, 1988.

256. Cooper B, Schafer AI, Puchalsky D, Handin RI: Platelet resistance to prostaglandin D2 in patients with myeloproliferative disorders. *Blood* 52(3):618–626, 1978.

257. Moore A, Nachman RL: Platelet Fc receptor. Increased expression in myeloproliferative disease. *J Clin Invest* 67(4):1064–1071, 1981.

258. Bolin RB, Okumura T, Jamieson GA: Changes in distribution of platelet membrane glycoproteins in patients with myeloproliferative disorders. *Am J Hematol* 3:63–71, 1977.

259. Eche N, Sie P, Caranobe C, et al: Platelets in myeloproliferative disorders. III: Glycoprotein profile in relation to platelet function and platelet density. *Scand J Haematol* 26(2):123–129, 1981.

260. Thibert V, Bellucci S, Cristofari M, et al: Increased platelet CD36 constitutes a common marker in myeloproliferative disorders. *Br J Haematol* 91(3):618–624, 1995.

261. Moliterno AR, Hankins WD, Spivak JL: Impaired expression of the thrombopoietin receptor by platelets from patients with polycythemia vera. *N Engl J Med* 338(9):572–580, 1998.

262. Humbert M, Nurden P, Bihour CP, et al: Ultrastructural studies of platelet aggregates from human subjects receiving clopidogrel and from a patient with an inherited defect of an ADP-dependent pathway of platelet activation. *Arterioscler Thromb Vasc Biol* 16(12):1532–1543, 1996.

263. Rocca B, Ciabattoni G, Tartaglione R, et al: Increased thromboxane biosynthesis in essential thrombocythemia. *Thromb Haemost* 74(5):1225–1230, 1995.

264. Landolfi R, Ciabattoni G, Patrignani P, et al: Increased thromboxane biosynthesis in patients with polycythemia vera: Evidence for aspirin-suppressible platelet activation *in vivo*. *Blood* 80(8):1965–1971, 1992.

265. Tripodi A, Chantarangkul V, Gianniello F, et al: Global coagulation in myeloproliferative neoplasms. *Ann Hematol* 92(12):1633–1639, 2013.

266. Marchetti M, Tartari CJ, Russo L, et al: Phospholipid-dependent procoagulant activity is highly expressed by circulating microparticles in patients with essential thrombocythemia. *Am J Hematol* 89(1):68–73, 2014.

267. Cazzola M, Kralovics R: From Janus kinase 2 to calreticulin: The clinically relevant genomic landscape of myeloproliferative neoplasms. *Blood* 123(24):3714–3719, 2014.

268. Baxter EJ, Scott LM, Campbell PJ, et al: Acquired mutation of the tyrosine kinase JAK2 in human myeloproliferative disorders. *Lancet* 365(9464):1054–1061, 2005.

269. Levine RL, Wadleigh M, Cools J, et al: Activating mutation in the tyrosine kinase JAK2 in polycythemia vera, essential thrombocythemia, and myeloid metaplasia with myelofibrosis. *Cancer Cell* 7(4):387–397, 2005.

270. James C, Ugo V, Le Couedic JP, et al: A unique clonal JAK2 mutation leading to constitutive signalling causes polycythaemia vera. *Nature* 434(7037):1144–1148, 2005.

271. Kralovics R, Passamonti F, Buser AS, et al: A gain-of-function mutation of JAK2 in myeloproliferative disorders. *N Engl J Med* 352(17):1779–1790, 2005.

272. Scott LM, Tong W, Levine RL, et al: JAK2 exon 12 mutations in polycythemia vera and idiopathic erythrocytosis. *N Engl J Med* 356(5):459–468, 2007.

273. Pardanani AD, Levine RL, Lasho T, et al: MPL515 mutations in myeloproliferative and other myeloid disorders: A study of 1182 patients. *Blood* 108(10):3472–3476, 2006.

274. Schnittger S, Bacher U, Haferlach C, et al: Characterization of 35 new cases with four different MPLW515 mutations and essential thrombocytosis or primary myelofibrosis. *Haematologica* 94(1):141–144, 2009.

275. Nangalia J, Massie CE, Baxter EJ, et al: Somatic CALR mutations in myeloproliferative neoplasms with nonmutated JAK2. *N Engl J Med* 369(25):2391–2405, 2013.

276. Klampfl T, Gisslinger H, Harutyunyan AS, et al: Somatic mutations of calreticulin in myeloproliferative neoplasms. *N Engl J Med* 369(25):2379–2390, 2013.

277. Arellano-Rodrigo E, Alvarez-Larran A, Reverter JC, et al: Increased platelet and leukocyte activation as contributing mechanisms for thrombosis in essential thrombocythemia and correlation with the JAK2 mutational status. *Haematologica* 91(2):169–175, 2006.

278. Falanga A, Marchetti M, Vignoli A, et al: V617F JAK-2 mutation in patients with essential thrombocythemia: Relation to platelet, granulocyte, and plasma hemostatic and inflammatory molecules. *Exp Hematol* 35(5):702–711, 2007.

279. Robertson B, Urquhart C, Ford I, et al: Platelet and coagulation activation markers in myeloproliferative diseases: Relationships with JAK2 V617 F status, clonality, and antiphospholipid antibodies. *J Thromb Haemost* 5(8):1679–1685, 2007.

280. Coucelo M, Caetano G, Sevivas T, et al: JAK2V617F allele burden is associated with thrombotic mechanisms activation in polycythemia vera and essential thrombocythemia patients. *Int J Hematol* 99(1):32–40, 2014.

281. Pemmaraju N, Moliterno AR, Williams DM, et al: The quantitative JAK2 V617F neutrophil allele burden does not correlate with thrombotic risk in essential thrombocytosis. *Leukemia* 21(10):2210–2212, 2007.

282. Rumi E, Harutyunyan AS, Pietra D, et al; Associazione Italiana per la Ricerca sul Cancro Gruppo Italiano Malattie Mieloproliferative I: CALR exon 9 mutations are somatically acquired events in familial cases of essential thrombocythemia or primary myelofibrosis. *Blood* 123(15):2416–2419, 2014.

283. Andrikovics H, Krahling T, Balassa K, et al: Distinct clinical characteristics of myeloproliferative neoplasms with calreticulin mutations. *Haematologica* 99(7):1184–1190, 2014.

284. Tefferi A, Wassie EA, Guglielmelli P, et al: Type 1 versus Type 2 calreticulin mutations in essential thrombocythemia: A collaborative study of 1027 patients. *Am J Hematol* 89(8):E121–E124, 2014.

285. Rotunno G, Mannarelli C, Guglielmelli P et al; Associazione Italiana per la Ricerca sul Cancro Gruppo Italiano Malattie Mieloproliferative I: Impact of calreticulin mutations on clinical and hematological phenotype and outcome in essential thrombocythemia. *Blood* 123(10):1552–1555, 2014.

286. Mitchell MC, Boitnott JK, Kaufman S, et al: Budd-Chiari syndrome: Etiology, diagnosis and management. *Medicine (Baltimore)* 61(4):199–218, 1982.

287. Murphy S: Thrombocytosis and thrombocythaemia. *Clin Haematol* 12(1):89–106, 1983.

288. Schafer AI: Bleeding and thrombosis in the myeloproliferative disorders. *Blood* 64(1):1–12, 1984.

289. Gangat N, Wolanskyj AP, Tefferi A: Abdominal vein thrombosis in essential thrombocythemia: Prevalence, clinical correlates, and prognostic implications. *Eur J Haematol* 77(4):327–333, 2006.

290. Yonal I, Pinarbasi B, Hindilerden F, et al: The clinical significance of JAK2V617F mutation for Philadelphia-negative chronic myeloproliferative neoplasms in patients with splanchnic vein thrombosis. *J Thromb Thrombolysis* 34(3):388–396, 2012.

291. Smalberg JH, Arends LR, Valla DC, et al: Myeloproliferative neoplasms in Budd-Chiari syndrome and portal vein thrombosis: A meta-analysis. *Blood* 120(25):4921–4928, 2012.

292. Valla D, Casadevall N, Huisse MG, et al: Etiology of portal vein thrombosis in adults. A prospective evaluation of primary myeloproliferative disorders. *Gastroenterology* 94(4):1063–1069, 1988.

293. Hoekstra J, Janssen HL: Vascular liver disorders (II): Portal vein thrombosis. *Neth J Med* 67(2):46–53, 2009.

294. Hoekstra J, Janssen HL: Vascular liver disorders (I): Diagnosis, treatment and prognosis of Budd-Chiari syndrome. *Neth J Med* 66(8):334–339, 2008.

295. Frewin R, Dowson A: Headache in essential thrombocythaemia. *Int J Clin Pract* 66(10):976–983, 2012.

296. Singh AK, Wetherley-Mein G: Microvascular occlusive lesions in primary thrombocythaemia. *Br J Haematol* 36(4):553–564, 1977.

297. van Genderen PJ, Terpstra W, Michiels JJ, et al: High-dose intravenous immunoglobulin delays clearance of von Willebrand factor in acquired von Willebrand disease. *Thromb Haemost* 73(5):891–892, 1995.

298. Michiels JJ, Berneman ZN, Schroyens W, Van Vliet HH: Pathophysiology and treatment of platelet-mediated microvascular disturbances, major thrombosis and bleeding complications in essential thrombocythaemia and polycythaemia vera. *Platelets* 15(2):67–84, 2004.

299. Rinder HM, Schuster JE, Rinder CS, et al: Correlation of thrombosis with increased platelet turnover in thrombocytosis. *Blood* 91(4):1288–1294, 1998.

300. Besses C, Cervantes F, Pereira A, et al: Major vascular complications in essential thrombocythemia: A study of the predictive factors in a series of 148 patients. *Leukemia* 13(2):150–154, 1999.

301. Barbui T, Barosi G, Grossi A, et al: Practice guidelines for the therapy of essential thrombocythemia. A statement from the Italian Society of Hematology, the Italian Society of Experimental Hematology and the Italian Group for Bone Marrow Transplantation. *Haematologica* 89(2):215–232, 2004.

302. De Stefano V, Za T, Rossi E, et al: Recurrent thrombosis in patients with polycythemia vera and essential thrombocythemia: Incidence, risk factors, and effect of treatments. *Haematologica* 93(3):372–380, 2008.

303. Finazzi G, Carobbio A, Thiele J, et al: Incidence and risk factors for bleeding in 1104 patients with essential thrombocythemia or prefibrotic myelofibrosis diagnosed according to the 2008 WHO criteria. *Leukemia* 26(4):716–719, 2012.

304. Schafer AI: Molecular basis of the diagnosis and treatment of polycythemia vera and essential thrombocythemia. *Blood* 107(11):4214–4222, 2006.

305. Beer PA, Erber WN, Campbell PJ, Green AR: How I treat essential thrombocythemia. *Blood* 117(5):1472–1482, 2011.

306. Vannucchi AM: How I treat polycythemia vera. *Blood* 124(22):3212–3220, 2014.

307. Spivak J: Daily aspirin—Only half the answer. *N Engl J Med* 350(2):99–101, 2004.

308. Marchioli R, Finazzi G, Specchia G, et al; CYTO-PV Collaborative Group: Cardiovascular events and intensity of treatment in polycythemia vera. *N Engl J Med* 368(1):22–33, 2013.

309. Kaplan ME, Mack K, Goldberg JD, et al: Long-term management of polycythemia vera with hydroxyurea: A progress report. *Semin Hematol* 23(3):167–171, 1986.

310. Gilbert HS: Modern treatment strategies in polycythemia vera. *Semin Hematol* 40(1 Suppl 1):26–29, 2003.

311. Barbui T, Finazzi G: Treatment indications and choice of a platelet-lowering agent in essential thrombocythemia. *Curr Hematol Rep* 2(3):248–256, 2003.

312. Cortelazzo S, Finazzi G, Ruggeri M, et al: Hydroxyurea for patients with essential thrombocythemia and a high risk of thrombosis. *N Engl J Med* 332(17):1132–1136, 1995.

313. Pescatore SL, Lindley C: Anagrelide: A novel agent for the treatment of myeloproliferative disorders. *Expert Opin Pharmacother* 1(3):537–546, 2000.

314. Emadi A, Spivak JL: Anagrelide: 20 years later. *Expert Rev Anticancer Ther* 9(1):37–50, 2009.

315. Solberg LA Jr, Tefferi A, Oles KJ, et al: The effects of anagrelide on human megakaryocytopoiesis. *Br J Haematol* 99(1):174–180, 1997.

316. Fruchtman SM, Petitt RM, Gilbert HS, et al: Anagrelide: Analysis of long-term efficacy, safety and leukemogenic potential in myeloproliferative disorders. *Leuk Res* 29(5):481–491, 2005.

317. Wagstaff AJ, Keating GM: Anagrelide: A review of its use in the management of essential thrombocythaemia. *Drugs* 66(1):111–131, 2006.

318. Campbell PJ, Scott LM, Buck G, et al: Definition of subtypes of essential thrombocythaemia and relation to polycythaemia vera based on JAK2 V617F mutation status: A prospective study. *Lancet* 366(9501):1945–1953, 2005.

319. Hultdin M, Sundstrom G, Wahlin A, et al: Progression of bone marrow fibrosis in patients with essential thrombocythemia and polycythemia vera during anagrelide treatment. *Med Oncol* 24(1):63–70, 2007.

320. Gisslinger H, Gotic M, Holowiecki J, et al; ANAHYDRET Study Group: Anagrelide compared with hydroxyurea in WHO-classified essential thrombocythemia: The ANAHYDRET Study, a randomized controlled trial. *Blood* 121(10):1720–1728, 2013.

321. Mohri H, Noguchi T, Kodama F, et al: Acquired von Willebrand disease due to inhibitor of human myeloma protein specific for von Willebrand factor. *Am J Clin Pathol* 87(5):663–668, 1987.

322. Michiels JJ, Abels J, Steketee J, et al: Erythromelalgia caused by platelet-mediated arteriolar inflammation and thrombosis in thrombocythemia. *Ann Intern Med* 102(4):466–471, 1985.

323. van Genderen PJ, Prins FJ, Lucas IS, et al: Decreased half-life time of plasma von Willebrand factor collagen binding activity in essential thrombocythaemia: Normalization after cytoreduction of the increased platelet count. *Br J Haematol* 99(4):832–836, 1997.

324. Pascale S, Petrucci G, Dragani A, et al: Aspirin-insensitive thromboxane biosynthesis in essential thrombocythemia is explained by accelerated renewal of the drug target. *Blood* 119(15):3595–3603, 2012.

325. Cavalca V, Rocca B, Squellerio I, et al: *in vivo* prostacyclin biosynthesis and effects of different aspirin regimens in patients with essential thrombocythaemia. *Thromb Haemost* 112(1):118–127, 2014.

326. Landolfi R, Marchioli R, Kutti J, et al: Efficacy and safety of low-dose aspirin in polycythemia vera. *N Engl J Med* 350(2):114–124, 2004.

327. Gangat N, Wolanskyj AP, Schwager S, Tefferi A: Predictors of pregnancy outcome in essential thrombocythemia: A single institution study of 63 pregnancies. *Eur J Haematol* 82(5):350–353, 2009.

328. Passamonti F, Randi ML, Rumi E, et al: Increased risk of pregnancy complications in patients with essential thrombocythemia carrying the JAK2 (617V>F) mutation. *Blood* 110(2):485–489, 2007.

329. Barbui T, Finazzi G: Myeloproliferative disease in pregnancy and other management issues. *Hematology Am Soc Hematol Educ Program* 246–252, 2006.

330. Sultan Y, Caen JP: Platelet dysfunction in preleukemic states and in various types of leukemia. *Ann N Y Acad Sci* 201:300–306, 1972.

331. Cowan DH, Haut MJ: Platelet function in acute leukemia. *J Lab Clin Med* 79(6):893–905, 1972.

332. Cowan DH, Graham RC Jr, Baunach D: The platelet defect in leukemia. Platelet ultrastructure, adenine nucleotide metabolism, and the release reaction. *J Clin Invest* 56(1):188–200, 1975.

333. Foss B, Bruserud O: Platelet functions and clinical effects in acute myelogenous leukemia. *Thromb Haemost* 99(1):27–37, 2008.

334. Leinoe EB, Hoffmann MH, Kjaersgaard E, et al: Prediction of haemorrhage in the early stage of acute myeloid leukaemia by flow cytometric analysis of platelet function. *Br J Haematol* 128(4):526–532, 2005.

335. Glembotsky AC, Bluteau D, Espasandin YR, et al: Mechanisms underlying platelet function defect in a pedigree with familial platelet disorder with a predisposition to acute myelogenous leukemia: Potential role for candidate RUNX1 targets. *J Thromb Haemost* 12(5):761–772, 2014.

336. Kaur G, Jalagadugula G, Mao G, Rao AK: RUNX1/core binding factor A2 regulates platelet 12-lipoxygenase gene (ALOX12): Studies in human RUNX1 haplodeficiency. *Blood* 115(15):3128–3135, 2010.

337. Quintas-Cardama A, Han X, Kantarjian H, Cortes J: Tyrosine kinase inhibitor-induced platelet dysfunction in patients with chronic myeloid leukemia. *Blood* 114(2):261–263, 2009.

338. Neelakantan P, Marin D, Laffan M, et al: Platelet dysfunction associated with ponatinib, a new pan BCR-ABL inhibitor with efficacy for chronic myeloid leukemia resistant to multiple tyrosine kinase inhibitor therapy. *Haematologica* 97(9):1444, 2012.

339. Meschengieser S, Blanco A, Maugeri N, et al: Platelet function and intraplatelet von Willebrand factor antigen and fibrinogen in myelodysplastic syndromes. *Thromb Res* 46(4):601–606, 1987.

340. Zeidman A, Sokolover N, Fradin Z, et al: Platelet function and its clinical significance in the myelodysplastic syndromes. *Hematol J* 5(3):234–238, 2004.

341. Bellucci S, Huisse MG, Boval B, et al: Defective collagen-induced platelet activation in two patients with malignant haemopathies is related to a defect in the GPVI-coupled signalling pathway. *Thromb Haemost* 93(1):130–138, 2005.

342. Girtovitis FI, Ntaios G, Papadopoulos A: Defective platelet aggregation in myelodysplastic syndromes. *Acta Haematol* 118(2):117–122, 2007.

343. Burbury KL, Seymour JF, Dauer R, Westerman DA: Under-recognition of platelet dysfunction in myelodysplastic syndromes: Are we only seeing the tip of the iceberg? *Leuk Lymphoma* 54(1):11–13, 2013.

344. Frigeni M, Galli M: Childhood myelodysplastic syndrome associated with an acquired Bernard-Soulier-like platelet dysfunction. *Blood* 124(16):2609, 2014.

345. Pui CH, Jackson CW, Chesney C: Normal platelet function after therapy for acute lymphocytic leukemia. *Arch Intern Med* 143(1):73–74, 1983.

346. Andre JM, Galambrun C, Trzeciak MC, et al: Acquired Glanzmann's thrombasthenia associated with acute lymphoblastic leukemia. *J Pediatr Hematol Oncol* 27(10):554–557, 2005.

347. Raman V, Quillen K, Sloan JM: Acquired Glanzmann thrombasthenia associated with Hodgkin lymphoma: Rapid reversal of functional platelet defect with ABVD (Adriamycin/bleomycin/vinblastine/dacarbazine) chemotherapy. *Clin Lymphoma Myeloma Leuk* 14(2):e51–e54, 2014.

348. Westbrook CA, Golde DW: Clinical problems in hairy cell leukemia: Diagnosis and management. *Semin Oncol* 11(4 Suppl 2):514–522, 1984.

349. Rosove MH, Naeim F, Harwig S, Zighelboim J: Severe platelet dysfunction in hairy cell leukemia with improvement after splenectomy. *Blood* 55(6):903–906, 1980.

350. Roussi JH, Houbouyan LL, Alterescu R, et al: Acquired von Willebrand's syndrome associated with hairy cell leukaemia. *Br J Haematol* 46(3):503–506, 1980.

351. Lackner H: Hemostatic abnormalities associated with dysproteinemias. *Semin Hematol* 10(2):125–133, 1973.

352. Coppola A, Tufano A, Di Capua M, Franchini M: Bleeding and thrombosis in multiple myeloma and related plasma cell disorders. *Semin Thromb Hemost* 37(8):929–945, 2011.

353. Perkins HA, MacKenzie MR, Fudenberg HH: Hemostatic defects in dysproteinemias. *Blood* 35(5):695–707, 1970.

354. Rapoport M, Yona R, Kaufman S, et al: Unusual bleeding manifestations of amyloidosis in patients with multiple myeloma. *Clin Lab Haematol* 16(4):349–353, 1994.

355. Furie B, Greene E, Furie BC: Syndrome of acquired factor X deficiency and systemic amyloidosis in vivo studies of the metabolic fate of factor X. *N Engl J Med* 297(2):81–85, 1977.

356. McPherson RA, Onstad JW, Ugoretz RJ, Wolf PL: Coagulopathy in amyloidosis: Combined deficiency of factors IX and X. *Am J Hematol* 3:225–235, 1977.

357. Palmer RN, Rick ME, Rick PD, Zeller JA, Gralnick HR: Circulating heparan sulfate anticoagulant in a patient with a fatal bleeding disorder. *N Engl J Med* 310(26):1696–1699, 1984.

358. Chapman GS, George CB, Danley DL: Heparin-like anticoagulant associated with plasma cell myeloma. *Am J Clin Pathol* 83(6):764–766, 1985.

359. Torjemane L, Guermazi S, Ladeb S, et al: Heparin-like anticoagulant associated with multiple myeloma and neutralized with protamine sulfate. *Blood Coagul Fibrinolysis* 18(3):279–281, 2007.

360. Liebman H, Chinowsky M, Valdin J, et al: Increased fibrinolysis and amyloidosis. *Arch Intern Med* 143(4):678–682, 1983.

361. Meyer K, Williams EC: Fibrinolysis and acquired alpha-2 plasmin inhibitor deficiency in amyloidosis. *Am J Med* 79(3):394–396, 1985.

362. McGrath KM, Stuart JJ, Richards F 2nd: Correlation between serum IgG, platelet membrane IgG, and platelet function in hypergammaglobulinaemic states. *Br J Haematol* 42(4):585–591, 1979.

363. Kasturi J, Saraya AK: Platelet functions in dysproteinaemia. *Acta Haematol* 59(2):104–113, 1978.

364. Vigliano EM, Horowitz HI: Bleeding syndrome in a patient with IgA myeloma: Interaction of protein and connective tissue. *Blood* 29(6):823–836, 1967.

365. Shinagawa A, Kojima H, Berndt MC, et al: Characterization of a myeloma patient with a life-threatening hemorrhagic diathesis: Presence of a lambda dimer protein inhibiting shear-induced platelet aggregation by binding to the A1 domain of von Willebrand factor. *Thromb Haemost* 93(5):889–896, 2005.

366. DiMinno G, Coraggio F, Cerbone AM, et al: A myeloma paraprotein with specificity for platelet glycoprotein IIIa in a patient with a fatal bleeding disorder. *J Clin Invest* 77:157–164, 1986.

367. Mannucci PM, Lombardi R, Bader R, et al: Studies of the pathophysiology of acquired von Willebrand's disease in seven patients with lymphoproliferative disorders or benign monoclonal gammopathies. *Blood* 64(3):614–621, 1984.

368. Takahashi H, Nagayama R, Tanabe Y, et al: DDAVP in acquired von Willebrand syndrome associated with multiple myeloma. *Am J Hematol* 22(4):421–429, 1986.

369. Lamboley V, Zabraniecki L, Sie P, et al: Myeloma and monoclonal gammopathy of uncertain significance associated with acquired von Willebrand's syndrome. Seven new cases with a literature review. *Joint Bone Spine* 69(1):62–67, 2002.

370. Federici AB: Acquired von Willebrand syndrome: Is it an extremely rare disorder or do we see only the tip of the iceberg? *J Thromb Haemost* 6(4):565–568, 2008.

371. Voisin S, Hamidou M, Lefrancois A, et al: Acquired von Willebrand syndrome associated with monoclonal gammopathy: A single-center study of 36 patients. *Medicine (Baltimore)* 90(6):404–411, 2011.

372. Howard CR, Lin TL, Cunningham MT, Lipe BC: IgG kappa monoclonal gammopathy of undetermined significance presenting as acquired type III von Willebrand syndrome. *Blood Coagul Fibrinolysis* 25(6):631–633, 2014.

373. Coucke L, Marcelis L, Deeren D, et al: Lymphoplasmacytic lymphoma exposed by haemoptysis and acquired von Willebrand syndrome. *Blood Coagul Fibrinolysis* 25(4):395–397, 2014.

374. Scepansky E, Othman M, Smith H: Acquired von Willebrand syndrome with a type 2B phenotype: Diagnostic and therapeutic dilemmas. *Acta Haematol* 131(4):213–217, 2014.

375. Wallace MR, Simon SR, Ershler WB, Burns SL: Hemorrhagic diathesis in multiple myeloma. *Acta Haematol* 72(5):340–342, 1984.

376. Hyman BT, Westrick MA: Multiple myeloma with polyneuropathy and coagulopathy. A case report of the polyneuropathy, organomegaly, endocrinopathy, M-protein, and skin change (POEMS) syndrome. *Arch Intern Med* 146(5):993–994, 1986.

377. Bovill EG, Ershler WB, Golden EA, et al: A human myeloma-produced monoclonal protein directed against the active subpopulation of von Willebrand factor. *Am J Clin Pathol* 85(1):115–123, 1986.

378. Silberstein LE, Abrahm J, Shattil SJ: The efficacy of intensive plasma exchange in acquired von Willebrand's disease. *Transfusion* 27(3):234–237, 1987.

379. Federici AB, Stabile F, Castaman G, et al: Treatment of acquired von Willebrand syndrome in patients with monoclonal gammopathy of uncertain significance: Comparison of three different therapeutic approaches. *Blood* 92(8):2707–2711, 1998.

380. Federici AB: Use of intravenous immunoglobulin in patients with acquired von Willebrand syndrome. *Hum Immunol* 66(4):422–430, 2005.

381. Federici AB, Budde U, Castaman G, et al: Current diagnostic and therapeutic approaches to patients with acquired von Willebrand syndrome: A 2013 update. *Semin Thromb Hemost* 39(2):191–201, 2013.

382. Mazoyer E, Fain O, Dhote R, Laurian Y: Is rituximab effective in acquired von Willebrand syndrome? *Br J Haematol* 144(6):967–968, 2009.

383. Michiels JJ, Budde U, van der Planken M, et al: Acquired von Willebrand syndromes: Clinical features, aetiology, pathophysiology, classification and management. *Best Pract Res Clin Haematol* 14(2):401–436, 2001.

384. Kumar S, Pruthi RK, Nichols WL: Acquired von Willebrand disease. *Mayo Clin Proc* 77(2):181–187, 2002.

385. Hong S, Lee J, Chi H, et al: Systemic lupus erythematosus complicated by acquired von Willebrand's syndrome. *Lupus* 17(9):846–848, 2008.

386. Pruthi RK: Hypertrophic obstructive cardiomyopathy, acquired von Willebrand syndrome, and gastrointestinal bleeding. *Mayo Clin Proc* 86(3):181–182, 2011.

387. Casonato A, Sponga S, Pontara E, et al: von Willebrand factor abnormalities in aortic valve stenosis: Pathophysiology and impact on bleeding. *Thromb Haemost* 106(1):58–66, 2011.

388. Heilmann C, Geisen U, Beyersdorf F, et al: Acquired von Willebrand syndrome in patients with extracorporeal life support (ECLS). *Intensive Care Med* 38(1):62–68, 2012.

389. Meyer AL, Malehsa D, Budde U, et al: Acquired von Willebrand syndrome in patients with a centrifugal or axial continuous flow left ventricular assist device. *JACC Heart Fail* 2(2):141–145, 2014.

390. Morrison KA, Jorde UP, Garan AR, et al: Acquired von Willebrand disease during CentriMag support is associated with high prevalence of bleeding during support and after transition to heart replacement therapy. *ASAIO J* 60(2):241–242, 2014.

391. Mitrovic M, Elezovic I, Miljic P, Suvajdzic N: Acquired von Willebrand syndrome in patients with Gaucher disease. *Blood Cells Mol Dis* 52(4):205–207, 2014.

392. Federici AB: Acquired von Willebrand syndrome associated with hypothyroidism: A mild bleeding disorder to be further investigated. *Semin Thromb Hemost* 37(1):35–40, 2011.

393. Stuijver DJ, Piantanida E, van Zaane B, et al: Acquired von Willebrand syndrome in patients with overt hypothyroidism: A prospective cohort study. *Haemophilia* 20(3):326–332, 2014.

394. Wiegand G, Hofbeck M, Zenker M, et al: Bleeding diathesis in Noonan syndrome: Is acquired von Willebrand syndrome the clue? *Thromb Res* 130(5):e251–e254, 2012.

395. Mazurier C, Parquet-Gernez A, Descamps J, et al: Acquired von Willebrand's syndrome in the course of Waldenström's disease. *Thromb Haemost* 44(3):115–118, 1980.

396. Handin RI, Martin V, Moloney WC: Antibody-induced von Willebrand's disease: A newly defined inhibitor syndrome. *Blood* 48(3):393–405, 1976.

397. Van Genderen PJ, Papatsonis DN, Michiels JJ, et al: High-dose intravenous gamma-globulin therapy for acquired von Willebrand disease. *Postgrad Med J* 70(830):916–920, 1994.

398. Goudemand J, Samor B, Caron C, et al: Acquired type II von Willebrand's disease: Demonstration of a complexed inhibitor of the von Willebrand factor-platelet interaction and response to treatment. *Br J Haematol* 68(2):227–233, 1988.

399. Mohri H, Hisanaga S, Mishima A, et al: Autoantibody inhibits binding of von Willebrand factor to glycoprotein Ib and collagen in multiple myeloma: Recognition sites present on the A1 loop and A3 domains of von Willebrand factor. *Blood Coagul Fibrinolysis* 9(1):91–97, 1998.

400. Igarashi N, Miura M, Kato E, et al: Acquired von Willebrand's syndrome with lupus-like serology. *Am J Pediatr Hematol Oncol* 11(1):32–35, 1989.

401. Agrawal AK, Golden C, Matsunaga A: Acquired von Willebrand disease in an osteosarcoma patient. *J Pediatr Hematol Oncol* 33(8):622–623, 2011.

402. Scott JP, Montgomery RR, Tubergen DG, Hays T: Acquired von Willebrand's disease in association with Wilms' [sic] tumor: Regression following treatment. *Blood* 58(4):665–669, 1981.

403. Rao KP, Kizer J, Jones TJ, et al: Acquired von Willebrand's syndrome associated with an extranodal pulmonary lymphoma. *Arch Pathol Lab Med* 112(1):47–50, 1988.

404. Baxter PA, Nuchtern JG, Guillerman RP, et al: Acquired von Willebrand syndrome and Wilms tumor: Not always benign. *Pediatr Blood Cancer* 52(3):392–394, 2009.

405. Levesque H, Borg JY, Cailleux N, et al: Acquired von Willebrand's syndrome associated with decrease of plasminogen activator and its inhibitor during hypothyroidism. *Eur J Med* 2(5):287–288, 1993.

406. Aylesworth CA, Smallridge RC, Rick ME, Alving BM: Acquired von Willebrand's disease: A rare manifestation of postpartum thyroiditis. *Am J Hematol* 50(3):217–219, 1995.

407. Tiede A, Priesack J, Werwitzke S, et al: Diagnostic workup of patients with acquired von Willebrand syndrome: A retrospective single-centre cohort study. *J Thromb Haemost* 6(4):569–576, 2008.

408. Joist JH, Cowan JF, Zimmerman TS: Acquired von Willebrand's disease. Evidence for a quantitative and qualitative factor VIII disorder. *N Engl J Med* 298(18):988–991, 1978.

409. Cushing M, Kawaguchi K, Friedman KD, Mark T: Factor VIII/von Willebrand factor concentrate therapy for ventricular assist device-associated acquired von Willebrand disease. *Transfusion* 52(7):1535–1541, 2012.

410. Jimenez AR, Vallejo ES, Cruz MZ, et al: Rituximab effectiveness in a patient with juvenile systemic lupus erythematosus complicated with acquired von Willebrand syndrome. *Lupus* 22(14):1514–1517, 2013.

411. Sucker C, Scharf RE, Zotz RB: Use of recombinant factor VIIa in inherited and acquired von Willebrand disease. *Clin Appl Thromb Hemost* 15(1):27–31, 2009.

412. Macik BG, Gabriel DA, White GC 2nd, et al: The use of high-dose intravenous gamma-globulin in acquired von Willebrand syndrome. *Arch Pathol Lab Med* 112(2):143–146, 1988.

413. Rinder MR, Richard RE, Rinder HM: Acquired von Willebrand's disease: A concise review. *Am J Hematol* 54(2):139–145, 1997.

414. Franchini M, Lippi G: Recent acquisitions in acquired and congenital von Willebrand disorders. *Clin Chim Acta* 377(1–2):62–69, 2007.

415. Biondo F, Matturro A, Santoro C, et al: Remission of acquired von Willebrand syndrome after successful treatment of gastric MALT lymphoma. *Haemophilia* 18(1):e34–e35, 2012.

416. Oliveira MC, Kramer CK, Marroni CP, et al: Acquired factor VIII and von Willebrand factor (aFVIII-VWF) deficiency and hypothyroidism in a case with hypopituitarism. *Clin Appl Thromb Hemost* 16(1):107–109, 2010.

417. Manfredi E, van Zaane B, Gerdes VE, et al: Hypothyroidism and acquired von Willebrand's syndrome: A systematic review. *Haemophilia* 14(3):423–433, 2008.

418. Budde U, Scharf RE, Franke P, et al: Elevated platelet count as a cause of abnormal von Willebrand factor multimer distribution in plasma. *Blood* 82:1749–1757, 1993.

419. Franchini M, Mannucci PM: von Willebrand disease-associated angiodysplasia: A few answers, still many questions. *Br J Haematol* 161(2):177–182, 2013.

420. Solomon C, Budde U, Schneppenheim S, et al: Acquired type 2A von Willebrand syndrome caused by aortic valve disease corrects during valve surgery. *Br J Anaesth* 106(4):494–500, 2011.

421. Rao AK: Uraemic platelets. *Lancet* 1:913, 1986.

422. Boccardo P, Remuzzi G, Galbusera M: Platelet dysfunction in renal failure. *Semin Thromb Hemost* 30(5):579–589, 2004.

423. Rosenbaum R, Hoffstein PE, Stanley RJ, Klahr S: Use of computerized tomography to diagnose complications of percutaneous renal biopsy. *Kidney Int* 14:87–92, 1978.

424. Diaz-Buxo JA, Donadio JVJ: Complications of percutaneous renal biopsy: An analysis of 1000 consecutive biopsies. *Clin Nephrol* 4:223, 1975.

425. Mannucci PM, Tripodi A: Hemostatic defects in liver and renal dysfunction. *Hematology Am Soc Hematol Educ Program* 168–173, 2012.

426. Valeri CR, Cassidy G, Pivacek LE, et al: Anemia-induced increase in the bleeding time: Implications for treatment of nonsurgical blood loss. *Transfusion* 41(8):977–983, 2001.

427. Castillo R, Lozano T, Escolar G, et al: Defective platelet adhesion on vessel subendothelium in uremic patients. *Blood* 68(2):337–342, 1986.

428. Livio M, Gotti E, Marchesi D, et al: Uraemic bleeding: Role of anaemia and beneficial effect of red cell transfusions. *Lancet* 2(8306):1013–1015, 1982.

429. Fernandez F, Goudable C, Sie P, et al: Low haematocrit and prolonged bleeding time in uraemic patients: Effect of red cell transfusions. *Br J Haematol* 59:139–148, 1985.

430. Moia M, Mannucci PM, Vizzotto L, et al: Improvement in the haemostatic defect of uraemia after treatment with recombinant human erythropoietin. *Lancet* 2:1227–1229, 1987.

431. Tang WW, Stead RA, Goodkin DA: Effects of epoetin alfa on hemostasis in chronic renal failure. *Am J Nephrol* 18:263–273, 1998.

432. Turrito VT, Weiss HJ: Red blood cells: Their dual role in thrombus formation. *Science* 207:541, 1980.

433. Casonato A, Pontara E, Vertolli UP, et al: Plasma and platelet von Willebrand factor abnormalities in patients with uremia: Lack of correlation with uremic bleeding. *Clin Appl Thromb Hemost* 7(2):81–86, 2001.

434. Zwaginga JJ, Ijsseldijk MJ, Beeser-Visser N, et al: High von Willebrand factor concentration compensates a relative adhesion defect in uremic blood. *Blood* 75:1498–1508, 1990.

435. Sloand EM, Sloand JA, Prodouz K, et al: Reduction of platelet glycoprotein Ib in uremia. *Br J Haematol* 77:375–381, 1991.

436. Gralnick HR, McKeown LP, Williams SB, et al: Plasma and platelet von Willebrand factor defects in uremia. *Am J Med* 85:806–810, 1988.

437. Escolar G, Cases A, Bastida E, et al: Uremic platelets have a functional defect affecting the interaction of von Willebrand factor with glycoprotein IIb-IIIa. *Blood* 76:1336–1340, 1990.

438. Di Minno G, Cerbone A, Usberti M, et al: Platelet dysfunction in uremia. II. Correction by arachidonic acid of the impaired exposure of fibrinogen receptors by adenosine diphosphate or collagen. *J Lab Clin Med* 108:246–252, 1986.

439. Rabiner SF, Hrodek O: Platelet factor 3 in normal subjects and patients with renal failure. *J Clin Invest* 47(4):901–912, 1968.

440. Ware JA, Clark BA, Smith M, Salzman EW: Abnormalities of cytoplasmic $Ca^{2+}$ in platelets from patients with uremia. *Blood* 73:172–176, 1989.

441. Mannucci PM, Remuzzi G, Pusineri F, et al: Deamino-8-arginine vasopressin shortens the bleeding time in uremia. *N Engl J Med* 308(1):8–12, 1983.

442. Winter M, Frampton G, Bennett A, et al: Synthesis of thromboxane $B_2$ in uraemia and the effects of dialysis. *Thromb Res* 30:265–272, 1983.

443. Neirynck N, Vanholder R, Schepers E, et al: An update on uremic toxins. *Int Urol Nephrol* 45(1):139–150, 2013.

444. Bazilinski N, Shaykh M, Dunea G, et al: Inhibition of platelet function by uremic middle molecules. *Nephron* 40:423–428, 1985.

445. Remuzzi G, Livio M, Marchiaro G, et al: Bleeding in renal failure: Altered platelet function in chronic uraemia only partially corrected by haemodialysis. *Nephron* 22:347–353, 1978.

446. Livio M, Benigni A, Remuzzi G: Coagulation abnormalities in uremia. *Semin Neprhol* 5:82–90, 1985.

447. Siqueira MA, Brunini TM, Pereira NR, et al: Increased nitric oxide production in platelets from severe chronic renal failure patients. *Can J Physiol Pharmacol* 89(2):97–102, 2011.

448. Meenakshi SR, Agarwal R: Nitric oxide levels in patients with chronic renal disease. Journal of clinical and diagnostic research: *J Clin Diagn Res* 7(7):1288–1290, 2013.

449. Remuzzi G, Perico N, Zoja C, et al: Role of endothelium-derived nitric oxide in the bleeding tendency of uremia. *J Clin Invest* 86(5):1768–1771, 1990.

450. Aiello S, Noris M, Todeschini M, et al: Renal and systemic nitric oxide synthesis in rats with renal mass reduction. *Kidney Int* 52:171–181, 1997.

451. Noris M, Remuzzi G: Uremic bleeding: Closing the circle after 30 years of controversies? *Blood* 94(8):2569–2574, 1999.

452. Mendes Ribeiro AC, Brunini TM, Ellory JC, Mann GE: Abnormalities in L-arginine transport and nitric oxide biosynthesis in chronic renal and heart failure. *Cardiovasc Res* 49(4):697–712, 2001.

453. Brunini TM, Yaqoob MM, Novaes Malagris LE, et al: Increased nitric oxide synthesis in uraemic platelets is dependent on L-arginine transport via system y(+)L. *Pflugers Arch* 445(5):547–550, 2003.

454. Linthorst GE, Avis HJ, Levi M: Uremic thrombocytopathy is not about urea. *J Am Soc Nephrol* 21(5):753–755, 2010.

455. Remuzzi G: Bleeding disorders in uremia: Pathophysiology and treatment. *Adv Nephrol Necker Hosp* 18:171–186, 1989.

456. Andrassy K, Ritz E: Uremia as a cause of bleeding. *Am J Nephrol* 5:313, 1985.

457. Ando M, Iwamoto Y, Suda A, et al: New insights into the thrombopoietic status of patients on dialysis through the evaluation of megakaryocytopoiesis in bone marrow and of endogenous thrombopoietin levels. *Blood* 97(4):915–921, 2001.

458. George CRP, Slichter SJ, Quadracci LJ: A kinetic evaluation of hemostasis in renal disease. *N Engl J Med* 291:1111, 1974.

459. Linthorst GE, Folman CC, van Olden RW, von dem Borne AE: Plasma thrombopoietin levels in patients with chronic renal failure. *Hematol J* 3(1):38–42, 2002.

460. A comparison of two doses of aspirin (30 mg vs. 283 mg a day) in patients after a transient ischemic attack or minor ischemic stroke. The Dutch TIA Trial Study Group. *N Engl J Med* 325(18):1261–1266, 1991.

461. Peterson P, Hayes TE, Arkin CF, et al: The preoperative bleeding time test lacks clinical benefit. *Arch Surg* 133:134–139, 1998.

462. Stewart JH, Castaldi PA: Uraemic bleeding: A reversible platelet defect corrected by dialysis. *Q J Med* 36(143):409–423, 1967.

463. Lindsay RM, Friesen M, Koens F, et al: Platelet function in patients on long-term peritoneal dialysis. *Clin Nephrol* 6:335–339, 1976.

464. Weigert AL, Schafer AI: Uremic bleeding: Pathogenesis and therapy. *Am J Med Sci* 316:94–104, 1998.

465. Vigano G, Benigni A, Mendogni D, et al: Recombinant human erythropoietin to correct uremic bleeding. *Am J Kidney Dis* 18:44–49, 1991.

466. Tassies D, Reventer JC, Cases A, et al: Effect of recombinant human erythropoietin treatment on circulating reticulated platelets in uremic patients: Association with early improvement in platelet function. *Am J Hematol* 59(2):105–109, 1998.

467. Mannucci PM: Desmopressin: A non-transfusional form of treatment for congenital and acquired bleeding disorders. *Blood* 72:1449, 1988.

468. Rose EH, Aledort LM: Nasal spray desmopressin (DDAVP) for mild hemophilia A and von Willebrand disease. *Ann Intern Med* 114:563, 1991.

469. Canavese C, Salomone M, Pacitti A, et al: Reduced response of uraemic bleeding time to repeated doses of desmopressin. *Lancet* 1:867, 1985.

470. Byrnes JJ, Larcada A, Moake JL: Thrombosis following desmopressin for uremic bleeding. *Am J Hematol* 28:63, 1988.

471. Mannucci PM, Lusher JM: Desmopressin and thrombosis. *Lancet* 2(8664):675–676, 1989.

472. Liu YK, Kosfeld RE, Marcum SG: Treatment of uremic bleeding with conjugated estrogen. *Lancet* 2(8408):887–890, 1984.

473. Vigano G, Gaspari F, Locatelli M, et al: Dose-effect and pharmacokinetics of estrogens given to correct bleeding time in uremia. *Kidney Int* 34:853–858, 1988.

474. Heistinger M, Stockenhuber F, Schneider B, et al: Effect of conjugated estrogens on platelet function and prostacyclin generation in CRF. *Kidney Int* 38:1181–1186, 1990.

475. Bronner MH, Pate MD, Cunningham JT, Marsh WH: Estrogen-progesterone therapy for bleeding of gastrointestinal telangiectasias in chronic renal failure. *Ann Intern Med* 105(3):371–374, 1986.

476. Vigano G, Zoja C, Corna D, et al: 17 Beta-estradiol is the most active component of the conjugated estrogen mixture active on uremic bleeding by a receptor mechanism. *Mol Pharmacol* 252(1):344–348, 1990.

477. Triulzi DJ, Blumber N: Variability in response to cryoprecipitate treatment for hemostatic defects in uremia. *Yale J Biol Med* 63:1–7, 1990.

478. Thompson AR, Harker LA: Approach to bleeding disorders, in *Manual of Hemostasis and Thrombosis*, 3rd ed, pp 57–64. FA Davis, Philadelphia, 1983.

479. Bloor AJ, Smith GA, Jaswon M, et al: Acquired thrombasthenia due to GPIIbIIIa platelet autoantibodies in a 4-yr-old child. *Eur J Haematol* 76(1):89–90, 2006.

480. Porcelijn L, Huiskes E, Maatman R, et al: Acquired Glanzmann's thrombasthenia caused by glycoprotein IIb/IIIa autoantibodies of the immunoglobulin G$_1$ (IgG$_1$), IgG$_2$ or IgG$_4$ subclass: A study in six cases. *Vox Sang* 95(4):324–330, 2008.

481. Blickstein D, Dardik R, Rosenthal E, et al: Acquired thrombasthenia due to inhibitory effect of glycoprotein IIbIIIa autoantibodies. *Isr Med Assoc J* 16(5):307–310, 2014.

482. Solh M, Mescher C, Klappa A, et al: Acquired Glanzmann's thrombasthenia with optimal response to rituximab therapy. *Am J Hematol* 86(8):715–716, 2011.

483. George JN, Woolf SH, Raskob GE, et al: Idiopathic thrombocytopenic purpura: A practice guideline developed by explicit methods for the American Society of Hematology. *Blood* 88(1):3–40, 1996.

484. George JN, El-Harake MA, Raskob GE: Chronic idiopathic thrombocytopenic purpura. *N Engl J Med* 331:1207–1215, 1994.

485. McMillan R: Antiplatelet antibodies in chronic adult immune thrombocytopenic purpura: Assays and epitopes. *J Pediatr Hematol Oncol* 25(Suppl 1):S57–S61, 2003.

486. Meyer M, Kirchmaier CM, Schirmer A, et al: Acquired disorder of platelet function associated with autoantibodies against membrane glycoprotein IIb-IIIa complex-1. Glycoprotein analysis. *Thromb Haemost* 65:491–496, 1991.

487. Balduini CL, Grignani G, Sinigaglia F, et al: Severe platelet dysfunction in a patient with autoantibodies against membrane glycoproteins IIb-IIIa. *Haemostasis* 7:98–104, 1987.

488. Balduini CL, Bertolino G, Noris P, et al: Defect of platelet aggregation and adhesion induced by autoantibodies against platelet glycoprotein IIIa. *Thromb Haemost* 68:208–213, 1992.

489. Fuse I, Higuchi W, Narita M, et al: Overproduction of antiplatelet antibody against glycoprotein IIb after splenectomy in a patient with Evans syndrome resulting in acquired thrombasthenia [see comments]. *Acta Haematol* 99(2):83–88, 1998.

490. Stricker RB, Wong D, Saks SR, et al: Acquired Bernard-Soulier syndrome: Evidence for the role of a 210,000-molecular weight protein in the interaction of platelets with von Willebrand factor. *J Clin Invest* 76:1274–1278, 1985.

491. Devine DV, Currie MS, Rosse WF, Greenberg CS: Pseudo-Bernard-Soulier syndrome: Thrombocytopenia caused by autoantibody to platelet glycoprotein Ib. *Blood* 70:428–431, 1987.

492. Deckmyn H, Zhang J, Van Houtte E, Vermylen J: Production and nucleotide sequence of an inhibitory human IgM autoantibody directed against platelet glycoprotein Ia/IIa. *Blood* 84(6):1968–1974, 1994.

493. Dromigny A, Triadou P, Lesavre P, et al: Lack of platelet response to collagen associated with autoantibodies against glycoprotein (GP) Ia/IIa and Ib/IX leading to the discovery of SLE. *Hematol Cell Ther* 38(4):355–357, 1996.

494. Boylan B, Chen H, Rathore V, et al: Anti-GPVI-associated ITP: An acquired platelet disorder caused by autoantibody-mediated clearance of the GPVI/FcRgamma-chain complex from the human platelet surface. *Blood* 104(5):1350–1355, 2004.

495. Wiedmer T, Ando B, Sims PJ: Complement C5b-9-stimulated platelet secretion is associated with a calcium-initiated activation of cellular protein kinases. *J Biol Chem* 262:13674, 1987.

496. Warkentin TE: Heparin-induced thrombocytopenia: Pathogenesis and management. *Br J Haematol* 121(4):535–555, 2003.

497. Lechner K, Pabinger I, Obermeier HL, Knoebl P: Immune-mediated disorders causing bleeding or thrombosis in lymphoproliferative diseases. *Semin Thromb Hemost* 40(3):359–370, 2014.

498. Giannini S, Mezzasoma AM, Guglielmini G, et al: A new case of acquired Glanzmann's thrombasthenia: Diagnostic value of flow cytometry. *Cytometry B Clin Cytom* 74(3):194–199, 2008.

499. Kannan M, Chatterjee T, Ahmad F, et al: Acquired Glanzmann's thrombasthenia associated with hairy cell leukaemia. *Eur J Clin Invest* 39(12):1110–1111, 2009.

500. Lackner H, Karpatkin S: On the "easy bruising" syndrome with normal platelet count: A study of 75 patients. *Ann Intern Med* 83(2):190–196, 1975.

501. Clancy R, Jenkins E, Firkin B: Qualitative platelet abnormalities in idiopathic thrombocytopenic purpura. *N Engl J Med* 286:622, 1972.

502. Heyns DA, Fraser J, Retief FP: Platelet aggregation in chronic idiopathic thrombocytopenic purpura. *J Clin Pathol* 31:1239, 1978.

503. Regan MG, Lackner H, Karpatkin S: Platelet function and coagulation profile in lupus erythematosus. *Am J Med* 81:462, 1974.

504. Dorsch CA, Meyerhoff J: Mechanisms of abnormal platelet aggregation in systemic lupus erythematosus. *Arthritis Rheum* 25:966, 1982.

505. Meyerhoff J, Dorsch CA: Decreased platelet serotonin levels in systemic lupus erythematosus. *Arthritis Rheum* 24:1495, 1981.

506. Stuart MJ, Kelton JG, Allen JB: Abnormal platelet function and arachidonate metabolism in chronic idiopathic thrombocytopenic purpura. *Blood* 58:326, 1981.

507. Harker LA, Malpass TW, Branson HE, et al: Mechanism of abnormal bleeding in patients undergoing cardiopulmonary bypass: Acquired transient platelet dysfunction associated with selective alpha-granule release. *Blood* 56:824–834, 1980.

508. Woodman RC, Harker LA: Bleeding complications associated with cardiopulmonary bypass. *Blood* 76:1680–1697, 1990.

509. Mammen EF, Koets MH, Washington BC, et al: Hemostasis changes during cardiopulmonary bypass surgery. *Semin Thromb Hemost* 11:281, 1985.

510. Khuri SF, Wolfe JA, Josa M, et al: Hematologic changes during and after cardiopulmonary bypass and their relationship to the bleeding time and nonsurgical blood loss. *J Thorac Cardiovasc Surg* 104:94–107, 1992.

511. Martin JF, Daniel TD, Trowbridge EA: Acute and chronic changes in platelet volume and count after cardiopulmonary bypass induced thrombocytopenia in man. *Thromb Haemost* 57(1):55–58, 1987.

512. Chandler AB, Hutson MS: Platelet plug formation in an extracorporeal unit. *Am J Clin Pathol* 64(1):101–107, 1975.

513. Lindon JN, McManama, Kushner L: Does the conformation of adsorbed fibrinogen dictate platelet interactions with artificial surfaces? *Blood* 68:355, 1986.

514. Singer RL, Mannion JD, Bauer TL, Armenti FR, Edie RN: Complications from heparin-induced thrombocytopenia in patients undergoing cardiopulmonary bypass. *Chest* 104(5):1436–1440, 1993.

515. Pouplard C, Leroux D, Rollin J, et al: Incidence of antibodies to protamine sulfate/heparin complexes in cardiac surgery patients and impact on platelet activation and clinical outcome. *Thromb Haemost* 109(6):1141–1147, 2013.

516. Bakchoul T, Zollner H, Amiral J, et al: Anti-protamine-heparin antibodies: Incidence, clinical relevance, and pathogenesis. *Blood* 121(15):2821–2827, 2013.

517. Panzer S, Schiferer A, Steinlechner B, et al: Serological features of antibodies to protamine inducing thrombocytopenia and thrombosis. *Clin Chem Lab Med* 53(2):249–255, 2015.

518. Bick RL: Hemostasis defects associated with cardiac surgery, prosthetic devices, and other extracorporeal circuits. *Semin Thromb Hemost* 11(3):249–280, 1985.

519. Bachmann F, McKenna R, Cole ER, Najafi H: The hemostatic mechanism after open heart surgery. I. Studies on plasma coagulation factors and fibrinolysis in 512 patients after extracorporeal circulation. *J Thorac Cardiovasc Surg* 70:76, 1975.

520. Beurling-Harbury C, Galvan CA: Acquired decrease in platelet secretory ADP associated with increased post-operative bleeding in post-cardiopulmonary bypass patients and in patients with severe valvular heart disease. *Blood* 52:13, 1978.

521. Abrams CS, Ellison N, Budzynski AZ, Shattil S: Direct detection of activated platelets and platelet-derived microparticles in humans. *Blood* 75:128–138, 1990.

522. Nannizzi-Alaimo L, Rubenstein MH, Alves VL, et al: Cardiopulmonary bypass induces release of soluble CD40 ligand. *Circulation* 105(24):2849–2854, 2002.

523. Wahba A, Rothe G, Lodes H, et al: The influence of the duration of cardiopulmonary bypass on coagulation, fibrinolysis and platelet function. *Thorac Cardiovasc Surg* 49(3):153–156, 2001.

524. George JN, Pickett EB, Saucerman S, et al: Platelet surface glycoproteins. Studies on resting and activated platelets and platelet membrane microparticles in normal subjects, and observations in patients during adult respiratory distress syndrome and cardiac surgery. *J Clin Invest* 78(2):340–348, 1986.

525. Gluszko P, Ricinski B, Musial J, et al: Fibrinogen receptors in platelet adhesion to surfaces of extracorporeal circuit. *Am J Physiol* 252:H615, 1987.

526. van den Dengen JJ, Karliczek GF, Brenken U, et al: Clinical study of blood trauma during perfusion with membrane and bubble oxygenators. *J Thorac Cardiovasc Surg* 83(1):108–116, 1982.

527. Edmunds LH Jr, Colman RW: Thrombin during cardiopulmonary bypass. *Ann Thorac Surg* 82(6):2315–2322, 2006.
528. Gabel J, Hakimi CS, Westerberg M, et al: Retransfusion of cardiotomy suction blood impairs haemostasis: *Ex vivo* and *in vivo* studies. *Scand Cardiovasc J* 47(6):368–376, 2013.
529. Kestin AS, Valeri CR, Khuri SF, et al: The platelet function defect of cardiopulmonary bypass. *Blood* 82:107–117, 1993.
530. Weksler BB, Pett SB, Alonso D, et al: Differential inhibition of aspirin of vascular prostaglandin synthesis in atherosclerotic patients. *N Engl J Med* 308:800–805, 1983.
531. Levy JH: Pharmacologic preservation of the hemostatic system during cardiac surgery. *Ann Thorac Surg* 72(5):S1814–S1820, 2001.
532. Tabuchi N, de Haan J, Boonstra PW, van Oeveren W: Activation of fibrinolysis in the pericardial cavity during cardiopulmonary bypass. *J Thorac Cardiovasc Surg* 106(5):828–833, 1993.
533. Hunt BJ, Parratt RN, Segal HC, et al: Activation of coagulation and fibrinolysis during cardiothoracic operations. *Ann Thorac Surg* 65(3):712–718, 1998.
534. Rapaport SI: Preoperative hemostatic evaluation: Which tests, if any? *Blood* 61(2):229–231, 1983.
535. Magovern JA, Sakert T, Benckart DH, et al: A model for predicting transfusion after coronary artery bypass grafting [see comments]. *Ann Thorac Surg* 61(1):27–32, 1996.
536. Simon TA, Akl BF, Murphy W: Controlled trial of routine administration of platelet concentrates in cardiopulmonary bypass surgery. *Ann Thorac Surg* 37:359, 1987.
537. Wasser MN, Houbiers JG, D'Amaro J, et al: The effect of fresh versus stored blood on post-operative bleeding after coronary bypass surgery: A prospective randomized study. *Br J Haematol* 72:81–84, 1989.
538. Sowade O, Warnke H, Scigalla P, et al: Avoidance of allogeneic blood transfusions by treatment with epoetin beta (recombinant human erythropoietin) in patients undergoing open-heart surgery. *Blood* 89(2):411–418, 1997.
539. Shimpo H, Mizumoto T, Onoda K, et al: Erythropoietin in pediatric cardiac surgery: Clinical efficacy and effective dose. *Chest* 111(6):1565–1570, 1997.
540. Schmoeckel M, Nollert G, Mempel M, et al: Effects of recombinant human erythropoietin on autologous blood donation before open heart surgery. *Thorac Cardiovasc Surg* 41(6):364–368, 1993.
541. Axford TC, Dearani JA, Ragno G, et al: Safety and therapeutic effectiveness of reinfused shed blood after open heart surgery [see comments]. *Ann Thorac Surg* 57(3):615–622, 1994.
542. Griffith LD, Billman GF, Daily PO, Lane TA: Apparent coagulopathy caused by infusion of shed mediastinal blood and its prevention by washing of the infusate [see comments]. *Ann Thorac Surg* 47(3):400–406, 1989.
543. Hsu LC: Heparin-coated cardiopulmonary bypass circuits: Current status. *Perfusion* 16(5):417–428, 2001.
544. Spijker HT, Graaff R, Boonstra PW, et al: On the influence of flow conditions and wettability on blood material interactions. *Biomaterials* 24(26):4717–4727, 2003.
545. Lappegard KT, Fung M, Bergseth G, et al: Effect of complement inhibition and heparin coating on artificial surface-induced leukocyte and platelet activation. *Ann Thorac Surg* 77(3):932–941, 2004.
546. Weerwind PW, Caberg NE, Reutelingsperger CP, et al: Exposure of procoagulant phospholipids on the surface of platelets in patients undergoing cardiopulmonary bypass using non-coated and heparin-coated extracorporeal circuits. *Int J Artif Organs* 25(8):770–776, 2002.
547. Johnell M, Elgue G, Larsson R, et al: Coagulation, fibrinolysis, and cell activation in patients and shed mediastinal blood during coronary artery bypass grafting with a new heparin-coated surface. *J Thorac Cardiovasc Surg* 124(2):321–332, 2002.
548. Linneweber J, Chow TW, Kawamura M, et al: *In vitro* comparison of blood pump induced platelet microaggregates between a centrifugal and roller pump during cardiopulmonary bypass. *Int J Artif Organs* 25(6):549–555, 2002.
549. Despotis GJ, Avidan MS, Hogue CW Jr: Mechanisms and attenuation of hemostatic activation during extracorporeal circulation. *Ann Thorac Surg* 72(5):S1821–S1831, 2001.
550. Nuttall GA, Erchul DT, Haight TJ, et al: A comparison of bleeding and transfusion in patients who undergo coronary artery bypass grafting via sternotomy with and without cardiopulmonary bypass. *J Cardiothorac Vasc Anesth* 17(4):447–451, 2003.
551. Mariani MA, Gu YJ, Boonstra PW, et al: Procoagulant activity after off-pump coronary operation: Is the current anticoagulation adequate? *Ann Thorac Surg* 67(5):1370–1375, 1999.
552. Paparella D, Galeone A, Venneri MT, et al: Activation of the coagulation system during coronary artery bypass grafting: Comparison between on-pump and off-pump techniques. *J Thorac Cardiovasc Surg* 131(2):290–297, 2006.
553. Vallely MP, Bannon PG, Bayfield MS, et al: Quantitative and temporal differences in coagulation, fibrinolysis and platelet activation after on-pump and off-pump coronary artery bypass surgery. *Heart Lung Circ* 18(2):123–130, 2009.
554. Hackmann T, Gascoyne R, Naiman SC, et al: A trial of desmopressin to reduce blood loss in uncomplicated cardiac surgery. *N Engl J Med* 321:1437–1444, 1989.
555. Seear MD, Wadsworth LD, Rogers PC, et al: The effect of desmopressin acetate (DDAVP) on postoperative blood loss after cardiac operations in children [see comments]. *J Thorac Cardiovasc Surg* 98(2):217–219, 1989.
556. Wademan BH, Galvin SD: Desmopressin for reducing postoperative blood loss and transfusion requirements following cardiac surgery in adults. *Interact Cardiovasc Thorac Surg* 18(3):360–370, 2014.
557. Walker ID, Davidson JF, Faichney A, et al: A double-blind study of prostacyclin in cardiopulmonary bypass surgery. *Br J Haematol* 49:415–423, 1981.
558. Society of Thoracic Surgeons Blood Conservation Guideline Task Force, Ferraris VA, Brown JR, Despotis GJ, et al: 2011 update to the Society of Thoracic Surgeons and the Society of Cardiovascular Anesthesiologists blood conservation clinical practice guidelines. *Ann Thorac Surg* 91(3):944–982, 2011.
559. O'Connell KA, Wood JJ, Wise RP, et al: Thromboembolic adverse events after use of recombinant human coagulation factor VIIa. *JAMA* 295(3):293–298, 2006.
560. Goodnough LT, Levy JH: Off-label use of recombinant human factor VIIa. *Ann Thorac Surg* 98(2):393–395, 2014.
561. Giannini E, Botta F, Borro P, et al: Relationship between thrombopoietin serum levels and liver function in patients with chronic liver disease related to hepatitis C virus infection. *Am J Gastroenterol* 98(11):2516–2520, 2003.
562. Nussmeier NA, Whelton AA, Brown MT, et al: Complications of the COX-2 inhibitors parecoxib and valdecoxib after cardiac surgery. *N Engl J Med* 352(11):1081–1091, 2005.
563. Mangano DT, Tudor IC, Dietzel C: The risk associated with aprotinin in cardiac surgery. *N Engl J Med* 354(4):353–365, 2006.
564. Schneeweiss S, Seeger JD, Landon J, Walker AM: Aprotinin during coronary-artery bypass grafting and risk of death. *N Engl J Med* 358(8):771–783, 2008.
565. Shaw AD, Stafford-Smith M, White WD, et al: The effect of aprotinin on outcome after coronary-artery bypass grafting. *N Engl J Med* 358(8):784–793, 2008.
566. Fergusson DA, Hebert PC, Mazer CD, et al: A comparison of aprotinin and lysine analogues in high-risk cardiac surgery. *N Engl J Med* 358(22):2319–2331, 2008.
567. Amitrano L, Guardascione MA, Brancaccio V, Balzano A: Coagulation disorders in liver disease. *Semin Liver Dis* 22(1):83–96, 2002.
568. Lisman T, Porte RJ: Rebalanced hemostasis in patients with liver disease: Evidence and clinical consequences. *Blood* 116(6):878–885, 2010.
569. Hugenholtz GC, Adelmeijer J, Meijers JC, et al: An unbalance between von Willebrand factor and ADAMTS13 in acute liver failure: Implications for hemostasis and clinical outcome. *Hepatology* 58(2):752–761, 2013.
570. Krauss JS, Jonah MH: Platelet dysfunction (thrombocytopathy) in extra-hepatic biliary obstruction. *South Med J* 75(4):506–507, 1982.
571. Hillbom M, Muuronen A, Neiman J: Liver disease and platelet function in alcoholics. *Br Med J* 295:581, 1987.
572. Stein SF, Harker LA: Kinetic and functional studies of platelets, fibrinogen, and plasminogen in patients with hepatic cirrhosis. *J Lab Clin Med* 99:217, 1982.
573. Violi F, Leo R, Vezza E, et al: Bleeding time in patients with cirrhosis: Relation with degree of liver failure and clotting abnormalities. Coagulation Abnormalities in Cirrhosis Study Group. *J Hepatol* 20(4):531–536, 1994.
574. Livio M, Mannucci PM, Vigano G, et al: Conjugated estrogens for the management of bleeding associated with renal failure. *N Engl J Med* 315:731, 1986.
575. Svensson PJ, Bergqvist PB, Juul KV, Berntorp E: Desmopressin in treatment of haematological disorders and in prevention of surgical bleeding. *Blood Rev* 28(3):95–102, 2014.
576. Pareti FI, Capitanio A, Mannucci L: Acquired storage pool disease in platelets during disseminated intravascular coagulation. *Blood* 48:511, 1976.
577. Pareti FI, Capitanio A, Mannucci L, Ponticelli C, Mannucci PM: Acquired dysfunction due to the circulation of "exhausted" platelets. *Am J Med* 69:235–240, 1980.
578. Solum NO, Rigollot C, Budzynski A, Marder VJ: A quantitative evaluation of the inhibition of platelet aggregation by low molecular weight degradation products of fibrinogen. *Br J Haematol* 24:619, 1973.
579. Stoff JS, Stemerman M, Steer M, Salzman E, Brown RS: A defect in platelet aggregation in Bartter's syndrome. *Am J Med* 68:171–180, 1980.
580. van Wersch J, Rodriques Pereira R: Platelet aggregation in six families with Bartter's syndrome. *Clin Chim Acta* 130:363–368, 1983.
581. Nusing RM, Reinalter SC, Peters M, et al: Pathogenetic role of cyclooxygenase-2 in hyperprostaglandin E syndrome/antenatal Bartter syndrome: Therapeutic use of the cyclooxygenase-2 inhibitor nimesulide. *Clin Pharmacol Ther* 70(4):384–390, 2001.
582. Hebert SC: Bartter syndrome. *Curr Opin Nephrol Hypertens* 12(5):527–532, 2003.
583. Zapata JC, Cox D, Salvato MS: The role of platelets in the pathogenesis of viral hemorrhagic fevers. *PLoS Negl Trop Dis* 8(6):e2858, 2014.
584. Lim SH, Tan CE, Agasthian T, Chew LS: Acquired platelet dysfunction with eosinophilia: Review of seven adult cases. *J Clin Pathol* 47:950–952, 2014.
585. Poon MC, Ng SC, Coppes MJ: Acquired platelet dysfunction with eosinophilia in white children. *J Pediatr* 126(6):959–961, 1995.
586. Laosombat V, Wongchanchailert M, Sattayasevana B, et al: Acquired platelet dysfunction with eosinophilia in children in the south of Thailand. *Platelets* 12(1):5–14, 2001.
587. Szczeklik A, Milner PC, Birch J, et al: Prolonged bleeding time, reduced platelet aggregation, altered PAF-acether sensitivity and increased platelet mass are a trait of asthma and hay fever. *Thromb Haemost* 56:283–287, 1986.
588. Carvalho AC, Quinn DA, DeMarinis SM, et al: Platelet function in acute respiratory failure. *Am J Hematol* 25:377–388, 1987.
589. Bracey AW, Wu AH, Aceves J, et al: Platelet dysfunction associated with Wilms tumor and hyaluronic acid. *Am J Hematol* 24:247–257, 1987.

# CHAPTER 12
# THE VASCULAR PURPURAS

Doru T. Alexandrescu and Marcel Levi

## SUMMARY

Purpura, the clinical manifestation of blood extravasation into mucosa or skin, results from various conditions, including rheumatologic, infectious, dermatologic, traumatic, and hematologic disorders. This chapter does not detail purpura resulting from quantitative or functional defects in hemostasis and coagulation, such as deficiencies of platelets or coagulation factors; these causes are discussed in other chapters (e.g., thrombocytopenia in Chap. 7; coagulation factor deficiencies in Chaps. 13 and 14).

The differential diagnosis of the disparate causes of noncoagulopathic purpura is best approached by stratifying purpura into three types of lesions: (1) palpable or retiform and noninflammatory, such as hyperglobulinemic purpura of Waldenström; (2) palpable or nonpalpable but inflammatory, such as Henoch-Schönlein purpura; and (3) nonpalpable and noninflammatory, such as senile purpura. By accounting for palpability, presence of inflammation, size, and shape, the differential diagnosis of a particular lesion can be significantly reduced.

## ● DEFINITION AND DIAGNOSTIC APPROACH

Purpura refers to visible hemorrhage into mucous membranes or skin, which corresponds to extravasation of red blood cells around small dermal vessels and chronic hemosiderin deposition.[1] Purpuric lesions, by definition, do not blanch completely upon compression, as opposed to erythema. Blanching is commonly tested by compression of skin lesions with a glass slide, referred to as diascopy (Fig. 12–1). Certain conditions give rise to lesions that mimic purpura with incomplete blanching upon diascopy, but are not purpura because no hemorrhage has occurred. Examples include disorders that impede on the red cell flow, such as tortuous veins.[1]

Assessing lesion palpability is the first step in evaluating purpuric lesions (Fig. 12–2). The causes for palpability are varied and include fibrin deposition, localized edema, significant cellular infiltration, and subcutaneous extravasation of red blood cells.

Inspecting the lesion for inflammatory changes is the next step in evaluating purpuric lesions. The presence of pain, erythema, and palpation for warmth and localized swelling are signs of inflammation and suggest a vasculitis or immune complex disorder.

Acronyms and Abbreviations: ANCA, antineutrophil cytoplasmic antibody; APS, antiphospholipid syndrome; CSS, Churg-Strauss syndrome; DIC, disseminated intravascular coagulation; HCV, hepatitis C virus; HHT, hereditary hemorrhagic telangiectasia; HP, hypergammaglobulinemic purpura; HSP, Henoch-Schönlein purpura; MELAS, mitochondrial encephalopathy, lactic acidosis, stroke-like; SLE, systemic lupus erythematosus; WG, Wegener granulomatosis.

The shape of a purpuric lesion, either round or retiform (branching), is important in assessing the lesion. In the absence of accompanying inflammation, retiform purpuric lesions suggest small-vessel occlusion. A retiform, inflammatory purpuric lesion supports the diagnosis of vasculitis as a result of immunoglobulin (Ig) complex formation.[2] Small, focal areas of hemorrhage are referred to as *petechiae* (≤4 mm). Larger lesions are referred to as *intermediate* or *midsize purpura* (>4 mm, <1 cm) or *ecchymosis* (≥1 cm).[3]

Purpuric lesions frequently appear purple; however, they can take on a variety of colors, according to the age of the lesion and the oxygen saturation of the hemoglobin in the extravasated blood. Ecchymosis usually starts as blue or purple, evolves to a greenish brown (a mixture of blue and yellow), and ultimately changes with variable speed to yellow as hemoglobin degrades to bilirubin.[4] These examples of hemorrhage into the dermis must be distinguished from telangiectasia, which are vascular anomalies that blanch with pressure (see Fig. 12–1). Tables 12–1 through 12–3 classify the etiologies for purpura discussed in this chapter.

## ● PALPABLE NONINFLAMMATORY PURPURIC LESIONS

See Table 12–1.

### DYSPROTEINEMIAS

*Cryoglobulinemia*

Cryoglobulinemia refers to the presence in plasma of cold-insoluble immunoglobulins[5] and is a secondary finding associated with several disease states. Cryoglobulins are commonly present in low concentrations; therefore, approximately 90 percent of patients are asymptomatic or have minimal symptoms.[6] Symptoms occur when the abnormal protein precipitates at the temperatures present in superficial venules in the skin and acral parts of the body. Cryoglobulinemia syndromes are divided into three main types based on the immunoglobulin composition of the precipitate. Type I cryoglobulinemia results from the accumulation of monoclonal IgG, IgM, or IgA. It is most commonly seen in association with lymphoproliferative disorders, such as myeloma, Waldenström macroglobulinemia, or lymphoma. Type II, or mixed cryoglobulinemia involves formation of complexes composed of polyclonal IgG with monoclonal immunoglobulins, typically IgM with anti-IgG specificity. Exposure to various exogenous antigens appears to cause polyclonal immunoglobulin production, with activity against bacteria, viruses, and fungi. Mixed cryoglobulinemia is commonly seen secondary to hepatitis C virus (HCV) infection,[7] HIV, collagen vascular disorders, and hematologic neoplasias.[8,9] In mixed cryoglobulinemia secondary to HCV infection, the presence of active cutaneous vasculitis correlates with increased levels of the B-cell–attracting chemokine 1 (CXCL13).[10] This process manifests with petechiae of the legs, palpable purpura, and necrotic skin ulcerations. First-line treatment includes use of interferon-α or other antiviral agents, often with adjunct glucocorticoids or plasmapheresis.[11] Direct treatment of the HCV infection with ribavirin, interferon, or other antiviral therapy, such as the protease inhibitors, ameliorates this associated lymphoproliferative disorder.[12] Deposition of immune complexes on vessel walls leads to tissue damage in the vasculature, nerves, joints, and skin leading to the hallmark findings of mixed cryoglobulinemia: weakness, arthralgia, and purpura. This purpura often is palpable and is accompanied by areas of hemorrhagic necrosis (Fig. 12–3) and occasionally follicular pustular purpura. Other cutaneous manifestations include lower-extremity ulcerations, urticaria, Raynaud phenomena, and subungual purpura (Fig. 12–4). Type III

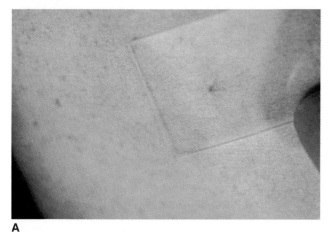

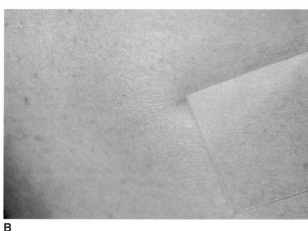

**Figure 12–1.** **A.** Spider telangiectasia. **B.** Blanching of spider telangiectasia. Note that spider telangiectasia blanches with diascopy.

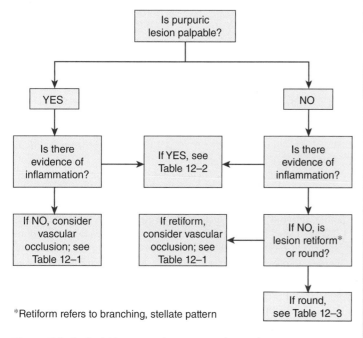

*Retiform refers to branching, stellate pattern

**Figure 12–2.** Bedside approach to purpuric lesion diagnosis.

---

**TABLE 12–1.** Palpable Noninflammatory Purpuric Lesions

A. Dysproteinemias
   1. Cryoglobulinemia (see Figs. 12–3 and 12–4)
   2. Waldenström hyperglobulinemic purpura (see Fig. 12–5)
   3. Light-chain vasculopathy
   4. Cryofibrinogenemia
B. Thrombotic
   1. Heparin necrosis
   2. Warfarin necrosis (see Fig. 12–6)
   3. Protein C and protein S deficiencies
   4. Paroxysmal nocturnal hemoglobinuria
   5. Antiphospholipid syndrome (see Fig. 12–8)
   6. Livedoid vasculitis
C. Embolic
   1. Cholesterol emboli (see Fig. 12–9)
   2. Cutaneous calciphylaxis
   3. Emboli from intracardiac thrombi
D. Arthropod bites

---

**TABLE 12–2.** Palpable and Nonpalpable Inflammatory Purpuric Lesions

A. Pyoderma gangrenosum (see Fig. 12–7)
B. Sweet syndrome (see Fig. 12–10)
C. Behçet disease
D. Serum sickness (Fig. 12–11)
E. Henoch-Schönlein purpura (see Fig. 12–12)
F. Infections
G. Erythema multiforme (see Fig. 12–20)
H. Cutaneous polyarteritis nodosum (see Fig. 12–21)
I. Paraneoplastic vasculitis
J. Drug-induced vasculitis
K. Antineutrophilic cytoplasmic antibody–associated vasculitides
   1. Wegener granulomatosis (see Fig. 12–23)
   2. Churg-Strauss

---

**TABLE 12–3.** Nonpalpable, Noninflammatory, Round Purpuric Lesions

A. Increased transmural pressure gradient and trauma
B. Drug reactions
C. Coagulation disorders
D. Decreased vessel integrity without trauma
   1. Senile purpura
   2. Excess glucocorticoid (Cushing syndrome, glucocorticoid treatment)
   3. Scurvy—vitamin C deficiency (see Fig. 12–25)
   4. Systemic amyloidosis
   5. Connective tissue disorders (Ehlers-Danlos syndrome, pseudoxanthoma elasticum)
   6. Mitochondrial encephalomyopathy with lactic acidosis and stroke-like syndrome (MELAS)
E. Waldenström hypergammaglobulinemic purpura (see Table 12–1 and Fig. 12–5)
F. Rendu-Osler-Weber disease (see Fig. 12–26)

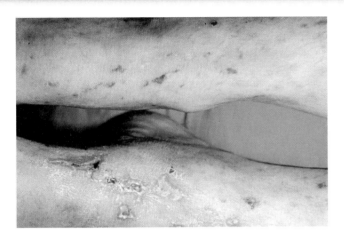

**Figure 12–3.** Cryoglobulinemia: peripheral purpura.

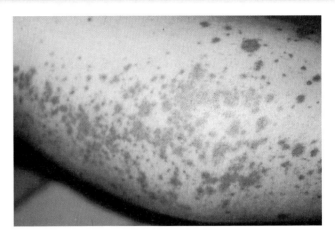

**Figure 12–5.** Waldenström hyperglobulinemic purpura. Note discrete and coalescing petechiae on lower limb.

cryoglobulinemia associates polyclonal IgG and IgM complexes, also resulting in symptoms of mixed cryoglobulinemia.[6] It is associated with a variety of infections, systemic lupus erythematous (SLE), and poststreptococcal glomerulonephritis.

### Waldenström Hyperglobulinemic Purpura

A polyclonal increase of immunoglobulins, most commonly $IgG_1$, appears to be responsible for the varied cutaneous findings seen in this hypergammaglobulinemic purpura (HP). Waldenström first described a hyperproteinemic syndrome characterized by hypergammaglobulinemia, recurrent purpura, elevated erythrocyte sedimentation rate, and anemia.[13] Most commonly seen in young women, this syndrome is associated with a large number of autoimmune disorders, including rheumatoid arthritis, Sjögren syndrome, SLE, hepatitis C, polymyositis, and sarcoidosis. Discrete to confluent collections of lower limb petechiae are its most common skin findings (Fig. 12–5), but lesions can occur in various body locations.[14] Although lesions are usually self-limited and resolve in 7 to 10 days, recurrence of purpura is common and is associated with exposure to cold temperatures or increases in hydrostatic pressure, such as with the use of tight stockings or prolonged standing.[15] Clinical manifestations consist of palpable purpura or diminutive macular erythematous lesions occurring on the lower legs. A reticulate pattern of purpura has been described.[16] Development of edema and arthralgia has also been described.[17]

Common histologic findings include perivascular infiltrates, hemorrhage, and vascular necrosis. In addition to a polyclonal increase in either IgA, IgM, or IgG, serology may reveal cryoglobulinemia, rheumatoid factor, or antinuclear antibodies.[18] Imbalances in IgG subclass expression, usually because of a decrease in $IgG_2$, appear to be associated with recurrent infections.[17] Development of antilymphocyte antibodies results in lymphopenia. Anti-Ro/SSA antibodies occur in up to 78 percent of HP patients, suggesting that screening for anti-Ro/SSA should be considered in cases suspicious for Waldenström.[19]

### Light-Chain Vasculopathy

Precipitates of immunoglobulin light chains that form crystalline deposits in the skin cause hemorrhagic palpable purpura. A nonamyloid monoclonal light chain of predominant $\kappa$ type is involved in two-thirds of the cases.[20,21] Crystalline deposits are present in the skin and other tissues. Although the clinical presentation may mimic a systemic vasculitis, no histologic signs of inflammation are seen. Light-chain vasculopathy with cutaneous findings has also been described in association with multiple myeloma. Intravascular deposition of crystals containing IgG and $\lambda$ light chains were found on immunohistochemical analysis and manifested with gangrene of the feet and intestinal perforation.[22]

### Cryofibrinogenemia

First described by Korst and Kratochvil in 1955, cryofibrinogenemia is a form of serum dysproteinemia characterized by formation of an abnormal cold-precipitable fibrinogen. Cutaneous manifestations include cyanosis, erythema, Raynaud phenomenon, and palpable purpura of the nose, ears, and distal extremities.[23] Tissue ischemia and gangrene may result. Pathogenesis of cryofibrinogenemia may involve an inhibition of normal fibrinolysis produced by a high plasma level of $\alpha_1$-antitripsin and $\alpha_2$-macroglobulin proteases.[24] Cryofibrinogenemia is commonly secondary to thromboembolic disorders, metastatic malignancies, infections, and collagen vascular disease.[25] Treatment modalities include avoidance of cold, plasmapheresis, and danazol, an anabolic glucocorticoid, or immunosuppression with glucocorticoids or cytotoxic agents.

## THROMBOTIC PURPURA

### Heparin Necrosis

Cutaneous reactions to heparin administration vary greatly from a type I urticarial rash to purpuric plaques with cutaneous ulceration or necrosis.[26] The syndrome occurs after both subcutaneous

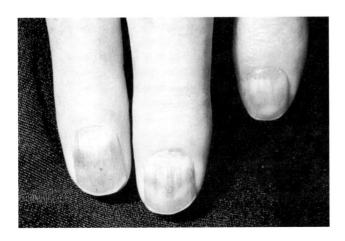

**Figure 12–4.** Cryoglobulinemia: subungual purpura.

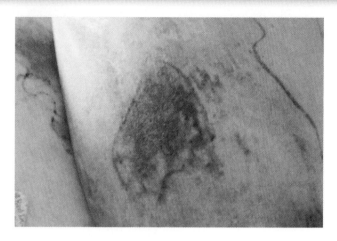

**Figure 12–6.** Coumadin necrosis. Develops in acral areas and areas of fat deposition such as buttocks or breast. Typically, lesions develop 3 to 10 days after initiation of anticoagulant treatment and are caused by rapid clearing of protein C. The lesions are characterized microscopically by small-vessel thrombosis.

and intravenous administration of unfractionated heparin, but it has also been rarely described after low-molecular-weight heparin.[27] A delayed-type hypersensitivity reaction to the medication is involved. Skin lesions appear within 1 to 2 weeks after treatment initiation and include necrotic purpuric lesions.[28] Development of cutaneous lesions is closely related to heparin-induced thrombocytopenia (Chap. 8), which involves anti–platelet factor 4 antibody–mediated platelet aggregation with development of thrombosis and microvascular occlusion.[27]

### Warfarin Necrosis

The development of painful erythematous plaques and nodules is a potential complication of warfarin therapy (Fig. 12–6). These lesions can rapidly become hemorrhagic and necrotic, leading to large areas of infarct with black eschar formation and subsequent skin sloughing. Purpura, vesicular, maculopapular, or urticarial eruptions can be encountered.[1] Warfarin-induced necrosis has a prevalence between 0.01 and 0.1 percent and presents typically 3 to 10 days after initiation of anticoagulant treatment.[29,30] However, an atypical presentation can occur much later, for example, in a patient with protein S deficiency.[31,32] Although warfarin necrosis tends to develop in areas of greatest fat deposition, such as breasts, thighs, and buttocks, acral areas, including penis, fingers, and toes, can also be involved.[33] Warfarin necrosis results from the rapid decrease of vitamin K–dependent coagulation factors of relatively short half-life, such as proteins C and S, while longer-lasting coagulation factors, such as factor II and factor X, are not yet decreased, resulting in a net procoagulant state. Microvascular occlusion of small dermal and subcutaneous vessels by fibrin deposits is seen on histologic analysis, but true vasculitis is infrequent.[29] Treatment involves prompt cessation of the vitamin K antagonist, along with administration of heparin and vitamin K, and occasionally surgical debridement. Because patients with protein C or S deficiency are at increased susceptibility to warfarin necrosis, heparin should always be administered in these patients prior to initiation of warfarin (Coumadin).[34]

### Proteins C and S Deficiencies

Clinical manifestations of proteins C and S deficiencies include venous thromboembolism, warfarin-induced skin necrosis, and neonatal purpura fulminans (Chap. 19). Congenital and acquired deficiencies in these proteins can lead to palpable necrotic purpura and ecchymosis.[35,36]

Erythematous purpuric lesions associated with homozygous protein C deficiency can develop within hours of birth and can rapidly progress to hemorrhagic necrosis.[37] Acquired deficiencies of protein C are associated with autoantibodies to protein C, antibiotics administration, septic shock, HIV, and liver disease (Chap. 17).[38] Acquired protein S deficiency may occur after varicella infection, when it is associated with the generation of antiprotein S immunoglobulins.[39] Protein repletion with fresh-frozen plasma or protein C concentrate is effective as initial treatment for protein C deficiency to help clear both cutaneous lesions and venous occlusion, while lifelong anticoagulant treatment is used to prevent recurrence.[34,40]

### Paroxysmal Nocturnal Hemoglobinuria

Paroxysmal nocturnal hemoglobinuria is a hematopoietic clonal disorder resulting in defective production of cell surface-binding proteins.[41] Cutaneous manifestations are secondary to a hypercoagulable state and include palpable purpura, petechiae, ecchymosis, leg ulcers, plaques, necrosis, and hemorrhagic bullae.[42] Parvovirus B19 may play an etiologic role in the development of cutaneous necrosis.[43] An association with pyoderma gangrenosum (Fig. 12–7)[44] and occurrence of purpura fulminans[45] have been described. Histology reveals formation of microvascular fibrin thrombi.[42]

### Antiphospholipid Syndrome

Antiphospholipid syndrome (APS) is a disease characterized by hypercoagulability associated with the presence of antibodies against phospholipids, such as anticardiolipin and lupus anticoagulant (Chap. 21).[46] Approximately 40 percent of patients with APS present with cutaneous lesions secondary to both large-vessel and microvascular thrombosis.[47] Skin manifestations include ecchymosis, livedo reticularis and racemosa, leg ulcerations, bullae, splinter hemorrhages, livedoid vasculopathy, superficial venous thrombosis, atrophie blanche, and extensive necrosis (Fig. 12–8).[47,48] Presence of livedo reticularis is frequently the presenting symptom of APS, most commonly when the syndrome is secondary to SLE, and its presence commonly precedes vascular events.[49] Development of acute bullous purpura has been described.[50] Treatment includes anticoagulant agents with immunosuppressant administration for associated thrombocytopenia. Prevention of thromboembolic events with aspirin is of uncertain value.[51]

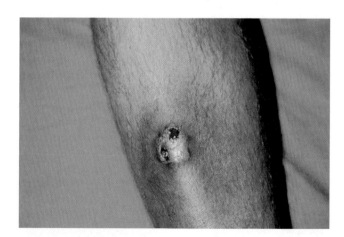

**Figure 12–7.** Pyoderma gangrenosum. A large number of systemic diseases are associated with pyoderma gangrenosum, including inflammatory bowel diseases, hematologic and solid malignancies, and rheumatologic disorders. Microscopically, the lesions are characterized by central necrotizing, neutrophilic infiltration, and a surrounding perivascular and intramural lymphocytic infiltration.

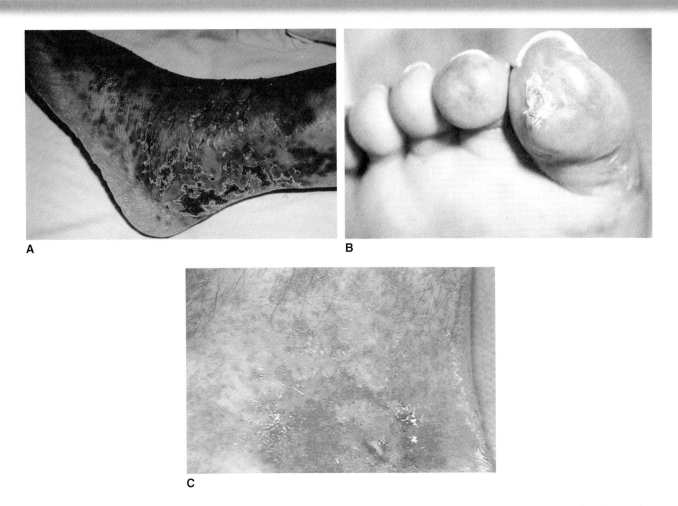

**Figure 12–8. A.** Antiphospholipid antibody syndrome. A number of skin lesions can be seen, including ecchymosis, livedo reticularis and racemosa, leg ulcerations, bullae, splinter hemorrhages, superficial venous thrombosis, atrophie blanche, and, as shown here, extensive necrosis. **B.** Anticardiolipin antibody. **C.** Lupus anticoagulant.

### Livedoid Vasculitis

Livedoid vasculitis (segmental hyalinizing vasculitis) is a chronic recurrent thrombo-occlusive disorder characterized by the initial development of erythematous purpuric lesions with telangiectasis and peripheral petechiae, and lower-extremity ulcerations. Subsequent healing leads to atrophie blanche, a term that refers to the appearance of ivory-white stellate scars commonly surrounded by hyperpigmented areas and telangiectasia. These lesions appear to be caused by small-vessel fibrin thrombi in the middle and lower dermis as a result of a procoagulant tendency.[52] Although most commonly arising without associated cause, livedoid vasculitis is associated with polyarteritis nodosa, APS, and SLE.[53,54] Although not consistently beneficial, common therapies include discontinuation of oral contraceptives, anticoagulation and antiplatelet medications, glucocorticoids, and dapsone. Ketanserin, an $S_2$ serotoninergic receptor blocker, psoralen plus ultraviolet A therapy, and intravenous immunoglobulins also have been used successfully.[55]

## EMBOLIC PURPURA

### Cholesterol Crystal Emboli

Also known as atheroemboli, cholesterol crystal emboli are responsible for a syndrome characterized by lower extremity pain and livedo reticularis with preservation of peripheral pulses. Other common cutaneous findings include gangrene, purpura, ulcerations, cyanosis, and nodules (Fig. 12–9).[56] Clinical symptoms include fever, myalgia, and altered mental status. Laboratory features include an elevated erythrocyte sedimentation rate, eosinophilia, and acute renal failure. Onset of symptoms varies from immediate after physical dislodgement of plaque, up to months later when caused by anticoagulant therapy.[1] A blue toe syndrome is, in fact, rare, and most atheroemboli are clinically silent.[57] Atherosclerotic lesions in the descending aorta are the most common source of cholesterol emboli. This explains the propensity for lower-extremity findings during intravascular procedures or initiation of thrombolytic or anticoagulant therapy.[56] Histologic evaluation can offer a definitive diagnosis with findings of intraluminal birefringent cholesterol crystals within blood vessel lumen, in the absence of vasculitis.[58] No effective treatment is available. Nevertheless, supportive care with proper hydration and dialysis may lessen the potential for end-organ damage.

### Cutaneous Calciphylaxis

Calciphylaxis (calcific uremic arteriolopathy)[59] is a thrombo-occlusive disorder involving formation of cutaneous, subcutaneous, and vascular calcifications. It is most commonly seen in patients with end-stage renal disease, classically caused by the development of secondary hyperparathyroidism.[60] Approximately 4 percent of hemodialysis-dependent patients suffer from calciphylaxis. Survival is less than 50 percent at 5 years after diagnosis.[61] Other etiologies include primary

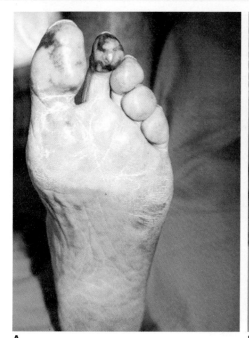
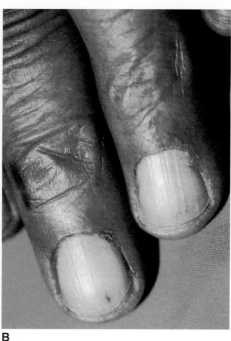

A          B

Figure 12–9. A. Cholesterol emboli. B. Rupture of an atherosclerotic plaque can result in showers of microemboli that lodge in distal arterioles, causing splinter hemorrhages.

hyperparathyroidism, malignancy, alcoholic liver disease, and collagen tissue disorders.[62] Cutaneous lesions present initially as reddish-purple plaques, evolving to tender, gangrenous ulcers or reticular hemorrhagic necrosis. Treatment involves a combination of medical and surgical interventions, such as parathyroidectomy, renal transplantation, wound debridement, and amputation.[61]

### Emboli from Intracardiac Thrombi

Acral purpuric lesions secondary to emboli arise from left atrial myxomas or right atrial clots through paradoxical embolization.[63] These purpuric lesions include palpable purpura, livedo reticularis, erythematous macules and papules, cyanosis, petechiae, splinter hemorrhages, ulcerations, and cutaneous necrosis. Cyanosis, livedo reticularis, and lower-extremity ulcerations can also be seen.[64]

## ARTHROPOD BITES

Purpuric lesions are not uncommon after arthropod bites. Bites from bed bugs, *Cimex lectularius*, can give rise to localized purpuric macules or papules, whereas bites from kissing bugs, Reduviidae, often manifest as urticaria with hemorrhagic bulla.[65] Cutaneous findings after envenomation from a brown recluse spider, *Loxosceles reclusa*, include purpuric necrosis with surrounding erythema evolving to ulcer formation.

## ⬤ PALPABLE AND NONPALPABLE INFLAMMATORY PURPURIC LESIONS

See Table 12–2.

## PYODERMA GANGRENOSUM

Pyoderma gangrenosum is an idiopathic inflammatory skin condition characterized by early follicular erythematous papules and pustules or tender, fluctuant nodules with surrounding erythema that spread peripherally and ulcerate, surrounded by a violaceous rim (see Fig. 12–7).[66] In 50 percent of cases of pyoderma gangrenosum, there is an associated disorder, such as inflammatory bowel disorders (classically ulcerative

colitis), arthritis, hematologic disorders, and solid tumors.[67] All four main clinical variants (ulcerative, pustular, bullous, and vegetative) share the histopathologic finding of a sterile abscess with central necrotizing neutrophilic infiltration and a surrounding perivascular and intramural lymphocytic infiltration. First-line treatment involves wound care and immunosuppressants, such as glucocorticoids, cyclosporine, dapsone, azathioprine, and infliximab.[68]

## SWEET SYNDROME

Also referred to as acute, febrile neutrophilic dermatosis, Sweet syndrome is characterized by the acute manifestation of painful erythematous and violaceous papules, nodules, and plaques accompanied by fever and elevated neutrophil count (Fig. 12–10).[69] These papules, which most commonly appear on the face, neck, and upper extremities, present a central yellowish discoloration and tend to coalesce, forming well-circumscribed, irregularly bordered plaques. Other organs can be involved, including the central nervous system, kidneys, lungs, and bones.[70] Classically more prominent in middle-aged women, this

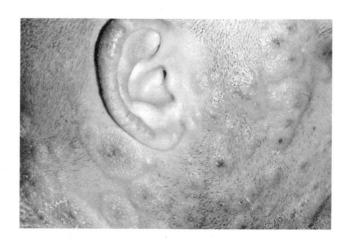

**Figure 12–10.** Sweet syndrome. The lesions are characterized by nonvasculitic neutrophilic infiltration, commonly on the face.

syndrome associates a complex cytokine dysregulation. Other manifestations include respiratory and urinary infections and autoimmune disorders (including rheumatoid arthritis, SLE, and inflammatory bowel disease). Histologic analysis shows a distinct nonvasculitic neutrophilic infiltrate in the superficial dermis with dermal edema. Systemic glucocorticoid treatment is the standard treatment, while clofazimine, dapsone, colchicine, indomethacin, and cyclosporine have also been used successfully.[71]

## BEHÇET DISEASE

Besides its classification as a neutrophilic dermatosis, Behçet disease is also an inflammatory disorder that affects multiple organ systems. Clinical features include chronic and relapsing cutaneous manifestations, such as palpable purpura, infiltrative erythema, and papulopustular lesions, as well as oral mucosal and genital ulcers, arthralgias, and gastrointestinal and central nervous system involvement.[72] Genetic studies show an association between Behçet disease and human leukocyte antigen B51.[73] Histologic features include leukocytoclastic or lymphocytic vasculitis, hence its previous classification as a vasculitis. Anti–tumor necrosis factor-$\alpha$ directed therapies (infliximab, etanercept), interferon-$\alpha$, immunosuppressive and immunomodulatory agents such as thalidomide, intravenous immunoglobulin, and even stem cell transplantation are used in Behçet disease.[74,75]

## SERUM SICKNESS

Serum sickness reflects the clinical manifestations of immune complex formation and deposition. Cutaneous lesions such as urticarial and morbilliform eruptions predominate, although palpable purpura and erythema multiforme can also be encountered. Serum sickness associated with infection or medical therapy can result in specific characteristic lesions. The use of antithymocyte globulin for marrow failure, for instance, results in 75 percent of patients developing serpiginous bands of erythema and purpura on the sides of their hands and feet (Fig. 12–11).[76] These characteristic lesions consistently appear 1 to 2 days prior to the onset of systemic symptoms of serum sickness, which include fever and malaise. Analysis of biopsies by direct immunofluorescence reveals deposition of IgM, IgE, IgA, and C3. This deposition appears to activate neutrophils, leading to release of lysosomal enzymes and the development of dermal vasculitis.[77]

## HENOCH-SCHÖNLEIN PURPURA

Henoch-Schönlein purpura (HSP) is a predominantly pediatric vasculitic syndrome characterized by the acute onset of abdominal pain and lower-extremity eruption of diffuse urticarial plaques and palpable purpura. It was first described in 1801 by Dr. William Heberden.[78] HSP predominantly affects patients 2 to 20 years of age, with 90 percent of patients being younger than 10 years old.[79] Several environmental triggers precede HSP onset, such as viral (upper respiratory infections, hepatitis B virus, HCV, parvovirus B19, and HIV) and bacterial (*Streptococcus* species, *Staphylococcus aureus*, and *Salmonella* species) infections in children. Adult disease may be precipitated by medications (nonsteroidal antiinflammatory drugs [NSAIDs], angiotensin-converting enzyme inhibitors, and antibiotics), food allergies, vaccinations, and insect bites.[80] The pathogenesis of HSP leukocytoclastic vasculitis is complex. It appears to involve IgA$_1$ immune complex and complement deposition on vessel walls. Elevated values of thrombomodulin, tissue plasminogen activator, and plasminogen activator inhibitor-1 appear to correlate with endothelial injury and fibrinolytic activity in the acute phase of HSP.[81]

Cutaneous eruptions often begin acutely as urticarial papules and plaques evolving to petechiae, ecchymoses, and palpable and nonpalpable purpura over the lower extremities and buttocks (Fig. 12–12). Palpable purpura is a universal finding, being present in one series in 98.6 percent of patients.[82] Clinically, lesions may take the form of retiform or patterned purpura, presence of a retiform edge of various inflammatory lesions, or skin necrosis.[83] Other common manifestations include localized subcutaneous edema, glomerulonephritis, arthritis, and (severe) abdominal pain.

Despite its chronic relapsing pattern, the long-term evolution is benign in the majority of patients.[82] The self-limited course of HSP may be contributed by an enhanced apoptosis of immune cells, which diminishes the severity of the acute inflammatory response.[84] Consequently, treatment is frequently supportive. Immunosuppressive drugs, including glucocorticoids, are typically reserved for cases with renal

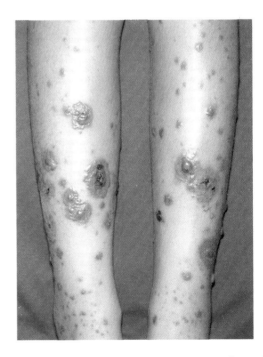

**Figure 12–12.** Henoch-Schönlein purpura. Urticarial papules and plaques can evolve into palpable purpura. The lesions are characterized by leukocytoclastic vasculitis.

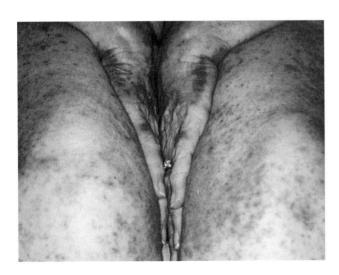

**Figure 12–11.** Serum sickness caused by antithymocyte globulin. The lesions consist of immunoglobulins and neutrophils.

involvement.[78] Persistent purpura, severe abdominal symptoms, and diminished plasma coagulation factor XIII activity are predictive of renal involvement, requiring initiation of glucocorticoids.[85]

## INFECTIONS

Careful analysis of skin lesions of infectious etiology can provide important hints toward identifying the responsible pathogen. Purpura can arise through a variety of pathophysiologic mechanisms associated with infection: (1) vascular effects of toxins, (2) septic emboli, (3) direct invasion of vessels with subsequent vascular occlusion, and (4) immune complex formation.[86] Although the morphology of such purpuric lesions may be nonspecific, many pathogens lead to characteristic findings.

### Bacterial

Gram-positive and gram-negative infections may give rise to a large array of purpuric patterns depending on organism virulence and patient immune status. Skin lesions range from simple macules and papules to bullae, ulcers, and necrosis.

Purpura fulminans, a hemorrhagic infarction syndrome consisting of disseminated intravascular coagulation (DIC), acral purpura, and shock may manifest in the setting of bacterial sepsis with encapsulated organisms (Chap. 19).[87] Most commonly seen in immunocompromised hosts, purpura fulminans can also be produced by bacterial pathogens in immunocompetent patients.[88] This syndrome can be associated with asplenism or functional hyposplenism.[89] Although most patients are younger than the age of 10 years, adults can also be affected.[90] Retiform purpuric lesions result from fibrin-induced microvascular occlusion and commonly have a rapid evolution toward necrosis and eschar formation. Adult patients with purpura fulminans as a result of meningococcemia have significantly depressed proteins C and S levels, which may explain the tendency toward fibrin deposition and development of cutaneous ischemic lesions, such as symmetrical peripheral gangrene.[91] Facial purpura and livedo reticularis may be seen during fulminant pneumococcal infection in asplenic patients.[92] Postinfectious purpura fulminans may also occur after infections with streptococci or varicella-zoster[39] and was associated with development of anti–protein S antibodies. Another characteristic lesion is the development of ecthyma gangrenosum in immunocompromised hosts (Fig. 12–13).

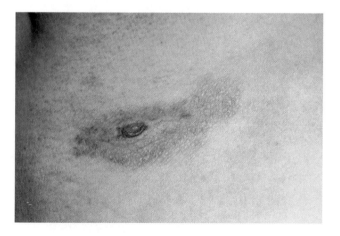

**Figure 12–13.** Ecthyma gangrenosum. Associated with gram-negative sepsis, disseminated fungal infection, or other serious infectious diseases, these hemorrhagic bullae evolve from erythematosus plaques, both of which are shown here.

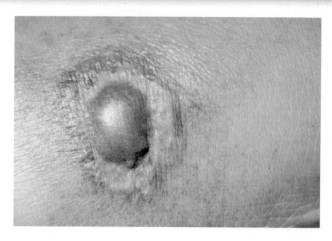

**Figure 12–14.** Lyme disease. Erythema migrans with a central hemorrhagic bulla is the characteristic lesion.

In children, more than 20 percent of cases admitted to the hospital with petechiae and fever were found to have invasive bacterial infections (*Neisseria meningitidis*, *Haemophilus influenzae* type B, and *Streptococcus pneumoniae*), and approximately 7 percent of cases were diagnosed with meningiococcemia.[93] Sepsis secondary to *N. meningitidis* can produce a characteristic pattern of purpuric lesions. Erythematous papules can quickly progress to numerous petechiae combined with violaceous reticular purpuric lesions.[94] A retiform aspect can be seen during progression of the infection to purpura fulminans. The finding of petechiae on a patient with symptoms and signs of bacterial meningitis is predictive of meningococcal meningitis.[95]

*Borrelia burgdorferi* infection gives rise to erythema migrans, the characteristic lesion of Lyme disease. Skin lesion is classically a nonpruritic annular erythematous expanding plaque, occasionally including a central hemorrhagic bullae (Fig. 12–14). Other reported cutaneous findings associated with this infection include papular urticaria, Henoch-Schönlein–like purpura, and morphea.[96]

### Viral

Purpuric lesions can also be a manifestation of a viral infection. For example, the adenoviruses and enteroviruses have been associated with fever and petechiae in children.[97] Similarly, parvovirus B19 can produce a syndrome of petechiae or purpuric papules progressing to confluent purpuric papules or plaques in a sharply demarcated glove-and-sock distribution.[98] In addition to the cutaneous findings, the "gloves-and-socks syndrome" is characterized by fever and occasionally leukopenia and can also be produced by the measles virus.[99] Purpura in the axilla and chest also has been described during parvovirus B19 infection (Fig. 12–15).[100] Histopathologic analysis of these purpuric lesions show an evolution from superficial perivascular lymphocytic infiltrate to a dermatitis accompanied by necrotic keratinocytes and hemorrhage.[101] *Hantavirus* causes a syndrome of hemorrhagic fever and renal failure accompanied by headache, cutaneous and mucosal petechiae, and purpuric lesions.[102]

### Fungal

Fungal infections in the immunocompromised population are a growing medical issue, given the increasing number of patients receiving immunosuppressants for organ transplantation or malignancy. Disseminated or locally invasive infections can give rise to petechiae and hemorrhagic necrosis. Common fungal pathogens in disseminated disease includes *Candida* (Fig. 12–16), *Aspergillus* (Fig. 12–17), *Histoplasma*, and *Fusarium*.[103] Disseminated candidiasis can manifest as ecthyma gangrenosum in immunocompromised patients, suggesting consideration for

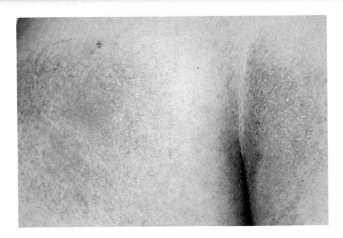

**Figure 12–15.** Parvovirus B19 erythema and petechiae. The classic slapped-cheek rash on the face can appear on other areas of the body, sometimes punctuated with petechiae of unclear etiology.

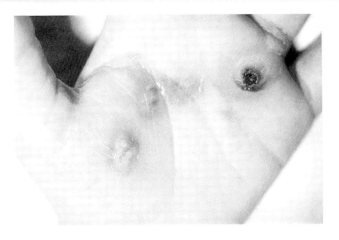

**Figure 12–17.** Aspergillosis: primary cutaneous inoculation from contaminated armboard.

a skin biopsy.[104] Cutaneous aspergillosis can also occur in immunocompetent individuals and manifest as eruptive maculopapules, necrotizing plaques, or subcutaneous granulomas.[105]

### Parasitic

Immunocompromised patients are at risk of developing purpuric lesions secondary to parasitic infections, such as *Pneumocystis jiroveci*. Disseminated strongyloidiasis is characterized by larva currens, a serpiginous urticarial eruption caused by the migration of filiform larvae through the dermis.[106] Other cutaneous lesions include generalized petechiae and widespread reticular purpura of the arms, legs, and abdomen (Fig. 12–18), with a characteristic *thumbprint* periumbilical distribution.[107]

### Rickettsial

Infections caused by *Rickettsia* species can also lead to purpuric lesions as a result of their direct invasion of endothelial cells. This is followed by medial and intimal necrosis with subsequent thrombosis and hemorrhage.[86] Cutaneous lesions in Rocky Mountain spotted fever range from petechiae to acral purpuric lesions and hemorrhagic necrosis (Fig. 12–19). Maculopapular and vesicular rashes along with

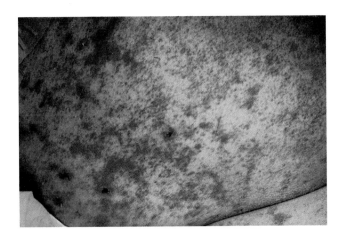

**Figure 12–18.** Disseminated strongyloidiasis.

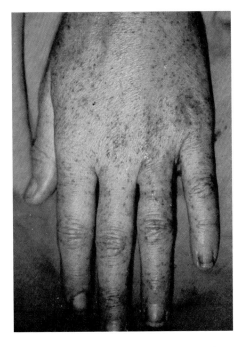

**Figure 12–19.** Rocky Mountain spotted fever. This rickettsial disorder can present with petechiae on the dorsum of the hand.

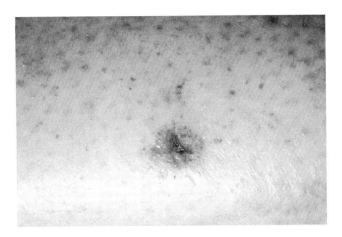

**Figure 12–16.** Disseminated candidiasis. Purpuric nodules in a patient with acute myelogenous leukemia. Ecthyma gangrenosum can also occur in this disease.

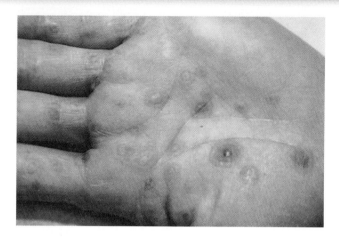

**Figure 12–20.** Erythema multiforme. This hypersensitivity reaction, usually to one of various drugs, characteristically presents with targetoid lesions.

lower-extremity eschars produced by *Rickettsia africae* may also occur in travelers to sub-Saharan Africa.[108]

## ERYTHEMA MULTIFORME

Erythema multiforme (EM) is a cutaneous disorder characterized by the development of crops of well-demarcated, erythematous target lesions with central clearing,[109] most commonly representing a hypersensitivity reaction triggered by infection or drug exposure (Fig. 12–20). The severity of this disorder ranges from mild (EM minor) to severe (EM major or Stevens-Johnson syndrome). EM has been reported to be triggered by a number of viruses (most commonly herpes simplex, but also adenovirus, cytomegalovirus, and HIV)[110,111] and medications (sulfonamides, penicillins, bupropion, phenylbutazone, phenytoin, NSAIDs, adalimumab).[112] A cellular allergic reaction coupled with impaired histamine metabolism because of a decrease in histamine-*N*-methyltransferase activity may be causative.[113] Treatment for mild cases is supportive, while the use of glucocorticoids is warranted in severe cases.

## CUTANEOUS POLYARTERITIS NODOSA

Classic polyarteritis nodosa represents a systemic small- and medium-size vessel vasculitis most commonly involving the skin, heart, liver, and kidneys. A relatively benign cutaneous form exists that lacks significant systemic involvement[114] and consistently involves the deep dermis and panniculus.[115] Lesions develop as tender erythematous nodules[116] with occasional retiform purpura and livedo reticularis localized to the upper and lower extremities, but the trunk, neck, and face can also be involved (Fig. 12–21). The duration of lesions varies from days to a few months.[115] Histologic analysis of involved skin shows deep dermal artery necrosis with infiltration of neutrophils and eosinophils, and fibrin deposition. Treatment typically involves the use of NSAIDs and glucocorticoids, alone or in combination. Some cases of cutaneous polyarteritis nodosa are reported to have progressed on long-term follow-up,[117] hence the need for close monitoring of patients diagnosed with an apparently benign, cutaneous form of disease.[118]

## PARANEOPLASTIC VASCULITIS

Most common vasculitides associated with neoplasia are cutaneous leukocytoclastic vasculitis, paraneoplastic vasculitis, and HSP.[119,120]

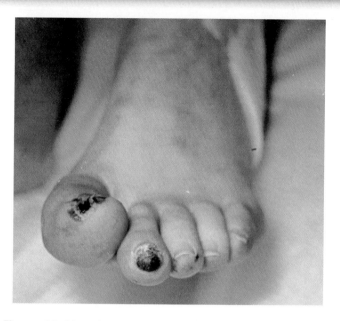

**Figure 12–21.** Polyarteritis nodosa. Acral purpura accompanying tender erythematous nodules.

Paraneoplastic vasculitis is most commonly associated with hematologic neoplasia[121] and is commonly a result of paraproteinemia. However, an association with carcinomas of the lung, colon, breast, and cervix has been observed.[122–124] Solid tumors predominate in certain types of paraneoplastic vasculitis, such as the HSP.[125] Cutaneous manifestations include petechiae, urticaria, and palpable purpura and are often intensely pruritic. In hematologic disorders, these lesions often precede the development of malignancy by an average of 10 months.[126] Histologic examination shows necrotizing leukocytoclastic vasculitis with neutrophilic infiltration.

## DRUG-INDUCED VASCULITIS

A long list of drugs are reported to cause a vasculitis resulting in erythematous purpuric lesions. One-fifth of all cutaneous vasculitis are produced by drugs, including allopurinol, cefaclor, colony-stimulating factors, D-penicillamine, furosemide (Fig. 12–22), hydralazine, isotretinoin, methotrexate, phenytoin, minocycline, and propylthiouracil.[127]

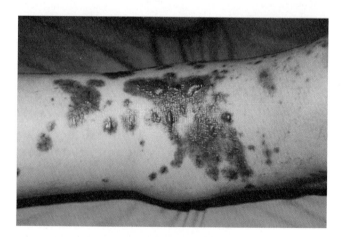

**Figure 12–22.** Leukocytoclastic vasculitis secondary to furosemide.

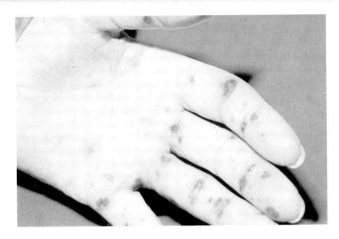

**Figure 12–23.** Wegener granulomatosis.

## ANTINEUTROPHIL CYTOPLASMIC ANTIBODY–ASSOCIATED VASCULITIS

### Wegener Granulomatosis

This small- to medium-vessel vasculitis most commonly affects upper and lower respiratory tracts and kidneys and is strongly associated with the development of circulating antineutrophil cytoplasmic antibodies (ANCAs).[128] Skin involvement has been reported in 35 to 50 percent of cases.[129] Cutaneous manifestations include a combination of palpable purpura, oral ulcers, and erythematous cutaneous and subcutaneous nodules (Fig. 12–23).[130] Necrotizing vasculitis, palisading granulomas, and granulomatous vasculitis are characteristic histologic findings.[131]

### Churg-Strauss Syndrome

Churg-Strauss syndrome (CSS) is characterized by granulomatous inflammation in the lungs associated with asthma and eosinophilia.[132] Cutaneous findings such as ulcers, papules, palpable purpura, cutaneous nodules, and infarcts of fingers and toes are encountered in 50 to 80 percent of cases.[130] CSS limited to the skin was described.[133] Eosinophilia accompanies elevated IgE levels and a positive perinuclear ANCA. Granulomatous inflammation and necrotizing vasculitis of small- to medium-size blood vessels are present histologically.[131]

## ● NONPALPABLE, NONINFLAMMATORY, ROUND PURPURIC LESIONS

See Table 12–3.

## INCREASED TRANSMURAL PRESSURE GRADIENT AND TRAUMA

Acute increases in vascular transmural pressure gradients lead to extravasation of red blood cells resulting in nonpalpable, noninflammatory petechial and larger purpuric lesions. Examples include postictal purpura,[134] weightlifting,[135] postemesis facial purpura,[136] prolonged Valsalva, and childbirth. Acute decreases in extravascular negative pressure, referred to as suction purpura from gas mask, kissing, or cupping, can also increase this gradient, resulting in well-circumscribed lesions in the shape of the causative device.[137] The development of petechiae in mountain climbers is presumably caused by significantly reduced atmospheric pressures at high elevations.[138] Lower-extremity venous incompetence, predominantly at the medial ankle, can result in macules or patches of yellowish-brown purpura.

Focal ecchymosis and other purpuric lesions can manifest as a result of trauma. Characteristic patterns of purpuric lesions are commonly used in forensic science. Traumatic asphyxia, for instance, is characterized by cervicofacial cyanosis and swelling, petechiae, and subconjunctival hemorrhage.[139] Factitious purpura, often related to deliberate suction purpura, should be considered in the differential for purpura.[140] Other physical causes of purpura consist of physical remedies, such as spooning (Quat Sha) or coin rubbing (Cao Gio). Exercise-induced purpura results in purpuric, erythematous, or urticarial lesions distributed on the lower legs.[141]

## THROMBOCYTOPENIAS

### Disseminated Intravascular Coagulation

DIC is defined as widespread, amplified, and uncontrolled intravascular coagulation with a range of causes including sepsis, trauma, and malignancy.[142] Petechiae and purpuric plaques result from thrombocytopenia and are common manifestations of DIC (Chap. 19).

### Immune Thrombocytopenia Purpura

Immune (or idiopathic) thrombocytopenia purpura is an acquired disease characterized by autoantibody-mediated platelet destruction commonly resulting in purpuric lesions of the skin and mucosa as well as other sites of abnormal bleeding (Chap. 17).[143]

### Thrombotic Thrombocytopenia Purpura

Thrombotic thrombocytopenia purpura is characterized by nonimmune platelet consumption, microvascular hemolysis, and organ damage. It is associated with a deficiency in the von Willebrand factor cleaving protease, ADAMTS-13 (a disintegrin and metalloproteinase with thrombospondin domain 13; Chap. 22).[144] Petechiae and purpuric plaques may occur.

## DRUG REACTIONS

A large number of medications are reported to result in vasculitic and nonvasculitic purpuric eruptions.[145] Nevertheless, *any* drug on the medication list of a patient with a purpuric lesion (within 2 weeks of starting a new drug or a few days if prior sensitization is suspected) may be involved.[146]

## COAGULATION DISORDERS

A large number of disorders manifest with thrombocytopenia or impaired thrombocyte function that results in increased bruising. In addition, impaired fibrin formation, resulting from coagulation factor deficiencies, the use of anticoagulants, vitamin K deficiency, or poor hepatic function, may cause bruising and hematomas.

## DECREASED VESSEL INTEGRITY WITHOUT TRAUMA

### Senile Purpura

Synonymous with actinic purpura, senile purpura refers to the easy bruising seen in the aged and sun-damaged skin, commonly appearing on the dorsal aspect of the hands and forearms (Fig. 12–24). One proposed etiology is the degeneration of skin extracellular matrix components that leaves dermal capillaries unsupported and vulnerable to shearing injuries,[147] but zinc deficiency is also suspected.[148]

### Excess Glucocorticoid

The presence of excess endogenous (Cushing syndrome) or exogenous (iatrogenic) glucocorticoid use can result in dermal thinning and vessel

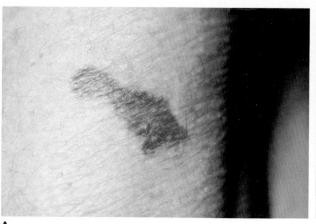

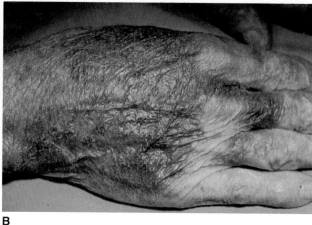

**A**    **B**

**Figure 12–24.** Senile purpura. Note accompanying skin atrophy.

fragility. Consequently, bright red, nonpalpable purpuric lesions tend to arise after slight or even undetected trauma and manifest in a linear or geometric pattern.[149]

### Scurvy—Vitamin C Deficiency

Vitamin C (ascorbic acid) deficiency occurs because of reduced dietary intake or absorption. A consequent disruption in normal collagen production results in blood vessel fragility leading to petechiae, perifollicular hemorrhage, and larger purpuric plaques, most commonly on the lower extremities (Fig. 12–25).[150] Thus, scurvy is usually a clinical diagnosis. Cutaneous features can also include follicular hyperkeratotic papules, poor wound healing, and bent or corkscrew-shaped body hairs.[151] Vitamin C supplementation is rapidly effective.

### Systemic Amyloidosis

Systemic amyloidosis is characterized by a clonal proliferation of plasma cells with consequent immunoglobulin light-chain deposition in vital organs. Microscopic 8- to 10-nm protofilaments aggregate to form fibrils.[152] It can present as a primary disorder or secondarily to multiple myeloma. Characteristic features are periorbital "pinch purpura," "raccoon eyes," and macroglosia.[153]

Waxy, purpuric cutaneous and mucocutaneous lesions manifest when light-chain aggregates deposit in dermal blood vessels. Although rare, palmodigital purpura has been reported as the sole cutaneous

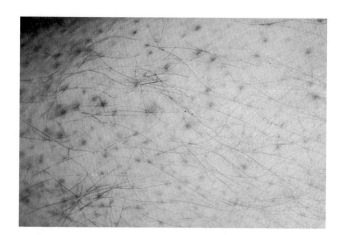

**Figure 12–25.** Parafollicular purpura characteristic of scurvy.

finding in a case of myeloma-associated systemic amyloidosis.[154] A distinct localized form, primary cutaneous amyloidosis, is caused by local dermal infiltration of plasma cells.[155]

## CONNECTIVE TISSUE DISORDERS

### Ehlers-Danlos Syndrome

A rare autosomal dominant syndrome, Ehlers-Danlos syndrome is a consequence of a mutation in collagen synthesis, tenascin X, or lysyl hydroxylase, and others. This leads to loss of skin elasticity, delayed wound healing, easy bruising, joint hypermobility, and systemic organ and tissue fragility.[156] Cutaneous findings include thin skin and a tendency to develop nonpalpable purpuric lesions.[157]

### Pseudoxanthoma Elasticum

Pseudoxanthoma elasticum is genetic disorder characterized by mineralization and fragmentation of elastin in the skin, retina, and blood vessels.[158] This autosomally inherited disease is associated with a mutation in the *ABCC6* gene, an ATP-binding cassette transporter, which may play an important role in connective tissue turnover.[159] Cutaneous lesions include small white or yellow papules classically appearing on the neck in a "gooseflesh" aspect,[160] but systemic hemorrhagic events are also encountered.

### Melas Syndrome

Nonpalpable purpuric lesions can occur on the palms and soles in *m*itochondrial *e*ncephalomyopathy with *l*actic *a*cidosis and *s*troke-like episodes (MELAS) syndrome.[161] MELAS syndrome, one of a family of mitochondrial encephalomyopathies, has been associated with a mutation in a mitochondrial transfer RNA (tRNA) or the reduced form of nicotinamide adenine dinucleotide (NADH) dehydrogenase complex I.[162] Skin manifestations can also include hypertrichosis, ichthyosis, and vitiligo.[163]

## RENDU-OSLER-WEBER DISEASE (HEREDITARY HEMORRHAGIC TELANGIECTASIA)

Rendu-Osler-Weber disease is an autosomal dominant hereditary disorder characterized by local angiodysplasia, mostly present in the skin, mucous membranes, and often in organs such as the lungs, liver, and brain.[164] It may lead to nose bleeding, acute and chronic digestive tract bleeding, and various problems resulting from the involvement of other organs. Vascular malformations may present as telangiectasias

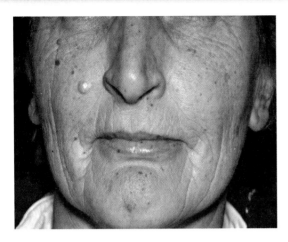

**Figure 12–26.** Rendu-Osler-Weber disease (hereditary hemorrhagic telangiectasia).

(small vascular malformations) in the skin (Fig. 12–26). Subcutaneous bleeding may occur as well, presenting as nonpalpable purpuric lesions. Angiodysplasia in Rendu-Osler-Weber disease is caused by a defect in angiogenesis. Five genetic types of hereditary hemorrhagic telangiectasia (HHT) are recognized. More than 80 percent of all cases of HHT are caused by mutations in either *ENG (endoglin, HHT1)* or *ALK1 (ACVRL1, HHT2)*.[165] Treatment of the disease is symptomatic, for example, by iron administration when iron-deficiency anemia occurs, or by laser treatment of small (bleeding) malformations in mucous membranes or embolization of larger arteriovenous malformations.

# REFERENCES

1. Carlson JA, Chen KR: Cutaneous pseudovasculitis. *Am J Dermatopathol* 29:44, 2007.
2. Piette WW: The differential diagnosis of purpura from a morphologic perspective. *Adv Dermatol* 9:3, discussion 24, 1994.
3. Piette WW: Hematologic diseases, in *Fitzpatrick's Dermatology in General Medicine*, 6th ed, edited by IM Freedburg, AZ Eisen, K Wolff, KF Austen, LA Goldsmith, SI Katz, p 1523. McGraw-Hill, New York, 2003.
4. Stephenson T: Ageing of bruising in children. *J R Soc Med* 90:312, 1997.
5. Winfield JB: Cryoglobulinemia. *Hum Pathol* 14:350, 1983.
6. Galossi A, Guarisco R, Bellis L, Puoti C: Extrahepatic manifestations of chronic HCV infection. *J Gastrointestin Liver Dis* 16:65, 2007.
7. Agnello V, Romain PL: Mixed cryoglobulinemia secondary to hepatitis C virus infection. *Rheum Dis Clin North Am* 22:1, 1996.
8. Braun GS, Horster S, Wagner KS, et al: Cryoglobulinaemic vasculitis: Classification and clinical and therapeutic aspects. *Postgrad Med J* 83:87, 2007.
9. Sansonno D, Dammacco F: Hepatitis C virus, cryoglobulinaemia, and vasculitis: Immune complex relations. *Lancet Infect Dis* 5:227, 2005.
10. Sansonno D, Tucci FA, Troiani L, et al: Increased serum levels of the chemokine CXCL13 and up-regulation of its gene expression are distinctive features of HCV-related cryoglobulinemia and correlate with active cutaneous vasculitis. *Blood* 112:1620, 2008.
11. Fabrizi F, Dixit V, Messa P: Antiviral therapy of symptomatic HCV-associated mixed cryoglobulinemia: Meta-analysis of clinical studies. *J Med Virol* 85:1019, 2013.
12. Casato M, Mecucci C, Agnello V, et al: Regression of lymphoproliferative disorder after treatment for hepatitis C virus infection in a patient with partial trisomy 3, Bcl-2 overexpression, and type II cryoglobulinemia. *Blood* 99:2259, 2002.
13. Waldenström J: Clinical methods for determination of hyperproteinemia and their practical value for diagnosis. *Nord Med* 20:2288, 1943.
14. Finder KA, McCollough ML, Dixon SL, et al: Hypergammaglobulinemic purpura of Waldenstrom. *J Am Acad Dermatol* 23:669, 1990.
15. Malaviya AN, Kaushik P, Budhiraja S, et al: Hypergammaglobulinemic purpura of Waldenström: Report of 3 cases with a short review. *Clin Exp Rheumatol* 18:518, 2000.
16. Tan E, Ng SK, Tan SH, Wong GC: Hypergammaglobulinaemic purpura presenting as reticulate purpura. *Clin Exp Dermatol* 24:469, 1999.
17. Al-Mayouf SM, Ghonaium A, Bahabri S: Hypergammaglobulinaemic purpura associated with IgG subclass imbalance and recurrent infection. *Clin Rheumatol* 19:499, 2000.
18. Oosterkamp HM, van der Pijl H, Derksen J, et al: Arthritis and hypergammaglobulinemic purpura in hypersensitivity pneumonitis. *Am J Med* 100:478, 1996.
19. Miyagawa S, Fukumoto T, Kanauchi M, et al: Hypergammaglobulinaemic purpura of Waldenstrom and Ro/SSA autoantibodies. *Br J Dermatol* 134:919, 1996.
20. Pozzi C, D'Amico M, Fogazzi GB, et al: Light chain deposition disease with renal involvement: Clinical characteristics and prognostic factors. *Am J Kidney Dis* 42:1154, 2003.
21. Stone GC, Wall BA, Oppliger IR, et al: A vasculopathy with deposition of lambda light chain crystals. *Ann Intern Med* 110:275, 1989.
22. Usuda H, Emura I, Naito M: Crystal globulin-induced vasculopathy accompanying ischemic intestinal lesions of a patient with myeloma. *Pathol Int* 46:165, 1996.
23. Sankarasubbaiyan S, Scott G, Holley JL: Cryofibrinogenemia: An addition to the differential diagnosis of calciphylaxis in end-stage renal disease. *Am J Kidney Dis* 32:494, 1998.
24. Amdo TD, Welker JA. An approach to the diagnosis and treatment of cryofibrinogenemia. *Am J Med* 116:332, 2004.
25. Blain H, Cacoub P, Musset L, et al: Cryofibrinogenaemia: A study of 49 patients. *Clin Exp Immunol* 120:253, 2000.
26. Wutschert R, Piletta P, Bounameaux H: Adverse skin reactions to low molecular weight heparins: Frequency, management and prevention. *Drug Saf* 20:515, 1999.
27. Moore A, Lau E, Yang C, et al: Dalteparin-induced skin necrosis in a patient with metastatic lung adenocarcinoma. *Am J Clin Oncol* 30:329, 2007.
28. Chong BH: Heparin-induced thrombocytopenia. *J Thromb Haemost* 1:1471, 2003.
29. Chan YC, Valenti D, Mansfield AO, Stansby G: Warfarin induced skin necrosis. *Br J Surg* 87:266, 2000.
30. Harenberg J, Hoffmann U, Huhle G, et al: Cutaneous reactions to anticoagulants. Recognition and management. *Am J Clin Dermatol* 2:69, 2001.
31. Scarff CE, Baker C, Hill P, Foley P: Late-onset warfarin necrosis. *Australas J Dermatol* 43:202, 2002.
32. Ward CT, Chavalitanonda N: Atypical warfarin-induced skin necrosis. *Pharmacotherapy* 26:1175, 2006.
33. Stone MS, Rosen T: Acral purpura: An unusual sign of coumarin necrosis. *J Am Acad Dermatol* 14:797, 1986.
34. Segel GB, Francis CA: Anticoagulant proteins in childhood venous and arterial thrombosis: A review. *Blood Cells Mol Dis* 26:540, 2000.
35. Marlar RA, Neumann A: Neonatal purpura fulminans due to homozygous protein C or protein S deficiencies. *Semin Thromb Hemost* 16:299, 1990.
36. Kemahli S, Alhenc-Gelas M, Gandrille S, et al: Homozygous protein C deficiency with a double variant His 202 to Tyr and Ala 346 to Thr. *Blood Coagul Fibrinolysis* 9:351, 1998.
37. Ezer U, Misirlioglu ED, Colba V, et al: Neonatal purpura fulminans due to homozygous protein C deficiency. *Pediatr Hematol Oncol* 18:453, 2001.
38. Gruber A, Blasko G, Sas G: Functional deficiency of protein C and skin necrosis in multiple myeloma. *Thromb Res* 42:579, 1986.
39. van Ommen CH, van Wijnen M, de Groot FG, et al: Postvaricella purpura fulminans caused by acquired protein s deficiency resulting from antiprotein s antibodies: Search for the epitopes. *J Pediatr Hematol Oncol* 24:413, 2002.
40. De Stefano V, Mastrangelo S, Schwarz HP, et al: Replacement therapy with a purified protein C concentrate during initiation of oral anticoagulation in severe protein C congenital deficiency. *Thromb Haemost* 70:247, 1993.
41. Hillman RS, Ault, KA: The dysplastic and sideroblastic anemias, in *Hematology in Clinical Practice*, 2nd ed, edited by J Morgan, P Hanley, p 151. McGraw-Hill, New York, 1998.
42. White JM, Watson K, Arya R, Du Vivier AW: Haemorrhagic bullae in a case of paroxysmal nocturnal haemoglobinuria. *Clin Exp Dermatol* 28:504, 2003.
43. Cholez C, Schmutz JL, Hulin C, et al: Cutaneous necrosis during paroxysmal nocturnal haemoglobinuria: Role of parvovirus B19? *J Eur Acad Dermatol Venereol* 19:381, 2005.
44. Goulden V, Bond L, Highet AS: Pyoderma gangrenosum associated with paroxysmal nocturnal haemoglobinuria. *Clin Exp Dermatol* 19:271, 1994.
45. Watt SG, Winhoven S, Hay CR, Lucas GS: Purpura fulminans in paroxysmal nocturnal haemoglobinuria. *Br J Haematol* 137:271, 2007.
46. Blume JE, Miller CC: Antiphospholipid syndrome: A review and update for the dermatologist. *Cutis* 78:409, 2006.
47. DiFrancesco LM, Burkart P, Hoehn JG: A cutaneous manifestation of antiphospholipid antibody syndrome. *Ann Plast Surg* 51:517, 2003.
48. Weinstein S, Piette W: Cutaneous manifestations of antiphospholipid antibody syndrome. *Hematol Oncol Clin North Am* 22:67, 2008.
49. Uthman IW, Khamashta MA: Livedo racemosa: A striking dermatological sign for the antiphospholipid syndrome. *J Rheumatol* 33:2379, 2006.
50. Martin L, Armingaud P, Georgescu V, et al: Acute bullous purpura associated with hyperhomocysteinemia and antiphospholipid antibodies. *J Am Acad Dermatol* 49:S161, 2003.
51. Hereng T, Lambert M, Hachulla E, et al: Influence of aspirin on the clinical outcomes of 103 anti-phospholipid antibodies-positive patients. *Lupus* 17:11, 2008.
52. Hairston BR, Davis MD, Pittelkow MR, Ahmed I: Livedoid vasculopathy: Further evidence for procoagulant pathogenesis. *Arch Dermatol* 142:1413, 2006.
53. Mimouni D, Ng PP, Rencic A, et al: Cutaneous polyarteritis nodosa in patients presenting with atrophie blanche. *Br J Dermatol* 148:789, 2003.
54. Acland KM, Darvay A, Wakelin SH, Russell-Jones R: Livedoid vasculitis: A manifestation of the antiphospholipid syndrome? *Br J Dermatol* 140:131, 1999.
55. Ravat FE, Evans AV, Russell-Jones R: Response of livedoid vasculitis to intravenous immunoglobulin. *Br J Dermatol* 147:166, 2002.

56. Donohue KG, Saap L, Falanga V: Cholesterol crystal embolization: An atherosclerotic disease with frequent and varied cutaneous manifestations. *J Eur Acad Dermatol Venereol* 17:504, 2003.

57. Jucgla A, Moreso F, Muniesa C, et al: Cholesterol embolism: Still an unrecognized entity with a high mortality rate. *J Am Acad Dermatol* 55:786, 2006.

58. Meyrier A: Cholesterol crystal embolism: Diagnosis and treatment. *Kidney Int* 69:1308, 2006.

59. Floege J: When man turns to stone: Extraosseous calcification in uremic patients. *Kidney Int* 65:2447, 2004.

60. Parker RW, Mouton CP, Young DW, Espino DV: Early recognition and treatment of calciphylaxis. *South Med J* 96:53, 2003.

61. Hayashi M: Calciphylaxis: Diagnosis and clinical features. *Clin Exp Nephrol* 17:498, 2013.

62. Nigwekar SU, Wolf M, Sterns RH, Hix JK: Calciphylaxis from nonuremic causes: A systematic review. *Clin J Am Soc Nephrol* 3:1139, 2008.

63. Alexandrescu DT, Wiernik PH: Cutaneous manifestations of a catheter-related thrombus. *Arch Dermatol* 141:1049, 2005.

64. García-F-Villalta MJ, Sanz-Sánchez T, Aragüés M, et al: Cutaneous embolization of cardiac myxoma. *Br J Dermatol* 147:379, 2002.

65. Zhu YI, Stiller MJ: Arthropods and skin diseases. *Int J Dermatol* 41:533, 2002.

66. Shankar S, Sterling JC, Rytina E: Pustular pyoderma gangrenosum. *Clin Exp Dermatol* 28:600, 2003.

67. Crowson AN, Mihm MC Jr, Magro C: Pyoderma gangrenosum: A review. *J Cutan Pathol* 30:97, 2003.

68. Gettler S, Rothe M, Grin C, Grant-Kels J: Optimal treatment of pyoderma gangrenosum. *Am J Clin Dermatol* 4:597, 2003.

69. Cohen PR, Kurzrock R: Sweet's syndrome: A neutrophilic dermatosis classically associated with acute onset and fever. *Clin Dermatol* 18:265, 2000.

70. Nobeyama Y, Kamide R: Sweet's syndrome with neurologic manifestation: Case report and literature review. *Int J Dermatol* 42:438, 2003.

71. Cohen PR, Kurzrock R: Sweet's syndrome: A review of current treatment options. *Am J Clin Dermatol* 3:117, 2002.

72. Chen KR, Kawahara Y, Miyakawa S, Nishikawa T: Cutaneous vasculitis in Behçet disease: A clinical and histopathologic study of 20 patients. *J Am Acad Dermatol* 36:689, 1997.

73. Yurdakul S, Hamuryudan V, Yazici H: Behçet syndrome. *Curr Opin Rheumatol* 16:38, 2004.

74. Olivieri I, Latanza L, Siringo S, et al: Successful treatment of severe Behçet's disease with infliximab in an Italian Olympic athlete. *J Rheumatol* 35:930, 2008.

75. Curigliano V, Giovinale M, Fonnesu C, et al: Efficacy of etanercept in the treatment of a patient with Behçet's disease. *Clin Rheumatol* 27:933, 2008.

76. Bielory L, Gascon P, Lawley TJ, et al: Human serum sickness: A prospective analysis of 35 patients treated with equine anti-thymocyte globulin for bone marrow failure. *Medicine (Baltimore)* 67:40, 1988.

77. Jegasothy BV: Immune complexes in the reactive inflammatory vascular dermatoses. *Dermatol Clin* 3:185, 1985.

78. Ballinger S: Henoch-Schönlein purpura. *Curr Opin Rheumatol* 15:591, 2003.

79. Saulsbury FT: Henoch-Schönlein purpura. *Curr Opin Rheumatol* 13:35, 2001.

80. Eftychiou C, Samarkos M, Golfinopoulou S, et al: Henoch-Schönlein purpura associated with methicillin-resistant *Staphylococcus aureus* infection. *Am J Med* 119:85, 2006.

81. Besbas N, Saatci U, Ruacan S, et al: The role of cytokines in Henoch-Schönlein purpura. *Scand J Rheumatol* 26:456, 1997.

82. Fretzayas A, Sionti I, Moustaki M, et al: Henoch-Schönlein purpura: A long-term prospective study in Greek children. *J Clin Rheumatol* 14:324, 2008.

83. Carlson JA, Chen KR: Cutaneous vasculitis update: Small vessel neutrophilic vasculitis syndromes. *Am J Dermatopathol* 28:486, 2006.

84. Ozaltin F, Besbas N, Uckan D, et al: The role of apoptosis in childhood Henoch-Schönlein purpura. *Clin Rheumatol* 22:265, 2003.

85. Kaku Y, Nohara K, Honda S: Renal involvement in Henoch-Schönlein purpura: A multivariate analysis of prognostic factors. *Kidney Int* 53:1755, 1998.

86. Kingston ME, Mackey D: Skin clues in the diagnosis of life-threatening infections. *Rev Infect Dis* 8:1, 1986.

87. Childers BJ, Cobanov B: Acute infectious purpura fulminans: A 15-year retrospective review of 28 consecutive cases. *Am Surg* 69:86, 2003.

88. Cnota JF, Barton LL, Rhee KH: Purpura fulminans associated with *Streptococcus pneumoniae* infection in a child. *Pediatr Emerg Care* 15:187, 1999.

89. Ward KM, Celebi JT, Gmyrek R, Grossman ME: Acute infectious purpura fulminans associated with asplenism or hyposplenism. *J Am Acad Dermatol* 47:493, 2002.

90. Betrosian AP, Berlet T, Agarwal B: Purpura fulminans in sepsis. *Am J Med Sci* 332:339, 2006.

91. Rintala E, Kauppila M, Seppala OP, et al: Protein C substitution in sepsis-associated purpura fulminans. *Crit Care Med* 28:2373, 2000.

92. Rusonis PA, Robinson HN, Lamberg SI: Livedo reticularis and purpura: Presenting features in fulminant pneumococcal septicemia in an asplenic patient. *J Am Acad Dermatol* 15:1120, 1986.

93. Baker RC, Seguin JH, Leslie N, et al: Fever and petechiae in children. *Pediatrics* 84:1051, 1989.

94. Baselga E, Drolet BA, Esterly NB: Purpura in infants and children. *J Am Acad Dermatol* 37:673, quiz 706, 1997.

95. Mancebo J, Domingo P, Blanch L, et al: The predictive value of petechiae in adults with bacterial meningitis. *JAMA* 256:2820, 1986.

96. Berger BW: Dermatologic manifestations of Lyme disease. *Rev Infect Dis* 11(Suppl 6):S1475, 1989.

97. Nielsen HE, Andersen EA, Andersen J, et al: Diagnostic assessment of haemorrhagic rash and fever. *Arch Dis Child* 85:160, 2001.

98. McNeely M, Friedman J, Pope E: Generalized petechial eruption induced by parvovirus B19 infection. *J Am Acad Dermatol* 52:S109, 2005.

99. Perez-Ferriols A, Martinez-Aparicio A, Aliaga-Boniche A: Papular-purpuric "gloves and socks" syndrome caused by measles virus. *J Am Acad Dermatol* 30:291, 1994.

100. Shiraishi H, Umetsu K, Yamamoto H, et al: Human parvovirus (HPV/B19) infection with purpura. *Microbiol Immunol* 33:369, 1989.

101. Smith SB, Libow LF, Elston DM, et al: Gloves and socks syndrome: Early and late histopathologic features. *J Am Acad Dermatol* 47:749, 2002.

102. Bruno P, Hassell LH, Brown J, et al: The protean manifestations of hemorrhagic fever with renal syndrome. A retrospective review of 26 cases from Korea. *Ann Intern Med* 113:385, 1990.

103. Helm TN, Longworth DL, Hall GS, et al: Case report and review of resolved fusariosis. *J Am Acad Dermatol* 23:393, 1990.

104. Fine JD, Miller JA, Harrist TJ, Haynes HA: Cutaneous lesions in disseminated candidiasis mimicking ecthyma gangrenosum. *Am J Med* 70:1133, 1981.

105. Galimberti R, Kowalczuk A, Hidalgo Parra I, et al: Cutaneous aspergillosis: A report of six cases. *Br J Dermatol* 139:522, 1998.

106. von Kuster LC, Genta RM: Cutaneous manifestations of strongyloidiasis. *Arch Dermatol* 124:1826, 1988.

107. Ly MN, Bethel SL, Usmani AS, et al: Cutaneous *Strongyloides stercoralis* infection: An unusual presentation. *J Am Acad Dermatol* 49:S157, 2003.

108. Jensenius M, Fournier PE, Kelly P, et al: African tick bite fever. *Lancet Infect Dis* 3:557, 2003.

109. Lamoreux MR, Sternbach MR, Hsu WT: Erythema multiforme. *Am Fam Physician* 74:1883, 2006.

110. Ng PP, Sun YJ, Tan HH, Tan SH: Detection of herpes simplex virus genomic DNA in various subsets of erythema multiforme by polymerase chain reaction. *Dermatology* 207:349, 2003.

111. Schechner AJ, Pinson AG: Acute human immunodeficiency virus infection presenting with erythema multiforme. *Am J Emerg Med* 22:330, 2004.

112. Yang YH, Tsai MJ, Tsau YK, et al: Clinical observations of erythema multiforme in children. *Acta Paediatr Taiwan* 40:107, 1999.

113. Imamura S, Horio T, Yanase K, et al: Erythema multiforme: Pathomechanism of papular erythema and target lesion. *J Dermatol* 19:524, 1992.

114. Siberry GK, Cohen BA, Johnson B: Cutaneous polyarteritis nodosa. Reports of two cases in children and review of the literature. *Arch Dermatol* 130:884, 1994.

115. Díaz-Pérez JL, De Lagrán ZM, Díaz-Ramón JL, Winkelmann RK: Cutaneous polyarteritis nodosa. *Semin Cutan Med Surg* 26:77, 2007.

116. Kluger N, Pagnoux C, Guillevin L, et al: Comparison of cutaneous manifestations in systemic polyarteritis nodosa and microscopic polyangiitis. *Br J Dermatol* 159:615, 2008.

117. Minkowitz G, Smoller BR, McNutt NS: Benign cutaneous polyarteritis nodosa. Relationship to systemic polyarteritis nodosa and to hepatitis B infection. *Arch Dermatol* 127:1520, 1991.

118. Chen KR: Cutaneous polyarteritis nodosa: A clinical and histopathological study of 20 cases. *J Dermatol* 16:429, 1989.

119. Diez-Porres L, Rios-Blanco JJ, Robles-Marhuenda A, et al: ANCA-associated vasculitis as paraneoplastic syndrome with colon cancer: A case report. *Lupus* 14:632, 2005.

120. Ayob S, McDonagh AJ: Paraneoplastic leucocytoclastic vasculitis heralding a solid-organ tumour. *Clin Exp Dermatol* 40:206, 2015.

121. Farrell AM, Stern SC, El-Ghariani K, et al: Splenic lymphoma with villous lymphocytes presenting as leucocytoclastic vasculitis. *Clin Exp Dermatol* 24:19, 1999.

122. Carlson JA, Ng BT, Chen KR: Cutaneous vasculitis update: Diagnostic criteria, classification, epidemiology, etiology, pathogenesis, evaluation and prognosis. *Am J Dermatopathol* 27:504, 2005.

122a. Ponge T, Boutoille D, Moreau A, et al: Systemic vasculitis in a patient with small-cell neuroendocrine bronchial cancer. *Eur Respir J* 12:1228, 1998.

123. Pertuiset E, Lioté F, Launay-Russ E, et al: Adult Henoch-Schönlein purpura associated with malignancy. *Semin Arthritis Rheum* 29:360, 2000.

124. Nakajima H, Ikeda M, Yamamoto Y, Kodama H: Large annular purpura and paraneoplastic purpura in a patient with Sjögren's syndrome and cervical cancer. *J Dermatol* 27:40, 2000.

125. El Tal AK, Tannous Z: Cutaneous vascular disorders associated with internal malignancy. *Dermatol Clin* 26:45, 2008.

126. Greer JM, Longley S, Edwards NL, et al: Vasculitis associated with malignancy. Experience with 13 patients and literature review. *Medicine (Baltimore)* 67:220, 1988.

127. Radić M, Martinović Kaliterna D, Radić J: Drug-induced vasculitis: A clinical and pathological review. *Neth J Med* 70:12, 2012.

128. Seo P, Stone JH: The antineutrophil cytoplasmic antibody-associated vasculitides. *Am J Med* 117:39, 2004.

129. Daoud MS, Gibson LE, DeRemee RA, et al: Cutaneous Wegener's granulomatosis: Clinical, histopathologic, and immunopathologic features of thirty patients. *J Am Acad Dermatol* 31:605, 1994.

130. Puéchal X: Antineutrophil cytoplasmic antibody-associated vasculitides. *Joint Bone Spine* 74:427, 2007.
131. Csernok E, Gross WL: Primary vasculitides and vasculitis confined to skin: Clinical features and new pathogenic aspects. *Arch Dermatol Res* 292:427, 2000.
132. Keogh KA, Specks U: Churg-Strauss syndrome. *Semin Respir Crit Care Med* 27:148, 2006.
133. Khan NA, Shenoy PK, McClymont L, Palmer TJ: Exophthalmos and facial swelling: A case of limited Churg-Strauss syndrome. *J Laryngol Otol* 110:578, 1996.
134. Reis JJ, Kaplan PW: Postictal hemifacial purpura. *Seizure* 7:337, 1998.
135. Pierson JC, Suh PS: Powerlifter's purpura: A Valsalva-associated phenomenon. *Cutis* 70:93, 2002.
136. Alcalay J, Ingber A, Sandbank M: Mask phenomenon: Postemesis facial purpura. *Cutis* 38:28, 1986.
137. Metzker A, Merlob P: Suction purpura. *Arch Dermatol* 128:822, 1992.
138. Forster PJ: Microvascular fragility at high altitude. *Br Med J (Clin Res Ed)* 296:1004, 1988.
139. Kondo T, Betz P, Eisenmenger W: Retrospective study on skin reddenings and petechiae in the eyelids and the conjunctivae in forensic physical examinations. *Int J Legal Med* 110:204, 1997.
140. Urkin J, Katz M: Suction purpura. *Isr Med Assoc J* 2:711, 2000.
141. Ramelet AA: Exercise-induced purpura. *Dermatology* 208:293, 2004.
142. Levi M, ten Cate H: Disseminated intravascular coagulation. *N Engl J Med* 341:586, 2001.
143. Beardsley DS: Pathophysiology of immune thrombocytopenic purpura. *Blood Rev* 16:13, 2002.
144. Tsai HM: Advances in the pathogenesis, diagnosis, and treatment of thrombotic thrombocytopenic purpura. *J Am Soc Nephrol* 14:1072, 2003.
145. Bruinsma W: The file of side effects to the skin: A guide to drug eruptions. *Semin Dermatol* 8:141, 1989.
146. Stern RS, Shear NH: Cutaneous reactions to drugs and biological modifiers, in *Cutaneous Medicine and Surgery*, vol 1, edited by KA Arndt, PE LeBoit, JK Robinson, BU Wintroub, p 412. WB Saunders, Philadelphia, 1996.
147. Feinstein RJ, Halprin KM, Penneys NS, et al: Senile purpura. *Arch Dermatol* 108:229, 1973.
148. Haboubi NY, Haboubi NA, Gyde OH, et al: Zinc deficiency in senile purpura. *J Clin Pathol* 38:1189, 1985.
149. Del Rosso J, Friedlander SF: Corticosteroids: Options in the era of steroid-sparing therapy. *J Am Acad Dermatol* 53:S50, 2005.
150. Nguyen RT, Cowley DM, Muir JB: Scurvy: A cutaneous clinical diagnosis. *Australas J Dermatol* 44:48, 2003.
151. Olmedo JM, Yiannias JA, Windgassen EB, Gornet MK: Scurvy: A disease almost forgotten. *Int J Dermatol* 45:909, 2006.
152. Goldsbury C, Green J: Time-lapse atomic force microscopy in the characterization of amyloid-like fibril assembly and oligomeric intermediates. *Methods Mol Biol* 299:103, 2005.
153. Eder L, Bitterman H: Image in clinical medicine. Amyloid purpura. *N Engl J Med* 356:2406, 2007.
154. Vella FS, Simone B, Antonaci S: Palmodigital purpura as the only skin abnormality in myeloma-associated systemic amyloidosis. *Br J Haematol* 120:917, 2003.
155. Breathnach SM: Amyloid and amyloidosis. *J Am Acad Dermatol* 18:1, 1988.
156. Fernandes NF, Schwartz RA: A "hyperextensive" review of Ehlers-Danlos syndrome. *Cutis* 82:242, 2008.
157. Germain DP: Clinical and genetic features of vascular Ehlers-Danlos syndrome. *Ann Vasc Surg* 16:391, 2002.
158. Bercovitch L, Terry P: Pseudoxanthoma elasticum 2004. *J Am Acad Dermatol* 51:S13, 2004.
159. Hu X, Plomp AS, Van Soest S, et al: Pseudoxanthoma elasticum: A clinical, histopathological, and molecular update. *Surv Ophthalmol* 48:424, 2003.
160. Laube S, Moss C: Pseudoxanthoma elasticum. *Arch Dis Child* 90:754, 2005.
161. Horiguchi Y, Fujii T, Imamura S: Purpuric cutaneous manifestations in mitochondrial encephalomyopathy. *J Dermatol* 18:295, 1991.
162. Kubota Y, Ishii T, Sugihara H, et al: Skin manifestations of a patient with mitochondrial encephalomyopathy with lactic acidosis and strokelike episodes (MELAS syndrome). *J Am Acad Dermatol* 41:469, 1999.
163. Sproule DM, Kaufmann P: Mitochondrial encephalopathy, lactic acidosis, and strokelike episodes: Basic concepts, clinical phenotype, and therapeutic management of MELAS syndrome. *Ann N Y Acad Sci* 1142:133, 2008.
164. Dupuis-Girod S, Bailly S, Plauchu H: Hereditary hemorrhagic telangiectasia (HHT): From molecular biology to patient care. *J Thromb Haemost* 8:1447, 2010.
168. Duffau P, Lazarro E, Viallard JF: Hereditary hemorrhagic telangiectasia. *Rev Med Intern* 35:21, 2014.

# CHAPTER 13
# HEMOPHILIA A AND HEMOPHILIA B

Miguel A. Escobar and Nigel S. Key

## SUMMARY

Hemophilias A and B are the only two bleeding disorders inherited in a sex-linked fashion. The gene for both disorders is on the long arm of the X chromosome. Both disorders appear as otherwise clinically indistinguishable hemorrhagic diseases of mild, moderate, or life-threatening severity. In the most severe form, both hemophilias A and B are characterized by multiple bleeding episodes into joints and other tissues leading to chronic crippling hemarthropathy and internal organ hemorrhage unless treated early or prophylactically with factor VIII or IX concentrates, respectively. Even though phenotypically similar, both diseases are genetically heterogeneous, with more than 1000 mutations leading to the absence of or dysfunctional factor VIII or IX molecules that do not support normal thrombin generation or adequate fibrin clot formation.

Despite similarities in hemorrhagic symptoms, there are major differences between hemophilias A and B. Hemophilia A is about five times more common than hemophilia B and is caused by defects in the factor VIII gene, a large 186-kb gene with 26 exons. A common mutation results from inversion and crossing over of intron 22 during meiosis. This mutation leads to severe hemophilia, and because no factor VIII protein is made, these patients are prone to developing antibody inhibitors to therapeutically administered factor VIII that neutralize its coagulant function, making adequate therapy problematic. Approximately 20 percent of severely affected hemophilia A patients develop such inhibitors, whereas only 3 percent or fewer of severely affected hemophilia B patients develop inhibitors against factor IX. About one-third of the mutations in hemophilias A and B arise *de novo* at CpG "hotspots." These mutations are apt to occur in the germ cells of a maternal grandfather whose daughters will be carriers and whose grandsons will have a 50 percent chance of having hemophilia.

Replacement therapy is available for both hemophilia A and hemophilia B patients. Safe, effective, and highly purified factor VIII and factor IX concentrates derived from plasma or made by recombinant technology are available for prophylactic therapy to prevent bleeding episodes or prompt treatment of

Acronyms and Abbreviations: AAV, adeno-associated virus; aPTT, activated partial thromboplastin time; BT, bleeding time; BU, Bethesda unit; CGA, cytosine, guanine, adenine; CJD, Creutzfeldt-Jakob disease; COX, cyclooxygenase; CRM, cross-reacting material; CT, computed tomography; DDAVP, 1-desamino-8-D-arginine vasopressin (desmopressin); DVT, deep vein thrombosis; EACA, ε-aminocaproic acid; FEIBA, factor VIII inhibitor bypassing activity; GLA, γ-carboxyglutamic acid; Ig, immunoglobulin; PT, prothrombin time; PTC, plasma thromboplastin component (factor IX); RFLP, restriction fragment length polymorphism; TCT, thrombin clotting time; VWD, von Willebrand disease; VWF, von Willebrand factor.

hemorrhagic events. Prophylaxis is the treatment of choice and can prevent disabling joint disease and other hemorrhagic events such that patients can expect a relatively normal life span provided that adequate replacement therapy is available. For patients with inhibitors, factor VIIa and factor VIII inhibitor bypassing activity can be used to "bypass" the factor VIII or factor IX deficiency. Both disorders are good candidates for gene therapy that may eventually lead to their cure.

## ● HEMOPHILIA A (CLASSIC HEMOPHILIA, FACTOR VIII DEFICIENCY)

### DEFINITION AND HISTORY

Hemophilia A is an X-linked hereditary disorder caused by defective synthesis of factor VIII. Hemophilia A is less common than von Willebrand disease (VWD; Chap. 16), but it is more common than other inherited clotting factor abnormalities. The estimated incidence of hemophilia A is one in every 5000 to 7000 live male births. It occurs in all ethnic groups in all parts of the world.[1]

Sex-linked hemophilia was recognized at least as early as the 2nd century, when a rabbi correctly deduced that sons of hemophilic carriers were at risk for bleeding following circumcision.[2] In the 19th century, several authors noted the sex-linked inheritance pattern of the disease and ascribed the hemorrhagic episodes to delayed blood coagulation. Morawitz[3] developed the classic theory of blood coagulation, which recognized two major reactions: (1) conversion of prothrombin to thrombin by a tissue substance that Morawitz termed *thrombokinase*, and (2) conversion of fibrinogen to fibrin by thrombin. In 1911, Addis[4] demonstrated that thrombin formed more slowly in hemophilic blood than in normal blood and that the defect could be corrected by small amounts of normal plasma. However, he incorrectly theorized that hemophilia resulted from prothrombin deficiency. As protein purification techniques improved throughout the 1930s and 1940s, thrombokinase was resolved into several distinct components. Brinkhous[5] demonstrated that the prothrombin content of hemophilic plasma was normal and that the basic defect in hemophilia was the delayed conversion of prothrombin to thrombin. The defect could be corrected by a fraction of normal plasma containing the antihemophilic factor, later named *factor VIII*. In 1947, Pavlovsky[6] observed that when blood from one patient with hemophilia was transfused into another patient with a similar clinical phenotype, the prolonged clotting time in the recipient was corrected. At the time, Pavlovsky did not recognize that he was dealing with two different types of hemophilia. This fact was recognized by Aggeler and coworkers[7] in 1952, when they described a patient deficient in "plasma thromboplastin component," a blood clotting factor different from factor VIII. A deficiency of "plasma thromboplastin component," later termed *factor IX*, was identified as the cause of hemophilia B. A month later, Biggs and colleagues described a similar patient whose surname was Christmas, thus the synonym "Christmas disease."[8] Hemophilias A and B are the only two hereditary clotting factor defects inherited in a sex-linked pattern, and they are clinically indistinguishable, although data suggest that on the whole, hemophilia B may be less severe than hemophilia A.[9] However, in an individual patient, the disorders cannot be distinguished without a specific assay for factor VIII or IX.

In 1964, a proposal to organize the growing number of coagulation factors into a cascade or waterfall mechanism was put forth by Davie and Ratnoff and by Macfarlane.[10,11] In this scheme, each zymogen clotting factor was sequentially activated to a protease that subsequently activated the next zymogen until thrombin ultimately was produced. In this scheme, factors VIII and IX were considered to be proenzymes. Later, however, factor VIII, when activated by thrombin, was shown not to be a proenzyme but rather an essential cofactor for factor IXa. The waterfall hypothesis has been modified so that the primary role of the tissue factor–factor VII complex in the initiation of coagulation is emphasized (Chap. 3).[12]

## ETIOLOGY AND PATHOGENESIS

Hemophilia A is a heterogeneous disorder resulting from defects in the factor VIII gene that leads to absent or reduced circulating levels of functional factor VIII. The reduced activity can result from a decreased amount of factor VIII protein, the presence of a functionally abnormal protein, or a combination of both. For factor VIII to be an effective cofactor for factor IXa, it must first be activated by thrombin, a reaction that results in the formation of a heterotrimer composed of the $A_1$, $A_2$, $A_3$, $C_1$, and $C_2$ domains of factor VIII in a complex with calcium (Chap. 3).[13] Activated factor VIII (factor VIIIa) and activated factor IX (factor IXa) associate on the surface of activated platelets, forming a functional factor X–activating complex ("tenase" or "Xase").[14] In the presence of factor VIIIa, the rate of factor X activation by factor IXa is dramatically enhanced. That hemophilia A and hemophilia B have similar clinical manifestations is not surprising, because both factor VIIIa and factor IXa are required to form the Xase complex. The lack of either activated protein leads to a similar lack of platelet surface Xase activity with subsequent decreased thrombin generation. In patients with hemophilia, clot formation is delayed because of the decreased thrombin generation. The clot that is formed is friable, easily dislodged, and highly susceptible to fibrinolysis, all of which lead to excessive bleeding and poor wound healing.[15]

## GENETICS

Hemophilia A results when mutations occur in the factor VIII gene located on the long arm of the X chromosome (X-q28). The disease occurs almost exclusively in males. Figure 13–1 shows the inheritance pattern of hemophilia A and hemophilia B. All the sons of affected hemophilic males are normal, whereas all the daughters are obligatory carriers of the factor VIII defect. Sons of carriers have a 50 percent chance of being affected, whereas daughters of carriers have a 50 percent chance of being carriers themselves.

The factor VIII gene is very large, approximately 186 kb, with approximately 9 kb of exons. The gene contains 26 exons and 25 introns.[16] Based on the sequence of the factor VIII gene in normal individuals and patients with hemophilia A, numerous specific mutations have been described[16,17]; as of 2015, more than 2000 specific variants in the factor VIII gene resulting in classic hemophilia have been described.[17]

Hemophilia A can result from multiple alterations in the factor VIII gene. These include gene rearrangements; missense mutations, in which a single base substitution leads to an amino acid change in the molecule; nonsense mutations, which result in a stop codon; abnormal splicing of the gene; deletions of all or portions of the gene; and insertions of genetic elements.[18] The genetic defects leading to hemophilia have been reviewed.[17]

One of the most common mutations, accounting for 40 to 50 percent of severe hemophilia A patients, is a unique "combined gene inversion and crossing over" that disrupts the factor VIII gene.[19,20] Figures 13–2 and 13–3 schematically depict the factor VIII gene and the mechanism of the "inversion–crossing over."[21] Within intron 22 are two other genes: (1) $F8A(a_1)$, which is transcribed in the 5′ direction, and (2) $F8B$, which is transcribed in the 3′ direction of the factor VIII gene. The hatched boxes in Figure 13–3 show two other extragenic homologous sequences ($a_2$,$a_3$) 5′ to the $F8A$ gene that lies within intron 22 ($a_1$). The presence of extragenic $F8A$ sequences 5′ to the $F8A$ gene within intron 22 is central to the inversion and translocation of part of the factor VIII gene from exon 1 to exon 22. The mechanism is homologous recombination between the $F8A$ sequence that lies within intron 22 and one of the homologous extragenic sequences of the $F8A$ gene 5′ to the factor VIII gene. During meiosis, crossing over of homologous sequences occurs between the $F8A$ gene lying within intron 22 and one of the extragenic homologous $F8A$ sequences 5′ to intron 22. Thus, the transcription of the complete factor VIII sequence is interrupted (Fig. 13–3). Figure 13–3 shows a common inversion and crossing over, but homologous recombinations can occur with either of the extragenic genes. Approximately 2 to 5 percent of the severe cases of hemophilia A carry the intron 1 inversion resulting in the separation of the F8 promoter–exon 1 sequence from the remainder of the F8 gene.[22] The "inversion–crossing over" mutations result in severe hemophilia, and approximately 20 percent of these patients are susceptible to developing antibody inhibitors that neutralize factor VIII coagulant function.

Of the different insertions in the factor VIII gene that have been reported, a few are long interspersed elements (LINEs) that are transposon sequences; that is, sequences that have been inserted frequently throughout the genome.[23] Most of these insertions result in severe hemophilia.

In many cases of hemophilia, there is no family history of the disease, and at least 30 percent of the cases of hemophilia are a result of spontaneous (*de novo*) mutations. Most of these occur at CpG dinucleotides in the factor VIII gene.[23] *De novo* occurrences of hemophilia usually result from a mutation in the gamete of a normal male; for example, a mutation in the germ cell of a maternal grandfather will give rise to the hemophilia gene in his daughters such that his grandsons may have hemophilia.[18] Codons for the amino acid arginine (CGA [cytosine, guanine, adenine]) are frequently affected by mutations at CG doublets. A C→T transition often results in a stop codon with synthesis of a truncated factor VIII molecule and usually is associated with severe hemophilia A. However, a G→A transition results in a missense mutation, which often leads to a dysfunctional factor VIII molecule that may be associated with mild, moderate, or severe hemophilia. Some missense

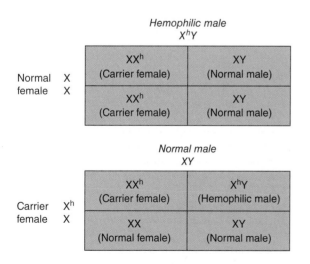

**Figure 13–1.** Inheritance pattern of hemophilia. All daughters of a hemophilic male are carriers of hemophilia, whereas all sons are normal. Daughters of carriers have a 50 percent chance of being a carrier, whereas sons of carriers have a 50 percent chance of having hemophilia. X, normal; X$^h$, abnormal X chromosome with the hemophilic gene; X$^h$Y, hemophilic male; XX, normal female; XX$^h$, carrier female; XY, normal male; Y, normal.

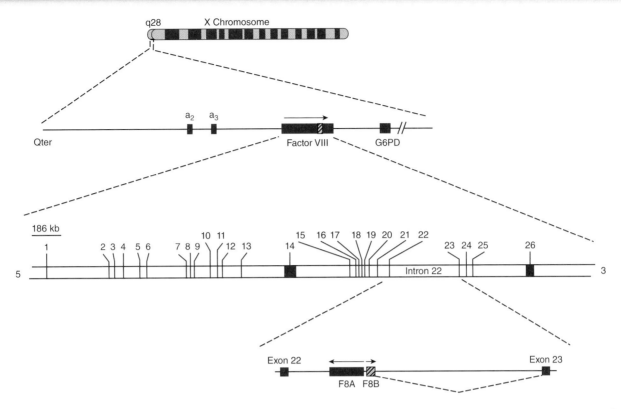

**Figure 13–2.** Schematic of the factor VIII gene *(FVIII)*. The *FVIII* gene is located at q28 on the long arm of the X chromosome. The region of the *FVIII* gene is enlarged on the *second line*. Note that two genes, designated a₂ and a₃, are 5′ to the *FVIII* gene. The *hatched area* indicated on *FVIII* corresponds to intron 22 shown on the *third line*. Within intron 22 *(fourth line)* are two nested genes, one designated *F8A*, which is transcribed in a direction opposite to that of the whole *FVIII* and is homologous to the a₂ and a₃ genes shown on *line 2*. G6PD, glucose-6-phosphate dehydrogenase. *(Reproduced with permission from Scriver CR, Beaudet AL, Sly WS et al: Metabolic and Molecular Basis of Inherited Diseases, 8th ed. New York: McGraw-Hill; 1995.)*

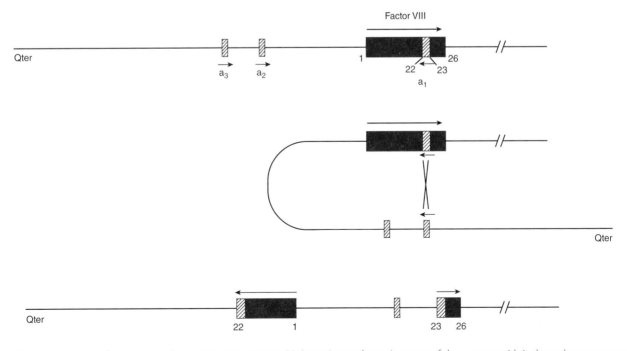

**Figure 13–3.** Schematic of inversion and crossing over at intron 22. Inversion and crossing-over of the a₃ gene with its homologous sequence a₁ nested within intron 22 are shown. *Middle panel:* When crossing over of the a₁ gene nested within intron 22 and the a₃ gene extragenic to *FVIII* occurs, a portion of *FVIII* is transcribed in a reverse manner from exon 1 through exon 22. Homologous recombination with the extragenic a₂ gene is also possible. In some individuals there are two a₂ or a₃ extragenic sequences giving rise to four possible types of the "inversion–crossing over" mechanism. *(Reproduced with permission from Antonarakis SE, Kazazian HH, Tuddenham EG: Molecular etiology of factor VIII deficiency in hemophilia A. Hum Mutat 1995;5(1):1–22.)*

mutations result in the production of normal or near-normal amounts of factor VIII antigen, while the coagulant activity may be dramatically or only slightly reduced. Many other single-base substitutions have been described, resulting in hemophilia of varying degrees of severity.

Large deletions in the factor VIII gene almost always are associated with severe hemophilia. On the other hand, a small deletion that does not change the reading frame of the gene may result in milder disease. Patients with large deletions who have no detectable factor VIII antigen are more susceptible to the development of anti–factor VIII antibodies, although antibodies clearly also occur in patients without deletions.[16,23]

Hemophilia A in females is extremely rare, although an affected female offspring from a hemophilic father and carrier mother have been reported. Hemophilia A may occur in females with X chromosomal abnormalities such as Turner syndrome, X chromosomal mosaicism, and other X chromosomal defects.[23,24] If the normal X chromosome is inactivated disproportionately ("imbalanced X inactivation") in a carrier female, factor VIII levels may be sufficiently low to cause bleeding manifestations. Usually these manifestations are mild, but they may be serious during surgical procedures or following significant trauma.

## PRENATAL DIAGNOSIS AND CARRIER DETECTION

A careful and complete family history is important for carrier detection.[25] All daughters of a hemophilic father are obligatory carriers of the hemophilic defect. If a known carrier has a daughter, that daughter has a 50 percent chance of being a carrier.

Carrier detection is important when a daughter of a known carrier or a female offspring of a hemophilic patient wishes to become pregnant. At times, the history of hemophilia in the family is in a distant blood relative, and the gene for hemophilia may skip several generations. The current standard for identifying carrier status is through direct gene sequencing. Carriers who harbor the intron 22 inversion or intron 1 inversion can be identified using the Southern blot technique and polymerase chain reaction, respectively.[22,25] If these mutations are found to be absent, sequencing of the complete coding region is performed.[26]

Use of markers for restriction fragment length polymorphism (RFLP) is simpler than direct sequencing of the coding region of the factor VIII gene, but use of the RFLP technique requires that the pedigree analyses include at least one hemophilic male whose mother is heterozygous for one or more RFLP markers.[27,28] This technique is no longer considered to be the optimal approach in genotyping of affected males or carrier females.

Prenatal diagnosis of hemophilia now can be performed almost routinely.[29] If a carrier female has a fetus that can be identified as a female by chromosomal analysis of cells obtained by amniocentesis (at approximately 16 weeks of gestation), analysis of free fetal DNA, ultrasound, or chorionic villus sampling at week 10 of gestation, little concern exists regarding whether the female fetus is a carrier because carriers usually have no bleeding tendency. If the fetus is a male, sufficient cells can be obtained to perform DNA analysis using the methods described above. The decision on whether to carry an affected male fetus to term should be decided by the parents after they are appropriately counseled and provided with all the necessary genetic, clinical, and therapeutic information about hemophilia. As the treatment for hemophilia A improves, the decision to continue an affected pregnancy should become far easier.

## CLINICAL FEATURES

Hemophilia A is characterized by excessive bleeding into various tissues of the body, including soft tissue hematomas and hemarthroses that can lead to severe crippling hemarthropathy. Recurrent hemarthroses are

| TABLE 13–1. Clinical Classification of Hemophilia | | |
|---|---|---|
| **Classification** | **Factor VIII Level** | **Clinical Features** |
| Severe | ≤1% of normal (≤0.01 U/mL) | 1. Spontaneous hemorrhage from early infancy 2. Frequent spontaneous hemarthroses and other hemorrhages, requiring clotting factor replacement |
| Moderate | 1–5% of normal (0.01–0.05 U/mL) | 1. Hemorrhage secondary to trauma or surgery 2. Occasional spontaneous hemarthroses |
| Mild | 6–40% of normal (0.06–0.40 U/mL) | 1. Hemorrhage secondary to trauma or surgery 2. Rare spontaneous hemorrhage |

characteristic of the disease. The disease has been broadly classified as mild, moderate, and severe, although overlap exists between these categories. Table 13–1 shows a classification based on the severity of clinical manifestations. A range of plasma factor VIII concentrations in percentages of normal and in units per milliliter is given for each category. Approximately 10 percent of individuals with factor VIII levels compatible with severe hemophilia may exhibit milder symptoms.[30] Among other explanations, this phenotypic heterogeneity could be a result of coinheritance of thrombophilic mutations, such as the factor V Leiden mutation (R506Q).[31] Severely affected patients (<1 percent factor VIII) frequently experience "spontaneous" bleeding without known trauma other than that associated with the usual day-to-day activities. Without effective treatment, recurrent hemarthroses, resulting in chronic hemophilic arthropathy, occur by young adulthood and are highly characteristic of the severe form of the disorder. However, bleeding episodes are intermittent, and some patients do not bleed for weeks or months. Except for intracranial bleeding, sudden death because of hemorrhage is rare in societies where clotting factor concentrates are freely available.

Moderately affected patients with hemophilia may have occasional hematomas. Hemarthroses, usually associated with a known trauma, may occur as well. These patients have greater than 1 percent but less than 5 percent of normal factor VIII activity.

Mildly affected patients with hemophilia, who have factor VIII levels between 6 to 40 percent, have infrequent bleeding episodes. The disease may go undiagnosed and be discovered only because of excessive hemorrhage postoperatively, following trauma, or after the toss and tumble of contact sports.

Most carriers have approximately 50 percent factor VIII activity and experience no bleeding symptoms, even with surgical procedures. Carriers with factor VIII levels significantly less than 50 percent, as a result of imbalanced X chromosome inactivation, may experience excessive bleeding after trauma (e.g., childbirth or surgery). Therefore, measurement of factor VIII level is recommended in all carriers.

### Hemarthroses

Bleeding into joints accounts for approximately 75 percent of bleeding episodes in severely affected patients with hemophilia A.[32,33] The normal synovium has few cells, but numerous capillaries beneath the synovial layer can be damaged by the mechanical trauma associated with daily use of joints. The joints most frequently involved, in decreasing order of frequency, are knees, elbows, ankles, shoulders, wrists, and hips. Hinge joints are much more likely to be involved than are ball-and-socket joints. Hemarthroses usually occur when an affected child begins to walk.

Hemarthroses are heralded by an aura of mild discomfort that, over a period of minutes to hours, becomes progressively painful. The joint usually swells, becomes warm, and exhibits limited motion. Occasionally, the patient experiences a mild fever. Significant and sustained fever, however, suggests an infected joint. When joint bleeding does not respond to replacement therapy, one should suspect the presence of an inhibitor of factor VIII or an infected joint. Bleeding into the knee joint is more easily detected by physical findings than is bleeding into either the elbow or shoulder. When bleeding stops, the blood resorbs, and the symptoms gradually subside over a period of several days. If hemarthroses are treated early, pain usually subsides in 6 to 8 hours and disappears in 12 to 24 hours. However, repeated hemorrhage into the joints eventually results in extensive destruction of articular cartilage, synovial hyperplasia, and other reactive changes in the adjacent bone and tissues. Iron deposits from residual blood are a major factor in the pathogenesis of hemophilic arthropathy.[33] Acute bleeding into a chronically affected joint may be difficult to distinguish from the pain of degenerative arthritis.

A major complication of repeated hemarthroses is joint deformity complicated by muscle atrophy and soft tissue contractures (Fig. 13–4). Figure 13–5 shows the various radiologic stages of progressive destruction of joint cartilage and adjacent bone. Osteoporosis and cystic areas in the subchondral bone may develop, and progressive loss of joint space occurs. Figure 13–6 shows a magnetic resonance image (MRI) of a normal knee in comparison to a knee from an individual with severe hemophilia with arthropathy. Figure 13–7 depicts bleeding into a hemophilic ankle.

Repeated bleeding into a joint results in synovial hypertrophy and inflammation. The synovium is thickened and folded, leading to limited joint motion. The result is a tendency for repeated hemorrhages leading to a so-called target joint.[32] Indeed, a target joint is defined by the occurrence of three or more spontaneous bleeds within a 6-month period. The joints most often involved are the knees, ankles, and elbows, which become chronically swollen. Chronic synovitis may persist for months or years unless the condition is adequately treated.

Infection of hemophilic joints is not common but must be suspected in all patients with fever, leukocytosis, or other systemic manifestations. Rapid diagnosis is mandatory, because infection of such joints leads to rapid loss of joint architecture and function. A painful and swollen joint may require aspiration, which should be performed by experienced personnel using meticulous aseptic techniques and appropriate factor replacement therapy prior to aspiration.

### Hematomas

Soft tissue hematomas are also characteristic of hemophilia A. Hemorrhage into subcutaneous connective tissues or into muscles may occur with or without a known trauma. Hematomas, once formed, may stabilize and slowly resorb. However, in moderately and severely affected patients, hematomas have a tendency to enlarge progressively and to dissect in all directions, unless appropriately treated. Rarely, retroperitoneal hematomas, after beginning in the iliopsoas muscle, can dissect superiorly through the diaphragm, into the chest, and sometimes even into the soft tissues of the neck, compromising the airway. A retroperitoneal hematoma is more likely to compromise renal function by causing ureteral obstruction. Figure 13–8 shows the computed tomography (CT) scan of a patient with a retroperitoneal hemorrhage. Other hematomas

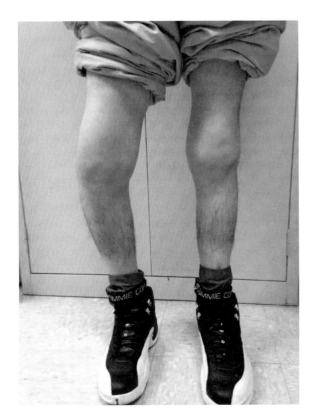
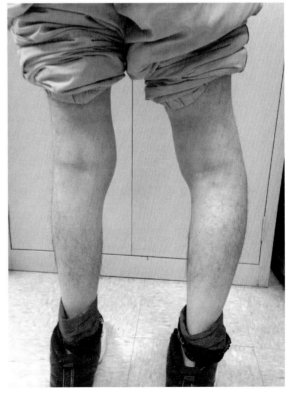

**Figure 13–4.** Hemophilic arthropathy. The chronic effects of repeated hemorrhage into the knees of a severely affected hemophilic patient are seen. Note contractures and deformity with atrophy of muscle tissue.

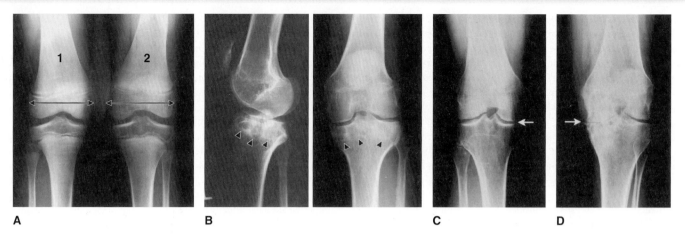

**Figure 13–5.** Various radiologic stages of hemophilic arthropathy. Stages 0 (normal joint) and 1 (fluid in the joint) are not shown. **A.** Stage 2. Some osteoporosis and epiphyseal overgrowth are present in knee 2. Epiphysis is wider in knee 2 than in knee 1 *(arrows)*. **B.** Stage 3. Subchondral bone cysts *(arrowheads)*. Joint spaces exhibit irregularities. **C.** Stage 4. Prominent bone cysts with marked narrowing of joint space *(arrow)*. **D.** Stage 5. Obliteration of joint space with epiphyseal overgrowth *(arrow)*.

expand locally and may compress adjacent organs, blood vessels, and nerves. A rare, and often fatal, complication of an abdominal hematoma is perforation and drainage into the colon. Subcutaneous hematomas may dissect into muscle. Pharyngeal and retropharyngeal hematomas, sometimes complicating simple colds, may enlarge and obstruct the airway. Hemorrhage in or around the airway is a potentially life-threatening situation that requires prompt administration of factor VIII.

Hemorrhages occur into muscle in the following order of frequency: calf, thigh, buttocks, and forearm. Recurrent or unresolved hematomas may lead to muscle contractures, nerve palsies, and muscle

atrophy. Bleeding into the tongue (Fig. 13–9) or frenulum is particularly frequent in young children and usually is caused by trauma.

Bleeding into fascia and muscle can result in a so-called compartment syndrome. This results when hemorrhage in a confined space compresses the arterial vasculature resulting in ischemic muscle injury. Compartment syndrome tends to occur in the distal part of the extremities, particularly in the flexor muscles, and sometimes requires urgent fasciotomy under cover of clotting factor replacement therapy. Bleeding into the myocardium or erect penis is very unusual, perhaps explained by the high concentration of tissue factor in these tissues.

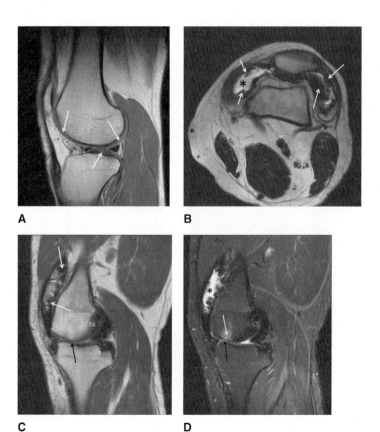

**Figure 13–6.** Magnetic resonance imaging (MRI) of normal and hemophilic knees. **A.** MRI of normal knee. **B.** A transverse T2-weighted spin-echo image of the knee shows an effusion (*) and multiple foci of hemosiderin deposition *(arrows)* along the synovium lining the suprapatellar bursa. **C.** A sagittal T2-weighted spin-echo image of the knee shows dark foci of synovial hemosiderin deposition *(white arrows)* accompanied by narrowing of the femorotibial joint *(black arrow)*. **D.** A sagittal STIR (short tau inversion recovery) image of the knee (in the same patient as **B**) demonstrates an effusion in the suprapatellar bursa (*). The irregular, lumpy surface of the bursa represents thickened, hemosiderin-laden synovium. Femorotibial joint narrowing *(black arrow)* is associated with edema in the subchondral bone of the femoral condyle *(white arrow)*. *(Used with permission of Dr. Jordan Renner, University of North Carolina.)*

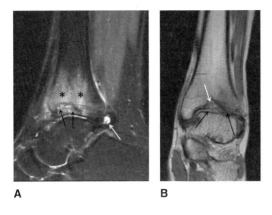

**Figure 13–7. A.** A sagittal STIR (short tau inversion recovery) image of an ankle shows an effusion *(white arrow)*. Edema in the distal tibia (∗) surrounds a debris-filled defect in the subchondral bone of the distal tibia *(black arrows)*. **B.** A coronal proton density of the ankle in the same patient as in **A** shows the defect in the subchondral bone of the distal tibia *(white arrow)*. Mild narrowing of the tibiotalar joint *(black arrows)* is more apparent laterally.

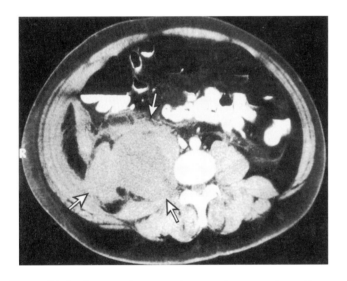

**Figure 13–8.** Computed tomography scan of a retroperitoneal hematoma in a patient with severe hemophilia A. Extent of the hematoma is indicated by the arrows.

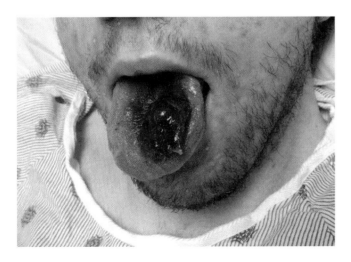

**Figure 13–9.** Photograph of a tongue hematoma caused by trauma.

## Pseudotumors (Blood Cysts)

Pseudotumors are blood cysts that occur in soft tissues or bone. They are rare but dangerous complications of hemophilia (Fig. 13–10).[34] They are classified into three types. One type is a simple cyst that is confined by tendinous attachments within the fascial envelope of a muscle. The second type initially develops as a simple cyst in soft tissues such as a tendon, but it interferes with the vascular supply to the adjacent bone and periosteum, resulting in cyst formation and resorption of bone. The third type is thought to result from subperiosteal bleeding that separates the periosteum from the bony cortex. Most pseudotumors are not associated with pain unless rapid growth or nerve compression occurs. As the volume of the cyst increases, the cyst compresses and destroys the adjacent muscle, nerve, and/or bone or expands around structures like ureters causing renal failure. Pseudotumors usually contain either serosanguineous fluid or a viscous brownish material surrounded by a fibrous membrane (Fig. 13–10). Pseudotumors have a tendency to expand over several years and eventually become multiloculated. Some reach enormous size and involve so many structures that they become inoperable. Erosion through surrounding tissues and penetration into viscera or through the skin can occur, usually as a late event. Sinus tracts from the pseudotumor predispose to infection and septicemia. Pseudotumors often develop in the lower half of the body, usually in the thigh, buttock, or pelvis, but they can occur anywhere, including the temporal bone. CT or MRI is useful for diagnosis. Needle biopsies of pseudotumors should be avoided because of the risk of infection and hemorrhage. A reliable treatment is operative removal of the entire mass because the pseudotumor likely will reform if it is not completely removed. Embolization, percutaneous drainage, and radiotherapy of a pseudotumor have been reported and may be of value in hemophiliacs with inhibitors when surgery is not possible.[35] Surgical treatment of patients with large pseudotumors should be done in a hemophilia treatment center with a specialized multidisciplinary team of experts.[36]

## Hematuria

Many severely affected patients with hemophilia experience episodes of spontaneous and asymptomatic hematuria. The urine may be brown or red, depending on the rate of bleeding. Most bleeding arises from the renal pelvis, usually from one kidney but occasionally from both. Appropriate studies to exclude a structural lesion in the kidneys should be performed. Administration of factor replacement and hydration is usually sufficient to arrest the bleeding. Antifibrinolytic agents, such as aminocaproic acid and tranexamic acid, should be avoided in individuals with hematuria because of the risk of forming clots and producing obstructing clots in the ureter.

## Neurologic Complications

Intracranial bleeding is one of the most dangerous hemorrhagic events in hemophilic patients.[37] Currently, bleeding into the brain is a leading cause of death in hemophilic patients. Hemorrhage into the central nervous system may be "spontaneous" but usually follows trauma, which may be trivial. Symptoms often occur soon after trauma, but sometimes are delayed. For example, symptoms of a subdural hematoma may be delayed for days or several weeks. Hemorrhage into the brain parenchyma or a subdural or epidural hematoma should always be suspected in hemophilic patients with unusual headaches. When intracranial bleeding is suspected, the patient should be treated immediately with factor VIII, and diagnostic procedures, such as CT scans or MRI studies, should be delayed until after treatment is initiated. Although lumbar puncture has been performed safely in severe hemophilic patients without replacement therapy, replacing factor VIII to a level of approximately 50 percent of normal prior to the procedure is advisable.

Hemorrhage into the spinal canal is an uncommon neurologic complication in hemophilia, mostly related to trauma that can result

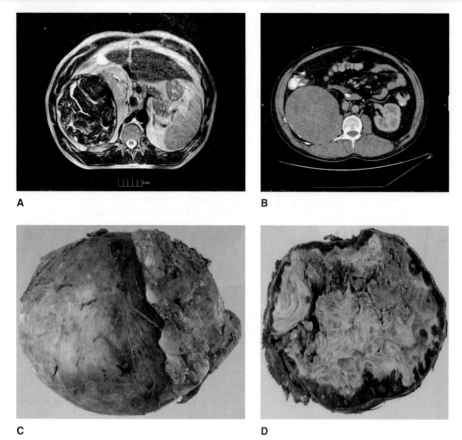

**Figure 13–10.** Retroperitoneal pseudotumor. **A** and **B.** Magnetic resonance imaging and computed tomography scan of pseudotumor arising from the iliopsoas muscle compressing the kidney and other adjacent structures. Loculations and calcifications can be seen. **C.** Gross specimen after surgical removal, weighting approximately 6 pounds. **D.** Cross-section of pseudotumor shows peripheral red hemorrhage, centrally caseified blood and necrosis. Note the thick capsule that surrounds the tumor.

in paraplegia. Bleeding may occur within the spinal cord itself, but epidural bleeding compressing the cord is more common.

Peripheral nerve compression is a frequent complication of muscle hematomas, particularly in the extremities. Compression of the femoral nerve by a hematoma in the iliopsoas muscle can result in sensory loss over the lateral and anterior thigh, weakness and atrophy of the quadriceps, and loss of the patellar reflex. The ulnar nerve is the next most frequently involved peripheral nerve. Bleeding may occur in any muscle and may compress local neural blood supply. This situation can be followed by permanent neuromuscular defects and multiple contractures.

### Mucous Membrane Hemorrhage

Mucous membrane bleeding is common in hemophilia. Epistaxis and hemoptysis, often resulting from allergic reactions or trauma, can be associated with local structural lesions involving the upper and/or lower respiratory tract. Treatment of epistaxis by cautery or nasal packing sometimes is followed by recurrent bleeding because of sloughing of the cauterized area or dislodging of a poorly formed clot when the packing is removed. Gastrointestinal hemorrhage has a 1.3 percent annual incidence and is mostly associated with older age and complications of advanced liver disease. Ingestion of antiinflammatory drugs for relief of pain of hemophilic arthropathy is a frequent cause of upper gastrointestinal hemorrhage, and a history of ingestion of aspirin and other antiinflammatory drugs should be specifically addressed (and proscribed) when assessing the etiology of such bleeding.[38]

### Dental and Surgical Bleeding

Hemophilic patients are treated with clotting factor preoperatively and postoperatively to prevent bleeding. Mildly or sometimes moderately affected patients may go unrecognized until surgery results in excessive bleeding at the surgical site. Bleeding may be delayed for several hours or, occasionally, for several days. Surgery in such patients is characterized by delayed wound healing because of poor clot formation.[15] Prolonged bleeding and subsequent infection of the wound hematoma may further complicate healing. Appropriate factor VIII replacement therapy, sometimes supplemented by antifibrinolytic agents, can prevent intraoperative and postoperative hemorrhages.

Dental extraction is the most frequent surgical procedure performed on hemophilic patients. Loss of deciduous teeth seldom causes excessive bleeding, but extraction of permanent teeth may result in excessive hemorrhage that can persist intermittently for several days to weeks unless appropriate treatment is administered. In the untreated patient with severe hemophilia, life-threatening, dissecting pharyngeal and/or sublingual hematomas may result from dental procedures or from administration of regional block anesthesia.

## LABORATORY FEATURES

Patients with severe hemophilia A have a prolonged activated partial thromboplastin time (aPTT). The prothrombin time (PT) and thrombin clotting time (TCT) are normal. Different combinations of aPTT reagents and instrumentation exhibit varying sensitivities to factor VIII levels. In mild hemophilia, the aPTT may be only slightly prolonged or at the upper limit of normal, especially if factor VIII activity is 20 percent or greater. The aPTT is corrected when hemophilic plasma is mixed with an equal volume of normal plasma. If the hemophilic plasma contains an anti–factor VIII inhibitor antibody, the aPTT on a similar mixture is prolonged, but incubation of the mixture for 1 or 2 hours at 37°C is sometimes required to detect the prolongation. A definitive diagnosis of hemophilia A should be based on a specific assay for factor VIII activity.

Functional factor VIII coagulant activity is measured by one-stage clotting assays based on the aPTT. Chromogenic assays for factor VIII activity also are used widely but do not always agree with one-stage assays.[39] Although infrequently measured in practice, factor VIII antigen is measured by immunologic assays, which detect normal and most abnormal factor VIII molecules. If the factor VIII antigen level is normal but the clotting activity is reduced, the patient has a dysfunctional factor VIII molecule. Such patients have antigen-positive hemophilia, also referred to as cross-reacting material (CRM) positive.[40] Patients in whom both the factor VIII antigen level and activity are nearly undetectable are said to be CRM negative.

## DIFFERENTIAL DIAGNOSIS

VWD sometimes is confused with hemophilia A. The basic defect in VWD is reduced activity of von Willebrand factor (VWF), which acts as a carrier of factor VIII *in vivo* (Chap. 16). Thus, in VWD, factor VIII levels are reduced, although considerable variability exists. Although factor VIII is synthesized normally in patients with VWD, the half-life of factor VIII is markedly shortened because the VWF "carrier" molecule is decreased or absent. Other abnormalities in VWD that distinguish VWD from hemophilia A are decreased VWF antigen level and decreased VWF activity, often measured using the ristocetin cofactor activity assay and a prolonged closure time using the platelet function analyzer PFA-100. In type III VWD, factor VIII levels may be very low (<5 percent of normal), making it difficult to distinguish from classical hemophilia. The lack of a sex-linked pattern of inheritance in the family will help in the differential diagnosis.

Another variant of VWD that is particularly difficult to distinguish from hemophilia A is VWD-Normandy, in which VWF multimers are normal but plasma factor VIII levels are low.[41] Several mutations causing VWD-Normandy have been described, but all of them result in decreased binding of factor VIII to VWF.[42] The result is shortening of the intravascular survival of factor VIII and thus reduced factor VIII activity. The Normandy variant of VWD should be suspected in patients with mild hemophilia A who do not exhibit a sex-linked recessive inheritance pattern.

Hemophilia A must be distinguished from other hereditary blood clotting factor deficiencies that exhibit a prolonged aPTT, including deficiencies of factors IX, XI, and XII, prekallikrein, and high-molecular-weight kininogen. Only deficiencies of factors VIII and IX cause chronic crippling hemarthroses with a family history suggestive of an X-linked bleeding disorder. Only specific assays can distinguish hemophilia A from factor IX deficiency (hemophilia B). Factor XI deficiency occurs in males and females and is a milder hemorrhagic disorder compared to severe hemophilia A or B. Factor XI deficiency can be confused with mild hemophilia A or B on screening laboratory tests, but specific assays distinguish them. Deficiencies of factor XII, prekallikrein, and high-molecular-weight kininogen can be distinguished from hemophilia because they are not associated with bleeding. Mild hemophilia A, with factor VIII levels of approximately 10 to 20 percent of normal, must be distinguished from combined deficiency of factors V and VIII.[43,44] Both the PT and aPTT are moderately prolonged in the combined disorder.[44]

## THERAPY

### General

General principles applicable to therapy for hemophilia A include avoidance of aspirin, nonsteroidal antiinflammatory drugs, and other agents that interfere with platelet aggregation. Acetaminophen or relatively specific cyclooxygenase (COX)-2 inhibitors such as celecoxib have been recommended, but these drugs can be harmful when taken in excessive doses or for prolonged periods. Patients should be advised of the numerous nonprescription analgesics and herbals that contain aspirin or other antiplatelet agents. Addictive narcotic agents should be used with great caution and only when clearly indicated, because drug dependency can be a major problem for patients with hemophilia. In general, intramuscular injections should be avoided unless the patient receives adequate replacement therapy. In the absence of prophylactic therapy, patients with hemophilia A must be treated as early as possible to avoid bleeding complications. Surgical procedures in hemophilic patients should be scheduled early in the week to avoid "weekend crises." Ample supplies of factor VIII should be available in the blood bank or pharmacy to ensure rapid access to treatment when needed. All hemophilic patients should have access to home treatment and periodic examinations at a comprehensive hemophilia treatment center. Prophylactic therapy is recommended in all severely affected patients, and it should be initiated before the onset of recurrent hemarthroses (primary prophylaxis) or as directed. Secondary prophylaxis for an established "target" joint may be necessary.[45]

### Factor VIII Replacement Therapy

Hemorrhagic episodes in patients with hemophilia A can be managed by replacing factor VIII. Several products are available for use in raising factor VIII to hemostatic levels (Table 13–2). Fresh-frozen plasma and

**TABLE 13–2.** Currently Available Factor VIII Products[a]

| | Origin | Viral Inactivation |
|---|---|---|
| **Intermediate purity** | | |
| Humate P[b] | Plasma | Pasteurization[c] |
| **High purity** | | |
| Koate DVI[b] | Plasma | Solvent-detergent[d], heat treated[i] |
| Alphanate[b] | Plasma | Solvent-detergent, heat treated[i] |
| **Ultrapure**[e] | | |
| Hemofil M | Plasma | Solvent-detergent[d] |
| Monoclate P | Plasma | Pasteurization[c] |
| **Recombinant** | | |
| Advate[h] | CHO cells[f] | Solvent-detergent |
| Recombinate[e] | CHO cells[f] | |
| Kogenate FS[e] | BHK cells[g] | Solvent-detergent |
| Novoeight[h] | CHO cells[f] | Solvent-detergent, nanofiltration |
| Xyntha[h] | CHO cells[f] | Solvent-detergent, nanofiltration |
| Afstyla[h] | CHO cells[f] | Solvent-detergent, nanofiltration |
| Nuwiq[h] | HEK cells[j] | Solvent-detergent, nanofiltration |
| Eloctate*[h] | HEK cells[j] | Solvent-detergent, nanofiltration |
| Adynovate*[h] | CHO cells[f] | Solvent-detergent |

*Extended half-life factor VIII product.

[a]Additional concentrates are available in Europe.

[b]Contains von Willebrand factor (VWF).

[c]Pasteurization at 60°C for 10 hours.

[d]Solvent-detergent: tri-n-butyl phosphate (TNBP) + polysorbate 80.

[e]Human albumin added; insignificant VWF.

[f]Chinese hamster ovarian cells (recombinant product).

[g]Baby hamster kidney cells (recombinant product).

[h]Not exposed to human or animal protein during manufacture.

[i]Heat treated at 80°C for 72 hours.

[j]Human embryonic kidney cells (recombinant product).

cryoprecipitate both contain factor VIII and once were the only products available for treatment. A disadvantage of plasma is that large volumes must be infused to achieve and maintain even minimal factor VIII levels. The highest factor VIII level that can be achieved with plasma is approximately 20 percent of normal, which is not always attainable or sufficient for hemostasis. Cryoprecipitate, containing approximately 80 U of factor VIII in 10 mL of solution, can be used to attain normal factor VIII levels, but individual bags of cryoprecipitate must be pooled; the factor VIII dose can only be estimated; and the product must be stored frozen. Several commercial lyophilized factor VIII concentrates, using cryoprecipitate of pooled normal human plasmas as starting material (2000 to 20,000 donors), are available and do not have the disadvantages of plasma and cryoprecipitate (Table 13–2). Factor VIII concentrates have been sterilized by heating in solution, by superheating to 80°C after lyophilization, and by exposure to organic solvent-detergents that inactivate lipid-enveloped viruses, including HIV and hepatitides B and C viruses, but do not inactivate parvovirus or hepatitis A.[46,47] Parvovirus infection does not occur frequently in hemophilia A patients because parvovirus is transmitted by cellular elements of the blood. Nevertheless, seroconversion to B19 parvovirus has been observed in patients receiving plasma-derived concentrates undergoing solvent-detergent extraction or pasteurization.

Some of these products contain significant amounts of VWF (see Table 13–2). Plasma-derived factor VIII concentrates prepared by monoclonal antibody techniques and subjected to viral inactivation techniques are highly purified and, barring breakdown in manufacturing procedures, are considered to be safe in terms of transmission of viral diseases.

Factor VIII produced by recombinant DNA techniques is available, safe, and effective. There are new "third-generation" factor VIII products that are manufactured without exposure to animal or human protein. Although all factor VIII products, both recombinant and plasma-derived, are currently safe and effective, some physicians and patients prefer products that are not exposed to human or animal proteins during the manufacturing process.

The dose of factor VIII can be determined as follows. If 1 U of factor VIII per milliliter of plasma is considered 100 percent of normal, the dose required to raise the level to a given value depends on the patient's plasma volume (approximately 5 percent of body weight in kilograms) and the level to which factor VIII is to be raised. Thus, the plasma volume of a 70-kg adult is approximately equivalent to 3500 mL (5 percent × 70 kg = 3.5 kg = 3500 g, approximately equivalent to 3500 mL). To achieve normal factor VIII levels of 1 U/mL (100 percent), 3500 U of factor VIII should be given. This scenario assumes a 100 percent recovery of the administered dose. Recovery has approached 100 percent in studies but depends on the method of assay and the factor VIII standard used for comparison.[48] After the initial dose of factor VIII, further doses of factor VIII are based on a half-life of 8 to 12 hours. Thus, after a loading dose of 3500 U of factor VIII, a dose of 1750 U could be given in 12 hours. However, for practical purposes, the dose of factor VIII is based on the knowledge that 1 U of factor VIII per kilogram of body weight raises the circulating factor VIII level by approximately 0.02 U/mL. Thus, to raise the factor VIII level to 100 percent, that is, 1 U/mL, the dose of factor VIII required is approximately 50 U per kilogram of body weight, assuming the patient's baseline factor VIII level is less than 1 percent of normal. The site and severity of hemorrhage determine the frequency and dose of factor VIII to be infused.

Table 13–3 summarizes the recommended doses of factor VIII for various types of hemorrhage.[48] These doses are not based on rigorous randomized studies, and recommendations vary among hemophilia centers. Given the high cost of factor VIII, some physicians prefer to use lower doses.

Factor VIII can be given as a constant infusion to hospitalized patients. Following a loading dose to raise factor VIII to the desired level, 150 to 300 U of factor VIII per hour can be infused. Factor VIII levels can be conveniently monitored in blood obtained from veins other than the vein into which factor VIII was infused intravenously.[49] In selected patients, factor VIII can be given outside the hospital in a continuous infusion using pump devices.[50]

## DDAVP (Desmopressin)

During the 1970s, 1-desamino-8-D-arginine vasopressin (DDAVP; desmopressin) was found to cause a transient increase in factor VIII in normal subjects and in patients with mild to moderate hemophilia. After a dose of DDAVP (0.3 mcg per kilogram body weight), given intravenously or subcutaneously, factor VIII levels increase two- to

**TABLE 13–3.** Doses of Factor VIII for Treatment of Hemorrhage*

| Site of Hemorrhage | Desired Factor VIII Level (% of Normal) | Factor VIII Dose† (U/kg Body Weight) | Frequency of Dose‡ (Every No. of Hours) | Duration (Days) |
|---|---|---|---|---|
| Hemarthroses | 30–50 | ~25 | 12–24 | 1–2 |
| Superficial intramuscular hematoma | 30–50 | ~25 | 12–24 | 1–2 |
| Gastrointestinal tract | 50–100 | 50 | 12 | 7–10 |
| Epistaxis | 30–50 | ~25 | 12 | Until resolved |
| Oral mucosa | 30–50 | ~25 | 12 | Until resolved |
| Hematuria | 30–100 | ~25–50 | 12 | Until resolved |
| Central nervous system | 50–100 | 50 | 12 | At least 7–10 days |
| Retropharyngeal | 50–100 | 50 | 12 | At least 7–10 days |
| Retroperitoneal | 50–100 | 50 | 12 | At least 7–10 days |

*Mild or moderately affected patients may respond to 1-deamino-8-D-arginine vasopressin (DDAVP), which should be used in lieu of blood or blood products whenever possible.

†Factor VIII may be administered in a continuous infusion if the patient is hospitalized. After initial bolus, a dose of approximately 2 to 5 U/kg/h of factor VIII usually is sufficient in an average-size adult. Bolus doses are given every 12 to 24 hours.

‡The frequency of dosing and duration of therapy can be adjusted, depending on the severity and duration of the patient's bleeding episode.

threefold above baseline in most, but not all, mildly or moderately affected hemophilia A patients. Patients with severe hemophilia A do not respond to DDAVP.[51] A concentrated intranasal spray of DDAVP also can be used (150 mcg in each nostril for adults and 150 mcg in one nostril for children weighing less than 50 kg). The degree of response to the drug should always be determined in patients before a bleeding episode, because occasionally mildly or moderately affected patients do not respond. The peak response to DDAVP usually occurs 30 to 60 minutes after dosing. In patients with mild or moderate hemophilia A and in carriers whose baseline factor VIII levels are less than 0.5 U/mL, DDAVP may be used in lieu of blood products. The mechanism by which DDAVP increases factor VIII is unknown.

Repeated administration of DDAVP results in a diminished response to the agent (tachyphylaxis). In many patients, the response to the second DDAVP dose averages 30 percent less than the response to the first dose, and the response rate may be even less after additional doses.[52] DDAVP is a potent antidiuretic. As a result, hyponatremia has been reported in some patients whose water intake exceeds approximately 1 L per 24 hours after dosing. There is no convincing evidence to indicate that DDAVP administration is associated with thrombosis in hemophilic patients.

### Antifibrinolytic Agents

Antifibrinolytic agents, such as $\varepsilon$-aminocaproic acid (EACA) and tranexamic acid, have been used to enhance hemostasis in patients with hemophilia A.[53,54] Fibrinolytic inhibitors may be given as adjunctive therapy for bleeding from mucous membranes and are particularly valuable as adjunctive therapy for dental procedures. The usual oral dose of tranexamic acid for adults is 1 g four times per day. EACA can be given as a loading dose of 4 to 5 g followed by 1 g/h by continuous IV infusion in adults. Another regimen of EACA is 4 g every 4 to 6 hours orally for 2 to 8 days, depending on the severity of the bleeding episode. Antifibrinolytic therapy is contraindicated in the presence of hematuria because clots resistant to lysis may obstruct the ureters.

### Fibrin Glue

Fibrin glue, otherwise known as fibrin tissue adhesive, has been used as adjunctive therapy to factor VIII in hemophilic patients.[55] Briefly, fibrin glue contains fibrinogen, thrombin, and factor XIII. Fibrinolytic inhibitors are added to some commercial products. The fibrinogen–factor XIII mixture is placed on the injury site and clotted with a human thrombin solution containing calcium. As a result, the fibrin clot is crosslinked and anchored to tissue. It is especially useful for hemostasis in patients undergoing dental surgery who receive a preextraction bolus of factor VIII followed by application of fibrin glue to the tooth socket. Fibrin glue also has been used as adjunctive therapy to factor VIII following orthopedic procedures and circumcision. It is very valuable for controlling bleeding when applied to the bed of a surgical wound following removal of large pseudotumors. Some hemophilia centers prepare their own "homemade" fibrin glue using cryoprecipitate as a source of fibrinogen and factor XIII.

### Treatment of Minor or Moderate Hemorrhage

On occasion, superficial cuts and abrasions are managed with local measures, that is, application of pressure sometimes suffices to control bleeding, although oozing may continue intermittently for several hours. Topical thrombin is of little value in this type of bleeding. In general, cautery should be avoided because bleeding may restart when the cauterized area is sloughed.

When replacement therapy for epistaxis is needed, the factor VIII level should be raised to approximately 30 to 50 percent of normal. For treatment of hematuria, patients should be instructed to drink large quantities of fluids. If hematuria is mild, uncomplicated, and painless, factor VIII replacement may not be necessary unless the hematuria persists. Gross or protracted hematuria requires replacement therapy. In these patients, factor VIII levels of at least 50 percent of normal or higher are needed, probably because urine is rich in urokinase that rapidly lyses clots.

Hemophilic patients requiring endoscopic procedures first should be treated with factor VIII to raise levels to at least 0.5 U/mL before the procedure. Only one dose may be necessary if endoscopy is uncomplicated. In cases of biopsies, severe abrasions, or perforations following endoscopy, factor VIII replacement should be continued until healing of the lesion is complete. For expanding soft tissue hematomas, factor VIII therapy should be started immediately and maintained until the hematoma begins to resolve. With effective therapy, the patient usually experiences rapid relief from pain. For treatment of acute hemarthroses, prompt administration of factor VIII decreases the occurrence of extensive degencrative joint changes, deformity, and muscle wasting. For chronic synovitis and for bleeding into "target" joints, daily administration of factor VIII to raise levels to 100 percent of normal for 6 to 8 weeks ("secondary prophylaxis") is usually indicated.

### Treatment of Major Nonsurgical Hemorrhages

Any hemorrhage in a patient with hemophilia A may become major, but the following hemorrhages are common and frequently life-threatening: retropharyngeal, retroperitoneal, and central nervous system bleeding, whether subdural, subarachnoid, or into the brain parenchyma.[56]

For treatment of retropharyngeal bleeding, particularly that associated with a sensation of tightness in the throat, pain in the neck, dysphagia, or difficulty breathing, patients should receive factor VIII immediately in doses sufficient to raise factor VIII levels to normal (1.0 U/mL). Near-normal levels should be maintained until bleeding ceases and the hematoma begins to resolve. For retroperitoneal hemorrhage, early treatment is required, and therapy should be continued for 7 to 10 days; otherwise, bleeding may recur upon resumption of activity.

Immediate administration of factor VIII, sufficient to raise the level to normal, should be started upon the first sign of an intracranial hemorrhage or following a history of head trauma. Even asymptomatic patients with a history of head trauma should receive at least one dose of factor VIII as a prophylactic measure, and this dose should be given before diagnostic procedures such as a CT scan. Treatment of a known intracranial hemorrhage should be maintained for a minimum of 7 to 10 days, and the circulating factor VIII level should be kept normal throughout this period. Prolonged secondary prophylaxis is often indicated following an intracerebral hemorrhage, particularly in patients with HIV disease, who seem to have a high recurrence rate. Evacuation of subdural hematomas and surgical removal of hematomas involving the brain parenchyma can be performed, depending on location. Despite aggressive replacement therapy, however, mortality from central nervous system bleeding is high.

### Replacement of Factor VIII for Surgical Procedures

For major surgical procedures, factor VIII should be raised to normal levels before operation and maintained for 7 to 10 days or until healing is complete. Treatment can be started a few hours before surgery and continued intraoperatively using a continuous infusion or boluses every 8 to 12 hours. Postoperatively, factor VIII levels should be monitored at least one or two times per day to ensure that adequate levels are maintained. Because factor VIII may be "consumed" during surgery, factor VIII levels should be monitored intraoperatively and doses of factor VIII higher than normal may be required. Bone and joint surgery may require longer periods of factor VIII coverage. Replacement of knee, hip, ankle, and elbow joints may be required for intractable pain associated with loss of function, and several weeks of replacement therapy may be needed postoperatively.[57]

### Home Therapy

Home therapy using available factor VIII concentrates was introduced in the United States in 1977 and was a major advance in the treatment of all forms of hemophilia.[58,59] Current practice for home therapy is to treat patients at home using a regular prophylactic regimen. Patients, age 6 years and older, can be taught to treat themselves with factor VIII. The training of patients and their families for home therapy is best accomplished in a regional comprehensive hemophilia diagnostic and treatment center or an affiliate of one of these centers. Patients are given an adequate quantity of factor concentrates and the supplies required for intravenous administration. Prompt treatment of hemarthroses and hematomas made possible by home therapy has markedly improved the morbidity and mortality associated with hemophilia. In addition, the quality of life of hemophilia A patients has improved dramatically.[59,60]

### Prophylactic Therapy

The advent of stable and safe factor VIII concentrates has made prophylactic therapy for hemophilia A in severely affected patients feasible. Such therapy is now the treatment of choice for all severely affected hemophilia patients (unfortunately, such treatment is not available or affordable for all patients). Administration of 25 to 40 U of factor VIII per kilogram of body weight three times per week or every other day markedly decreases the frequency of hemophilic arthropathy and other long-term effects of hemorrhagic episodes.[60-62] Primary prophylaxis is usually initiated before the age of 2 years or after the first joint bleed, which is usually when the child begins to walk. Central venous catheters may be required sometimes for very young children; however, they are associated with a risk of infections and thrombosis.[63] Secondary prophylaxis is started after the onset of hemarthrosis and can be used for short periods of time or to manage target joints. The consumption of factor concentrate is higher when patients are on prophylaxis when compared to on-demand therapy, but analysis of the economic impact of prophylactic therapy, weighing the benefits against the high costs of factor VIII concentrates, suggests the clinical benefit of prophylaxis is warranted, as evidenced by significant improvement in the clinical condition of patients and improvement in the quality of life.[62,64]

## COURSE AND PROGNOSIS

After the advent of factor VIII concentrates in the 1960s, the morbidity and mortality from bleeding in hemophilia were significantly reduced, and by the late 1970s, the life expectancy of hemophilia A patients began to approach that of normal individuals in those populations. However, use of replacement therapy has not been without significant complications. Prior to 1985, common and serious adverse side effects of treatment included chronic liver disease resulting from hepatitides B and C and, from about 1978, infection with HIV.[65] Factor VIII concentrates were prepared from many thousands of donors, making contamination of factor VIII concentrates by bloodborne viruses highly likely. With the introduction of heat- or solvent-detergent–treated concentrates in 1985, contamination of blood products with these viruses has been eliminated for all practical purposes. However, AIDS became a leading cause of death in older patients with hemophilia.[65] Chronic liver disease in hemophilia A patients resulting from transfusion-related hepatitides B and C may be accelerated by HIV infection and by the associated hepatotoxicity of antiviral drug therapy.[66] Fortunately, patients treated prophylactically after 1985 can expect almost normal life spans free of the complications of hepatitis, AIDS, and other currently recognized bloodborne viral diseases. However, the development of inhibitor

antibodies against factor VIII has been, and continues to be, one of the more serious complications of replacement therapy.

### Factor VIII Inhibitors

Other than the transmission of viral diseases by factor VIII infusions, the main complication of hemophilia A replacement therapy is the development of specific inhibitor antibodies that neutralize factor VIII.[67] The reported prevalence of anti–factor VIII inhibitors in severe hemophilia A patients is variable, ranging from 3.6 percent to 27 percent. In the white population, the estimated prevalence is approximately 13 percent, compared to 27 percent and 25 percent in the black and Hispanic population, respectively.[68] The risk of inhibitor development is higher in patients with large deletions and nonsense mutations when compared to small deletions/insertions and missense mutations. Frequent testing for inhibitors in previously untreated patients receiving newer highly purified factor VIII products from plasma or by recombinant technology revealed the frequent occurrence of transient inhibitors to factor VIII, many of which were of low titer and did not necessitate cessation of treatment with the same product. Although still controversial, some believe that the risk of inhibitors does not appear to be higher with the use of highly purified products than the risk reported in earlier studies using products of intermediate purity that contain VWF.[69-74] Some studies have reported that VWF is immunomodulatory, so that products containing VWF may be less likely to induce inhibitors compared to highly purified products. One outbreak of inhibitors in Europe appeared to be related to the neoantigenicity of an intermediate-purity plasma-derived factor VIII concentrate. Fortunately, inhibitors disappeared from affected patients when use of the product was stopped.[75]

Table 13–4 lists the risk factors that have been associated with the development of inhibitors. They arise most frequently in severely affected patients, following treatment at an early age. Many have gross gene rearrangements or the intron 22 inversion abnormality of the factor VIII gene.

Factor VIII inhibitors are antibodies, most often of the immunoglobulin (Ig) G class and frequently restricted to the IgG$_4$ subclass.[67] Antibodies against the A$_2$ and C domains of factor VIII are most common. These antibodies interfere with the interactions of factor VIII with other hemostatic components.[67,76]

Early diagnosis of factor VIII inhibitors is essential. Although the presence of an inhibitor can be suspected on clinical grounds, as when a patient does not respond to conventional doses of factor VIII, laboratory diagnosis is required for confirmation. Factor VIII inhibitors are time and temperature dependent *in vitro*. The prolonged aPTT of the

---

**TABLE 13–4.** Risk Factors for Development of Anti–Factor VIII Antibodies in Hemophilia A Patients

Disease severity: 80% of hemophilia A patients with inhibitors have <1% factor VIII activity

Early exposure to factor VIII concentrates: majority of high-titer inhibitors develop after <90 days of exposure to factor VIII

Genetic factors

1. Family history of inhibitor development

2. Ethnic background: Blacks > Hispanics > Whites

3. Molecular defects: inversion and crossing over defect in intron 22, gene deletions, and nonsense point mutations resulting in patients without factor VIII antigen

Method of purification of factor VIII concentrate

Data from Rizza CR, Lowe G: *Hemophilia & Other Bleeding Disorders.* New York: WB Saunders; 1997.

plasma of a patient without an inhibitor is corrected when mixed 1:1 with normal plasma even after incubation at 37°C for 1 to 2 hours. In contrast, the aPTT of a 1:1 mixture of plasma from a patient with an inhibitor and normal plasma is significantly prolonged after incubation at 37°C for 1 to 2 hours. Specific diagnosis rests upon demonstrating that an appropriate dilution of the patient's plasma, when added to normal plasma, specifically neutralizes factor VIII and not other blood clotting factors that influence the aPTT (i.e., factors IX, XI, XII, prekallikrein, high-molecular-weight kininogen). The demonstration that the inhibitor is specific for factor VIII distinguishes it from inhibitors of other clotting factors, for example, the lupus anticoagulant, and nonspecific inhibitors. A common assay used for inhibitor detection and quantification is the Bethesda assay.[77] In the Bethesda assay, the patient's plasma is diluted such that, when the plasma is mixed with an equal volume of normal pooled human plasma and incubated for 2 hours at 37°C, the factor VIII activity in the mixture is decreased by 50 percent. A modification of the Bethesda assay is the Nijmegen assay, in which buffer is used instead of factor VIII–deficient plasma. This method has been shown to be more dependable at detecting low concentrations of inhibitors.[78]

Several approaches to treatment of factor VIII inhibitors are available (Table 13–5). Use of these treatments requires knowledge of whether the patient with an inhibitor is a "high" or "low" responder and whether the bleeding episode requiring treatment is minor or major.[67]

**High-Responder Patients**  Approximately 60 percent of patients who have inhibitors are high responders. High responders are defined as patients whose inhibitor titer is higher than 5 Bethesda units (BU) at baseline or whose initial inhibitor titer is less than 5 BU but rises to greater than 5 BU after administration of factor VIII. Thus, high responders who are not treated with factor VIII for long periods may have a sustained high level of inhibitor, or they may have a very low to undetectable level of inhibitor until they are challenged with factor VIII.

Major bleeding episodes in a high-responder patient whose initial inhibitor titer is less than 5 BU can be treated with human factor VIII concentrate (see Table 13–5). When the initial titer is low, sufficient factor VIII can be administered in high doses to neutralize the inhibitor and attain adequate factor VIII levels for hemostasis. Although factor VIII inhibitor bypassing agents can be used (see below), they are not as reliable as factor VIII in achieving hemostasis, and their effect cannot be adequately monitored with specific laboratory tests. If factor VIII is used, a loading dose of 10,000 to 15,000 U may be required, followed by up to 1000 U of factor VIII per hour, depending on the factor VIII level. One can expect an anamnestic response approximately 5 days after administration of factor VIII.

In high-responder patients whose initial inhibitor titer is less than 5 BU and who experience a minor bleeding episode, the agent of choice is a factor VIII inhibitor bypassing agent. Recombinant factor VIIa in doses of 90 to 120 mcg per kilogram of body weight or higher every 2 to 3 hours is safe and effective in most hemorrhagic episodes.[79] The dosing frequency is based on a factor VIIa plasma half-life of approximately 2 to 3 hours. The mechanisms of action of factor VIIa have been investigated using *in vitro* techniques. After coagulation is initiated by the tissue factor–factor VIIa pathway, factor VIIa at recommended doses is hypothesized to activate factor X on the surface of activated platelets, even in the absence of additional tissue factor activity.[80] Factor Xa then can associate with factor Va and convert prothrombin to thrombin. Because activated platelets are localized to the site of vessel injury, thrombin generation by factor VIIa is localized to the site of bleeding. This process may account for the reported safety of factor VIIa.[80] Factor VIII inhibitor bypassing activity (FEIBA), a plasma-derived agent, has also been used successfully to treat bleeding episodes in inhibitor patients and is both safe and effective[81] given at a recommended dose of 50 to 100 U per kilogram body weight every 8 to 12 hours (not to exceed 200 U per kilogram per day).

High-responder patients whose initial inhibitor titer is greater than 5 BU usually do not respond to even very high doses of human factor VIII. Thus, recombinant factor VIIa or FEIBA should be used.[81] If these agents are not available, nonactivated prothrombin complex concentrates or plasma exchange with high-dose replacement factor VIII can be considered.

**Low-Responder Patients**  Low-responder patients are arbitrarily defined as patients whose inhibitor titer is less than 5 BU even after a challenge with factor VIII. For major bleeding episodes, high doses of human factor VIII can be used as recommended above. For minor bleeds, recombinant factor VIIa or FEIBA is recommended because some "low" responders may convert to high responders when they are challenged repeatedly with factor VIII.

Nonactivated or activated prothrombin complex concentrates both contain variable amounts of activated factors, including factors VIIa, IXa, and Xa. The activated products have higher concentrations of activated factors than do nonactivated products. FEIBA contains a complex of prothrombin and factor Xa that can bind to membrane surfaces and enhance thrombin generation in the absence of factors VIII or IX.[80,81]

**Surgery in Inhibitor Patients**  The question of whether major surgery can be performed in patients with hemophilia A or B with inhibitors arises now that joint replacement is possible.[82] Knee, ankle, hip, and elbow replacements have been carried out successfully in patients with inhibitor antibodies using bypassing agents. Basically, the patient is given a loading dose of factor VIIa followed by bolus doses of factor VIIa and use of fibrin sealant and antifibrinolytic therapy until healing is complete. FEIBA has also been successfully used in surgery in hemophilic patients with inhibitors.[83]

**TABLE 13–5.** Treatment of Inhibitors in Hemophilia A Patients

| Type of Patient | Initial Titer | Minor Hemorrhage* | Major Hemorrhage* |
|---|---|---|---|
| High responder | <5 BU | Recombinant factor VIIa; FEIBA | Factor VIII[†]; recombinant factor VIIa; FEIBA |
| High responder | >5 BU | Recombinant factor VIIa; FEIBA | Recombinant factor VIIa; FEIBA; plasma exchange |
| Low responder | <5 BU | Recombinant factor VIIa; FEIBA | High-dose factor VIII; recombinant factor VIIa; FEIBA |

BU, Bethesda unit; FEIBA, factor VIII inhibitor bypassing activity.

*Agents for treatment of major and minor hemorrhage are listed. Some physicians will choose the first product listed as the agent of choice, but the choice varies among physicians.

†High dose of factor VIII may overcome an initial low-titer inhibitor, although an anamnestic response can be expected in high responders.

Data from Hoffman M, Dargaud Y: Mechanisms and monitoring of bypassing agent therapy, *J Thromb Haemost* 2012 Aug;10(8):1478–1485.

**TABLE 13–6.** Examples of Tolerance Protocols for Hemophilia A Inhibitor Patients with Good-Risk Factors

| Immune Tolerance Protocols | Dose | Time to Negative Inhibitor |
|---|---|---|
| High-dose regimen | 200 U/kg factor VIII per day | 4.6 months |
| Low-dose regimen | 50 U/kg factor VIII three times per week | 9.2 months |

Data from DiMichele DM: Immune tolerance in haemophilia: the long journey to the fork in the road, *Heamophilia* 2012 Oct;159(2):123–134.

**Immune Tolerance** Removal of the antibody is the definitive goal of inhibitor management. Plasmapheresis, adsorption of the antibody on an affinity column during plasma exchange, and administration of intravenous γ-globulin have been used in patients with an inhibitor. The Malmö protocol uses nearly all of these approaches in combination, including extracorporeal adsorption of antibody to a Sepharose A column, administration of cyclophosphamide, daily administration of factor VIII, and intravenous γ-globulin.[84]

The most promising approach to eradication of an inhibitor is use of immune tolerance regimens. The basis of this approach is administration of frequent (daily or thrice weekly) doses of factor VIII until the inhibitor titer is undetectable.[85] Low- and high-dose regimens have been described (Table 13–6). Predictors of success have been described in clinical studies in patients with high titer inhibitors and include young age at detection of inhibitor; inhibitor titer less than 10 BU before starting immune tolerance induction (ITI); peak titer less than 100 BU after starting ITI; historical peak titer less than 200 BU; age less than 5 years old between diagnosis and start of ITI; and genotype (small deletions and insertions and missense mutations). Factor VIII inhibitor bypassing agents are used for prevention and treatment of acute bleeds that occur during immune tolerance induction.

Other approaches to treatment of factor VIII inhibitors include immunosuppressive drugs, like cyclosporine and rituximab.[85–87] However, these drugs, although occasionally successful, seem to be more effective in patients with acquired hemophilia resulting from autoantibodies against factor VIII.

### Infectious Complications

**Hepatitis** Almost all multitransfused patients with hemophilia treated before 1985 were infected with one or more viruses that caused hepatitis. Although many infected patients did not suffer acute symptoms, at least 50 percent developed chronic persistent or chronic active hepatitis that, in many cases, resulted in cirrhosis. Hepatitis C and B viruses are commonly associated with chronic liver disease. Many adult hemophilia patients treated with concentrates before 1985 have circulating antibodies to hepatitis B surface antigen and hepatitis C. Hepatitis C infection progresses more rapidly in the presence of HIV infection. Until recently, therapy with pegylated interferon and ribavirin reduced viral load and improved survival of many affected patients; however, newer approaches using serine protease inhibitors and nucleotide polymerase inhibitors have led to a high rate of sustained virologic responses.[88] All patients with hemophilia should be vaccinated against hepatitis A and hepatitis B.

**Human Immunodeficiency Virus** Many of the older, severely affected hemophilia A patients who were treated before 1985 have antibodies to HIV, indicating infection with the virus. The incidence of HIV antibodies in mildly affected patients is much lower and correlates with treatment with factor VIII concentrates before viral inactivation

procedures were used. In one study, 14 percent of patients treated only with cryoprecipitate from 1979 to 1985 were infected with HIV, whereas 88 percent of patients treated with factor VIII concentrates became infected.[89] Screening of donor populations and new techniques for preparing factor VIII concentrates since 1985 have eliminated the risk of HIV transmission.

**Risk of Viral Disease Transmission by New Factor VIII Products** All available factor VIII concentrates, both plasma-derived and recombinant products, are considered safe and effective with almost no risk of transmitting currently known viral diseases. However, occasional exceptions have been observed. For example, solvent-detergent treatment does not inactivate viruses without lipid envelopes, including the hepatitis A virus and parvovirus. As a result, outbreaks of hepatitis A have been reported in patients receiving some solvent-detergent–treated products. These outbreaks of viral diseases usually have been related to breakdowns in the manufacturing process.

**Prions** Prions are infectious particles consisting of proteinaceous material devoid of a nucleic acid genome.[90] They are thought to be variant forms of a normal protein with an altered conformation. The "infectious" nature of prions may result from their ability to bind to other proteins and induce similar conformational changes in them such that new "infectious" particles can be generated. Prions are responsible for several neurodegenerative disorders, including Creutzfeldt-Jakob disease (CJD) in humans, scrapie in sheep, and spongiform encephalopathy in cows. Prions are resistant to most currently available viral inactivation techniques. Removal of prion particles using iodine column chromatography has been claimed.[91] Although prion diseases generally are transmitted by ingestion of infected neural tissues, a new variant of CJD appears to occur in people who have eaten beef from cows infected with a form of prion causing bovine spongiform encephalopathy. This form of CJD has been reported mainly in the United Kingdom and in certain other European countries and has been related to the bovine disease.[92] For example, prions have been found in tonsillar tissue of patients with new-variant CJD, heightening concern about whether prions of this type might be transmitted by blood products.[93] Conclusive data about possible prion infection of hemophilic patients are lacking, so continued vigilance is necessary.

## ● HEMOPHILIA B (FACTOR IX DEFICIENCY, CHRISTMAS FACTOR DEFICIENCY)

### ETIOLOGY AND PATHOGENESIS

Hemophilia B occurs in one of every 25,000 to 30,000 live male births. As with hemophilia A, hemophilia B is found in all ethnic groups and has no geographic predilection.

Factor IX is a vitamin K–dependent, single-chain glycoprotein consisting of 415 amino acids. It is activated by the factor VIIa–tissue factor complex, or factor XIa, forming the active enzyme factor IXa (Chap. 3). Once activated, factor IXa activates factor X in the presence of factor VIIIa, phospholipid (activated platelets), and calcium. Factor VIIIa is a necessary cofactor for activity of factor IXa. Therefore, deficiency of either factor IX or VIII leads to a similar lack of factor X–activating activity on the platelet surface. Factor Xa converts prothrombin to thrombin in the presence of factor Va, activated platelets, and calcium. Hemophilia B can result from either the absence or the dysfunction of factor IX molecules. Clinical severity of hemophilia B is roughly correlated with factor IX functional activity.

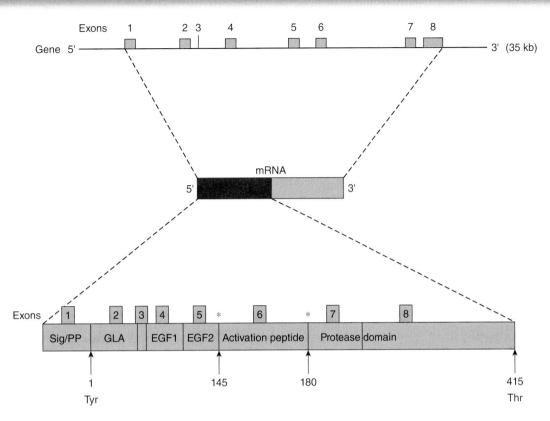

**Figure 13–11.** Schematic of the factor IX gene, the messenger RNA, and the protein. Exons are depicted by the tan boxes. The light 3′ portion of the mRNA is untranslated. The diagram of the protein shows the domains and the exons that encode each portion of the protein. The cleavage sites of factor XIa or factor VIIa–tissue factor complex are indicated by asterisks.

## GENETICS AND MOLECULAR BIOLOGY

The factor IX gene is located on the long arm of the X chromosome. It is approximately 33 kb long, which is much smaller than the gene for factor VIII.[94] Because it is less complex, the factor IX gene has been studied in greater detail than the factor VIII gene. Figure 13–11 is a schematic of the gene and the protein product. The protein consists of a signal peptide that targets the protein for secretion from the hepatocyte to the circulation. The propeptide is necessary for posttranslational modification of 12 aminoterminal glutamic acid residues by an intracellular vitamin K–dependent carboxylase. The propeptide is cleaved from the mature protein before it enters the circulation. The aminoterminus of factor IX contains 12 $\gamma$-carboxyglutamic acid (GLA) residues necessary for calcium-dependent lipid binding. The activation peptide is cleaved from the zymogen form of factor IX by either factor VIIa/tissue factor or factor XIa, resulting in the two-chain active enzyme, factor IXa$\beta$. The catalytic triad (His 221, Asp 229, ser 365) resides on the heavy chain (Chap. 3).[94]

There are more than 1000 distinct mutations or deletions in the factor IX gene reported in the factor IX database, including more than 900 distinct amino acid substitutions and numerous complete gene deletions.[95,96] More than 30 percent of factor IX mutations occur at CpG dinucleotides. These mutations often involve critical Arg residues that result in a dysfunctional molecule.[96–99] Many mutations have been reported in more than one kindred, and some of these mutations derive from the same "founder."[100] As predicted by genetic theory of X chromosome–linked recessive disorders, approximately one-third of mutations resulting in hemophilia B arise *de novo*.

Mutations in regulatory regions of the factor IX gene have been identified. Particularly interesting examples are mutations in the 5′ promoter region that lead to the hemophilia B Leyden phenotype.[101] This disorder is characterized by very low levels of factor IX antigen and activity at birth and during early childhood. The factor IX levels gradually rise to 60 percent of normal or greater following puberty, possibly caused by the age-related stability element/age-related increase element–mediated genetic mechanism.[102] Several different mutations in the promoter region of the factor IX gene disrupt binding of transcription factors, resulting in reduced transcription of the factor IX gene.[101,103] The hormonal changes occurring at puberty apparently can overcome the transcription defect and maintain hemostatic levels of factor IX.

Hemophilia B inheritance is similar to that of hemophilia A. All daughters of affected males are obligate carriers, whereas all sons are normal. Female carriers may have factor IX levels ranging from less than 10 to 100 percent of normal, but the mean level is approximately 50 percent. Carriers of hemophilia B usually are asymptomatic, except in cases of extreme X chromosome inactivation, X mosaicism, Turner syndrome, or testicular feminization.[104] When the level of factor IX activity is less than 25 percent of normal, abnormal bleeding may occur, especially after trauma and surgery.

### Carrier Detection and Prenatal Diagnosis

Factor IX genotyping is achieved by direct sequencing. Prenatal diagnosis may be accomplished by analysis of DNA obtained by chorionic villus sampling as early as 8 to 10 weeks after conception.[105] This procedure also can be performed on fetal cells obtained by amniocentesis and is more accurate than fetal blood sampling for factor IX activity and factor IX antigen. Large deletions are relatively rare in severe hemophilia B, but are associated with a higher risk of factor IX inhibitors when present.

## CLINICAL FEATURES

Bleeding episodes in patients with hemophilia B are clinically indistinguishable from those in patients with hemophilia A, although as stated elsewhere, the hemophilia B population as a whole seems to have fewer and less severe complications than severely affected hemophilia A patients[9] (see "Clinical Features" under "Hemophilia A" above). When patients are inadequately treated, repeated hemarthroses leading to chronic, crippling hemarthropathy occur. Hematoma formation with dissection into surrounding tissues is possible. Hematuria, bleeding from mucous membranes, and other bleeding manifestations are as described in the section on hemophilia A. The physical, psychological, vocational, and social aspects of the disease are similar to those encountered with hemophilia A. Classification of hemophilia B is based on clinical severity and roughly correlates with the level of factor IX coagulant activity. Severe disease usually is associated with factor IX levels of less than 1 percent of normal; moderate disease is associated with factor IX levels of 1 to 5 percent; and mild disease is associated with factor IX levels ranging from 5 to 40 percent.

The occurrence of factor IX inhibitor antibodies is much less common in hemophilia B patients than in hemophilia A patients and is very rare in nonsevere disease. Only approximately 3 percent of severely affected patients develop inhibitors.

## LABORATORY FEATURES

The screening tests used in the diagnosis of hemophilia A also are used in the diagnosis of hemophilia B. In most cases of hemophilia B, PT is normal and aPTT is prolonged. However, specific assay of factor IX coagulant activity is required for definitive diagnosis. The most commonly used test is a one-stage clotting assay based on aPTT. Determination of factor IX antigen levels is valuable in further classifying the disorder.

## DIFFERENTIAL DIAGNOSIS

Hemophilia B must be distinguished from hemophilia A. Both forms are inherited as X-linked recessive disorders, and both have almost identical hemorrhagic and clinical manifestations. The only method for differentiating hemophilia B from hemophilia A is performing specific assays for factors VIII and IX on the patient's plasma.

Inherited and acquired deficiencies of other vitamin K–dependent factors, liver disease, and warfarin overdose must be distinguished from hemophilia B. In these cases, not only factor IX but all other vitamin K–dependent clotting factors, including prothrombin, factor VII, and factor X, are decreased. Acquired antibodies specific for factor IX occur in nonhemophilic patients but are very rare.

## THERAPY

### Factor IX Replacement

The basic treatment of hemophilia B is replacement of factor IX. Several products are available for use (Table 13–7). The older factor IX–containing products often are referred to as prothrombin complex concentrates. These products, which are prepared from large pools of human plasma (several thousand donors), contain not only factor IX but also prothrombin, factors VII and X, and proteins C and S. In addition, the products may contain small amounts of activated factors, such as factors VIIa, IXa, and Xa. Some of these products are associated with thromboembolic events, presumably resulting from contamination with the activated components. Deep venous thrombosis (DVT) and disseminated intravascular coagulation have been reported in some patients who receive large doses of prothrombin complex concentrates, but these complications seem to occur less frequently with currently available

**TABLE 13–7.** Currently Available Factor IX Products*

| | Origin | Viral Inactivation |
|---|---|---|
| **Intermediate purity (prothrombin complex concentrates)** | | |
| Profilnine SD | Plasma | Solvent-detergent |
| Bebulin VH | Plasma | Vapor heating |
| **High purity** | | |
| Mononine | Plasma | Ultrafiltration; chemical |
| AlphaNine | Plasma | Solvent-detergent; virus filtered |
| **Recombinant** | | |
| BeneFIX | CHO cells | Solvent-detergent Nanofiltration |
| Rixubis | CHO cells | Solvent-detergent Nanofiltration |
| Ixinity | CHO cells | Solvent-detergent Chromatography Nanofiltration |
| Alprolix[†] | HEK cells | Nanofiltration Chromatography |
| Idelvion[†] | CHO cells | Solvent-detergent Nanofiltration |

CHO, Chinese hamster ovary (recombinant product); HEK, human embryo kidney.

*Additional factor IX concentrates are available in Europe.

[†]Extended half-life factor IX product.

purified factor IX products than with earlier preparations. Prothrombin complex concentrates are no longer the optimal choice for replacement therapy in hemophilia B, even though they are much less expensive than the highly purified factor IX concentrates. When prothrombin complex concentrates are used for replacement therapy, factor IX levels greater than 50 percent of normal should not be exceeded in order to minimize the risk of thrombosis. Use of these products in factor IX–deficient patients with liver dysfunction may be hazardous because the activated factors contaminating these preparations may not be cleared efficiently by a diseased liver, and thrombosis might be induced.

Table 13–7 lists the highly purified factor IX products. Some products are prepared from human plasma; at present, three products are produced by recombinant DNA technology. Although all available factor IX concentrates are considered safe and effective, the recombinant product undergoes a final viral inactivation step. In addition, the recombinant products are not exposed to human albumin or bovine serum during preparation. Thus, even the theoretical risk of transmission of prion diseases is averted with this preparation. Some clinicians consider the recombinant product to be the agent of choice, although it has a major drawback in that the intravascular recovery of factor IX generally is lower than the recovery of highly purified factor IX product prepared from plasma.[106] The recombinant factor IX products are not thought to be thrombogenic. New factor IX products have been recently approved, and others are undergoing clinical trials or currently being developed, some of them with extended half-life (see Table 13–7).[107] Different technologies have been applied to extend the half-life of factor IX including Fc-fusion, recombinant albumin fusion, and PEGylation (glycoPEGylation), so one can expect the number of available factor IX products to increase in the near future.

## Dosing of Factor IX

The dose calculations for all factor IX products are different from those used in hemophilia A because intravascular recovery of factor IX is only approximately 50 percent, and the recovery is even lower with the recombinant product. The reason for this finding is unclear, but as factor IX binds to type IV collagen, a component of the vascular wall, infused factor IX adsorption, may contribute to the reduced recovery.[108] The dose of factor IX can be estimated by assuming that 1 U of factor IX per kilogram body weight increases circulating factor IX by 1 percent of normal or 0.01 U/mL.[109] Thus, to achieve 100 percent of normal (using only highly purified factor IX products) in a severely affected patient, 100 U of factor IX per kilogram body weight should be given as a bolus, followed by half this amount every 12 to 18 hours. Dosing should be monitored by assays of factor IX before and after bolus administration. Factor IX also can be administered as a constant infusion in hospitalized patients after the bolus administration. The dose of factor IX to be infused per hour can be estimated based on a factor IX half-life of 18 to 24 hours. Thus, in a 60-kg adult who receives highly purified factor IX, 6000 U of the factor should raise the factor IX level to approximately 100 percent of normal. Over the next 12 to 18 hours, the level decreases by approximately 50 percent. Thus, the patient needs approximately 3000 U of factor IX during that period or 250 U of factor IX per hour as an infusion.[109] These calculations are only estimates of average responses, so factor IX dosing should be monitored by factor IX assays and the dose adjusted appropriately. Prophylactic therapy for hemophilia B also can be attempted in individuals selected in the same manner as that described for hemophilia A patients. The prophylactic dose of factor IX is 25 to 40 U/kg of body weight two times per week or 50 to 100 U/kg every 7 to 10 days if using extended half-life products.

Although currently available factor IX concentrates are safe in terms of transmission of HIV and hepatitides B and C viruses, patients treated prior to 1985 may have been infected with these agents.

## COURSE AND PROGNOSIS

Unless treated properly, severe hemophilia B is fraught with the same complications of recurrent hemorrhages as hemophilia A. Thus, hemarthroses and chronic hemophilic arthropathy are common in inadequately treated patients. In addition to joint deformities, chronic active hepatitis is common in patients treated before 1985. Approximately 50 percent of older and severely affected patients now are HIV-positive. Patients treated after 1985, when HIV testing became available, are not likely to have contracted HIV.

Patients with severe hemophilia B may develop inhibitory antibodies against factor IX, making treatment very difficult.[110,111] Approximately 3 percent of patients with severe hemophilia B develop specific inhibitor antibodies, frequently restricted in immunoglobulin composition to the $IgG_4$ subclass and $\kappa$ light chains.[111] Most inhibitors can be detected when the aPTT of a mixture of normal plasma and the patient's plasma is prolonged. In contrast to the inhibitors in hemophilia A patients, inhibitor antibodies against factor IX are not time and temperature dependent; thus, incubating the mixtures for 2 hours at 37°C usually is unnecessary. Inhibitors to factor IX can be quantitated by modifying the Bethesda method for detecting factor VIII inhibitors. Many patients with inhibitors have mutations that result in the absence of circulating factor IX antigen, most commonly because of deletions and nonsense mutations.

## TREATMENT OF PATIENTS WITH FACTOR IX INHIBITOR ANTIBODIES

When the inhibitor titer is less than 5 BU/mL, the factor IX inhibitor possibly can be neutralized using large doses of highly purified factor IX concentrates. However, when the inhibitor titer is greater than 5 BU/mL,

acute bleeding in patients should be treated with the same agents used to bypass factor VIII inhibitors (see Table 13–5). Recombinant factor VIIa in doses of 90 to 120 mcg per kilogram body weight administered intravenously every 2 to 3 hours can be used. Alternatively, FEIBA at a dose of 50 to 100 U per kilogram body weight every 8 to 12 hours (not to exceed 200 U/kg per day) or nonactivated prothrombin complex concentrates can be used.

Induction of immune tolerance can be attempted in hemophilia B patients using daily infusions of purified factor IX preparations. However, significant adverse reactions, including anaphylaxis and nephrotic syndrome, have been reported in severely affected patients with inhibitors.[112] Of the reported cases, many patients were younger than 12 years of age and suffered from severe hemophilia B as a result of large deletions of the factor IX gene. The nephrotic syndrome may be transient and remit upon cessation of factor IX replacement. The pathogenesis of the nephrotic syndrome is not known. Patients with hemophilia B and factor IX antibodies who experience anaphylaxis with factor IX infusions and have hemorrhage should be treated with factor VIIa concentrates because both unactivated prothrombin complex concentrates and FEIBA contain factor IX.[112]

## Curative Approaches for Hemophilia: Liver Transplantation and Gene Therapy

Normal livers have been transplanted successfully into patients with hemophilia A or B, with resulting cure of the hemophilic condition.[113,114] The procedure is most often performed for end-stage chronic viral hepatitis that afflicts many older hemophilic patients. However, given the obvious limitations of this approach, it cannot be considered a viable treatment option to treat hemophilia *per se.*

On the other hand, gene replacement therapy for hemophilia offers an ideal theoretical approach for prophylactic therapy or even for a definitive cure. Proof of concept of gene therapy as a viable long-term option for the treatment of hemophilia B has been established, as discussed below. Currently, however, the challenges associated with gene transfer of the much larger *FVIII* gene have slowed down progress in the development of gene therapy for hemophilia A, although these limitations are being addressed.

There are several approaches by which the defective gene encoding factor VIII or factor IX can be introduced into a congenitally deficient host. Viruses have evolved to introduce genetic material into target cells and are usually employed as the vector, or "Trojan Horse," to allow transfection or transduction of the genetic information.[115,116] Several potential vectors have been used in clinical gene therapy studies for hemophilia and other single-gene disorders over the past 2 decades, including adenoviruses, recombinant adeno-associated viral vectors (rAAVs), and retroviral vectors, which include the lentiviral vectors based on HIV-1. At present, rAAVs are favored by the majority of ongoing trials in hemophilia, although preexisting immunity to some of these naturally occurring serotypes, which limits their use, is quite prevalent (up to 40 percent) in human populations. Although concerns exist about oncogenic genotoxicity (also known as insertional mutagenesis) associated with the earlier generation lentiviral vectors, they also have theoretical benefits; specifically, they are capable of infecting both dividing and nondividing cells with resultant persistent expression after integration into the host cell genome. In addition, they avoid the vector-mediated cytotoxicity (such as hepatic transaminitis) and immunologic reactions associated with rAAV.[117]

Certain vectors (such as rAAV) can be injected intravenously—usually on a single occasion—with resultant tropism of the vector and its payload to the liver. Previously, gene transfer via multiple intramuscular injections was also evaluated, and while not unduly toxic, sustained levels of factor IX greater than 1 percent were not maintained long-term.

These "*in vivo*" gene transfer protocols vary from "*ex vivo*" gene therapy, in which a specific type of cell is targeted before being reintroduced into the host. Target cells used for gene transfer in hemophilia have included human fibroblasts, hematopoietic stem cells, and platelets.

Despite a number of early-phase clinical trials over 20+ years, it was not until 2011 that the first report was released of predictable and consistent maintenance of factor IX levels (in the range of 1 to 6 percent of normal) being achieved in six subjects with hemophilia B. The bleeding frequency and clotting factor usage were reduced by 90 percent in these patients. This experience, from the groups at University College London and St. Jude's Research Hospital in Memphis, Tennessee, was updated with a follow-up of up to 3 years in the original cohort of six patients, together with an additional four treated individuals.[118] The protocol consisted of a single intravenous injection of a self-complementary rAAV-8; at the highest vector doses used, biochemical transaminitis occurred in some of the patients. This hepatotoxicity was mediated by a host cytotoxic T-lymphocyte response to viral capsid antigens expressed on transfected hepatocytes. Fortunately, however, there was a consistently beneficial and prompt response to modest doses of oral prednisolone.

This milestone study has prompted a resurgent interest in gene therapy for hemophilia, with several phase I studies now under way. Remaining challenges include the use of purer vector preparations (with fewer empty capsids) and strategies to circumvent the natural immunity to AAV.[116] These modifications should permit this approach to be applicable in a greater proportion of patients and result in even higher long-term expression of factor IX.

Finally, utilization of the same approach to hemophilia A is limited by the inefficient expression of factor VIII, as well as the large size of the coding sequence, even in the absence of the B domain. However, the use of B-domain–deleted codon optimized factor VIII molecules has produced encouraging results in animal models of gene therapy. It is hoped that these preclinical data translate into persistent factor VIII expression levels in patients with hemophilia A. It remains to be seen how often inhibitors to factor VIII occur in these patients.

# ●SPECIAL PROBLEMS ASSOCIATED WITH HEMOPHILIAS A AND B

Unusual problems are occasionally encountered in both hemophilia A and B. Some of these are discussed in a brief publication.[119] For example, scuba diving can be dangerous in severely affected hemophiliacs and should be avoided. Hemophilic patients requiring laser treatment for visual problems may not require replacement therapy provided that a surgical incision is not required during such therapy. Carriers of either hemophilia A or B may have bleeding problems during delivery or surgery and will require replacement therapy. Carriers whose fetuses have hemophilia may require cesarean section if vaginal delivery is found to be difficult. Forceps and mechanical devices should be avoided during delivery of infants who are hemophilic. Some patients with hemophilia may also have another familial bleeding disorder, such as VWD.

Hemophilic patients who survived the HIV epidemic are aging and are developing comorbidities similar to nonhemophilia males, including hypertension, cardiovascular disease, renal failure, and dyslipidemias. The deficiency of either factor VIII or IX seems to provide some protection against thrombosis.[120] However, myocardial infarction has been reported in hemophilic patients even without treatment.[121] DVT has also been reported following replacement therapy in both hemophilia A and hemophilia B. Acute DVT can be treated with heparin for 7 to 10 days as long as the patient receives factor replacement therapy. Thereafter, anticoagulation is not recommended. Thromboembolic episodes in

hemophilia B are much less common since the advent of highly purified factor IX products.

The management of cardiovascular disease in the hemophilia population is a challenge.[122,123] The use of antiplatelet therapy seems safe in mild and moderate individuals; for the severely deficient patient, however, prophylaxis with factor VIII or factor IX should be used. For anticoagulation with heparin or vitamin K antagonists, factor trough levels above 0.25 U/L are recommended. For the management of acute coronary syndromes and arrhythmias requiring intervention, replacement with adequate factor concentrate should be done without exceeding levels above 80 to100 percent of normal. Radial artery access rather than femoral and bare metal stents are preferred over drug-eluting stents. Individuals requiring valve replacement should receive a biologic rather than a mechanical valve when possible.

Hemophilia patients who have atrial fibrillation should undergo cardioversion when possible. If cardioversion is not successful, some physicians recommend treatment with aspirin, but anticoagulants should be used with caution taking into consideration the severity of the hemophilia and the risk of stroke.

# REFERENCES

1. Brinkhous KM: A short history of hemophilia, with some comments on the word "hemophilia," in *Handbook of Hemophilia*, edited by KM Brinkhous, HC Hemker, p 3. Elsevier, New York, 1975.
2. Katznelson JL: Hemophilia, with special reference to the Talmud. *Harofe Haivri Heb Med J* 1:165, 1958.
3. Morawitz P: Die Chemie der Blutgerinnung. *Ergeb Physiol* 4:307, 1905.
4. Addis T: The pathogenesis of hereditary haemophilia. *J Pathol Bacteriol* 15:427, 1911.
5. Brinkhous KM: A study of the clotting defect in hemophilia. The delayed formation of thrombin. *Am J Med Sci* 198:509, 1939.
6. Pavlovsky A: Contribution to the pathogenesis of hemophilia. *Blood* 2:185, 1947.
7. Aggeler PM, White SG, Glendenning MB: Plasma thromboplastin component (PTC) deficiency: A new disease resembling hemophilia. *Proc Soc Exp Biol Med* 79:692, 1952.
8. Biggs R, Douglas AS, Macfarlane AG, et al: Christmas disease: A condition previously mistaken for hemophilia. *Br Med J* 2:1378, 1952.
9. Escobar M, Sallah S: Hemophilia A and hemophilia B: Focus on arthropathy and variables affecting bleeding and prophylaxis. *J Thromb Haemost* 11:1449, 2013.
10. Davie EW, Ratnoff OD: Waterfall sequence for intrinsic blood clotting. *Science* 145:1310, 1964.
11. Macfarlane RG: An enzyme cascade in the blood clotting mechanism, and its function as a biological amplifier. *Nature* 202:498, 1964.
12. Broze GR Jr: Tissue factor pathway inhibitor and the revised theory of coagulation. *Annu Rev Med* 46:103, 1995.
13. Fay PJ: Reconstitution of human factor VIII from isolated subunits. *Arch Biochem Biophys* 262:525, 1988.
14. Roberts HR: Contributions to the evolution of knowledge about hereditary hemorrhagic disorders. *Cell Mol Life Sci* 64:517, 2007.
15. Hoffman M, Hargen A, Lewkowski A, et al: Cutaneous wound healing is impaired in hemophilia B. *Blood* 108:3053, 2006.
16. Tuddenham EG: Factor VIII, in *Molecular Basis of Thrombosis and Hemostasis*, edited by KA High, HR Roberts, p 167. Marcel Dekker, New York, 1995.
17. Factor VIII variant database. Available at: http://www.factorviii-db.org.
18. Tuddenham EG, Cooper DN, Gitschier J, et al: Haemophilia A: Database of nucleotide substitutions, deletions, insertions and rearrangements of the factor VIII gene. *Nucleic Acids Res* 22:4851, 1996.
19. Antonarakis SE, Rossiter JP, Young M, et al: Factor VIII gene inversions in severe hemophilia A: Results of an international consortium study. *Blood* 86:2206, 1995.
20. Higuchi M, Kazazian HH Jr, Kasch L, et al: Molecular characterization of severe hemophilia A suggests that about half the mutations are not within the coding regions and splice junctions of the factor VIII gene. *Proc Natl Acad Sci U S A* 88:7405, 1991.
21. Gitschier J, Kogan S, Diamond C, Levinson B: Genetic basis of hemophilia A. *Thromb Haemost* 66:37, 1991.
22. Bagnall RD, Waseem N, Green PM, Giannelli F: Recurrent inversion breaking intron 1 of the factor VIII gene is a frequent cause of severe hemophilia A. *Blood* 99:168, 2002.
23. Kazazian HH, Wong C, Youssoufian H, et al: Hemophilia A resulting from de novo insertion of L1 sequences represents a novel mechanism for mutation in man. *Nature* 332:164, 1998.
24. Mori PG, Pasino M, Vadala CR, et al: Haemophilia "A" in a 46Xi(Xq) female. *Br J Haematol* 43:143, 1979.
25. Lakich D, Kazazian HH, Antonarakis SE, Gitschier J: Inversions disrupting the factor VIII gene are a common cause of severe hemophilia A. *Nat Genet* 5:236, 1993.

26. Peake IR, Lillicrap DP, Boulyjenkov V, et al: Report of a joint WHO/WFH meeting on control of haemophilia: Carrier detection and prenatal diagnosis. *Blood Coagul Fibrinolysis* 4:313, 1993.

27. Ljung RC: Prenatal diagnosis of haemophilia. *Haemophilia* 5:84, 1999.

28. Poon MC, Hoar DI, Low S, et al: Hemophilia A carrier detection by restriction fragment length polymorphism analysis and discriminant analysis based on ELISA of factor VIII and vWf. *J Lab Clin Med* 119:751, 1992.

29. Chi C, Lee CA, Shiltagh N, et al: Pregnancy in carriers of hemophilia. *Haemophilia* 14:56, 2008.

30. Brummel-Ziedins KE, Orfeo T, Rosendaal FR, et al: Empirical and theoretical phenotypic discrimination. Phenotypic discrimination models. *J Thromb Haemost* 7(1):181, 2009.

31. Nichols WC, Amano K, Cacheris PM, et al: Moderation of hemophilia A phenotype by the factor V R506Q mutation. *Blood* 88:1183, 1996.

32. Gilbert MS: Musculoskeletal complications of haemophilia: The joint. *Haemophilia* 6:34, 2000.

33. Jansen NA, Rosendaal G, Lafeber FP: Understanding haemophilic arthropathy: An exploration of current issues. *Br J Haematol* 143:632, 2008.

34. Rodriguez Merchan EC: The hemophilic pseudotumour. *Int Orthop* 19:255, 1995.

35. Caviglia H, Candela M, Landro ME, et al: Haemophilia pseudotumours in patients with inhibitors. *Haemophilia* 2015;21(5):681-685.

36. Hein M, Martinowitz U: Pseudotumors in patients with hemophilia, in *Textbook of Hemophilia*, 3rd ed, edited by CA Lee, EE Berntorp, WK Hoots, p 233. Wiley Blackwell, Hoboken, NJ, 2014.

37. Zanon E, Iorio A, Rocino A, et al: Intracraneal haemorrhage in the Italian population of haemophilia patients with and without inhibitors. *Haemophilia* 18:39, 2012.

38. Eyster ME, Asaad SM, Gold BD, et al: Upper gastrointestinal bleeding in haemophiliacs: Incidence and relation to use of non-steroidal anti-inflammatory drugs. *Haemophilia* 13:279, 2007.

39. Moser KA, Funk DM: Chromogenic factor VIII activity assay. *Am J Hematol* 89:781, 2014.

40. McGinniss MJ, Kazazian HH Jr, Hoyer LW, et al: Spectrum of mutations in CRM-positive and CRM-reduced hemophilia A. *Genomics* 15:392, 1993.

41. Tully EA, Gaucher C, Jorieux S, et al: Expression of von Willebrand factor "Normandy." An autosomal mutation that mimics hemophilia A. *Proc Natl Acad Sci U S A* 88:6377, 1991.

42. Michiels JJ, Gadisseur A, Vangenegten I, et al: Recessive von Willebrand disease type 2 Normandy: Variable expression of mild hemophilia and VWD type 1. *Acta Haematol* 121:119, 2009.

43. Seligsohn U, Zwang E, Zivelin A: Combined factor V and factor VIII deficiency among non-Ashkenazi Jews. *N Engl J Med* 307:1191, 1982.

44. Ginsberg D: Identifying novel genetic determinants of hemostatic balance. *J Thromb Haemost* 8:1561, 2005.

45. Srivastava A, Brewer AK, Mauser-Bunschoten EP, et al: Guidelines for the management of hemophilia. *Haemophilia* 19:e1, 2013.

46. Santagostino E, Mannucci PM, Gringeri A, et al: Transmission of parvovirus B19 by coagulation factor concentrates exposed to 100 degrees C of heat after lyophilization. *Transfusion* 37:517, 1997.

47. Robertson BH, Alter MJ, Bell BP, et al: Hepatitis A virus sequence detected in clotting factor concentrates associated with disease transmission. *Biologicals* 26:95, 1998.

48. Escobar MA: Treatment on demand—*In vivo* dose finding studies. *Haemophilia* 9:360, 2003.

49. McMillan CW, Webster WP, Roberts HR, Blythe WB: Continuous intravenous infusion of factor VIII in classic hemophilia. *Br J Haematol* 18:659, 1972.

50. Schulman S: Continuous infusion. *Haemophilia* 9:368, 2003.

51. Rodeghiero F, Castaman G, Di Bona E, Ruggeri M: Consistency of responses to repeated DDAVP infusions in patients with von Willebrand's disease and hemophilia A. *Blood* 74:1997, 1989.

52. Mannucci PM, Bettega D, Cattaneo M: Patterns of development of tachyphylaxis in patients with haemophilia and von Willebrand disease after repeated doses of desmopressin (DDAVP). *Br J Haematol* 82:87, 1992.

53. Coppola A, Windyga J, Tufano A, et al: Treatment for preventing bleeding in people with haemophilia or other congenital bleeding disorders undergoing surgery. *Cochrane Database Syst Rev* 2:CD009961, 2015.

54. Ghosh K, Shetty S, Jijina F, Mohanty D: Role of epsilon amino caproic acid in the management of haemophilic patients with inhibitors. *Haemophilia* 10:58, 2004.

55. Martinowitz U, Saltz R: Fibrin sealant. *Curr Opin Hematol* 3:395, 1996.

56. Revel-Vilk S, Golomb MR, Achonu C, et al: Effect of intracranial bleeds on the health and quality of life of boys with hemophilia. *J Pediatr* 144:490, 2004.

57. Rodriguez-Merchan EC: Orthopaedic surgery in persons with haemophilia. *Thromb Haemost* 89:34, 2003.

58. Rabiner SF, Telfer MC: Home transfusion for patients with hemophilia A. *N Engl J Med* 283:1011, 1977.

59. Teitel JM, Barnard D, Israels S, et al: Home management of haemophilia. *Haemophilia* 10:118, 2004.

60. Manco-Johnson MJ, Riske B, Kasper CK: Advances in care of children with hemophilia. *Semin Thromb Hemost* 29:585, 2003.

61. Nilsson IM, Berntorp E, Lofqvist T, Pettersson H: Twenty-five years' experience of prophylactic treatment in severe haemophilia A and B. *J Intern Med* 232:25, 1992.

62. Manco-Johnson MJ, Abshire TC, Shapiro AD et al: Prophylaxis versus episodic treatment to prevent joint disease in boys with severe hemophilia. *N Engl J Med* 357:535, 2007.

63. Price VE, Carcao M, Connolly B, et al: A prospective, longitudinal study of central venous catheter-related deep venous thrombosis in boys with hemophilia. *J Thromb Haemost* 2:737, 2004.

64. Globe DR, Curtis RG, Koerper MA: Utilization of care in haemophilia: A resource-based method for cost analysis from the Haemophilia Utilization Group Study (HUGS). *Haemophilia* 10(Suppl 1):63, 2004.

65. Levetow LB, Sox HC, Stoto MA: *HIV and the Blood Supply: An Analysis of Crisis Decision Making, Institute of Medicine*, p 1. National Academy Press, Washington, DC, 1994.

66. Santagostino E, De Filippi F, Rumi MG, et al: Sustained suppression of hepatitis C virus by high doses of interferon and ribavirin in adult hemophilic patients. *Transfusion* 44:790, 2004.

67. Lollar P: Pathogenic antibodies to coagulation factors: I. Factor VIII and factor IX. *J Thromb Haemost* 2:1082, 2004.

68. Iorio A: Epidemiology of inhibitors in hemophilia, in *Textbook of Hemophilia*, 3rd ed, edited by CA Lee, EE Berntorp, WK Hoots, p 53. Wiley Blackwell, Hoboken, NJ, 2014.

69. Hoots WK, Lusher J: High-titer inhibitor development in hemophilia A: Lack of product specificity. *J Thromb Haemost* 2:358, 2004.

70. Gouw SC, van den Berg HM, le Cessie S, van der Bom JG: Treatment characteristics and the risk of inhibitor development: A multicenter cohort study among previously untreated patients with severe hemophilia A. *Blood* 109:4648, 2007.

71. Gouw SC, van der Bom JG, Auerswald G, et al: Recombinant versus plasma-derived factor VIII products and the development of inhibitors in previously untreated patients with severe hemophilia A: The CANAL cohort study. *Blood* 109:4693, 2007.

72. Gouw SC, van der Bom JG, Ljung R, et al: Factor VIII products and inhibitor development in severe hemophilia A. *N Engl J Med* 17:231, 2013.

73. Iorio A, Halimeh S Holzhauer S, et al: Rate of inhibitor development in previously untreated hemophilia A patients treated with plasma-derived or recombinant VIII concentrates: A systematic review. *J Thromb Haemost* 8:1256, 2010.

74. Gouw SC, van der Berg HM, Oldenberg J, et al: F8 gene mutation type and inhibitor development in patients with severe hemophilia A: Systematic review and meta-analysis. *Blood* 119:2922, 2012.

75. Peerlinck K, Arnout J, Gilles JH, et al: A higher than expected incidence of factor VIII inhibitors in multitransfused haemophilia A patients treated with an intermittent purity pasteurized factor VIII concentrate. *Thromb Haemost* 69:115, 1993.

76. Parker ET, Healey JF, Barrow RT, et al: Reduction of the inhibitory antibody response to human factor VIII in hemophilia A mice by mutagenesis of the A2 domain B cell epitope. *Blood* 104:704, 2004.

77. Kasper CK: Laboratory tests for factor VIII inhibitors, their variation, significance and interpretation. *Blood Coagul Fibrinolysis* 2:S7, 1991.

78. Verbruggen B, Novakova I, Wessels H, et al: The Nijmegen modification of the Bethesda assay for factor VIII:C inhibitors: Improved specificity and reliability and specificity. *Thromb Haemost* 73:247, 1995.

79. Ananyeva NM, Lee TK, Jain N, et al: Inhibitors in hemophilia A: Advances in elucidation of inhibitory mechanisms and in inhibitor management with bypassing agents. *Semin Thromb Hemost* 35:735, 2009.

80. Monroe DM, Roberts HR: Mechanism of action of high-dose factor VIIa: Points of agreement and disagreement. *Arterioscler Thromb Vasc Biol* 23:8, 2003.

81. Hoffman M, Dargaud Y: Mechanisms and monitoring of bypassing agent therapy. *J Thromb Haemost* 10:1478, 2012.

82. Escobar M, Maahs J, Hellman E, et al: Multidisciplinary management of patients with haemophilia with inhibitors undergoing surgery in the United States: Perspectives and best practices derived from experienced treatment centers. *Haemophilia* 18:971, 2012.

83. Rangarajan S, Austin S, Goddard NJ, et al: Consensus recommendations for the use of FEIBA in hemophilia A patients with inhibitors undergoing elective orthopedic and non-orthopedic surgery. *Haemophilia* 19:294, 2013.

84. DiMichele DM: Immune tolerance in haemophilia: The long journey to the fork in the road. *Haemophilia* 159:123, 2012.

85. DiMichele DM, Hoots WK, Pipe SW, et al: International workshop on immune tolerance induction: Consensus recommendations. *Haemophilia* 13:1, 2007.

86. Kempton CL, Meeks SL: Toward optimal therapy for inhibitors in hemophilia. *Blood* 124:3365, 2014.

87. Collins PN, Mathias M, Hanley J, et al: Rituximab and immune tolerance in severe hemophilia A: A consecutive national cohort. *J Thromb Haemost* 7:787, 2009.

88. Kohli A, Shaffer A, Sherman A, et al: Treatment of hepatitis C: A systematic review. *JAMA* 312:631, 2014.

89. Gjerset GF, Clements MJ, Counts RB, et al: Treatment type and amount influenced human immunodeficiency virus seroprevalence of patients with congenital bleeding disorders. *Blood* 78:1623, 1991.

90. Aguzzi A, Nuvolone M, Zhu C: The immunobiology of prion diseases. *Nat Rev Immunol* 13:888, 2013.

91. Shanbrom E, Owens W: Cascade iodination: A novel method to enhance the safety and efficacy of therapeutic proteins. *J Thromb Haemost* 2:836, 2004.

92. Ironside JW: Variant Creutzfeldt-Jakob disease. *Folia Neuropathol* 50:50, 2012.

93. Dolan G: Clinical implications of emerging pathogens in haemophilia: The variant Creutzfeldt-Jakob disease experience. *Haemophilia* 12:16, 2006.

94. Kurachi K, Davie EW: Isolation and characterization of a cDNA coding for factor IX. *Proc Natl Acad Sci U S A* 79:6461, 1982.

95. Rallapalli PM, Kemball-Cook G, Tuddenham EG, et al: An interactive mutation database for human coagulation factor IX provides novel insights into the phenotypes and genetics of hemophilia B. *J Thromb Haemost* 11:1329, 2013.

96. F9 Mutation database. Available at http://www.factorix.org.

97. Monroe DM, McCord DM, Huang MN, et al: Functional consequences of an arginine 180 to glutamine mutation in factor IX Hilo. *Blood* 73:1540, 1989.

98. Bertina RM, van der Linden IK, Mannucci PM, et al: Mutations in hemophilia Bm occur at the Arg180-Val activation site or in the catalytic domain of factor IX. *J Biol Chem* 265:10876, 1990.

99. Bottema CD, Ketterling RP, Ii S, et al: Missense mutations and evolutionary conservation of amino acids: Evidence that many of the amino acids in factor IX function as "spacer" elements. *Am J Hum Genet* 49:820, 1991.

100. Ketterling RP, Bottema CD, Phillips JA III, Sommer SS: Evidence that descendants of three founders constitute about 25% of hemophilia B in the United States. *Genomics* 10:1093, 1991.

101. Briet E, Bertina RM, van Tilburg NH, Veltkamp JJ: Hemophilia B Leyden: A sex-linked hereditary disorder that improves after puberty. *N Engl J Med* 306:788, 1982.

102. Kurachi S, Huo JS, Ameri A, et al: An age-related homeostasis mechanism is essential for spontaneous amelioration of hemophilia B Leyden. *Proc Natl Acad Sci U S A* 106:7921, 2009.

103. Reijnen MJ, Sladek FM, Bertina RM, Reitsma PH: Disruption of a binding site for hepatocyte nuclear factor 4 results in hemophilia B Leyden. *Proc Natl Acad Sci U S A* 89:6300, 1992.

104. Lusher JM, McMillan CW: Severe factor VIII and factor IX deficiency in females. *Am J Med* 65:637, 1978.

105. Goodeve AC: Laboratory methods for the genetic diagnosis of bleeding disorders. *Clin Lab Haematol* 20:3, 1998.

106. White GC, Bebe A, Nielsen B: Recombinant factor IX. *Thromb Haemost* 78:261, 1997.

107. Escobar MA: Advances in the treatment of inherited coagulation disorders. *Haemophilia* 19:648, 2013.

108. Wolberg AS, Stafford DW, Erie DA: Human factor IX binds to specific sites on the collagenous domain of collagen IV. *J Biol Chem* 272:16717, 1997.

109. Kim HC, McMillan CW, White GC, et al: Purified factor IX using monoclonal immunoaffinity technique: Clinical trials in hemophilia B and comparison to prothrombin complex concentrates. *Blood* 79:568, 1992.

110. Puetz J, Soucie JM, Kempton CL, et al: Prevalent inhibitors in haemophilia B subjects enrolled in the Universal Data Collection database. *Haemophilia* 20:25, 2014.

111. High KA: Factor IX: Molecular structure, epitopes, and mutations associated with inhibitor formation, in *Inhibitors to Coagulation Factors*, edited by LM Aledort, LW Hoyer, JM Lusher, HM Reisner, CG White, p 79. Plenum, New York, 1995.

112. Warrier I, Ewenstein BM, Koerper MA, et al: Factor IX inhibitors and anaphylaxis in hemophilia B. *J Pediatr Hematol Oncol* 19:23, 1997.

113. Bontempo FA, Lewis JH, Gorenc TJ, et al: Liver transplantation in hemophilia A. *Blood* 69:1721, 1987.

114. Wilde J, Teixeira P, Bramhall SR, et al: Liver transplantation in haemophilia. *Br J Haematol* 117:952, 2002.

115. High KA, Nathwani A, Spencer T, Lillicrap D: Current status of haemophilia gene therapy. *Haemophilia* 20:43, 2014.

116. Monahan PE, Gui T: Gene therapy for hemophilia: Advancing beyond the first clinical success. *Curr Opin Hematol* 20:410, 2013.

117. Chuah MK, Evens H, VandenDriessche T: Gene therapy for hemophilia. *J Thromb Haemost* 11:99, 2013.

118. Nathwani AC, Reiss UM, Tuddenham EG, at al: Long-term safety and efficacy of factor IX gene therapy in hemophilia B. *N Engl J Med* 371:1994, 2014.

119. Ma A, Roberts HR, Escobar MA, editors: *Haemophilia and Haemostasis: A Case-Based Approach to Management*, 2nd ed. Blackwell, Oxford, 2012.

120. Girolami A, Ruzzon E, Fabris F, et al: Myocardial infarction and other arterial occlusions in hemophilia A patients. A cardiological evaluation of all 42 cases reported in the literature. *Acta Haematol* 116:120, 2006.

121. Kulkarni R, Soucie JM, Evatt BL: Prevalence and risk factors for heart disease among males with hemophilia. *Am J Hematol* 79:36, 2005.

122. Mannucci PM, Schutgens RE, Santagostino E, et al: How I treat age-related morbidities in elderly persons with hemophilia. *Blood* 114:5256, 2009.

123. Tuinenburg A, Damen SA, Ypma PF, et al: Cardiac catheterization and intervention in haemophilia patients: Prospective evaluation of the 2009 institutional guideline. *Haemophilia* 19:370, 2013.

# CHAPTER 14

# INHERITED DEFICIENCIES OF COAGULATION FACTORS II, V, V+VIII, VII, X, XI, AND XIII

Flora Peyvandi and Marzia Menegatti*

## SUMMARY

Rare bleeding disorders (RBDs), accounting for the 3 to 5 percent of patients with abnormal hemostasis, include the nonhemophilia inherited deficiencies of coagulation factor II (prothrombin), factor V, combined factor V/VIII, factor VII, factor X, factor XI, factor XIII, and fibrinogen. The prevalence of RBDs is variable, both the relative frequency among the different factors and frequency in different regions of the world. The genetic transmission of these disorders is usually autosomal recessive. Bleeding manifestations caused by these inherited deficiencies are of variable severity and usually related to the extent of the decreased activity of the particular coagulation factor. Usually, only homozygous and compound heterozygous patients are symptomatic, although occasionally heterozygotes display a bleeding tendency. On the whole, the most typical symptom, common to all RBDs, is the occurrence of mucosal bleeding, whereas life-endangering bleeding, such as central nervous system or umbilical cord bleeding, is more frequent only in the some deficiencies, such as afibrinogenemia and severe factor XIII and factor X deficiencies, characterized by very low or undetectable coagulant activity. Treatment of patients affected with the various coagulation factor deficiencies could be (1) on demand for spontaneous bleeding episodes, (2) after surgical procedures, and (3) for prevention (prophylaxis). Because of the rarity of these disorders and the technical limitations of laboratory testing and the lack of specific concentrates, a unified, evidence-based therapeutic approach to many such patients is not always clear. To overcome these limitations, new strategies, such as the creation of global partnerships and networking between treatment centers, have been developed to increase our knowledge and create platforms for researchers and clinicians to exchange information.

**Acronyms and Abbreviations:** aPTT, activated partial thromboplastin time; COPII, coat protein complex II; EGF, epidermal growth factor; ELISA, enzyme-linked immunosorbent assay; ERGIC, endoplasmic reticulum–Golgi intermediate compartment; FFP, fresh-frozen plasma; GGCX, γ-glutamyl carboxylase; Gla, γ-carboxyglutamic acid; LMAN, mannose-binding lectin; MCFD, multiple combined-factor deficiency; PAR, protease-activated receptor; PCC, prothrombin complex concentrate; PPH, postpartum hemorrhage; PT, prothrombin time; TAFI, thrombin-activatable fibrinolysis inhibitor; TF, tissue factor; TT, thrombin time; VKORC1, vitamin K epoxide reductase–oxidase complex.

*The authors would like to thank Dr. U. Selighson and Dr. O. Salomon for their contributions to this chapter.

Rare congenital deficiencies of plasma proteins involved in blood coagulation, such as fibrinogen, prothrombin, and factors V, V+VIII, VII, X, XI, and XIII, generally lead to lifelong bleeding disorders. These disorders have been described in most populations with an incidence varying from one case in 500,000 for factor VII deficiency, to one case in 2 to 3 million for prothrombin and factor XIII deficiency.[1,2] However, their relative frequency varies among populations, being higher in regions where consanguineous or endogamous marriages are common, partly as a result of increased high frequencies of specific mutant genes in these inbred populations.[3–8] Two large surveys were made by the World Federation of Hemophilia (WFH; www.wfh.org) and the European Network of the Rare Bleeding Disorders (EN-RBD; www.rbdd.eu), with the aim of collecting epidemiologic data and providing information to hemophilia organizations and treatment centers to reduce and prevent complications of bleeding. Data collected by these surveys showed that factor VII and factor XI deficiencies are the most prevalent rare bleeding disorders (RBDs), each accounting for approximately one-third of all RBDs, while the rarest disorders are factor II (prothrombin) deficiency and combined deficiency of factors V and VIII (Table 14–1). The severity of bleeding manifestations in affected patients is variable. The most typical symptom, common to all RBDs, is bleeding from the mucosal tracts or at the site of invasive procedures; life- and limb-endangering symptoms, such as umbilical cord and central nervous system bleeding, recurrent hemarthroses, and soft tissue hematomas, occur with higher frequency only in some severe deficiencies.[9–15] Although heterozygotes for the coagulation factor deficiencies usually do not manifest a bleeding tendency, some cases of postdelivery and post–dental-extraction bleeding in heterozygotes for factor X deficiency have been reported.[16]

## ● LABORATORY DIAGNOSIS

The complexity of blood coagulation and the large number of proteins and nonprotein substances involved necessitate that a global test be used to simply and reproducibly assess its function: the screening tests such as prothrombin time (PT) and activated partial thromboplastin time (aPTT) are the first step in evaluating patients reporting a clinical and family history of bleeding. The PT interrogates the extrinsic coagulation pathway, and its prolongation is indicative of the deficiency of factor VII; a normal aPTT is highly dependent on the intrinsic coagulation pathway, so that its prolongation is indicative of deficiencies of factors XI, VIII, IX, and XII. However, all patients homozygous or compound heterozygous for factor XI deficiency have aPTT values longer than 2 SD above the normal mean,[17] while heterozygotes substantially overlap the normal range.[17,18] The prolongation of both the PT and aPTT indicates the lack of a factor belonging to the common pathway, including prothrombin, factor V, or factor X. However, patients with factor X deficiency harboring mutations that cause a defect only in the tissue factor (TF) pathway will only display a prolonged PT, and their aPTT will be normal. Other patients who carry mutations that only affect the intrinsic pathway activity of factor X will exhibit a normal PT and prolonged aPTT.[19] Abnormal results of either of these screening tests should be followed by mixing studies where equal amounts of patient plasma and normal plasma are mixed and retested; the relevant test time is normalized in patients with factor deficiencies but is not corrected or only minimally corrected in patients with factor inhibitors. In case of correction, specific coagulation assays are then performed to make the diagnosis of the specific factor deficiency. To evaluate fibrinogen deficiency, all coagulation tests that depend on the formation of fibrin as the end point are necessary; hence, in addition to PT and aPTT, thrombin time (TT) has to also be performed. In factor XIII deficiency, PT and aPTT are normal. Diagnosis of factor XIII deficiency is established by

**TABLE 14–1.** Worldwide Distribution of Rare Bleeding Disorders Derived from the World Federation of Hemophilia and the European Network of Rare Bleeding Disorders Surveys

| Deficiency | WFH Survey (%) | EN-RBD Database (%) |
|---|---|---|
| Fibrinogen | 7 | 8 |
| Factor II | 1 | 1 |
| Factor V | 9 | 10 |
| Factor V + factor VIII | 3 | 3 |
| Factor VII | 36 | 39 |
| Factor X | 8 | 8 |
| Factor XI | 30 | 24 |
| Factor XIII | 6 | 7 |

EN-RBD, European Network of the Rare Bleeding Disorders (www.rbdd.eu); WFH, World Federation of Hemophilia (www.wfh.org).

demonstrating increased clot solubility in 5 M urea, dilute monochloroacetic acid, or acetic acid. However, this method, quantitative and not yet standardized, detects only severe factor XIII deficiency (with activity <5 percent), thus leading to a possible underdiagnosis of factor XIII deficiency. The factor XIII deficiency diagnosis protocol requires a number of assays, which test for both activity as well as antigen levels. In the case of estimation of factor XIII activity using quantitative (e.g., photometric assays, which measure the ammonia released during a transglutaminase reaction) or incorporation assays (dansylcadaverine-casein assay, which measures the level of incorporation of a labeled amine into a protein substrate) during transglutaminase-mediated cross linking,[20] the plasma blanking procedure is mandatory to avoid the factor XIIIa–independent ammonia release that could lead to incorrect results in the low-activity range (below 5 to 10 percent).[21,22] Factor XIII A-subunit antigen can be measured by enzyme-linked immunosorbent assay (ELISA).[23] Factor antigen assays are not strictly necessary for diagnosis and treatment but are necessary to distinguish type I from type II deficiencies that become very important in fibrinogen or prothrombin deficiency, where normal antigen levels and reduced coagulant activity (dysfibrinogenemia and dysprothrombinemia) are associated with higher risk of thrombosis. Hereditary factor V deficiency is also a peculiar case that can be confused with combined deficiency of factor V + factor VIII because the two entities have similar manifestations and are characterized by prolonged PT and aPTT. Consequently, assays of factor V and factor VIII are mandatory for making the distinction.

## CLASSIFICATION

The development of guidelines for classification of RBDs has been historically hampered by a lack of sufficient knowledge about epidemiology and clinical outcomes, the difficulty in recognizing affected patients and collecting longitudinal clinical data, the limits of laboratory assays, and a lack of consensus concerning the criteria by which these disorders are classified. Classification of RBDs based on the residual level of plasma coagulant activity of the missing factor has considered for many years all RBDs as a single entity, and a mild, moderate, or severe classification as in hemophilia was adopted (except for some disorders such as afibrinogenemia and factor XIII deficiency). In 2012, the Rare Bleeding Disorders Working Group, under the umbrella of the Factor VIII & Factor IX Scientific and Standardisation Committee (SSC)

of the International Society on Thrombosis and Haemostasis (ISTH), analyzed the results of data coming from four registries (EN-RBD, the United Kingdom Haemophilia Centre Doctors' Organization registry, the North American Rare Bleeding Disorders Registry, and the Indian registry) including a total of 4359 patients. Despite the large number of patients evaluated in this overview (both from the literature and the aforementioned registries), there is a large heterogeneity in the pre-assigned severity definitions for both coagulant activity and bleeding symptoms.[24] At the same time, the EN-RBD, based on a cross-sectional study using data from 489 patients and involving 13 European treatment centers, for the first time evaluated the correlation between the coagulant residual plasma activity level and clinical bleeding severity in each RBD. Clinical bleeding episodes were classified into four categories of severity based on the location and the potential clinical impact, as well as the trigger of bleeding (spontaneous, after trauma, or drug induced). By means of linear regression analysis, this study found a strong association between coagulant activity level and clinical bleeding severity for fibrinogen, combined factors V + VIII, X, and XIII deficiencies. A weak association with clinical bleeding severity was present for factors V and VII deficiencies, while coagulation activity level of factor XI did not predict clinical bleeding severity. From the same study, it also clear that the minimum level to ensure complete absence of clinical symptoms is different for each disorder, leading to the conclusion that RBDs should not be considered as a single class of disorders, but instead studies should focus on the evaluation of specific aspects of each single RBD and different from hemophilia.[25]

## MOLECULAR ANALYSIS

The molecular diagnosis of RBDs is based on the mutation search in the genes encoding the corresponding coagulation factor. Exceptions are the combined deficiency of coagulation factors V+VIII, caused by mutations in genes encoding proteins involved in the factor V and factor VIII intracellular transport (multiple combined-factor deficiency [MCFD] 2 and mannose-binding lectin [LMAN] 1) and the combined deficiency of vitamin K–dependent proteins (prothrombin and factors VII, IX, and X), caused by mutations in genes that encode enzymes involved in posttranslational modifications[26] and in vitamin K metabolism ($\gamma$-glutamyl carboxylase [GGCX] and vitamin K epoxide reductase–oxidase complex [VKORC1]).[27] Coagulant factors genes are located on different chromosomes except for the genes of factor VII (F7), factor X (F10), fibrinogen (FGA, FGB, FGG), and factor XI (F11) (Table 14–2). In particular, F10 lays only 2.8 kb downstream of F7; thus, the combined deficiency of the two factors can be also the result of chromosomal abnormalities of the long arm of chromosome 13.[28–30] The strategy for molecular analysis is generally based on polymerase chain reaction amplification followed by Sanger sequencing of all exons, flanking intronic sequence and 5′ and 3′ untranslated regions. In contrast with hemophilia A, caused in approximately half of the patients by an inversion mutation involving introns 1 or 22 of the factor VIII gene, RBDs are often caused by mutations unique for each kindred and scattered throughout the genes. Information on already identified mutations causing RBDs is traceable from the mutation database on the ISTH website (http://www.isth.org/?MutationsRareBleedin). Missense mutations are the most frequent gene abnormalities, representing 50 to 80 percent of all identified mutations, except for LMAN1 variants where the most frequent mutations are insertions/deletions (50 percent). Insertion/deletion mutations represent 20 to 30 percent of the gene variations of the fibrinogen, factor V (F5), MCFD2, and factor XIII (F13A) genes, and less than 15 percent of the remaining coagulation factor gene mutations. Splicing and nonsense mutations comprise 5 to 15 percent of all identified mutations in all coagulation factors, with a maximum

**TABLE 14–2.** General Genetic Features of Coagulation Factors

| Deficiency | Gene | Chromosome | Reference |
|---|---|---|---|
| Factor II | F2 | 11p11–q12 | 56 |
| Factor V | F5 | 1q21–25 | 82 |
| Factors V + VIII | LMAN1 | 18q21.3–q22 | 110,111,124 |
| | MCFD2 | 2p21–p16.3 | 26 |
| Factor VII | F7 | 13q34 | 30,149 |
| Factor X | F10 | 13q34–qter | 192 |
| Factor XI* | F11 | 4q34–35 | 238,239 |
| Factor XIII | F13A | 6p24–p25 | 294,295 |
| | F13B | 1q31–q32.1 | 297,298 |

*F11 gene is located on the same chromosome of fibrinogen genes (fibrinogen deficiency is not discussed in this chapter).

rate of 20 percent in the LMAN1 gene. Variants located in the 3′ and 5′ untranslated regions of the genes are the least-frequent types of mutation (<5 percent), found only at the fibrinogen, factor VII, factor XI, and factor XIII loci. The combined presence of more than one recessively transmitted coagulation factor defect may also rarely occur, resulting in combined deficiency of factors VII and X[31–33] and combined deficiency of factors VII and V, VIII, X, or XI.[34] Despite significant advances in our knowledge of the genetic basis of the RBDs, in 5 to 10 percent of patients affected with severe clotting factor deficiencies, no genetic defect can be found. In these patients, the use of next-generation sequencing might help to identify novel pathways in coagulation disorders.

# TREATMENT

Treatment of RBDs is a difficult task because the absence of longitudinal clinical data and the limitations of available laboratory assays make it difficult to develop evidenced-based guidelines for the diagnosis and treatment of RBDs. A patient's personal and family history of bleeding is an important guide for management. Dosages and frequency of treatment depend on the minimal hemostatic level of the deficient factor, its plasma half-life (see Table 14–3), and the type of bleeding episode. At variance with patients affected with hemophilia A or B who have vastly improved the quality of life from advances in the manufacture of safe and effective products,[35] patients with RBDs have seen less progress. The main treatments in RBDs are represented by replacement therapy of the deficient coagulation factor and nontransfusional adjuvant therapies (antifibrinolytic amino acids, estrogen/progestin). Fresh-frozen plasma (FFP) and cryoprecipitate are the backbone of RBD treatment, particularly in those countries with low economic resources. However, specific plasma-derived concentrates are currently available only for fibrinogen and factors VII, XI, and XIII, and they are licensed only in some European countries; replacement therapy of coagulation factors may require the prescription of unlicensed products that are not readily available.

Prothrombin and factor X deficiencies are often treated with prothrombin complex concentrates (PCCs), which often also contain uncontrolled amounts of factor II, factor VII, and factor X. Products to cover the need for a dedicated therapy of patients with factor V deficiency and to facilitate the prophylaxis scheme in patients with factor X deficiency are of recent production. Finally, only two recombinant products are currently available for treatment of RBDs: recombinant factor VIIa (rFVIIa;) and recombinant factor XIII (rFXIII) (see "Factor VII Deficiency" and "Factor XIII Deficiency"). Although there are a number of reports available in the literature reporting on treatment

on demand and by prophylaxis in RBDs,[36,37] no clear-cut guidelines are yet available apart from those of the United Kingdom Haemophilia Centre Doctors' Organization.[38] Table 14–3 shows available treatment for each deficiency and suggested dosages.

# WOMEN WITH RARE BLEEDING DISORDERS

Women with RBDs require specific attention and care because in addition to experiencing the common associated bleeding symptoms, they may also experience bleeding complications from regular hemostatic challenges during menstruation, pregnancy, and childbirth, as well as from other gynecologic conditions, such as hemorrhagic ovarian cysts, endometriosis, hyperplasia, polyps, and fibroids. Menorrhagia, defined as blood loss of more than 80 mL per menstruation, is reported to be one of the most important symptoms in women with RBDs.[39,40] Menstruation may be quite problematic for women with coagulation disorders who have excessive blood loss, which can have a major impact on their quality of life and employment.

Pregnancy and childbirth pose particular clinical challenges to women with RBDs, because, apart from factor XI deficiency, detailed information about these issues and their management is very scarce and limited to just a few case reports.[41,42] Pregnancy is accompanied by increased concentrations of fibrinogen, factor VII, factor VIII, factor X, and von Willebrand factor, which are particularly marked in the third trimester.[43–47] In contrast, prothrombin, factor V, factor IX, and factor XIII are relatively unchanged.[43] All of these changes contribute to the hypercoagulable state of pregnancy; however, women with coagulation factor deficiencies do not achieve the same factor levels as those of women without deficiencies,[39] increasing the possibility of pregnancy loss or bleeding complications, especially if the defect is severe.

# PROTHROMBIN DEFICIENCY

## DEFINITION

Inherited prothrombin deficiency is one of the rarest coagulation factor deficiencies. It presents in two forms: type I, true deficiency (hypoprothrombinemia), and type II, in which a dysfunctional prothrombin is produced (dysprothrombinemia). These autosomal recessive disorders are genetically heterogeneous and characterized by a mild to moderate bleeding tendency. Both types of prothrombin deficiency impair the generation or function of thrombin, the central enzyme of the blood coagulation system.

**TABLE 14–3.** Treatment of Inherited Coagulation Disorders

| Deficient Factor | Plasma Half-Life | Recommended Trough Levels | On-Demand Dosages | Recommended Trough Levels After Publication of the EN-RBD Results to Maintain Patient Asymptomatic |
|---|---|---|---|---|
| Fibrinogen | 2–4 days | 0.5–1.0 g/L | Cryoprecipitate (5–10 bags) <br> SD-treated plasma (15–30 mL/kg) <br> Fibrinogen concentrate (50–100 mg/kg) | 1 g/L |
| Prothrombin | 3–4 days | 20–30% | SD-treated plasma (15–20 mL/kg) <br> PCC (20–30 units/kg) with dosing based on labeled factor IX units | >10% |
| Factor V | 36 hours | 10–20% | SD-treated plasma (15–20 mL/kg) | 10% |
| Factors V and VIII | Factor V 36 hours <br> Factor VIII 10–14 hours | 10–15% | As for factor V | 40% |
| Factor VII | 4–6 hours | 10–15% | Factor VII concentrate (30–40 mL/kg) <br> PCC (20–30 units/kg) <br> rFVIIa (15–30 mcg/kg every 4–6 hours) | >20% |
| Factor X | 40–60 hours | 10–20% | SD-treated plasma (10–20 mL/kg) <br> PCC (20–30 units/kg) <br> Factor X/factor IX concentrate (10–20 units/kg) | >40% |
| Factor XI | 50 hours | 15–20% | SD-treated plasma (15–20 mL/kg) <br> Factor XI concentrate (15–20 units/kg) | 15–20% |
| Factor XIII | 9–12 days | 2–5% | Cryoprecipitate (2–3 bags) <br> SD-treated plasma (3 mL/kg) <br> Factor XIII concentrate (50 units/kg for high hemorrhagic events) | 30% |

PCC, prothrombin complex concentrate; rFVIIa, recombinant factor VIIa; SD, solvent-detergent.

## PROTEIN

Prothrombin, approximate Mr 72,000, is structurally homologous with other members of the vitamin K–dependent proteins, factors VII, IX, and X, proteins C, S, and Z, and bone γ-carboxyglutamic acid (Gla) protein. Prothrombin is synthesized in the liver as a prepropeptide of 622 amino acids, and its plasma concentration is 100 to 150 mcg/mL. The circulating protein in its mature form is a single-chain glycoprotein of 579 residues, composed of the Gla domain (residues 1 to 37) and the catalytic domain (residues 272 to 579), where a light A chain is disulfide-bonded to the heavy B chain containing the catalytic triad. In the zymogen molecule, there are several exodomains, such as two kringle domains—kringle 1 (F1; residues 38 to 155), kringle 2 (F2; residues 156 to 271)—and the prepropeptide region.[48,49] The prepropeptide domain is responsible for protein processing, targeting, and carboxylation, and it is removed prior to secretion from the cell. The Gla domain constitutes the aminoterminus of the mature prothrombin molecule and contains the 10 glutamic acid residues that are posttranslationally modified through action of vitamin K–dependent carboxylase to Gla. As a result of this modification, prothrombin acquires the capacity to bind calcium and membranes containing acidic phospholipids. The kringle domain contains two extensively folded, disulfide-bonded "kringle" motifs. They are present in diverse proteins and are thought to mediate protein–protein interactions. For example, the kringle 2 domain of prothrombin mediates interaction of prothrombin with activated factor V (Va).[50] The catalytic domain contains the enzyme active site, which is responsible for fibrinogen cleavage. The residues characteristic

for the serine protease family, His363, Asp419, and Ser525, constitute a charge relay system responsible for bond cleavage. The crystal structure of prothrombin has not been determined, but the crystal structure of human α-thrombin complexed with *D-Phe-Pro-Arg chloromethylketone* (an inhibitor that is a transition state analogue covalently bound to the enzyme) has been determined.[51]

Prothrombin plays a central role in coagulation, functioning in both TF and contact activation pathways. Prothrombin is converted to its proteolytically active form, thrombin, by the prothrombinase complex consisting of activated factor X (Xa), factor Va, and phospholipid surface of platelets and other cells. Two forms of thrombin are generated: meizothrombin, if prothrombin is cleaved at residue 320, and α-thrombin, if cleavage occurs first at residue 271, removing prothrombin fragment 1.2, and subsequently cleaved at residue 320. Thrombin is a multifunctional serine protease. In addition to converting fibrinogen to fibrin, thrombin also exerts functions in the coagulation cascade, consisting of both pro- and anticoagulant effects[52] and activates platelets by cleavage of the protease-activated receptor (PAR)-1 and PAR-4, initiating signals leading to platelet adhesion and aggregation.[53,54] Thrombin also stimulates wound healing through its action as a growth factor and its proangiogenic activity.[55]

## GENETICS

The prothrombin gene is located on the short (p) arm of chromosome 11.[56] It is 20-kb long and consists of 14 exons separated by 13 introns. Fifty-four mutations that cause prothrombin deficiency have been identified, of which 42 are missense, three nonsense, seven deletions/insertions, and two splicing mutations (see mutation database on the ISTH website, http://www.isth.org/?MutationsRareBleedin and Ref. 9). Type II deficiency (dysprothrombinemia) results from missense mutations that are located throughout the gene. As expected, many mutations are in the catalytic domain, imparting catalytic dysfunction on thrombin. Other mutations give rise to abnormally slow activation of prothrombin. Only about 10 mutations were identified in patients with type I deficiency, of which five were present in homozygotes. Globally, there is a clear prevalence of patients with a Latin/Hispanic origin, as nearly 70 percent of all patients with thrombin gene defects come from such areas (Barcelona, Padua, Segovia, and Puerto Rico).[9]

A number of polymorphisms have been identified in the prothrombin gene. One of these polymorphisms, a G>A change at nucleotide 20210 in the 3′ untranslated region of the prothrombin gene, is associated with increased plasma levels of prothrombin and an increased tendency to venous thrombosis (Chap. 20).[57]

## CLINICAL MANIFESTATIONS

According to a recent classification by the SSC of the ISTH, prothrombin deficiency may be classified as severe, moderate, and mild, corresponding to blood levels of less than 5 percent, 5 to 10 percent, and greater than 10 percent, respectively.[24] In severely prothrombin-deficient patients, bleeding may be marked, including spontaneous hemarthroses; less severe patients may show mild to moderate mucocutaneous and soft tissue bleeding that usually correlates with the degree of functional prothrombin deficiency. Heterozygous subjects, having plasma prothrombin levels between 30 and 60 percent of normal, are usually asymptomatic; however, occasionally, excessive bleeding after moderate-intensity trauma, tooth extractions, or surgical procedures may occur. Patients with dysprothrombinemia show a variable bleeding tendency that is usually less severe than in type I deficiency. Women with prothrombin deficiency may suffer from menorrhagia. Because of the extreme rarity of such deficiency, reports on events during pregnancy/delivery are very scarce, with only one described in four of eight pregnancies in a hypoprothrombinemic woman.[58] In the same report, one postpartum hemorrhage (PPH) episode in the four term pregnancies was reported, despite administration of clotting factor concentrate. However, these data were not confirmed by a following Iranian series, including a total of 14 patients with the same deficiency (coagulant activity levels 4 to 10 percent).[59]

Undetectable plasma prothrombin probably is incompatible with life, as inferred from the partial embryonic and neonatal lethality of prothrombin knockout mice, which do not survive to adulthood.[60,61]

## THERAPY

Replacement therapy is needed only in severe patients, in case of bleeding or to ensure adequate prophylaxis before surgical procedures. In severe clinical settings, higher levels of prothrombin may be achieved with FFP, or with PCCs, which avoids the risk of volume overload sometimes associated with the use of FFP.[62] However, PCCs contain other vitamin K–dependent coagulation factors (VII, IX, and X) and small amounts of their activated forms, which could potentially induce thrombotic complications; those containing an amount of factor VII below 10 percent are commonly known as three-factor PCCs. These concentrates are heated or treated with solvent–detergent, processes that remove HIV, hepatitis B, hepatitis C, and other viruses but that do not remove parvovirus B19 or hepatitis A virus[63–65]; the latter viruses can be effectively removed by dry heat and nanofiltration.[66] However, transmission of other possible bloodborne agents, such as prions causing Creutzfeldt-Jakob disease and its new variant, has not been totally eliminated.

Bruises and mild superficial bleeding generally do not require replacement therapy. Antifibrinolytic agents (tranexamic acid and gabexate mesylate) have also been used for minor surgical procedures. The oral contraceptives have been shown to exert beneficial effects on menometrorrhagia in women characterized by prothrombin coagulant levels less than 3 percent.[9] Thromboprophylaxis in dysprothrombinemic patients considered at high risk for a thrombotic event (e.g., orthopedic surgery) is a controversial issue. It is likely that administering low-molecular-weight heparin prophylactically to surgical patients at the same doses and schedules as those recommended for nondefect patients having similar procedures may be a valuable and safe procedure after correction of factor II deficiency by FFP or PCC infusion.

## ● FACTOR V DEFICIENCY

### DEFINITION AND HISTORY

Hereditary factor V deficiency was initially termed parahemophilia because of its similarities with classical hemophilia.[67] In most of the affected individuals, the phenotype is characterized by the concomitant deficiency of factor V activity and antigen (type I deficiency); however, approximately 25 percent of patients have normal antigen levels (type II deficiency), thus indicating the presence of a dysfunctional protein.[68]

### PROTEIN

Factor V is synthesized by the liver,[69] and its plasma concentration is approximately 20 nM (7 mcg/mL).[70–72] Factor V is a high-molecular-weight (Mr ~330,000), single-chain, large glycoprotein that consists of 2196 amino acids that bears significant, regional sequence homology to factor VIII. Analysis of the approximately 7-kb factor V complementary DNA showed that the protein is organized according to the following domain structure: $A_1$-$A_2$-B-$A_3$-$C_1$-$C_2$. The A and C domains have approximately 40 percent homology with analogous domains in factor VIII.[72,73] The large B domain shows no homology with the corresponding B domain of factor VIII. Factor V is converted to its activated form following several proteolytic cleavages by thrombin[74] or factor Xa.[75] These cleavages remove the B domain and yield factor Va, which consists of a heavy chain ($A_1$-$A_2$ domains) associated by $Ca^{2+}$ with a light chain ($A_3$-$C_1$-$C_2$ domains). The light chain contains the binding sites for membrane phospholipids, prothrombin, and activated protein C; both light and heavy chains probably are necessary for factor Xa binding. Assembly of factors Va and Xa on the phospholipid membrane of platelets in the presence of calcium ions forms the prothrombinase complex, which catalyzes the conversion of prothrombin to thrombin. The contribution of factor Xa in the absence of factor Va to overall thrombin generation is relatively minor. Importantly, incorporation of the cofactor into the macromolecular enzyme complex enhances prothrombin activation by several orders of magnitude.[76]

In addition to hepatocytes, the primary site of factor V secretion, approximately 20 percent of the protein in whole blood is localized in the α granules of platelets, where it is complexed with an extremely large protein, multimerin.[77] Megakaryocytes do not synthesize factor V; rather, endocytosis of plasma-derived factor V accounts for the platelet factor V pool.[78] Following endocytosis, factor V is modified intracellularly; these changes to platelet factor V appear to provide the cofactor with unique physical and functional characteristics, which render it more procoagulant compared with its plasma counterpart.[79] Platelet degranulation and release of platelet factor V at the site of vascular injury is thought to be a critical contributor to the local factor V concentration. Furthermore, there is some evidence that, because platelet factor V is locally released in high concentrations, it is less susceptible to inhibition and may function normally in hemostasis. Factor Va is inactivated by activated protein C through limited proteolysis at Arg506, Arg306, and Arg679 in the presence of protein S, calcium ions, and either platelet or endothelial cell membrane phospholipids.[80] Partial protection from this cleavage is provided by factor Xa when bound to factor Va on the surface of platelets.[81]

## GENETICS

The factor V gene maps to chromosome 1q21–25.[82] It is greater than 80 kb in length, and the coding sequence is divided into 25 exons, ranging in size from 72 to 2820 base pairs (bp), and 24 introns, varying between 0.4 kb and 11 kb.[83]

A total of 132 distinct mutations of the factor V gene have been identified, of which 64 are missense, 36 are insertions/deletions, 17 are nonsense, 15 are splice site mutations, and one is a deletion of the whole gene (see http://www.isth.org/?MutationsRareBleedin and Ref. 10). Most mutations cause truncations and are localized throughout the gene. Several mutations have interesting features. One, a Tyr1702Cys transition, was identified in eight unrelated families, of whom six were Italian. The frequency of this mutant allele in Italy is 0.002.[84] Another mutation, an Ala221Val (New Brunswick) alteration, characterized in the homozygous state by activity and antigen levels of 29 and 39 percent of normal, respectively, displays decreased stability of the expressed protein and was the first genetic defect reported to be associated with type II deficiency.[85] Additional mutations exhibit decreased secretion of the protein from producing cells.[86,87] Remarkably, the Gln773ter and Arg1133ter mutations and a 4-bp deletion mutation, all present in exon 13 and predicted to result in partial truncation of the B-domain and complete truncation of the A3-, C1-, and C2-domains, cause no bleeding or only a mild bleeding tendency in affected patients having factor V antigen and activity levels 1 percent of normal.[88–90]

Factor V Leiden (Arg506Gln) is a highly prevalent (up to 5 percent in some populations) polymorphism in the factor V gene that decreases the efficiency of factor Va inactivation by activated protein C.[91] Patients with factor V Leiden are at increased risk of unprovoked thrombosis, with homozygotes at greater risk than heterozygotes. The *trans* association of factor V Leiden and a mutation in factor V that causes factor V deficiency results in a prothrombotic state comparable to factor V Leiden homozygosity. This is sometimes termed "pseudohomozygous" activated protein C resistance and does not cause bleeding despite low factor V antigen levels.[92] Among several polymorphisms detected in the factor V gene, His1299Arg in exon 13 is particularly interesting because it is associated with a reduced plasma factor V level and mild activated protein C resistance.[93] His1299Arg co-segregates with several other polymorphisms encoding several amino acid changes, together named R2 haplotype.[94] In two heterozygotes for factor V Arg506Gln mutation who presented with venous thrombosis, reduced factor V activity resulting from the His1299Arg polymorphism harbored by the non-Leiden chromosome, imparted a pseudohomozygous phenotype for activated protein C resistance.[95] Additional polymorphisms or mutations in the factor V gene have been observed to increase the risk of venous thrombosis.[96]

In addition, there are at least two examples in which platelet factor V is reduced. In the Quebec platelet disorder, initially described as an autosomal dominant disorder with severe bleeding manifestations, platelet factor V levels are reduced because of enhanced proteolysis resulting from overexpression of urokinase-type plasminogen activator,[97] as they are in factor V New York.[98]

## CLINICAL MANIFESTATIONS

Factor V deficiency is inherited as an autosomal recessive trait. Heterozygotes, whose plasma factor V activity ranges between 25 and 60 percent of normal, usually are asymptomatic, although an American

registry recorded mild bleeding in 50 percent of the cases.[99] According to a recent classification by the SSC of the ISTH, factor V deficiency may be classified as severe, moderate, and mild when factor V levels are undetectable, less than 10 percent, and 10 percent or greater, respectively.[24]

Common manifestations include ecchymoses, epistaxis, gingival bleeding, hemorrhage following minor lacerations, and menorrhagia.[99–101] Severe deficiency typically presents at birth or in early childhood, but depending on factor levels, some patients remain asymptomatic. Bleeding from other sites is less common, but instances of hemarthroses unrelated to trauma and intracerebral hemorrhage have been reported.[100] Trauma, dental extractions, and surgery confer a high risk of excessive bleeding.

PPH occurs in more than 50 percent of pregnancies in women with factor V deficiency,[102,103] especially those with low factor V activity levels. Venous and arterial thromboses have been described in patients with factor V levels ranging between 2 and 14 percent of normal.[104] Factor V deficiency deprives activated protein C of one of its essential substrates, thereby downregulating the inhibitory function of the protein C system.

Factor V is indispensable for life, as was demonstrated by experimental knockout mice lacking the factor V gene, which die either in utero at embryonic day 9 or 10 because of defects in yolk-sac vasculature and somite formation; the remaining half develop to term but die of massive hemorrhage within hours of birth.[105] The expression of a minimal factor V activity because of the introduction of a liver-specific transgene, below the sensitivity threshold of the detection assay (<0.1 percent), leads to the survival of mice.[106]

## THERAPY

Patients with epistaxis and gingival bleeding may respond to tranexamic acid (1 g four times daily), and local hemostatic measures may suffice for minor lacerations. Menorrhagia can also be managed directly using oral contraceptives, progestin-containing intrauterine devices, endometrial ablation, or hysterectomy. If these measures fail, severe spontaneous bleeding occurs, or surgery is performed, treatment option is limited to FFP replacement as no specific factor V concentrate is yet available on the market and factor V is not present in cryoprecipitate or PCCs. Development of a functional factor V inhibitor after receiving plasma transfusions was reported in only two patients with hereditary deficiency; the inhibitor disappeared in one patient, but a low titer of the inhibitor persisted in the other patient.[107,108]

A new factor V concentrate has been developed for clinical use in patients deficient in factor V, and preclinical studies are currently being performed for the orphan drug designation application to the European Medicines Agency (EMA) and the Food and Drug Administration (FDA) so as to make it available on the market as soon as possible.

## ● COMBINED DEFICIENCY OF FACTORS V AND VIII

### DEFINITION AND HISTORY

Combined deficiency of factors V and VIII (F5F8D) is completely separate from factor V deficiency and factor VIII deficiency. The latter two are transmitted with different patterns of inheritance (autosomal recessive for factor V, X-linked for factor VIII) and involve proteins encoded by two different genes (*F5* gene and *F8* gene). F5F8D was first described in 1954[109]; however, the molecular mechanism of the association of the combined factor deficiency was not understood until the late 1990s,[110,111] when null mutations in the endoplasmic reticulum–Golgi intermediate compartment (*ERGIC*)-53 gene, now called *LMAN1*, were determined to be causative. In 2003, a second locus associated with the deficiency in approximately 15 percent of affected families with no mutation in LMAN1 was identified[26]: the *MCFD2* gene encoding for a cofactor for LMAN1. Even if a debate were carried out on the possible existence of other loci involved in the intracellular transport of factors V and VIII and associated with the disease, until now, previous biochemical studies failed to identify additional components of the LMAN1–MCFD2 receptor complex,[112] supporting the idea that F5F8D might be limited to the *LMAN1* and *MCFD2* genes.[113] The disorder has been detected in many populations, but a relatively high frequency occurs among Tunisian and Middle Eastern Jews residing in Israel[114] and among Iranians.[115]

## PROTEIN

Factors V and VIII are essential coagulation factors that circulate in plasma as precursors. Upon limited proteolysis by thrombin or factor Xa and in concert with negatively charged phospholipid surfaces, factors VIIIa and Va exhibit profound cofactor activities for activation of factor X by factor IXa and for activation of prothrombin by factor Xa, respectively. Inactivation of factors Va and VIIIa is accomplished by activated protein C in the presence of protein S and phospholipids through several proteolytic cleavages at distinct sites. Factor V and factor VIII have similar domain organizations with partial homology (see "Factor V Deficiency" above).

The pathogenesis of combined deficiency of factors V and VIII puzzled investigators for more than 40 years. The enigma was resolved by the finding that the disease stems from the deficiency of either one of two interacting proteins, LMAN1 and MCFD2, which play a role in the intracellular transport of factors V and VIII. LMAN1 is a 53-kDa type 1 transmembrane nonglycosylated protein with homology to leguminous lectin proteins.[116] It displays different oligomerization states—monomer, dimer, and hexamer—which have been implicated in its exit/retention within the endoplasmic reticulum (ER), and is thought to bind correctly folded glycosylated cargo proteins, including factors V and VIII in the ER, recruiting the cargo for package into coat protein complex II (COPII)–coated vesicles and to transport them first to the ERGIC and then to the Golgi. MCFD2 is a small (146 residues) soluble protein of 16 kDa with a signal sequence mediating translocation into the ER and two EF-hand motifs that may bind $Ca^{2+}$ ions in the C-terminal region.[117] MCFD2 forms a $Ca^{2+}$-dependent 1:1 stoichiometric complex with LMAN1, which works as a cargo receptor for efficient ER–Golgi transfer of coagulation factors V and VIII during their secretion. Although several proteins have been identified as cargo of LMAN1 (factor V, factor VIII, cathepsin C, cathepsin Z, nicastrin, and $\alpha_1$-antitrypsin),[118–121] MCFD2 is only known to be required for transport of the blood coagulation factors, suggesting a possible role for MCFD2 as a specific recruitment factor for this subset of LMAN1 cargo proteins.[122] The three-dimensional structure of the complex between MCFD2 and the carbohydrate recognition domain (CRD) of LMAN1 was determined, and a model of functional coordination between the two proteins was proposed: MCFD2 is converted into the active form upon complex formation with LMAN1, thereby becoming able to capture polypeptide segments of factors V and VIII. The coagulation factors bind the LMAN1 oligomer in the ER but are released upon arrival in the acidic post-ER compartments because the sugar binding of ERGIC-53 is pH-dependent.[123]

## GENETICS

Homozygosity mapping and positional cloning in nine unrelated Jewish families demonstrated that *LMAN1*, composed of 13 exons, localizes on the long arm of chromosome 18.[110,111,124] Using a similar approach in other families with the combined factors V and VIII deficiency, the short *MCFD2*, made up of four exons, was localized on the short arm of chromosome 2.[26] Thirty-four mutations identified in *LMAN1*

predicted either a truncated protein product or no protein at all, being more than 90 percent deletion/insertion, null, or splicing mutations. In contrast, of the 22 mutations identified in the *MCFD2*, 11 are missense and 11 are null mutations. Missense mutations are located at the EF-2 domains, giving rise to defective binding to LMAN1.[125] A distinct founder haplotype was found in patients belonging to six unrelated families of Tunisian-Jewish origin bearing a donor splice-site mutation in intron 9 of *LMAN1*.[110,125] All six families originated from an ancient Jewish community that has resided on the island of Djerba for more than 2 millennia. A survey of this community, which presently lives in Israel, disclosed that the mutation is prevalent at an allele frequency of 0.0107.[126] Another founder effect for a G insertion in exon 1 of *LMAN1* was observed in eight unrelated Jewish families of Middle Eastern origin.[110,125] A Met to Thr mutation in *LMAN1* has been detected in several unrelated Italian families, implying another founder effect.[125]

## CLINICAL MANIFESTATIONS

Symptoms of combined factors V and VIII deficiency are generally mild. Comparison of relatively large cohorts of patients with such disorder in India, Iran, and Israel indicates that bleeding from trauma/surgery is the most frequently reported clinical manifestation.[114,115,127,128] This observation likely reflects the fact that often the combined factors V and VIII deficiency is brought to the attention of physicians following excessive bleeding during and after trauma, surgery, and labor. Homozygous patients exhibit spontaneous and posttraumatic bleeding. Menorrhagia, epistaxis, easy bruising, hemarthrosis, and gingival hemorrhage are commonly observed and are unrelated to trauma in approximately 20 percent of cases.[115,129] Hematuria, gastrointestinal tract bleeding, and spontaneous central nervous system bleeding are less common.[115] There are insufficient data on the incidence of bleeding during pregnancy and PPH in women with combined factor V and VIII deficiency.

Heterozygotes exhibit slight but significantly reduced mean levels of factors V and VIII.[114] In a literature survey of 161 heterozygotes, 22 reported having significant bleeding manifestations.[130] However, no correlation between the factor V or factor VIII levels and bleeding tendency was noted.[25]

*LMAN1* gene knockout mice duplicate the F5F8-deficient phenotype in humans, albeit with a milder presentation, resulting from a lesser reduction in plasma levels of factors V and VIII.[131] The partial perinatal lethality observed in LMAN1-deficient mice on some genetic backgrounds was unexpected and has been explained as the result of a further drop in the level of LMAN1-dependent protein(s) below a critical threshold or as a result of a strain-specific difference in another cargo receptor whose function overlaps with LMAN1.

## THERAPY

Because of the mild-to-moderate bleeding symptoms, treatment is on demand, depending on the severity of bleeding. According to a recent result from the EN-RBD project, however, the level of both factors to ensure the absence of bleeding symptoms should be greater than 40 percent.[25] The recommended therapy includes FFP, which provides factor V, and factor VIII concentrate, which compensates for the shorter half-life of plasma factor VIII. An antifibrinolytic agent such as tranexamic acid or ε-aminocaproic acid can be helpful in patients exhibiting menorrhagia, epistaxis, or gingival bleeding. DDAVP (1-deamino-8-D-arginine vasopressin, desmopressin) could be administered for less severe bleeding. Patients with severe bleeding episodes or patients undergoing surgical procedures, including dental extractions, should receive FFP as replacement for factor V and cryoprecipitate or factor VIII concentrate as a source of factor VIII. DDAVP can be used to increase factor VIII level, but this treatment sometimes fails.[132]

# ● FACTOR VII DEFICIENCY

## DEFINITION AND HISTORY

Factor VII was first identified as serum prothrombin conversion accelerator or proconvertin and its hereditary deficiency described by Alexander and colleagues in 1951.[133] Among the rare clotting factor deficiencies, the relative frequency of factor VII deficiency is high (see Table 14–1).[99,100] A presumptive diagnosis can be easily made because, except for very rare cases of factor X deficiency only affecting the TF pathway of coagulation (see "Laboratory Diagnosis"), factor VII deficiency is the only coagulation disorder that produces a prolonged PT and a normal aPTT.

## PROTEIN

Human factor VII is a single-chain glycoprotein (Mr ~50,000) that is secreted from the liver parenchymal cells as a zymogen. The mature protein consists of 406 amino acids organized in three main domains: a Gla domain at the N-terminus containing 10 Gla residues, an epidermal growth factor (EGF) domain in the center, and a serine protease domain at the C-terminus.[134] Factor VII zymogen circulates in blood at an extremely low concentration (~500 ng/mL)[135] and has the shortest half-life of all coagulation factors (4 to 6 hours; see Table 14–3). Factor VII is converted to the activated form, factor VIIa, by cleavage of an Arg152-Ile153 bond, resulting in a two-chain molecule held together by a disulfide bond. This conversion is mediated by factor Xa,[136] factor IXa,[137] factor XIIa,[138] thrombin,[136] and factor VIIa in the presence of TF, in an autoactivation reaction.[139] Binding of factor VII to TF strikingly enhances these reactions.[140-144]

The initial generation of thrombin that heralds blood coagulation occurs when blood is exposed to TF present in the subendothelium in tissues or on the surface of stimulated monocytes or microparticles. The exposed TF forms a complex with circulating factor VIIa and supports the initiation of coagulation by converting factors IX and X into their active forms (factor IXa and factor Xa).[145,146] Hence, the TF–factor VIIa complex has two roles: to increase the conversion of factor VII to factor VIIa and to increase the proteolytic activity of factor VIIa toward its substrates, factors IX and X. Factors IXa and Xa may remain associated with cells that display the TF or disseminate in the blood and bind to the surface of activated platelets, which form the initial platelet plug.[147]

## GENETICS

The factor VII gene (F7) spans approximately 12.8 kb[148] and is located on chromosome 13q34,[30,149] 2.8 kb upstream from the factor X gene (F10).[150] The gene contains a prepro leader sequence and eight exons that encode the mature protein.

More than 240 mutations have been reported (see http://www.isth.org/?MutationsRareBleedin and Ref. 12). The mutations are distributed throughout the gene, and most are missense mutations (62.2 percent); other type of mutations are equally present (ranging from approximately 6.2 percent of mutations in 3′-5′ untranslated region [UTR] to 12.3 percent of deletions/insertions [del/ins]). Most mutations causing factor VII deficiency have been observed in individual patients. However, one missense mutation (Ala244Val) was detected in 102 (84 percent) of 121 independent mutant alleles discerned in 88 unrelated patients in Israel.[151] Most subjects were of Iranian and Moroccan-Jewish origin and shared an identical haplotype, consistent with a founder effect. In the general Iranian-Jewish and Moroccan-Jewish populations, the prevalence values of the Ala244Val allele are 0.023 and 0.025, respectively.[152] Several additional clusters of patients with a specific mutation were reported: (1) Ala294Val, with or without a deletion of nt C, at position 11128,

prevails in patients from Poland and Germany but has also been identified in other Europeans[153,154]; (2) 12 unrelated families from Norway who carry Gln100Arg[155]; (3) IVS75G>A, which was detected in six unrelated patients from the Lazio region in Italy, all of whom bear the same haplotype, suggesting a founder effect[156]; and (4) Gly331Ser, which was identified in 10 Italian and four German patients on one haplotype.[157] The widely distributed and common Arg304Gln mutation probably is a recurrent mutation.[158]

Three polymorphisms in the factor VII gene are also associated with reduced plasma levels of the factor: (1) an Arg353Gln substitution, which results in impaired secretion of factor VII from cells[159] and gives rise to a 20 to 25 percent decrease in plasma factor VII level in heterozygotes and a 40 to 50 percent decrease in homozygotes[160,161]; (2) a decanucleotide insertion upstream from the 5′ end of the gene at −323, which confers a 33 percent decrease in the promoter activity[162]; and (3) a hypervariable region 4 polymorphism (HVR4) in intron 7.[163] The variable number of tandem repeats (five to eight copies of 37 bp) apparently influences the splicing efficiency. The effect of the variable repeats on factor VII level is less conspicuous than the decanucleotide insertion at the promoter region and the Arg353Gln polymorphism.

## CLINICAL FEATURES

Bleeding manifestations occur in homozygotes and in compound heterozygotes for factor VII deficiency. However, a typical feature of this disease is its clinical heterogeneity: some patients do not bleed at all after major hemostatic challenge, while others with similar levels report frequent bleeding episodes. Life- or limb-endangering bleeding manifestations are relatively rare, with the most frequent symptoms being epistaxis and menorrhagia. However, central nervous system bleeding was also reported to have high incidence (16 percent) in a series of 75 infants,[164] and the authors concluded that the greatest risk factor for this development was trauma related to the birth process. In addition, heterozygotes who have partial factor VII deficiency may present with bleeding; a recent survey of 499 heterozygotes revealed that 19 percent reported pathologic bleeding.[165] Dental extractions, tonsillectomy, and surgical procedures involving the urogenital tracts frequently are accompanied by bleeding when no prior therapy is instituted. Normal pregnancy is accompanied by increased concentrations of fibrinogen and factor VII; nonetheless, cases of miscarriages and PPH, albeit at relatively low rates, have been observed in patients with factor VII deficiency.[166,167]

Thrombotic episodes have also been reported in 3 to 4 percent of patients with factor VII deficiency, particularly in the presence of surgery and replacement treatment, but spontaneous thrombosis may also occur. A survey of 514 cases with severe or partial factor VII deficiency recorded seven patients with venous thrombosis and one patient with arterial thrombosis.[168] Most of the cases presented with associated risk factors, mainly surgery, prolonged immobilization, and treatment with PCCs.[169]

When factor VII is completely lacking, as in knockout mice, there is no embryonic lethality; however, fatal hemorrhage occurs perinatally.[170,171]

## THERAPY

As for all the other congenital bleeding disorders, replacement therapy is essential in patients who present with severe hemorrhage, such as hemarthrosis or intracerebral bleeding or surgical hemostasis, and for individuals with a bleeding history. Factor replacement therapy may also be used for prophylaxis in children with severe factor VII deficiency.[172] The EN-RBD study suggests a trough factor VII activity level of 25 percent is needed for patients to remain asymptomatic[25]; prophylactic treatment is usually recommended for patients with major bleeding episodes such as central nervous system and gastrointestinal tract bleeding and hemarthroses. A number of replacement therapeutic options have been administered to patients with factor VII deficiency, including FFP, PCCs, plasma-derived factor VII concentrates (volume overload should be expected if plasma is used as the replacement material), and rFVIIa. rFVIIa has been used in managing patients with hemarthroses and during surgery[173,174] (see Table 14–3). The main limitation of this drug is its short half-life; therefore, it requires at least two to three infusions per week in regular prophylaxis.[38] To improve rFVIIa half-life, longer-acting rFVIIa molecules were recently generated by fusion protein or conjugation technologies[175]: the rFVIIa molecule fused to albumin (rVIIa-FP) is the only molecule under clinical trial, to study its pharmacokinetics and safety, in patients with inherited coagulation FVII deficiency.[176] The pegylated rFVIIa derivative (N7-GP) and the FVIIa-CTP with a carboxyl terminal peptide addition have been studied in patients with hemophilia A or B with inhibitor.[177,178]

A significant rise in the factor VII level is observed during pregnancy in women with mild/moderate forms of factor VII deficiency (heterozygotes), but not in women with severe deficiency.[179–182] Therefore, in women with mild/moderate deficiency, replacement therapy may not be required during labor and delivery, while it would be required in women with low factor VII coagulant activity levels or a positive bleeding history who are more likely to be at risk of PPH.[181,183–185] A recent review of the literature noted that hemorrhage rates were equivalent in women with and without prophylaxis, thus concluding that use of hemostatic prophylaxis should not be considered mandatory, but as part of an individualized discussion taking into consideration response to previous hemostatic challenges and mode of delivery.[186] Replacement therapy is unnecessary for minor bleeding episodes. Local hemostasis for skin lacerations and administration of an antifibrinolytic agent for menorrhagia, epistaxis, and gingival hemorrhage usually are sufficient to arrest bleeding. Asymptomatic patients undergoing minimally invasive surgery, such as dental procedures, can be successfully treated with tranexamic acid given both orally or intravenously at the usual dosages.

# ●FACTOR X DEFICIENCY

## DEFINITION AND HISTORY

Inherited factor X deficiency was identified by two independent groups, each of which described a patient with a bleeding diathesis that could not be attributed to deficiencies in other known coagulation factors. The factor in both patients was subsequently named factor X.[187–189]

## PROTEIN

Factor X is mainly synthesized by the liver as a 488-amino-acid protein and circulates in plasma at a concentration of 8 to 10 mcg/mL.[190] Its primary structure is homologous to that of other vitamin K–dependent proteins, such as prothrombin, factor VII, factor IX, protein C, and protein S.[191] The first 40-amino-acid residues, the prepropeptide, contain the hydrophobic signal sequences targeting the protein for secretion.[192] The Gla domain forms the N-terminus of the mature protein and contains 11 Gla residues that are responsible for calcium and phospholipid binding.[193] Adjacent to the Gla domain is a short aromatic amino acid stack of predominantly hydrophobic amino acids, followed by the EGF domain, believed to mediate protein–protein interactions. The heavily glycosylated 52-amino-acid activation peptide of factor X separates the EGF domain from the C-terminal catalytic domain. Factor X undergoes proteolytic processing in the ER so that circulating factor is a two-chain, disulfide-linked protein consisting of a 17-kDa light chain made up of the Gla and EGF domains and a 40-kDa heavy chain made up of the

activation and catalytic domains.[194] The heavy chain contains the activation peptide (residues 143 to 195) and the catalytic serine protease domain, structurally homologous to that of other coagulation serine proteases containing the catalytic site formed by residues His236, Asp282, and Ser379. The 52-residue activation peptide is released after factor X is converted to its active form factor Xa by the cleavage between residues Arg194 and Ile195. Physiologically factor X is activated by TF/factor VIIa (extrinsic pathway) and factor IXa/factor VIIIa (intrinsic pathway),[195] but it can also be activated *in vitro* by Russel viper venom.[196] In turn, factor Xa catalyzes thrombin formation. In presence of factor Va, $Ca^{2+}$, and phospholipid membrane, factor Xa forms the prothrombinase complex that accelerates to 280,000-fold thrombin formation.[197]

## GENETICS

The *F10* gene spans approximately 25 kb and is made up of eight exons.[192] It shows significant homology with the genes of other vitamin K–dependent serine proteases, which suggests all of these multidomain genes evolved from a common ancestral gene.[198]

The currently described 105 mutations that cause factor X deficiency include large deletions, small frameshift deletions, and nonsense and missense mutations; the missense mutations group is the largest (80 percent), while mutations in the 3'- and 5'-UTRs are completely absent (see http://www.isth.org/?MutationsRareBleedin and Ref. 13). Activation through the TF pathway may be affected when the mutations are located, for example, in the Gla domain, as in Glu7Gly (St. Louis II) or Glu19Ala.[19,199,200] Activation through factor IXa is affected by, for example, Thr318Met (Roma).[201] Activation of factor X through Russell viper venom is almost intact in the Pro343Ser (Friuli) mutation.[202] Two interesting clusters of unrelated families were described in Algeria, with Phe31Ser mutation,[203] and in the border region between Turkey and Iran, with the Gly222Asp mutation.[204]

## CLINICAL MANIFESTATIONS

The clinical manifestations of factor X deficiency are related to the functional levels of the protein. According to the recent results of the EN-RBD study, strong associations between clinical bleeding severity and coagulation factor activity level were shown in factor X deficiency; consequently, patients with factor X activity levels less than 10 percent of normal have a higher occurrence of spontaneous major bleeding.[25] Bleeding occurs primarily into joints and soft tissues, from the umbilical cord and mucous membranes.[205] The bleeding tendency may appear at any age, although patients with factor X activity less than 2 percent present early in life with, for instance, umbilical-stump or central nervous system hemorrhage.[13,205,206]

In an analysis of 102 patients from Europe and Latin America, three mutations were associated with intracerebral hemorrhage (Gly380Arg, IVS7–1G>A, and Tyr163delAT), and Gly$^{-20}$Arg mutation was associated with severe hemarthrosis.[205] The most common bleeding symptom reported at all levels of severity of the deficiency is epistaxis. Patients with severe deficiencies commonly experience hemarthrosis and hematomas, but gastrointestinal and umbilical cord bleeding, hematuria, and central nervous system bleeding also occur. In a small group of patients with factor X deficiency, one-third of heterozygous patients who had dental extraction, surgery, or delivery without prophylactic replacement therapy showed postoperative bleeding that required treatment.[16] Menorrhagia is a common symptom affecting women with all degrees of severity, and PPH was also reported in four of 14 pregnancies.[207] Two successful pregnancies out of four were reported in a woman only when receiving regular prophylaxis; the other two pregnancies, without regular prophylaxis, resulted in preterm labor (both babies died in the neonatal period).[208] Other case reports, however, have described successful term pregnancies in women with severe factor X deficiency without antenatal prophylaxis.[207,209] Knockout mice show partial embryonic lethality (E11.5–E12.5); complete absence of factor X is incompatible with murine survival to adulthood, but minimal factor X activity (range: 1 to 3 percent) is sufficient to rescue the lethal phenotype.[210–212]

## THERAPY

Recently, a novel, high-purity, high-potency, specifically labelled, plasma-derived factor X concentrate has been developed and has received marketing authorization from the EMA and FDA for the treatment and prophylaxis of bleeding episodes and for perioperative management in patients with hereditary factor X deficiency.[213–215] However, where the specific therapy is not available, heated and solvent–detergent–treated PCCs containing factor X, in addition to factors II, VII, and IX, are administered. Use of these concentrates carries a low risk of transmission of bloodborne viruses. However, a risk of thrombosis, including venous thromboembolism, diffuse intravascular coagulation, and myocardial infarction, has been reported.

For soft tissue, mucous membrane, and joint hemorrhage, the aim of treatment should be maintaining a factor X level that is at least 10 to 20 percent of normal. For more serious hemorrhage, a factor X level that is greater than 40 percent of normal should be the goal.[25] In patients with particularly severe bleeding manifestations, prophylactic therapy should be considered. FFP can be used to treat patients with factor X deficiency; however, the administration of FFP can be associated with complications, particularly in children and elderly patients with cardiac disease, because of fluid overload.[38] The arrival on the market of a new freeze-dried human factor X concentrate has facilitated prophylaxis in patients with factor X deficiency (Factor X P Behring)[216]; however, factor X P Behring also contains factor IX, although in a known amount.

## ⬤ FACTOR XI DEFICIENCY

### DEFINITION AND HISTORY

Factor XI deficiency initially was described as a "new hemophilia" in two sisters and their maternal uncle by Rosenthal and colleagues in 1953.[217] Because it manifested in both sexes—two sisters and their maternal uncle—the clinical features were not consistent with hemophilia A or B, and it was called hemophilia C.[218] The deficiency was erroneously thought to be transmitted as an autosomal dominant disorder with variable expressivity. Later studies clearly established that, in most cases, the mode of transmission of factor XI deficiency is autosomal recessive.[215] Affected subjects have been described in most populations, but the disorder is common in Jews, particularly those of Ashkenazi origin.[219]

Factor XI deficiency as a result of a dysfunctional protein is rare, as only a few patients with deficiency of factor XI activity and seemingly normal antigen levels have been described thus far.[220–223]

### PROTEIN

Factor XI is a glycoprotein that consists of two identical 80-kDa polypeptide chains linked by a disulfide bond.[224] Each subunit contains 607 amino acids with a serine protease domain at the C-terminus and four tandem repeats of 90 or 91 amino acids, designated "apple domains," at the N-terminus. The described crystal structure of factor XI dimer[225] defined the interface of the monomers in apple 4 domains in which three residues—Leu284, Ile290, and Tyr329—are essential for noncovalent binding between the monomers. This binding enables the formation of a disulfide bond between Cys321 residues in the fourth apple domain of each monomer.[226,227]

Although factor XI is synthesized by the liver, very low levels of factor XI transcript can also be detected in megakaryocytes and platelets, renal tubules, and pancreatic islet cells.[228] Factor XI circulates in blood as an equimolar complex with high-molecular-weight kininogen (HK)[229] at a concentration of 3 to 7 mcg/mL, but the importance of the factor XI–HK interaction is not fully understood. Activation of factor XI involves cleavage of an Arg369-Ile370 bond, yielding a heavy chain containing the four apple domains linked by a disulfide bond to a light chain that contains the catalytic domain.[224] The physiologic activator of factor XI during hemostasis has long been debated. The original scheme of the coagulation cascade—according to which factor XI is activated by factor XIIa through the intrinsic pathway (the "contact phase")—was challenged by the observation that deficiencies of factor XII as well as of the other contact factors (HK and prekallikrein) are not associated with a bleeding diathesis.[14]

The major activator of factor XI in vivo is thrombin.[230,231] Factor XI binds through its apple 3 domain to lipid rafts on platelets containing glycoprotein Ib–IX–V complex. This glycoprotein complex also binds thrombin; thus, both substrate and enzyme are colocalized at the same site.[232] Factor XI activation also can occur on the fibrin surface after a clot forms.[233] Factor XIa, once generated, activates factor IX by limited proteolysis of two peptide bonds in the presence of calcium ions.[234] The presence of factor XI contributes to the activation of thrombin-activatable fibrinolysis inhibitor (TAFI) that, once activated, removes terminal lysine residues from fibrin, which impairs binding of certain forms of plasminogen to fibrin and disrupts tissue plasminogen activator–induced plasmin generation in the blood clot.[235] Large amounts of thrombin are necessary for TAFI activation, but the reaction is substantially augmented when thrombin is bound to thrombomodulin.[236] It follows that impaired generation of thrombin, for example, in inherited deficiency of factor VIII, IX, or XI, not only delays clot formation but also enhances premature lysis of clots.[237] These data fit well with clinical observations in factor XI–deficient patients who are particularly susceptible to bleeding following injury at sites exhibiting local fibrinolytic activity.[18]

### GENETICS

The 23-kb gene encoding for factor XI consists of 15 exons and 14 introns and is located on chromosome 4q34–35.[238,239]

Three mutations, designated types I, II, and III, were first described in six Ashkenazi-Jewish patients with severe factor XI deficiency.[240] The types II and III, a change in exon 5 at Glu117 leading to a stop codon and a change in exon 9 that results in a substitution of Phe283 by Leu, respectively, account for 95 percent of cases in Ashkenazi-Jewish patients.[240] A recent study indicated that both type II and type III mutations are also prevalent in the Italian population, although at a much lower rate.[241] In patients belonging to different ethnic groups, a significantly higher level of allelic heterogeneity has been reported. Remarkable exceptions are represented by some "closed populations" harboring mutations compatible with a founder effect: Cys38Arg in French Basques,[242] Gln88Stop in French families from Nantes,[222] Cys128Stop in Britons,[6] Ile436Lys in Northeastern Italy,[243] and Q263X in Korean patients.[244]

As of this writing, 220 mutations have been reported in non-Jewish and Jewish patients of various origins, including 154 missense, 23 nonsense, and 23 del/ins mutations, with the remaining being splice site (18 mutations) and 5'- and 3'-UTR (two mutations). Inheritance of factor XI deficiency is usually autosomal recessive, as in other RBDs, although some missense mutations exert a dominant negative effect through heterodimer formation between the mutant and wild-type polypeptides, resulting in a pattern of dominant transmission.[245]

## CLINICAL FEATURES

Factor XI deficiency is the only RBD in which the EN-RBD study showed no association between clinical bleeding severity and coagulation factor activity level.[25] This disorder manifests as a mild to moderate bleeding manifestations, and most bleeding episodes of patients with severe FXI deficiency are injury-related. Some patients with severe factor XI deficiency may not bleed at all following trauma.[246] The phenotype of bleeding is not correlated with the genotype but frequently with site of injury.[18,246,247] Surgical procedures involving tissues with high fibrinolytic activity (urinary tract, tonsils, nose, tooth sockets) frequently are associated with excessive bleeding in patients with severe factor XI deficiency, irrespective of the genotype.[248]

Most women with severe factor XI deficiency are asymptomatic or minimally so. During 93 deliveries (85 vaginal, eight cesarean), 43 of 62 women did not experience PPH despite no prophylactic treatment,[41] which was confirmed not to be mandatory for these women by a subsequent study of 33 women who had approximately 70 uneventful pregnancies out of 105 pregnancies. In the subsequent study, only three women had factor XI activity less than 15 IU/dL, and none of them had PPH.[42]

Whether heterozygotes exhibit a bleeding tendency (except for those bearing mutations causing a dominant negative effect) is controversial because there are reports on both heterozygotes with no bleeding complications following a variety of surgical procedures and reports that 20 to 48 percent of heterozygotes do bleed.[218,245,247,249,250]

In regard to venous thrombosis, it was reported that in five patients, two developed pulmonary embolism following infusion of factor XI concentrate,[251–253] and a third patient developed thrombus in the inferior vena cava following cryptococcal infection. In contrast, severe factor XI deficiency was shown to confer protection against ischemic stroke.[254]

Mice homozygous for a knockout factor XI allele show a tendency for slightly prolonged tail transection bleeding times and are protected from vessel-occluding fibrin formation after transient ischemic brain injury.[255,256]

## THERAPY

Available treatments for patients with the severe form of factor XI deficiency are FFP and factor XI concentrate. Factor XI concentrates currently available (Bio Products Laboratory, United Kingdom, and LFB Biomedicaments, France) are associated with thrombosis even after adding heparin to the antithrombin in the Bio Products Laboratory product and antithrombin and heparin to the C1 esterase in the LFB Biomedicaments product.[14,257] Therefore, it is advisable to monitor patients for clinical and laboratory signs of coagulation activation, in particular in elderly patients, in those with cardiovascular disease, and in those undergoing surgery with thrombotic potential, especially when factor XI concentrate[258] or rFVIIa is considered.[259,260] In addition, the presence of an inhibitor, particularly in patients with less than 1 percent of factor XI activity and previously exposed to plasma, factor XI concentrates, or immunoglobulins, should be evaluated. Low doses of rFVIIa along with tranexamic acid seem promising in the treatment of patients with inhibitors. When procedures are planned at tissues exhibiting fibrinolytic activity, which is associated with higher risk of bleeding in comparison to sites without fibrinolytic activity, the use of antifibrinolytic agents alone or in combination with other treatments is recommended. Patients undergoing dental extractions do not require replacement therapy. No plasma replacement therapy is necessary during or after labor unless excessive bleeding occurs. Patients with factor XI deficiency and inhibitor do not bleed spontaneously. Acquired inhibitors that neutralize the activity of factor XI have been described in patients with severe factor XI deficiency and baseline activity of less than 1 IU/dL after being exposed to plasma,[261]

after injections of Rh immunoglobulin and without previous exposure to blood products,[262] or after exposure to factor XI concentrates. Use of rFVIIa has been successful for major surgical procedures,[14] and an *in vitro* study revealed that abnormal thrombin generation in the plasma of patients with an inhibitor was corrected by adding moderate amounts of rFVIIa.[263]

## ● FACTOR XIII DEFICIENCY

### DEFINITION AND HISTORY

The first clinical report of factor XIII deficiency was in 1960[264]; since then, more than 500 cases of factor XIII deficiency have been identified worldwide, with an incidence of one individual in 1 to 3 million population.[22,265] Congenital factor XIII deficiency is characterized by severe delayed spontaneous bleeding and recurrent abortion with normal coagulation screening tests.

### PROTEIN

Factor XIII (fibrin-stabilizing factor) is a plasma transglutaminase that crosslinks $\gamma$-glutamyl–$\varepsilon$-lysine residues of fibrinogen chains, thereby stabilizing the fibrin clot. Plasma factor XIII is an Mr 340,000 heterotetramer composed of two catalytic A subunits and two carrier B subunits linked by noncovalent bonds. The average concentration of the $A_2B_2$ tetramer in plasma is approximately 22 mcg/mL, and its half-life is 9 to 14 days.[266] Intracellularly, factor XIII is found as a homodimer composed of two A subunits ($A_2$).[267,268] Factor XIII A subunit is mainly synthesized in macrophages and megakaryocytes.[267,268] Because factor XIII A subunit lacks a signal sequence, it cannot be released by the classic secretory pathway through the Golgi apparatus. Conceivably, factor XIII A subunit is released into the circulation from cells as a consequence of cell injury.[269] Structurally, each A monomeric subunit (Mr ~82,000) is composed of an activation peptide, which is removed by thrombin cleavage of an Arg37-Gly38 bond in the presence of calcium ions, and four distinct domains: $\beta$-sandwich, central core, barrel 1, and barrel 2 regions. The central core domain contains a catalytic triad (common to the transglutaminase family) formed through hydrogen bond interactions between Cys314, His373, and Asp396.[270–272] It is structurally homologous with the $\alpha$ chain of tissue transglutaminase,[273] the $\alpha$ chain of keratinocyte transglutaminase,[274] and band 4.2 of erythrocytes,[275] although the latter lacks transglutaminase activity.

The site of synthesis for factor XIII B subunit has been suggested to be the liver.[276] The B subunit (Mr 76,500) is composed of 10 tandem repeats of complement control protein (CCP) modules designated as Sushi domains, which are also observed in proteins of the complement system.[277,278] The two B subunits of factor XIII function as carrier proteins for the A subunits,[279,280] stabilizing them in the circulation and regulating the calcium-dependent activation of factor XIII.

On activation by thrombin and $Ca^{2+}$, the A and B subunits dissociate. Proteolytic activation by thrombin involves the cleavage of a N-terminal 37-residue activation peptide. The cleavage and the calcium binding both serve to induce structural changes that open up the catalytic triad to substrate access[281]; this process is accelerated by fibrin.[282–284] The clot-stabilizing effect of factor XIII is achieved by the crosslinking of fibrinogen chains, between the $\gamma$-carbonyl group of glutamine and the $\varepsilon$-amino group of lysine. In fibrin, this amide bond is located between A$\alpha$-chain sequences and between $\gamma$-chain sequences[285–289]; factor XIII A also crosslinks $\alpha_2$ antiplasmin to the $\alpha$-chain fibrin,[290] thereby increasing the resistance of fibrin to plasmin degradation, and crosslinks fibronectin to the $\alpha$-chain of fibrin,[291] affecting the mechanical properties of the clot and increasing cell adhesion.[292]

In addition to fibrinogen and $\alpha_2$-antiplasmin, factor XIII has many other substrates, including fibronectin, vitronectin, collagen, factor V, von Willebrand factor, $\alpha_2$-antiplasmin, actin, myosin, vinculin, thrombospondin, plasminogen-activating inhibitor (PAI), TAFI 2, and AT1 receptor dimers of monocytes, implicating multiple and different roles for factor XIII in various systems other than coagulation.[293]

## GENETICS

The gene for the factor XIII A subunit is located on chromosome 6p24-p25.[294,295] It spans more than 170 kb and is composed of 15 exons.[296] The B-subunit gene is located on chromosome 1q31-q32.1,[297,298] spans 28 kb, and is composed of 12 exons.[298]

One hundred twenty-one mutations causing factor XIII A-subunit deficiency have been reported as of this writing, of which only one maps to the promoter region, 57 are missense, 11 are nonsense, 17 are splice-site, and 35 are del/ins mutants (http://www.isth.org/?MutationsRareBleedin and Ref. 299). A homozygous four-base insertion in exon 14 (c.2116insAAGA) introducing a frameshift that after seven altered amino acids results in a stop codon and a protein with AQ3 truncated second $\beta$-barrel domain (p.Pro675TyrfsX7)[300] has been reported to cause an extremely rare type II variant. The mutant protein lost its activity, but the plasma factor XIII antigen level was at the lower limit of the reference interval. This finding suggests that the C-terminal part of $\beta$-barrel 2 is essential for the expression of factor XIII activity.

Splice-site mutation in intron 5 (IVS5–1 G>A) seems to be the most common mutation as it has already been reported in six unrelated families from six different European countries, whereas the Arg660Pro was found in Palestinian Arabs, consistently with founder effects.[265,301] It is likely that the Arg661stop mutation in Finnish patients and the Arg77Cys mutation in Swiss patients are also a result of founder effects, although both are at CpG dinucleotides and therefore can be considered recurrent mutations.[265,302,303] Another mutation, Ser295Arg, was identified in six Pakistani families and may also stem from a common founder, but this remains to be established.[304] Six nonsynonymous/coding polymorphisms in the factor XIIIA1 (*F13A1*) gene,[25] Val34Leu in exon 2, Tyr204Phe in exon 5, Pro(CCA)331(CCC)Pro in exon 8, Glu(GAA)567Glu(GAG) and Pro564Leu in exon 12, and Val650Ile and Glu651Gln in exon 14, have been analyzed in an association study. The study showed that only the Val34Leu is a true functional polymorphism and the rest are in linkage disequilibrium with it. In this study, only haplotypes containing the "34L" allele affected factor XIII function.[299,305] However, a larger number of synonymous/noncoding polymorphisms (>500) are known for the *F13A1* gene.[305] Only 16 different mutations have been reported so far for the *FXIIIB* gene.[299]

## CLINICAL MANIFESTATIONS

Factor XIII deficiency causes formation of blood clots that are unstable and susceptible to fibrinolytic degradation by plasmin. As a result, affected individuals have an increased tendency to bleed and rebleed. Delayed umbilical cord bleeding reported in 80 percent of patients with factor XIII deficiency can be considered as a diagnostic symptom of the deficiency. Central nervous system bleeding is reported in approximately 30 percent of cases,[306,307] making primary prophylaxis mandatory in patients affected with severe factor XIII deficiency. Ecchymoses; intramuscular and subcutaneous hematomas; oral cavity, mouth, and gingival bleeding; and prolonged bleeding following trauma are also characteristic symptoms.[306] Delayed wound healing occurs in approximately 15 percent of patients deficient in factor XIII. The exact mechanism by which factor XIII, or factor XIIIa, exerts its beneficial effect on wound healing is unknown. A proangiogenic effect of factor XIIIa was described, suggesting that decreased vascularization of wounds results in improper repair.[307]

In a review of the literature on 121 women with factor XIII deficiency, menorrhagia and ovulation bleeding were found to be common gynecologic problems, affecting 26 and 8 percent of women, respectively.[308] Of a total of 192 pregnancies, 127 (66 percent) resulted in a miscarriage and 65 (34 percent) reached viability stage; among the 136 pregnancies without prophylactic therapy, 124 (91 percent) resulted in a miscarriage and 12 (9 percent) progressed to viability stage. In affected women, formation of the cytotrophoblastic shell is impaired.[309] Conceivably, factor XIII A-subunit deficiency at the implantation site abrogates fibrin/fibronectin crosslinking, which is essential for attachment of the placenta to the uterus.[310]

Placental abruption, preterm delivery, and PPH could be also a problem if not adequately treated.[310]

No large clinical reports on heterozygous patients with factor XIII deficiency are available, thus not allowing one to draw evidence-based conclusions on the prevalence of clinical symptoms in this group of patients. Recently, a subset of 28 heterozygotes for factor XIII deficiency among 350 carriers of an autosomal recessive inherited coagulation disorder showed an association with prolonged or massive bleeding after minor trauma.[311] However, these data need to be confirmed in other cohorts of patients.

Factor XIII A-subunit knockout mice manifest no excess embryonic lethality or bleeding into the thoracic cavity, peritoneum, or skin, compatible with survival to adulthood. However, the survival rate of knockout males was markedly lower than that of the wild-types.[312] Female factor XIII knockout mice show intrauterine bleeding during pregnancy, similar to women with severe factor XIII A-subunit deficiency who experience the same problem, as well as recurrent abortions. Factor XIIIB knockout mice show a prolonged bleeding time at variance with patients with a complete factor XIII B-subunit deficiency, who report only mild bleeding symptoms and display normal bleeding times.[313,314]

## THERAPY

According to the EN-RBD results, blood levels of factor XIII that are 30 percent of normal are necessary to assure an asymptomatic state; the study also showed that patients with a coagulant activity under this level might bleed with a heterogeneous clinical presentation.[25] Therefore, a cutoff level of factor XIII coagulant activity that could discriminate patients with severe bleeding manifestations from those with minor or no bleeding could be helpful. A recent prospective data collection project (PRO-RBDD; www.rbdd.org) followed 57 patients with factor XIII deficiency and showed that a level of 15 percent of factor XIII clotting activity could indicate a good therapeutic target to maintain patients with no bleeding.[315] This goal may be reached via a number of options. Many case reports show improved bleeding symptoms in patients on prophylactic therapy.[316] Plasma replacement therapy is highly satisfactory because of the long half-life of factor XIII (9 to 12 days). Plasma-derived, virus-inactivated concentrates of factor XIII are available[317] and are the treatment of choice. The development of adverse events after treatment is rare. The most dreaded adverse event is the development of inhibitors, although its incidence is rare.[318] An RBD registry created in North America discovered that 3 percent of factor XIII–deficient patients who received FFP or factor XIII concentrate treatment developed inhibitors.[100] A new rFXIIIA$_2$ concentrate has become available. Its efficacy and safety have been shown in a multinational prophylaxis trial demonstrating that a single dose of 35 IU/kg of rFXIII A maintained plasma factor XIII levels above 10 percent in patients for ≥6 years with deficiency of factor XIII A subunit.[319] Pharmacokinetics results for younger patients were also recently reported.[320]

# ACQUIRED DEFICIENCIES

Acquired coagulation factor deficiencies may occur in patients with liver disease, amyloidosis (specifically factor X),[321,322] autoimmune disorders, patients on oral anticoagulant therapy, and, rarely, patients who develop nonneutralizing antibodies that remove the protein from the circulation. Such antibodies directed against prothrombin[323] and factor VII[324] have been described in patients with lupus anticoagulants. Rare instances of an acquired factor V inhibitor as a result of exposure to bovine thrombin preparations and drugs, or because of an unknown cause, should also be considered.[325] Acquired isolated factor X deficiency with severe bleeding manifestations occurs rarely because of the formation of specific antibodies with no underlying autoimmune disorder[326] or in association with upper respiratory tract infections, burns, and leprosy.[327–329] Inhibitors of factor X with no known precipitating factors have also been described.[330] Acquired factor XIII deficiency with significant reductions in factor XIII levels (down to as low as 20 percent of normal) as a result of decreased synthesis or increased consumption has been reported in several medical conditions, including pulmonary embolism, Crohn disease, ulcerative colitis, Henoch-Schönlein purpura, liver cirrhosis, and sepsis. There are several case reports of an autoimmune bleeding disorder, designated as autoimmune/acquired hemorrhaphilia, being caused by anti–factor XIII inhibitors.[331] The anti–factor XIII inhibitors tend to be more severe than regular hemorrhagic-acquired factor XIII deficiency and require both immunosuppressive therapy to eradicate autoantibodies and factor XIII replacement therapy to stop the bleeding.[332]

# REFERENCES

1. Tuddenham EGD, Cooper DN: *The Molecular Genetics of Haemostasis and Its Inherited Disorders.* Oxford University Press, New York, 1994.
2. Peyvandi F, Palla R, Menegatti M, Mannucci PM: Introduction. Rare bleeding disorders: General aspects of clinical features, diagnosis, and management. *Semin Thromb Hemost* 35:349, 2009.
3. Borhany M, Pahore Z, Ul Qadr Z, et al: Bleeding disorders in the tribe: Result of consanguineous in breeding. *Orphanet J Rare Dis* 5:23, 2010.
4. Jaouad IC, Elalaoui SC, Sbiti A, et al: Consanguineous marriages in Morocco and the consequence for the incidence of autosomal recessive disorders. *J Biosoc Sci* 41:575, 2009.
5. Saadat M, Ansari-Lari M, Farhud DD: Consanguineous marriage in Iran. *Ann Hum Biol* 31:263, 2004.
6. Peretz H, Mulai A, Usher S, et al: The two common mutations causing factor XI deficiency in Jews stem from distinct founders: One of ancient Middle Eastern origin and another of more recent European origin. *Blood* 90:2654, 1997.
7. Karimi M, Haghpanah S, Amirhakimi A, et al: Spectrum of inherited bleeding disorders in southern Iran, before and after the establishment of comprehensive coagulation laboratory. *Blood Coagul Fibrinolysis* 20:642, 2009.
8. Viswabandya A, Baidya S, Nair SC, et al: Correlating clinical manifestations with factor levels in rare bleeding disorders: A report from Southern India. *Haemophilia* 18:e195, 2012.
9. Lancellotti S, Basso M, De Cristofaro R: Congenital prothrombin deficiency: An update. *Semin Thromb Hemost* 39:596, 2013.
10. Thalji N, Camire RM: Parahemophilia: New insights into factor V deficiency. *Semin Thromb Hemost* 39:607, 2013.
11. Zheng C, Zhang B: Combined deficiency of coagulation factors V and VIII: An update. *Semin Thromb Hemost* 39:613, 2013.
12. Mariani G, Bernardi F: Factor VII deficiency. *Semin Thromb Hemost* 35:400, 2009.
13. Menegatti M, Peyvandi F: Factor X deficiency. *Semin Thromb Hemost* 35:407, 2009.
14. Duga S, Salomon O: Congenital factor XI deficiency: An update. *Semin Thromb Hemost* 39:621, 2013.
15. Schroeder V, Kohler HP: Factor XIII deficiency: An update. *Semin Thromb Hemost* 39:632, 2013.
16. Karimi M, Menegatti M, Afrasiabi A, et al: Phenotype and genotype report on homozygous and heterozygous patients with congenital factor X deficiency. *Haematologica* 93:934, 2008.
17. Seligsohn U, Modan M: Definition of the population at risk of bleeding due to factor XI deficiency in Ashkenazic Jews and the value of activated partial thromboplastin time in its detection. *Isr J Med Sci* 17:413, 1981.
18. Asakai R, Chung DW, Davie EW, Seligsohn U: Factor XI deficiency in Ashkenazi Jews in Israel. *N Engl J Med* 325:153, 1991.
19. Girolami A, Scarparo P, Scandellari R, Allemand E: Congenital factor X deficiencies with a defect only or predominantly in the extrinsic or in the intrinsic system: A critical evaluation. *Am J Hematol* 83:668, 2008.
20. Katona E, Penzes K, Molnar E, Muszbek L: Measurement of factor XIII activity in plasma. *Clin Chem Lab Med* 50:1191, 2012.
21. Kohler HP, Ichinose A, Seitz R, et al: Diagnosis and classification of factor XIII deficiencies. *J Thromb Haemost* 9:1404, 2011.
22. Muszbek L, Bagoly Z, Cairo A, Peyvandi F: Novel aspects of factor XIII deficiency. *Curr Opin Hematol* 18:366, 2011.
23. Katona E, Haramura G, Karpati L, et al: A simple, quick one-step ELISA assay for the determination of complex plasma factor XIII (A2B2). *Thromb Haemost* 83:268, 2000.
24. Peyvandi F, Di Michele D, Bolton-Maggs PHB, et al: Classification of rare bleeding disorders (RBDs) based on the association between coagulant factor activity and clinical bleeding severity. *J Thromb Haemost* 10:1938, 2012.
25. Peyvandi F, Palla R, Menegatti M, et al: Coagulation factor activity and clinical bleeding severity in rare bleeding disorders: Results from the European Network of Rare Bleeding Disorders. *J Thromb Haemost* 10:615, 2012.
26. Zhang B, Cunningham MA, Nichols WC, et al: Bleeding due to disruption of a cargo-specific ER-to-Golgi transport complex. *Nat Genet* 34:220, 2003.
27. Sadler JE. Medicine: K is for koagulation. *Nature* 427:493, 2004.
28. Pfeiffer RA, Ott R, Gilgenkrantz S, Alexandre P: Deficiency of coagulation factors VII and X with deletion of a chromosome 13 (q34). Evidence from two cases with 46,XY,t(13;Y) (q11;q34). *Hum Genet* 62:358, 1982.
29. Scambler PJ, Williamson R: The structural gene for human coagulation factor X is located on chromosome 13q34. *Cytogenet Cell Genet* 39:231, 1985.
30. Gilgenkrantz S, Briquel M-E, Andre E, et al: Structural genes of coagulation factors VII and X located on 13q34. *Ann Genet* 29:32, 1986.
31. Boxus G, Slacmeulder M, Ninane J: Combined hereditary deficiency in factors VII and X revealed by a prolonged partial thromboplastin time. *Arch Pediatr* 4:44, 1997.
32. Menegatti M, Karimi M, Garagiola I, et al: A rare inherited coagulation disorder: Combined homozygous factor VII and factor X deficiency. *Am J Hematol* 77:90, 2004.
33. Girolami A, Ruzzon E, Tezza F, et al: Congenital FX deficiency combined with other clotting defects or with other abnormalities: A critical evaluation of the literature. *Haemophilia* 14:323, 2008.
34. Girolami A, Ruzzon E, Tezza F, et al: Congenital combined defects of factor VII: A critical review. *Acta Haematol* 117:51, 2007.
35. Carr ME Jr: Future directions in hemostasis: Normalizing the lives of patients with hemophilia. *Thromb Res* 125(Suppl 1):S78, 2010.
36. Hunt BJ: Bleeding and coagulopathies in critical care. *N Engl J Med* 370:847, 2014.
37. Kadir RA, Davies J, Winikoff R, et al: Pregnancy complications and obstetric care in women with inherited bleeding disorders. *Haemophilia* 19(Suppl 4):1, 2013.
38. Mumford AD, Ackroyd S, Alikhan R, et al: BCSH Committee. Guideline for the diagnosis and management of the rare coagulation disorders: A United Kingdom Haemophilia Centre Doctors' Organization guideline on behalf of the British Committee for Standards in Haematology. *Br J Haematol* 167:304, 2014.
39. James AH: More than menorrhagia: A review of the obstetric and gynaecological manifestations of bleeding disorders. *Haemophilia* 11:295, 2005.
40. Kadir RA, Economides DL, Sabin CA, et al: Frequency of inherited bleeding disorders in women with menorrhagia. *Lancet* 351:485, 1998.
41. Salomon O, Steinberg DM, Tamarin I, et al: Plasma replacement therapy during labor is not mandatory for women with severe factor XI deficiency. *Blood Coagul Fibrinolysis* 16:37, 2005.
42. Myers B, Pavord S, Kean L, et al: Pregnancy outcome in factor XI deficiency: Incidence of miscarriage, antenatal and postnatal haemorrhage in 33 women with factor XI deficiency. *BJOG* 114:643, 2007.
43. Stirling Y, Woolf L, North WR, et al: Haemostasis in normal pregnancy. *Thromb Haemost* 52:176, 1984.
44. Sanchez-Luceros A, Meschengieser SS, Marchese C, et al: Factor VIII and von Willebrand factor changes during normal pregnancy and puerperium. *Blood Coagul Fibrinolysis* 14:647, 2003.
45. Wickstrom K, Edelstam G, Lowbeer CH, et al: Reference intervals for plasma levels of fibronectin, von Willebrand factor, free protein S and antithrombin during third-trimester pregnancy. *Scand J Clin Lab Invest* 64:31, 2004.
46. Bremme KA: Haemostatic changes in pregnancy. *Best Pract Res Clin Haematol* 16:153, 2003.
47. Hellgren M, Blomback M: Studies on blood coagulation and fibrinolysis in pregnancy, during delivery and in the puerperium. Normal condition. *Gynecol Obstet Invest* 12:141, 1981.
48. Lanchantin GF, Hart DW, Friedmann JA, et al: Amino acid composition of human plasma prothrombin. *J Biol Chem* 243:5479, 1968.
49. Degen SJ, MacGillivray RT, Davie EW: Characterization of the complementary deoxyribonucleic acid and gene coding for human prothrombin. *Biochemistry* 22:2087, 1983.
50. Kotkow KJ, Deitcher SR, Furie B, Furie BC: The second kringle domain of prothrombin promotes factor Va-mediated prothrombin activation by prothrombinase. *J Biol Chem* 270:4551, 1995.
51. Bode W, Mayr I, Baumann U, et al: The refined 1.9 A crystal structure of human α-thrombin interaction with D-Phe-Pro-Arg chloromethylketone and significance of the Tyr-Pro-Pro-Trp insertion segment. *EMBO J* 8:3467, 1989.
52. Esmon CT: Regulation of blood coagulation. *Biochim Biophys Acta* 1477:349, 2000.

53. Lee H, Hamilton JR: Physiology, pharmacology, and therapeutic potential of protease-activated receptors in vascular disease. *Pharmacol Ther* 134:246, 2012.

54. Coughlin SR: Protease-activated receptors in hemostasis, thrombosis and vascular biology. *J Thromb Haemost* 3:1800, 2005.

55. Lane DA, Phillipu H, Huntington JA: Directing thrombin. *Blood* 106:2605, 2005.

56. Royle NJ, Irwin DM, Koschnsky ML, et al: Human genes encoding prothrombin and ceruloplasmin map to 11p11-q12, and 3q21–24, respectively. *Somat Cell Mol Genet* 13:285, 1987.

57. Poort SR, Rosendaal FR, Reitsma PH, Bertina RM: A common genetic variation in the 3′-untranslated region of the prothrombin gene is associated with elevated plasma prothrombin levels and an increase in venous thrombosis. *Blood* 88:3698, 1996.

58. Catanzarite VA, Novotny WF, Cousins LM, Schneider JM: Pregnancies in a patient with congenital absence of prothrombin activity: Case report. *Am J Perinatol* 14:135, 1997.

59. Peyvandi F, Mannucci PM: Rare coagulation disorders. *Thromb Haemost* 82:1207, 1999.

60. Sun WY, Witte DP, Degen JL, et al: Prothrombin deficiency results in embryonic and neonatal lethality in mice. *Proc Natl Acad Sci U S A* 95:7597, 1998.

61. Xue J, Wu Q, Westfield LA, et al: Incomplete embryonic lethality and fatal neonatal hemorrhage caused by prothrombin deficiency in mice. *Proc Natl Acad Sci U S A* 95:7603, 1998.

62. Lechler E: Use of prothrombin complex concentrates for prophylaxis and treatment of bleeding episodes in patients with hereditary deficiency of prothrombin, factor VII, factor X, protein C, protein S, or protein Z. *Thromb Res* 95(Suppl 1):S39, 1999.

63. Mannucci PM: Outbreak of hepatitis A among Italian patients with haemophilia. *Lancet* 339:819, 1992.

64. Gerritzen A, Schneweis KE, Brackmann HH, et al: Acute hepatitis A in haemophiliacs. *Lancet* 340:1231, 1992.

65. Ragni MV, Koch WC, Jorda JA: Parvovirus B19, infection in patients with hemophilia. *Transfusion* 36:238, 1996.

66. Jorquera JI: Safety procedures of coagulation factors. *Haemophilia* 13(Suppl 5):41, 2007.

67. Owren PA: Parahemophilia: Hemorrhagic diathesis due to absence of a previously unknown factor. *Lancet* 1:446, 1947.

68. Chiu HC, Whitaker E, Colman RW: Heterogeneity of human factor V deficiency. Evidence for the existence of an antigen-positive variant. *J Clin Invest* 72:493, 1983.

69. Wilson DB, Salem HH, Mruk JS, et al: Biosynthesis of coagulation factor V by human hepatocellular carcinoma cell line. *J Clin Invest* 73:654, 1983.

70. Mazzorana M, Baffet G, Kneip B, et al: Expression of coagulation factor V gene by normal adult human hepatocytes in primary culture. *Br J Haematol* 78:229, 1991.

71. Tracy PB, Eide LL, Bowie EJW, Mann KG: Radioimmunoassay of factor V in human plasma and platelets. *Blood* 60:59, 1982.

72. Mann KG, Kalafatis M: Factor V: A combination of Dr Jekyll and Mr Hyde. *Blood* 101:20, 2003.

73. Camire RM, Bos MHA: The molecular basis of factor V and VIII procofactor activation. *J Thromb Haemost* 7:1951, 2009.

74. Suzuki K, Dahlback B, Stenflo J: Thrombin-catalyzed activation of human coagulation factor V. *J Biol Chem* 257:6556, 1982.

75. Foster WB, Nesheim ME, Mann KG: The factor Xa-catalyzed activation of factor V. *J Biol Chem* 258:13970, 1983.

76. Mann KG, Nesheim ME, Church WR, et al: Surface-dependent reactions of the vitamin K-dependent enzyme complexes. *Blood* 76:1, 1990.

77. Hayward CP, Furmaniak-Kazmierczak E, Cieutat AM, et al: Factor V is complexed with multimerin in resting platelet lysates and colocalizes with multimerin in platelet alpha-granules. *J Biol Chem* 270:19217, 1995.

78. Camire RM, Pollak ES, Kaushansky K, Tracy PB: Secretable human platelet-derived factor V originates from the plasma pool. *Blood* 92:3035, 1998.

79. Gould WR, Silveira JR, Tracy PB: Unique in vivo modifications of coagulation factor V produce a physically and functionally distinct platelet-derived cofactor: Characterization of purified platelet-derived factor V/Va. *J Biol Chem* 279:2383, 2004.

80. Suzuki K, Stenflo J, Dahlback B, et al: Inactivation of human coagulation factor V by activated protein C. *J Biol Chem* 258:1914, 1983.

81. Nesheim ME, Canfield WM, Kisiel W, et al: Studies of the capacity of factor Xa to protect factor Va from inactivation by activated protein C. *J Biol Chem* 257:1443, 1982.

82. Wang H, Riddell DC, Guinto ER, et al: Localization of the gene encoding human factor V to chromosome 1q21–25. *Genomics* 2:324, 1988.

83. Cripe LD, Moore KD, Kane WH: Structure of the gene for human coagulation factor V. *Biochemistry* 31:3777, 1992.

84. Castoldi E, Lunghi B, Mingozzi F, et al: A missense mutation (Y1702C) in the coagulation factor V gene is a frequent cause of factor V deficiency in the Italian population. *Haematologica* 86:629, 2001.

85. Steen M, Miteva M, Villoutreix BO, et al: Factor V New Brunswick: Ala221Val associated with FV deficiency reproduced in vitro and functionally characterized. *Blood* 102:1316, 2003.

86. Duga S, Montefusco MC, Asselta R, et al: Arg2074Cys missense mutation in the C2, domain of factor V causing moderately severe factor V deficiency: Molecular characterization by expression of the recombinant protein. *Blood* 101:173, 2003.

87. Montefusco MC, Duga S, Asselta R, et al: Clinical and molecular characterization of 6 patients affected by severe deficiency of coagulation factor V: Broadening of the mutational spectrum of factor V gene and in vitro analysis of the newly identified missense mutations. *Blood* 102:3210, 2003.

88. Van Wijk R, Nieuwenhuis K, van den Berg M, et al: Five novel mutations in the gene for human blood coagulation factor V associated with type I factor V deficiency. *Blood* 98:358, 2001.

89. Van Wijk R, Montefusco MC, Duga S, et al: Coexistence of a novel homozygous nonsense mutation in exon 13, of the factor V gene with the homozygous Leiden mutation in two unrelated patients with severe factor V deficiency. *Br J Haematol* 114:871, 2001.

90. Guasch JF, Cannegieter S, Reitsma PH, et al: Severe coagulation factor V deficiency caused by a 4 bp deletion in the factor V gene. *Br J Haematol* 101:32, 1998.

91. Dahlbäck B, Villoutreix BO: Molecular recognition in the protein C anticoagulant pathway. *J Thromb Haemost* 1:1525, 2003.

92. Simioni P, Scudeller A, Radossi P, et al: "Pseudo homozygous" activated protein C resistance due to double heterozygous factor V defects (factor V Leiden mutation and type I quantitative factor V defect) associated with thrombosis: Report of two cases belonging to two unrelated kindreds. *Thromb Haemost* 75:422, 1996.

93. Lunghi B, Iacoviello L, Gemmati D, et al: Detection of new polymorphic markers in the factor V gene: Association with factor V levels in plasma. *Thromb Haemost* 75:45, 1996.

94. Yamazaki T, Nicolaes GA, Sorensen KW, et al: Molecular basis of quantitative factor V deficiency associated with factor V R2 haplotype. *Blood* 100:2515, 2002.

95. Castaman G, Lunghi B, Missiaglia E, et al: Phenotypic homozygous activated protein C resistance associated with compound heterozygosity for Arg506Gln (factor V Leiden) and His1299Arg substitutions in factor V. *Br J Haematol* 99:257, 1997.

96. Vos HL: Inherited defects of coagulation factor V: The thrombotic side. *J Thromb Haemost* 4:35, 2006.

97. Blavignac J, Bunimov N, Rivard GE, Hayward CP: Quebec platelet disorder: Update on pathogenesis, diagnosis, and treatment. *Semin Thromb Haemost* 37:713, 2011.

98. Weiss HJ, Lages B, Zheng S, Hayward CP: Platelet factor V New York: A defect in factor V distinct from that in factor V Quebec resulting in impaired prothrombinase generation. *Am J Hematol* 66:130, 2001.

99. Acharya SS, Coughlin A, Dimichele DM: Rare Bleeding Disorder Registry: Deficiencies of factors II V, VII X, XIII, fibrinogen and dysfibrinogenemias. *J Thromb Haemost* 2:248, 2004.

100. Peyvandi F, Duga S, Akhavan S, Mannucci PM: Rare coagulation deficiencies. *Haemophilia* 8:308, 2002.

101. Asselta R, Tenchini ML, Duga S: Inherited defects of coagulation factor V: The hemorrhagic side. *J Thromb Haemost* 4:26, 2006.

102. Girolami A, Scandellari R, Lombardi AM, et al: Pregnancy and oral contraceptives in factor V deficiency: A study of 22, patients (five homozygotes and 17 heterozygotes) and review of the literature. *Haemophilia* 11:26, 2005.

103. Noia G, De Carolis S, De Stefano V, et al: Factor V deficiency in pregnancy complicated by Rh immunization and placenta previa. A case report and review of the literature. *Acta Obstet Gynecol Scand* 76:890, 1997.

104. Girolami A, Ruzzon E, Tezza F: Arterial and venous thrombosis in rare congenital bleeding disorders: A critical review. *Haemophilia* 12:345, 2006.

105. Cui J, O'Shea KS, Purkayastha A, et al: Fatal haemorrhage and incomplete block to embryogenesis in mice lacking coagulation factor V. *Nature* 384:66, 1996.

106. Yang TL, Cui J, Taylor JM, et al: Rescue of fatal neonatal hemorrhage in factor V deficient mice by low transgene expression. *Thromb Haemost* 83:70, 2000.

107. Fratantoni JC, Hilgartner M, Nachman RL: Nature of the defect in congenital factor V deficiency: Study in a patient with an acquired circulating anticoagulant. *Blood* 39:751, 1972.

108. Mazzucconi MG, Solinas S, Chistolini A, et al: Inhibitor to factor V in severe factor V congenital deficiency: A case report. *Nouv Rev Fr Hematol* 27:303, 1985.

109. Oeri J, Matter M, Isenschmid H, et al: Congenital factor V deficiency (parahemophilia) with true hemophilia in two brothers. *Bibl Paediatr* 58:575, 1954.

110. Nichols WC, Seligsohn U, Zivelin A, et al: Linkage of combined factors V and VIII deficiency to chromosome 18q by homozygosity mapping. *J Clin Invest* 99:596, 1997.

111. Nichols WC, Seligsohn U, Zivelin A, et al: Mutations in the ER–Golgi intermediate compartment protein ERGIC-53 cause combined deficiency of coagulation factors V and VIII. *Cell* 93:61, 1998.

112. Zhang B, Kaufman RJ, Ginsburg D: LMAN1 and MCFD2 form a cargo receptor complex and interact with coagulation factor VIII in the early secretory pathway. *J Biol Chem* 280:25881, 2005.

113. Zhang B, McGee B, Yamaoka JS, et al: Combined deficiency of factor V and factor VIII is due to mutations in either LMAN1 or MCFD2. *Blood* 107:903, 2006.

114. Seligsohn U, Zivelin A, Zwang E: Combined factor V and factor VIII deficiency among non-Ashkenazi Jews. *N Engl J Med* 307:1191, 1982.

115. Peyvandi F, Tuddenham EG, Akhtari AM, et al: Bleeding symptoms in 27 Iranian patients with the combined deficiency of factor V and factor VIII. *Br J Haematol* 100:773, 1998.

116. Itin C, Roche AC, Monsigny M, et al: ERGIC-53 is a functional mannose-selective and calcium-dependent human homologue of leguminous lectins. *J Cell Biol* 107:483, 1996.

117. Guy JE, Wigren E, Svärd M, et al: New insights into multiple coagulation factor deficiency from the solution structure of human MCFD2. *J Mol Biol* 381:941, 2008.

118. Appenzeller C, Andersson H, Kappeler F, et al: The lectin ERGIC-53 is a cargo transport receptor for glycoproteins. *Nat Cell Biol* 1:330, 1999.

119. Vollenweider F, Kappeler F, Itin C, et al: Mistargeting of the lectin ERGIC-53 to the endoplasmic reticulum of HeLa cells impairs the secretion of a lysosomal enzyme. *J Cell Biol* 142:377, 1998.

120. Nyfeler B, Reiterer V, Wendeler MW, et al: Identification of ERGIC-53 as an intracellular transport receptor of alpha1-antitrypsin. *J Cell Biol* 180:705, 2008.

121. Morais VA, Brito C, Pijak DS, et al: N-glycosylation of human nicastrin is required for interaction with the lectins from the secretory pathway calnexin and ERGIC-53. *Biochim Biophys Acta* 1762:802, 2006.

122. Nyfeler B, Zhang B, Ginsburg D, et al: Cargo selectivity of the ERGIC-53/MCFD2 transport receptor complex. *Traffic* 7:1473, 2006.

123. Nishio M, Kamiya Y, Mizushima T, et al: Structural basis for the cooperative interplay between the two causative gene products of combined factor V and factor VIII deficiency. *Proc Natl Acad Sci U S A* 107:4034, 2010.

124. Neerman-Arbez M, Antonarakis SE, Blouin JL, et al: The locus for combined factor V-factor VIII deficiency (F5F8D) maps to 18q21, between D18S849, and D18S1103. *Am J Hum Genet* 61:143, 1997.

125. Zhang B, Spreafico M, Zheng C, et al: Genotype-phenotype correlation in combined deficiency of factor V and factor VIII. *Blood* 111:5592, 2008.

126. Segal A, Zivelin A, Rosenberg N, et al: A mutation in LMAN 1, (ERGIC-53) causing combined factor V and factor VIII deficiency is prevalent in Jews originating from the island of Djerba in Tunisia. *Blood Coagul Fibrinolysis* 15:99, 2004.

127. Viswabandya A, Baidya S, Nair SC, et al: Clinical manifestations of combined factor V and VIII deficiency: A series of 37 cases from a single center in India. *Am J Hematol* 85:538, 2010.

128. Mansouritorgabeh H, Rezaieyazdi Z, Pourfathollah AA, et al: Haemorrhagic symptoms in patients with combined factors V and VIII deficiency in north-eastern Iran. *Haemophilia* 10:271, 2004.

129. Seligsohn U: Combined factor V and factor VIII deficiency, in *Factor VIII: Von Willebrand Factor*, vol 2, edited by Seghatchian J, Savidge GT, p 89. CRC Press, Boca Raton, FL, 1989.

130. Fischer RR, Giddings JC, Roisenberg I: Hereditary combined deficiency of clotting factors V and VIII with involvement of von Willebrand factor. *Clin Lab Haematol* 10:53, 1988.

131. Zhang B, Zheng C, Zhu M, et al: Mice deficient in LMAN1 exhibit FV and FVIII deficiencies and liver accumulation of $\alpha_1$-antitrypsin. *Blood* 118:3384, 2011.

132. Sallah AS, Angchaisuksiri P, Roberts HR: Use of plasma exchange in hereditary deficiency of factor V and factor VIII. *Am J Hematol* 52:229, 1996.

133. Alexander B, Goldstein R, Landwehr G, Cook CD: Congenital SPCA deficiency: A hitherto unrecognized coagulation defect with hemorrhage rectified by serum and serum fractions. *J Clin Invest* 30:596, 1951.

134. Hagen FS, Gray CL, O'Hara P, et al: Characterization of a cDNA coding for human factor VII. *Proc Natl Acad Sci U S A* 83:2412, 1986.

135. Fair DS: Quantitation of factor VII in the plasma of normal and warfarin-treated individuals by radioimmunoassay. *Blood* 62:784, 1983.

136. Radcliffe R, Nemerson Y: Activation and control of factor VII by activated factor X and thrombin: Isolation and characterization of a single chain form of factor VII. *J Biol Chem* 250:388, 1975.

137. Seligsohn U, Osterud B, Brown SF, et al: Activation of human factor VII in plasma and in purified systems: Roles of activated factor IX, kallikrein, and activated factor XII. *J Clin Invest* 64:1056, 1979.

138. Radcliffe R, Bagdasarian A, Colman R, Nemerson Y: Activation of bovine factor VII by Hageman factor fragments. *Blood* 50:611, 1977.

139. Nakagaki T, Foster DC, Berkner KL, Kisiel W: Initiation of the extrinsic pathway of blood coagulation: Evidence for the tissue factor dependent autoactivation of human coagulation factor VII. *Biochemistry* 30:10819, 1991.

140. Rapaport SI, Rao LV: The tissue factor pathway: How it has become a "prima ballerina." *Thromb Haemost* 74:7, 1995.

141. Banner DW, D'Arcy A, Chene C, et al: The crystal structure of the complex of blood coagulation factor VIIa with soluble tissue factor. *Nature* 380:41, 1996.

142. Cooper DN, Millar DS, Wacey A, et al: Inherited factor VII deficiency: Molecular genetics and pathophysiology. *Thromb Haemost* 78:151, 1997.

143. Edgington TS, Dickinson CD, Ruf W: The structural basis of function of the TF-VIIa complex in the cellular initiation of coagulation. *Thromb Haemost* 78:401, 1997.

144. Morrissey JH, Neuenschwander PF, Huang Q, et al: Factor VIIa–tissue factor: Functional importance of protein-membrane interactions. *Thromb Haemost* 78:112, 1997.

145. Kirchhofer D, Nemerson Y: Initiation of blood coagulation: The tissue factor/factor VIIa complex. *Curr Opin Biotechnol* 7:386, 1996.

146. Mann KG, van't Veer C, Cawthern K, et al: The role of the tissue factor pathway in initiation of coagulation. *Blood Coagul Fibrinolysis* 9:S3, 1998.

147. Hoffman M, Monroe DM, Roberts HR: Cellular interactions in hemostasis. *Haemostasis* 1:12, 1996.

148. O'Hara PJ, Grant FJ, Haldeman BA, et al: Nucleotide sequence of the gene coding for human factor VII, a vitamin K-dependent protein participating in blood coagulation. *Proc Natl Acad Sci U S A* 84:5158, 1987.

149. Ott R, Pfeiffer RA: Evidence that activities of coagulation factors VII and X are linked to chromosome 13, (q34). *Hum Hered* 34:123, 1984.

150. Miao CH, Leytus SP, Chung DW, Davie EW: Liver-specific expression of the gene coding for human factor X, a blood coagulation factor. *J Biol Chem* 267:7395, 1992

151. Fromovich-Amit Y, Zivelin A, Rosenberg N, et al: Characterization of mutations causing factor VII deficiency in 61, unrelated Israeli patients. *J Thromb Haemost* 2:1774, 2004.

152. Tamary H, Fromovich Y, Shalmon L, et al: Ala244Val is a common, probably ancient mutation causing factor VII deficiency in Moroccan and Iranian Jews. *Thromb Haemost* 76:283, 1996.

153. Wulff K, Herrmann FH: Twenty-two novel mutations of the factor VII gene in factor VII deficiency. *Hum Mutat* 15:489, 2000.

154. Giansily-Blaizot M, Aguilar-Martinez P, Biron-Andreani C, et al: Analysis of the genotypes and phenotypes of 37, unrelated patients with inherited factor VII deficiency. *Eur J Hum Genet* 9:105, 2001.

155. Chaing S, Clarke B, Sridhara S, et al: Severe factor VII deficiency caused by mutations abolishing the cleavage site for activation and altering binding to tissue factor. *Blood* 83:3524, 1994.

156. Bernardi F, Patracchini P, Gemmati D, et al: Molecular analysis of factor VII deficiency in Italy: A frequent mutation (FVII Lazio) in a repeated intronic region. *Hum Genet* 92:446, 1993.

157. Etro D, Pinotti M, Wulff K, et al: The Gly331Ser mutation in factor VII in Europe and the Middle East. *Haematologica* 88:1434, 2003.

158. Bernardi F, Liney DL, Patracchini P, et al: Molecular defects in CRM+ factor VII deficiencies: Modeling of missense mutations in the catalytic domain of FVII. *Br J Haematol* 86:610, 1994.

159. Hunault M, Arbini AA, Lopaciuk S, et al: The Arg353, Gln polymorphism reduces the level of coagulation factor VII: In vivo and in vitro studies. *Arterioscler Thromb Vasc Biol* 17:2825, 1997.

160. Green F, Kelleher C, Wilkes H, et al: A common genetic polymorphism associated with lower coagulation factor VII levels in healthy individuals. *Arterioscler Thromb* 11:540, 1991.

161. Bernardi F, Marchetti G, Pinotti M, et al: Factor VII gene polymorphisms contribute about one-third of the factor VII level variation in plasma. *Arterioscler Thromb Vasc Biol* 16:72, 1996.

162. Pollak ES, Hung HL, Godin W, et al: Functional characterization of the human factor VII 5'-flanking region. *J Biol Chem* 271:1738, 1996.

163. Marchetti G, Gemmati D, Patracchini P, et al: PCR detection of a repeat polymorphism within the F7, gene. *Nucleic Acids Res* 19:4570, 1991.

164. Ragni MV, Lewis JH, Spero JA, Hasiba U: Factor VII deficiency. *Am J Hematol* 10:79–88, 1981.

165. Herrmann FH, Wulff K, Auerswald G, et al: Factor VII deficiency: Clinical manifestation of 717, subjects from Europe and Latin America with mutations in the factor 7, gene. *Haemophilia* 15:267, 2008.

166. Kulkarni AA, Lee CA, Kadir RA: Pregnancy in women with congenital factor VII deficiency. *Haemophilia* 12:413, 2006.

167. Rizk DE, Castella A, Shaheen H, Deb P: Factor VII deficiency detected in pregnancy: A case report. *Am J Perinatol* 16:223, 1999.

168. Mariani G, Herrmann FH, Schulman S, et al: Thrombosis in inherited factor VII deficiency. *J Thromb Haemost* 1:2153, 2003.

169. Girolami A, Berti de Marinis G, Vettore S, Girolami B: Congenital FVII deficiency and pulmonary embolism: A critical appraisal of all reported cases. *Clin Appl Thromb Hemost* 19:55, 2013.

170. Rosen ED, Chan JC, Idusogie E, et al: Mice lacking factor VII develop normally but suffer fatal perinatal bleeding. *Nature* 390:290, 1997.

171. Chan JC, Carmeliet P, Moons L, et al: Factor VII deficiency rescues the intrauterine lethality in mice associated with a tissue factor pathway inhibitor deficit. *J Clin Invest* 103:475, 1999.

172. Napolitano M, Giansily-Blaizot M, Dolce A, et al: Prophylaxis in congenital factor VII deficiency: Indications, efficacy and safety. Results from the Seven Treatment Evaluation Registry (STER). *Haematologica* 98:538, 2013.

173. Mariani G, Konkle BA, Ingerslev J: Congenital factor VII deficiency: Therapy with recombinant activated factor VII—A critical appraisal. *Haemophilia* 12:19, 2006.

174. Tcheng WY, Donkin J, Konzal S, Wong WY: Recombinant factor VIIa in a patient with severe congenital factor VII deficiency. *Haemophilia* 10:295, 2004.

175. Carr ME, Tortella BJ: Emerging and future therapies for hemophilia. *J Blood Med* 6:245, 2015.

176. Zollner S, Schuermann D, Raquet E, et al: Pharmacological characteristics of a novel, recombinant fusion protein linking coagulation factor VIIa with albumin (rVIIa-FP). *J Thromb Haemost* 12:220, 2014.

177. Moss J, Rosholm A, Lauren A: Safety and pharmacokinetics of a glycoPEGylated recombinant activated factor VII derivative: A randomized first human dose trial in healthy subjects. *J Thromb Haemost* 9:1368, 2011.

178. Binder L, Bar-Ilan A, Hoffman M, Hart G: Mod-5014, a long-acting FVIIa-CTP, proposing a novel prophylactic treatment supporting less frequent subcutaneous or intravenous injections with a similar mechanism of action to rFVIIa: Proof-of-concept in hemophilic animal models. *Blood* 126:4670, 2015 (abstract).

179. Robertson LE, Wasserstrum N, Banez E, et al: Hereditary factor VII deficiency in pregnancy: Peripartum treatment with factor VII concentrate. *Am J Hematol* 40:38, 1992.

180. Aynaoğlu G, Durdağ GD, Ozmen B, Söylemez F: Successful treatment of hereditary factor VII deficiency presented for the first time with epistaxis in pregnancy: A case report. *J Matern Fetal Neonatal Med* 23:1053, 2010.

181. Braun MW, Triplett DA: Case report: Factor VII deficiency in an obstetrical patient. *J Indiana State Med Assoc* 72:900, 1979.

182. Fadel HE, Krauss JS: Factor VII deficiency and pregnancy. *Obstet Gynecol* 73:453, 1989.

183. Eskandari N, Feldman N, Greenspoon JS: Factor VII deficiency in pregnancy treated with recombinant factor VIIa. *Obstet Gynecol* 99:935, 2002.

184. Jimenez-Yuste V, Villar A, Morado M, et al: Continuous infusion of recombinant activated factor VII during caesarean section delivery in a patient with congenital factor VII deficiency. *Haemophilia* 6:588, 2000.

185. Pike GN, Bolton-Maggs PH: Factor deficiencies in pregnancy. *Hematol Oncol Clin North Am* 25:359, 2011.

186. Baumann Kreuziger LM, Morton CT, Reding MT: Is prophylaxis required for delivery in women with factor VII deficiency? *Haemophilia* 19:827, 2013.

187. Duckert F, Fluckinger P, Matter M, Koller F: Clotting factor X. Physiologic and physico-chemical properties. *Proc Soc Exp Biol Med* 90:17, 1955.

188. Telfer TP, Denson KW, Wright DR: A "new" coagulation defect. *Br J Haematol* 2:308, 1956.

189. Hougie C, Barrow EM, Graham JB: Stuart clotting defect. I. Segregation of an hereditary hemorrhagic state from the heterogeneous group heretofore called "stable factor" (SPCA, proconvertin, factor VII) deficiency. *J Clin Invest* 36:485, 1957.

190. Bajaj SP, Mann KG: Simultaneous purification of bovine prothrombin and factor X. Activation of prothrombin by trypsin-activated factor X. *J Biol Chem* 248:7729, 1973.

191. Ichinose A, Takeya H, Espling E, et al: Amino acid sequence of human protein Z, a vitamin K-dependent plasma glycoprotein. *Biochem Biophys Res Commun* 172:1139, 1990.

192. Leytus SP, Foster DC, Kurachi K, Davie EW: Gene for human factor X: A blood coagulation factor whose gene organization is essentially identical with that of factor IX and protein C. *Biochemistry* 25:5098, 1986.

193. McMullen BA, Fujikawa K, Kisiel W, et al: Complete amino acid sequence of the light chain of human blood coagulation factor X: Evidence for identification of residue 63, as beta-hydroxyaspartic acid. *Biochemistry* 22:2875, 1983.

194. Jackson CM: Characterization of two glycoprotein variants of bovine factor X and demonstration that the factor X zymogen contains two polypeptide chains. *Biochemistry* 11:4873, 1972.

195. Fujikawa K, Coan MH, Legaz ME, Davie EW: The mechanism of activation of bovine factor X (Stuart factor) by intrinsic and extrinsic pathways. *Biochemistry* 13:5290, 1974.

196. Kisiel W, Hermodson MA, Davie EW: Factor X activating enzyme from Russell's viper venom: Isolation and characterization. *Biochemistry* 15:4901, 1976.

197. Furie B, Furie BC: The molecular basis of blood coagulation. *Cell* 53:505, 1988.

198. Neurath H: Evolution of proteolytic enzymes. *Science* 224:350, 1984.

199. Rudolph AE, Mullane MP, Porche-Sorbet R, et al: Factor X St. Louis II. Identification of a glycine substitution at residue 7, and characterization of the recombinant protein. *J Biol Chem* 271:28601, 1996.

200. Pinotti M, Marchetti G, Baroni M, et al: Reduced activation of the Gla19Ala FX variant via the extrinsic coagulation pathway results in symptomatic CRMred FX deficiency. *Thromb Haemost* 88:236, 2002.

201. De Stefano V, Leone G, Ferrelli R, et al: Factor X Roma: A congenital factor X variant defective at different degrees in the intrinsic and the extrinsic activation. *Br J Haematol* 69:387, 1988.

202. James HL, Girolami A, Fair DS: Molecular defect in coagulation factor X Friuli results from a substitution of serine for proline at position 343. *Blood* 77:317, 1991.

203. Akhavan S, Chafa O, Obame FN, et al: Recurrence of a Phe31Ser mutation in the Gla domain of blood coagulation factor X, in unrelated Algerian families: A founder effect? *Eur J Haematol* 78:405, 2007.

204. Epcacan S, Menegatti M, Akbayram S, Cairo A, Peyvandi F, Oner AF: Frequency of the p.Gly262Asp mutation in congenital factor X deficiency. *Eur J Clin Invest* 45:1087, 2015.

205. Herrmann FH, Auerswald G, Ruiz-Saez A, et al: Factor X deficiency: Clinical manifestation of 102 subjects from Europe and Latin America with mutations in the factor 10 gene. *Haemophilia* 12:479, 2006.

206. Peyvandi F, Mannucci PM, Lak M, et al: Congenital Factor X deficiency: Spectrum of bleeding symptoms in 32 Iranian patients. *Br J Haematol* 102:626, 1998.

207. Romagnolo C, Burati S, Ciaffoni S, et al: Severe factor X deficiency in pregnancy: Case report and review of the literature. *Haemophilia* 10:665, 2004.

208. Kumar M, Mehta P: Congenital coagulopathies and pregnancy: Report of four pregnancies in a factor X-deficient woman. *Am J Hematol* 46:241, 1994.

209. Larrain C: Congenital blood coagulation factor X deficiency. Successful result of the use prothrombin concentrated complex in the control of caesarean section hemorrhage in 2 pregnancies. *Rev Med Chil* 122:1178, 1994.

210. Dewerchin M, Liang Z, Moons L, et al: Blood coagulation factor X deficiency causes partial embryonic lethality and fatal neonatal bleeding in mice. *Thromb Haemost* 83:185, 2000.

211. Rosen ED, Cornelissen I, Liang Z, et al: In utero transplantation of wild-type fetal liver cells rescues factor X-deficient mice from fatal neonatal bleeding diatheses. *J Thromb Haemost* 1:19, 2003.

212. Tai SJ, Herzog RW, Margaritis P, et al: A viable mouse model of factor X deficiency provides evidence for maternal transfer of factor X. *J Thromb Haemost* 6:339, 2008.

213. Escobar MA, Auerswald G, Austin S, Huang JN, Norton M, Millar CM: Experience of a new high-purity factor X concentrate in subjects with hereditary factor X deficiency undergoing surgery. *Haemophilia* 22:713, 2016.

214. Austin SK, Kavakli K, Norton M, Peyvandi F, Shapiro A; FX Investigators Group: Efficacy, safety and pharmacokinetics of a new high-purity factor X concentrate in subjects with hereditary factor X deficiency. *Haemophilia* 22:419, 2016.

215. Austin SK, Brindley C, Kavakli K, Norton M, Shapiro A; FX Investigators Group: Pharmacokinetics of a high-purity plasma-derived factor X concentrate in subjects with moderate or severe hereditary factor X deficiency. *Haemophilia* 22:426, 2016.

216. Karimi M, Vafafar A, Haghpanah S, et al: Efficacy of prophylaxis and genotype-phenotype correlation in patients with severe factor X deficiency in Iran. *Haemophilia* 18:211, 2012.

217. Rosenthal RL, Dreskin OH, Rosenthal N: A new hemophilia like disease caused by deficiency of a third plasma thromboplastic factor. *Proc Soc Exp Biol Med* 82:171, 1953.

218. Rapaport SI, Proctor RR, Patch NJ, Yettra M: The mode of inheritance of PTA deficiency: Evidence for the existence of major PTA deficiency and minor PTA deficiency. *Blood* 18:149, 1961.

219. Seligsohn U: High gene frequency of factor XI (PTA) deficiency in Ashkenazi-Jews. *Blood* 51:1223, 1978.

220. Mannhalter C, Hellstern P, Deutsch E: Identification of a defective factor XI cross-reacting material in a factor XI-deficient patient. *Blood* 70:31, 1987.

221. Zivelin A, Ogawa T, Bulvik S, et al: Severe factor XI deficiency caused by a Gly$^{555}$ to Glu mutation (factor XI-Glu555): A cross-reactive material positive variant defective in factor IX activation. *J Thromb Haemost* 2:1782, 2004.

222. Quelin F, Trossaert M, Sigaud M, et al: Molecular basis of severe factor XI deficiency in seven families from the west of France. Seven novel mutations, including an ancient Q88X mutation. *J Thromb Haemost* 2:71, 2004.

223. Martincic D, Zimmerman SA, Ware RE, et al: Identification of mutations and polymorphisms in the factor XI genes of an African-American family by dideoxy fingerprinting. *Blood* 92:3309, 1998.

224. McMullen BA, Fujikawa K, Davie EW: Location of the disulfide bonds in human coagulation factor XI: The presence of tandem apple domains. *Biochemistry* 30:2056, 1991.

225. Papagrigoriou E, McEwan PA, Walsh PN, Emsley J: Crystal structure of the factor XI zymogen reveals a pathway for transactivation. *Nat Struct Mol Biol* 13:557, 2006.

226. Zucker M, Zivelin A, Landau M, et al: Three residues at the interface of factor XI monomers augment covalent dimerization of factor XI. *J Thromb Haemost* 7:970, 2009.

227. Wu W, Sinha D, Shikov S, et al: Factor XI homodimer structure is essential for normal proteolytic activation by factor XIIa, thrombin, and factor XIa. *J Biol Chem* 283:18655, 2008.

228. Cheng Q, Kantz J, Poffenberger G, et al: Factor XI protein in human pancreas and kidney. *Thromb Haemost* 100:158, 2008.

229. Thompson RE, Mandle R Jr, Kaplan AP: Association of factor XI and high molecular weight kininogen in human plasma. *J Clin Invest* 60:1376, 1997.

230. Gailani D, Broze GJ Jr: Factor XI activation in a revised model of blood coagulation. *Science* 253:909, 1991.

231. Naito K, Fujikawa K: Activation of human blood coagulation factor XI independent of factor XII: Factor XI is activated by thrombin and factor XIa in the presence of negatively charged surfaces. *J Biol Chem* 266:7353, 1991.

232. Baglia FA, Shrimpton CN, Lopez JA, Walsh PN: The glycoprotein Ib-IX-V complex mediates localization of factor XI to lipid rafts on the platelet membrane. *J Biol Chem* 278:21744, 2003.

233. Von dem Borne PA, Meijers JC, Bouma BN: Effect of heparin on the activation of factor XI by fibrin-bound thrombin. *Thromb Haemost* 76:347, 1996.

234. Osterud B, Bouma BN, Griffin JH: Human blood coagulation factor IX: Purification, properties, and mechanism of activation by activated factor XI. *J Biol Chem* 253:5946, 1978.

235. Bouma BN, Meijers JC: Thrombin-activatable fibrinolysis inhibitor (TAFI, plasma procarboxypeptidase B, procarboxypeptidase R, procarboxypeptidase U). *J Thromb Haemost* 1:1566, 2003.

236. Bajzar L, Morser J, Nesheim M: TAFI, or plasma procarboxypeptidase B, couples the coagulation and fibrinolytic cascades through the thrombin-thrombomodulin complex. *J Biol Chem* 271:16603, 1996.

237. Broze GJ Jr, Higuchi DA: Coagulation-dependent inhibition of fibrinolysis: Role of carboxypeptidase-U and the premature lysis of clots from hemophilic plasma. *Blood* 88:3815, 1996.

238. Asakai R, Davie EW, Chung DW: Organization of the gene for human factor XI. *Biochemistry* 26:7221, 1987.

239. Kato A, Asakai R, Davie EW, Aoki N: Factor XI gene (F11) is located on the distal end of the long arm of human chromosome 4. *Cytogenet Cell Genet* 52:77, 1989.

240. Asakai R, Chung DW, Ratnoff OD, Davie EW: Factor XI (plasma thromboplastin antecedent) deficiency in Ashkenazi Jews is a bleeding disorder that can result from three types of point mutations. *Proc Natl Acad Sci U S A* 86:7667, 1989.

241. Zadra G, Asselta R, Tenchini ML, et al: Simultaneous genotyping of coagulation factor XI type II and type III mutations by multiplex real-time polymerase chain reaction to determine their prevalence in healthy and factor XI-deficient Italians. *Haematologica* 93:715, 2008.

242. Zivelin A, Bauduer F, Ducout L, et al: Factor XI deficiency in French Basques is caused predominantly by an ancestral Cys38Arg mutation in the factor XI gene. *Blood* 99:2448, 2002.

243. Girolami A, Scarparo P, Bonamigo E, et al: A cluster of factor XI-deficient patients due to a new mutation (Ile 436 Lys) in northeastern Italy. *Eur J Haematol* 88:229, 2012.

244. Kim J, Song J, Lyu CJ, et al: Population-specific spectrum of the F11 mutations in Koreans: Evidence for a founder effect. *Clin Genet* 82:180, 2012.

245. Kravtsov DV, Wu W, Meijers JC, et al: Dominant factor XI deficiency caused by mutations in the factor XI catalytic domain. *Blood* 104:128, 2004.

246. Bolton-Maggs PH, Patterson DA, Wensley RT, Tuddenham EG: Definition of the bleeding tendency in factor XI-deficient kindreds: A clinical and laboratory study. *Thromb Haemost* 73:194, 1995.

247. Bolton-Maggs PH, Young Wan-Yin B, McCraw AH, et al: Inheritance and bleeding in factor XI deficiency. *Br J Haematol* 69:521, 1988.

248. Salomon O, Steinberg DM, Seligsohn U: Variable bleeding manifestations characterize different types of surgery in patients with severe factor XI deficiency enabling parsimonious use of replacement therapy. *Haemophilia* 12:490, 2006.

249. Sidi A, Seligsohn U, Jonas P, Many M: Factor XI deficiency: Detection and management during urological surgery. *J Urol* 119:528, 1978.

250. Brenner B, Laor A, Lupo H, et al: Bleeding predictors in factor-XI deficient patients. *Blood Coagul Fibrinolysis* 8:511, 1997.

251. Bolton-Maggs PH, Peretz H, Butler R, et al: A common ancestral mutation (C128X) occurring in 11 non-Jewish families from the UK with factor XI deficiency. *J Thromb Haemost* 2:918, 2004.

252. Brodsky JB, Burgess GE III: Pulmonary embolism with factor XI deficiency. *JAMA* 234:1156, 1975.

253. Evans G, Pasi KJ, Mehta A, et al: Recurrent venous thromboembolic disease and factor XI concentrate in a patient with severe factor XI deficiency, chronic myelomonocytic leukaemia, factor V Leiden and heterozygous plasminogen deficiency. *Blood Coagul Fibrinolysis* 8:437, 1997.

254. Salomon O, Steinberg DM, Koren-Morag N, et al: Reduced incidence of ischemic stroke in patients with severe factor XI deficiency. *Blood* 111:4113, 2008.

255. Luo D, Szaba FM, Kummer LW, et al: Factor XI deficient mice display reduced inflammation, coagulopathy, and bacterial growth during listeriosis. *Infect Immun* 80:91, 2012.

256. Gailani D, Lasky NM, Broze GJ Jr: A murine model of factor XI deficiency. *Blood Coagul Fibrinolysis* 8:134, 1997.

257. James P, Salomon O, Mikovic D, Peyvandi F: Rare bleeding disorders-bleeding assessment tools, laboratory aspects and phenotype and therapy of FXI deficiency. *Haemophilia* 20(Suppl 4):71, 2014.

258. Mannucci PM, Bauer KA, Santagostino E, et al: Activation of the coagulation cascade after infusion of a factor XI concentrate in congenitally deficient patients. *Blood* 84:1314, 1994.

259. O'Connell NM, Riddell AF, Pascoe G, et al: Recombinant factor VIIa to prevent surgical bleeding in factor XI deficiency. *Haemophilia* 14:775, 2008.

260. Schulman S, Németh: An illustrative case and a review on the dosing of recombinant factor VIIa in congenital factor XI deficiency. *Haemophilia* 12:223, 2006.

261. Salomon O, Zivelin A, Livnat T, et al: Prevalence, causes, and characterization of factor XI inhibitors in patients with inherited factor XI deficiency. *Blood* 101:4783, 2003.

262. Zucker M, Zivelin A, Teitel J, Seligsohn U: Induction of an inhibitor antibody to factor XI in a patient with severe inherited factor XI deficiency by Rh immune globulin. *Blood* 111:1306, 2008.

263. Livnat T, Zivelin A, Martinowitz U, et al: Prerequisites for recombinant factor VIIa-induced thrombin generation in plasmas deficient in factors VIII, IX or XI. *J Thromb Haemost* 4:192, 2006.

264. Duckert F, Jung E, Sherling DH: An undescribed congenital haemorrhagic diathesis probably due to fibrin stabilizing factor deficiency. *Thromb Diath Haemorrh* 5:179, 1960.

265. Ivaskevicius V, Seitz R, Kohler HP et al: International registry on factor XIII deficiency: A basis informant mostly on European data. *Thromb Haemost* 97:914, 2007.

266. Muszbek L, Adany R, Mikkola H: Novel aspects of blood coagulation factor XIII: I. Structure, distribution, activation, and function. *Crit Rev Clin Lab Sci* 33:357, 1996.

267. Schwartz ML, Pizzo SV, Hill RL, McKee PA: Human factor XIII from plasma and platelets. Molecular weights, subunit structures, proteolytic activation, and cross-linking of fibrinogen and fibrin. *J Biol Chem* 248:1395, 1973.

268. Muszbek L, Ariens RA, Ichinose A, ISTH SSC Subcommittee on Factor X: Factor XIII: Recommended terms and abbreviations. *J Thromb Haemost* 5:181, 2007.

269. Weiss MS, Metzner HJ, Hilgenfeld R: Two nonproline cis peptide bonds may be important for factor XIII function. *FEBS Lett* 423:291, 1998.

270. Yee VC, Pedersen LC, Le Trong I, et al: Three-dimensional structure of a transglutaminase: Human blood coagulation factor XIII. *Proc Natl Acad Sci U S A* 91:7296, 1994.

271. Lorand L, Graham RM: Transglutaminases: Crosslinking enzymes with pleiotropic functions. *Nat Rev Mol Cell Biol* 4:140, 2003.

272. Yee VC, Le Trong I, Bishop PD, et al: Structure and function studies of factor XIIIa by X-ray crystallography. *Semin Thromb Hemost* 22:377, 1996.

273. Gentile V, Saydak M, Chiocca EA, et al: Isolation and characterization of cDNA clones to mouse macrophage and human endothelial cell tissue transglutaminases. *J Biol Chem* 266:478, 1991.

274. Phillips MA, Stewart BE, Qin Q, et al: Primary structure of keratinocyte transglutaminase. *Proc Natl Acad Sci U S A* 87:9333, 1990.

275. Sung LA, Chien S, Chang LS, et al: Molecular cloning of human protein 4.2: A major component of the erythrocyte membrane. *Proc Natl Acad Sci U S A* 87:955, 1990.

276. Ichinose A, McMullen BA, Fujikawa K, Davie EW: Amino acid sequence of the b subunit of human factor XIII, a protein composed of ten repetitive segments. *Biochemistry* 25:4633, 1986.

277. Souri M, Kaetsu H, Ichinose A: Sushi domains in the B subunit of factor XIII responsible for oligomer assembly. *Biochemistry* 47:8656, 2008.

278. Lorand L, Gray AJ, Brown K, et al: Dissociation of the subunit structure of fibrin stabilizing factor during activation of the zymogen. *Biochem Biophys Res Commun* 56:914, 1974.

279. Mary A, Achyuthan KE, Greenberg CS: B-chains prevent the proteolytic inactivation of the a-chains of plasma factor XIII. *Biochim Biophys Acta* 966:328, 1988.

280. Biswas A, Ivaskevicius V, Thomas A, Oldenburg J: Coagulation factor XIII deficiency. *Hamostaseologie* 34:160, 2014.

281. Komaromi I, Bagoly Z, Muszbek L: Factor XIII: Novel structural and functional aspects. *J Thromb Haemost* 9:9, 2011.

282. Kohler HP: Interaction between FXIII and fibrinogen. *Blood* 121:1934, 2013.

283. Smith KA, Adamson PJ, Pease RJ, et al: Interactions between factor XIII and the alpha C region of fibrinogen. *Blood* 117:3460–3460, 2011.

284. Ariens RA, Lai TS, Weisel JW, et al: Role of factor XIII in fibrin clot formation and effects of genetic polymorphisms. *Blood* 100:743, 2002.

285. Varadi A, Scheraga HA: Localization of segments essential for polymerization and for calcium binding in the gamma-chain of human fibrinogen. *Biochemistry* 25:519, 1986.

286. Smith KA, Adamson PJ, Pease RJ et al: Interactions between factor XIII and the alpha C region of fibrinogen. *Blood* 117:3460, 2011.

287. Smith KA, Pease RJ, Avery CA et al: The activation peptide cleft exposed by thrombin cleavage of FXIII-A(2) contains a recognition site for the fibrinogen alpha chain. *Blood* 121:2117, 2013.

288. Doolittle RF, Hong S, Wilcox D: Evolution of the fibrinogen gamma' chain: Implications for the binding of factor XIII, thrombin and platelets. *J Thromb Haemost* 7:1431, 2009.

289. Sakata Y, Aoki N: Cross-linking of alpha 2-plasmin inhibitor to fibrin by fibrin-stabilizing factor. *J Clin Invest* 65:290, 1980.

290. Mosher DF, Schad PE, Vann JM: Cross-linking of collagen and fibronectin by factor XIIIa: Localization of participating glutaminyl residues to a tryptic fragment of fibronectin. *J Biol Chem* 255:1181, 1980.

291. Fraser SR, Booth NA, Mutch NJ: The antifibrinolytic function of factor XIII is exclusively expressed through alpha(2)-antiplasmin cross-linking. *Blood* 117:6371, 2011.

292. Van Giezen JJ, Minkema J, Bouma BN, Jansen JW: Cross-linking of alpha 2-antiplasmin to fibrin is a key factor in regulating blood clot lysis: Species differences. *Blood Coagul Fibrinolysis* 4:869, 1993.

293. Richardson VR, Cordell P, Standeven KF, Carter AM: Substrates of factor XIII-A: Roles in thrombosis and wound healing. *Clin Sci (Lond)* 124:123, 2013.

294. Board PG, Webb GC, McKee J, Ichinose A: Localization of the coagulation factor XIII A subunit gene (F13A) to chromosome bands 6p24-p25. *Cytogenet Cell Genet* 48:25, 1988.

295. Weisberg LJ, Shiu DT, Greenberg CS, et al: Localization of the gene for coagulation factor XIII a-chain to chromosome 6, and identification of sites of synthesis. *J Clin Invest* 79:649, 1987.

296. Ichinose A, Davie EW: Characterization of the gene for the a subunit of human factor XIII (plasma transglutaminase), a blood coagulation factor. *Proc Natl Acad Sci U S A* 85:5829, 1988.

297. Webb GC, Coggan M, Ichinose A, Board PG: Localization of the coagulation factor XIII B subunit gene (F13B) to chromosome bands 1q31–32.1, and restriction fragment length polymorphism at the locus. *Hum Genet* 81:157, 1989.

298. Bottenus RE, Ichinose A, Davie EW: Nucleotide sequence of the gene for the b subunit of human factor XIII. *Biochemistry* 29:11195, 1990.

299. Biswas A, Ivaskevicius V, Seitz R, et al: An update of the mutation profile of Factor 13A and B genes. *Blood Rev* 25:193, 2011.

300. Morange P, Trigui N, Frere C, et al: Molecular characterization of a novel mutation in the factor XIII a subunit gene associated with a severe defect: Importance of prophylactic substitution. *Blood Coagul Fibrinolysis* 20:605, 2009.

301. Inbal A, Yee VC, Kornbrot N, et al: Factor XIII deficiency due to a Leu660Pro mutation in the factor XIII subunit-A gene in three unrelated Palestinian Arab families. *Thromb Haemost* 77:1062, 1997.

302. Mikkola H, Syrjala M, Rasi V, et al: Deficiency in the A-subunit of coagulation factor XIII: Two novel point mutations demonstrate different effects on transcript level. *Blood* 84:517, 1994.

303. Schroeder V, Durrer D, Meili E, et al: Congenital factor XIII deficiency in Switzerland: From the worldwide first case in 1960, to its molecular characterisation in 2005. *Swiss Med Wkly* 137:272, 2007.

304. Aslam S, Standen GR, Khurshid M, Bilwani F: Molecular analysis of six factor XIII-A-deficient families in Southern Pakistan. *Br J Haematol* 109:463, 2000.

305. Hsieha L, Nugent D: Rare factor deficiencies. *Curr Opin Hematol* 19:380, 2012.

306. Karimi M, Bereczky Z, Cohan N, Muszbek L: Factor XIII deficiency. *Semin Thromb Hemost* 35:426, 2009.

307. Dardik R, Loscalzo J, Inbal A: Factor XIII (FXIII) and angiogenesis. *J Thromb Haemost* 4:19, 2006.

308. Sharief LAT, Kadir RA: Congenital factor XIII deficiency in women: A systematic review of literature. *Haemophilia* 19:e349, 2013.

309. Asahina T, Kobayashi T, Okada Y, et al: Maternal blood coagulation factor XIII is associated with the development of cytotrophoblastic shell. *Placenta* 21:388, 2000.

310. Inbal A, Muszbek L: Coagulation factor deficiencies and pregnancy loss. *Semin Thromb Hemost* 29:171, 2003.

311. Mahmoodi M, Peyvandi F, Afrasiabi A, et al: Bleeding symptoms in heterozygous carriers of inherited coagulation disorders in southern Iran. *Blood Coagul Fibrinolysis* 22:396, 2011.

312. Koseki-Kuno S, Yamakawa M, Dickneite G, Ichinose A: Factor XIII A subunit-deficient mice developed severe uterine bleeding events and subsequent spontaneous miscarriages. *Blood* 102:4410, 2003.

313. Lauer P, Metzner HJ, Zettlmeissl G, et al: Targeted inactivation of the mouse locus encoding coagulation factor XIIIA: Hemostatic abnormalities in mutant mice and characterization of the coagulation deficit. *Thromb Haemost* 88:967, 2002.

314. Souri M, Koseki-Kuno S, Takeda N, et al: Male specific cardiac pathologies in mice lacking either the A or B subunit of factor XIII. *Thromb Haemost* 99:401, 2008.

315. Peyvandi F, Palla R, Menegatti M, Bucciarelli P, Boscarino M, Muszbek L: Minimal residual FXIII coagulant activity to prevent spontaneous major bleeding, on behalf of the PRO-RBDD group. *Haemophilia* 22(Suppl 4):17, 2016 (abstract).

316. Dreyfus M, Barrois D, Borg JY, et al: Successful long-term replacement therapy with FXIII concentrate (Fibrogammin1 P) for severe congenital factor XIII deficiency: A prospective multicentre study. *J Thromb Haemost* 9:1264, 2011.

317. Gootenberg JE: Factor concentrates for the treatment of factor XIII deficiency. *Curr Opin Hematol* 5:372, 1998.

318. Odame JE, Chan AK, Wu JK, Breakey VR: Factor XIII deficiency management: A review of the literature. *Blood Coagul Fibrinolysis* 25:199, 2014.

319. Inbal A, Oldenburg J, Carcao M, Rosholm A, Tehranchi R, Nugent D: Recombinant factor XIII: A safe and novel treatment for congenital factor XIII deficiency. *Blood* 119:5111, 2012.

320. Williams M, Will A, Stenmo C, Rosholm A, Tehranchi R: Pharmacokinetics of rFXIII A in young children with congenital FXIII deficiency and comparison with older patients. *Haemophilia* 20:99, 2014.

321. Furie B, Voo L, McAdam KP, Furie BC: Mechanism of factor X deficiency in systemic amyloidosis. *N Engl J Med* 304:827, 1981.

322. Fair DS, Edgington TS: Heterogeneity of hereditary and acquired factor X deficiencies by combined immunochemical and functional analyses. *Br J Haematol* 59:235, 1985.

323. Bajaj SP, Rapaport SI, Fierer DS, et al: A mechanism for the hypoprothrombinemia of the acquired hypoprothrombinemia-lupus anticoagulant syndrome. *Blood* 61:684, 1983.

324. Lim S, Zuha R, Burt T, et al: Life-threatening bleeding in a patient with a lupus inhibitor and probable acquired factor VII deficiency. *Blood Coagul Fibrinolysis* 17:867, 2006.

325. Wiwanitkit V: Spectrum of bleeding in acquired factor V inhibitor: A summary of 33 cases. *Clin Appl Thromb Hemost* 12:485, 2006.

326. Rao LV, Zivelin A, Iturbe I, Rapaport SI: Antibody-induced acute factor X deficiency: Clinical manifestations and properties of the antibody. *Thromb Haemost* 72:363, 1994.

327. Mulhare PE, Tracy PB, Golden EA, et al: A case of acquired factor X deficiency with in vivo and in vitro evidence of inhibitor activity directed against factor X. *Am J Clin Pathol* 96:196, 1991.

328. Matsunaga AT, Shafer FE: An acquired inhibitor to factor X in a pediatric patient with extensive burns. *J Pediatr Hematol Oncol* 18:223, 1996.

329. Gallais V, Bredoux H, leRoux G, Laroche L: Acquired and transient factor X deficiency associated with sodium valproate treatment. *Eur J Haematol* 57:330, 1996.

330. Lankiewicz MW, Bell WR: A unique circulating inhibitor with specificity for coagulation factor X. *Am J Med* 93:343, 1992.

331. Ichinose A, Souri M: Japanese Collaborative Research Group on Acquired Haemorrhaphilia Due to Factor XIII Deficiency: As many as 12 cases with haemorrhagic acquired factor XIII deficiency due to its inhibitors were recently found in Japan. *Thromb Haemost* 105:925, 2011.

332. Ichinose A: Factor XIII as a key molecule at the intersection of coagulation and fibrinolysis as well as inflammation and infection control. *Int J Hematol* 95:362, 2012.

# CHAPTER 15
# HEREDITARY FIBRINOGEN ABNORMALITIES

Marguerite Neerman-Arbez and Philippe de Moerloose*

## SUMMARY

Hereditary fibrinogen abnormalities make up two classes of plasma fibrinogen defects: (1) type I, afibrinogenemia or hypofibrinogenemia, in which there are low or absent plasma fibrinogen antigen levels (quantitative fibrinogen deficiencies), and (2) type II, dysfibrinogenemia or hypodysfibrinogenemia, in which there are normal or reduced antigen levels associated with disproportionately low functional activity (qualitative fibrinogen deficiencies). In afibrinogenemia, most mutations of the three encoding genes of fibrinogen chains are null. In some cases, missense or late-truncating nonsense mutations allow synthesis of the corresponding fibrinogen chain, but intracellular fibrinogen assembly and/or secretion is impaired. In certain hypofibrinogenemic cases, the mutant fibrinogen molecules are produced and retained in the rough endoplasmic reticulum of hepatocytes in the form of inclusion bodies, causing endoplasmic reticulum storage disease. Afibrinogenemia is associated with mild to severe bleeding, whereas hypofibrinogenemia is often asymptomatic. Thromboembolism may also occur, and affected women may suffer from recurrent pregnancy loss. Hereditary dysfibrinogenemias are characterized by biosynthesis of a structurally abnormal fibrinogen molecule that exhibits reduced functional properties. Dysfibrinogenemia is commonly associated with bleeding, thrombosis, or both thrombosis and bleeding, but in many patients, it is asymptomatic. Hypodysfibrinogenemia is a subcategory of this disorder. Certain mutations involving the C-terminus of the fibrinogen *a* chain are associated with amyloidosis, in which an abnormal fragment from the fibrinogen *a* C domain is deposited in the kidneys. The cause for thrombophilia in type II fibrinogen abnormalities often is uncertain but may involve defective calcium binding, impaired tissue-type plasminogen activator–mediated fibrinolysis, resistance to fibrinolysis, or reduced thrombin binding to fibrin. Replacement therapy with fibrinogen concentrates has proven to be useful for management of fibrinogen disorders but should be adapted to each patient, based on the personal and family history.

**Acronyms and Abbreviations:** FFP, fresh-frozen plasma; *FGA*, fibrinogen Aα-chain gene; *FGB*, fibrinogen Bβ-chain gene; *FGG*, fibrinogen γ-chain gene; FpA, fibrinopeptide A; FpB, fibrinopeptide B; LMWH, low-molecular-weight heparin; PCR, polymerase chain reaction; TAFI, thrombin-activatable fibrinolysis inhibitor; t-PA, tissue-type plasminogen activator.

Several detailed and thoroughly annotated reviews of mutations causing inherited fibrinogen disorders have been published,[1-3] and tables compiling causative mutations identified before 2009 have been published previously.[4] In addition, a registry for hereditary fibrinogen abnormalities[5] can be accessed at http://site.geht.org/base-de-donnees-fibrinogene/ that lists variants reported in publications, conference abstracts, and submitted online, with original references. This chapter discusses the major molecular mechanisms leading to disease, as well as the laboratory and clinical aspects of fibrinogen disorders and their treatment, without listing all fibrinogen gene anomalies.

## ● INTRODUCTION

Fibrinogen plays a major role in hemostasis as the precursor molecule for the insoluble fibrin clot (Fig. 15–1). In addition fibrinogen participates in numerous other biologic processes, such as inflammation, wound healing, and angiogenesis. Fibrinogen binds plasminogen, α-antiplasmin, fibronectin, and factor XIII, among other proteins. It also binds to platelets and supports platelet aggregation. After fibrinogen is converted to fibrin by thrombin, it provides nonsubstrate binding sites for thrombin; consequently, fibrinogen is sometimes termed *antithrombin I*.[6] Fibrinogen also binds to vascular endothelial and other cells, plasma or tissue matrix components such as fibronectin and glycosaminoglycans, and peptide growth factors. Fibrin provides a template for assembly and activation of the fibrinolytic system components and is the major substrate for the enzyme plasmin (Chap. 25). Both fibrinogen and fibrin serve as substrates for plasma factor XIIIa that catalyzes covalent crosslinking/ligation.

## ● STRUCTURE AND SYNTHESIS

Fibrinogen is a 340-kDa glycoprotein synthesized in hepatocytes[7] that circulates in plasma at a concentration of 1.5 to 3.5 mg/mL (~4 to 10 $\mu$M). Each fibrinogen molecule is approximately 45 nm in length. The core structure consists of two outer D regions (or D domains) and a central E region (or E domain) connected through coiled-coil connectors (Fig. 15–2).[8] The molecule exhibits a twofold axis of symmetry perpendicular to the long axis, consisting of two sets of three polypeptide chains (Aα, Bβ, γ) that are joined in their aminoterminal regions by disulfide bridges to form the E region. The outer D regions contain the globular C terminal domains of the Bβ chain (βC) and γ chain (γC). The βC and γC domains, which are highly conserved in vertebrates, are members of the FreD (fibrinogen-related domain) family of proteins. Unlike the βC and γC domains, the C-terminal domains of the Aα chain (αC) are intrinsically unfolded and flexible and tend to be noncovalently tethered in the vicinity of the central E region (Fig. 15–2). The three genes encoding fibrinogen Bβ *(FGB)*, Aα *(FGA)*, and γ *(FGG)*, ordered from centromere to telomere, are clustered in a region of approximately 50 kb on human chromosome 4.[9] *FGA* and *FGG* are transcribed from the reverse strand, in the opposite direction to *FGB*. Alternative splicing[10] results in two isoforms for the fibrinogen α chain: the common Aα chain, encoded by exons 1 to 5, and an extended Aα-E isoform, encoded by exons 1 to 6, which represents only 1 to 2 percent of transcripts. Alternative splicing for *FGG* also produces two transcripts: the major mRNA species contains all 10 exons and encodes the common γ chain (or γA), while the minor product (γ′) does not splice out intron 9 and the corresponding open reading frame replaces the four codons of exon 10 with 20 alternative codons. *FGB* encodes a single 1.9-kb transcript with a 1.5-kb coding sequence. Each gene is separately transcribed and translated to produce nascent polypeptides of 644 amino acids (Aα), 491 amino acids (Bβ), and 437 amino acids (γ).

*The authors thank Dr. Alessandro Casini for helpful comments and suggestions.

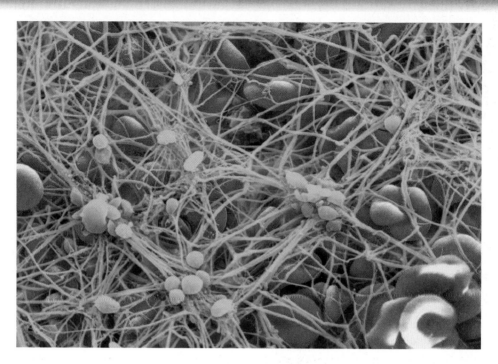

**Figure 15–1.** Colorized scanning electron micrograph of a whole blood clot. The fibrin mesh is shown in green, and trapped platelets and erythrocytes are colored violet and red, respectively. *(Used with permission of Yuri Veklich and John W. Weisel, University of Pennsylvania School of Medicine.)*

During translocation of the single chains into the lumen of the endoplasmic reticulum (ER), a signal peptide is cotranslationally cleaved from each chain. The resulting chains have 625 amino acids (Aα), 461 amino acids (Bβ), and 411 amino acids (γ). Assembly proceeds in the ER with the formation of an Aα-γ or Bβ-γ intermediate. The addition of either a Bβ or Aα chain gives rise to a [AαBβγ] half-molecule, which dimerizes to form the functional hexamer.[11] The protein undergoes several posttranslational modifications in the Golgi complex, including maturation of $N$-linked oligosaccharides, phosphorylation, hydroxylation, and sulfation.[12]

Following assembly, which is completed within minutes, the mature molecule is constitutively secreted into the circulation, where it exhibits a half-life of approximately 4 days.[13] In addition to plasma fibrinogen, blood contains an internalized intracellular fibrinogen pool that is stored within platelet α granules. Both megakaryocytes and platelets are capable of internalizing plasma fibrinogen via the fibrinogen integrin $α_{IIb}β_3$ receptor,[14] which binds to a C-terminal platelet recognition sequence that is present on γA chains but is absent from γ′ chains. Consequently, internalized platelet fibrinogen molecules contain only γA chains.[15]

## ●FIBRINOGEN CONVERSION TO FIBRIN AND NETWORK ASSEMBLY

Fibrin polymerization consists of several consecutive reactions, each affecting the ultimate structure and properties of the fibrin scaffold, which, in turn, determines the development and outcome of numerous diseases including coagulopathies and thrombosis.[16,17] Conversion of fibrinogen to a fibrin clot[18] occurs in three distinct phases: (1) enzymatic cleavage by thrombin to produce fibrin monomers; (2) self-assembly of fibrin units to form an organized polymeric structure; and (3) covalent crosslinking of fibrin by factor XIIIa. In the first phase of conversion to

fibrin, cleavage of fibrinogen at AαR35/G36 (R16/G17)* and later Bβ R44/G45 (R14/G15) results in release of fibrinopeptides A (FpA) and B (FpB), respectively, thus exposing "A" knobs and "B" knobs (Fig. 15–3). The "A" knob located at the new aminoterminal end of the fibrin α chain starts with the GPRV amino acid sequence. The "A" knob in fibrin interacts with the constitutive complementary association site known as hole "a" in another molecule to initiate the fibrin assembly process. Hole "a" is encompassed by residues 363 to 405 (337 to 379) of the γ chain.

A knob-hole a (A:a) interaction results in formation of double-stranded fibrils in which fibrin molecules become aligned in an end-to-middle, staggered, overlapping arrangement (see Fig. 15–3).[16–18] Fibrils subsequently undergo branching by lateral fibril associations in which two fibrils converge to form a four-stranded "bilateral" fibril junction. Progressive lateral associations among fibrils result in larger fibril bundles or fibers. A second type of junction, termed *equilateral branching*, is formed by three fibrils converging to form a three-member junction.[19] Both types of branch junctions provide scaffolding for the clot network, the ultimate

*The recommendation of the Human Genome Variation Society (HGVS) is to number amino acid residues from the initiator Met, with the protein reference sequences representing the primary translation product, not the processed, mature protein. This is the standard nomenclature used by geneticists. For fibrinogen, however, as for many other secreted proteins, such as the coagulation factors, this is not the nomenclature used in earlier publications (historically fibrinogen residues are numbered according to the secreted product lacking the signal peptide). In this text both nomenclatures are used: amino acid residues and substitutions are described first according to HGVS guidelines followed in brackets by the corresponding amino acid in the mature chain lacking the signal peptide. To convert from the HGVS nomenclature to the mature protein nomenclature, subtract 19 for Aα, 30 for Bβ, or 26 for γ. A one-letter abbreviation for amino acids is used in this chapter. A, alanine; C, cysteine; D, aspartic acid; E, glutamic acid; F, phenylalanine; G, glycine; H, histidine; I, isoleucine; K, lysine; L, leucine; M, methionine; N, asparagine; P, proline; Q, glutamine; R, arginine; S, serine; T, threonine; V, valine; W, tryptophan; Y, tyrosine.

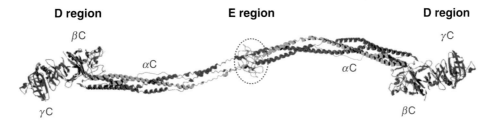

**D region**   **E region**   **D region**

βC   γC

αC   αC

γC   βC

**Figure 15–2.** Ribbon representation of native chicken fibrinogen[22] modified from PDB file 1M1J (www.pdb.org/pdb/). α Chains are in green, β chains are in purple, and γ chains are in blue. The globular C-terminal domains of the Bβ and γ chains forming the D regions are shown, as well as the central E region, which contains the N-terminal portions of all three chains. Unlike the βC and γC domains, the C-terminal domains of the Aα chain (αC) are flexible and tend to be noncovalently tethered in the vicinity of the central E region.

structure of which is governed by several variables, including salt concentration, pH, fibrinogen concentration, and thrombin concentration.[16,17,20]

Fibrinopeptide B (FpB) release occurs more slowly than fibrinopeptide A (FpA) release and exposes another polymerization site known as the "B" knob beginning with the amino acid sequence GHRP. GHRP interacts with a constitutive hole "b" in the β chain encompassed by residues 427 to 462 (397 to 432). FpB cleavage is accelerated by fibrin polymerization, whereas FpA cleavage is independent of fibrin polymerization. B:b interactions are not required for lateral fibril associations, but they contribute to lateral association by inducing rearrangements in βC that allow βC:βC contacts to occur.[21,22]

The flexible αC domains also participate in fibrin polymerization.[23] Fibrin clots made from plasma fibrinogen molecules lacking more than 100 C-terminal residues from the αC domain display prolonged thrombin times, reduced turbidity, and produce thinner fibers, indicating that αC domains participate in lateral fibril associations. In addition, αC domains become dissociated as a result of FpB cleavage. This allows αC domains to participate in noncovalent interactions with other αC domains, thereby promoting lateral fibril associations and fibrin network assembly. Finally, additional self-associating sites in the D region participate in fibrin assembly. These are the D:D sites and $\gamma_{XL}$ sites that promote end-to-end alignment of assembling fibrin units and factor XIIIa crosslinking, respectively.[24,25]

# CROSSLINKING BY FACTOR XIII

The clot formed by fibrin polymerization requires further stabilization to increase its mechanical strength and resist immediate degradation by the fibrinolytic pathway. Factor XIIIa (a heterotetramer FXIII-A2B2) is a transglutaminase that stabilizes the elongating protofibril by crosslinking adjacent γ chains through the formation of ε-(γ-glutamyl) lysine isopeptide bonds.[26] These occur between lysine 432 (406) of one γ chain and glutamine 424 (398) or 425 (399) of another chain. Crosslinking increases the resistance of the clot to deformation. The same process occurs, but at lower rate, between α chains and also between α chains and γ chains. In the presence of factor XIIIa, α-antiplasmin becomes covalently bound to the distal α chains of fibrin or fibrinogen.[26] The factor XIII binding site for fibrin has been characterized: residues in the Aα-C domain, that is, 408 to 421 (389 to 402), bind a cleft in FXIII-A2 that is exposed only after cleavage of the activation peptide by thrombin.[27] Fibronectin is also incorporated into the fibrin clot. This occurs by noncovalent interactions between the two proteins through specific binding sites, followed by their covalent crosslinking with factor XIIIa.[28] Fibronectin incorporation appears to affect the adhesion and migration of cells at sites of fibrin deposition, thereby contributing to wound healing and other cell-dependent processes.

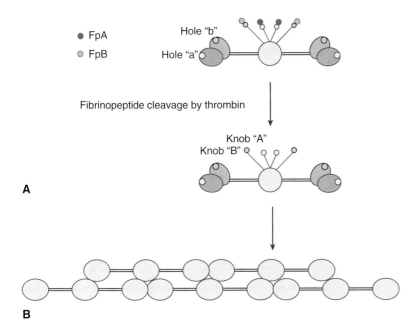

- ● FpA
- ○ FpB

Hole "b"

Hole "a"

Fibrinopeptide cleavage by thrombin

Knob "A"
Knob "B"

**A**

**B**

**Figure 15–3.** First steps of fibrinogen conversion to fibrin and fibrin assembly. **A.** Schematic of fibrinogen showing fibrinopeptides A (FpA) and B (FpB), the constitutive holes "a" and "b" in the globular C-terminal domains of the γ chains and β chains, respectively, and the "A" and "B" knobs, which are exposed only after FpA and FpB cleavage by thrombin. Here the globular βC and γC domains are shown separately, βC in purple, γC in blue as in Fig. 15–2. **B.** Self-assembly of fibrin units to form an organized polymeric structure. Here, for simplicity, the D regions are represented as a single globular unit.

# FIBRINOLYSIS

Plasminogen and tissue-type plasminogen activator (t-PA) binding sites in the D regions (i.e., $\gamma$ 337 to 350) (312 to 324) and $\alpha$C domains (i.e., A$\alpha$ 167 to 179) (148 to 160) are cryptic in fibrinogen and become exposed during fibrin assembly or during formation of crosslinked fibrinogen fibrils (Chap. 25).[29,30] Two phases can be distinguished in the t-PA–induced lysis of a fibrin clot.[31] In the first slow phase, t-PA activates plasminogen on the intact fibrin surface. The generation of C-terminal lysine residues in partially degraded fibrin (by plasmin) in the second phase of clot lysis may result in accumulation of plasminogen at the clot surface and a concomitant increase in lysis rate. Thrombin-activatable fibrinolysis inhibitor (TAFI) removes C-terminal lysine residues, resulting in a strongly reduced binding of plasminogen and in an inhibition of the second phase of clot lysis by a reduction of the activation of plasminogen on the fibrin surface. TAFI, $\alpha$-antiplasmin, lipoprotein(a), and histidine-rich glycoprotein bind to fibrin and all have an inhibitory effect on fibrinolysis through various mechanisms.

# ANTITHROMBIN ACTIVITY OF FIBRIN

Thrombin binds to its substrate, fibrinogen, through a fibrinogen recognition site in thrombin, referred to as exosite 1. The fibrin clot itself also exhibits significant thrombin-binding potential; this nonsubstrate binding potential of fibrin for thrombin is referred to as antithrombin activity I.[6] This activity is defined by two classes of nonsubstrate thrombin-binding sites in fibrin, one of "low affinity" in the E-region and the other of "high affinity" in D regions of fibrin(ogen) molecules containing the variant $\gamma'$ chain. Altogether, heterodimeric $\gamma$A/$\gamma'$ and homodimeric molecules $\gamma'$/$\gamma'$ chains make up 8 to 15 percent of the total $\gamma$-chain population.[10] Low-affinity thrombin-binding activity reflects thrombin exosite 1 binding in the E region of fibrin, whereas high-affinity thrombin binding to $\gamma'$ chains takes place through exosite 2. The binding affinity of thrombin for $\gamma'$-containing fibrin molecules is increased by concomitant fibrin binding to thrombin exosite 1. Antithrombin I (fibrin) is an important inhibitor of thrombin generation that functions by sequestering thrombin in the forming fibrin clot and also by reducing the catalytic activity of fibrin-bound thrombin. Vascular thrombosis may result from absence of antithrombin I (as in afibrinogenemia; see "Afibrinogenemia and Hypofibrinogenemia" below), reduced plasma $\gamma'$-chain content,[32] or defective thrombin binding to fibrin as found in certain dysfibrinogenemias (see "Dysfibrinogenemia and Hypodysfibrinogenemia" below). In contrast, an increased susceptibility to arterial thrombosis has been reported when $\gamma'$-chain levels are significantly elevated. Moreover, thrombin bound to $\gamma_A$/$\gamma'$-fibrin is protected from inhibition by antithrombin to a greater extent than thrombin bound to $\gamma_A$/$\gamma_A$-fibrin. Thus, $\gamma_A$/$\gamma'$-fibrin serves as a reservoir of active thrombin, which may contribute to the prothrombotic nature of thrombi.[33]

# AFIBRINOGENEMIA AND HYPOFIBRINOGENEMIA

## DEFINITION, HISTORY, AND EPIDEMIOLOGY

Type I disorders (afibrinogenemia and hypofibrinogenemia) affect the quantity of fibrinogen in circulation. Type II disorders (dysfibrinogenemia and hypodysfibrinogenemia) affect the quality of circulating fibrinogen.[1] While the first dysfibrinogenemia mutation was identified as early as 1968,[34] the molecular basis of afibrinogenemia was elucidated much later.[35] This disorder is characterized by autosomal recessive inheritance and the complete absence of fibrinogen in plasma.

The disease, originally described in 1920,[36] has an estimated prevalence of approximately one in 1,000,000. In populations where consanguineous marriages are common, the prevalence of afibrinogenemia is increased.[37] Because hypofibrinogenemia (fibrinogen levels below 1.5 g L$^{-1}$) is often caused by heterozygosity for a fibrinogen gene mutation, this is much more frequent than afibrinogenemia. If one applies the Hardy-Weinberg binomial distribution of alleles in the population to afibrinogenemia, carriers of fibrinogen deficiency–causing mutations could be as frequent as one in 500.

## ETIOLOGY AND PATHOGENESIS

Since the identification of the first causative mutation for congenital afibrinogenemia in 1999,[35] approximately 100 distinct mutations, the majority in *FGA*, have been identified in patients with afibrinogenemia (in homozygosity or in compound heterozygosity) or in patients with hypofibrinogenemia. Causative mutations can be divided into two main classes: null mutations with no protein production at all and mutations producing abnormal protein chains that are retained inside the cell.[1]

### Large Deletions

The first causative mutation for afibrinogenemia was identified in a nonconsanguineous Swiss family with two pairs of afibrinogenemic brothers.[35] In a first step toward establishing whether or not the disease was linked to the fibrinogen gene cluster on chromosome 4, haplotype data were obtained for five microsatellite markers surrounding this locus. One of these, FGAi3, a (TCTT)n polymorphic marker located in intron 3 of the *FGA* gene, was found to be deleted in all four affected individuals and was hemizygous in the obligate carriers, implying that homozygous deletion of at least part of the *FGA* gene was responsible for the congenital afibrinogenemia in this family. Indeed, the genetic defect was found to be a recurrent deletion of approximately 11 kb of DNA, with breakpoints in *FGA* intron 1 and the *FGA–FGB* intergenic region, resulting in an absence of fibrinogen.

Three other large deletions in the fibrinogen gene cluster have been identified, all involving part of the *FGA* gene. These are a deletion of 1.2 kb eliminating the entire *FGA* exon 4 in a Japanese patient[38]; a deletion of 15 kb, with breakpoints situated in *FGA* intron 4 and in the *FGA–FGB* intergenic region in a Thai patient[39]; and a 4.1-kb deletion encompassing *FGA* exon 1 in an Italian patient.[40] All patients were homozygous for the identified deletions except for the Thai patient, for whom complete maternal uniparental disomy was confirmed for the deleted chromosome 4.[39]

### Splice-Site Mutations

Several splice-site mutations have been identified in all three fibrinogen genes. In afibrinogenemic patients of European origin, the most common mutation is a donor splice mutation in intron 4, c.510+1G→T (previously described as IVS4+1 G→T).[1,41] Haplotype data suggest that this mutation, like the *FGA* 11-kb deletion, is also recurrent, or a very ancient mutation, because the c.510+1G→T mutation is found on multiple discrete haplotypes.

### Frameshift Mutations

Frameshift mutations have been identified in all three fibrinogen genes. *FGA* exon 5, the largest fibrinogen-coding exon, has the most frameshift mutations. Interestingly, seven single base-pair deletions in *FGA* exon 5 result in usage of the same new reading frame. All seven mutations are predicted to encode a long stretch of aberrant amino acids before terminating at the same premature stop codon, 69 to 158 codons downstream.[42] The aberrant amino acid sequence (if the abnormal protein is synthesized and stable, which remains to be determined) may lead to abnormal folding of the A$\alpha$ chain, thus affecting fibrinogen chain assembly or secretion.

### Nonsense Mutations

Many nonsense mutations accounting for afibrinogenemia and hypofibrinogenemia have been identified. Of the nine nonsense mutations identified in *FGB*, four are located in *FGB* exon 8.[43] In particular, two *FGB* nonsense mutations—W467X (W437X) and W470X (W440X)—are localized very close to the β-chain C-terminus and are expected to cause the synthesis of βC chains truncated of only 25 and 22 residues, respectively.[44,45] Expression studies in transfected COS cells performed for both mutations showed that the mutations allowed individual chain synthesis and intracellular assembly of the hexamer but impaired secretion, suggesting that an intact *FGB* C-terminal domain is necessary for fibrinogen secretion into the circulation.[46]

### Missense Mutations

Null mutations, that is, large deletions, frameshift, early truncating nonsense, and splice-site mutations, account for the majority of afibrinogenemia alleles, as expected. Missense mutations leading to complete fibrinogen deficiency are therefore particularly interesting, revealing the functional importance of individual residues or three-dimensional structures. Missense mutations are clustered in the highly conserved C-terminal globular domains of the γ and Bβ chains.[1,43] Expression studies in transfected cells for five *FGB* missense mutations, all identified in homozygosity or compound heterozygosity in afibrinogenemic patients, showed that these mutations, like the late-truncating nonsense mutations discussed previously, allowed individual chain synthesis and intracellular assembly of the hexamer but again impaired secretion.[47–50] Further characterization of the *FGB* G444S (G414S) mutant using immunostaining for fibrinogen and visualization by confocal microscopy revealed that the secretion-impaired mutant was retained in the ER, proving the existence of an efficient quality control mechanism for fibrinogen secretion.[46]

Several missense mutations have been identified in *FGG* in heterozygosity in patients with hypofibrinogenemia. For the majority of these mutations, analysis of patient plasma fibrinogen by mass spectrometry confirmed absence of the mutant γ chain in the circulation. Others have been studied at the functional level in transfected cells: fibrinogen Matsumoto IV C179R (C153R) was found to impair intracellular hexamer assembly,[51] whereas fibrinogen Bratislava W253C (W227C) was found to impair fibrinogen secretion.[52]

### Mutations Causing Hepatic Endoplasmic Reticulum Retention and Hypofibrinogenemia

In the majority of patients with afibrinogenemia or hypofibrinogenemia, there is no evidence of intracellular accumulation of the mutant fibrinogen chain. This implies the existence of an efficient degradation pathway for fibrinogen mutants that allows individual chain synthesis and assembly but not secretion. Four mutations, all in *FGG*, are known to cause hypofibrinogenemia accompanied by hepatic storage disease. These are three missense mutations (fibrinogen Brescia, Aguadilla, and Al duPont)[53–55] and a 15-bp deletion at the end of *FGG* exon 8 (fibrinogen Angers),[56] which creates a new *FGG* exon 8–intron 8 junction and donor splice site. All four mutations cause fibrinogen deficiency in the heterozygous state because of the absence of the mutant γ chain in patient plasma, but also progressive liver disease associated with hepatocellular cytoplasmic inclusions. The molecular mechanism by which these mutations, localized in the five-stranded β-sheet of γC and hole "a," which are crucial for fibrin polymerization, lead to impaired secretion, retention in the ER, and formation of aggregates remains to be determined.

## CLINICAL FEATURES

### Afibrinogenemia

Bleeding because of afibrinogenemia usually manifests in the neonatal period, with 85 percent of cases presenting umbilical cord bleeding, but a later age of onset is not unusual. Bleeding may occur in the skin, gastrointestinal tract, genitourinary tract, or central nervous system, with intracranial hemorrhage being the major cause of death. Joint bleeding, which is common in patients with severe hemophilia, is less frequent: in a series of 72 patients with severe fibrinogen deficiency, hemarthrosis was observed in 25 percent of cases.[57] There is an intriguing susceptibility of spontaneous rupture of the spleen in afibrinogenemic patients. Bone cysts have also been described as a rare complication of afibrinogenemia and appear to benefit from prophylactic therapy with fibrinogen concentrate.[58]

Menstruating women may experience menometrorrhagia, but some have normal menses. First-trimester abortion is usual in afibrinogenemic women. The importance of fibrinogen in pregnancy was demonstrated in studies with fibrinogen knockout mice that cannot carry fetuses to term.[59] Women may also have antepartum and postpartum hemorrhage. Hemoperitoneum after rupture of the corpus luteum has also been observed.

Paradoxically, both arterial and venous thromboembolic complications are observed in afibrinogenemic patients. These complications can occur in the presence of concomitant risk factors such as a coinherited thrombophilic risk factor or after replacement therapy. However, in many patients, no known risk factors are present. Many hypotheses have been put forward to explain this predisposition to thrombosis. One explanation is that even in the absence of fibrinogen platelet aggregation is possible because of the action of von Willebrand factor and, in contrast to patients with severe hemophilia, afibrinogenemic patients are able to generate thrombin, both in the initial phase of limited production and also in the secondary burst of thrombin generation. In some patients, an increase of prothrombin activation fragments or thrombin–antithrombin complexes has been observed, which may reflect enhanced thrombin generation.[60] These abnormal levels can be normalized by fibrinogen infusions.

As previously mentioned, fibrin also acts as antithrombin I by both sequestering and downregulating thrombin activity.[6] Thrombin that is not trapped by the clot is available for platelet activation and smooth muscle cell migration and proliferation, particularly in the arterial vessel wall. Thrombus formation is maintained in fibrinogen-deficient mice[61] and in fibrinogen-deficient zebrafish,[62] but the thrombus is unstable and has a tendency to embolize. Similarly, the absence of fibrinogen in human plasma results in large but loosely packed thrombi under flow conditions.[63]

### Hypofibrinogenemia

Hypofibrinogenemia patients are very often heterozygous carriers of afibrinogenemia mutations.[1] These patients are usually asymptomatic with fibrinogen levels of approximately 1.0 g L$^{-1}$, levels that are in theory high enough to protect against bleeding and maintain pregnancy. However, these patients can bleed when exposed to trauma or if they have a second associated hemostatic abnormality. Hypofibrinogenemic women may also suffer from pregnancy loss.

## LABORATORY FEATURES

The clinical diagnosis is established by functional and immunologic measurements of fibrinogen concentration backed by genetic analyses.

### Phenotype Analysis

Absence of immunoreactive fibrinogen is essential for the diagnosis of congenital afibrinogenemia. All coagulation tests that depend on the formation of fibrin as the end point—that is, prothrombin time (PT), partial thromboplastin time (PTT), or thrombin time (TT)—are infinitely prolonged. Plasma activity of all other clotting factors is usually normal. Some abnormalities in platelet functions tests can be observed, which can be reversed upon addition of fibrinogen. Because fibrinogen is one of the main determinants of erythrocyte sedimentation, it is not surprising that afibrinogenemic patients have very low erythrocyte sedimentation rates. When skin testing is performed for delayed hypersensitivity, there is no induration because of the lack of fibrin deposition.

Hypofibrinogenemia is defined as a proportional decrease of functional and immunoreactive fibrinogen. Coagulation tests depending on the formation of fibrin as well as the assays used are variably prolonged, with the most sensitive assay being the TT.

### Genotype Analysis

The large number of mutations identified in patients with afibrinogenemia allows the design of an efficient flowchart for mutation detection in new cases.[64] Two common mutations are found in individuals of European origin, both in *FGA*: the c.510+1G→T intron 4 donor splice-site mutation and the *FGA* 11-kb deletion, both found on multiple haplotypes. In all new patients of European origin, the *FGA* c.510+1G→T should be the first mutation to be screened. Southern blot or polymerase chain reaction (PCR) analysis of the *FGA* 11 kb deletion should also be performed, because it is the second most common mutation in patients of European origin and because of the risk of diagnostic error: a nonconsanguineous patient who appears to be homozygous for a mutation in *FGA* exons 2 to 6 may in reality be a heterozygous carrier of the large 11-kb deletion.[65] Given the high frequency of mutations in *FGA*, the other *FGA* exons (starting with exon 5) should then be studied for mutations before screening *FGB* (starting with exon 8) and *FGG* (starting with exons 7 and 8). The same strategy can also be applied to afibrinogenemic patients of non-European origin for whom recurrent mutations have yet to be identified. If the patient comes from a geographical region or population in which a mutation has already been identified, that mutation should be the first to be screened for. Screening of patients with hypofibrinogenemia can follow the same strategy apart from patients with ER fibrinogen-positive liver inclusions, for which four mutations in *FGG* are known so far to cause hepatic storage disease.

Prenatal diagnosis has been performed in a few cases.[66] This is important for families with afibrinogenemia and access to adequate treatment because the prenatal diagnosis of an affected infant allows initiation of treatment immediately after birth before the first bleeding manifestation.

### Genotype–Phenotype Correlations: Potential Importance of Global Assays

Current diagnostic tests are appropriate for establishing the diagnosis, but clearly additional tests are required for a more accurate prediction of the clinical phenotype of a patient and consequently the appropriate treatment. Indeed, although in afibrinogenemia all patients have unmeasurable functional fibrinogen, the severity of bleeding is highly variable among patients, even among those with the same genotype. Similarly, there is no clear relationship between the molecular defect and the risk of thrombosis.

One possible explanation for the observed variability of clinical manifestations is the existence of modifier genes/alleles: some variants may increase the severity of bleeding while others may ameliorate the phenotype. Such modifiers have yet to be identified. However, the common thrombophilias (e.g., factor V Leiden) most certainly play a role in decreasing the severity of bleeding. The existence of modifying genes/polymorphisms is also strongly suspected in the previously discussed cases of hypofibrinogenemia associated with fibrinogen inclusion bodies in hepatocytes. Indeed, all individuals heterozygous for one of the four *FGG* causative mutations have hypofibrinogenemia, but not all have fibrinogen aggregates and associated liver disease.

Global assays, such as thromboelastography and thrombin generation test, may provide a complementary and, in some cases, a better evaluation of an individual's hemostatic state. Such global assays could be useful for the design of individual therapeutic strategies.[67]

## DIFFERENTIAL DIAGNOSIS

Inherited afibrinogenemia and hypofibrinogenemia have to be distinguished from acquired disorders. These include disseminated intravascular coagulation, primary fibrinolysis, liver disease, and disorders caused by certain drugs (e.g., thrombolytic agents and L-asparaginase). In addition, one should be aware that artifactually low levels of fibrinogen can be observed with samples that have clotted as a result of improper collection. In most cases, the clinical context and the association with other laboratory abnormalities will allow differentiation of inherited from acquired disorders. Identification of a causative mutation in one of the three fibrinogen genes will confirm the diagnosis.

## THERAPY

### Available Treatments and Modalities

Replacement therapy is effective in treating bleeding episodes in congenital fibrinogen disorders. Depending on the country of residence, patients receive fresh-frozen plasma (FFP), cryoprecipitate, or fibrinogen concentrates.[64] Fibrinogen concentrate preparations include safety steps for inactivation or removal of viruses, which make them safer than cryoprecipitate or FFP. Furthermore, more precise dosing can be accomplished with fibrinogen concentrates because their potency is known, in contrast to FFP or cryoprecipitates.

The conventional treatment is on demand, in which fibrinogen is administered as soon as possible after onset of bleeding. Another approach is primary prophylaxis that includes administration of fibrinogen concentrates from an early age to prevent bleeding and, in the case of pregnancy, to prevent miscarriage. Effective long-term secondary prophylaxis with administration of fibrinogen every 7 to 14 days (particularly after central nervous system bleeds) has been advocated. The frequency and dose of fibrinogen concentrates should be adjusted to maintain a level above $0.5 \text{ g L}^{-1}$.[64]

The United Kingdom guidelines on therapeutic products for coagulation disorders[68] provide recommendations about the best treatment options (dosage, management of bleeding, surgery, and pregnancy, as well as prophylaxis). According to these guidelines, in case of bleeding, fibrinogen levels should be increased to $1.0 \text{ g L}^{-1}$ and maintained above this threshold until hemostasis is secured, and above $0.5 \text{ g L}^{-1}$ until wound healing is complete. To increase the fibrinogen concentration of $1 \text{ g L}^{-1}$, a dose of approximately 50 mg/kg is required. The doses and duration of treatment also vary depending on the type of injury or operative procedure and on the patient's personal and familial history of bleeding and thrombosis.

Women with congenital afibrinogenemia are able to conceive, and embryonic implantation is normal, but the pregnancy usually results in spontaneous abortion at 5 to 8 weeks of gestation unless fibrinogen replacement is given.[69] Maintaining the fibrinogen level above $0.6 \text{ g L}^{-1}$ and, if possible, higher than $1.0 \text{ g L}^{-1}$ is recommended. Lower fibrinogen concentrations ($<0.4 \text{ g L}^{-1}$) have proven adequate to maintain pregnancy but not to avoid hemorrhagic complications. Continuous infusion of fibrinogen concentrate should be performed during labor to maintain fibrinogen higher than $1.5 \text{ g L}^{-1}$ (ideally greater than $2.0 \text{ g L}^{-1}$).[70] Thromboembolic events can occur, particularly with the use of cryoprecipitates that contain appreciable quantities of factor VIII and von Willebrand factor in addition to fibrinogen.

In addition to fibrinogen substitution, antifibrinolytic agents may be given, particularly to treat mucosal bleeding or to prevent bleeding following procedures such as dental extraction. Fibrin glue is useful to treat superficial wounds or following dental extractions. Oral contraceptive preparations are useful in case of menorrhagia. Oral iron preparations can be given in cases with associated iron-deficiency anemia. Routine vaccination against hepatitis, as well as a regular surveillance for both the disease and treatment-related complications in a comprehensive care setting, is highly recommended.[64]

Finally, orthotopic liver transplantation is a possible rescue treatment for failure of fibrinogen replacement therapy. This procedure successfully restored normal hemostasis in an afibrinogenemic patient with severe Budd-Chiari syndrome and inferior cava vein thrombosis[71] and in one of the four afibrinogenemic patients homozygous for the 11-kb *FGA* mutation.[35,72]

### Complications of Therapy

In many countries, only FFP or cryoprecipitate is available, which is problematic because the viral inactivation process is in general not as efficient as it is for fibrinogen concentrates (although emerging nonviral pathogens such as the prion responsible for variant Creutzfeldt-Jacob disease must be considered, even for concentrates). Even if viral inactivation steps are performed, these preparations (particularly FFP) can induce volume overload. There is also a risk of transfusion-related acute lung injury, because of the presence of cytotoxic antibodies in the infused plasma.

Acquired inhibitors to fibrinogen after replacement therapy have been reported in only two cases. It is not clear why afibrinogenemic patients do not develop inhibitors more frequently. One explanation for some cases is that minute amounts of fibrinogen, which can only be detected by highly sensitive immunoassays, are present in the circulation.

One of the major complications in afibrinogenemic patients is thrombosis, which can occur spontaneously following blood component therapy. Some clinicians give small doses of heparin or low-molecular-weight heparin (LMWH) during administration of fibrinogen. Before surgery, patients with a thrombotic phenotype should be treated with compression stockings and LMWH. Successful use of lepirudin has been reported for an afibrinogenemic patient who suffered recurrent arterial thrombosis despite treatment with heparin and aspirin.[73] Thromboembolic complications are difficult to manage because both anticoagulants and fibrinogen preparations have to be administered.

### New Preparations

The increasing need for fibrinogen preparations in congenital but also in acquired deficiencies has stimulated some companies to improve existing preparations or to develop new ones. A recombinant fibrinogen molecule is also under development.[74]

## ⬤DYSFIBRINOGENEMIA AND HYPODYSFIBRINOGENEMIA

### DEFINITION, HISTORY, AND EPIDEMIOLOGY

The second class of hereditary fibrinogen abnormalities comprises the type II disorders, that is, dysfibrinogenemia and hypodysfibrinogenemia. Dysfibrinogenemia is defined by the presence of normal levels of functionally abnormal plasma fibrinogen. Hypodysfibrinogenemia is defined by low levels of a dysfunctional protein. As in afibrinogenemia and hypofibrinogenemia, both are heterogeneous disorders caused by many different mutations in the three fibrinogen-encoding genes. Dysfibrinogenemias

and hypodysfibrinogenemias are autosomal dominant disorders. Most affected patients are heterozygous for missense mutations in the coding region of one of the three fibrinogen genes. Because the secreted fibrinogen hexamer contains two copies of each of the three fibrinogen chains, and the resulting fibrin network contains multiple copies of the molecule, heterozygosity for one mutant allele is sufficient to impair the structure and function of the fibrin clot (Fig. 15–4).

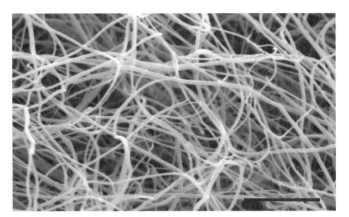
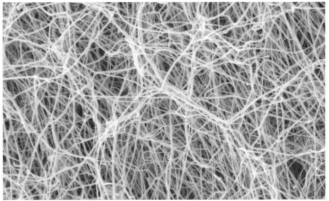
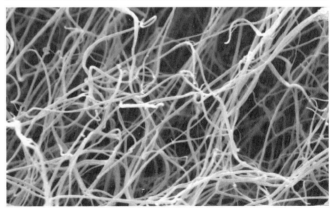

**Figure 15–4.** Scanning electron micrographs showing structural variations in clots formed from dysfibrinogens. **Top.** Control clot from normal purified fibrinogen clotted with thrombin showing relatively uniform distribution of fibers forming a branched network. **Middle.** Clot from fibrinogen Caracas I[96] showing very thin fibers, indicating a defect in lateral aggregation. **Bottom.** Clot from fibrinogen Caracas VI[97] showing a nonuniform distribution of thin and thick fibers in the clot, with bundles of fibers, larger pores, and more fiber ends than control clots. Magnification bar: 5 μm. (*Used with permission of John W. Weisel and Rita Marchi.*)

As of this writing, more than 100 distinct mutations have been identified in patients with dysfibrinogenemia and hypodysfibrinogenemia. The described mutants are very often named after the city of origin of the family or the city of the laboratory characterizing the mutation. Many cases are asymptomatic and are only identified as a result of routine coagulation screening. Indeed, a compilation of approximately 250 cases revealed that 55 percent of patients were asymptomatic, 25 percent had a history of bleeding, and 20 percent had a tendency toward thrombosis.[75] However, our retrospective multicentric study of the long-term outcomes of 101 genotyped patients suggests that bleeding and thrombotic events are more frequent.[76]

## ETIOLOGY AND PATHOGENESIS

Dysfibrinogenemic abnormalities usually are reflected in one or more phases of the fibrinogen-fibrin conversion and fibrin assembly process, notably impaired release of fibrinopeptides and defective fibrin polymerization or factor XIIIa–mediated crosslinking.[77,78] Other abnormalities involve abnormal tissue deposition such as in renal amyloidosis,[79] defective fibrinolysis,[80] abnormal interactions with platelets,[77,80] and defective calcium binding.[81]

### Mutations Resulting in Abnormal "A" Knobs or Deficient Fibrinopeptide Release

Fibrinogen Detroit was the first abnormal fibrinogen in which the specific mutation was identified at the protein level.[34] This *FGA* R38S (R19S) mutation is located in the "A" knob (i.e., GPRV), resulting in impaired fibrin polymerization and a bleeding tendency. Other substitutions involving residue R38 (R19) have been found to be associated with bleeding in some cases, for example, Munich I, R38N (R19N), and Mannheim I, R38G (R19G), and with thrombosis in other cases, for example, Aarhus and Kumamoto, which are also a result of R38G (R19G). The mechanism for thrombophilia remains unclear, but coexisting risk factors may contribute to the clinical manifestations. Furthermore, the inability of a mutant fibrin to effectively bind and sequester thrombin may play a role in such a clinical presentation. Bleeding that occurs under conditions involving defective fibrinopeptide release or production of a defective "A" knob is most likely related to the reduced polymerization potential of the mutant fibrins that are produced, with resulting defective clot formation.[82]

Missense mutations at residue *FGA* R35 (R16), which is part of the thrombin cleavage site in the fibrinogen α chain, appear to be the most common causative mutations accounting for dysfibrinogenemia, based on information compiled in the French Study Group on Hemostasis and Thrombosis registry for hereditary fibrinogen abnormalities.[5] The R35 (R16) residue can be mutated to either H (CGT→CAT) or C (CGT→TGT), leading to delayed or absent FpA release, respectively, and subsequent delayed polymerization. A prolonged reptilase time is observed for both variants. Most patients do not have a bleeding tendency. Some patients have been found to be homozygous for these mutations or phenotypically homozygous,[65] as a result of compound heterozygosity for an R35 (R16) missense mutation and the large 11-kb *FGA* deletion first characterized in afibrinogenemia. In these cases, a mild bleeding tendency is observed.

Missense mutations in *FGB* affecting FpB release have been identified[83] but are much less common than those affecting FpA release.

### Mutations Leading to Polymerization Defects in the D Region

Sites in the D region important for fibrin polymerization are affected in many dysfibrinogenemias. Mutations affecting hole "a" in the γ chain are numerous, while no naturally occurring mutation involving hole "b" in the Bβ chain has been described, compatible with the view that A:a

interactions are the driving force of fibrin polymerization.[16] The interface for the end-to-end D:D site in the γ chain lies between R301 (R275) and S326 (S300), with T306 (T280) contacting R301 (R275) at the D:D interface. Mutations at the R301 (R275) residue to C (CGT→TGT) or H (CGT→CAT) are the second most common cause of dysfibrinogenemia, accounting for around 10 percent of fibrinogen variants.[5] Impaired polymerization has been observed for all substitutions at this position. Most of these cases are asymptomatic, but some patients heterozygous for R301C (R275C) have thrombophilia, sometimes in association with an additional thrombotic risk factor such as factor V Leiden.[84]

### Mutations Accounting for Hypodysfibrinogenemia

Hypodysfibrinogenemia, which is defined by low levels of a dysfunctional protein, can be caused by different molecular mechanisms. One mechanism is heterozygosity for a single mutation that leads to synthesis of an abnormal fibrinogen chain that is secreted less efficiently than normal fibrinogen, for example, fibrinogen Kyoto IV.[85] Another mechanism is the presence of two different mutations with one mutation responsible for the fibrinogen deficiency (the "hypo phenotype") and one mutation responsible for the abnormal function of the molecule (the "dys phenotype"). For example, in fibrinogen Keokuk,[86] there is compound heterozygosity for the common afibrinogenemia splice-site mutation c.510G→T and a premature truncating nonsense mutation in *FGA* Q347X (Q328X). Another example is fibrinogen Leipzig II in which the common hypofibrinogenemia mutations *FGG* A108G (A82G) and *FGG* G377S (G351S) are located on the same allele.[87] Homozygosity for a single mutation, which allows reduced secretion of a functionally impaired molecule, has been described in fibrinogens Otago[88] and Marburg.[89] Finally, maternal uniparental disomy for a nonsense mutation in *FGB*, W323X (W293X), was found to be the cause of severe hypodysfibrinogenemia in a Chinese patient.[90]

## CLINICAL FEATURES

Patients with inherited dysfibrinogenemia are frequently asymptomatic and can be discovered incidentally because of abnormal coagulation tests. A compilation of more than 260 cases of dysfibrinogenemia revealed that 55 percent of the patients had no clinical complications while 25 percent exhibited bleeding, and 20 percent had a tendency to thrombosis, mainly venous.[75] However, when 2376 patients with deep vein thrombosis were screened for thrombophilia, the prevalence of dysfibrinogenemia was very low (0.8 percent), and hence testing for dysfibrinogenemia in patients with deep vein thrombosis is not recommended.[91] Patients with dysfibrinogenemia associated with hemorrhage bleed most often after trauma, surgery, or during the puerperium.[76] Thrombosis may also occur during pregnancy and in the postpartum period. Women with dysfibrinogenemia can also suffer from spontaneous abortions. The problems during and after pregnancy are not necessarily correlated to the fibrinogen concentration.

Some mutations in the Aα chain of fibrinogen are associated with a particular form of hereditary amyloidosis.[79,92] The E545V (E526V) amino acid substitution is the most common of these mutations.[92] The abnormal fibrinogen fragments form amyloid fibrils, and the extracellular deposition of these fibrils leads to renal failure. Chronic renal dialysis is performed for managing renal failure. Renal transplantation can be envisaged as an alternative to chronic dialysis. However, continuous fibrinogen-related amyloid deposition ultimately results in allograft destruction. Combined liver and kidney transplantation prevents further amyloid deposition in the renal allograft and elsewhere but is associated with additional perioperative and subsequent risks.

## LABORATORY FEATURES

### Phenotype Analysis

Initial screening tests for fibrinogen dysfunction should include fibrinogen concentration, measured functionally and immunochemically, TT, and reptilase time. Dysfibrinogenemia is diagnosed by a discrepancy between clottable and immunoreactive fibrinogen. However, even in specialized laboratories, this diagnosis can be difficult because the sensitivity of the tests depends on the specific mutation, reagents, and techniques.[93,94]

In classical dysfibrinogenemias, the functional assay of fibrinogen yields low levels compared with the immunologic assays, but levels are sometimes concordant, and the functional level may even be normal (as well as TT). The determination of the precise nature of a fibrinogen defect has to be performed in highly specialized laboratories since it involves purification of fibrinogen, measurement of the rate of fibrinopeptide cleavage, analysis of fibrin monomer polymerization, and fibrinolysis. Thromboelastography, commonly used for decision making for fibrinolytic and anticoagulant therapy, may be particularly useful for investigation of dysfibrinogenemia. The thromboelastography signal is fibrin dependent, and its amplitude is enhanced by platelets and reflects the stretch and recovery of the clot during its formation.[95]

### Genotype Analysis

The gold standard for the diagnosis of dysfibrinogenemia is the characterization of the molecular defect. However, although advances in DNA analysis have made mutation detection easier, it is not always clear whether the identified mutation is the cause of the presenting phenotype. Family studies showing segregation of the mutation with the phenotype, exclusion that the DNA alteration is a common polymorphism in the general population, and structural correlations are necessary for establishing the link between the DNA alteration and the disorder. As previously mentioned, two mutation "hotspots" are of prime interest in screening for dysfibrinogenemia mutations: residue R35 (R16) situated in *FGA* exon 2, and residue R301 (R275) in *FGG* exon 8. Other causative mutations are common in the surrounding residues. Thus, it is recommended to initially screen *FGA* exon 2 and *FGG* exon 8 in cases of dysfibrinogenemia. In our recent study of 101 dysfibrinogenemia cases,[76] 87 percent of the causative mutations were located in these two exons. Here, mutations of *FGG* R301 (R275) were more common than mutations of *FGA* R35 (R16) (52 percent and 23 percent, respectively).

### Genotype–Phenotype Correlations

As previously discussed, the clinical manifestations of dysfibrinogenemia are highly variable and may relate in some cases to differences in clot strength, structure, and stability.[1,17] In a few cases, mutations are predictive of the clinical phenotype, such as the R573C (R554C) substitution in the Aα chain (e.g., fibrinogens Chapel Hill III, Paris V, and Dusart) that predisposes patients to thrombosis. Impaired fibrinolysis exhibited by this dysfibrinogen appears to be responsible for the thrombotic complications. Other examples associated with thrombosis include dysfibrinogens Barcelona III, Haifa I, or Bergamo II as a result of the common γ R301H (R275H) mutation and Cedar Rapids I caused by γ R301C (R275C). However, in fibrinogen Cedar Rapids I, only patients heterozygous for both factor V Leiden and the *FGG* R301C (R275C) substitutions were symptomatic, suggesting that this mutation causes thrombosis when associated with another defect. On the other hand, several mutations in the aminoterminal region of the Aα chain, such as fibrinogen Detroit R38S (R19S) and Mannheim I R38G (R19G), are associated with bleeding.

## DIFFERENTIAL DIAGNOSIS

Inherited dysfibrinogenemia has to be distinguished from acquired dysfibrinogenemia. Liver diseases (e.g., cirrhosis, chronic active liver disease, hepatoma, liver failure) are the main causes of acquired dysfibrinogenemia. L-Asparaginase treatment also may result in the production of abnormal fibrinogen. In addition, there are a few case reports of acquired dysfibrinogenemia secondary to pancreatitis, paraneoplastic syndrome, and renal carcinoma. The acquired dysfibrinogenemias represent a heterogeneous group of disorders with multiple pathogenetic mechanisms, the most clearly defined fibrinogen abnormalities being an increase in carbohydrate content in patients with liver disease. These abnormal fibrinogens are usually characterized by prolonged thrombin and reptilase times, abnormal fibrin monomer polymerization, but normal fibrinopeptide release. Fibrinogen concentration is variable.

In some cases, no underlying disease is found, and to determine whether a fibrinogen abnormality is congenital or acquired may be difficult. The demonstration of the same fibrinogen abnormality in another family member is a strong argument for a congenital disorder. When measured in newborns, fibrinogen levels should be interpreted with caution because neonatal fibrinogen has an altered content of carbohydrate that can mimic dysfibrinogenemia in certain laboratory tests.

Rare cases of circulating autoantibodies to fibrinogen, for example in systemic lupus erythematosus and in patients receiving surgical sealants containing bovine fibrinogen, have also been reported.

## THERAPY

Any treatment considered in patients with dysfibrinogenemia should be based on the personal and family history. Indeed, as already discussed, subjects with hereditary dysfibrinogenemias may be asymptomatic throughout their whole life or may suffer from bleeding and/or thrombotic complications.[1,75,76] In patients who bleed, functional levels of fibrinogen should be raised above 1.0 g L$^{-1}$ and maintained above this threshold until hemostasis is secured and above 0.5 g L$^{-1}$ until wound healing is complete. Topical fibrin glue or antifibrinolytic agents may be used for superficial bleeds. In pregnant women with a bleeding phenotype, the recommendations for afibrinogenemia and hypofibrinogenemia can be followed. With a personal or familial history of thrombosis, thromboprophylaxis and antithrombotic treatments may be proposed after a careful analysis of each particular situation. Long-term management strategies for thrombophilic dysfibrinogenemia are the same as the strategies for patients with recurrent thromboembolism and may include long-term anticoagulant therapy.

## REFERENCES

1. de Moerloose P, Casini A, Neerman-Arbez M: Congenital fibrinogen disorders: An update. *Semin Thromb Hemost* 39:585, 2013.
2. Asselta R, Duga S, Tenchini ML: The molecular basis of quantitative fibrinogen disorders. *J Thromb Haemost* 4:2115, 2006.
3. Galanakis DK: Afibrinogenemias and dysfibrinogenemias, in *Hemostasis and Thrombosis: Basic Principles and Clinical Practice*, 6th ed, edited by JS Bennett, WC Aird, VJ Marder, S Schulman, GC White. Lippincott Williams and Wilkins, Baltimore, 2012.
4. Neerman-Arbez M, de Moerloose P: Hereditary fibrinogen abnormalities, in *Williams Hematology*, 8th ed, edited by M Lichtman, E Beutler, TJ Kipps, U Seligsohn, K Kaushansky, J Prchal, p 2051. McGraw-Hill, New York, 2010.
5. Hanss M, Biot F: A database for human fibrinogen variants. *Ann N Y Acad Sci* 936:89, 2001.
6. Mosesson MW: Update on antithrombin I (fibrin). *Thromb Haemost* 98:105, 2007.
7. Tennent GA, Brennan SO, Stangou AJ, et al: Human plasma fibrinogen is synthesized in the liver. *Blood* 109:1971, 2007.
8. Medved L, Weisel JW: Recommendations for nomenclature on fibrinogen and fibrin. *J Thromb Haemost* 7:355, 2009.
9. Kant J, Fornace AJ Jr, Saxe D, et al: Organization and evolution of the human fibrinogen locus on chromosome four. *Proc Natl Acad Sci U S A* 82:2344, 1985.
10. de Maat M, Verschuur M: Fibrinogen heterogeneity: Inherited and noninherited. *Curr Opin Hematol* 12:377, 2005.
11. Huang S, Mulvihill ER, Farrell DH, et al: Biosynthesis of human fibrinogen. Subunit interactions and potential intermediates in the assembly. *J Biol Chem* 268:8919, 1993.
12. Henschen-Edman AH: On the identification of beneficial and detrimental molecular forms of fibrinogen. *Haemostasis* 29:179, 1999.

13. Collen D, Tytgat GN, Claeys H, Piessens R: Metabolism and distribution of fibrinogen I. *Br J Haematol* 22:681, 1972.

14. Handagama P, Scarborough RM, Shuman MA, Bainton DF: Endocytosis of fibrinogen into megakaryocytes and platelet alpha-granules is mediated by alpha IIb beta 3 (glycoprotein IIb-IIIa). *Blood* 82:135, 1993.

15. Francis CW, Nachman RL, Marder VJ: Plasma and platelet fibrinogen differ in gamma chain content. *Thromb Haemost* 51:84, 1984.

16. Weisel JW, Litvinov RI: Mechanisms of fibrin polymerization and clinical implications. *Blood* 121:1712, 2013.

17. Ariëns RA: Fibrin(ogen) and thrombotic disease. *J Thromb Haemost* 11(Suppl 1):294, 2013.

18. Mosesson MW: The structure and biological features of fibrinogen and fibrin. *Ann N Y Acad Sci* 936:11, 2001.

19. Mosesson MW, DiOrio JP, Siebenlist KR, et al: Evidence for a second type of fibril branch point in fibrin polymer networks, the trimolecular junction. *Blood* 82:1517, 1993.

20. Lord ST: Fibrinogen and fibrin: Scaffold proteins in hemostasis. *Curr Opin Hematol* 14:236, 2007.

21. Medved LV, Litvinovich SV, Ugarova TP, et al: Localization of a fibrin polymerization site complimentary to Gly-His-Arg sequence. *FEBS Lett* 320:239, 1993.

22. Yang Z, Mochalkin I, Doolittle RF: A model of fibrin formation based on crystal structures of fibrinogen and fibrin fragments complexed with synthetic peptides. *Proc Natl Acad Sci U S A* 97:14156, 2000.

23. Weisel JW, Medved LV: The structure and function of the alpha C domains of fibrinogen. *Ann N Y Acad Sci* 936:312, 2001.

24. Mosesson MW, Siebenlist KR, Hainfeld JF, Wall JS: The covalent structure of factor XIIIa crosslinked fibrinogen fibrils. *J Struct Biol* 115:88, 1995.

25. Siebenlist KR, Meh D, Mosesson MW: Protransglutaminase (factor XIII) mediated crosslinking of fibrinogen and fibrin. *Thromb Haemost* 86:1221, 2001.

26. Mosesson MW, Siebenlist KR, Hernandez I, et al: Evidence that alpha2-antiplasmin becomes covalently ligated to plasma fibrinogen in the circulation: A new role for plasma factor XIII in fibrinolysis regulation. *J Thromb Haemost* 6:1565, 2008.

27. Smith KA, Pease RJ, Avery CA, et al: The activation peptide cleft exposed by thrombin cleavage of FXIII-A(2) contains a recognition site for the fibrinogen α chain. *Blood* 121:2117, 2013.

28. Makogonenko E, Ingham KC, Medved L: Interaction of the fibronectin COOH-terminal Fib-2 regions with fibrin: Further characterization and localization of the Fib-2-binding sites. *Biochemistry* 46:5418, 2006.

29. Mosesson MW, Siebenlist KR, Voskuilen M, Nieuwenhuizen W: Evaluation of the factors contributing to fibrin-dependent plasminogen activation. *Thromb Haemost* 79:796, 1998.

30. Medved L, Niewenhuizen W: Molecular mechanisms of initiation of fibrinolysis by fibrin. *Thromb Haemost* 89:409, 2003.

31. Rijken DC, Lijnen HR: New insights into the molecular mechanisms of the fibrinolytic system. *J Thromb Haemost* 7:4, 2009.

32. Uitte de Willige S, de Visser MC, Houwing-Duistermaat JJ, et al: Genetic variation in the fibrinogen gamma gene increases the risk for deep venous thrombosis by reducing plasma fibrinogen gamma' levels. *Blood* 106:4176, 2005.

33. Fredenburgh JC, Stafford AR, Leslie BA, Weitz JI: Bivalent binding to gammaA/gamma'-fibrin engages both exosites of thrombin and protects it from inhibition by the antithrombin-heparin complex. *J Biol Chem* 283:2470, 2008.

34. Blomback M, Blomback B, Mammen EF, Prasad AS: Fibrinogen Detroit—A molecular defect in the N-terminal disulphide knot of human fibrinogen? *Nature* 218:134, 1968.

35. Neerman-Arbez M, Honsberger A, Antonarakis SE, Morris MA: Deletion of the fibrinogen alpha-chain gene (FGA) causes congenital afibrinogenemia. *J Clin Invest* 103:215, 1999.

36. Rabe F, Salomon E: Ueber-faserstoffmangel im Blute bei einem Falle von Hämophilie. *Arch Intern Med* 95:2, 1920.

37. Peyvandi F, Mannucci PM: Rare coagulation disorders. *Thromb Haemost* 82:1207, 1999.

38. Watanabe K, Shibuya A, Ishii E, et al: Identification of simultaneous mutation of fibrinogen alpha chain and protein C genes in a Japanese kindred. *Br J Haematol* 120:101, 2003.

39. Spena S, Duga S, Asselta R, et al: Congenital afibrinogenaemia caused by uniparental isodisomy of chromosome 4 containing a novel 15-kb deletion involving fibrinogen A alpha-chain gene. *Eur J Hum Genet* 12:891, 2004.

40. Monaldini L, Asselta R, Duga S, et al: Mutational screening of six afibrinogenemic patients: Identification and characterization of four novel molecular defects. *Thromb Haemost* 97:546, 2007.

41. Neerman-Arbez M, de Moerloose P: Mutations in the fibrinogen gene cluster accounting for congenital afibrinogenemia: An update and report of 10 novel mutations. *Hum Mutat* 28:540, 2006.

42. Robert-Ebadi H, de Moerloose P, El Khorassani M, et al: A novel frameshift mutation in FGA accounting for congenital afibrinogenemia predicted to encode an aberrant peptide terminating 158 amino acids downstream. *Blood Coagul Fibrinolysis* 20:385, 2009.

43. Casini A, Lukowski S, Quintard VL, et al: FGB mutations leading to congenital quantitative fibrinogen deficiencies: An update and report of four novel mutations. *Thromb Res* 133:868, 2014.

44. Homer VM, Brennan SO, Ockelford P, George PM: Novel fibrinogen truncation with deletion of Bbeta chain residues 440–461 causes hypofibrinogenaemia. *Thromb Haemost* 88:427, 2002.

45. Neerman-Arbez M, Vu D, Abu-Libdeh B, et al: Prenatal diagnosis for congenital afibrinogenemia caused by a novel nonsense mutation in the FGB gene in a Palestinian family. *Blood* 101:3492, 2003.

46. Vu D, Di Sanza C, Caille D, et al: Quality control of fibrinogen secretion in the molecular pathogenesis of congenital afibrinogenemia. *Hum Mol Genet* 14:3271, 2005.

47. Duga S, Asselta R, Santagostino E, et al: Missense mutations in the human beta fibrinogen gene cause congenital afibrinogenemia by impairing fibrinogen secretion. *Blood* 95:1336, 2000.

48. Vu D, Bolton-Maggs PH, Parr JR, et al: Congenital afibrinogenemia: Identification and expression of a missense mutation in FGB impairing fibrinogen secretion. *Blood* 102:4413, 2003.

49. Spena S, Asselta R, Duga S, et al: Congenital afibrinogenemia: Intracellular retention of fibrinogen due to a novel W437G mutation in the fibrinogen B beta-chain gene. *Biochim Biophys Acta* 1639:87, 2003.

50. Monaldini L, Asselta R, Duga S, et al: Fibrinogen Mumbai: Intracellular retention due to a novel G434D mutation in the Bbeta-chain gene. *Haematologica* 91:628, 2006.

51. Terasawa F, Okumura N, Kitano K, et al: Hypofibrinogenemia associated with a heterozygous missense mutation gamma153Cys to Arg (Matsumoto IV): In vitro expression demonstrates defective secretion of the variant fibrinogen. *Blood* 94:4122, 1999.

52. Vu D, de Moerloose P, Batorova A, et al: Hypofibrinogenaemia caused by a novel FGG missense mutation (W253C) in the gamma chain globular domain impairing fibrinogen secretion. *J Med Genet* 42:e57, 2005.

53. Brennan SO, Wyatt J, Medicina D, et al: Fibrinogen Brescia: Hepatic endoplasmic reticulum storage and hypofibrinogenemia because of a gamma284 Gly→Arg mutation. *Am J Pathol* 157:189, 2000.

54. Brennan SO, Maghzal G, Shneider BL, et al: Novel fibrinogen gamma375 Arg→Trp mutation (fibrinogen Aguadilla) causes hepatic endoplasmic reticulum storage and hypofibrinogenemia. *Hepatology* 36:652, 2002.

55. Brennan SO, Davis RL, Conard K, et al: Novel fibrinogen mutation γ314Thr→Pro (fibrinogen AI duPont) associated with hepatic fibrinogen storage disease and hypofibrinogenaemia. *Liver Int* 30:1541, 2010.

56. Dib N, Quelin F, Ternisien C, et al: Fibrinogen Angers with a new deletion gamma GVYYQ 346–350 causes hypofibrinogenemia with hepatic storage. *J Thromb Haemost* 5:1999, 2007.

57. Peyvandi F, Kaufman RJ, Seligsohn U, et al: Rare bleeding disorders. *Haemophilia* 12(Suppl 3):137, 2006.

58. Van Meegeren ME, de Rooy JW, Schreuder HW, Brons PP: Bone cysts in patients with afibrinogenaemia: A literature review and two new cases. *Haemophilia* 20:244, 2014.

59. Iwaki T, Sandoval-Cooper MJ, Paiva M, et al: Fibrinogen stabilizes placental-maternal attachment during embryonic development in the mouse. *Am J Pathol* 160:1021, 2002.

60. Korte W, Feldges A: Increased prothrombin activation in a patient with congenital afibrinogenemia is reversible by fibrinogen substitution. *Clin Investig* 72:396, 1994.

61. Ni H, Denis CV, Subbarao S, et al: Persistence of platelet thrombus formation in arterioles of mice lacking both von Willebrand factor and fibrinogen. *J Clin Invest* 106:385, 2000.

62. Fish RJ, Di Sanza C, Neerman-Arbez M: Targeted mutation of zebrafish FGA models human congenital afibrinogenemia. *Blood* 123:2278, 2014.

63. Remjin JA, Wu Y-P, Ijsseldijk W, et al: Absence of fibrinogen in afibrinogenemia results in large but loosely packed thrombi under flow conditions. *Thromb Haemost* 85:736, 2001.

64. de Moerloose P, Neerman-Arbez M: Treatment of congenital fibrinogen disorders. *Expert Opin Biol Ther* 8:979, 2008.

65. Galanakis DK, Neerman-Arbez M, Scheiner T, et al: Homophenotypic A-alpha R16H fibrinogen (Kingsport): Uniquely altered polymerization associated with slower fibrinopeptide A than fibrinopeptide B release. *Blood Coagul Fibrinolysis* 18:731, 2007.

66. Neerman-Arbez M, Vu D, Abu-Libdeh B, et al: Prenatal diagnosis for congenital afibrinogenemia caused by a novel nonsense mutation in the FGB gene in a Palestinian family. *Blood* 101:3492, 2003.

67. Kalina U, Stöhr HA, Bickhard H, et al: Rotational thromboelastography for monitoring of fibrinogen concentrate therapy in fibrinogen deficiency. *Blood Coagul Fibrinolysis* 19:777, 2008.

68. Bolton-Maggs PH, Perry DJ, Chalmers EA, et al: The rare coagulation disorders—Review with guidelines for management from the United Haemophilia Centre Doctor's Organisation. *Haemophilia* 10:593, 2004.

69. Grech H, Majumdar G, Lawrie AS, Savidge GF: Pregnancy in congenital afibrinogenaemia: Report of a successful case and review of the literature. *Br J Haematol* 78:571, 1991.

70. Kobayashi T, Kanayama N, Tokunaga N, et al: Prenatal and peripartum management of congenital afibrinogenaemia. *Br J Haematol* 109:364, 2000.

71. Fuchs RJ, Levin J, Tadel M, Merritt W: Perioperative coagulation management in a patient with afibrinogenemia undergoing liver transplantation. *Liver Transpl* 13:752, 2007.

72. Stroka D, Keogh A, Vu D, et al: In vitro rescue of FGA deletion by lentiviral transduction of afibrinogenemic patient's hepatocytes. *J Thromb Haemost* 12:1874, 2014.

73. Schuepbach RA, Meili EO, Schneider E, et al: Lepirudin therapy for thrombotic complications in congenital afibrinogenaemia. *Thromb Haemost* 91:1044, 2004.

74. Radulovic V, Baghaei F, Blixter IF, et al: Comparable effect of recombinant and plasma-derived human fibrinogen concentrate on ex vivo clot formation after cardiac surgery. *J Thromb Haemost* 10:1696, 2012.

75. Haverkate F, Samama M: Familial dysfibrinogenemia and thrombophilia. Report on a study of the SSC Subcommittee on Fibrinogen. *Thromb Haemost* 73:151, 1995.

76. Casini A, Blondon M, Lebreton A, et al: Natural history of patients with congenital dysfibrinogenemia. *Blood* 125:553, 2015.

77. Rosenberg JB, Newman PJ, Mosesson MW, et al: Paris I dysfibrinogenemia: A point mutation in intron 8 results in insertion of a 15 amino acid sequence in the fibrinogen gamma-chain. *Thromb Haemost* 69:217, 1993.
78. Hamano A, Mimuro J, Aoshima M, et al: Thrombophilic dysfibrinogen Tokyo V with the amino acid substitution of gammaAla327Thr: Formation of fragile but fibrinolysis-resistant fibrin clots and its relevance to arterial thromboembolism. *Blood* 103:3045, 2004.
79. Uemichi T, Liepnieks JJ, Benson MD: Hereditary renal amyloidosis with a novel variant fibrinogen. *J Clin Invest* 93:731, 1994.
80. Miesbach W, Scharrer I, Henschen A, et al: Inherited dysfibrinogenemia: Clinical phenotypes associated with five different fibrinogen structure defects. *Blood Coagul Fibrinolysis* 21:35–40, 2010.
81. Koopman J, Haverkate F, Briet E, Lord ST: A congenitally abnormal fibrinogen (Vlissingen) with a 6-base deletion in the gamma-chain gene, causing defective calcium binding and impaired fibrin polymerization. *J Biol Chem* 266:13456, 1991.
82. Casini A, De Maistre E, Casini-Stuppi V, et al: Fibrinogen Geneva II: A new congenitally abnormal fibrinogen alpha chain (Gly17Asp) with a review of similar mutations resulting in abnormal knob A. *Blood Coagul Fibrinolysis* 25:280, 2014.
83. Hirota-Kawadobora M, Terasawa F, Yonekawa O, et al: Fibrinogens Kosai and Ogasa: Bbeta15Gly→Cys (GGT→TGT) substitution associated with impairment of fibrinopeptide B release and lateral aggregation. *J Thromb Haemost* 1:275, 2003.
84. Siebenlist KR, Mosesson MW, Meh DA, et al: Coexisting dysfibrinogenemia (gammaR275C) and factor V Leiden deficiency associated with thromboembolic disease (fibrinogen Cedar Rapids). *Blood Coagul Fibrinolysis* 11:293, 2000.
85. Okumura N, Terasawa F, Hirota-Kawadobora M, et al: A novel variant fibrinogen, deletion of Bbeta111Ser in coiled-coil region, affecting fibrin lateral aggregation. *Clin Chim Acta* 365:160, 2006.
86. Lefebvre P, Velasco PT, Dear A, et al: Severe hypodysfibrinogenemia in compound heterozygotes of the fibrinogen AalphaIVS4 + 1G→T mutation and an AalphaGln328 truncation (fibrinogen Keokuk). *Blood* 103:2571, 2004.
87. Meyer M, Dietzel H, Kaetzel R, et al: Fibrinogen Leipzig II (gamma351Gly→Ser and gamma82Ala→Gly): Hypodysfibrinogenaemia due to two independent amino acid substitutions within the same polypeptide chain. *Thromb Haemost* 98:903, 2007.
88. Ridgway HJ, Brennan SO, Faed JM, George PM: Fibrinogen Otago: A major alpha chain truncation associated with severe hypofibrinogenaemia and recurrent miscarriage. *Br J Haematol* 98:632, 1997.
89. Koopman J, Haverkate F, Grimbergen J, et al: Fibrinogen Marburg: A homozygous case of dysfibrinogenemia, lacking amino acids A alpha 461–610 (Lys 461 AAA→stop TAA). *Blood* 80:1972, 1992.
90. Ding Q, Ouyang Q, Xi X, et al: Maternal chromosome 4 heterodisomy/isodisomy and Bβ chain Trp323X mutation resulting in severe hypodysfibrinogenaemia. *Thromb Haemost* 108:654, 2012.
91. Hayes T: Dysfibrinogenemia and thrombosis. *Arch Pathol Lab Med* 126:1387, 2002.
92. Uemichi T, Liepnieks JJ, Benson MD: Hereditary renal amyloidosis with a novel variant fibrinogen. *J Clin Invest* 93:731, 1994.
93. Shapiro SE, Phillips E, Manning RA, et al: Clinical phenotype, laboratory features and genotype of 35 patients with heritable dysfibrinogenaemia. *Br J Haematol* 160:220, 2013.
94. Miesbach W, Schenk J, Alesci S, Lindhoff-Last E: Comparison of the fibrinogen Clauss assay and the fibrinogen PT derived method in patients with dysfibrinogenemia. *Thromb Res* 126:e428, 2010.
95. Galanakis DK, Neerman-Arbez M, Brennan S, et al: Thromboelastographic phenotypes of fibrinogen and its variants: Clinical and non-clinical implications. *Thromb Res* 133:1115, 2014.
96. Marchi R, Meyer M, de Bosch N, et al: Biophysical characterization of fibrinogen Caracas I with an Aalpha-chain truncation at Aalpha-466 Ser: Identification of the mutation and biophysical characterization of properties of clots from plasma and purified fibrinogen. *Blood Coagul Fibrinolysis* 15:285, 2004.
97. Marchi RC, Meyer MH, de Bosch NB, et al: A novel mutation (deletion of Aalpha-Asn 80) in an abnormal fibrinogen: Fibrinogen Caracas VI. Consequences of disruption of the coiled-coil for the polymerization of fibrin: Peculiar clot structure and diminished stiffness of the clot. *Blood Coagul Fibrinolysis* 15:559, 2004.

# CHAPTER 16
# VON WILLEBRAND DISEASE

Jill Johnsen and David Ginsburg

## SUMMARY

von Willebrand factor (VWF) is a central component of hemostasis, serving both as an adhesive link between platelets and the injured blood vessel wall and as a carrier for clotting factor VIII (FVIII). Abnormalities in VWF function result in von Willebrand disease (VWD), the most common inherited bleeding disorder in humans. The overall prevalence of VWD has been estimated to be as high as 1 percent of the general population, although the prevalence of clinically significant disease is probably closer to 1:1000. VWD is associated with either quantitative deficiency (type 1 and type 3) or qualitative abnormalities of VWF (type 2). The uncommon type 3 variant is the most severe form of VWD and is characterized by very low or undetectable levels of VWF, a severe bleeding diathesis, and a generally autosomal recessive pattern of inheritance. Type 1 VWD, the most common variant, is characterized by VWF that is normal in structure and function but decreased in quantity (in the range of 20 to 50 percent of normal). In type 2 VWD, the VWF is abnormal in structure and/or function. Type 2A VWD is associated with selective loss of the largest and most functionally active VWF multimers. Type 2A is further subdivided into group 1, as a result of mutations that interfere with biosynthesis and secretion, and group 2, in which the mutant VWF exhibits an increased sensitivity to proteolysis in plasma. Type 2B VWD is caused by mutations clustered within the VWF A1 domain, in a segment critical for binding to the platelet glycoprotein Ib receptor. These mutations produce a "gain of function" resulting in spontaneous VWF binding to platelets and clearance of the resulting platelet complexes, leading to thrombocytopenia and loss of the most active (large) VWF multimers. Type 2N VWD is characterized by mutations within the FVIII binding domain of VWF, leading to disproportionately decreased factor VIII and a disorder resembling mild to moderate hemophilia A, but with autosomal rather than X-linked inheritance. Type 1 VWD can often be effectively managed by treatment with DDAVP (1-deamino-8-D-arginine vasopressin, desmopressin), which produces a two- to threefold increase in plasma VWF level due to release from endothelial storage sites in the vessel wall. Response to DDAVP is generally poor in type 3 and some type 2 VWD variants. These disorders often require treatment with factor replacement in the form of VWF/FVIII concentrates containing large quantities of intact VWF multimers.

Acronyms and Abbreviations: ADAMTS13, a disintegrin and metalloprotease with thrombospondin type 1 motifs; aPTT, activated partial thromboplastin time; DDAVP, 1-desamino-8-D-arginine vasopressin or desmopressin; ER, endoplasmic reticulum; GP, glycoprotein; HHT, hereditary hemorrhagic telangiectasia; ISTH, International Society on Thrombosis and Haemostasis; PCR, polymerase chain reaction; RIPA, ristocetin-induced platelet aggregation; VWD, von Willebrand disease; VWF, von Willebrand factor.

## DEFINITION AND HISTORY

In 1926, Eric von Willebrand described a bleeding disorder in 24 of 66 members of a family from the Åland Islands.[1] Both sexes were afflicted, and the bleeding time was prolonged despite normal platelet counts and normal clot retraction. von Willebrand distinguished this condition from the other hemostatic diseases known at the time and recognized its genetic basis, calling the disorder "hereditary pseudohemophilia," but incorrectly characterizing the inheritance as X-linked dominant. von Willebrand's confusion about the inheritance pattern was probably the result of, at least in part, the greater recognition of bleeding symptoms in women because of the hemostatic stresses of menstruation and parturition. The proband in the original family, Hjördis, was 5 years old at the time of von Willebrand's initial evaluation and ultimately died at age 13 years during her fourth menstrual cycle. Four of Hjördis' sisters died between the ages of 2 and 4 years, and deaths in the family were also noted during childbirth.

An apparently similar disorder was independently reported in the United States by Minot and others in 1928. The original family in the Åland Islands was reexamined by von Willebrand and Jürgens in 1933, leading to the conclusion that the defect in this disorder was caused by an impairment of platelet function. It was not until 1953 that Alexander and Goldstein demonstrated reduced levels of coagulation factor VIII (FVIII) in von Willebrand disease (VWD) patients, along with prolonged bleeding time. This observation was confirmed by others, including studies of the original von Willebrand pedigree by Nilsson and coworkers. In the late 1950s, Nilsson and coworkers demonstrated that a fraction of plasma referred to as "I-O" could correct the FVIII deficiency and normalize the bleeding time, indicating that the defect in VWD was a result of the deficiency of a plasma factor rather than an intrinsic platelet abnormality. Infusion of fraction I-O promptly increased the FVIII level in a hemophilic patient, while in VWD, the FVIII level rose gradually, peaking at 5 to 8 hours. Fraction I-O prepared from a hemophilia A patient was also shown to correct the defect in VWD, demonstrating that these disorders were caused by deficiencies of distinct plasma factors (reviewed in Refs. 2 and 3).

It was not until 1971 that Zimmerman, Ratnoff, and Powell prepared the first antibodies against what was thought to be a highly purified form of FVIII.[4] This FVIII-related antigen was found to be normal in hemophilia A patients but decreased in VWD. This puzzle was finally resolved with the demonstration that von Willebrand factor (VWF) and FVIII are closely associated, with more than 98 percent of the mass of the complex made up of VWF (see section "The Function of von Willebrand Factor" below). Thus, antibodies raised against this complex predominantly recognize VWF. The first direct assay of VWF function was based on the observation that the antibiotic ristocetin induced thrombocytopenia and the demonstration by Howard and Firkin[5] that ristocetin-induced platelet aggregation (RIPA) was absent in some VWD patients. Weiss and coworkers[6] used this observation to develop a quantitative assay for VWF function that remains a mainstay of laboratory evaluation for VWD to this day. In 1973, several groups succeeded in dissociating VWF from FVIII procoagulant activity.[7,8]

Final proof that VWF and FVIII are independent proteins encoded by distinct genes came with the complementary DNA (cDNA) cloning of the two molecules in 1984 and 1985.[9-14] These discoveries also marked the beginning of the molecular genetic era for the study of VWF and FVIII, leading to the identification of gene mutations in many patients with hemophilia and VWD, as well as considerable insight into the structure and function of these related proteins.

Table 16-1 summarizes the current nomenclature and terminology for FVIII and VWF. VWD is a heterogeneous disorder with more

**TABLE 16–1.** von Willebrand Factor and Factor VIII Terminology

**Factor VIII**

Antihemophilic factor, the protein that is reduced in plasma of patients with classic hemophilia A and most von Willebrand disease (VWD) and is measured in standard coagulation assays

**Factor VIII activity (factor VIII:C)**

The coagulant property of the factor VIII protein (this term is sometimes used interchangeably with factor VIII)

**Factor VIII antigen (VIII:Ag)**

The antigenic determinant(s) on factor VIII measured by immunoassays, which may employ polyclonal or monoclonal antibodies

**von Willebrand factor (VWF)**

The large multimeric glycoprotein that is necessary for normal platelet adhesion, a normal bleeding time, and stabilizing factor VIII

**von Willebrand factor antigen (VWF:Ag)**

The antigenic determinant(s) on VWF measured by immunoassays, which may employ polyclonal or monoclonal antibodies; *inaccurate designations of historical interest only* include factor VIII-related antigen (VIIIR:Ag), factor VIII antigen, AHF antigen, and AHF-like antigen

**Ristocetin cofactor activity (VWF:RCo)**

The property of VWF that supports ristocetin-induced agglutination of washed or fixed normal platelets

**von Willebrand factor collagen-binding activity (VWF:CB)**

The property of VWF that supports binding to collagen, measured by enzyme-linked immunosorbent assay (ELISA)

than 20 variants described. The previous complex and confusing classification has been consolidated and simplified into six distinct types,[15] as summarized in Table 16–2. Type 3 VWD is associated with very low or undetectable levels of VWF and severe bleeding. Type 1 VWD is characterized by concordant reductions in FVIII activity, VWF antigen, and ristocetin cofactor activity, generally to the range of 20 to 30 percent of normal, but sometimes up to 50 percent of normal, in association with a normal VWF multimer distribution. Type 2 VWD is heterogeneous and further divided into four subtypes (2A, 2B, 2M, and 2N) by the nature of the VWF qualitative dysfunction. Type 2A VWD results from abnormal VWF secretion or proteolysis and is characterized by a disproportionately low level of ristocetin cofactor activity relative to VWF antigen and absence of large and intermediate-sized multimers. Type 2B VWD results from an abnormal VWF molecule with increased affinity for platelet glycoprotein Ib (GPIb) and can also be associated with reduced high-molecular-weight VWF multimers and thrombocytopenia. Functional abnormalities in VWF can also result in defective interactions with platelets, as in type 2M VWD, or decreased FVIII binding to VWF, designated type 2N VWD and characterized by mild to moderate FVIII deficiency. Many other subtypes have been reported, including platelet-type (pseudo-) VWD, which is actually an intrinsic platelet disorder caused by mutations in GPIb (Chap. 10). Finally, acquired forms of VWD also occur, such as in patients with antibodies to VWF or thrombocytosis secondary to myeloproliferative neoplasms, resulting in accelerated loss of circulating VWF.

# ETIOLOGY AND PATHOGENESIS

VWF is synthesized exclusively in endothelial cells and megakaryocytes. The VWF monomer is assembled into higher-order multimers, a structure required for optimal adhesive function, and performs two major functions in hemostasis. First, VWF serves as the initial critical bridge between circulating platelets and the injured blood vessel wall, accounting for the apparent defect in platelet function and prolonged bleeding times historically observed in VWD patients. Second, VWF serves as the carrier in plasma for FVIII, ensuring its stability and localizing it to the initial platelet plug for participation in thrombin generation and fibrin clot formation (Chap. 3). This tight, noncovalent interaction between VWF and FVIII accounts for the copurification of these two molecules and the resulting initial confusion as to the origin of hemophilia and VWD. FVIII is encoded by the *F8* gene on the X chromosome (Chaps. 3 and 13), while VWF is encoded by the *VWF* gene on human chromosome 12.

## THE VON WILLEBRAND FACTOR GENE AND COMPLEMENTARY DNA

The VWF cDNA was initially cloned from endothelial cells[11–14] and the corresponding gene mapped to the short arm of chromosome 12 (12p13.3).[11] The VWF mRNA is approximately 9 kb in length, encoding a primary translation product of 2813 amino acid residues with an estimated $M_r$ of 310,000. Comparison of the primary peptide sequence obtained from plasma VWF[16] with the VWF cDNA sequence established the prepropolypeptide nature of VWF.[17] Prepropolypeptide VWF is composed of a 22-amino-acid signal peptide, a 741-amino-acid precursor polypeptide known as the VWF propeptide (VWFpp), and the mature subunit.[11,17–20] Cleavage of the 741-amino-acid propeptide from the amino terminus produces the mature VWF monomer subunit of 2050 amino acids (Fig. 16–1).

Analysis of the VWF sequence identifies four distinct types of repeated domains: three A domains, three B domains, two C domains, and four D domains,[18,21] within which appear additional repeating motifs (schematic in Ref. 22). The first pair of D domains is tandemly arranged in the VWFpp, followed by a partial and full D domain at the N terminus of the mature subunit. The final complete D domain is separated by a segment of more than 600 amino acids containing the triplicated A domains. The repeated domain structure of VWF suggests that the gene may have evolved via a complex series of partial duplications, although exon structure is not highly conserved between homologous domains.

Comparison of the VWF amino acid sequence to other proteins identifies a superfamily of related proteins that share sequence similarity with the VWF A domains.[23] The common theme among these potentially evolutionarily related genes is a role in extracellular matrix or adhesive function. Consistent with this notion, VWF functional domains for binding to the platelet receptor GPIb and specific ligands within the extracellular matrix have been localized to the VWF A repeats. A potential relationship between the VWF C domains and portions of thrombospondin and procollagen has also been proposed.[24]

The *VWF* gene spans 178 kb and is divided into 52 exons.[25] Exons range in size from 40 bases to 1.4 kb (exon 28). Exon 28 is unusually large, encoding the entire A1 and A2 domains and containing most of the known type 2A and all of the type 2B VWD mutations. The concentration of these defects within one exon has facilitated the identification of human mutations responsible for these VWD variants (see "Molecular Genetics of von Willebrand Disease," below). A partial, nonfunctional duplication of the *VWF* gene, termed a pseudogene, is located on human chromosome 22.[26] The pseudogene, known as *VWFP1*, duplicates the

**TABLE 16-2.** Classification of von Willebrand Disease

| Type | Molecular Characteristics | Inheritance | Frequency | Factor VIII Activity | VWF Antigen | Ristocetin Cofactor Activity | RIPA | Plasma VWF Multimer Structure |
|------|---------------------------|-------------|-----------|----------------------|-------------|------------------------------|------|-------------------------------|
| Type 1 | Partial quantitative VWF deficiency | Autosomal dominant, incomplete penetrance | 1–30:1000; most common VWD variant (>70% of VWD) | Decreased | Decreased | Decreased | Decreased or normal | Normal distribution (mutant subunits permitted) |
| Type 3 | Severe quantitative reduction or absence of VWF | Autosomal recessive (or codominant) | 1–5:1,000,000 | Markedly decreased | Very low or absent | Very low or absent | Absent | Usually absent |
| Type 2A | Qualitative VWF defect; loss of large VWF multimers, decreased VWF-dependent platelet adhesion | Usually autosomal dominant | ~10–15% of clinically significant VWD | Decreased to normal | Usually low | Markedly decreased | Decreased | Largest and intermediate multimers absent |
| Type 2B | Qualitative VWF defect; increased VWF–platelet interaction (GPIb) | Autosomal dominant | Uncommon variant (<5% of clinical VWD) | Decreased to normal | Usually low | Decreased to normal | Increased to low concentrations of ristocetin | Largest multimers reduced/absent |
| Type 2M | Qualitative VWF defect; decreased VWF–platelet interaction, no loss of large VWF multimers | Usually autosomal dominant | Rare (case reports) | Variably decreased | Variably decreased | Decreased | Variably decreased | Normal and occasionally ultralarge forms |
| Type 2N | Qualitative VWF defect; decreased VWF–factor VIII binding capacity | Autosomal recessive | Uncommon; heterozygotes may be prevalent in some populations | Decreased | Normal | Normal | Normal | Normal |
| Platelet-type (pseudo-) | Platelet defect; increased platelet–VWF interactions | Autosomal dominant | Rare | Decreased to normal | Decreased to normal | Decreased | Increased to low concentrations of ristocetin | Largest multimers absent |

GPIb, glycoprotein Ib; RIPA, ristocetin-induced platelet aggregation; VWD, von Willebrand disease; VWF, von Willebrand factor.

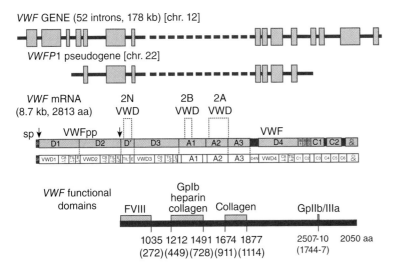

VWF GENE (52 introns, 178 kb) [chr. 12]

VWFP1 pseudogene [chr. 22]

VWF mRNA (8.7 kb, 2813 aa)

2N VWD   2B VWD   2A VWD

sp   VWFpp   VWF

D1   D2   D'   D3   A1   A2   A3   D4   C1   C2

VWF functional domains

FVIII   GpIb heparin collagen   Collagen   GpIIb/IIIa

1035 1212 1491 1674 1877   2507-10   2050 aa
(272) (449) (728) (911) (1114)   (1744-7)

**Figure 16–1.** Schematic of the human *VWF* gene, mRNA, and protein. The *VWF* gene and *VWFP1* pseudogene are depicted at the top, with boxes representing exons and the solid black line representing introns. Schematics of the VWF mRNA encoding the full prepro-VWF subunit are depicted in the middle as bar and lettered boxes. The upper schematic denotes commonly annotated regions of internally repeated sequences; the lower schematic illustrates the multiple repeating motifs of VWF. The locations of signal peptide (sp) and VWF propeptide (VWFpp) cleavage sites are indicated by *arrowheads*. The approximate localizations for known VWF functional domains within the mature VWF subunit are indicated at the bottom. Numbers underneath the domains refer to amino acid residues numbered from the ATG start site; numbers in parentheses indicate the amino acid residue position in the mature VWF subunit. aa, amino acids; chr, chromosome. *(Adapted with permission from Ginsburg D, Bowie EJW. Molecular genetics of von Willebrand disease, Blood 1992 May 15; 79(10):2507–2519.)*

middle portion of the *VWF* structural gene, spanning exons 23 to 34 and the intervening noncoding sequences. *VWFP1* is approximately 97 percent identical in sequence to the authentic *VWF* gene, indicating that it is of fairly recent evolutionary origin.[27] Gene conversion involving the *VWFP1* pseudogene, possibly through recombination with the large homologous exon 28 sequence, has been proposed as a mechanism for introducing mutations into the *VWF* gene.[28–31]

VWF is synthesized exclusively in megakaryocytes and endothelial cells and, as a result, has frequently been used as a specific histochemical marker to identify cells of endothelial cell origin. Although generally assumed to mark all endothelial cells, VWF is expressed at widely varying levels among endothelial cells, depending on the size and location of the associated blood vessel.[32,33] A careful survey in the mouse identified wide differences in the level of VWF mRNA, with 5 to 50 times higher concentrations in the lung and brain, particularly in small vessels, than in comparable vessels in the liver and kidney. In general, the higher levels of VWF mRNA and antigen were found in the endothelial cells of large vessels rather than in microvasculature and in venous rather than arterial endothelial cells.[33]

Specific DNA sequences within or near the proximal promoter of the *VWF* gene appear to be required for endothelial-specific gene expression,[34–39] although it is likely that additional important regulatory elements exist outside of this region, some of which may lie at a great distance.[40] VWF is expressed in most, but not all, endothelial cells,[41] and this vascular-bed specific gene expression program is likely a result of the concerted action of multiple regulatory elements. Endothelial *VWF* gene expression also appears to be upregulated by exposure to shear stress. The length of a polymorphic GT repeat in the proximal *VWF* promoter correlates with the magnitude of this response, and several other more distal DNA sequences are predicted to be involved in a shear stress response.[42] However, this GT repeat does not appear to influence circulating VWF levels.[43]

## VON WILLEBRAND FACTOR BIOSYNTHESIS

The processing steps involved in the biosynthesis of VWF are similar in megakaryocytes and endothelial cells (reviewed in Refs. 44 and 45). VWF is first synthesized as a large precursor monomer polypeptide, depicted schematically in Fig. 16–1. VWF is unusually rich in cysteine, which accounts for 8.3 percent of its amino acid content. All cysteines in the mature VWF molecule are thought to be involved in disulfide bonds,[46] although these bonds may be exposed in circulating mature VWF by shear stress.[47] Pro-VWF monomers are assembled into dimers through disulfide bonds at both C termini, and only dimers are exported from the endoplasmic reticulum (ER).[46,48,49]

Glycosylation begins in the ER, with 12 potential *N*-linked glycosylation sites present on the mature subunit and three on the propeptide. Extensive additional posttranslational modification of VWF occurs in the Golgi apparatus, including the addition of multiple *O*-linked carbohydrate structures, sulfation, and multimerization through the formation of disulfide bonds at the N termini of adjacent dimers. It is unusual for a protein to undergo extensive disulfide bond formation at this late stage, and this process appears to be catalyzed by disulfide isomerase activity present within the VWFpp.[50] Mutation at either of two specific cysteines within the propeptide that are thought to be critical for disulfide isomerase activity, or a shift in the spacing between them, results in loss of multimer formation.[50] An intermediate species with disulfide bonds between the propeptide and VWF D'D3 domain appears briefly in either the late ER or early Golgi,[51] which may position these domains for subsequent multimerization. The multimerization process appears to require the slightly acidic environment of the distal Golgi.[52] The VWFpp self-associates and may also serve to align VWF

subunits for multimer assembly.[53] However, the propeptide facilitates multimer assembly even when coexpressed as a separate molecule from the mature VWF monomer.[54,55]

Propeptide cleavage occurs late in VWF synthesis or just prior to secretion. Cleavage occurs adjacent to two basic amino acids, Lys-Arg at positions –2 and –1. An Arg at position –4 is also required for recognition by the intracellular protease responsible for propeptide cleavage.[56] Multimerization and propeptide cleavage are not linked to each other. The multimers secreted by cultured endothelial cells contain both pro-VWF and mature subunits,[57,58] and recombinant VWF with a point mutation inhibiting propeptide cleavage is still assembled into normal multimer structures.[59] Although propeptide cleavage appears to occur primarily intracellularly, cleavage may also occur after secretion.

VWF is stored in tubular structures within the α granules of platelets and within the Weibel-Palade bodies in endothelial cells[60,61] (reviewed in Ref. 62). These large VWF structures form by tubular packing of the VWF N-terminal domains within the secretory granules.[63] Weibel-Palade bodies are derived from the Golgi apparatus and are found in most endothelial cells, although the number varies considerably between endothelial cell beds. It has been shown that VWF and FVIII colocalize in storage granules. Although VWF is not required to traffic FVIII to platelets,[64] VWF appears to play a role in trafficking FVIII to Weibel-Palade bodies in endothelial cells.[65,66] Weibel-Palade bodies mature as they move to the periphery of the cell in an ordered process dependent on Rab proteins and Rab effector proteins, which act as chaperones and organizers of the various stages of Weibel-Palade body maturity and subsequent exocytosis (reviewed in Ref. 67). The transmembrane glycoprotein P-selectin is also found in the membranes of both the α granule and the Weibel-Palade body.[68] The VWF D'D3 domain has been shown *in vitro* to associate with P-selectin and to be necessary for the recruitment of P-selectin to Weibel-Palade bodies.[69] There appears to be heterogeneity within Weibel-Palade body populations both in relative content of VWF and P-selectin and in response to regulated secretion by different stimuli.[70] In addition to VWF and P-selectin, the Weibel-Palade body also contains tissue-type plasminogen activator (t-PA), a thrombolytic secreted protein that also may be released distinctly from VWF,[71] and several other proteins that are known to participate in inflammation or angiogenesis (for a complete list of Weibel-Palade contents, see Ref. 72).

VWF is secreted from endothelial cells continuously via constitutive and constitutive-like (or basal) pathways and upon stimulated release of storage granules via a classic regulated pathway.[44,73] Regulated secretion of VWF from its storage site in the Weibel-Palade body is triggered by a number of secretagogues, including thrombin,[74] fibrin,[75] histamine,[76] the C5b-9 complement complex,[77] and several inflammatory cytokines.[78] Recent *in vitro* data suggest that there may also be suppression of regulated VWF secretion by statins.[79,80] The secretagogue desmopressin acetate (DDAVP), a vasopressin analogue, is used clinically for its capacity to cause a marked release of VWF and FVIII *in vivo* by acting through type 2 vasopressin receptors to induce secretion from the Weibel-Palade bodies in endothelial cells.[81] Constitutive-like secretion of VWF occurs evenly at the luminal and abluminal surface, while regulated secretion from the Weibel-Palade body is highly polarized in the luminal direction (Fig. 16–2).[73,82] While constitutively secreted multimers are of relatively small size, the multimers stored within the Weibel-Palade body are the largest, most biologically potent form.[83,84] The VWF stored in platelet α granules is also enriched for large multimers.[85] The N-terminal D domains appear to be required for VWF storage, with deletion of any of the individual domains resulting in constitutive secretion.[86,87] It also appears that cleavage of the VWFpp is required for efficient formation of storage granules.[88]

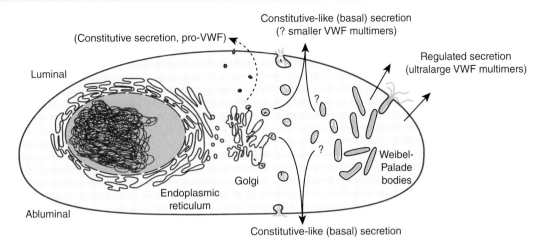

**Figure 16–2.** Schematic of von Willebrand factor (VWF) processing and secretion from endothelial cells. VWF dimers are formed in the endoplasmic reticulum, where VWF begins to be glycosylated. VWF dimers are transported to the Golgi, where the VWF undergoes further glycosylation and sulfation. Multimerization begins in the Golgi and continues within the secretory granules (Weibel-Palade bodies). A small amount of immature VWF is released constitutively (i.e., without regulation or storage) from endothelial cells as dimers or very small multimers. VWF is also released continuously from both the luminal and abluminal endothelial cell surfaces by constitutive-like (or basal) secretion. This VWF has been processed in the Golgi and may be transiently stored in an intermediate secretory granule or Weibel-Palade bodies. Mature VWF is packaged and stored as ultralarge multimers in Weibel-Palade bodies. This ultralarge VWF is released from the luminal surface of stimulated endothelial cells by regulated secretion. Once in circulation, VWF multimers undergo proteolysis by ADAMTS13 (a disintegrin and metalloprotease with a thrombospondin type 1 motif member 13) under moderate to high shear conditions. *(Adapted with permission from Johnsen J, Lopez JA. VWF secretion: what's in a name?* Blood *2008 Aug 15;112(4):926–927.)*

The concentration of VWF in plasma is approximately 10 mcg/mL, with approximately 15 percent of circulating VWF localized to the platelet compartment.[89] Marrow transplants between normal and VWD pigs demonstrate that platelet VWF is derived entirely from synthesis within marrow megakaryocytes and does not contribute to the normal plasma VWF pool.[90–92] These studies also demonstrate that both the plasma and the platelet VWF pools are required for full hemostasis, although the plasma pool appears to be more critical.

Plasma VWF is further processed in the circulation through cleavage by a specific protease, ADAMTS13 (*a d*isintegrin *a*nd *m*etalloprotease with *t*hrombospondin type 1 motifs–13), resulting in reduction in the size of the largest multimers (reviewed in Ref. 93). After regulated secretion *in vitro*, ultralarge VWF multimers may anchor to the endothelial cell surface via P-selectin,[94,95] resulting in shear stress and VWF cleavage by ADAMTS13. The major proteolytic cleavage site maps to the peptide bond between Tyr1605 and Met1606 in the VWF A2 domain,[96] and recombinant VWF missing the A2 domain is resistant to proteolysis.[97] VWF carrying a subgroup of type 2A VWD mutations exhibits increased susceptibility to cleavage by this protease,[98] and this is the proposed mechanism for the selective loss of large VWF multimers in this group of patients (see "Molecular Genetics of von Willebrand Disease," below). Increased VWF susceptibility to proteolysis by ADAMTS13 has also been described in a subset of type 1 VWD patients, but the clinical significance of this is unclear as increased proteolysis appears to only occur under certain conditions.[99] Decreased ADAMTS13 activity, either because of congenital deficiency or acquired inhibitors, plays a central role in the pathophysiology of thrombotic thrombocytopenic purpura (Chap. 22).

## THE FUNCTION OF VON WILLEBRAND FACTOR

VWF is a large multivalent adhesive protein that plays an important role in platelet attachment to subendothelial surfaces, platelet aggregation at sites of vessel injury, and stabilization of coagulation FVIII in the circulation. Not only is the interaction of VWF and FVIII important for the protection of FVIII from inactivation or degradation, FVIII bound to VWF may localize to cells and/or sites where it can more readily participate in the promotion of blood coagulation and/or thrombus formation.

VWF is required for the adhesion of platelets to the subendothelium, particularly at moderate to high shear force. VWF performs this bridging function by binding to two platelet receptors, GPIb and GPIIb/IIIa, as well as to specific ligands within the exposed subendothelium at sites of vascular injury (reviewed in Ref. 100). Binding of VWF to its platelet receptors generally does not occur in the circulation under normal conditions. However, the interaction of VWF with exposed ligands in the vessel wall, combined with high shear stress conditions, facilitates VWF binding to platelet GPIb and subsequent platelet adhesion and activation. Activation of platelets leads to the exposure of the GPIIb/IIIa complex, an integrin receptor that can bind to fibrinogen, VWF, and other ligands, to form the platelet–platelet bridges required for thrombus propagation. Platelet adhesion to VWF immobilized at a site of injury appears to be a two-step process, with the initial tethering of the rapidly moving platelet dependent on the VWF–GPIb interaction and subsequent firm adhesion occurring through GPIIb/IIIa after platelet activation.[101] VWF may also play a role in inflammation by directly interacting with leukocytes,[102] but the clinical significance of this observation is not clear.

### von Willebrand Factor Binding to the Vessel Wall

VWF binds to the vessel wall at sites of vascular endothelial injury (reviewed in Ref. 103). VWF binds to several different types of collagens, including types I through VI. Distinct binding domains for the fibrillar collagens, types I and III, have been localized to specific segments within the VWF A1 and A3 repeats (see Fig. 16–1),[104,105] and a potential third domain has been identified in the VWFpp.[106] Studies of recombinant VWF suggest that the A3 collagen-binding domain may be the most important,[107,108] although the VWF A1 domain has been shown to be critical to binding type IV collagen under shear in studies of VWD patients and recombinant VWF.[109] VWF has also been shown to bind to the nonfibrillar collagen type VI, which is resistant to collagenase[110] and colocalizes with VWF in the subendothelium.[111] Type VI collagen supports the binding of VWF under high shear through cooperative interactions between binding domains within the VWF A1 and A3 repeat.[112] Although VWF binding has also been demonstrated to a number of other potential components of the subendothelium, including glycosaminoglycans,[113,114] sulfatides,[115] and VWF itself,[116] the biologic significance of these interactions remains to be demonstrated.

### von Willebrand Factor Binding to Platelets

VWF interacts with platelets both to mediate platelet aggregation and platelet localization to sites of vascular injury (reviewed in Ref. 103). Circulating VWF does not spontaneously interact with platelets, but once bound to an injured vessel wall, VWF is subjected to higher shear stresses and a platelet-binding site in the VWF A1 domain is uncovered. VWF interacts with a receptor complex on the surface of platelets composed of the disulfide-linked GPIbα and GPIbβ chains noncovalently associated with GPIX and GPV. The binding site for VWF is within a 293-amino-acid segment at the N-terminus of GPIb and requires sulfation of several key tyrosine residues for optimal binding.[117] The GPIb binding domain within VWF lies within the A1 segment, within the disulfide loop formed between the cysteine residues at 1272 (amino acid 509 in mature VWF) and 1458 (695) (see Fig. 16–1).[118,119] GPIb binding to the A1 domain enhances proteolysis of recombinant VWF fragments by ADAMTS13 and suggests a feedback mechanism for limiting thrombus propagation in vivo.[120] Scanning mutagenesis studies of recombinant VWF characterized a number of amino acid residues within the VWF A1 domain that are critical for binding to GPIb and for interaction with botrocetin.[121] Several mutations were also identified that increase platelet binding, an effect similar to that of mutations associated with type 2B VWD (see "Molecular Genetics of von Willebrand Disease," below). These natural and synthetic mutations cluster in a small area on the surface of the VWF A1 domain structure, as revealed by x-ray crystallographic studies.[122] The complexity of the VWF A1–GPIb interaction is evidenced by the ability of gain-of-function and loss-of-function VWF A1 mutants to counterbalance each other in mice.[123] The structure of the A1 domain closely resembles that of other previously studied A domains, including the VWF A3 domain.[124,125] The structure of GPIb in complex with the VWF A1 domain provides insight into the structural basis for the gain-of-function mutations associated with type 2B VWD.[126] The abundant plasma protein $\beta_2$-glycoprotein I can bind the VWF A1 domain when VWF is structurally open to GPIbα binding. This may result in biologically relevant inhibition of the VWF–platelet interaction, as inhibitory anti-$\beta_2$-glycoprotein I autoantibodies found in some patients with antiphospholipid antibody syndrome are associated with thrombosis.[127]

Ristocetin binds to both VWF and platelets, but the mechanism by which it enhances the VWF/GPIb interaction is still poorly understood.[128,129] The snake venom botrocetin appears to induce GPIb binding through a different alteration in the VWF A1 domain and is also used to study this interaction.[130] Heparin binds the VWF A1 domain within the loop formed by the disulfide bond formed between the residues Cys1272 and Cys1458,[131] where it appears to competitively inhibit VWF binding to GPIb[132,133] and enhance VWF proteolysis by ADAMTS13 in vitro.[120] Although it has been suggested that this may account for hemorrhage not predicted by conventional heparin monitoring, the clinical significance of the VWF–heparin interaction is not clear.

The arg-gly-asp-ser (RGDS) sequence at amino acids 2507 to 2510 of the mature VWF subunit serves as the binding site within VWF for GPIIb/IIIa. The GPIIb/IIIa complex, also known as integrin $\alpha_{IIb}\beta_3$, is a member of the integrin family of cell surface receptors. GPIIb/IIIa

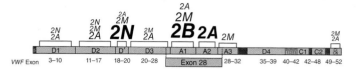

**Figure 16–3.** von Willebrand disease (VWD) mutations. The von Willebrand factor domain locations of all reported mutations associated with type 2A, 2B, 2M, and 2N VWD. Lettering size represents the proportion of total mutations reported within the designated VWF domain for that subtype, with larger letters indicating more mutations. Shown below are the relative positions of the VWF gene exons. Type 1 and type 3 VWD-associated mutations have been reported throughout the VWF gene. (*Mutation data from Nichols WC and Ginsburg D: von Willebrand disease. Medicine (Baltimore) 76(1):1–20, 1997 and the VWD mutation database at www.vwf.group.shef.ac.uk.*)

undergoes a conformational change to a high-affinity ligand-binding state following platelet activation, which, in addition to VWF, can bind a number of other adhesive proteins, including fibrinogen. Although VWF is present in blood at much lower concentrations than is fibrinogen, evidence suggests that VWF may be a critical ligand. VWF participates in platelet tethering and adhesion to fibrin under flow conditions,[101,134] where the C1C2 domains of VWF are required for fibrin binding.[134] An RGD sequence is also present in the VWFpp, although its functional significance is unknown.

### The Interaction of von Willebrand Factor with Factor VIII

The noncovalent interaction between FVIII and VWF is required for the stability of FVIII in the circulation, as is evident from the FVIII levels of less than 10 percent that are observed in most severe VWD patients. Although each VWF subunit appears to carry a binding site for FVIII, the stoichiometry for the VWF–FVIII complex found in normal plasma is approximately one to two FVIII molecules per 100 VWF monomers.[135] FVIII bound to VWF is also protected from proteolytic degradation by activated protein C (reviewed in Ref. 136). FVIII also appears to increase the susceptibility of VWF to proteolysis by ADAMTS13 under shear conditions.[137]

The FVIII binding domain within VWF has been localized to the first 272 N-terminal amino acids of the mature subunit.[138] In mice, expression of the VWF D'D3 domains alone has been shown to be sufficient to stabilize FVIII levels.[139] Antibody studies suggest a particularly critical role for amino acids 841 to 859.[140,141] The mutations identified in patients with type 2N VWD, in which VWF binding to FVIII is specifically affected (see "Molecular Genetics of von Willebrand Disease," below), are all clustered in this region, including the most common type 2N mutation Arg854Gln.[142] The corresponding binding site for VWF on FVIII includes an acidic region at the N-terminus of the light chain (residues 1669 to 1689)[143] and requires sulfation of Tyr1680 for optimal binding.[144] Overlay of VWD 2N mutations with the crystal structure of the VWF A1–FVIII domains shows the 2N mutations clustered in a dynamic VWF TIL' domain (shown in Fig. 16–3), implicating a need for flexibility in this domain for normal FVIII binding.[145] Thrombin cleavage after Arg1689 in FVIII activates and releases FVIII from VWF. Thus, VWF may serve to efficiently deliver FVIII to the sites of clot formation, where it can complex with factor IXa on the platelet surface.

## MOLECULAR GENETICS OF VON WILLEBRAND DISEASE

VWD is an extremely heterogeneous and complex disorder, with more than 20 distinct subtypes reported (referenced in Ref. 146). A large number of mutations within the *VWF* gene have been identified (see Fig. 16–3). However, because of both the genetic complexity of VWD and the practical considerations of *VWF* gene sequencing in most clinical settings, a *VWF* gene mutation is not required for the diagnosis of VWD.[147] A list is maintained by a consortium of VWD investigators and can be accessed through the Internet at http://www.vwf.group.shef.ac.uk/. These findings form the basis for the simplified classification of VWD outlined in Table 16–2[147] and used throughout this chapter. Types 1 and 3 VWD are defined as pure quantitative deficiencies of VWF that are either partial (type 1) or complete (type 3). Type 2 VWD is characterized by qualitative abnormalities of VWF structure and/or function. The quantity of VWF found in type 2 VWD may be normal, but it is usually mildly to moderately decreased (see Table 16–2).

The diagnosis of VWD, particularly type 1 VWD, can be confounded by the incomplete penetrance of the disease and the wide range of VWF levels in normal populations (see "Laboratory Features" below). Nonpathogenic variation can impact laboratory assays *in vitro*, as is the case with Asp1472His, which alters VWF–ristocetin interactions but has no impact on hemostasis *in vivo*.[148] Ethnicity should also be considered. European ancestries were overrepresented in the studies that informed laboratory cutoffs, while African Americans exhibit generally higher VWF and FVIII levels. Additionally, there are numerous *VWF* gene "mutations" previously thought to be causative of VWD that are now known to be common in African Americans[149,150] who have normal VWF and FVIII levels,[149] including the Asp1472His variant.[151]

### Type 1 von Willebrand Disease

Type 1 VWD is the most common form, accounting for approximately 70 percent of patients with the disease. Type 1 VWD is generally autosomal dominant in inheritance and is associated with coordinate reductions in FVIII, ristocetin cofactor activity, and VWF antigen with maintenance of the full complement of multimers (Fig. 16–4). Subgroups

within type 1 VWD have been proposed based on the relative levels of VWF present in the plasma and platelet pools,[152-155] but with the exception in some circumstances for an accelerated VWF clearance phenotype (unofficially termed VWF type 1C[156]), subtype distinctions in type 1 VWD are not generally used in clinical practice.

Type 1 VWF was previously assumed to simply represent the heterozygous form of type 3 VWD. However, in a large Canadian study, 48 percent of heterozygous carriers of type 3 VWD gene mutations carried a diagnosis of type 1 VWD, while the remainder were asymptomatic.[157] Furthermore, in two large studies of type 1 VWD families, numerous putative *VWF* mutations were identified, but very few were predictive of *VWF* null alleles.[31,158] Thus, some, but probably not all (see section "Clinical Features" below), type 1 VWD is the result of defects within the *VWF* gene. Studies of type 1 VWD mutations in patients, *in vitro*, and in animal models have characterized diverse mechanisms underlying type 1 VWD, including decreased VWF production,[159] retention of VWF in the ER,[160,161] impaired VWF secretion,[161,162] and decreased VWF survival.[159,162,163] Mutations that give rise to defective VWF subunits that interfere in a dominant negative way with the normal allele may be particularly likely to cause symptomatic VWD in the heterozygote[164]; for example, mutations at several cysteine residues in the VWF D3 domain and in the VWFpp of patients with moderately severe type 1 VWD. VWF carrying one of these mutations is retained in the ER, where it is proposed to exert a dominant negative effect on VWF derived from the normal allele via heterodimerization and degradation.[165,166]

To date, most mutation studies and genetic linkage analysis of type 1 VWD have been consistent with defects within the *VWF* gene. Although no single mutation can explain the majority of type 1 VWD, common *VWF* founder mutations can occur within populations, such as Tyr1584Cys identified in 14 percent of Canadian type 1 VWD patients, and possibly a similar proportion of patients in Europe.[158,167] The Tyr1584Cys mutation is associated with decreased VWF survival, likely a result of increased susceptibility to proteolysis by ADAMTS13.[168-171] These large multicenter studies of type 1 VWD families found candidate *VWF* mutations in 63 to 70 percent of families with type 1 VWD, leaving 37 to 40 percent of type 1 VWD index cases without a putative mutation in *VWF*.[158,167] Cases with *VWF* gene mutations tend to be more severe and highly heritable, while cases without an identifiable *VWF* mutation generally have higher VWF antigen (VWF:Ag) levels (>30 IU/dL).[31] In a large, multicenter European study of 150 type 1 VWD families, about one-third of cases historically diagnosed to have type 1 VWD were found to have abnormal multimers, and of these, nearly all (95 percent) had a putative *VWF* gene mutation and significantly lower VWF:Ag, VWF ristocetin cofactor activity (VWF:RCo), assay of FVIII activity (FVIII:C), and VWF collagen-binding assay (VWF:CB) levels. Conversely, index cases with normal multimers had higher laboratory VWF values and fewer identifiable *VWF* mutations (55 percent), suggesting that the pathogenic mechanism(s) underlying this cohort of "true" type 1 VWD patients is more genetically complex.[158] Given the complex biosynthesis and processing of VWF, defects at a number of other loci could also be expected to result in quantitative VWF abnormalities (reviewed in Ref. 172). This concept is supported by families with type 1 VWD in which bleeding histories and low ristocetin cofactor activities do not always cosegregate with genetic markers at the VWF locus,[31,173] while one or more genetic factors outside the *VWF* locus may be associated with the variation in bleeding severity observed within VWD pedigrees.[174,175] It is interesting to note that a spontaneous mouse model of type 1 VWD exhibits up to 20-fold reductions in plasma VWF as a result of an unusual mutation in a glycosyltransferase gene, leading to aberrant posttranslational processing of VWF and accelerated clearance from plasma.[176] Similar mechanisms affecting VWF survival, perhaps combined with altered proteolysis,[177-179] may

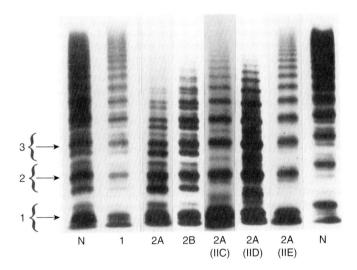

**Figure 16–4.** Agarose gel electrophoresis of plasma von Willebrand factor (VWF). VWF multimers from plasma of patients with various subtypes of von Willebrand disease (VWD) are shown. The brackets to the left encompass three individual multimer subunits, including the main band and its associate satellite bands. *N* indicates normal control lanes. Lanes 5 through 7 are rare variants of type 2A VWD. The former designations for these variants are indicated in parentheses below the lanes (IIC through E). *(Adapted with permission from Zimmerman TS, Dent JA, Ruggeri ZM, Nannini LH: Subunit composition of plasma von Willebrand factor. Cleavage is present in normal individuals, increased in IIA and IIB von Willebrand disease, but minimal in variants with aberrant structure of individual oligomers (types IIC, IID, and IIE). J Clin Invest 77(3):947–951, 1986.)*

explain the observed modifying effect of the ABO blood group glyco-syltransferases on plasma VWF survival.[180] Additional genetic factors have been implicated to influence VWF via altered survival, including the clearance receptors CLEC4M and LRP1 (CD91) (reviewed in Ref. 181). The biologic consequences of VWF modifiers identified in normal populations are unclear, and studies are needed to determine their significance in VWD.

### Type 3 von Willebrand Disease

Patients with type 3 VWD account for 1 to 5 percent of clinically significant VWD, have very low or undetectable levels of plasma and platelet VWF:Ag and VWF:RCo, and generally present early in life with severe bleeding.[182] FVIII coagulant activity is markedly reduced but usually detectable at levels of 3 to 10 percent of normal. Type 3 VWD has generally been considered an autosomal recessive disorder, but in a recent Canadian study of 100 individuals in 34 families, 48 percent of "carriers" had a diagnosis of type 1 VWD,[157] suggesting the dominant type 1 VWD pattern of inheritance is common in type 3 VWD families.

Mutations associated with type 3 VWD have been reported throughout the VWF gene (http://www.vwf.group.shef.ac.uk/). Gross VWF gene deletion detectable by Southern blot[26,183-186] or multiple ligation-probe amplification[157,187] is the molecular mechanism for type 3 VWD in only a small subset of families. However, large deletions may confer an increased risk for the development of alloantibodies against VWF.[26,185] A similar correlation between gene deletion and risk for alloantibody formation has been observed in hemophilia (Chap. 13). Comparative analysis of VWF genomic DNA and platelet VWF mRNA has identified nondeletion defects resulting in complete loss of VWF mRNA expression as a molecular mechanism in some patients with type 3 VWD.[188,189] A number of nonsense and frameshift mutations that would be predicted to result in loss of VWF protein expression or in expression of a markedly truncated or disrupted protein have been identified in some type 3 VWD families.[30,164,190,191] A frameshift mutation in exon 18 appears to be a particularly common cause of type 3 VWD in the Swedish population and has been shown to be the defect responsible for VWD in the original Åland Island pedigree.[28,192] This mutation results in a stable mRNA encoding a truncated protein that is rapidly degraded in the cell.[164] This mutation also appears to be common among type 3 VWD patients in Germany,[193] but not in the United States.[164]

### Type 2A von Willebrand Disease

Type 2A is the most common qualitative variant of VWD and is generally associated with autosomal dominant inheritance and selective loss of the large and intermediate VWF multimers from plasma (see Fig. 16–4). A 176-kDa proteolytic fragment present in normal individuals is markedly increased in quantity in many type 2A VWD patients. This fragment is consistent with proteolytic cleavage of the peptide bond between Tyr1605 and Met1606.[96,194] Based on this observation, initial DNA sequence analysis in patients centered on VWF exon 28, in the region encoding this segment of the VWF protein, leading to the identification of the first point mutations responsible for VWD.[195] Since that time, a large number of mutations have been identified, accounting for the majority of type 2A VWD patients.[190] Many of these mutations are clustered within a 134-amino-acid segment of the VWF A2 domain (between Gly1505 and Glu1638; see Fig. 16–3), and the most common, Arg1597Trp, appears to account for about one-third of type 2A VWD patients.[190,191,196]

Type 2A VWD mutations have been grouped by two distinct molecular mechanisms. In the first subset, classified as group 1, the type 2A VWD mutation has been commonly considered a defect in intracellular transport, with retention of mutant VWF in the ER. In addition to retention or degradation of mutant VWF in the ER, type 2A mutations can also disrupt intracellular processing and secretion via defective multimerization and/or loss of regulated storage.[197] In the second subset, or group 2, mutant VWF is normally processed and secreted in vitro, and thus loss of multimers in vivo is presumed to occur based on increased susceptibility to proteolysis in plasma[96,198-201] at the Tyr1605-Met1606 site cleaved by ADAMTS13.[99,202] The susceptibility of type 2A VWD mutations to proteolysis by ADAMTS13 in vitro supports accelerated proteolysis as a mechanism for the loss of high-molecular-weight VWF multimers in these patients.[196]

The multimer structure of platelet VWF correlates well with the underlying type 2A mechanisms. Group 1 patients show loss of large VWF multimers within platelets as a result of defective synthesis, while group 2 patients have normal VWF multimers within the protected environment of the α granule.[198] These observations confirm the earlier subclassification of type 2A VWD based on platelet multimers.[152] Subclassification into group 1 or 2 might be expected to predict response to DDAVP therapy, although this remains to be demonstrated.

In addition to the major classes of type 2A VWD described above, a number of rare variants historically classified as types IIC to IIH, type IB, and "platelet discordant" are included in the more general type 2A category. Most of these rare variants were distinguished on the basis of subtle differences in the multimer pattern (see Fig. 16–4; multimer changes relative to the location of type 2 mutations is reviewed in Ref. 203). The IIC variant is usually inherited as an autosomal recessive trait and is associated with loss of large multimers and a prominent dimer band. Several mutations have been identified in the VWFpp of these patients,[204-206] presumably interfering with multimer assembly and/or trafficking to storage granules. A mutation at the C terminus of VWF, interfering with dimer formation, was described in a patient with the IID variant.[207] Most of the other reported variants of type 2A VWD are quite rare, often limited to single case reports.

### Type 2B von Willebrand Disease

Type 2B VWD is usually inherited as an autosomal dominant disorder and is characterized by thrombocytopenia and loss of large VWF multimers. The plasma VWF in type 2B VWD binds to normal platelets in the presence of lower concentrations of ristocetin than does normal VWF and can aggregate platelets spontaneously. Accelerated clearance of the resulting complexes between platelets and the large, most adhesive forms of VWF accounts for the thrombocytopenia and the characteristic multimer pattern (see Fig. 16–4).

The peculiar functional abnormality characteristic of type 2B VWD suggested a molecular defect within the GPIb binding domain of VWF. For this reason, initial DNA sequence analysis focused on the corresponding portion of VWF exon 28.[208,209] Type 2B mutations are located within the VWF A1 domain at one surface of the described crystallographic structure.[122,126] The four most common mutations are clustered within a 36-amino-acid stretch between Arg1306 and Arg1341 (see Fig. 16–3); together, these account for more than 80 percent of type 2B VWD patients.[191] Functional analysis of mutant recombinant VWF[210-214] confirms that these single-amino-acid substitutions are sufficient to account for increased GPIb binding and the resulting characteristic type 2B VWD phenotype. Structural studies of type 2B VWD mutations show that these residues interact with the leucine-rich repeats of GPIb thought to be critical to the VWF A1–GPIb interactions under shear.[215] Type 2B mutations have now been modeled extensively in mice, all of which exhibited accelerated VWF clearance, as expected.[216] Type 2B VWD mice also had short-lived platelets, with evidence of macrophage-mediated platelet clearance.[217] In these models, platelets were observed to be coated by type 2B VWF,[217] a phenomenon that may contribute to a previously unsuspected acquired platelet function defect.[218] Interestingly, mice with the same type 2B mutations exhibit variable loss of large multimers[216] and varying degrees of thrombocytopenia,[219] similar to the variation observed in human pedigrees. Individual type 2B patients can also exhibit varying multimer structure and platelet counts over time. For example, two siblings with the Arg1306Trp mutation and abnormal multimers intermittently regained normal VWF multimer distribution during periods of thrombocytopenia.[220]

Families have been described that exhibit enhanced VWF binding to GPIb but a normal distribution of VWF multimers. These variants, previously referred to as type I New York, type I Malmö, and type I Sydney, are now all designated as type 2B VWD. Type I New York and type I Malmö are caused by the same *VWF* mutation, Pro1266Leu. This mutation is located within the cluster of type 2B mutations in the VWF A1 domain and results in a similar increase in platelet GPIb binding.[221]

### Type 2N von Willebrand Disease

As described in Chap. 13, hemophilia A results from defects in the FVIII gene and is inherited in an X-linked recessive manner. Distinct from hemophilia A, families have been reported in which the inheritance of low FVIII appeared to be autosomal, based on the occurrence of affected females or direct transmission from an affected father.[222,223] Several cases of an apparent autosomal recessive decrease in FVIII were shown to be caused by decreased VWF binding of FVIII,[224–226] now referred to as VWD type 2N, after the Normandy province of origin of the first patient. DNA sequence analysis has identified more than 37 distinct mutations[227] associated with this disorder, most located at the VWF N terminus (see Fig. 16–3) (curated in the Scientific and Standardisation Committee of the International Society on Thrombosis and Haemostasis VWF Database, http://www.vwf.group.shef.ac.uk/). One of these mutations, Arg854Gln, appears to be particularly common, may contribute to variability in the severity of type 1 VWD in some cases,[228] and may also cause a VWF secretion defect.[229] Rare cases of misdiagnosis of type 2N have led to treatment with recombinant FVIII for presumed hemophilia A, with poor responses and adverse clinical outcomes.[230]

### Type 2M von Willebrand Disease

This category was classically reserved for rare VWD variants in which a defect in VWF platelet-dependent function leads to significant bleeding but VWF multimer structure is not affected (although some have subtle multimer abnormalities). Most contemporary type 2M variants are indeed associated with absent ristocetin cofactor activity but normal platelet binding with other agonists. A total of 28 type 2M VWD mutations have been described,[227] including a number of other families with normal VWF multimers and disproportionately decreased ristocetin cofactor activity,[231,232] families with a combination of defects in VWF:CB and VWF–GPIb interactions of varying severities,[233,234] and mutations with isolated defects in VWF:CB with normal VWF:RCo activity.[231] Several families have also been described with a VWD variant (VWD Vicenza) characterized by larger-than-normal VWF multimers and classified as either type 1 or type 2M VWD.[235] Genetic linkage analysis indicates that the Vicenza defect lies within the VWF gene,[236] and mutations within the VWF gene have been reported to be associated with VWD Vicenza.[237] The underlying molecular mechanism responsible for the VWD Vicenza phenotype remains controversial,[238] although recent kinetic modeling suggests that altered VWF survival alone could account for the VWF perturbations observed in this disorder.[239]

## ● CLINICAL FEATURES

### INHERITANCE

Type 1 VWD is generally transmitted as an autosomal dominant disorder and accounts for approximately 70 percent of clinically significant VWD. However, disease expressivity is variable, and penetrance is incomplete.[164,240] Laboratory values and clinical symptoms can vary considerably, even within the same individual, and establishing a definite diagnosis of VWD is often difficult. In two large families with type 1 VWD, only 65 percent of individuals with both an affected parent and an affected descendent had significant clinical symptoms.[241] For comparison, 23 percent of the unrelated spouses of the patients, who presumably did not have a bleeding disorder, were judged to have a positive bleeding history.

A number of factors have long been known to modify VWF levels, including ABO blood group, secretor blood group, estrogens, thyroid hormones, age, and stress.[242–244] ABO blood group is the best characterized of these factors. Genome-wide linkage has repeatedly confirmed strong linkage between the ABO locus and VWF levels (reviewed in Ref. 245). Mean VWF:Ag levels are approximately 75 percent for type O individuals and 123 percent for type AB individuals when compared to a pool of normal donor plasmas. Thus, it may be difficult to differentiate between a low-normal VWF value and mild type 1 VWD in blood group O individuals. In recent years, additional modifiers of VWF have been identified in large genetic association studies,[246,247] including genes associated with VWF intracellular trafficking (*STXBP5*[248,249]) and VWF clearance (*CLEC4M*[250]). Additionally, a genome-wide association study identified a novel genetic locus on chromosome 2 contributing to variation in plasma VWF.[172] The variable expressivity and incomplete penetrance of type 1 VWD and overlap in VWF levels between mild type 1 VWD and normal populations has complicated the determination of accurate incidence figures for VWD, with estimates ranging from as high as 1 percent[251,252] to as low as 2 to 10 per 100,000 population.[253]

In general, the type 2 VWD variants, which comprise 20 to 30 percent of all VWD diagnoses,[254] are more uniformly penetrant. In a survey of 670 French families in which stricter criteria of VWF levels of <30 IU/dL were applied, type 2 VWD was more common, constituting 66 percent of diagnoses.[255] Type 2A and type 2B VWD account for the vast majority of patients with qualitative VWF abnormalities. Types 2A, 2B, and 2M are generally autosomal dominant in inheritance, although Type 2N and other rare cases of apparent recessive inheritance have been reported.

Estimates of prevalence for severe (type 3) VWD range from 0.5 to 5.3 per 1,000,000 population.[256–258] Although this variant is frequently defined as autosomal recessive in inheritance, this is not a consistent finding. As described above, one or both parents of a severe VWD patient can be clinically asymptomatic and have entirely normal laboratory test results, although in many families, one or both parents appear to be affected with classic type 1 VWD. Thus, in some families, severe VWD may represent the homozygous form of type 1 VWD. In this model, the apparent recessive inheritance in a subset of families could simply be the result of the incomplete penetrance of type 1 VWD. Alternatively, there may be a fundamental difference in the molecular mechanisms responsible for type 1 and type 3 VWD.[164]

Compound heterozygosity (the presence of more than one *VWF* gene mutation) can occur, and the clinical presentation in such cases can depend on the interaction between the different mutant VWF proteins. Compound heterozygosity can impact response to therapy because of a complex VWD phenotype and has implications for genetic counseling. If compound heterozygosity is deduced from the family history and/or laboratory studies or discovered during genetic testing, the most recent update to the VWD nomenclature represents both types separated by a slash (/), such as VWD type 2B/2N.[147]

## CLINICAL SYMPTOMS

Mucocutaneous bleeding is the most common symptom in patients with type 1 VWD.[241] It is important to note that more than 20 percent of normal individuals may give a positive bleeding history.[259] Bleeding assessment scores have evolved over many years,[260,261] leading the International

Society on Thrombosis and Haemostasis to propose a unified Bleeding Assessment Test (ISTH-BAT).[262] The ISTH-BAT,[262] which is administered by expert providers, and the derivative Self-BAT,[263] which can be self-administered by patients, permit quantitative scoring and a more objective bleeding history for screening for VWD. In general, high bleeding scores are suggestive of a bleeding diathesis and can predict future bleeding,[264] and low bleeding scores have good negative predictive value,[261] but no bleeding questionnaire as yet is clearly diagnostic for VWD. These observations, together with the limited sensitivity and specificity of the currently available laboratory tests (see below), make the diagnosis of mild VWD quite difficult and probably contributes to the wide range of prevalence figures for type 1 VWD currently in the literature. A National Heart, Lung, and Blood Institute Expert Panel has proposed clinical guidelines for evaluating patients to determine whether laboratory testing for VWD or other bleeding disorders is warranted.[146]

Epistaxis occurs in approximately 60 percent of type 1 VWD patients, 40 percent have easy bruising and hematomas, 35 percent have menorrhagia, and 35 percent have gingival bleeding. Gastrointestinal bleeding occurs in approximately 10 percent of patients.[146] An apparent association between hereditary hemorrhagic telangiectasia (HHT) and VWD has been reported in several families. The causative genes in HHT were identified and are located on chromosomes 9q33–34 and 12q13[265] (Chap. 12), distinct from the VWF gene on chromosome 12p13. However, because inheriting VWD is likely to increase the severity of bleeding from HHT, the diagnosis is more likely to be made in patients inheriting both defects.[266] Mucocutaneous bleeding is common after trauma, with approximately 50 percent of patients reporting bleeding after dental extraction, approximately 35 percent after trauma or wounds, 25 percent postpartum, and 20 percent postoperatively. Hemarthroses in patients with moderate disease are extremely rare and are generally only encountered after major trauma. The bleeding symptoms can be quite variable among patients within the same family and even in the same patient over time. An individual may experience postpartum bleeding with one pregnancy but not with others, and clinical symptoms in mildly to moderately affected type 1 individuals often ameliorate by the second or third decade of life. Aside from an infrequent type 3 patient, death from bleeding rarely occurs in VWD.

Thrombocytopenia is a common feature of type 2B VWD and is not seen in any other form of VWD. Most patients only experience thrombocytopenia at times of increased VWF production or secretion, such as during physical effort, in pregnancy, in newborn infants, postoperatively, or if an infection develops. The platelet count rarely drops to levels thought to contribute to clinical bleeding.[267,268] Infants with type 2B VWD may present with neonatal thrombocytopenia, which could be confused with neonatal alloimmune thrombocytopenia, neonatal sepsis, or congenital thrombocytopenia.

Patients who are homozygous or compound heterozygous for type 2N VWD generally have normal levels of VWF:Ag and VWF:RCo and normal VWF platelet adhesive function. However, FVIII levels are moderately decreased, resulting in a mild to moderate hemophilia-like phenotype.[142] In contrast to patients with classic hemophilia A (FVIII deficiency), these patients do not respond to infusion of purified FVIII and should be treated with VWF-containing concentrates.[230] Heterozygotes for this disorder may have mildly decreased FVIII levels but are generally asymptomatic. Although type 2N VWD appears to be considerably less common than classic hemophilia A, it should be considered in the differential diagnosis of FVIII deficiency, particularly if any features suggest an autosomal pattern of inheritance. Although the FVIII level rarely drops below 5 percent, type 2N VWD mutation can be associated with FVIII levels as low as 1 percent, when co-inherited with a type 3 VWD allele.[269] The latter observation further suggests that a diagnosis of type 2N VWD should also be considered in patients with marked reductions of FVIII.

Patients with type 3 VWD can suffer from severe clinical bleeding and experience hemarthroses and muscle hematomas, as in severe hemophilia A (Chap. 13). After infusion of VWF-containing plasma fractions, some of these patients develop anti-VWF antibodies that neutralize VWF (reviewed in Ref. 270).[271]

Other heritable coagulopathies can coexist with VWF deficiency. An evaluation for other factor deficiencies or platelet disorders should be considered in patients who have a suggestive family history, a bleeding phenotype out or proportion or inconsistent with an expected VWD pattern, or a poor response to therapy. In VWD patients with combination coagulopathies, treatment of both disorders may be necessary to achieve a good clinical result.[272]

## ● LABORATORY FEATURES

In the initial laboratory evaluation of patients suspected by history of having VWD, the following tests are routinely performed: assay of FVIII:C and VWF:Ag and a measure of platelet-dependent VWF activity, typically the ristocetin cofactor activity (VWF:RCo), although VWF:RCo as the standard for VWF functional assay is changing[273] (see section "Ristocetin Cofactor Activity" below). Other tests that are commonly used include RIPA, VWF:CB, and VWF multimer analysis. Routine coagulation studies, such as prothrombin time (PT) or activated partial thromboplastin time (aPTT), are generally not useful in the evaluation of VWD. However, the aPTT can be prolonged in subjects with VWF deficiency[274] or in patients with homozygous type 2N VWD, because of the reduction in FVIII level. The wide range of normal and the considerable overlap with the levels observed in type 1 VWD make borderline levels difficult to interpret. A variety of concurrent diseases and drugs may modify the results of individual tests. Many conditions, such as recent exercise, age, pregnancy, time of the menstrual cycle, estrogen therapy, hypo- or hyperthyroidism, diabetes, uremia, liver disease, infection, myeloproliferative neoplasms, or malignancy can affect the FVIII activity, VWF:Ag, and ristocetin cofactor activity levels. These values can be regarded as acute-phase reactants, and even minor illnesses can increase the levels in a VWD patient to normal. Appropriate processing of laboratory specimens is also critical as VWF parameters can be artifactually skewed (either high or low) by phlebotomy conditions or specimen handling (reviewed in Ref. 146). Even controlling for many of these factors, the coefficients of variation of repeated VWF:Ag and ristocetin cofactor assays in a single person are quite large[275] and can be influenced by numerous factors including diurnal variation.[276] For this reason, repeated measurements are usually necessary, and the diagnosis of VWD or its exclusion should generally not be based on a single set of laboratory values.

The laboratory diagnosis of type 1 VWD can be confounded by the wide range of VWF levels in "normals" and borderline laboratory results. An alternative strategy is to classify some patients for whom the diagnosis of VWD is ambiguous as "low VWF," recognizing that these patients may have an increased risk of bleeding without labeling them as type 1 VWD.[253,277] In response to this need to distinguish patients with VWD from nonbleeding individuals with moderately low levels of VWF (30 to 50 IU/dL), a threshold of less than 30 IU/dL has been recommended.[146] In clinical practice, there remains wide variation in the assignment of normal VWF ranges and in the interpretation of laboratory results to make a VWD diagnoses.[278–280]

### FACTOR VIII

FVIII levels in VWD patients are generally coordinately decreased along with plasma VWF, although skewing of FVIII-to-VWF ratios can be observed.[281] Levels in type 3 VWD generally range from 3 to 10 percent. In contrast, the levels in type 1 and the type 2 VWD variants (other than 2N) are variable and usually only mildly or moderately decreased. The FVIII level in type 2N VWD is more severely decreased, but rarely to less than 5 percent.

## VON WILLEBRAND FACTOR ANTIGEN

Plasma VWF:Ag is usually quantitated by electroimmunoassay or an enzyme-linked immunosorbent assay (ELISA) technique. In type 1 VWD, the VWF:Ag assay usually parallels VWF:RCo, but it has lower specificity and sensitivity than the VWF:RCo assay. In patients with type 2 VWD, the VWF:Ag is variably decreased but can be normal (see Table 16–2).

## RISTOCETIN COFACTOR ACTIVITY

The standard measure of VWF platelet-dependent activity, VWF:RCo quantitates the ability of plasma VWF to agglutinate platelets via platelet membrane GPIbα in the presence of ristocetin.[282] In the most common method, normal platelets washed free of plasma VWF are used either as fresh platelets or after formaldehyde fixation.

The ristocetin cofactor assay has long been reported to be the most sensitive and specific single test for the detection of VWD.[283] The assay is limited, though, by high coefficients of variation and low sensitivity, drawbacks that were somewhat improved with automation.[261,273] Ristocetin cofactor assays are also uninformative in the presence of the VWF Pro1467Ser or Asp1472His variants, which interfere with the VWF–ristocetin interaction in vitro but do not reflect a bleeding diathesis in vivo.[151,284] Numerous alternative methods have been proposed as adjuncts or replacements of the standard platelet-based ristocetin cofactor activity assay.[273,285] A nomenclature for categories of platelet-dependent VWF activity methods has recently been proposed by the Scientific and Standardisation Committee of the ISTH as follows: VWF:RCo refers to all assays that use platelets and ristocetin; VWF:GPIbR assays use a recombinant GPIb fragment to bind VWF in the presence of ristocetin; VWF:GPIbM assays are based on VWF binding to a gain-of-function mutant recombinant GPIb fragment; and VWF:Ab assays measure binding of a monoclonal antibody to a VWF A1 domain epitope.[273] Assays in each of the latter categories will require further study to support adoption into routine VWD diagnostic algorithms as a VWF:RCo alternative.[273]

## RISTOCETIN-INDUCED PLATELET AGGLUTINATION

Similar to the ristocetin cofactor assay above, the RIPA assay also measures platelet agglutination caused by ristocetin-mediated VWF binding to platelet membrane GPIbα. In the case of RIPA, ristocetin is added directly to patient platelet-rich plasma, and platelet aggregation is measured. Hyperresponsiveness to RIPA results either from a type 2B VWD mutation or an intrinsic defect in the platelet (platelet-type or pseudo-VWD). In these disorders, patient platelet-rich plasma agglutinates spontaneously or at low ristocetin concentrations of only 0.2 to 0.7 mg/mL. At these concentrations, normal platelet-rich plasma does not agglutinate. Type 2B and platelet-type VWD can be distinguished by RIPA experiments performed with separated patient platelets or plasma mixed with the corresponding component from a normal individual or paraformaldehyde-fixed platelets. The RIPA is generally reduced in most other subtypes of VWD (see Table 16–2).

## MULTIMER ANALYSIS

Analysis of plasma VWF multimers is critical for the proper diagnosis and subclassification of VWD (see Fig. 16–4). This is generally accomplished by agarose gel electrophoresis of plasma VWF to separate VWF multimers on the basis of molecular size, with the largest multimers migrating more slowly than the intermediate or smaller multimers. The multimers may be visualized by autoradiography after incubation with [125]I-monospecific antihuman VWF antibody or, more commonly, by nonradioactive immunologic techniques. The normal multimeric distribution is an orderly ladder of major protein bands of increasing molecular weight, going from the smallest to the largest VWF multimers (see Fig. 16–4). Each normal multimer has a fine structure consisting of one major component and two to four satellite bands.[286] Type 2B and most of the type 2A variants were initially distinguished from each other on the basis of subtle variations in the satellite band pattern. In a large, European, multicenter, type 1 VWD study, careful analysis of VWF multimers in subjects historically diagnosed as type 1 VWD, including patients diagnosed at experienced centers, found one-third of "type 1" VWD patients had subtly abnormal multimers.[287] Although this previously would have required reclassification of these patients as type 2 VWD, the most recent update on the classification of VWD by the International Society on Thrombosis and Haemostasis Subcommittee on von Willebrand Factor expanded the category of type 1 VWD to permit subtle VWF multimer abnormalities.[147] The authors of the European type 1 VWD study note that having samples from the index case, affected family members, and unaffected family members on one gel made qualitative defects more readily detectable and that intermediate-resolution multimer gels were superior to low-resolution multimer gels in detecting abnormalities in this population. VWF tests sensitive to VWF multimer structure have been proposed by some experts as proxies for VWF multimer testing, such as the VWF:RCo-to-VWF:Ag ratio (VWF RCo:Ag ratio) or VWF:CB assay.[288] In studies comparing these approaches as surrogates for VWF multimer assays, the VWF RCo:Ag ratio was found to be less sensitive than multimer gel techniques in identifying qualitative VWF defects,[287] whereas VWF:CB can detect some type 2M VWD patients who have normal VWF multimers.[289,290] These observations support a continued important role for VWF multimer analysis in the laboratory evaluation of VWD.

## ADDITIONAL LABORATORY TESTS

As a result of the variable sensitivity and specificity of laboratory testing for VWD, additional diagnostic studies may be useful in the classification of VWD patients. The VWF:CB measures VWF binding to collagen (type I, type III, or mixed) by ELISA.[261] As above, assays based on VWF:CB can complement the VWF:RCo in detecting type 2 VWD variants,[291-294] and an abnormal VWF:CB-to-VWF:Ag ratio (VWF CB:Ag ratio) is suggestive of a qualitative VWF defect.[147] Abnormalities in VWF:CB can reflect loss of high-molecular-weight multimers and/or the discrete loss of collagen binding caused by a type 2M mutation. Use of VWF:CB assays is expanding in clinical practice, with select sites including this test routinely in initial VWD diagnostic laboratory testing.

Another group of tests are included in the term VWF "activity" (VWF:Act). These tests seek to assess VWF-GPIb binding capacity independent of ristocetin, usually by using antibodies to the VWF A1 domain in ELISAs. These tests are easily confused with the VWF:RCo, which has also been referred to as "VWF activity." None of these tests measures activity; rather, both VWF:RCo and VWF:Act are sensitive to VWF conformation. The VWF:Act does not always provide the same results as VWF:RCo, particularly with regard to type 2M VWD, and is not considered a substitute for the VWF:RCo (reviewed in Ref. 284).

When type 2N VWD is suspected, VWF:FVIII binding capacity can be measured.[226] Specific assays of FVIII binding to VWF (VWF:FVIIIB) have been developed and can be used to confirm the diagnosis of type 2N VWD.[295,296] Type 2N carriers do not always exhibit a decrease in

VWF:FVIIIB, but a decreased VWF:FVIIIB-to-VWF:Ag ratio may correlate with heterozygosity for a type 2N *VWF* mutation.[297] Although this assay is widely used in European hemostasis laboratories, its availability in the United States is currently limited to a few specialized reference laboratories.

An assay measuring the VWFpp can be used to calculate the VWFpp:antigen ratio (VWFpp:Ag ratio) to detect a subset of VWD patients with decreased VWF survival. Good correlation has been reported between subjects with significantly shortened VWF half-life after DDAVP challenge and an increased VWFpp:Ag ratio.[156,281,298] The presence of detectable VWFpp can also help distinguish severe type 1 from type 3 VWD.[299] This assay is currently available in a few reference laboratories. A normal platelet VWF:Ag in the setting of decreased plasma VWF laboratory parameters also suggests an accelerated clearance phenotype such as that seen in VWD type Vicenza,[300] but platelet VWF:Ag testing also is not widely available in clinical laboratories.

A number of other assays for VWF activity have been developed. The PFA-100 system, which measures platelet binding under high shear,[301,302] is controversial in the diagnosis or monitoring of VWD. Although the PFA-100 is usually abnormal in type 2 VWD and in more severe type 1 and type 3 VWD cases, milder type 1 VWD and some type 2 VWD patients can have normal results.[146] Other VWF assays can measure binding of an antibody to the GPIb binding site on VWF as a proposed screening test for VWD.[303–306] Additional assays can measure platelet agglutination induced by botrocetin (which is no longer commercially available) and other snake venom proteins.[307] In the National Heart, Lung, and Blood Institute Expert Panel guidelines (http://www.nhlbi.nih.gov/files/docs/guidelines/vwd.pdf), none of these tests are recommended for screening for VWD.[146]

With advances in understanding the molecular genetics of VWD, it is now possible to precisely diagnose and subclassify many variants of VWD on the basis of DNA mutations (reviewed in Ref. 308). DNA testing, particularly for type 2 VWD mutations that cluster within specific regions of the *VWF* gene (see Fig. 16–3), can be used to confirm the diagnosis and is available in specialized reference laboratories. The analysis of type 3 and type 1 VWD is more complex, as the currently known mutations are scattered throughout the gene[227] and account only for a subset of patients.

The bleeding time is mentioned here for historical purposes only, as it was used as a screening test for VWD and other abnormalities of platelet function. Bleeding time varied considerably with the experience of the operator and a variety of other factors, did not prolong with FVIII deficiency, and correlated poorly with bleeding risk. Thus, the bleeding time is no longer recommended in the evaluation of VWD.[146]

# PRENATAL TESTING

Given the mild clinical phenotype of most patients with the common variants of VWD, prenatal diagnosis for the purpose of deciding on terminating a pregnancy is rarely performed. However, type 3 VWD patients often have a profound bleeding disorder, similar to or more severe than classic hemophilia, and some families may request prenatal diagnosis. In those cases of VWD in which the precise mutation is known, DNA diagnosis can be performed rapidly and accurately by polymerase chain reaction (PCR) from amniotic fluid or chorionic villus biopsies (reviewed in Ref. 308) and would be expected to be compatible with new noninvasive prenatal testing methods.[309] In those cases where the mutation is unknown, diagnosis can still be attempted by genetic linkage analysis using the large panel of known polymorphisms within the VWF gene.[308] Although all cases of VWD analyzed to date appear to be linked to the VWF gene, the possibility of locus heterogeneity (i.e., a similar phenotype caused by a mutation in a gene other than VWF) should be considered.[310] As with all DNA testing, if prenatal testing is

being considered, genetic counseling should be provided before the decision to test is made as well as after the procedure.

# DIFFERENTIAL DIAGNOSIS

## PLATELET-TYPE (PSEUDO-) VON WILLEBRAND DISEASE

Platelet-type (pseudo-) VWD is a platelet defect that phenotypically mimics VWD (Chap. 10). Patients have mucocutaneous bleeding, plasma VWF often lacks the largest multimers, RIPA is enhanced at low concentrations of ristocetin, and thrombocytopenia of variable degree is often present. Molecular analysis has identified missense mutations within the GPIbα gene as the molecular basis for pseudo-VWD. These mutations are located within the segment of GPIb that encodes the VWF binding domain and appear to induce the conformational change complementary to that produced in VWF by type 2B VWD mutations (reviewed in Ref. 311).

The specialized RIPA test should be performed at low ristocetin concentrations to distinguish type 2B and platelet type VWD from type 2A VWD. In this test, purified normal plasma VWF or cryoprecipitate added to platelet preparations from patients with platelet-type VWD causes platelet aggregation, distinguishing this disorder from type 2B VWD where patient platelets aggregate only at higher ristocetin concentrations. In addition, type 2B VWD plasma transfers the enhanced RIPA to normal platelets, whereas plasma from patients with platelet-type VWD interacts normally with control platelets.

## ACQUIRED VON WILLEBRAND SYNDROME

Acquired VWD, or acquired von Willebrand syndrome (AVWS), is a relatively rare acquired bleeding disorder that usually presents as a late-onset bleeding diathesis in a patient with no prior bleeding history and a negative family history of bleeding (reviewed in Ref. 312). Decreased levels of FVIII, VWF:Ag, and VWF:RCo are common, and VWF multimers can be abnormal. AVWS is usually associated with another underlying disorder and has been reported to occur in patients with myeloproliferative neoplasms,[313] amyloidosis,[314] benign or malignant B-cell disorders,[315] hypothyroidism,[316] autoimmune disorders,[317] several solid tumors (particularly Wilms tumor),[318] cardiac or vascular defects (such as aortic stenosis),[319] ventricular assist devices,[320] or in association with several drugs, including ciprofloxacin and valproic acid.[321,322]

The mechanisms that cause AVWS can generally be attributed to an associated medical condition. A variety of B-cell disorders have been associated with the development of anti-VWF autoantibodies. In most cases, the AVWS appears to be due to rapid clearance of VWF induced by the circulating inhibitor, although these antibodies may also interfere with VWF function. Hypothyroidism results in decreased VWF synthesis.[316] In some cases of malignancy, AVWS is thought to be due to selective adsorption of VWF to the tumor cells or, in myeloproliferative neoplasms, clearance/alterations of VWF by the high circulating platelet mass. In AVWS associated with valvular heart disease, ventricular assist devices, or certain drugs, VWF may be lost by accelerated destruction or proteolysis under shear.[320–322]

Although the VWF multimers in AVWS usually exhibit a type 2A pattern with relative depletion of the large multimer forms, AVWS can manifest as a wide range of VWD phenotypes.[317,323] Distinguishing AVWS from genetic VWD can be difficult, as testing for the associated autoantibodies is generally not available in the clinical setting. The diagnosis often rests on the late onset of the disease, the absence of a family history, and the identification of an associated underlying disorder.

Management of AVWS is generally aimed at treating the underlying disorder. VWF levels and bleeding symptoms often improve with successful treatment of hypothyroidism or an associated malignancy. Refractory patients have been treated with glucocorticoids, plasma exchange, intravenous gamma globulin, rituximab, DDAVP, and VWF-containing FVIII concentrates.[312,324]

# ●THERAPY, COURSE, AND PROGNOSIS

The mainstays of therapy for VWD are DDAVP, which induces secretion of both VWF and FVIII (reviewed in Ref. 325), and replacement therapy with VWF-containing plasma concentrates. The choice of treatment in any given patient depends on the type and severity of VWD, the clinical setting, and the type of hemostatic challenge that must be met. Type 1 patients are most often treated with DDAVP alone, types 2A and 2B patients with a combination of DDAVP and a VWF-containing FVIII product, and type 2N and type 3 patients with VWF-containing concentrates.[146] A previous history of trauma or surgery and the success of previous treatment are important parameters to include in assessing the risk of bleeding. Prophylaxis is used in anticipation of hemostatic challenges,[146] such as dental extractions, and is efficacious in preventing recurrent bleeding in severe VWD patients.[326,327] Although in general there is a correlation between normal hemostasis and correction of VWF and FVIII activity, this does not occur in all cases.

## DESMOPRESSIN

DDAVP is an analogue of antidiuretic hormone that acts through type 2 vasopressin receptors to induce secretion of FVIII and VWF, likely via cyclic adenosine monophosphate–mediated secretion from the Weibel-Palade bodies in endothelial cells.[81] When DDAVP is administered to healthy subjects, it causes sustained increases of FVIII and ristocetin cofactor activity for approximately 4 hours.[328] Patients with type 1 VWD treated with DDAVP release unusually high-molecular-weight VWF multimers into the circulation for 1 to 3 hours after the infusion.[85,328] Therapy with DDAVP often increases the FVIII activity, VWF:Ag, and ristocetin cofactor activity to two to five times the basal level.

DDAVP has become a mainstay for the treatment of mild hemophilia and VWD[329] because it is relatively inexpensive, widely available, and avoids the risks of plasma-derived products. Approximately 80 percent of type 1 VWD patients have excellent responses to DDAVP, although this figure may be substantially lower depending on the criteria for diagnosis and response.[330] It is regularly used in the setting of mild to moderate bleeding and for prophylaxis of patients undergoing surgical procedures. DDAVP is administered at a dose of 0.3 mcg/kg continuous intravenous infusion over 30 minutes. DDAVP is also available for subcutaneous injection (at the same 0.3 mcg/kg dose) and in intranasal form (at a fixed dose of 300 mcg for adults and 150 mcg for children), which appears to be similar in efficacy to intravenous administration,[331,332] although the response may be more variable.

The response to DDAVP in any given individual with VWD is generally reproducible and predicts response to future doses as long as the follow-up doses are at least 2 to 4 days later. In one study, 22 type 1 VWD patients showed a departure of less than 20 percent from the mean FVIII peak level calculated from two separate infusions. In addition, the consistency of response in one patient reliably predicted the future response of that patient and other affected family members.[333] In a study of 77 type 1 VWD patients, DDAVP response was associated both with *VWF* mutation and baseline multimeric pattern, although subtle abnormalities in VWF multimers did not preclude a patient response to DDAVP. Interestingly, patients with the same *VWF* mutation did not

necessarily exhibit the same degree of responsiveness to DDAVP, implying the influence of other factors in the magnitude of DDAVP effect.[334] For patients requiring repeated infusions of DDAVP, the FVIII activity and VWF responses may not be of the same magnitude as after the first infusion. Although this decay in response has considerable individual variability, after one infusion of DDAVP per day for 4 days, it was found that the responses on days 2 to 4 were reduced approximately 30 percent compared to day 1.[331–333,335]

Therefore, in patients for whom DDAVP is potentially the treatment of choice, a test dose should be given at the planned therapeutic dose and route in advance of the first required course of treatment with measurements of before and after VWF and FVIII:C levels to ensure an adequate therapeutic response. Sampling additional time points after DDAVP infusion should be considered as some type 1 and type 2 VWD patients have a significantly shortened VWF half-life and it may be more appropriate to treat with VWF replacement therapy in clinical scenarios requiring more durable therapy to maintain hemostasis. For patients with type 1 VWD who are undergoing surgical procedures, DDAVP can be administered 1 hour before surgery and approximately every 12 hours thereafter for up to two to four doses before loss of clinically significant response. Patients should be monitored for response of FVIII and ristocetin cofactor activity and side effects, particularly hyponatremia (and then should be water restricted), when DDAVP is administered at frequent intervals. VWF-containing FVIII concentrates should be available for infusion as backup.

Approximately 20 to 25 percent of patients with VWD do not respond adequately to DDAVP. Type 2 VWD patients are less likely to have a response than type 1 patients,[330] and virtually no patients with type 3 VWD respond. The response to DDAVP of patients with type 2A VWD is variable. Although most patients respond only transiently, some patients exhibit complete hemostatic correction after DDAVP infusion.[336,337] It has been hypothesized that the differences in DDAVP efficacy among type 2A patients may correspond to the type of mutation, with better responses predicted in patients with group 2 mutations. A prospective study of the biologic response to DDAVP in well-characterized VWD patients included type 2A VWD patients with both group 1 and group 2 defects. Although patients with group 2 mutations had greater improvements in VWF:RCo and shortening of bleeding times than patients with group 1 defects, neither group could be classified as responders.[330]

Common side effects of DDAVP administration are mild cutaneous vasodilation resulting in a feeling of heat, facial flushing, tachycardia, tingling, and headaches. The potential for dilutional hyponatremia, especially in elderly and very young patients and with repeat dosing, requires appropriate attention to fluid restriction,[338,339] as it may result in seizures. There have been isolated reports of acute arterial thrombosis associated with administration of DDAVP, but the risk appears to be very low when judged against the total number of patients treated. DDAVP is contraindicated in patients with unstable coronary artery disease because of increased risk of thrombotic events, such as myocardial infarction.[340] Patients receiving DDAVP at closely spaced intervals of less than 24 to 48 hours can develop tachyphylaxis.[335]

Many experts consider DDAVP to be contraindicated in the treatment of type 2B VWD, as the high-molecular-weight VWF released from storage sites has an increased affinity for binding to GPIb and might be expected to induce spontaneous platelet aggregation and worsening thrombocytopenia.[221] However, there are reports of DDAVP used successfully in type 2B VWD patients, with an associated shortening of bleeding times and variable thrombocytopenia.[341,342] Although type 2N patients can exhibit increased FVIII:C levels after DDAVP, in some cases the FVIII:C levels rapidly decline, likely a result of the absence of stabilizing normal VWF, attenuating clinical efficacy. Type 2M patients generally do not have a satisfactory response to DDAVP.[330,343]

## VON WILLEBRAND FACTOR REPLACEMENT THERAPY

It is important to determine the response to DDAVP for each individual so as to avoid the unnecessary use of plasma products. For type 3 VWD patients, other patients unresponsive to DDAVP, or patients with major bleeding or in situations requiring precise control over therapeutic levels, VWF replacement therapy is appropriate. The use of selected virus-inactivated, VWF-containing FVIII concentrates is generally safe and effective.[146] Humate-P, Alphanate, Wilate, and Koate are all acceptable commercial VWF-containing plasma concentrates that have been evaluated in VWD replacement therapy in clinical studies, and other VWF-containing FVIII concentrates may also be effective. A plasma-free recombinant VWF (rVWF), Vonvendi, was approved for adult VWD patients in 2015. rVWF has a similar or longer half-life than plasma-derived VWF and showed hemostatic efficacy in a phase III clinical trial of 22 VWD patients.[344,345] In the phase III trial, rVWF was intended to be coadministered with recombinant FVIII (rFVIII), but in a few cases, rVWF was inadvertently initially infused without rFVIII. In these cases, hemostasis was achieved and delayed stabilization of endogenous FVIII observed.[345] The precise role of rVWF-rFVIII (or rVWF alone) in future VWF replacement therapy remains to be defined, as experience is still limited,[346] and further studies are needed, particularly in special VWD populations who may benefit from a non–plasma-derived (FVIII-deficient) VWF replacement product. Cryoprecipitate was useful in the past, but because it is not generally treated to inactivate bloodborne pathogens, is less targeted to correcting the VWD hemostatic defect, and its administration is associated with a large volume load, it is less desirable. It is important to note that most standard FVIII concentrates and all recombinant FVIII products are not effective in VWD because they lack clinically significant quantities of VWF. Although such products can substantially increase circulating FVIII:C, the infused factor is short-lived in the circulation in the absence of stabilizing VWF.[347] Only preparations that contain large quantities of VWF with well-preserved multimer structure are suitable for use in VWD patients.

In practice, VWD replacement therapy dosing and timing have been largely empiric. Recommendations for therapy have been outlined based on the degree and nature of hemorrhage and experience in clinical practice.[146] The objective is to elevate FVIII:C and VWF:RCo until bleeding stops and healing is complete. In general, replacement goals of FVIII:C and VWF:RCo should be initial replacement to greater than 100 IU/dL and maintenance of greater than 50 IU/dL for 7 to 14 days for major trauma, surgery, or central nervous system hemorrhage; greater than 30 to 50 IU/dL for 3 to 5 days for minor surgery or bleeding; greater than 50 IU/dL for delivery and continued for at least 3 to 5 days in the postpartum period; greater than 30 to 50 IU/dL for 1 to 5 days for dental extractions and minor surgery; and greater than 20 to 50 IU/dL for mucous membrane bleeding or menorrhagia. Laboratory monitoring of posttreatment FVIII:C and VWF levels is important in guiding therapy and avoidance of supratherapeutic replacement doses (>200 IU/dL VWF:RCo, >250 IU/dL FVIII), which are associated with an increased risk of thrombosis.[146,348,349] Although thrombosis is rare overall, VWD patients on prolonged therapy or with central access catheters appear to be at higher risk.[350]

In patients who have concomitant thrombocytopenia associated with or in addition to VWD, it may be necessary to transfuse platelets in addition to factor concentrates. If clinical bleeding continues, additional replacement therapy must be given and searches undertaken for other hemostatic defects. Type 3 VWD patients receiving multiple transfusions can develop antibodies directed against VWF (reviewed in Ref. 270). Continued replacement with VWF-containing concentrates is contraindicated because of the risk of anaphylaxis. A variety of approaches to the management of VWD inhibitors, similar to the treatment of FVIII inhibitors in hemophilia A (Chap. 13), have been attempted. Immunosuppression, recombinant FVIII, and recombinant factor VIIa have been reported to be useful in patients with type 3 VWD who have developed anti-VWF antibodies.

## OTHER NONREPLACEMENT THERAPIES

Fibrinolytic inhibitors, such as $\varepsilon$-aminocaproic acid or tranexamic acid, have been used effectively in some VWD patients. Antifibrinolytics are commonly used alone or in conjunction with DDAVP or a plasma-derived VWF replacement product in patients with gynecologic bleeding, with mucous membrane bleeding, or undergoing dental procedures.[146] Fibrinolytic inhibitors can be delivered systemically or topically and are generally well tolerated, but rarely can cause nausea or diarrhea and are contraindicated in patients with gross hematuria.

Estrogens or oral contraceptives have been used empirically in treating menorrhagia. In addition to their effects on the ovaries and uterus, some estrogens can increase plasma VWF levels. Patients with VWD frequently normalize their levels of FVIII, VWF:Ag, and VWF:RCo during pregnancy. Postpartum hemorrhage within the first few days after parturition may be related to the relatively rapid return of FVIII and VWF activities to prepregnancy levels, and postpartum hemorrhage in all forms of VWD may occur as long as 1 month postpartum. In pregnant patients with type 1 VWD, the FVIII and ristocetin cofactor activities usually rise above 50 percent. These patients usually do not require any specific therapy at the time of parturition. In contrast, individuals who have 30 percent or less FVIII or variant forms of VWD are more likely to require prophylactic therapy before delivery. In a recent study, women receiving treatment for VWD postpartum were unexpectedly found not to have corrected to target levels.[351] Therefore, laboratory testing is recommended at term and should be considered in the postpartum period in patients at risk for immediate and/or delayed bleeding complications or receiving therapy.

Recombinant activated factor VII (rFVIIa, or NovoSeven) has also been successfully used in VWD patients with severe hemorrhage refractory to VWF replacement therapy and in bleeding patients with anti-VWF antibodies (reviewed in Ref. 352). In the case of minor accessible bleeding, topical drugs such as fibrin sealants or topical bovine thrombin may also be considered when standard VWD therapies fail to provide adequate local hemostasis.[146]

## REFERENCES

1. von Willebrand EA: Hereditar Pseudohemofili. *Finska Lakarsallskapetes Handl* 67:7–112, 1926.
2. Hoyer LW: von Willebrand's disease. *Prog Hemost Thromb* 3:231–287, 1976.
3. Nilsson IM: von Willebrand's disease–Fifty years old. *Acta Med Scand* 201:497–508, 1977.
4. Zimmerman TS, Ratnoff OD, Powell AE: Immunologic differentiation of classic hemophilia (factor VIII deficiency) and von Willebrand disease. *J Clin Invest* 50:244–254, 1971.
5. Howard MA, Firkin BG: Ristocetin: A new tool in the investigation of platelet aggregation. *Thromb Diath Haemorrh* 76:362–369, 1971.
6. Weiss HJ, Rogers J, Brand H: Defective ristocetin-induced platelet aggregation in von Willebrand's disease and its correction by factor VIII. *J Clin Invest* 52:2697–2707, 1973.
7. Weiss HJ, Hoyer LW: von Willebrand factor: dissociation from antihemophilic factor procoagulant activity. *Science* 182(117):1149–1151, 1973.
8. Zimmerman TS, Edgington TS: Factor VIII coagulant activity and factor VIII-like antigen: independent molecular entities. *J Exp Med* 138:1015–1020, 1973.
9. Gitschier J, Wood WI, Goralka TM, et al: Characterization of the human factor VIII gene. *Nature* 312:326–330, 1984.
10. Toole JJ, Knopf JL, Wozney JM, et al: Molecular cloning of a cDNA encoding human antihaemophilic factor. *Nature* 312:342–347, 1984.

11. Ginsburg D, Handin RI, Bonthron DT, et al: Human von Willebrand factor (vWF): Isolation of complementary DNA (cDNA) clones and chromosomal localization. *Science* 228(4706):1401–1406, 1985.

12. Lynch DC, Zimmerman TS, Collins CJ, et al: Molecular cloning of cDNA for human von Willebrand factor: Authentication by a new method. *Cell* 41:49–56, 1985.

13. Sadler JE, Shelton-Inloes BB, Sorace JM, Harlan JM, Titani K, Davie EW: Cloning and characterization of two cDNAs coding for human von Willebrand factor. *Proc Natl Acad Sci USA* 82:6394–6398, 1985.

14. Verweij CL, de Vries CJM, Distel B, et al: Construction of cDNA coding for human von Willebrand factor using antibody probes for colony-screening and mapping of the chromosomal gene. *Nucleic Acids Res* 13:4699–4717, 1985.

15. Sadler JE, Budde U, Eikenboom JC, et al: Update on the pathophysiology and classification of von Willebrand disease: A report of the Subcommittee on von Willebrand Factor. *J Thromb Haemost* 4(10):2103–2114, 2006.

16. Titani K, Kumar S, Takio K, et al: Amino acid sequence of human von Willebrand factor. *Biochemistry* 25:3171–3184, 1986.

17. Fay PJ, Kawai Y, Wagner DD, et al: Propopeptide of von Willebrand factor circulates in blood and is identical to von Willebrand antigen II. *Science* 232:995–998, 1986.

18. Bonthron DT, Handin RI, Kaufman RJ, et al: Structure of pre-pro-von Willebrand factor and its expression in heterologous cells. *Nature* 324(6094):270–273, 1986.

19. Bonthron D, Orr EC, Mitsock LM, Ginsburg D, Handin RI, Orkin SH: Nucleotide sequence of pre-pro-von Willebrand factor cDNA. *Nucleic Acids Res* 14(17):7125–7127, 1986.

20. Shelton-Inloes BB, Titani K, Sadler JE: cDNA sequences for human von Willebrand factor reveal five types of repeated domains and five possible protein sequence polymorphisms. *Biochemistry* 25(11):3164–3171, 1986.

21. Shelton-Inloes BB, Broze GJ Jr, Miletich JP, Sadler JE: Evolution of human von Willebrand factor: cDNA sequence polymorphisms, repeated domains, and relationship to von Willebrand antigen II. *Biochem Biophys Res Commun* 144(2):657–665, 1987.

22. Springer TA: von Willebrand factor, Jedi knight of the bloodstream. *Blood* 124(9):1412–1425, 2014.

23. Colombatti A, Bonaldo P: The superfamily of proteins with von Willebrand factor type A-like domains: One theme common to components of extracellular matrix, hemostasis, cellular adhesion, and defense mechanisms. *Blood* 77(11):2305–2315, 1991.

24. Hunt LT, Barker WC: von Willebrand factor shares a distinctive cysteine-rich domain with thrombospondin and procollagen. *Biochem Biophys Res Commun* 144(2):876–882, 1987.

25. Mancuso DJ, Tuley EA, Westfield LA, et al: Structure of the gene for human von Willebrand factor. *J Biol Chem* 264(33):19514–19527, 1989.

26. Shelton-Inloes BB, Chehab FF, Mannucci PM, Federici AB, Sadler JE: Gene deletions correlate with the development of alloantibodies in von Willebrand disease. *J Clin Invest* 79(5):1459–1465, 1987.

27. Mancuso DJ, Tuley EA, Westfield LA, et al: Human von Willebrand factor gene and pseudogene: Structural analysis and differentiation by polymerase chain reaction. *Biochemistry* 30(1):253–269, 1991.

28. Zhang ZP, Blomback M, Nyman D, Anvret M: Mutations of von Willebrand factor gene in families with von Willebrand disease in the Aland Islands. *Proc Natl Acad Sci U S A* 90(17):7937–7940, 1993.

29. Eikenboom JC, Vink T, Briet E, Sixma JJ, Reitsma PH: Multiple substitutions in the von Willebrand factor gene that mimic the pseudogene sequence. *Proc Natl Acad Sci U S A* 91(6):2221–2224, 1994.

30. Eikenboom JC, Castaman G, Vos HL, Bertina RM, Rodeghiero F: Characterization of the genetic defects in recessive type 1 and type 3 von Willebrand disease patients of Italian origin. *Thromb Haemost* 79(4):709–717, 1998.

31. James PD, Notley C, Hegadorn C, et al: The mutational spectrum of type 1 von Willebrand disease: Results from a Canadian cohort study. *Blood* 109(1):145–154, 2007.

32. Rand JH, Badimon L, Gordon RE, Uson RR, Fuster V: Distribution of von Willebrand factor in porcine intima varies with blood vessel type and location. *Arteriosclerosis* 7(3):287–291, 1987.

33. Yamamoto K, de Waard V, Fearns C, Loskutoff DJ: Tissue distribution and regulation of murine von Willebrand factor gene expression in vivo. *Blood* 92(8):2791–2801, 1998.

34. Jahroudi N, Lynch DC: Endothelial-cell-specific regulation of von Willebrand factor gene expression. *Mol Cell Biol* 14(2):999–1008, 1994.

35. Harvey PJ, Keightley AM, Lam YM, Cameron C, Lillicrap D: A single nucleotide polymorphism at nucleotide -1793 in the von Willebrand factor (VWF) regulatory region is associated with plasma VWF:Ag levels. *Br J Haematol* 109(2):349–353, 2000.

36. Guan J, Guillot PV, Aird WC: Characterization of the mouse von Willebrand factor promoter. *Blood* 94(10):3405–3412, 1999.

37. Hough C, Cuthbert CD, Notley C, et al: Cell type-specific regulation of von Willebrand factor expression by the E4BP4 transcriptional repressor. *Blood* 105(4):1531–1539, 2005.

38. Kleinschmidt AM, Nassiri M, Stitt MS, et al: Sequences in intron 51 of the von Willebrand factor gene target promoter activation to a subset of lung endothelial cells in transgenic mice. *J Biol Chem* 283(5):2741–2750, 2008.

39. Aird WC, Jahroudi N, Weiler-Guettler H, Rayburn HB, Rosenberg RD: Human von Willebrand factor gene sequences target expression to a subpopulation of endothelial cells in transgenic mice. *Proc Natl Acad Sci U S A* 92(10):4567–4571, 1995.

40. Bernat JA, Crawford GE, Ogurtsov AY, Collins FS, Ginsburg D, Kondrashov AS: Distant conserved sequences flanking endothelial-specific promoters contain tissue-specific DNase-hypersensitive sites and over-represented motifs. *Hum Mol Genet* 15(13):2098–2105, 2006.

41. Pusztaszeri MP, Seelentag W, Bosman FT: Immunohistochemical expression of endothelial markers CD31, CD34, von Willebrand factor, and Fli-1 in normal human tissues. *J Histochem Cytochem* 54(4):385–395, 2006.

42. Hough C, Cameron CL, Notley CR, et al: Influence of a GT repeat element on shear stress responsiveness of the VWF gene promoter. *J Thromb Haemost* 6(7):1183–1190, 2008.

43. Daidone V, Cattini MG, Pontara E, et al: Microsatellite (GT)(n) repeats and SNPs in the von Willebrand factor gene promoter do not influence circulating von Willebrand factor levels under normal conditions. *Thromb Haemost* 101(2):298–304, 2009.

44. Wagner DD: Cell biology of von Willebrand factor. *Annu Rev Cell Biol* 6:217–246, 1990.

45. de Wit TR, van Mourik JA: Biosynthesis, processing and secretion of von Willebrand factor: Biological implications. *Best Pract Res Clin Haematol* 14(2):241–255, 2001.

46. Marti T, Rosselet SJ, Titani K, Walsh KA: Identification of disulfide-bridged substructures within human von Willebrand factor. *Biochemistry* 26(25):8099–8109, 1987.

47. Choi H, Aboulfatova K, Pownall HJ, Cook R, Dong JF: Shear-induced disulfide bond formation regulates adhesion activity of von Willebrand factor. *J Biol Chem* 282(49):35604–35611, 2007.

48. Wagner DD, Lawrence SO, Ohlsson-Wilhelm BM, Fay PJ, Marder VJ: Topology and order of formation of interchain disulfide bonds in von Willebrand factor. *Blood* 69(1):27–32, 1987.

49. Voorberg J, Fontijn R, Calafat J, Janssen H, van Mourik JA, Pannekoek H: Assembly and routing of von Willebrand factor variants: The requirements for disulfide-linked dimerization reside within the carboxy-terminal 151 amino acids. *J Cell Biol* 113(1):195–205, 1991.

50. Mayadas TN, Wagner DD: Vicinal cysteines in the prosequence play a role in von Willebrand factor multimer assembly. *Proc Natl Acad Sci U S A* 89(8):3531–3535, 1992.

51. Purvis AR, Sadler JE: A covalent oxidoreductase intermediate in propeptide-dependent von Willebrand factor multimerization. *J Biol Chem* 279(48):49982–49988, 2004.

52. Mayadas TN, Wagner DD: In vitro multimerization of von Willebrand factor is triggered by low pH. Importance of the propolypeptide and free sulfhydryls. *J Biol Chem* 264(23):13497–13503, 1989.

53. Wagner DD, Fay PJ, Sporn LA, Sinha S, Lawrence SO, Marder VJ: Divergent fates of von Willebrand factor and its propolypeptide (von Willebrand antigen II) after secretion from endothelial cells. *Proc Natl Acad Sci U S A* 84(7):1955–1959, 1987.

54. Verweij CL, Hart M, Pannekoek H: Expression of variant von Willebrand factor (vWF) cDNA in heterologous cells: Requirement of the pro-polypeptide in vWF multimer formation. *EMBO J* 6(10):2885–2890, 1987.

55. Wise RJ, Pittman DD, Handin RI, Kaufman RJ, Orkin SH: The propeptide of von Willebrand factor independently mediates the assembly of von Willebrand multimers. *Cell* 52(2):229–236, 1988.

56. Rehemtulla A, Kaufman RJ: Preferred sequence requirements for cleavage of pro-von Willebrand factor by propeptide-processing enzymes. *Blood* 79(9):2349–2355, 1992.

57. Wagner DD, Marder VJ: Biosynthesis of von Willebrand protein by human endothelial cells: Processing steps and their intracellular localization. *J Cell Biol* 99(6):2123–2130, 1984.

58. Lynch DC, Zimmerman TS, Ling EH, Browning PJ: An explanation for minor multimer species in endothelial cell-synthesized von Willebrand factor. *J Clin Invest* 77(6):2048–2051, 1986.

59. Verweij CL, Hart M, Pannekoek H: Proteolytic cleavage of the precursor of von Willebrand factor is not essential for multimer formation. *J Biol Chem* 263(17):7921–7924, 1988.

60. Weibel ER, Palade GE: New cytoplasmic components in arterial endothelia. *J Cell Biol* 23:101–112, 1964.

61. Wagner DD, Olmsted JB, Marder VJ: Immunolocalization of von Willebrand protein in Weibel-Palade bodies of human endothelial cells. *J Cell Biol* 95(1):355–360, 1982.

62. Metcalf DJ, Nightingale TD, Zenner HL, Lui-Roberts WW, Cutler DF: Formation and function of Weibel-Palade bodies. *J Cell Sci* 121(Pt 1):19–27, 2008.

63. Huang RH, Wang Y, Roth R, et al: Assembly of Weibel-Palade body-like tubules from N-terminal domains of von Willebrand factor. *Proc Natl Acad Sci U S A* 105(2):482–487, 2008.

64. Yarovoi H, Nurden AT, Montgomery RR, Nurden P, Poncz M: Intracellular interaction of von Willebrand factor and factor VIII depends on cellular context: Lessons from platelet-expressed factor VIII. *Blood* 105(12):4674–4676, 2005.

65. Rosenberg JB, Foster PA, Kaufman RJ, et al: Intracellular trafficking of factor VIII to von Willebrand factor storage granules. *J Clin Invest* 101(3):613–624, 1998.

66. van den Biggelaar M, Bierings R, Storm G, Voorberg J, Mertens K: Requirements for cellular co-trafficking of factor VIII and von Willebrand factor to Weibel-Palade bodies. *J Thromb Haemost* 5(11):2235–2242, 2007.

67. Nightingale T, Cutler D: The secretion of von Willebrand factor from endothelial cells: An increasingly complicated story. *J Thromb Haemost* 11(Suppl 1):192–201, 2013.

68. Bonfanti R, Furie BC, Furie B, Wagner DD: PADGEM (GMP140) is a component of Weibel-Palade bodies of human endothelial cells. *Blood* 73(5):1109–1112, 1989.

69. Michaux G, Pullen TJ, Haberichter SL, Cutler DF: P-selectin binds to the D′-D3 domains of von Willebrand factor in Weibel-Palade bodies. *Blood* 107(10):3922–3924, 2006.

70. Cleator JH, Zhu WQ, Vaughan DE, Hamm HE: Differential regulation of endothelial exocytosis of P-selectin and von Willebrand factor by protease-activated receptors and cAMP. *Blood* 107(7):2736–2744, 2006.

71. Knop M, Aareskjold E, Bode G, Gerke V: Rab3D and annexin A2 play a role in regulated secretion of vWF, but not tPA, from endothelial cells. *EMBO J* 23(15):2982–2992, 2004.

72. Rondaij MG, Bierings R, Kragt A, van Mourik JA, Voorberg J: Dynamics and plasticity of Weibel-Palade bodies in endothelial cells. *Arterioscler Thromb Vasc Biol* 26(5):1002–1007, 2006.

73. Giblin JP, Hewlett LJ, Hannah MJ: Basal secretion of von Willebrand factor from human endothelial cells. *Blood* 112(4):957–964, 2008.

74. Levine JD, Harlan JM, Harker LA, Joseph ML, Counts RB: Thrombin-mediated release of factor VIII antigen from human umbilical vein endothelial cells in culture. *Blood* 60(2):531–534, 1982.

75. Ribes JA, Francis CW, Wagner DD: Fibrin induces release of von Willebrand factor from endothelial cells. *J Clin Invest* 79(1):117–123, 1987.

76. Hamilton KK, Sims PJ: Changes in cytosolic Ca2+ associated with von Willebrand factor release in human endothelial cells exposed to histamine. Study of microcarrier cell monolayers using the fluorescent probe indo-1. *J Clin Invest* 79(2):600–608, 1987.

77. Hattori R, Hamilton KK, McEver RP, Sims PJ: Complement proteins C5b-9 induce secretion of high molecular weight multimers of endothelial von Willebrand factor and translocation of granule membrane protein GMP-140 to the cell surface. *J Biol Chem* 264(15):9053–9060, 1989.

78. Bernardo A, Ball C, Nolasco L, Moake JF, Dong JF: Effects of inflammatory cytokines on the release and cleavage of the endothelial cell-derived ultralarge von Willebrand factor multimers under flow. *Blood* 104(1):100–106, 2004.

79. Fish RJ, Yang H, Viglino C, Schorer R, Dunoyer-Geindre S, Kruithof EK: Fluvastatin inhibits regulated secretion of endothelial cell von Willebrand factor in response to diverse secretagogues. *Biochem J* 405(3):597–604, 2007.

80. Yamakuchi M, Greer JJ, Cameron SJ, et al: HMG-CoA reductase inhibitors inhibit endothelial exocytosis and decrease myocardial infarct size. *Circ Res* 96(11):1185–1192, 2005.

81. Kaufmann JE, Oksche A, Wollheim CB, Gunther G, Rosenthal W, Vischer UM: Vasopressin-induced von Willebrand factor secretion from endothelial cells involves V2 receptors and cAMP. *J Clin Invest* 106(1):107–116, 2000.

82. Sporn LA, Marder VJ, Wagner DD: Differing polarity of the constitutive and regulated secretory pathways for von Willebrand factor in endothelial cells. *J Cell Biol* 108(4):1283–1289, 1989.

83. Ewenstein BM, Warhol MJ, Handin RI, Pober JS: Composition of the von Willebrand factor storage organelle (Weibel-Palade body) isolated from cultured human umbilical vein endothelial cells. *J Cell Biol* 104(5):1423–1433, 1987.

84. Sporn LA, Marder VJ, Wagner DD: Inducible secretion of large, biologically potent von Willebrand factor multimers. *Cell* 46(2):185–190, 1986.

85. Fernandez MF, Ginsberg MH, Ruggeri ZM, Battle FJ, Zimmerman TS: Multimeric structure of platelet factor VIII/von Willebrand factor: The presence of larger multimers and their reassociation with thrombin-stimulated platelets. *Blood* 60(5):1132–1138, 1982.

86. Wagner DD, Saffaripour S, Bonfanti R, et al: Induction of specific storage organelles by von Willebrand factor propolypeptide. *Cell* 64(2):403–413, 1991.

87. Voorberg J, Fontijn R, Calafat J, Janssen H, van Mourik JA, Pannekoek H: Biogenesis of von Willebrand factor-containing organelles in heterologous transfected CV-1 cells. *EMBO J.* 12(2):749–758, 1993.

88. Journet AM, Saffaripour S, Cramer EM, Tenza D, Wagner DD: von Willebrand factor storage requires intact prosequence cleavage site. *Eur J Cell Biol* 60(1):31–41, 1993.

89. Nachman RL, Jaffe EA: Subcellular platelet factor VIII antigen and von Willebrand factor. *J Exp Med* 141(5):1101–1113, 1975.

90. Bowie EJ, Solberg LA Jr, Fass DN, et al. Transplantation of normal bone marrow into a pig with severe von Willebrand's disease. *J Clin Invest* 78(1):26–30, 1986.

91. Nichols TC, Samama CM, Bellinger DA, et al: Function of von Willebrand factor after crossed bone marrow transplantation between normal and von Willebrand disease pigs: Effect on arterial thrombosis in chimeras. *Proc Natl Acad Sci U S A* 92(7):2455–2459, 1995.

92. Andre P, Brouland JP, Roussi J, et al: Role of plasma and platelet von Willebrand factor in arterial thrombogenesis and hemostasis in the pig. *Exp Hematol* 26(7):620–626, 1998.

93. Bowen DJ, Collins PW: Insights into von Willebrand factor proteolysis: Clinical implications. *Br J Haematol* 133(5):457–467, 2006.

94. Padilla A, Moake JL, Bernardo A, et al: P-selectin anchors newly released ultralarge von Willebrand factor multimers to the endothelial cell surface. *Blood* 103(6):2150–2156, 2004.

95. Lopez JA, Dong JF: Shear stress and the role of high molecular weight von Willebrand factor multimers in thrombus formation. *Blood Coagul Fibrinolysis* 16(Suppl 1):S11–S16, 2005.

96. Dent JA, Berkowitz SD, Ware J, Kasper CK, Ruggeri ZM: Identification of a cleavage site directing the immunochemical detection of molecular abnormalities in type IIA von Willebrand factor. *Proc Natl Acad Sci U S A* 87(16):6306–6310, 1990.

97. Lankhof H, Damas C, Schiphorst ME, et al: von Willebrand factor without the A2 domain is resistant to proteolysis. *Thromb Haemost* 77(5):1008–1013, 1997.

98. Tsai HM, Sussman, II, Ginsburg D, Lankhof H, Sixma JJ, Nagel RL: Proteolytic cleavage of recombinant type 2A von Willebrand factor mutants R834W and R834Q: Inhibition by doxycycline and by monoclonal antibody VP-1. *Blood* 89(6):1954–1962, 1997.

99. Bowen DJ, Collins PW: An amino acid polymorphism in von Willebrand factor correlates with increased susceptibility to proteolysis by ADAMTS13. *Blood* 103(3):941–947, 2004.

100. Reininger AJ: Function of von Willebrand factor in haemostasis and thrombosis. *Haemophilia* 14(Suppl 5):11–26, 2008.

101. Savage B, Almus-Jacobs F, Ruggeri ZM: Specific synergy of multiple substrate-receptor interactions in platelet thrombus formation under flow. *Cell* 94(5):657–666, 1998.

102. Pendu R, Terraube V, Christophe OD, et al: P-selectin glycoprotein ligand 1 and beta2-integrins cooperate in the adhesion of leukocytes to von Willebrand factor. *Blood* 108(12):3746–3752, 2006.

103. Ruggeri ZM, Ware J: von Willebrand factor, in *Thrombosis and Hemorrhage*, edited by Loscalzo J, Schafer AI, pp 246–265. Lippincott Williams& Wilkins, Philadelphia, 2003.

104. Kalafatis M, Takahashi Y, Girma JP, Meyer D: Localization of a collagen-interactive domain of human von Willebrand factor between amino acid residues Gly 911 and Glu 1365. *Blood* 70(5):1577–1583, 1987.

105. Pareti FI, Niiya K, McPherson JM, Ruggeri ZM: Isolation and characterization of two domains of human von Willebrand factor that interact with fibrillar collagen types I and III. *J Biol Chem* 262(28):13835–13841, 1987.

106. Takagi J, Sekiya F, Kasahara K, Inada Y, Saito Y: Inhibition of platelet-collagen interaction by propolypeptide of von Willebrand factor. *J Biol Chem* 264(11):6017–6020, 1989.

107. Cruz MA, Yuan H, Lee JR, Wise RJ, Handin RI: Interaction of the von Willebrand factor (vWF) with collagen. Localization of the primary collagen-binding site by analysis of recombinant vWF A domain polypeptides. *J Biol Chem* 270(18):10822–10827, 1995.

108. Lankhof H, van Hoeij M, Schiphorst ME, et al: A3 domain is essential for interaction of von Willebrand factor with collagen type III. *Thromb Haemost* 75(6):950–958, 1996.

109. Flood VH, Schlauderaff AC, Haberichter SL, et al: Crucial role for the VWF A1 domain in binding to type IV collagen. *Blood* 125(14):2297–2304, 2015.

110. Rand JH, Patel ND, Schwartz E, Zhou SL, Potter BJ: 150-kD von Willebrand factor binding protein extracted from human vascular subendothelium is type VI collagen. *J Clin Invest* 88(1):253–259, 1991.

111. Rand JH, Wu XX, Potter BJ, Uson RR, Gordon RE: Co-localization of von Willebrand factor and type VI collagen in human vascular subendothelium. *Am J Pathol* 142(3):843–850, 1993.

112. Mazzucato M, Spessotto P, Masotti A, et al: Identification of domains responsible for von Willebrand factor type VI collagen interaction mediating platelet adhesion under high flow. *J Biol Chem* 274(5):3033–3041, 1999.

113. Fretto LJ, Fowler WE, McCaslin DR, Erickson HP, McKee PA: Substructure of human von Willebrand factor. Proteolysis by V8 and characterization of two functional domains. *J Biol Chem* 261(33):15679–15689, 1986.

114. Fujimura Y, Titani K, Holland LZ, et al: A heparin-binding domain of human von Willebrand factor. Characterization and localization to a tryptic fragment extending from amino acid residue Val-449 to Lys-728. *J Biol Chem* 262(4):1734–1739, 1987.

115. Christophe O, Obert B, Meyer D, Girma JP: The binding domain of von Willebrand factor to sulfatides is distinct from those interacting with glycoprotein Ib, heparin, and collagen and resides between amino acid residues Leu 512 and Lys 673. *Blood* 78(9):2310–2317, 1991.

116. Yuan H, Deng N, Zhang S, et al: The unfolded von Willebrand factor response in bloodstream: the self-association perspective. *J Hematol Oncol* 5:65, 2012.

117. Marchese P, Murata M, Mazzucato M, et al: Identification of three tyrosine residues of glycoprotein Ib alpha with distinct roles in von Willebrand factor and alpha-thrombin binding. *J Biol Chem* 270(16):9571–9578, 1995.

118. Fujimura Y, Titani K, Holland LZ, et al: von Willebrand factor. A reduced and alkylated 52/48-kDa fragment beginning at amino acid residue 449 contains the domain interacting with platelet glycoprotein Ib. *J Biol Chem* 261(1):381–385, 1986.

119. Mohri H, Fujimura Y, Shima M, et al: Structure of the von Willebrand factor domain interacting with glycoprotein Ib. *J Biol Chem* 263(34):17901–17904, 1988.

120. Nishio K, Anderson PJ, Zheng XL, Sadler JE: Binding of platelet glycoprotein Ibalpha to von Willebrand factor domain A1 stimulates the cleavage of the adjacent domain A2 by ADAMTS13. *Proc Natl Acad Sci USA* 101(29):10578–10583, 2004.

121. Matsushita T, Sadler JE: Identification of amino acid residues essential for von Willebrand factor binding to platelet glycoprotein Ib. Charged-to-alanine scanning mutagenesis of the A1 domain of human von Willebrand factor. *J Biol Chem* 270(22):13406–13414, 1995.

122. Emsley J, Cruz M, Handin R, Liddington R: Crystal structure of the von Willebrand factor A1 domain and implications for the binding of platelet glycoprotein Ib. *J Biol Chem* 273(17):10396–10401, 1998.

123. Chen J, Zhou H, Diacovo A, Zheng XL, Emsley J, Diacovo TG: Exploiting the kinetic interplay between GPIbalpha-VWF binding interfaces to regulate hemostasis and thrombosis. *Blood* 124(25):3799–3807, 2014.

124. Bienkowska J, Cruz M, Atiemo A, Handin R, Liddington R: The von willebrand factor A3 domain does not contain a metal ion-dependent adhesion site motif. *J Biol Chem* 272(40):25162–25167, 1997.

125. Huizinga EG, Martijn van der Plas R, Kroon J, Sixma JJ, Gros P: Crystal structure of the A3 domain of human von Willebrand factor: Implications for collagen binding. *Structure* 5(9):1147–1156, 1997.

126. Huizinga EG, Tsuji S, Romijn RA, et al: Structures of glycoprotein Ibalpha and its complex with von Willebrand factor A1 domain. *Science* 297(5584):1176–1179, 2002.

127. Hulstein JJ, Lenting PJ, de LB, Derksen RH, Fijnheer R, de Groot PG: beta2-Glycoprotein I inhibits von Willebrand factor dependent platelet adhesion and aggregation. *Blood* 110(5):1483–1491, 2007.

128. Scott JP, Montgomery RR, Retzinger GS: Dimeric ristocetin flocculates proteins, binds to platelets, and mediates von Willebrand factor-dependent agglutination of platelets. *J Biol Chem* 266(13):8149–8155, 1991.

129. Berndt MC, Du XP, Booth WJ: Ristocetin-dependent reconstitution of binding of von Willebrand factor to purified human platelet membrane glycoprotein Ib-IX complex. *Biochemistry* 27(2):633–640, 1988.

130. Fukuda K, Doggett TA, Bankston LA, Cruz MA, Diacovo TG, Liddington RC: Structural basis of von Willebrand factor activation by the snake toxin botrocetin. *Structure* 10(7):943–950, 2002.

131. Adachi T, Matsushita T, Dong Z, et al: Identification of amino acid residues essential for heparin binding by the A1 domain of human von Willebrand factor. *Biochem Biophys Res Commun* 339(4):1178–1183, 2006.

132. Sobel M, McNeill PM, Carlson PL, et al: Heparin inhibition of von Willebrand factor-dependent platelet function in vitro and in vivo. *J Clin Invest* 87(5):1787–1793, 1991.

133. Sobel M, Bird KE, Tyler-Cross R, et al: Heparins designed to specifically inhibit platelet interactions with von Willebrand factor. *Circulation* 93(5):992–999, 1996.

134. Keuren JF, Baruch D, Legendre P, et al: von Willebrand factor C1C2 domain is involved in platelet adhesion to polymerized fibrin at high shear rate. *Blood* 103(5):1741–1746, 2004.

135. Vlot AJ, Koppelman SJ, van den Berg MH, Bouma BN, Sixma JJ: The affinity and stoichiometry of binding of human factor VIII to von Willebrand factor. *Blood* 85(11):3150–3157, 1995.

136. Terraube V, O'Donnell JS, Jenkins PV. Factor VIII and von Willebrand factor interaction: Biological, clinical and therapeutic importance. *Haemophilia* 16(1):3–13, 2010.

137. Cao W, Krishnaswamy S, Camire RM, Lenting PJ, Zheng XL: Factor VIII accelerates proteolytic cleavage of von Willebrand factor by ADAMTS13. *Proc Natl Acad Sci USA* 105(21):7416–7421, 2008.

138. Foster PA, Fulcher CA, Marti T, Titani K, Zimmerman TS: A major factor VIII binding domain resides within the amino-terminal 272 amino acid residues of von Willebrand factor. *J Biol Chem* 262(18):8443–8446, 1987.

139. Yee A, Gildersleeve RD, Gu S, et al: A von Willebrand factor fragment containing the D'D3 domains is sufficient to stabilize coagulation factor VIII in mice. *Blood* 124(3):445–452, 2014.

140. Bahou WF, Ginsburg D, Sikkink R, Litwiller R, Fass DN: A monoclonal antibody to von Willebrand factor (vWF) inhibits factor VIII binding. Localization of its antigenic determinant to a nonadecapeptide at the amino terminus of the mature vWF polypeptide. *J Clin Invest* 84(1):56–61, 1989.

141. Ginsburg D, Bockenstedt PL, Allen EA, et al: Fine mapping of monoclonal antibody epitopes on human von Willebrand factor using a recombinant peptide library. *Thromb Haemost* 67(1):166–171, 1992.

142. Mazurier C: von Willebrand disease masquerading as haemophilia A. *Thromb Haemost* 67(4):391–396, 1992.

143. Lollar P, Hill-Eubanks DC, Parker CG: Association of the factor VIII light chain with von Willebrand factor. *J Biol Chem* 263(21):10451–10455, 1988.

144. Leyte A, van Schijndel HB, Niehrs C, et al: Sulfation of Tyr1680 of human blood coagulation factor VIII is essential for the interaction of factor VIII with von Willebrand factor. *J Biol Chem* 266(2):740–746, 1991.

145. Shiltagh N, Kirkpatrick J, Cabrita LD, et al: Solution structure of the major factor VIII binding region on von Willebrand factor. *Blood* 123(26):4143–4151, 2014.

146. National Heart, Lung, and Blood Institute: *The Diagnosis, Evaluation, and Management of von Willebrand Disease.* Available at https://www.nhlbi.nih.gov/health-pro/guidelines/current/von-willebrand-guidelines.

147. Sadler JE, Budde U, Eikenboom JC, et al: Update on the pathophysiology and classification of von Willebrand disease: A report of the Subcommittee on von Willebrand Factor. *J Thromb Haemost* 4(10):2103–2114, 2006.

148. Flood VH, Friedman KD, Gill JC, et al: No increase in bleeding identified in type 1 VWD subjects with D1472H sequence variation. *Blood* 121(18):3742–3744, 2013.

149. Johnsen JM, Auer PL, Morrison AC, et al: Common and rare von Willebrand factor (VWF) coding variants, VWF levels, and factor VIII levels in African Americans: The NHLBI Exome Sequencing Project. *Blood* 122(4):590–597, 2013.

150. Wang QY, Song J, Gibbs RA, Boerwinkle E, Dong JF, Yu FL: Characterizing polymorphisms and allelic diversity of von Willebrand factor gene in the 1000 genomes. *J Thromb Haemost* 11(2):261–269, 2013.

151. Flood VH, Gill JC, Morateck PA, et al: Common VWF exon 28 polymorphisms in African Americans affecting the VWF activity assay by ristocetin cofactor. *Blood* 116(2):280–286, 2010.

152. Weiss HJ, Pietu G, Rabinowitz R, Girma JP, Rogers J, Meyer D: Heterogeneous abnormalities in the multimeric structure, antigenic properties, and plasma-platelet content of factor VIII/von Willebrand factor in subtypes of classic (type I) and variant (type IIA) von Willebrand's disease. *J Lab Clin Med* 101(3):411–425, 1983.

153. Hoyer LW, Rizza CR, Tuddenham EG, Carta CA, Armitage H, Rotblat F: von Willebrand factor multimer patterns in von Willebrand's disease. *Br J Haematol* 55(3):493–507, 1983.

154. Mannucci PM, Lombardi R, Bader R, et al: Heterogeneity of type I von Willebrand disease: Evidence for a subgroup with an abnormal von Willebrand factor. *Blood* 66(4):796–802, 1985.

155. Mannucci PM: Platelet von Willebrand factor in inherited and acquired bleeding disorders. *Proc Natl Acad Sci U S A* 92(7):2428–2432, 1995.

156. Haberichter SL, Balistreri M, Christopherson P, et al: Assay of the von Willebrand factor (VWF) propeptide to identify patients with type 1 von Willebrand disease with decreased VWF survival. *Blood* 108(10):3344–3351, 2006.

157. Bowman M, Tuttle A, Notley C, et al: The genetics of Canadian type 3 von Willebrand disease: Further evidence for co-dominant inheritance of mutant alleles. *J Thromb Haemost* 11(3):512–520, 2013.

158. Goodeve A, Eikenboom J, Castaman G, et al: Phenotype and genotype of a cohort of families historically diagnosed with type 1 von Willebrand disease in the European study, Molecular and Clinical Markers for the Diagnosis and Management of Type 1 von Willebrand Disease (MCMDM-1VWD). *Blood* 109(1):112–121, 2007.

159. Robertson JD, Yenson PR, Rand ML, et al: Expanded phenotype-genotype correlations in a pediatric population with type 1 von Willebrand disease. *J Thromb Haemost* 9(9):1752–1760, 2011.

160. Eikenboom J, Hilbert L, Ribba AS, et al: Expression of 14 von Willebrand factor mutations identified in patients with type 1 von Willebrand disease from the MCMDM-1VWD study. *J Thromb Haemost* 7(8):1304–1312, 2009.

161. Wang JW, Valentijn KM, de Boer HC, et al: Intracellular storage and regulated secretion of von Willebrand factor in quantitative von Willebrand disease. *J Biol Chem* 286(27):24180–24188, 2011.

162. Pruss CM, Golder M, Bryant A, et al: Pathologic mechanisms of type 1 VWD mutations R1205H and Y1584C through in vitro and in vivo mouse models. *Blood* 117(16):4358–4366, 2011.

163. Millar CM, Riddell AF, Brown SA, et al: Survival of von Willebrand factor released following DDAVP in a type 1 von Willebrand disease cohort: Influence of glycosylation, proteolysis and gene mutations. *Thromb Haemost* 99(5):916–924, 2008.

164. Mohlke KL, Ginsburg D: von Willebrand disease and quantitative variation in von Willebrand factor. *J Lab Clin Med* 130(3):252–261, 1997.

165. Eikenboom JC, Matsushita T, Reitsma PH, et al: Dominant type 1 von Willebrand disease caused by mutated cysteine residues in the D3 domain of von Willebrand factor. *Blood* 88(7):2433–2441, 1996.

166. Bodo I, Katsumi A, Tuley EA, Eikenboom JC, Dong Z, Sadler JE: Type 1 von Willebrand disease mutation Cys1149Arg causes intracellular retention and degradation of heterodimers: A possible general mechanism for dominant mutations of oligomeric proteins. *Blood* 98(10):2973–2979, 2001.

167. O'Brien LA, James PD, Othman M, et al: Founder von Willebrand factor haplotype associated with type 1 von Willebrand disease. *Blood* 102(2):549–557, 2003.

168. Bowen D: Type 1 von Willebrand disease: A possible novel mechanism. *Blood Coagul Fibrinolysis* 15(Suppl 1):S21–S23, 2004.

169. Bowen DJ, Collins PW, Lester W, et al: The prevalence of the cysteine1584 variant of von Willebrand factor is increased in type 1 von Willebrand disease: Co-segregation with increased susceptibility to ADAMTS13 proteolysis but not clinical phenotype. *Br J Haematol* 128(6):830–836, 2005.

170. Davies JA, Collins PW, Hathaway LS, Bowen DJ: von Willebrand factor: Evidence for variable clearance in vivo according to Y/C1584 phenotype and ABO blood group. *J Thromb Haemost* 6(1):97–103, 2008.

171. Keeney S, Grundy P, Collins PW, Bowen DJ: C1584 in von Willebrand factor is necessary for enhanced proteolysis by ADAMTS13 in vitro. *Haemophilia* 13(4):405–408, 2007.

172. Desch KC, Ozel AB, Siemieniak D, et al: Linkage analysis identifies a locus for plasma von Willebrand factor undetected by genome-wide association. *Proc Natl Acad Sci U S A* 110(2):588–593, 2013.

173. Castaman G, Eikenboom JC, Bertina RM, Rodeghiero FL: Inconsistency of association between type 1 von Willebrand disease phenotype and genotype in families identified in an epidemiological investigation. *Thromb Haemost* 82(3):1065–1070, 1999.

174. Kunicki TJ, Federici AB, Salomon DR, et al: An association of candidate gene haplotypes and bleeding severity in von Willebrand disease (VWD) type 1 pedigrees. *Blood* 104(8):2359–2367, 2004.

175. Kunicki TJ, Baronciani L, Canciani MT, et al: An association of candidate gene haplotypes and bleeding severity in von Willebrand disease type 2A, 2B, and 2M pedigrees. *J Thromb Haemost* 4(1):137–147, 2006.

176. Mohlke KL, Purkayastha AA, Westrick RJ, et al: Mvwf, a dominant modifier of murine von Willebrand factor, results from altered lineage-specific expression of a glycosyltransferase. *Cell* 96(1):111–120, 1999.

177. McKinnon TA, Chion AC, Millington AJ, Lane DA, Laffan MA: N-linked glycosylation of VWF modulates its interaction with ADAMTS13. *Blood* 111(6):3042–3049, 2008.

178. O'Donnell JS, McKinnon TA, Crawley JT, Lane DA, Laffan MA: Bombay phenotype is associated with reduced plasma-VWF levels and an increased susceptibility to ADAMTS13 proteolysis. *Blood* 106(6):1988–1991, 2005.

179. Bowen DJ: An influence of ABO blood group on the rate of proteolysis of von Willebrand factor by ADAMTS13. *J Thromb Haemost* 1(1):33–40, 2003.

180. Gallinaro L, Cattini MG, Sztukowska M, et al: A shorter von Willebrand factor survival in O blood group subjects explains how ABO determinants influence plasma von Willebrand factor. *Blood* 111(7):3540-3545, 2008.

181. Casari C, Lenting PJ, Wohner N, Christophe OD, Denis CV: Clearance of von Willebrand factor. *J Thromb Haemost* 11:202-211, 2013.

182. Zimmerman TS, Abildgaard CF, Meyer D: The factor VIII abnormality in severe von Willebrand's disease. *N Engl J Med* 301(24):1307-1310, 1979.

183. Ngo KY, Glotz VT, Koziol JA, et al: Homozygous and heterozygous deletions of the von Willebrand factor gene in patients and carriers of severe von Willebrand disease. *Proc Natl Acad Sci U S A* 85(8):2753-2757, 1988.

184. Peake IR, Liddell MB, Moodie P, et al: Severe type III von Willebrand's disease caused by deletion of exon 42 of the von Willebrand factor gene: Family studies that identify carriers of the condition and a compound heterozygous individual. *Blood* 75(3):654-661, 1990.

185. Mancuso DJ, Tuley EA, Castillo R, de Bosch N, Mannucci PM, Sadler JE: Characterization of partial gene deletions in type III von Willebrand disease with alloantibody inhibitors. *Thromb Haemost* 72(2):180-185, 1994.

186. Xie F, Wang X, Cooper DN, et al: A novel Alu-mediated 61-kb deletion of the von Willebrand factor (VWF) gene whose breakpoints co-locate with putative matrix attachment regions. *Blood Cells Mol Dis* 36(3):385–391, 2006.

187. Cabrera N, Casa Ýa P, Cid AR, et al: First application of MLPA method in severe von Willebrand disease. Confirmation of a new large VWF gene deletion and identification of heterozygous carriers. *Br J Haematol* 152(2):240–242, 2011.

188. Nichols WC, Lyons SE, Harrison JS, Cody RL, Ginsburg D: Severe von Willebrand disease due to a defect at the level of von Willebrand factor mRNA expression: Detection by exonic PCR-restriction fragment length polymorphism analysis. *Proc Natl Acad Sci U S A* 88(9):3857–3861, 1991.

189. Eikenboom JC, Ploos van Amstel HK, Reitsma PH, Briet E: Mutations in severe, type III von Willebrand's disease in the Dutch population: Candidate missense and nonsense mutations associated with reduced levels of von Willebrand factor messenger RNA. *Thromb Haemost* 68(4):448–454, 1992.

190. Nichols WC, Ginsburg D: von Willebrand disease. *Medicine (Baltimore)* 76(1):1–20, 1997.

191. Ginsburg D, Sadler JE: von Willebrand disease: A database of point mutations, insertions, and deletions. For the Consortium on von Willebrand Factor Mutations and Polymorphisms, and the Subcommittee on von Willebrand Factor of the Scientific and Standardization Committee of the International Society on Thrombosis and Haemostasis. *Thromb Haemost* 69(2):177–184, 1993.

192. Zhang ZP, Falk G, Blomback M, Egberg N, Anvret M: A single cytosine deletion in exon 18 of the von Willebrand factor gene is the most common mutation in Swedish vWD type III patients. *Hum Mol Genet* 1(9):767–768, 1992.

193. Schneppenheim R, Krey S, Bergmann F, et al: Genetic heterogeneity of severe von Willebrand disease type III in the German population. *Hum Genet* 94(6):640–652, 1994.

194. Berkowitz SD, Dent J, Roberts J, et al: Epitope mapping of the von Willebrand factor subunit distinguishes fragments present in normal and type IIA von Willebrand disease from those generated by plasmin. *J Clin Invest* 79(2):524–531, 1987.

195. Ginsburg D, Konkle BA, Gill JC, et al: Molecular basis of human von Willebrand disease: Analysis of platelet von Willebrand factor mRNA. *Proc Natl Acad Sci U S A* 86(10):3723–3727, 1989.

196. Hassenpflug WA, Budde U, Obser T, et al: Impact of mutations in the von Willebrand factor A2 domain on ADAMTS13-dependent proteolysis. *Blood* 107(6):2339–2345, 2006.

197. Jacobi PM, Gill JC, Flood VH, Jakab DA, Friedman KD, Haberichter SL: Intersection of mechanisms of type 2A VWD through defects in VWF multimerization, secretion, ADAMTS-13 susceptibility, and regulated storage. *Blood* 119(19):4543–4553, 2012.

198. Lyons SE, Bruck ME, Bowie EJ, Ginsburg D: Impaired intracellular transport produced by a subset of type IIA von Willebrand disease mutations. *J Biol Chem* 267(7):4424–4430, 1992.

199. Dent JA, Galbusera M, Ruggeri ZM: Heterogeneity of plasma von Willebrand factor multimers resulting from proteolysis of the constituent subunit. *J Clin Invest* 88(3):774–782, 1991.

200. Gralnick HR, Williams SB, McKeown LP, et al: In vitro correction of the abnormal multimeric structure of von Willebrand factor in type IIa von Willebrand's disease. *Proc Natl Acad Sci U S A* 82(17):5968–5972, 1985.

201. Kunicki TJ, Montgomery RR, Schullek J: Cleavage of human von Willebrand factor by platelet calcium-activated protease. *Blood* 65(2):352–356, 1985.

202. Chung DW, Fujikawa K: Processing of von Willebrand factor by ADAMTS-13. *Biochemistry* 41(37):11065–11070, 2002.

203. Budde U: Diagnosis of von Willebrand disease subtypes: Implications for treatment. *Haemophilia* 14(Suppl 5):27–38, 2008.

204. Gaucher C, Dieval J, Mazurier C: Characterization of von Willebrand factor gene defects in two unrelated patients with type IIC von Willebrand disease. *Blood* 84(4):1024–1030, 1994.

205. Haberichter SL, Budde U, Obser T, Schneppenheim S, Wermes C, Schneppenheim R: The mutation N528S in the von Willebrand factor (VWF) propeptide causes defective multimerization and storage of VWF. *Blood* 115(22):4580–4587, 2010.

206. Schneppenheim R, Thomas KB, Krey S, et al: Identification of a candidate missense mutation in a family with von Willebrand disease type IIC. *Hum Genet* 95(6):681–686, 1995.

207. Schneppenheim R, Brassard J, Krey S, et al: Defective dimerization of von Willebrand factor subunits due to a Cys-> Arg mutation in type IID von Willebrand disease. *Proc Natl Acad Sci U S A* 93(8):3581–3586, 1996.

208. Cooney KA, Nichols WC, Bruck ME, et al: The molecular defect in type IIB von Willebrand disease. Identification of four potential missense mutations within the putative GpIb binding domain. *J Clin Invest* 87(4):1227–1233, 1991.

209. Ribba AS, Lavergne JM, Bahnak BR, Derlon A, Pietu G, Meyer D: Duplication of a methionine within the glycoprotein Ib binding domain of von Willebrand factor detected by denaturing gradient gel electrophoresis in a patient with type IIB von Willebrand disease. *Blood* 78(7):1738–1743, 1991.

210. Cooney KA, Ginsburg D: Comparative analysis of type 2b von Willebrand disease mutations: implications for the mechanism of von Willebrand factor binding to platelets. *Blood* 87(6):2322–2328, 1996.

211. Cooney KA, Lyons SE, Ginsburg D: Functional analysis of a type IIB von Willebrand disease missense mutation: Increased binding of large von Willebrand factor multimers to platelets. *Proc Natl Acad Sci U S A* 89(7):2869–2872, 1992.

212. Ware J, Dent JA, Azuma H, et al: Identification of a point mutation in type IIB von Willebrand disease illustrating the regulation of von Willebrand factor affinity for the platelet membrane glycoprotein Ib-IX receptor. *Proc Natl Acad Sci U S A* 88(7):2946–2950, 1991.

213. Kroner PA, Kluessendorf ML, Scott JP, Montgomery RR: Expressed full-length von Willebrand factor containing missense mutations linked to type IIB von Willebrand disease shows enhanced binding to platelets. *Blood* 79(8):2048–2055, 1992.

214. Randi AM, Jorieux S, Tuley EA, Mazurier C, Sadler JE: Recombinant von Willebrand factor Arg578-->Gln. A type IIB von Willebrand disease mutation affects binding to glycoprotein Ib but not to collagen or heparin. *J Biol Chem* 267(29):21187–21192, 1992.

215. Blenner MA, Dong X, Springer TA: Structural basis of regulation of von Willebrand factor binding to glycoprotein Ib. *J Biol Chem* 289(9):5565–5579, 2014.

216. Rayes J, Hollestelle MJ, Legendre P, et al: Mutation and ADAMTS13-dependent modulation of disease severity in a mouse model for von Willebrand disease type 2B. *Blood* 115(23):4870–4877, 2010.

217. Casari C, Du V, Wu YP, et al: Accelerated uptake of VWF/platelet complexes in macrophages contributes to VWD type 2B-associated thrombocytopenia. *Blood* 122(16):2893–2902, 2013.

218. Casari C, Berrou E, Lebret M, et al: von Willebrand factor mutation promotes thrombocytopathy by inhibiting integrin alphaIIbbeta3. *J Clin Invest* 123(12):5071–5081, 2013.

219. Golder M, Pruss CM, Hegadorn C, et al: Mutation-specific hemostatic variability in mice expressing common type 2B von Willebrand disease substitutions. *Blood* 115(23):4862–4869, 2010.

220. Ozeki M, Kunishima S, Kasahara K, et al: A family having type 2B von Willebrand disease with an R1306W mutation: Severe thrombocytopenia leads to the normalization of high molecular weight multimers. *Thromb Res* 125(2):e17–e22, 2010.

221. Holmberg L, Dent JA, Schneppenheim R, Budde U, Ware J, Ruggeri ZM: von Willebrand factor mutation enhancing interaction with platelets in patients with normal multimeric structure. *J Clin Invest* 91(5):2169–2177, 1993.

222. Graham JB, Barrow ES, Roberts HR, et al: Dominant inheritance of hemophilia A in three generations of women. *Blood* 46(2):175–188, 1975.

223. Veltkamp JJ, van Tilburg NH: "Autosomal haemophilia": A variant of von Willebrand's disease. *Br J Haematol* 26(1):141–152, 1974.

224. Mazurier C, Dieval J, Jorieux S, Delobel J, Goudemand M: A new von Willebrand factor (vWF) defect in a patient with factor VIII (FVIII) deficiency but with normal levels and multimeric patterns of both plasma and platelet vWF. Characterization of abnormal vWF/FVIII interaction. *Blood* 75(1):20–26, 1990.

225. Mazurier C, Gaucher C, Jorieux S, Parquet-Gernez A, Goudemand M: Evidence for a von Willebrand factor defect in factor VIII binding in three members of a family previously misdiagnosed mild haemophilia A and haemophilia A carriers: Consequences for therapy and genetic counselling. *Br J Haematol* 76(3):372–379, 1990.

226. Nishino M, Girma JP, Rothschild C, Fressinaud E, Meyer D: New variant of von Willebrand disease with defective binding to factor VIII. *Blood* 74(5):1591–1599, 1989.

227. Hampshire D, Goodeve A: The International Society on Thrombosis and Haematosis von Willebrand Disease Database: An update. *Semin Thromb Hemost* 37(05):470–479, 2011.

228. Eikenboom JC, Reitsma PH, Peerlink KM, Briet E: Recessive inheritance of von Willebrand's disease type I. *Lancet* 341(8851):982–986, 1993.

229. Castaman G, Giacomelli SH, Jacobi P, et al: Homozygous type 2N R854W von Willebrand factor is poorly secreted and causes a severe von Willebrand disease phenotype. *J Thromb Haemost* 8(9):2011–2016, 2010.

230. Gupta M, Lillicrap D, Stain AM, Friedman KD, Carcao MD: Therapeutic consequences for misdiagnosis of type 2N von Willebrand disease. *Pediatr Blood Cancer* 57(6):1081–1083, 2011.

231. Nichols WC, Ginsburg D, Ruggeri ZM: von Willebrand disease, in *Thrombosis and Hemorrhage*, edited by Loscalzo J, Schafer AI, pp 539–559. Lippincott Williams& Wilkins, Philadelphia, 2003.

232. Meyer D, Fressinaud E, Gaucher C, et al: Gene defects in 150 unrelated French cases with type 2 von Willebrand disease: from the patient to the gene. INSERM Network on Molecular Abnormalities in von Willebrand Disease. *Thromb Haemost* 78(1):451–456, 1997.

233. Larsen DM, Haberichter SL, Gill JC, Shapiro AD, Flood VH: Variability in platelet- and collagen-binding defects in type 2M von Willebrand disease. *Haemophilia* 19(4):590–594, 2013.

234. McKinnon TA, Nowak AA, Cutler J, Riddell AF, Laffan MA, Millar CM: Characterisation of von Willebrand factor A1 domain mutants I1416N and I1416T: Correlation of clinical phenotype with flow-based platelet adhesion. *J Thromb Haemost* 10(7):1409–1416, 2012.

235. Mannucci PM, Lombardi R, Castaman G, et al: von Willebrand disease "Vicenza" with larger-than-normal (supranormal) von Willebrand factor multimers. *Blood* 71(1):65–70, 1988.

236. Randi AM, Sacchi E, Castaman GC, Rodeghiero F, Mannucci PM: The genetic defect of type I von Willebrand disease "Vicenza" is linked to the von Willebrand factor gene. *Thromb Haemost* 69(2):173–176, 1993.

237. Casonato A, Pontara E, Sartorello F, et al: Reduced von Willebrand factor survival in type Vicenza von Willebrand disease. *Blood* 99(1):180–184, 2002.

238. Eikenboom JC, Castaman G, Kamphuisen PW, Rosendaal FR, Bertina RM: The factor VIII/von Willebrand factor ratio discriminates between reduced synthesis and increased clearance of von Willebrand factor. *Thromb Haemost* 87(2):252–257, 2002.

239. Gezsi A, Budde U, Deak I, et al: Accelerated clearance alone explains ultra-large multimers in von Willebrand disease Vicenza. *J Thromb Haemost* 8(6):1273–1280, 2010.

240. Berkowitz SD, Ruggeri ZM, Zimmerman TS: von Willebrand disease, in *Coagulation and Bleeding Disorders: The Role of Factor VIII and von Willebrand Factor*, edited by Zimmerman TS, Ruggeri ZM, pp 215–259. Marcel Dekker, New York, 1989.

241. Miller CH, Graham JB, Goldin LR, Elston RC: Genetics of classic von Willebrand's disease. I. Phenotypic variation within families. *Blood* 54(1):117–136, 1979.

242. Gill JC, Endres-Brooks J, Bauer PJ, Marks WJ Jr, Montgomery RR: The effect of ABO blood group on the diagnosis of von Willebrand disease. *Blood* 69(6):1691–1695, 1987.

243. Orstavik KH, Kornstad L, Reisner H, Berg K: Possible effect of secretor locus on plasma concentration of factor VIII and von Willebrand factor. *Blood* 73(4):990–993, 1989.

244. O'Donnell J, Boulton FE, Manning RA, Laffan MA: Genotype at the secretor blood group locus is a determinant of plasma von Willebrand factor level. *Br J Haematol* 116(2):350–356, 2002.

245. Franchini M, Crestani S, Frattini F, Sissa C, Bonfanti C: ABO blood group and von Willebrand factor: Biological implications. *Clin Chem Lab Med* 52(9):1273–1276, 2014.

246. Antoni G, Oudot-Mellakh T, Dimitromanolakis A, et al: Combined analysis of three genome-wide association studies on vWF and FVIII plasma levels. *BMC Med Genet* 12:102, 2011.

247. Smith NL, Chen MH, Dehghan A, et al: Novel associations of multiple genetic loci with plasma levels of factor VII, factor VIII, and von Willebrand factor: The CHARGE (Cohorts for Heart and Aging Research in Genome Epidemiology) Consortium. *Circulation* 121(12):1382–1392, 2010.

248. Ye S, Huang Y, Joshi S, et al: Platelet secretion and hemostasis require syntaxin-binding protein STXBP5. *J Clin Invest* 124(10):4517–4528, 2014.

249. Zhu Q, Yamakuchi M, Ture S, et al: Syntaxin-binding protein STXBP5 inhibits endothelial exocytosis and promotes platelet secretion. *J Clin Invest* 124(10):4503–4516, 2014.

250. Rydz N, Swystun LL, Notley C, et al: The C-type lectin receptor CLEC4M binds, internalizes, and clears von Willebrand factor and contributes to the variation in plasma von Willebrand factor levels. *Blood* 121(26):5228–5237, 2013.

251. Rodeghiero F, Castaman G, Dini E: Epidemiological investigation of the prevalence of von Willebrand's disease. *Blood* 69(2):454–459, 1987.

252. Werner EJ, Broxson EH, Tucker EL, Giroux DS, Shults J, Abshire TC: Prevalence of von Willebrand disease in children: a multiethnic study. *J Pediatr* 123(6):893–898, 1993.

253. Sadler JE: von Willebrand disease type 1: A diagnosis in search of a disease. *Blood* 101(6):2089–2093, 2003.

254. Lillicrap D: von Willebrand disease: Advances in pathogenetic understanding, diagnosis, and therapy. *Hematology Am Soc Hematol Educ Program* 2013:254–260, 2013.

255. Veyradier A, Boisseau P, Fressinaud E, et al: A laboratory phenotype/genotype correlation of 1167 French patients from 670 families with von Willebrand disease: A new epidemiologic picture. *Medicine (Baltimore)* 95(11):e3038, 2016.

256. Berliner SA, Seligsohn U, Zivelin A, Zwang E, Sofferman G: A relatively high frequency of severe (type III) von Willebrand's disease in Israel. *Br J Haematol* 62(3):535–543, 1986.

257. Mannucci PM, Bloom AL, Larrieu MJ, Nilsson IM, West RR: Atherosclerosis and von Willebrand factor. I. Prevalence of severe von Willebrand's disease in western Europe and Israel. *Br J Haematol* 57(1):163–169, 1984.

258. Weiss HJ, Ball AP, Mannucci PM: Incidence of severe von Willebrand's disease. *N Engl J Med* 307(2):127, 1982.

259. Nosek-Cenkowska B, Cheang MS, Pizzi NJ, Israels ED, Gerrard JM: Bleeding/bruising symptomatology in children with and without bleeding disorders. *Thromb Haemost* 65(3):237–241, 1991.

260. Rydz N, James PD: The evolution and value of bleeding assessment tools. *J Thromb Haemost* 10(11):2223–2229, 2012.

261. De Jong A, Eikenboom J: Developments in the diagnostic procedures for von Willebrand disease. *J Thromb Haemost* 14(3):449–460, 2016.

262. Elbatarny M, Mollah S, Grabell J, et al: Normal range of bleeding scores for the ISTH-BAT: Adult and pediatric data from the merging project. *Haemophilia* 20(6):831–835, 2014.

263. Deforest M, Grabell J, Albert S, et al: Generation and optimization of the self-administered bleeding assessment tool and its validation as a screening test for von Willebrand disease. *Haemophilia* 21(5):e384–388, 2015.

264. Federici AB, Bucciarelli P, Castaman G, et al: The bleeding score predicts clinical outcomes and replacement therapy in adults with von Willebrand disease. *Blood* 123(26):4037–4044, 2014.

265. van den Driesche S, Mummery CL, Westermann CJ: Hereditary hemorrhagic telangiectasia: An update on transforming growth factor beta signaling in vasculogenesis and angiogenesis. *Cardiovasc Res* 58(1):20–31, 2003.

266. Iannuzzi MC, Hidaka N, Boehnke M, et al: Analysis of the relationship of von Willebrand disease (vWD) and hereditary hemorrhagic telangiectasia and identification of a potential type IIA vWD mutation (IIe865 to Thr). *Am J Hum Genet* 48(4):757–763, 1991.

267. Rick ME, Williams SB, Sacher RA, McKeown LP: Thrombocytopenia associated with pregnancy in a patient with type IIB von Willebrand's disease. *Blood* 69(3):786–789, 1987.

268. Mazurier C, Parquet-Gernez A, Goudemand J, Taillefer MF, Goudemand M: Investigation of a large kindred with type IIB von Willebrand's disease, dominant inheritance and age-dependent thrombocytopenia. *Br J Haematol* 69(4):499–505, 1988.

269. Schneppenheim R, Budde U, Krey S, et al: Results of a screening for von Willebrand disease type 2N in patients with suspected haemophilia A or von Willebrand disease type 1. *Thromb Haemost* 76(4):598–602, 1996.

270. James PD, Lillicrap D, Mannucci PM: Alloantibodies in von Willebrand disease. *Blood* 122(5):636–640, 2013.

271. Selvam S, James P: Angiodysplasia in von Willebrand Disease: Understanding the clinical and basic science. *Semin Thromb Hemost* doi:10.1055/s-0037-1599145, 2017.

272. Asatiani E, Kessler CM: Multiple congenital coagulopathies co-expressed with von Willebrand's disease: The experience of Hemophilia Region III Treatment Centers over 25 years and review of the literature. *Haemophilia* 13(6):685–696, 2007.

273. Bodo I, Eikenboom J, Montgomery R, Patzke J, Schneppenheim R, Di Paola J: Platelet-dependent von Willebrand factor activity. Nomenclature and methodology: communication from the SSC of the ISTH. *J Thromb Haemost* 13(7):1345–1350, 2015.

274. Lippi G, Franchini M, Poli G, Salvagno GL, Montagnana M, Guidi GC: Is the activated partial thromboplastin time suitable to screen for von Willebrand factor deficiencies? *Blood Coagul Fibrinolysis* 18(4):361–364, 2007.

275. Abildgaard CF, Suzuki Z, Harrison J, Jefcoat K, Zimmerman TS: Serial studies in von Willebrand's disease: Variability versus "variants." *Blood* 56(4):712–716, 1980.

276. Timm A, Fahrenkrug J, Jorgensen HL, Sennels HP, Goetze JP: Diurnal variation of von Willebrand factor in plasma: The Bispebjerg study of diurnal variations. *Eur J Haematol* 93(1):48–53, 2014.

277. Sadler JE: New concepts in von Willebrand disease. *Annu Rev Med* 56:173–191, 2005.

278. Favaloro EJ, Bonar R, Chapman K, Meiring M, Funk AD: Differential sensitivity of von Willebrand factor (VWF) 'activity' assays to large and small VWF molecular weight forms: a cross-laboratory study comparing ristocetin cofactor, collagen-binding and mAb-based assays. *J Thromb Haemost* 10(6):1043–1054, 2012.

279. Hayward CP, Moffat KA, Plumhoff E, Van Cott EM: Approaches to investigating common bleeding disorders: An evaluation of North American coagulation laboratory practices. *Am J Hematol* 87(Suppl 1):S45–S50, 2012.

280. Quiroga T, Goycoolea M, Belmont S, et al: Quantitative impact of using different criteria for the laboratory diagnosis of type 1 von Willebrand disease. *J Thromb Haemost* 12(8):1238–1243, 2014.

281. Eikenboom J, Federici AB, Dirven RJ, et al: VWF propeptide and ratios between VWF, VWF propeptide, and FVIII in the characterization of type 1 von Willebrand disease. *Blood* 121(12):2336–2339, 2013.

282. Weiss HJ, Hoyer LW, Rickles FR, Varma A, Rogers J: Quantitative assay of a plasma factor deficient in von Willebrand's disease that is necessary for platelet aggregation. Relationship to factor VIII procoagulant activity and antigen content. *J Clin Invest* 52(11):2708–2716, 1973.

283. Rodeghiero F, Castaman G, Tosetto A: von Willebrand factor antigen is less sensitive than ristocetin cofactor for the diagnosis of type I von Willebrand disease: Results based on an epidemiological investigation. *Thromb Haemost* 64(3):349–352, 1990.

284. Flood VH, Friedman KD, Gill JC, et al: Limitations of the ristocetin cofactor assay in measurement of von Willebrand factor function. *J Thromb Haemost* 7(11):1832–1839, 2009.

285. Favaloro EJ: Diagnosis and classification of von Willebrand disease: A review of the differential utility of various functional von Willebrand factor assays. *Blood Coagul Fibrinolysis* 22(7):553–564, 2011.

286. Ruggeri ZM, Zimmerman TS: The complex multimeric composition of factor VIII/vWF. *Blood* 57:1140–1143, 1981.

287. Budde U, Schneppenheim R, Eikenboom J, et al: Detailed von Willebrand factor multimer analysis in patients with von Willebrand disease in the European study, molecular and clinical markers for the diagnosis and management of type 1 von Willebrand disease (MCMDM-1VWD). *J Thromb Haemost* 6(5):762–771, 2008.

288. Flood VH, Gill JC, Friedman KD, et al: Collagen binding provides a sensitive screen for variant von Willebrand disease. *Clin Chem* 59(4):684–691, 2013.

289. Flood VH, Gill JC, Christopherson PA, et al: Critical von Willebrand factor A1 domain residues influence type VI collagen binding. *J Thromb Haemost* 10(7):1417–1424, 2012.

290. Flood VH, Lederman CA, Wren JS, et al: Absent collagen binding in a VWF A3 domain mutant: Utility of the VWF:CB in diagnosis of VWD. *J Thromb Haemost* 8(6):1431–1433, 2010.

291. Favaloro EJ, Dean M, Grispo L, Exner T, Koutts J: von Willebrand's disease: Use of collagen binding assay provides potential improvement to laboratory monitoring of desmopressin (DDAVP) therapy. *Am J Hematol* 45(3):205–211, 1994.

292. Riddell AF, Jenkins PV, Nitu-Whalley IC, McCraw AH, Lee CA, Brown SA: Use of the collagen-binding assay for von Willebrand factor in the analysis of type 2M von Willebrand disease: A comparison with the ristocetin cofactor assay. *Br J Haematol* 116(1):187–192, 2002.

293. Popov J, Zhukov O, Ruden S, Zeschmann T, Sferruzza A, Sahud M: Performance and clinical utility of a commercial von Willebrand factor collagen binding assay for laboratory diagnosis of von Willebrand disease. *Clin Chem* 52(10):1965–1967, 2006.

294. Meiring M, Badenhorst PN, Kelderman M: Performance and utility of a cost-effective collagen-binding assay for the laboratory diagnosis of von Willebrand disease. *Clin Chem Lab Med* 45(8):1068–1072, 2007.

295. Mazurier C, Meyer D: Factor VIII binding assay of von Willebrand factor and the diagnosis of type 2N von Willebrand disease: Results of an international survey. On behalf of the Subcommittee on von Willebrand Factor of the Scientific and Standardization Committee of the ISTH. *Thromb Haemost* 76(2):270–274, 1996.

296. Zhukov O, Popov J, Ramos R, et al: Measurement of von Willebrand factor-FVIII binding activity in patients with suspected von Willebrand disease type 2N: Application of an ELISA-based assay in a reference laboratory. *Haemophilia* 15(3):788–796, 2009.

297. Casonato A, Pontara E, Sartorello F, et al: Identifying carriers of type 2N von Willebrand disease: Procedures and significance. *Clin Appl Thromb Hemost* 13(2):194–200, 2007.

298. Haberichter SL, Castaman G, Budde U, et al: Identification of type 1 von Willebrand disease patients with reduced von Willebrand factor survival by assay of the VWF propeptide in the European study: Molecular and clinical markers for the diagnosis and management of type 1 VWD (MCMDM-1VWD). *Blood* 111(10):4979–4985, 2008.

299. Sanders YV, Groeneveld D, Meijer K, et al: von Willebrand factor propeptide and the phenotypic classification of von Willebrand disease. *Blood* 125(19):3006–3013, 2015.

300. Casonato A, Pontara E, Sartorello F, et al: Identifying type Vicenza von Willebrand disease. *J Lab Clin Med* 147(2):96–102, 2006.

301. Fressinaud E, Veyradier A, Truchaud F, et al: Screening for von Willebrand disease with a new analyzer using high shear stress: A study of 60 cases. *Blood* 91(4):1325–1331, 1998.

302. Cattaneo M, Federici AB, Lecchi A, et al: Evaluation of the PFA-100 system in the diagnosis and therapeutic monitoring of patients with von Willebrand disease. *Thromb Haemost* 82(1):35–39, 1999.

303. De Vleeschauwer A, Devreese K: Comparison of a new automated von Willebrand factor activity assay with an aggregation von Willebrand ristocetin cofactor activity assay for the diagnosis of von Willebrand disease. *Blood Coagul Fibrinolysis* 17(5):353–358, 2006.

304. Salem RO, Van Cott EM: A new automated screening assay for the diagnosis of von Willebrand disease. *Am J Clin Pathol* 127(5):730–735, 2007.

305. Pinol M, Sales M, Costa M, Tosetto A, Canciani MT, Federici AB: Evaluation of a new turbidimetric assay for von Willebrand factor activity useful in the general screening of von Willebrand disease. *Haematologica* 92(5):712–713, 2007.

306. Sucker C, Senft B, Scharf RE, Zotz RB: Determination of von Willebrand factor activity: Evaluation of the HaemosIL assay in comparison with established procedures. *Clin Appl Thromb Hemost* 12(3):305–310, 2006.

307. Fujimura Y, Kawasaki T, Titani K: Snake venom proteins modulating the interaction between von Willebrand factor and platelet glycoprotein Ib. *Thromb Haemost* 76(5):633–639, 1996.

308. Keeney S, Bowen D, Cumming A, Enayat S, Goodeve A, Hill M: The molecular analysis of von Willebrand disease: A guideline from the UK Haemophilia Centre Doctors' Organisation Haemophilia Genetics Laboratory Network. *Haemophilia* 14(5):1099–1111, 2008.

309. Snyder MW, Simmons LE, Kitzman JO, et al: Noninvasive fetal genome sequencing: A primer. *Prenat Diagn* 33(6):547–554, 2013.

310. James PD, Lillicrap D: The molecular characterization of von Willebrand disease: Good in parts. *Br J Haematol* 161(2):166–176, 2013.

311. Othman M, Kaur H, Emsley J: Platelet-type von Willebrand disease: New insights into the molecular pathophysiology of a unique platelet defect. *Semin Thromb Hemost* 39(6):663–673, 2013.

312. Federici AB, Budde U, Castaman G, Rand JH, Tiede A: Current diagnostic and therapeutic approaches to patients with acquired von Willebrand syndrome: A 2013 update. *Semin Thromb Hemost* 39(2):191–201, 2013.

313. Budde U, Schaefer G, Mueller N, et al: Acquired von Willebrand's disease in the myeloproliferative syndrome. *Blood* 64(5):981–985, 1984.

314. Kos CA, Ward JE, Malek K, et al: Association of acquired von Willebrand syndrome with AL amyloidosis. *Am J Hematol* 82(5):363–367, 2007.

315. Mannucci PM, Lombardi R, Bader R, et al: Studies of the pathophysiology of acquired von Willebrand's disease in seven patients with lymphoproliferative disorders or benign monoclonal gammopathies. *Blood* 64(3):614–621, 1984.

316. Rogers JS 2nd, Shane SR, Jencks FS: Factor VIII activity and thyroid function. *Ann Intern Med* 97(5):713–716, 1982.

317. Viallard JF, Pellegrin JL, Vergnes C, et al: Three cases of acquired von Willebrand disease associated with systemic lupus erythematosus. *Br J Haematol* 105(2):532–537, 1999.

318. Scott JP, Montgomery RR, Tubergen DG, Hays T: Acquired von Willebrand's disease in association with Wilm's tumor: regression following treatment. *Blood* 58(4):665–669, 1981.

319. Warkentin TE, Moore JC, Morgan DG: Aortic stenosis and bleeding gastrointestinal angiodysplasia: Is acquired von Willebrand's disease the link? *Lancet* 340(8810):35–37, 1992.

320. Geisen U, Heilmann C, Beyersdorf F, et al: Non-surgical bleeding in patients with ventricular assist devices could be explained by acquired von Willebrand disease. *Eur J Cardiothorac Surg* 33(4):679–684, 2008.

321. Castaman G, Lattuada A, Mannucci PM, Rodeghiero F: Characterization of two cases of acquired transitory von Willebrand syndrome with ciprofloxacin: Evidence for heightened proteolysis of von Willebrand factor. *Am J Hematol* 49(1):83–86, 1995.

322. Tefferi A, Nichols WL: Acquired von Willebrand disease: Concise review of occurrence, diagnosis, pathogenesis, and treatment. *Am J Med* 103(6):536–540, 1997.

323. Kumar S, Pruthi RK, Nichols WL: Acquired von Willebrand disease. *Mayo Clin Proc* 77(2):181–187, 2002.

324. Kanakry JA, Gladstone DE: Maintaining hemostasis in acquired von Willebrand syndrome: A review of intravenous immunoglobulin and the importance of rituximab dose scheduling. *Transfusion* 53(8):1730–1735, 2013.

325. Svensson PJ, Bergqvist PB, Juul KV, Berntorp E: Desmopressin in treatment of haematological disorders and in prevention of surgical bleeding. *Blood Rev* 28(3):95–102, 2014.

326. Abshire TC, Federici AB, Alvarez MT, et al: Prophylaxis in severe forms of von Willebrand's disease: Results from the von Willebrand Disease Prophylaxis Network (VWD PN). *Haemophilia* 19(1):76–81, 2013.

327. Abshire T, Cox-Gill J, Kempton CL, et al: Prophylaxis escalation in severe von Willebrand disease: A prospective study from the von Willebrand Disease Prophylaxis Network. *J Thromb Haemost* 13(9):1585–1589, 2015.

328. Mannucci PM, Ruggeri ZM, Pareti FI, Capitanio A: 1-Deamino-8-d-arginine vasopressin: A new pharmacological approach to the management of haemophilia and von Willebrands' diseases. *Lancet* 1(8017):869–872, 1977.

329. Mannucci PM: Desmopressin (DDAVP) in the treatment of bleeding disorders: The first 20 years. *Blood* 90(7):2515–2521, 1997.

330. Federici AB, Mazurier C, Berntorp E, et al: Biologic response to desmopressin in patients with severe type 1 and type 2 von Willebrand disease: Results of a multicenter European study. *Blood* 103(6):2032–2038, 2004.

331. Lethagen S, Harris AS, Nilsson IM: Intranasal desmopressin (DDAVP) by spray in mild hemophilia A and von Willebrand's disease type I. *Blut* 60(3):187–191, 1990.

332. Rose EH, Aledort LM: Nasal spray desmopressin (DDAVP) for mild hemophilia A and von Willebrand disease. *Ann Intern Med* 114(7):563–568, 1991.

333. Rodeghiero F, Castaman G, Di Bona E, Ruggeri M: Consistency of responses to repeated DDAVP infusions in patients with von Willebrand's disease and hemophilia A. *Blood* 74(6):1997–2000, 1989.

334. Castaman G, Lethagen S, Federici AB, et al: Response to desmopressin is influenced by the genotype and phenotype in type 1 von Willebrand disease (VWD): Results from the European Study MCMDM-1VWD. *Blood* 111(7):3531–3539, 2008.

335. Mannucci PM, Bettega D, Cattaneo M: Patterns of development of tachyphylaxis in patients with haemophilia and von Willebrand disease after repeated doses of desmopressin (DDAVP). *Br J Haematol* 82(1):87–93, 1992.

336. de la Fuente B, Kasper CK, Rickles FR, Hoyer LW: Response of patients with mild and moderate hemophilia A and von Willebrand's disease to treatment with desmopressin. *Ann Intern Med* 103(1):6–14, 1985.

337. Gralnick HR, Williams SB, McKeown LP, et al: DDAVP in type IIa von Willebrand's disease. *Blood* 67(2):465–468, 1986.

338. Sharma R, Stein D: Hyponatremia after desmopressin (DDAVP) use in pediatric patients with bleeding disorders undergoing surgeries. *J Pediatr Hematol Oncol* 36(6):e371–375, 2014.

339. Mason JA, Robertson JD, McCosker J, Williams BA, Brown SA: Assessment and validation of a defined fluid restriction protocol in the use of subcutaneous desmopressin for children with inherited bleeding disorders. *Haemophilia* 22(5):700–705, 2016.

340. Mannucci PM: Treatment of von Willebrand's disease. *N Engl J Med* 351(7):683–694, 2004.

341. Casonato A, Sartori MT, de Marco L, Girolami A: 1-Desamino-8-D-arginine vasopressin (DDAVP) infusion in type IIB von Willebrand's disease: Shortening of bleeding time and induction of a variable pseudothrombocytopenia. *Thromb Haemost* 64(1):117–120, 1990.

342. McKeown LP, Connaghan G, Wilson O, Hansmann K, Merryman P, Gralnick HR: 1-Desamino-8-arginine-vasopressin corrects the hemostatic defects in type 2B von Willebrand's disease. *Am J Hematol* 51(2):158–163, 1996.

343. Mazurier C, Gaucher C, Jorieux S, Goudemand M: Biological effect of desmopressin in eight patients with type 2N ('Normandy') von Willebrand disease. Collaborative Group. *Br J Haematol* 88(4):849–854, 1994.

344. Mannucci PM, Kempton C, Millar C, et al: Pharmacokinetics and safety of a novel recombinant human von Willebrand factor manufactured with a plasma-free method: A prospective clinical trial. *Blood* 122(5):648–657, 2013.

345. Gill JC, Castaman G, Windyga J, et al: Hemostatic efficacy, safety, and pharmacokinetics of a recombinant von Willebrand factor in severe von Willebrand disease. *Blood* 126(17):2038–2046, 2015.

346. Brown R: Recombinant von Willebrand factor for severe gastrointestinal bleeding unresponsive to other treatments in a patient with type 2A von Willebrand disease: A case report. *Blood Coagul Fibrinolysis* doi:10.1097/MBC.0000000000000632, 2017.

347. Morfini M, Mannucci PM, Tenconi PM, et al: Pharmacokinetics of monoclonally purified and recombinant factor VIII in patients with severe von Willebrand disease. *Thromb Haemost* 70(2):270–272, 1993.

348. Makris M, Colvin B, Gupta V, Shields ML, Smith MP: Venous thrombosis following the use of intermediate purity FVIII concentrate to treat patients with von Willebrand's disease. *Thromb Haemost* 88(3):387–388, 2002.

349. Mannucci PM, Chediak J, Hanna W, et al: Treatment of von Willebrand disease with a high-purity factor VIII/von Willebrand factor concentrate: A prospective, multicenter study. *Blood* 99(2):450–456, 2002.

350. Coppola A, Franchini M, Makris M, Santagostino E, Di Minno G, Mannucci PM: Thrombotic adverse events to coagulation factor concentrates for treatment of patients with haemophilia and von Willebrand disease: a systematic review of prospective studies. *Haemophilia* 18(3):e173–187, 2012.

351. James AH, Konkle BA, Kouides P, et al: Postpartum von Willebrand factor levels in women with and without von Willebrand disease and implications for prophylaxis. *Haemophilia* 21(1):81–87, 2015.

352. Sucker C, Scharf RE, Zotz RB: Use of recombinant factor VIIa in inherited and acquired von Willebrand disease. *Clin Appl Thromb Hemost* 15(1):27–31, 2009.

# CHAPTER 17
# ANTIBODY-MEDIATED COAGULATION FACTOR DEFICIENCIES

Sean R. Stowell, John S. (Pete) Lollar, and Shannon L. Meeks

## SUMMARY

Clinically significant autoantibodies to coagulation factor deficiencies are uncommon but can produce life-threatening bleeding and death. The most commonly targeted coagulation factor in autoimmunity is factor VIII. Acquired hemophilia A, which results from these antibodies, can either be idiopathic or associated with older age, other autoimmune disorders, malignancy, the postpartum period, or the use of drugs such as penicillin and sulfonamides. Bleeding in acquired hemophilia A is treated with factor VIII–bypassing agents. The underlying autoimmune disorder frequently responds to immunosuppressive medication. Antiprothrombin antibodies usually are found in patients with lupus anticoagulant and are associated with bleeding. Antibodies of von Willebrand factor are found in patients with type 3 von Willebrand disease in response to infusion of plasma concentrates containing von Willebrand factor. Antibodies to factor V can occur as autoantibodies or as cross-reacting antibovine factor V antibodies that develop after exposure to bovine thrombin products that are contaminated with factor V. Pathogenic autoantibodies also have been described that target thrombin, factor IX, factor XI, factor XIII, protein C, protein S, and the endothelial cell protein C receptor.

## DEFINITION AND HISTORY

Antibodies directed against coagulation factors can develop as an acquired, autoimmune phenomenon. These "circulating anticoagulants" or "inhibitors" were recognized as early as 1906 as a cause of an acquired bleeding disorder.[1] The most common coagulation factor targeted in autoimmunity is factor VIII. The key feature that distinguishes antibody-mediated from other acquired coagulation factor deficiencies, such as impaired synthesis (e.g., a result of vitamin K deficiency) or increased consumption (e.g., in disseminated intravascular coagulation), is the ability of the patient's plasma to inhibit the coagulation of normal plasma. Inhibitors also can develop in response to replacement therapy in patients with congenital coagulation factor deficiencies, as discussed in Chap. 13.

Acronyms and Abbreviations: APC, activated protein C; aPCC, activated prothrombin complex concentrate; aPTT, activated partial thromboplastin time; BU, Bethesda units; CTLA4, cytotoxic T-lymphocyte associated protein 4; DAMP, damage-associated molecular patters; EACH, European Acquired Hemophilia Registry; FEIBA, factor VIII inhibitor–bypassing agent; PAPP, pathogen-associated molecular patterns; rVIIa, recombinant activated factor VII.

## ACQUIRED HEMOPHILIA A

### DEFINITIONS AND EPIDEMIOLOGY

The incidence of autoantibodies to factor VIII, which is the most commonly targeted coagulation factor in autoimmunity, is 1.4 per million people per year.[2-4] The associated clinical condition is called acquired hemophilia A. Approximately 40 to 50 percent of acquired hemophilia A patients have underlying conditions, including other autoimmune disorders (e.g., rheumatoid arthritis, systemic lupus erythematosus), malignancy, pregnancy, or a history consistent with a drug reaction.[5] The remaining idiopathic cases most commonly occur in elderly patients of either sex, with the median age at diagnosis being in the mid-70s.

### MECHANISMS OF ANTIBODY DEVELOPMENT

Even though adaptive immunity provides a unique ability to recognize a nearly infinite range of antigenic determinants, mechanisms of immunologic tolerance exist that reduce the probability of autoimmunity.[6] Self–nonself discrimination provides the key foundation upon which immune activity can be specifically directed toward potential pathogens.[6] However, self–nonself discrimination alone does not possess the capacity to distinguish innocuous antigens from antigens associated with a real threat of infection.[7] As a result, an elaborate network of innate immune factors also exists, which recognize potential danger in the form of cellular injury or conserved determinants on pathogens themselves, often referred to as damage-associated molecular patterns (DAMPs) and pathogen-associated molecular patterns (PAMPs), respectively.[7,8] Activation of immune cell function following exposure to PAMPs or DAMPs provides the necessary signals required for an efficient immunologic response to foreign antigen.[7-9]

The development of anti–factor VIII antibodies following factor VIII infusion in individuals with hemophilia A provides a classic example of the deleterious outcome of alloantibody formation following exposure to alloantigen. In this scenario, the factor VIII protein is foreign to the patients; consequently, central tolerance to the factor VIII protein does not occur. In contrast, acquired hemophilia results from loss of previous tolerance to a self antigen.[10-12]

For alloantibody development in patients with hemophilia A, individual variability in factor VIII levels accounts for some of the divergent level of tolerance to factor VIII observed. However, some individuals with undetectable levels of factor VIII antigen fail to generate factor VIII inhibitors, regardless of factor VIII exposure. Although these individuals would not be predicted to be tolerized to factor VIII, 70 to 80 percent of patients with baseline factor VIII levels of less than 1 percent do not develop an immune response to repeated dosing and are considered tolerized.[13-16] For the 20 to 30 percent of patients who develop inhibitors, there are both genetic and nongenetic risk factors for inhibitor development. Patients with a positive family history of inhibitors, those who have large factor VIII gene deletions, and nonwhites have a higher risk of inhibitor development.[17-20] The non–factor VIII genes—interleukin-10, tumor necrosis factor-α, and cytotoxic T-lymphocyte antigen 4–318 allele—are associated with inhibitor development.[17-20] Nongenetic risk factors, such as infusing factor at the time of a "danger" signal (e.g., a surgical procedure), intense factor exposure, and prophylaxis versus no prophylaxis, also are associated with inhibitor development.[16] Patients who receive factor at the time of a "danger" signal may experience sufficient tissue injury to provide the necessary immune activation through DAMPs. Furthermore, it remains possible that low-grade and potentially clinically undetectable infection may provide low levels of PAMPs that could likewise stimulate anti–factor VIII antibodies following factor VIII exposure. However, while PAMPs and/or DAMPs may provide the important immune activation signals,[21,22] several studies using animal models suggest that significant factor VIII antibody development can occur in the absence of known tissue injury or DAMP exposure.[23] Consistent with this, immune activation can occur in the apparent absence of DAMPs or PAMPs toward several model antigens.[24] Unique B-cell populations, especially those in the spleen, can rapidly respond to bloodborne antigens in the absence of any identifiable PAMPs or tissue injury, suggesting that these cells may be uniquely poised to respond to factor VIII.[25] Consistent with this, in experimental models, splenectomy can significantly inhibit factor VIII inhibitor development following factor VIII exposure,[26,27] suggesting that several of these unique B-cell populations may be involved in the development of factor VIII antibodies irrespective of DAMP or PAMP exposure.[25,26]

Although examples of antigens inducing B-cell activation in the absence of known DAMPs or PAMPs exist, most of these antigens require crosslinking of cell-surface B-cell receptors for efficient activation and therefore reflect highly repetitive antigenic structures.[28] In contrast, factor VIII represents a soluble antigen with little inherent predicted crosslinking ability. Most soluble antigen of this type actually induce tolerance following injection, likely because of the inability of soluble monovalent antigens to adequately crosslink and thereby stimulate B-cell receptors. Although factor VIII can exist in a soluble, monovalent form, it remains possible that factor VIII may form complexes with higher-molecular-weight species and thus form a network of factor VIII antigens that may serve as a suitable substrate for efficient B-cell receptor crosslinking and subsequent activation. Consistent with this, induction of tolerance to factor VIII by exposure to high levels of factor VIII may partially reflect a saturation of sites for factor VIII complex formation,[29] which may, in turn, result in B-cell exposure to high levels of soluble, monovalent factor VIII. However, if this occurs, studies suggest that it likely takes place independent of interactions with von Willebrand factor, the primary binding partner of factor VIII, or its own coagulant activity.[30] Clearly, there is much more to learn regarding the immunologic factors responsible for factor VIII inhibitor development.

In contrast to generating alloantibodies following factor VIII infusion, some patients generate autoantibodies against factor VIII, which can result in acquired factor VIII deficiency. As coagulation typically occurs at sites of inflammation and injury where DAMPs presumably are generated, tolerance to factor VIII may unfortunately be lost in these settings. Additionally, nonproteolytic and proteolytic degradation of coagulation proteins potentially could present neoepitopes. However, the fact that the development of acquired factor VIII deficiency is rare (1.4 per million population) provides a testimony to the ability of the immune system to discriminate efficiently between infectious nonself and noninfectious self.[12] Essentially, nothing is known about the breakdown of tolerance in patients who develop autoantibodies to coagulation factors.

## MOLECULAR PATHOLOGY

Factor VIII inhibitors in congenital and acquired hemophilia nearly always consist of a polyclonal immunoglobulin (Ig) G population. Although IgG$_4$ accounts for only 5 percent of the total IgG in normal plasma, it usually is a major, but not the sole, component of the anti–factor VIII antibody population.[31] IgG$_4$ antibodies do not fix complement, which has been cited as a reason that immune complex disease is not observed in factor VIII inhibitor patients. However, it is more likely that factor VIII simply is not present in sufficient quantity to form enough immune complex deposition to mediate tissue damage.

Factor VIII contains a sequence of domains designated A1-A2-B-ap-A3-C1-C2 (Chap. 13). During the activation of factor VIII by thrombin, the B and ap domains are released, producing an A1/A2/A3-C1-C2

activated factor VIII heterotrimer.[32] Anti–factor VIII antibodies in both congenital and acquired hemophilia A inhibitor are primarily directed to the A2 and C2 domains, although antibodies to all domains have been described.[33-35] The similarity in the properties of antibodies in congenital and acquired hemophilia, which represent very different immunologic settings, suggests that intrinsic structural features in the factor VIII molecule are an important determinant driving the immune response. Epitope spreading from a single "problem" epitope, which has been implicated in some autoantibody phenomena,[36] does not appear to be a property of factor VIII inhibitors because anti-C2 antibodies can occur in the absence of anti-A2 antibodies and vice versa.

The only known biologic function of factor VIII is to become proteolytically activated and participate as a cofactor for factor IXa during intrinsic pathway factor X activation on phospholipid membranes. Theoretically, antibodies could inhibit factor VIII procoagulant function in several ways, including blocking the binding of factor VIIIa to factor IXa, factor X, or phospholipid, or by interfering with the proteolytic activation of factor VIII. Some anti–A2 antibodies map to a region bounded by Arg484-Ile508[37] and inhibit activated factor VIII by blocking its ability to bind factor X.[38] Anti-C2 antibodies bind to the NH$_2$-terminal half of the C2 domain.[39] Anti-C2 antibodies have been identified that inhibit the binding of activated factor VIII to phospholipid membranes,[40] which is critical for its interaction with the platelet surfaces. However, the C2 domain also apparently contributes to the binding of factor VIII to its activators, thrombin and factor Xa.[41-43] Consistent with this, anti-C2 inhibitors have been identified that block factor VIII activation.[41,44]

Factor VIII inhibitors also have been identified in approximately 20 percent of normal healthy donors.[45] These inhibitors inhibit factor VIII activity in pooled normal plasma, but not autologous plasma, indicating that they are not autoantibodies, but rather alloantibodies directed against an unidentified polymorphism. Anti–factor VIII IgG also has been identified in all normal plasmas tested by affinity chromatography on immobilized factor VIII.[46] The increased sensitivity of the method is a consequence of its ability to resolve anti–factor VIII antibodies from anti–anti–factor VIII idiotypic antibodies that also are present. Idiotypic regulation has been proposed as a mechanism for controlling autoantibody activity in vivo.[47]

## CLINICAL FEATURES

Acquired hemophilia A patients usually present with spontaneous bleeding, which often is severe and life- or limb-threatening, although large cohort studies have shown that approximately 30 percent of patients do not require hemostatic management.[2,48] Patients with acquired hemophilia are more likely to have a severe bleeding diathesis than congenital hemophilia A inhibitor patients.[49] Additionally, in contrast to patients with congenital hemophilia A, hemarthrosis in these patients is rare. The reasons for these differences is puzzling, especially in light of the fact that the properties of factor VIII inhibitors in the two patient populations is similar. As noted above, inhibitors can block factor VIII function in several ways. Conceivably, unidentified mechanistic differences in inhibitor action account for the difference in clinical severity. Factor VIII inhibitors sometimes resolve spontaneously. However, it is not possible to predict in which subset of patients this will occur.

## LABORATORY FEATURES AND DIFFERENTIAL DIAGNOSIS

The new onset of an acquired bleeding disorder should immediately lead to screening tests that include an activated partial thromboplastin time (aPTT), a prothrombin time, and a platelet count. Patients with acquired hemophilia A have a prolonged aPTT resulting from decreased or absent factor VIII activity in the intrinsic pathway of blood coagulation. The autoantibody inhibits the factor VIII in the plasma from normal individuals, which forms the basis of the mixing study that is used to screen for inhibitors. The presence of a prolonged aPTT in a mixing study establishes the diagnosis of a circulating anticoagulant. Specific factor assays then are performed to determine whether a specific coagulation factor inhibitor or a lupus anticoagulant is present. The activity of other intrinsic pathway coagulation factors may be decreased in the presence of high titer factor VIII inhibitors. However, the levels of these factors normalize at increasing dilutions of patient plasma, whereas factor VIII activity remains decreased.

Once the identity of an inhibitor has been established, its titer is determined using the Bethesda assay.[50] Inhibitors frequently take minutes to hours to maximally inhibit factor VIII. Therefore, dilutions of patient plasma are preincubated with normal plasma for 2 hours at 37°C. The inhibitor titer is defined as the dilution of patient plasma that produces 50 percent inhibition of the factor VIII activity and is expressed in Bethesda units per milliliter (BU/mL). Inhibitors are classified informally as low titer or high titer when the titers are less than 5 BU/mL or greater than 5 to 10 BU/mL, respectively. The Bethesda assay has been modified by the addition of 0.1 M imidazole, pH 7.4, and by diluting test plasma into factor VIII–deficient plasma during the preincubation phase to prevent assay variation resulting from pH changes and adsorptive losses of factor VIII.[51] This "Nijmegen" modification of the Bethesda assay decreases false-positive low-titer inhibitors.[52] Patients with acquired hemophilia often have measurable residual factor VIII activity. This activity may cause an underestimate of the inhibitory titer. Preanalytical heat treatment has been proposed as a simple way to denature factor VIII to allow for more accurate determination of titer in both patients with acquired hemophilia A and patients with congenital hemophilia A who may have infused factor VIII.[53,54]

Factor VIII inhibitors are classified based on the kinetics and extent of inactivation of factor VIII in plasma.[55] Type I inhibitors follow second-order kinetics and inactivate factor VIII completely, which would be expected for a simple bimolecular antigen-antibody reaction. Type II inhibitors inactivate factor VIII incompletely and display more complex kinetics of inhibition. Hemophilia A inhibitor patients and acquired hemophilia A patients tend to have type I and type II inhibitors, respectively.[56] However, the borderline between type I and type II inhibitors is not always clear and the distinction is not useful clinically. Additionally, in a recent observational study of patients with acquired hemophilia in the United Kingdom, factor VIII levels and inhibitor titers at presentation were not predictive of the severity of bleeding events. The median factor VIII level and inhibitory titers were nearly identical for patients with fatal bleeding events compared to those who did not require treatment for their bleeding symptoms.[2]

## TREATMENT

The severe bleeding that often is the presenting feature of this disorder requires urgent action to establish a diagnosis and initiate therapeutic measures. Ideally, this is carried out in a setting where factor VIII inhibitors can be identified and quantitated and where there is subspecialty expertise in the management of bleeding disorders. Invasive procedures should be performed only if absolutely necessary, and venipuncture should be kept to a minimum given the risk of significant bleeding.[57]

Treatment of patients with acquired hemophilia A depends on the inhibitor titer. Although no prospective trials are available, clinical experience indicates that patients with a factor VIII inhibitor titer of less than 5 BU/mL often are treated successfully with sufficient doses of recombinant or plasma-derived factor VIII to neutralize the inhibitor. Patients with titers between 5 and 10 BU/mL also may respond to

factor VIII, whereas those with titers greater than 10 BU/mL generally do not respond. Formulas exist to calculate the amount of factor VIII needed to treat a patient, but these are rough estimates at best. The efficacy of factor VIII concentrates was lower than that of bypassing agents in a large registry study, which was likely secondary to challenges in appropriately dosing the factor VIII concentrate.[48]

Desmopressin can be administered by intravenous, subcutaneous, or intranasal routes and results in an increase in plasma von Willebrand factor levels and factor VIII activity.[58] Its potential use is in patients with baseline factor VIII levels greater than 5 IU/dL and minor bleeding. However, like factor VIII concentrates, response is not predictable and close monitoring of hemostatic efficacy and factor VIII levels is needed.

Factor VIII–bypassing agents, which drive the coagulation mechanism through the extrinsic pathway, are the mainstays of management of patients with a high titer of an inhibitor. Two agents, recombinant activated factor VII (rFVIIa; NovoSeven RT) and plasma-derived antiinhibitor coagulant complex (AICC; FEIBA VH Immuno, also called activated prothrombin complex concentrate [aPCC]), are commercially available and approved by the FDA for treatment of acquired hemophilia A. Although no comparative trials have been done, analysis of the European Acquired Haemophilia (EACH2) Registry showed similar hemostatic efficacy between rFVIIa and aPCC at approximately 90 percent.[48] Similar hemostatic efficacy between rFVIIa and aPCC has been seen in the treatment of congenital hemophilia A with inhibitors.[59] The recommended dose range of rFVIIa for the treatment of patients with acquired hemophilia is 70 to 90 mcg/kg repeated every 2 to 3 hours until hemostasis is achieved. aPCC is given at doses of 50 to 100 U/kg every 8 to 12 hours, but should not exceed 200 U/kg per day. Lower doses (50 to 75 U/kg) are used for mild bleeding, whereas higher doses (100 U/kg) are given for severe limb- or life-threatening bleeding. Treatment should be continued until there are clear signs of clinical improvement.

Although there are similar rates of efficacy between the two available bypassing agents, not all patients respond. Additionally, there are no widely accepted methods available for predicting response to therapy or monitoring patients on therapy. The use of thromboelastography and the thrombin generation assays as a predictor of response to therapy in congenital hemophilia A and inhibitors has been reported, but large clinical studies linking clinical data to outcome are lacking, leaving clinical response as the only available monitoring option.[60]

The major serious adverse event associated with bypassing agents is thrombosis. The EACH2 Registry reported similar rates in patients treated with rFVIIa or aPCC.[48] However, the risk of thrombosis is considered low when used for approved indications at the recommended doses. The incidence of thrombosis in patients with acquired hemophilia A treated with bypassing agents appears higher than that for patients with congenital hemophilia. This is probably because of cardiovascular risk factors in the acquired hemophilia population given their age and associated medical conditions. Escalating doses of either bypassing agent or a combination of the two agents should be done with caution, especially in older patients.

Factor VIII inhibitors usually cross-react poorly with porcine factor VIII.[61] A commercial plasma-derived porcine factor VIII concentrate was useful in the treatment of factor VIII inhibitor patients for approximately 20 years[62] but was discontinued in 2004 because of viral contamination of the product. Porcine factor VIII has the advantage of potentially being guided by laboratory monitoring of recovery of factor VIII activity in plasma. However, the development of antiporcine factor VIII antibodies may preclude its long-term use. A phase II/III clinical trial of a recombinant porcine factor VIII product has been completed in patients with acquired hemophilia A,[63] and a phase II trial has been completed in congenital hemophilia inhibitor patients.[64]

Although acquired inhibitors may remit spontaneously, fatal bleeding may occur up to several months after the initial diagnosis, even in patients who present with mild bleeding. Therefore, immunosuppressive therapy at the time of diagnosis to eradicate the inhibitor is recommended.[57] A variety of immunosuppressive agents have been used, including cyclophosphamide, azathioprine, cyclosporine, intravenous immunoglobulin, and rituximab. Immune tolerance induction using human factor VIII similar to what is done for patients with congenital hemophilia A and inhibitors has been used successfully. Additionally, plasmapheresis and immunoadsorption of the inhibitory antibody have been used.

First-line immunosuppressive regimens at many centers consist of glucocorticoids alone or glucocorticoids combined with cyclophosphamide.[65] No appropriately powered randomized studies have been performed, so the information available is from a single small randomized study, case reports, national surveys, and large registry data. The single randomized trial of 31 patients comparing prednisone and cyclophosphamide showed no difference in the treatment arms. A national registry study also showed no difference, with 76 percent of patients achieving complete remission in the steroid arm and 78 percent in the steroids plus cytotoxic agent arm.[66] The EACH2 Registry has the largest reported experience with 331 patients and reported a higher rate of stable complete remission at 70 percent for patients treated with steroids and cyclophosphamide compared with 48 percent for steroids alone and 59 percent for rituximab-containing regimens. Extensive analysis to control for potential confounding factors in this nonrandomized study confirmed that stable complete remission was more likely with a steroid plus cyclophosphamide than with steroids alone (odds ratio of 3.25). The median time to remission was 5 weeks in patients treated with steroids alone or steroids plus cyclophosphamide and 10 weeks in patients treated with rituximab. There have been no studies that have shown a difference in long-term outcomes including survival and sustained remission.[57,67]

The rarity of this disease, the severity of bleeding at onset, and the delay in diagnosis of these patients have all contributed to the lack of controlled trials. Given the lack of controlled trials, clinical management decisions are guided from the limited data available and clinical judgment.

# ● ACQUIRED ANTIBODIES TO OTHER COAGULATION FACTORS

## ANTI–FACTOR V AND ANTITHROMBIN ANTIBODIES

Thrombin and factor V inhibitors are discussed together because of their frequent coexistence in immune responses to commercial products that contain thrombin. Thrombin products have been used widely in surgical and endoscopic procedures. It has been estimated that more than 500,000 patients are treated annually with products containing thrombin.[68] Thrombin is used either alone or as a component of fibrin sealants, which consist of fibrinogen and thrombin preparations that are mixed together at the wound site to form a topical fibrin clot.[69] Additionally, factor XIII sometimes is added to crosslink and stabilize the clot.

Fibrin sealants contain thrombin and fibrinogen derived from human plasma, whereas stand-alone thrombin products are prepared from bovine plasma. Both types of products are heavily contaminated with other plasma proteins, including factor V and prothrombin.[70,71] Almost all patients exposed to bovine proteins develop a detectable immune response. In half of these patients, antibovine antibodies cross-react with human thrombin, factor V, or prothrombin.[68] Usually, these antibodies are subclinical.[72] However, mild to life-threatening hemorrhage can occur, especially if the titer of anti–human factor V antibodies is high. The risk of bleeding is higher in patients who receive bovine thrombin products more than once because of the development of a secondary immune response.

There have been no clinical trials comparing the safety and efficacy of fibrin sealants to stand-alone thrombin products. Because fibrin sealants are composed mainly of human proteins, they may be less immunogenic. However, anti–factor V antibodies have been reported in a patient receiving fibrin sealant.[73] There currently is no stand-alone human thrombin product. It seems likely that the development of highly purified plasma-derived or recombinant products containing human thrombin in the presence or absence of human fibrinogen would decrease the incidence of antithrombin and anti–factor V antibodies.[70]

Autoantibodies to thrombin are rare. However, the mechanisms of action of antithrombin antibodies have been studied extensively because of the wealth of information about thrombin structure and function.[74-77] In contrast, approximately half of the 105 cases of inhibitory anti–factor V antibodies reported and reviewed between 1955 and 1997 appeared to be autoantibodies not associated with the exposure to bovine thrombin products.[72] $\beta$-Lactam antibiotics also are associated with anti–factor V autoantibodies and may partly explain the increased incidence with surgery. In approximately 20 percent of cases of autoantibody formation, no underlying disease was identified. Anti–factor V autoantibodies have been identified rarely in patients with autoimmune diseases, solid tumors, and monoclonal gammopathies. In addition to autoantibody formation, alloantibodies to factor V have developed in patients with severe factor V deficiency in response to replacement therapy with fresh-frozen plasma.

Patients with inhibitory antibodies to factor V have prolonged prothrombin and aPTT, low factor V levels, and a normal thrombin time. The diagnosis of a factor V inhibitor is based on the specific loss of factor V coagulant activity when patient and normal plasma are mixed in a coagulation assay. The antibody titer can be defined as in the factor VIII Bethesda assay as the dilution of test plasma that produces 50 percent inhibition of factor V activity.

Not all patients with factor V inhibitors have hemorrhagic manifestations. Factor V inhibitors anecdotally produce a less serious bleeding disorder than factor VIII inhibitors. The relationship between inhibitor titer and bleeding has not been studied. The reported incidence of bleeding has been higher in patients with autoantibodies to factor V compared to anti–factor V antibodies in patients receiving bovine thrombin. However, this may reflect a bias resulting from the reason the patient sought medical attention.

Factor V contains an A1-A2-B-A3-C1-C2 domain structure that is homologous to factor VIII. Also, like factor VIII, the N-terminal half of the factor V C2 domain contains a phospholipid-binding site[78] that is necessary for normal procoagulant function[79] and is targeted by factor V inhibitors.[80,81]

## ANTIPROTHROMBIN ANTIBODIES

Antiprothrombin antibodies are most commonly associated with the antiphospholipid syndrome. The antiphospholipid syndrome is caused by lupus anticoagulants, which are defined as antibodies that produce phospholipid-dependent prolongation of *in vitro* coagulation assays. Anionic phospholipids participate as cofactors for the lupus anticoagulant binding to protein antigens, primarily $\beta_2$-glycoprotein I[82] and prothrombin.[83] The antibody–antigen complexes compete for the binding of coagulation factors to the phospholipid present in coagulation assays and produce the lupus anticoagulant phenomenon.

The role of prothrombin in the generation of lupus anticoagulant activity initially was suggested from studies of a bleeding patient with severe hypoprothrombinemia. However, in the absence of hypoprothrombinemia, lupus anticoagulants do not produce a bleeding diathesis and bleeding in patients with lupus anticoagulants is uncommon.[84] Antiprothrombin antibodies are associated with an increased incidence of thrombosis in these patients.[85] In patients with antiprothrombin antibodies and hypoprothrombinemia, precipitating, noninhibitory antibodies are present and prothrombin antigen levels are low, indicating that the hypoprothrombinemia is the result of rapid clearance of antigen–antibody complexes.[86] However, most patients with lupus anticoagulants have demonstrable antiprothrombin antibodies but do not have hypoprothrombinemia.[87] Thus, antibody-mediated hypoprothrombinemia appears to represent a relatively uncommon evolution of the autoimmune response to prothrombin in patients with lupus anticoagulants.

## ANTIBODIES TO COMPONENTS OF THE PROTEIN C SYSTEM

An acquired inhibitor to protein C associated with a fatal thrombotic disorder has been reported[88] but evidently is rare. In contrast, there is a relatively high prevalence of pathogenic anti–protein S antibodies. Inhibitory antibodies to protein S were detected in five of 15 patients with acquired protein S deficiency.[89] Anti–protein S antibodies, but not antibodies to cardiolipin, $\beta_2$-glycoprotein I, prothrombin, or protein C, appear to be a risk factor for acquired activated protein C (APC) resistance, defined as APC resistance in the absence of the factor V Leiden mutation, and for deep venous thrombosis.[90] Additionally, antibodies to the endothelial cell protein receptor have been identified that are associated with fetal death in patients with the antiphospholipid syndrome.[91]

## ACQUIRED ANTIBODIES TO OTHER COAGULATION FACTORS

Clinically significant antibodies to coagulation factors other than factor VIII, factor V, and prothrombin that produce acquired bleeding disorders are sufficiently rare that they merit case reports, which are only incompletely listed here. In contrast to acquired hemophilia A, acquired hemophilia B is extremely rare.[92,93] Patients with antifibrinogen antibodies have been identified either who are asymptomatic with abnormal laboratory values[94] or who have abnormal bleeding.[95] Patients with abnormal bleeding associated with acquired inhibitors to factor VII,[96] factor X,[97] factor XI,[98] or factor XIII[98–107] also have been described. The development of alloantibodies against von Willebrand factor occurs in patients with type 3 von Willebrand disease in response to treatment with plasma concentrates that contain von Willebrand factor.[108] Acquired von Willebrand disease can be caused by adsorption of von Willebrand factor to tumor cells, by loss of high-molecular-weight von Willebrand factor multimers, and by autoantibodies to von Willebrand factor.[109]

## REFERENCES

1. Margolius A Jr, Jackson DP, Ratnoff OD: Circulating anticoagulants: A study of 40 cases and a review of the literature. *Medicine (Baltimore)* 40:145–202, 1961.
2. Collins PW, Hirsch S, Baglin TP, et al: Acquired hemophilia A in the United Kingdom: A 2-year national surveillance study by the United Kingdom Haemophilia Centre Doctors' Organisation. *Blood* 109(5):1870–1877, 2007.
3. Borg JY, Guillet B, Le Cam-Duchez V, et al: Outcome of acquired haemophilia in France: The prospective SACHA (Surveillance des Auto antiCorps au cours de l'Hemophilie Acquise) registry. *Haemophilia* 19(4):564–570, 2013.
4. Knoebl P, Marco P, Baudo F, et al: Demographic and clinical data in acquired hemophilia A: Results from the European Acquired Haemophilia Registry (EACH2). *J Thromb Haemost* 10(4):622–631, 2012.
5. Green D, Lechner K: A survey of 215 non-hemophilic patients with inhibitors to factor VIII. *Thromb Haemost* 45(3):200–203, 1981.
6. Hogquist KA, Baldwin TA, Jameson SC: Central tolerance: Learning self-control in the thymus. *Nat Rev Immunol* 5(10):772–782, 2005.
7. Janeway CA Jr, Medzhitov R: Innate immune recognition. *Annu Rev Immunol* 20:197–216, 2002.
8. Matzinger P: Tolerance, danger, and the extended family. *Annu Rev Immunol* 12:991–1045, 1994.
9. Rubtsov AV, Swanson CL, Troy S, et al: TLR agonists promote marginal zone B cell activation and facilitate T-dependent IgM responses. *J Immunol* 180(6):3882–3888, 2008.
10. Lollar P: Pathogenic antibodies to coagulation factors. Part one: Factor VIII and factor IX. *J Thromb Haemost* 2(7):1082–1095, 2004.
11. Dunn AL, Abshire TC: Current issues in prophylactic therapy for persons with hemophilia. *Acta Haematol* 115(3–4):162–171, 2006.
12. Franchini M, Lippi G: Acquired factor VIII inhibitors. *Blood* 112(2):250–255, 2008.
13. White GC 2nd, Kempton CL, Grimsley A, et al: Cellular immune responses in hemophilia: Why do inhibitors develop in some, but not all hemophiliacs? *J Thromb Haemost* 3(8):1676–1681, 2005.
14. Lorenzo JI, Lopez A, Altisent C, Aznar JA: Incidence of factor VIII inhibitors in severe haemophilia: The importance of patient age. *Br J Haematol* 113(3):600–603, 2001.
15. Lusher JM, Arkin S, Abildgaard CF, Schwartz RS: Recombinant factor VIII for the treatment of previously untreated patients with hemophilia A. Safety, efficacy, and development of inhibitors. Kogenate Previously Untreated Patient Study Group. *N Engl J Med* 328(7):453–459, 1993.
16. Gouw SC, van der Bom JG, Marijke van den Berg H: Treatment-related risk factors of inhibitor development in previously untreated patients with hemophilia A: The CANAL cohort study. *Blood* 109(11):4648–4654, 2007.
17. Astermark J, Berntorp E, White GC, et al: The Malmo International Brother Study (MIBS): Further support for genetic predisposition to inhibitor development in hemophilia patients. *Haemophilia* 7(3):267–272, 2001.
18. Astermark J, Oldenburg J, Escobar M, et al: The Malmo International Brother Study (MIBS). Genetic defects and inhibitor development in siblings with severe hemophilia A [see comment]. *Haematologica* 90(7):924–931, 2005.
19. Goodeve A: The incidence of inhibitor development according to specific mutations—and treatment? [review] [8 refs]. *Blood Coagul Fibrinolysis* 14(Suppl 1):S17–S21, 2003.
20. Oldenburg J, Schroder J, Brackmann HH, et al: Environmental and genetic factors influencing inhibitor development [review] [44 refs]. *Semin Hematol* 41(1 Suppl 1):82–88, 2004.
21. Hendrickson JE, Desmarets M, Deshpande SS, et al: Recipient inflammation affects the frequency and magnitude of immunization to transfused red blood cells. *Transfusion* 46(9):1526–1536, 2006.
22. Hendrickson JE, Chadwick TE, Roback JD, et al: Inflammation enhances consumption and presentation of transfused RBC antigens by dendritic cells. *Blood* 110(7):2736–2743, 2007.
23. Meeks SL, Healey JF, Parker ET, et al: Antihuman factor VIII C2 domain antibodies in hemophilia A mice recognize a functionally complex continuous spectrum of epitopes dominated by inhibitors of factor VIII activation. *Blood* 110(13):4234–4242, 2007.
24. Stowell SR, Henry KL, Smith NH, et al: Alloantibodies to a paternally derived RBC KEL antigen lead to hemolytic disease of the fetus/newborn in a murine model. *Blood* 122(8):1494–1504, 2013.
25. Martin F, Kearney JF: Marginal-zone B cells. *Nat Rev Immunol* 2(5):323–335, 2002.
26. Navarrete A, Dasgupta S, Delignat S, et al: Splenic marginal zone antigen-presenting cells are critical for the primary allo-immune response to therapeutic factor VIII in hemophilia A. *J Thromb Haemost* 7(11):1816–1823, 2009.
27. Zhang AH, Skupsky J, Scott DW: Effect of B-cell depletion using anti-CD20 therapy on inhibitory antibody formation to human FVIII in hemophilia A mice. *Blood* 117(7):2223–2226, 2011.
28. Bachmann MF, Rohrer UH, Kundig TM, et al: The influence of antigen organization on B cell responsiveness. *Science* 262(5138):1448–1451, 1993.
29. Kempton CL, White GC 2nd: How we treat a hemophilia A patient with a factor VIII inhibitor. *Blood* 113(1):11–17, 2009.
30. Meeks SL, Cox CL, Healey JF, et al: A major determinant of the immunogenicity of factor VIII in a murine model is independent of its procoagulant function. *Blood* 120(12):2512–2520, 2012.
31. Hoyer LW, Gawryl MS, de la Fuente B: Immunochemical characterization of factor VIII inhibitors. *Prog Clin Biol Res* 150:73–85, 1984.
32. Lollar P, Parker CG: Subunit structure of thrombin-activated porcine factor VIII. *Biochemistry* 28(2):666–674, 1989.
33. Fulcher CA, de Graaf Mahoney S, Roberts JR, et al: Localization of human factor FVIII inhibitor epitopes to two polypeptide fragments. *Proc Natl Acad Sci U S A* 82(22):7728–7732, 1985.
34. Prescott R, Nakai H, Saenko EL, et al: The inhibitor antibody response is more complex in hemophilia A patients than in most nonhemophiliacs with factor VIII autoantibodies. Recombinate and Kogenate Study Groups. *Blood* 89(10):3663–3671, 1997.
35. Scandella D, Mattingly M, de Graaf S, Fulcher CA: Localization of epitopes for human factor VIII inhibitor antibodies by immunoblotting and antibody neutralization. *Blood* 74(5):1618–1626, 1989.
36. James JA, Harley JB: B-cell epitope spreading in autoimmunity. *Immunol Rev* 164:185–200, 1998.

37. Healey JF, Barrow RT, Tamim HM, et al: Residues Glu2181-Val2243 contain a major determinant of the inhibitory epitope in the C2 domain of human factor VIII. *Blood* 92(10):3701–3709, 1998.

38. Lollar P, Parker ET, Curtis JE, et al: Inhibition of human factor VIIIa by anti-A2 subunit antibodies. *J Clin Invest* 93(6):2497–2504, 1994.

39. Healey JF, Lubin IM, Nakai H, et al: Residues 484–508 contain a major determinant of the inhibitory epitope in the A2 domain of human factor VIII. *J Biol Chem* 270(24):14505–14509, 1995.

40. Arai M, Scandella D, Hoyer LW: Molecular basis of factor VIII inhibition by human antibodies. Antibodies that bind to the factor VIII light chain prevent the interaction of factor VIII with phospholipid. *J Clin Invest* 83(6):1978–1984, 1989.

41. Nogami K, Shima M, Hosokawa K, et al: Factor VIII C2 domain contains the thrombin-binding site responsible for thrombin-catalyzed cleavage at Arg1689. *J Biol Chem* 275(33):25774–25780, 2000.

42. Nogami K, Shima M, Hosokawa K, et al: Role of factor VIII C2 domain in factor VIII binding to factor Xa. *J Biol Chem* 274(43):31000–31007, 1999.

43. Saenko EL, Shima M, Rajalakshmi KJ, Scandella D: A role for the C2 domain of factor VIII in binding to von Willebrand factor. *J Biol Chem* 269(15):11601–11605, 1994.

44. Meeks SL, Healey JF, Parker ET, et al: Nonclassical anti-C2 domain antibodies are present in patients with factor VIII inhibitors. *Blood* 112(4):1151–1153, 2008.

45. Algiman M, Dietrich G, Nydegger UE, et al: Natural antibodies to factor VIII (anti-hemophilic factor) in healthy individuals. *Proc Natl Acad Sci U S A* 89(9):3795–3799, 1992.

46. Gilles JG, Saint-Remy JM: Healthy subjects produce both anti-factor VIII and specific anti-idiotypic antibodies. *J Clin Invest* 94(4):1496–1505, 1994.

47. Guilbert B, Dighiero G, Avrameas S: Naturally occurring antibodies against nine common antigens in human sera. I. Detection, isolation and characterization. *J Immunol* 128(6):2779–2787, 1982.

48. Baudo F, Collins P, Huth-Kuhne A, et al: Management of bleeding in acquired hemophilia A: Results from the European Acquired Haemophilia (EACH2) Registry. *Blood* 120(1):39–46, 2012.

49. Ludlam CA, Morrison AE, Kessler C: Treatment of acquired hemophilia. *Semin Hematol* 31(2 Suppl 4):16–19, 1994.

50. Kasper CK, Aledort L, Aronson D, et al: Proceedings: A more uniform measurement of factor VIII inhibitors. *Thromb Diath Haemorrh* 34(2):612, 1975.

51. Verbruggen B, Novakova I, Wessels H, et al: The Nijmegen modification of the Bethesda assay for factor VIII:C inhibitors: Improved specificity and reliability. *Thromb Haemost* 73(2):247–251, 1995.

52. Giles AR, Verbruggen B, Rivard GE, et al: A detailed comparison of the performance of the standard versus the Nijmegen modification of the Bethesda assay in detecting factor VIII:C inhibitors in the haemophilia A population of Canada. Association of Hemophilia Centre Directors of Canada. Factor VIII/IX Subcommittee of Scientific and Standardization Committee of International Society on Thrombosis and Haemostasis. *Thromb Haemost* 79(4):872–875, 1998.

53. Batty P, Platton S, Bowles L, et al: Pre-analytical heat treatment and a FVIII ELISA improve factor VIII antibody detection in acquired haemophilia A. *Br J Haematol* 166(6):953–956, 2014.

54. Soucie JM, Miller CH, Kelly FM, et al: A study of prospective surveillance for inhibitors among persons with haemophilia in the United States. *Haemophilia* 20(2):230–237, 2014.

55. Biggs R, Austen DE, Denson KW, et al: The mode of action of antibodies which destroy factor VIII. II. Antibodies which give complex concentration graphs. *Br J Haematol* 23(2):137–155, 1972.

56. Hoyer LW, Scandella D: Factor VIII inhibitors: Structure and function in autoantibody and hemophilia A patients. *Semin Hematol* 31(2 Suppl 4):1–5, 1994.

57. Collins PW, Chalmers E, Hart DP, et al: Diagnosis and treatment of factor VIII and IX inhibitors in congenital haemophilia (4th edition). UK Haemophilia Centre Doctors Organization. *Br J Haematol* 160(2):153–170, 2013.

58. Franchini M, Lippi G: The use of desmopressin in acquired haemophilia A: A systematic review. *Blood Transfus* 9(4):377–382, 2011.

59. Astermark J, Donfield SM, DiMichele DM, et al: A randomized comparison of bypassing agents in hemophilia complicated by an inhibitor: The FEIBA NovoSeven Comparative (FENOC) Study. *Blood* 109(2):546–551, 2007.

60. Young G, Sorensen B, Dargaud Y, et al: Thrombin generation and whole blood viscoelastic assays in the management of hemophilia: Current state of art and future perspectives. *Blood* 121(11):1944–1950, 2013.

61. Brettler DB, Forsberg AD, Levine PH, et al: The use of porcine factor VIII concentrate (Hyate:C) in the treatment of patients with inhibitor antibodies to factor VIII. A multicenter US experience. *Arch Intern Med* 149(6):1381–1385, 1989.

62. Hay CR: Porcine factor VIII: Past, present and future. *Haematologica* 85(10 Suppl):21–24; discussion 24–25, 2000.

63. Kruse-Jarres R, St-Louis J, Greist A, et al: Efficacy and safety of OBI-1, an antihaemophilic factor VIII (recombinant), porcine sequence, in subjects with acquired hemophilia A. *Haemophilia* 21(2):162–170, 2015.

64. Kempton CL, Abshire TC, Deveras RA, et al: Pharmacokinetics and safety of OBI-1, a recombinant B domain-deleted porcine factor VIII, in subjects with hemophilia A. *Haemophilia* 18(5):798–804, 2012.

65. Collins P, Baudo F, Huth-Kuhne A, et al: Consensus recommendations for the diagnosis and treatment of acquired hemophilia A. *BMC Res Notes* 3:161, 2010.

66. Green D, Rademaker AW, Briet E: A prospective, randomized trial of prednisone and cyclophosphamide in the treatment of patients with factor VIII autoantibodies. *Thromb Haemost* 70(5):753–757, 1993.

67. Collins P, Baudo F, Knoebl P, et al: Immunosuppression for acquired hemophilia A: Results from the European Acquired Haemophilia Registry (EACH2). *Blood* 120(1):47–55, 2012.

68. Schoenecker JG, Johnson RK, Lesher AP, et al: Exposure of mice to topical bovine thrombin induces systemic autoimmunity. *Am J Pathol* 159(5):1957–1969, 2001.

69. Ortel TL, Charles LA, Keller FG, et al: Topical thrombin and acquired coagulation factor inhibitors: Clinical spectrum and laboratory diagnosis. *Am J Hematol* 45(2):128–135, 1994.

70. Schoenecker JG, Johnson RK, Fields RC, et al: Relative purity of thrombin-based hemostatic agents used in surgery. *J Am Coll Surg* 197(4):580–590, 2003.

71. Zehnder JL, Leung LL: Development of antibodies to thrombin and factor V with recurrent bleeding in a patient exposed to topical bovine thrombin. *Blood* 76(10):2011–2016, 1990.

72. Knobl P, Lechner K: Acquired factor V inhibitors. *Baillieres Clin Haematol* 11(2):305–318, 1998.

73. Caers J, Reekmans A, Jochmans K, et al: Factor V inhibitor after injection of human thrombin (tissucol) into a bleeding peptic ulcer. *Endoscopy* 35(6):542–544, 2003.

74. Arnaud E, Lafay M, Gaussem P, et al: An autoantibody directed against human thrombin anion-binding exosite in a patient with arterial thrombosis: Effects on platelets, endothelial cells, and protein C activation. *Blood* 84(6):1843–1850, 1994.

75. La Spada AR, Skalhegg BS, Henderson R, et al: Brief report: Fatal hemorrhage in a patient with an acquired inhibitor of human thrombin. *N Engl J Med* 333(8):494–497, 1995.

76. Lian F, He L, Colwell NS, et al: Anticoagulant activities of a monoclonal antibody that binds to exosite II of thrombin. *Biochemistry* 40(29):8508–8513, 2001.

77. Sie P, Bezeaud A, Dupouy D, et al: An acquired antithrombin autoantibody directed toward the catalytic center of the enzyme. *J Clin Invest* 88(1):290–296, 1991.

78. Macedo-Ribeiro S, Bode W, Huber R, et al: Crystal structures of the membrane-binding C2 domain of human coagulation factor V. *Nature* 402(6760):434–439, 1999.

79. Ortel TL, Devore-Carter D, Quinn-Allen M, Kane WH: Deletion analysis of recombinant human factor V. Evidence for a phosphatidylserine binding site in the second C-type domain. *J Biol Chem* 267(6):4189–4198, 1992.

80. Izumi T, Kim SW, Greist A, et al: Fine mapping of inhibitory anti-factor V antibodies using factor V C2 domain mutants. Identification of two antigenic epitopes involved in phospholipid binding. *Thromb Haemost* 85(6):1048–1054, 2001.

81. Ortel TL, Moore KD, Quinn-Allen MA, et al: Inhibitory anti-factor V antibodies bind to the factor V C2 domain and are associated with hemorrhagic manifestations. *Blood* 91(11):4188–4196, 1998.

82. McNeil HP, Simpson RJ, Chesterman CN, Krilis SA: Anti-phospholipid antibodies are directed against a complex antigen that includes a lipid-binding inhibitor of coagulation: Beta 2-glycoprotein I (apolipoprotein H). *Proc Natl Acad Sci U S A* 87(11):4120–4124, 1990.

83. Fleck RA, Rapaport SI, Rao LV: Anti-prothrombin antibodies and the lupus anticoagulant. *Blood* 72(2):512–519, 1988.

84. Feinstein DI, Rapaport SI: Acquired inhibitors of blood coagulation. *Prog Hemost Thromb* 1:75–95, 1972.

85. Lakos G, Kiss E, Regeczy N, et al: Antiprothrombin and antiannexin V antibodies imply risk of thrombosis in patients with systemic autoimmune diseases. *J Rheumatol* 27(4):924–929, 2000.

86. Bajaj SP, Rapaport SI, Fierer DS, et al: A mechanism for the hypoprothrombinemia of the acquired hypoprothrombinemia-lupus anticoagulant syndrome. *Blood* 61(4):684–692, 1983.

87. Edson JR, Vogt JM, Hasegawa DK: Abnormal prothrombin crossed-immunoelectrophoresis in patients with lupus inhibitors. *Blood* 64(4):807–816, 1984.

88. Mitchell CA, Rowell JA, Hau L, et al: A fatal thrombotic disorder associated with an acquired inhibitor of protein C. *N Engl J Med* 317(26):1638–1642, 1987.

89. Sorice M, Arcieri P, Griggi T, et al: Inhibition of protein S by autoantibodies in patients with acquired protein S deficiency. *Thromb Haemost* 75(4):555–559, 1996.

90. Nojima J, Kuratsune H, Suehisa E, et al: Acquired activated protein C resistance associated with anti-protein S antibody as a strong risk factor for DVT in non-SLE patients. *Thromb Haemost* 88(5):716–722, 2002.

91. Hurtado V, Montes R, Gris JC, et al: Autoantibodies against EPCR are found in antiphospholipid syndrome and are a risk factor for fetal death. *Blood* 104(5):1369–1374, 2004.

92. Boggio LN, Green D: Acquired hemophilia. *Rev Clin Exp Hematol* 5(4):389–404; quiz following 431, 2001.

93. Krishnamurthy P, Hawche C, Evans G, Winter M: A rare case of an acquired inhibitor to factor IX. *Haemophilia* 17(4):712–713, 2011.

94. Nawarawong W, Wyshock E, Meloni FJ, et al: The rate of fibrinopeptide B release modulates the rate of clot formation: A study with an acquired inhibitor to fibrinopeptide B release. *Br J Haematol* 79(2):296–301, 1991.

95. Ruiz-Arguelles A: Spontaneous reversal of acquired autoimmune dysfibrinogenemia probably due to an antiidiotypic antibody directed to an interspecies cross-reactive idiotype expressed on antifibrinogen antibodies. *J Clin Invest* 82(3):958–963, 1988.

96. Aguilar C, Lucia JF, Hernandez P: A case of an inhibitor autoantibody to coagulation factor VII. *Haemophilia* 9(1):119–120, 2003.

97. Rao LV, Zivelin A, Iturbe I, Rapaport SI: Antibody-induced acute factor X deficiency: Clinical manifestations and properties of the antibody. *Thromb Haemost* 72(3):363–371, 1994.

98. Goodrick MJ, Prentice AG, Copplestone JA, et al: Acquired factor XI inhibitor in chronic lymphocytic leukaemia. *J Clin Pathol* 45(4):352–353, 1992.

99. Ajzner E, Schlammadinger A, Kerenyi A, et al: Severe bleeding complications caused by an autoantibody against the B subunit of plasma factor XIII: A novel form of acquired factor XIII deficiency. *Blood* 113(3):723–725, 2009.

100. Daly HM, Carson PJ, Smith JK: Intracerebral haemorrhage due to acquired factor XIII inhibitor—Successful response to factor XIII concentrate. *Blood Coagul Fibrinolysis* 2(4):507–514, 1991.

101. Fukue H, Anderson K, McPhedran P, et al: A unique factor XIII inhibitor to a fibrin-binding site on factor XIIIA. *Blood* 79(1):65–74, 1992.

102. Krumdieck R, Shaw DR, Huang ST, et al: Hemorrhagic disorder due to an isoniazid-associated acquired factor XIII inhibitor in a patient with Waldenström's macroglobulinemia. *Am J Med* 90(5):639–645, 1991.

103. Lopaciuk S, Bykowska K, McDonagh JM, et al: Difference between type I autoimmune inhibitors of fibrin stabilization in two patients with severe hemorrhagic disorder. *J Clin Invest* 61(5):1196–1203, 1978.

104. Lorand L, Maldonado N, Fradera J, et al: Haemorrhagic syndrome of autoimmune origin with a specific inhibitor against fibrin stabilizing factor (factor XIII). *Br J Haematol* 23(1):17–27, 1972.

105. Lorand L, Velasco PT, Murthy SN, et al: Autoimmune antibody in a hemorrhagic patient interacts with thrombin-activated factor XIII in a unique manner. *Blood* 93(3):909–917, 1999.

106. Lorand L, Velasco PT, Rinne JR, et al: Autoimmune antibody (IgG Kansas) against the fibrin stabilizing factor (factor XIII) system. *Proc Natl Acad Sci U S A* 85(1):232–236, 1988.

107. Tosetto A, Rodeghiero F, Gatto E, et al: An acquired hemorrhagic disorder of fibrin crosslinking due to IgG antibodies to FXIII, successfully treated with FXIII replacement and cyclophosphamide. *Am J Hematol* 48(1):34–39, 1995.

108. James PD, Lillicrap D, Mannucci PM: Alloantibodies in von Willebrand disease. *Blood* 122(5):636–640, 2013.

109. Federici AB: Acquired von Willebrand syndrome: Is it an extremely rare disorder or do we see only the tip of the iceberg? *J Thromb Haemost* 6(4):565–568, 2008.

# CHAPTER 18
# HEMOSTATIC ALTERATIONS IN LIVER DISEASE AND LIVER TRANSPLANTATION

Frank W. G. Leebeek and Ton Lisman

## SUMMARY

In patients with acute liver failure or chronic liver disease, many changes in the hemostatic system occur. The liver is the site of synthesis of nearly all coagulation factors, both pro- and anticoagulant proteins. A reduced synthesis function of the liver will lead to reduced levels of these factors in circulation. In addition, the liver is involved in the clearance of many activated coagulation factors and protein–inhibitor complexes from the circulation, which, in turn, can lead to activation of the coagulation system if liver function is impaired. Furthermore, the liver is involved in the synthesis and clearance of pro- and antifibrinolytic proteins, which may lead to a shift in the balance of the fibrinolytic system. Also primary hemostasis might be affected in liver disease because of thrombocytopenia and impaired platelet function, which is frequently encountered in these patients. It is evident that patients with liver disease have frequent bleeding episodes, mainly in the gastrointestinal tract, such as variceal bleeding. It has been a longstanding dogma that patients with liver disease are at a high risk of bleeding caused by the above mentioned hemostatic changes. However, in recent years, this cause of the bleeding tendency has been questioned because of the concomitant reductions of pro- and anticoagulant factors and pro- and antifibrinolytic factors. More recent studies using more sophisticated coagulation tests showed that thrombin generation is normal in patients with chronic liver failure and that some may even have a prothrombotic phenotype. This led to the development of a model of a rebalanced hemostatic system in these patients, which may have immediate implications for treatment. Hematologists and other clinicians taking care of patients with acute liver failure of chronic liver disease, such as cirrhosis, are still faced with the questions of whether these patients need correction of the changes in hemostasis before interventions such as paracentesis, biopsies, dental care, and surgery. It was generally believed that replacement therapy with frozen plasma or prothrombin complex concentrate was indicated. However, based on these new findings, physicians should now be more restrictive in the use of hemostatic agents and blood products in these patients both in liver disease and during liver transplantation.

**Acronyms and Abbreviations:** ADAMTS13, a disintegrin-like and metalloprotease with thrombospondin domain 13; aPTT, activated partial thromboplastin time; DDAVP, 1-deamino-8-D-arginine vasopressin; DIC, disseminated intravascular coagulation; FFP, fresh-frozen plasma; HAT, hepatic artery thrombosis; HSC, hepatic stellate cell; INR, international normalized ratio; ISI, international sensitivity index; LMWH, low-molecular-weight heparin; MELD, model of end-stage liver disease; PAI-1, plasminogen activator inhibitor 1; PFA, platelet function analyzer; PT, prothrombin time; PVT, portal vein thrombosis; TAFI, thrombin-activatable fibrinolysis inhibitor; t-PA, tissue-type plasminogen activator; VWF, von Willebrand factor.

The liver plays a central role in the hemostatic system. Liver parenchymal cells are the site of synthesis of most coagulation factors (except factor VIII), the natural inhibitors of coagulation, including protein C, protein S, and antithrombin, and essential components of the fibrinolytic system, such as plasminogen, $\alpha_2$-antiplasmin, and thrombin activatable fibrinolysis inhibitor (TAFI). The liver also regulates hemostasis and fibrinolysis by clearing activated coagulation factors and coagulation factor–inhibitor complexes from the circulation. In addition, changes in primary hemostasis mediated by platelets, von Willebrand factor (VWF), and ADAMTS13 (a disintegrin-like and metalloprotease with thrombospondin type 1 repeats) may occur. Therefore, when acute or chronic liver dysfunction is present in patients with liver disease, complicated hemostatic derangement may occur, which can lead to bleeding, thrombosis, or neither bleeding nor thrombosis.

# ● HEMOSTATIC ALTERATIONS IN CHRONIC LIVER DISEASE

## PRIMARY HEMOSTASIS

More than 75 percent of patients with chronic liver disease, especially in moderate to severe cirrhosis (Child B and C), have reduced levels of platelets (<150,000/$\mu$L), and 13 percent have platelet counts between 50,000 and 75,000/$\mu$L.[1] This may be caused by splenomegaly resulting in sequestration of platelets in the spleen, reduced synthesis of thrombopoietin by the diseased liver, or consumption coagulopathy.[2-5] In addition, it has been suggested that autoantibodies against platelets may reduce the half-life of platelets in cirrhosis.[6] Primary hemostasis may also be defective by a reduced platelet function. *In vitro* platelet aggregation studies in response to various agonists are frequently diminished in patients with liver disease. Defective platelet function may result from impaired signal transduction, acquired storage pool deficiency, proteolysis of platelet membrane proteins, and increased production of the endothelial-derived platelet inhibitors, nitric oxide and prostacyclin (reviewed in Ref. 7). A reduced hematocrit may contribute to defective platelet–vessel wall interaction. Platelet adhesion defects were also found under conditions of flow, but were in some studies attributed to thrombocytopenia and a low hematocrit.[8-10] Platelet procoagulant activity measured by a thrombin generation assay using platelet-rich plasma was similar in patients and healthy controls, which casts additional doubt on the extent of the functional defects of platelets in patients with liver disease.[11]

VWF antigen levels are strongly elevated in patients with liver disease. It has been suggested that this is the result of endothelial damage possibly mediated by endotoxemia (bacterial infection).[12,13] VWF mRNA and protein expression in the liver itself are substantially increased in cirrhosis, but VWF ristocetin cofactor activity is variable.[10,14-16] The high levels of VWF may ameliorate the hemostatic defect caused by thrombocytopenia and platelet function defects.[13] In a flow-based model, platelet adhesion to collagen was normalized in thrombocytopenia because of the high levels of VWF in cirrhotic plasma. In patients with liver disease, the regulation of VWF multimer size and activity can be impaired because of reduced synthesis of the VWF-cleaving protease ADAMTS13 by stellate cells in the liver.[17] Several studies showed, however, that the most active high-molecular-weight multimers of VWF are diminished in plasma of patients with cirrhosis, which may be mediated by plasmin or other proteases.[18,19] Classical tests of primary hemostasis, such as bleeding time, which is becoming obsolete as a result of its assay variability and inability to predict bleeding, may still be abnormal in patients with liver disease. Also, newer global tests of primary hemostasis, such as platelet function analyzer (PFA), show prolonged closure times with various agonists, but its value in prediction of bleeding in liver disease is unknown.[20]

## SECONDARY HEMOSTASIS: COAGULATION AND ANTICOAGULATION

The liver is the site of synthesis of most procoagulant proteins. As a result, decreased levels of coagulation factors II, V, VII, IX, X, and XI are commonly observed in patients with liver failure.[21] In contrast, factor VIII levels are increased, which may be related to the elevated level of its carrier protein VWF and to decreased clearance of factor VIII from the circulation by the liver low-density lipoprotein-related receptor.[14] Factor VIII is synthesized primarily in hepatic sinusoidal endothelial cells, whose function is preserved in liver disease.[14,22] Acquired vitamin K–dependent carboxylation deficiency may lead to qualitative defects in coagulation factors. Because of vitamin K deficiency or decreased production of γ-glutamyl carboxylase, circulating vitamin K–dependent coagulation factors II, VII, IX, and X may be deficient in γ-carboxylated glutamic acid residues in their GLA domains, giving rise to impaired function of these factors.[23] On the other hand, levels of anticoagulant protein C, protein S, antithrombin, heparin cofactor II, and $α_2$-macroglobulin are also decreased in patients with liver disease.[24] Fibrinogen levels are frequently in the normal range in patients with chronic liver disease, but may be decreased in patients with decompensated cirrhosis or acute liver failure.[25] A qualitative defect in fibrinogen may be found in patients with liver disease.[26] Screening tests of coagulation, such as the prothrombin time (PT) or activated partial thromboplastin time (aPTT), are frequently prolonged in patients with chronic liver disease. These results have been traditionally interpreted to reflect a hypocoagulable state. The PT and aPTT are sensitive to levels of procoagulant proteins in plasma, but not to the natural anticoagulants, protein C, protein S, and antithrombin. The use of a more sophisticated test of coagulation, such as total thrombin generation test, illustrates the limitation of PT and aPTT. In a thrombin-generation test measuring the total amount of thrombin generated during coagulation, decreased total thrombin generation is measured in patients with cirrhosis compared to controls.[11,27,28] Yet, when measured in the presence of thrombomodulin to enable protein C activation and thereby also taking into account the contribution of the main inhibitor of coagulation protein C, thrombin generation was indistinguishable from controls, despite abnormal conventional coagulation tests. Others found normal thrombin generation without addition of thrombomodulin and even increased thrombin generation with addition of thrombomodulin.[29,30] These results suggest that thrombin generation *in vivo* can be normal in patients with liver failure and that a prolonged PT does not *per se* indicate a bleeding risk. These findings indicate that a concomitant decrease of pro- and anticoagulant factors results in a rebalanced hemostatic system.[31]

Despite the limitations of the use of PT in patients with liver disease, the international normalized ratio (INR), which is a derivative of PT, is still used in prognostic scores for patients with acute or chronic liver disease. The model of end-stage liver disease (MELD) score is used to prioritize patients for liver transplantation. The INR was originally developed and validated only to monitor anticoagulant therapy with vitamin K antagonists. The interlaboratory variation of the INR in patients with liver disease is substantial, and its use results in significant differences in MELD scores when a single patient sample is tested in different laboratories using various PT reagents.[32,33] The use of alternative international sensitivity index (ISI) values obtained by calibration against plasma samples from patients with liver disease was shown to decrease this variability.[34,35]

## FIBRINOLYSIS

Except for tissue-type plasminogen activator (t-PA) and plasminogen-activator inhibitor (PAI)-1, all proteins involved in fibrinolysis, both pro- and antifibrinolytic, are synthesized by the liver.[36] Therefore, chronic liver disease leads to decreased plasma levels of plasminogen, $α_2$-antiplasmin, TAFI, and factor XIII. Plasma levels of t-PA are elevated as a result of increased secretion from endothelial cells and/or reduced clearance by the diseased liver. Plasma levels of PAI-1 also are increased but not to the same extent as t-PA, which may lead to a shift in balance in the fibrinolytic system.[37] It has long been assumed that most patients with chronic liver disease had accelerated fibrinolysis. This was based on *in vitro* assays, including various clot lysis assays, and on measurements of increased fibrin(ogen) degradation products, D-dimer, and plasmin-antiplasmin complexes (reviewed in Ref. 36). However, more recent studies found no evidence of hyperfibrinolysis in the majority of patients with cirrhosis despite decreased levels of TAFI and elevated D-dimer levels.[38,39] This conclusion was recently challenged by a study that used two assays to detect fibrinolysis in patients with various degrees of severity of cirrhosis. In both tests, approximately 40 percent of patients had evidence of hyperfibrinolysis, and in 60 percent of the patients, one of the tests revealed an increased fibrinolytic capacity, especially in those with severe liver dysfunction.[40] Hyperfibrinolysis in patients with cirrhosis may also occur secondary to low-grade disseminated intravascular coagulation (DIC) induced by endotoxemia and is manifested by concomitant increased levels of prothrombin fragment 1+2, fibrinopeptide A, D-dimer, thrombin-antithrombin complex, and plasmin-antiplasmin complex.[41] However, it has been argued that the increased levels of these markers may result from their decreased clearance by the liver rather than from DIC. In patients with liver disease who presented with gastrointestinal bleeding or soft tissue bleeding after trauma, *in vitro* signs of increased fibrinolysis have been reported.[42,43]

## ● A REBALANCED HEMOSTATIC SYSTEM IN CHRONIC LIVER DISEASE

It has been a longstanding dogma that patients with liver disease are at a high risk of bleeding due to reduction of synthesis of coagulation factors and other changes in hemostasis. More recent studies using more sophisticated coagulation tests have shown that thrombin generation is normal in patients with chronic liver failure and that some may even have a prothrombotic phenotype.[24,27,44] Because both procoagulant and anticoagulant proteins decline in patients with chronic liver diseases, it has been postulated that the hemostatic system is rebalanced (Table 18–1).[24,31,45] In addition, reductions of platelet number and impairment of platelet function are counteracted by high levels of VWF, and in many patients, the decline in profibrinolytic factors is balanced by the reduction of inhibitors of fibrinolysis.[13,38] This led to the model of a rebalanced hemostatic system in these patients, which has important implications for treatment.[24,31] This model also explains why most patients with liver disease usually do not exhibit severe bleeding manifestations—neither during minor invasive procedures, such as biopsies and paracentesis, nor during major surgeries, including liver transplantation.[46,47] Furthermore, patients with liver disease may even have increased risk of venous thromboembolism, not only liver-specific thrombosis, but also deep vein thrombosis.[48–50] The hemostatic balance in patients with liver disease is, however, quite delicate and vulnerable to be tipped toward bleeding or thrombosis. So far, it is impossible to identify which patients are more prone to bleeding or to thrombosis based on current laboratory assays. The complex changes in hemostasis encountered in patients with liver disease are depicted in Table 18-1. The delicate hemostatic balance in patients with liver disease may be changed by comorbidities, such as bacterial infections and renal failure frequently observed in these patients. It is of major importance to treat these comorbidities so as to reduce the risk of bleeding and thrombosis.[51]

**TABLE 18-1.** Changes in the Hemostatic System in Patients with Liver Disease That Contribute to Bleeding (Left) or Contribute to Thrombosis (Right)

| Changes That Impair Hemostasis | Changes That Promote Hemostasis |
|---|---|
| **Primary Hemostasis** | |
| Thrombocytopenia | Elevated levels of VWF |
| Platelet function defects | Decreased levels of ADAMTS13 |
| Enhanced production of nitric oxide and prostacyclin | |
| **Secondary Hemostasis** | |
| Low levels of factors II, V, VII, IX, X, and XI | Elevated levels of factor VIII |
| Vitamin K deficiency | Decreased levels of protein C, protein S, antithrombin, $a_2$-macroglobulin, and heparin cofactor II |
| Dysfibrinogenemia | |
| **Fibrinolysis** | |
| Low levels of $a_2$-antiplasmin, factor XIII, and TAFI | Low levels of plasminogen |
| | Increase in PAI-1 levels |
| Elevated t-PA levels | |

ADAMTS13, a disintegrin-like and metalloprotease with thrombospondin domain 13; PAI-1, plasminogen activator inhibitor 1; TAFI, thrombin-activatable fibrinolysis inhibitor; t-PA, tissue-type plasminogen activator; VWF, von Willebrand factor.

# HEMOSTATIC ALTERATIONS IN ACUTE LIVER FAILURE

Patients presenting with acute liver failure, for instance in acetaminophen intoxication, have profound changes in the hemostatic system. A severe decrease of coagulation factors is observed, with strongly increased INR.[52] However, an intact thrombin generation has been observed in acute liver failure patients, and hardly any changes were observed using thromboelastography.[53,54] In contrast to chronic liver disease, patients with acute liver failure frequently have normal platelet counts. Highly elevated levels of VWF and strongly decreased levels of ADAMTS13 are observed. This imbalance may lead to a prothrombotic state.[55] In patients with acute liver failure, there is an increased level of PAI-1 and reduced levels of plasminogen, which is consistent with a hypofibrinolytic state.[53,56] A strong increase of procoagulant microparticles has been observed in acute liver failure.[57] Spontaneous bleeding is not frequently encountered in patients with acute liver failure.[58]

# HEMOSTATIC ALTERATIONS DURING LIVER TRANSPLANTATION

Liver transplantation performed in patients in acute or chronic liver failure has always been complicated by significant and sometimes life-threatening bleeding problems requiring massive use of coagulation factors and erythrocyte transfusion.[59] Therefore, blood products were also transfused before and during transplantation to correct the hemostatic dysfunction. Improved surgical techniques and anesthesiologic care have led to a remarkable reduction of blood loss during liver transplantation. Currently,

no blood transfusion is given in up to 50 to 80 percent of patients undergoing a liver transplantation, depending on the center.[60,61] This improvement is also because of a better understanding of the coagulation profile during the various stages of the surgical intervention. During the first stage of liver transplantation, the removal of the diseased liver, no significant worsening of the preoperative hemostatic status occurs.[62] After removal of the diseased liver, the so-called anhepatic stage, significant hemostatic changes occur. Because activated coagulation factors are not cleared from the circulation, system activation of coagulation, in its most extreme form mimicking DIC, can develop, with consumption of platelets and coagulation factors and secondary hyperfibrinolysis. Moreover, hyperfibrinolysis may also occur as a result of defective clearance of t-PA.[63] The most severe hemostatic changes during liver transplantation occur immediately after reperfusion of the donor liver. Platelets are trapped in the graft, giving rise to an aggravation of thrombocytopenia and causing damage to the graft by induction of endothelial cell apoptosis.[64] Release of tissue factor and t-PA from the reperfused graft causes DIC with primary or secondary fibrinolysis.[63] Moreover, the graft also releases heparin-like substances that can inhibit coagulation.[65] In addition, other factors such as hypothermia, metabolic acidosis, and hemodilution adversely affect hemostasis during this phase.

During transplantation, the balance between VWF and ADAMTS13 changes because levels of VWF remain high, the functional properties of VWF improve, and the levels of ADAMTS13 decline (mostly due to impaired synthesis and possibly due to enhanced proteolytic degradation), which may partially compensate for the hemostatic dysfunction.[66] The platelet count and hemostatic proteins are at their nadir after reperfusion and rise gradually during the early postoperative period. However, the levels of procoagulant factors rise more rapidly than the levels of anticoagulant factors, which results in a temporary hypercoagulable state.[67] A transiently increased level of PAI-1 immediately after surgery can result in a hypofibrinolytic state that may aggravate the hypercoagulable status.

# CLINICAL PROBLEMS ENCOUNTERED IN PATIENTS WITH LIVER DISEASE

## BLEEDING IN PATIENTS WITH LIVER DISEASE

Although sophisticated hemostatic tests have now shown that disorders of primary hemostasis, a hypocoagulable status, and hyperfibrinolysis are generally not encountered or are only seen in a minority of patients with chronic liver disease, bleeding still may occur in these patients.[24] This is because individual patients still may have a compromised hemostatic function or because patients bleed for nonhemostatic reasons.[68] The most severe bleeding manifestation in patients with liver disease is bleeding from ruptured esophageal varices. This results from local vascular abnormalities and portal hypertension and not from deranged hemostasis. Occasionally, impaired hemostasis does cause easy bruising, purpura, epistaxis, gingival bleeding, menorrhagia, and gastrointestinal bleeding. Also, in acute liver failure, bleeding has frequently been reported in the past, but more recent studies clearly indicate that spontaneous bleeding occurs rarely.[58]

## HEMOSTATIC MANAGEMENT OF PATIENTS WITH LIVER DISEASE

### Hemostatic Management of Bleeding Episodes

Variceal bleeding in patients with liver disease should be immediately managed by local interventions, such as endoscopy and rubber band ligation or even shunt (transjugular intrahepatic portosystemic shunt [TIPS]) placement.[69] Fluid resuscitation should be given in case of hypotension and restricted blood transfusion in case of severe drop of hemoglobin level.[70] Because there is no evidence that changes in hemostasis are associated with the risk of variceal bleeding, treatment with coagulation factor concentrates is not indicated. Infusion of plasma may even lead to more bleeding as a result of an increase of portal pressure.[71,72] Treatment with vasoconstrictors such as terlipressin is recommended and should be started as soon variceal bleeding is suspected and continued until hemostasis is achieved or for up to 5 days. Upper gastrointestinal bleeding from peptic ulcer disease also occurs frequently in patients with liver disease. Infusion of recombinant factor VIIa did not result in reduction of blood loss or mortality in randomized clinical studies in patients with upper gastrointestinal bleeding and is not indicated.[72] Recently the use of hemostatic powder was used in patients who did not respond to other measures and was successfully used in some cases, but its value should be tested in larger randomized studies before it will be registered and can be recommended in this setting.[73,74] The most important intervention is to prevent variceal bleeding by prophylactic measures, such as rubber band ligation.

Minor bleeding, including bruising, purpura, and gingival bleeding, occur more frequently in patients with liver disease, but do not always need treatment or can be managed by local measures. Mucocutaneous bleeding, such as epistaxis, can be treated with fibrinolysis inhibitors, for instance tranexamic acid, and menorrhagia can be treated using oral contraceptives. In case of bleeding in patients with severe thrombocytopenia (<50,000/$\mu$L), platelet transfusion should be given, as would also be indicated in patients without underlying liver disease.

### Hemostatic Management Before Interventions and Surgical Procedures

Traditional guidelines have advised not to perform invasive procedures in patients with liver disease when routine hemostatic tests are abnormal unless they are corrected by blood products or pharmacologic prohemostatic agents. The rationale for such a prophylactic approach has been questioned for several reasons. First and most important is because abnormal coagulation tests in patients with liver disease are not necessarily associated with a bleeding risk.[24] As mentioned before, these results have been traditionally interpreted to reflect a hypocoagulable state, but appeared to have no impact on the bleeding risk after invasive procedures.[75-77] For instance, in a large prospective study, there was no evidence that prolongation of the PT was associated with bleeding after large-volume paracentesis in patients with liver disease and ascites.[75] Furthermore, normalization of traditional coagulation tests is rarely achieved by infusion of plasma products, and the efficacy of prophylactic treatment has not been proven.[78,79] In addition, transfusion of blood products carries a substantial risk of allergic reactions, volume overload, and potential transmission of pathogens.[80] Consequently, the current guideline of the American Association for the Study of Liver Diseases (AASLD) does not recommend the routine use of fresh-frozen plasma (FFP) transfusion for prophylactic correction of an abnormal PT before interventions, such as liver biopsy,[81] whereas other guidelines advise the use of FFP with a low grade of evidence.[82] Vitamin K is generally recommended in patients with liver disease and prolonged INR; however, its clinical benefit has been questioned.[83]

Thrombocytopenia in patients with cirrhosis is often mild and does not cause spontaneous bleeding or bleeding following minimally invasive procedures. There is little evidence that tests showing platelet dysfunction, including prolonged bleeding time or closure time measured with the PFA-100 thrombelastography, predict bleeding in patients with cirrhosis. Nevertheless, an early study showed that a prolonged bleeding time was associated with a fivefold increase in the risk of bleeding after liver biopsy.[84] Although shortening of the bleeding time was achieved by administration of 1-deamino-8-D-arginine vasopressin (DDAVP) in patients with liver disease,[85] no effect of DDAVP was observed in patients with bleeding from esophageal varices or on

the blood loss in patients undergoing hepatectomy[86] or liver transplantation.[87] Although this has not been addressed in many studies yet, it has been shown that bleeding complications during interventional procedures are associated with a low preprocedural platelet count.[88,89] If platelet counts are below $50 \times 10^9$/L, platelet transfusion is recommended before any intervention, as in other patients without underlying liver disease.[90] In case of neurosurgical interventions, platelets should be transfused up to a level of $100 \times 10^9$/L.[91] A relatively novel strategy to improve primary hemostasis in patients with hepatitis C is the administration of a thrombopoietin analogue (Eltrombopag). In the ELEVATE study, a short course of Eltrombopag was used to elevate the platelet count prior to invasive procedures. Use of Eltrombopag was associated with a higher rate of thrombosis, but no difference in bleeding was observed in this study, which may be related to the highly elevated VWF levels in patients with liver disease.[92,93] Eltrombopag is not indicated for the treatment of thrombocytopenia in patients with chronic liver disease before surgical interventions.

In individuals with generalized mucosal bleeding symptoms, which may be indicative of disorders of primary hemostasis or hyperfibrinolysis, treatment with fibrinolysis inhibitors such as tranexamic acid after the procedure should be considered.[68,89] Tranexamic acid is also advised in case of dental extractions because of the high fibrinolytic activity in the oral mucosa.

The use of fibrin sealant has been studied to reduce blood loss in patient undergoing liver surgery. Although these products reduce the time to hemostasis when applied on the transected liver surface, no improvement in postoperative complications was observed. Therefore, its value in these settings has not yet been established.[94]

### Hemostatic Management During Liver Transplantation

For many years, excessive blood loss during liver transplantation has been recognized as an important cause of morbidity and mortality; consequently, transfusion of a combination of blood products has been advocated for correction of the hemostatic derangements.[59] Experiments in experimental animal models have shown that the quality of the graft determines the extent of hemostatic changes following reperfusion.[94a] Indeed, blood loss following graft reperfusion is substantially increased in recipients of "extended criteria" donor livers (i.e., grafts with poorer quality because of, e.g., elevated donor age or prolonged cold ischemia times).[94b]

Because prophylactic transfusion of blood products may be associated with serious side effects, many centers have discontinued to attempt to improve hemostatic functions by administration of blood products prior to liver transplantation.[60] Liver transplantation procedures can now be performed without a requirement for transfusion of blood products in a substantial proportion of patients. One study reported that 79 percent of patients could be transplanted without the use of any blood product, provided the patient's central venous pressure was controlled through restriction of volume replacement and by using intraoperative phlebotomy during the transplantation.[61] Increased experience and improvements in surgical technique, anesthesiologic care, and better graft preservation methods have contributed to a steady decrease in blood transfusion requirements. When uncontrolled bleeding does occur, packed red cells, platelets, FFP, or fibrinogen concentrate can be transfused guided by laboratory values or thromboelastography.[95] Hyperfibrinolysis is thought to contribute significantly to impaired hemostasis during the anhepatic and reperfusion phases.[63] Use of synthetic antifibrinolytic agents, such as tranexamic acid (a lysine analogue) and aprotinin (a serine protease inhibitor), have reduced red cell and plasma transfusion.[96,97] Aprotinin was taken off the market in 2008 because of severe adverse events and mortality in patients undergoing cardiac surgery.[98]

# THROMBOSIS IN PATIENTS WITH LIVER DISEASE

## Deep Vein Thrombosis and Pulmonary Embolism

The reappraisal of changes in the hemostatic system in patients with liver disease has indicated that the coagulopathy of liver disease may not only reflect a reduced bleeding risk, but may even lead to a prothrombotic state.[99] Studies indicate that deep vein thrombosis and pulmonary embolism can occur in patients with cirrhosis.[48,100] A large nationwide population-based case-control study in Denmark indicated that patients with liver disease have a substantially increased risk for venous thromboembolism compared to controls with an odds ratio of 1.7 for patients with cirrhosis and an odds ratio of 1.9 for patients with other liver diseases.[48] Between 0.5 and 1.8 percent of all hospitalized patients with cirrhosis developed venous thrombosis. Therefore, liver disease should not be considered a contraindication for thromboprophylaxis with low-molecular-weight heparin (LMWH). Thromboprophylaxis is warranted in patients who are immobilized or undergo surgery and in hospitalized patients with active cancer. Treatment of venous thromboembolism in patients with liver disease is difficult, because of a higher risk of bleeding associated with anticoagulant treatment than in healthy individuals, although recent data suggest that therapeutic-dose LMWH is safe.[101–104] This, again, indicates that the balanced hemostatic system in patients with cirrhosis involves a narrow safety margin. Furthermore, the choice of anticoagulant may be difficult. LMWH or unfractionated heparin may be difficult to monitor as a result of low levels of antithrombin. Anti–factor Xa measurement seems to be unreliable in patients with liver disease because of analytical problems.[102,105] Also monitoring of treatment with vitamin K antagonists is difficult and may not be reliable based on the preexistent prolongation of the PT as a result of the underlying disease.[44] Considering the lack of studies, it is advised to maintain the INR between 2.0 and 3.0.[24] Recently, newer direct-acting oral anticoagulants have become available for the treatment of venous thrombosis, including factor IIa and factor Xa inhibitors, which do not require laboratory monitoring. Although these drugs have not yet been studied extensively in patients with liver disease, several reports have now been published on the use of these agents in patients with cirrhosis and vascular liver disorders.[105a] Future studies have to reveal whether these drugs are effective and can be used safely in this patient group.

## Portal Vein Thrombosis

Patients with advanced liver disease may develop thrombosis in the portal and mesenteric veins. These complications are not only related to decreased levels of the natural inhibitors of coagulation, antithrombin, protein C, and protein S, but also occur more often in individuals carrying common inherited thrombophilias such as factor V Leiden mutation and prothrombin G20210A variant.[106,107] A decreased blood flow in the splanchnic venous circulation because of portal hypertension has also been indicated as a risk factor for portal vein thrombosis (PVT). The prevalence of PVT in patients with cirrhosis increases with the progression of the disease, being less than 1 percent in patients with compensated cirrhosis and 8 to 25 percent in liver transplantation candidates.[44,108] Prophylactic treatment of patients with cirrhosis with low-dose LMWH reduced the risk of PVT and even increased survival.[101] The optimal treatment of PVT in cirrhosis patients remains to be established. Although randomized trials are still lacking, treatment with anticoagulants, such as LMWH or vitamin K antagonists, may prevent progression of thrombosis and may achieve recanalization in patients with PVT with or without cirrhosis.[109,110] However, not all patients with cirrhosis and PVT will benefit, and an individualized approach seems warranted.[111] Recently, the new direct oral anticoagulants have been approved for use in patients with venous thrombosis. Their use is not yet recommended in patients with liver disease, but recently, some case reports have been published in patients with splanchnic vein thrombosis.[112]

## Thrombosis Following Liver Transplantation

Following liver transplantation, both immediate and delayed thrombotic complications frequently occur.[113] Hepatic artery thrombosis (HAT) occurs in 1.6 to 8.9 percent of patients and may lead to graft failure, requiring retransplantation.[114,115] Thrombosis of the portal vein or inferior caval vein is much less common.[116] Although HAT has been considered a surgical complication, recent evidence suggests that excessive coagulation activation or inherited thrombophilia also may contribute to HAT.[117] Postoperative use of anticoagulants has been limited in liver transplant recipients as a result of the perceived bleeding risk. However, thrombotic complications do occur, and liver-related thrombosis in particular, such as HAT and PVT, is of concern as it often leads to graft loss. A single, uncontrolled, retrospective study showed that aspirin substantially reduces the risk of posttransplantation HAT, without an increase of bleeding.[118] Pulmonary emboli and intracardiac thrombosis may occur during liver transplantation, indicating that the hemostatic system may also tip toward thrombus formation during this procedure.[119] Whether or not other anticoagulants will prevent postoperative thrombosis remains to be established.

## Role of Coagulation in Fibrosis of the Liver

Thrombin, the key mediator of coagulation, also has several cellular effects mediated by protease-activated receptors (PARs). These PARs are expressed on hepatic stellate cells (HSCs), which are mediators of liver fibrosis. Thrombin generation leads to activation of HSCs and fibrogenesis.[120] Indeed, patients with prothrombotic phenotypes, such as carriers of the factor V Leiden mutation or antithrombin-deficient individuals, were shown to have enhanced progression of liver fibrosis in viral hepatitis.[121,122] In line with these observations, fibrogenesis may be reduced by using anticoagulant treatment; however, this has to be established in clinical studies.[44]

# REFERENCES

1. Afdhal N, McHutchison J, Brown R, et al: Thrombocytopenia associated with chronic liver disease. *J Hepatol* 48(6):1000–1007, 2008.
2. Aster RH: Pooling of platelets in the spleen: Role in the pathogenesis of "hypersplenic" thrombocytopenia. *J Clin Invest* 45(5):645–657, 1966.
3. Schmidt KG, Rasmussen JW, Bekker C, Madsen PE: Kinetics and in vivo distribution of 111-In-labelled autologous platelets in chronic hepatic disease: Mechanisms of thrombocytopenia. *Scand J Haematol* 34(1):39–46, 1985.
4. Goulis J, Chau TN, Jordan S, et al: Thrombopoietin concentrations are low in patients with cirrhosis and thrombocytopenia and are restored after orthotopic liver transplantation. *Gut* 44(5):754–758, 1999.
5. Ben-Ari Z, Osman E, Hutton RA, Burroughs AK: Disseminated intravascular coagulation in liver cirrhosis: Fact or fiction? *Am J Gastroenterol* 94(10):2977–2982, 1999.
6. Kajihara M, Kato S, Okazaki Y, et al: A role of autoantibody-mediated platelet destruction in thrombocytopenia in patients with cirrhosis. *Hepatology* 37(6):1267–1276, 2003.
7. Witters P, Freson K, Verslype C, et al: Review article: Blood platelet number and function in chronic liver disease and cirrhosis. *Aliment Pharmacol Ther* 27(11):1017–1029, 2008.
8. Ordinas A, Escolar G, Cirera I, et al: Existence of a platelet-adhesion defect in patients with cirrhosis independent of hematocrit: Studies under flow conditions. *Hepatology* 24(5):1137–1142, 1996.
9. Lisman T, Adelmeijer J, de Groot PG, et al: No evidence for an intrinsic platelet defect in patients with liver cirrhosis—Studies under flow conditions. *J Thromb Haemost* 4(9):2070–2072, 2006.
10. Escolar G, Cases A, Vinas M, et al: Evaluation of acquired platelet dysfunctions in uremic and cirrhotic patients using the platelet function analyzer (PFA-100): Influence of hematocrit elevation. *Haematologica* 84(7):614–619, 1999.
11. Tripodi A, Primignani M, Chantarangkul V, et al: Thrombin generation in patients with cirrhosis: The role of platelets. *Hepatology* 44(2):440–445, 2006.
12. Ferro D, Quintarelli C, Lattuada A, et al: High plasma levels of von Willebrand factor as a marker of endothelial perturbation in cirrhosis: Relationship to endotoxemia. *Hepatology* 23(6):1377–1383, 1996.

13. Lisman T, Bongers TN, Adelmeijer J, et al: Elevated levels of von Willebrand factor in cirrhosis support platelet adhesion despite reduced functional capacity. *Hepatology* 44(1):53–61, 2006.

14. Hollestelle MJ, Thinnes T, Crain K, et al: Tissue distribution of factor VIII gene expression *in vivo*—A closer look. *Thromb Haemost* 86(3):855–861, 2001.

15. Beer JH, Clerici N, Baillod P, et al: Quantitative and qualitative analysis of platelet GPIb and von Willebrand factor for liver cirrhosis. *Thromb Haemost* 73(4):601–609, 1995.

16. Hollestelle MJ, Geertzen HG, Straatsburg IH, et al: Factor VIII expression in liver disease. *Thromb Haemost* 91(2):267–275, 2004.

17. Mannucci PM, Canciani MT, Forza I, et al: Changes in health and disease of the metalloprotease that cleaves von Willebrand factor. *Blood* 98(9):2730–2735, 2001.

18. Federici AB, Berkowitz SD, Lattuada A, Mannucci PM: Degradation of von Willebrand factor in patients with acquired clinical conditions in which there is heightened proteolysis. *Blood* 81(3):720–725, 1993.

19. Tersteeg C, de Maat S, De Meyer SF, et al: Plasmin cleavage of von Willebrand factor as an emergency bypass for ADAMTS13 deficiency in thrombotic microangiopathy. *Circulation* 129(12):1320–1331, 2014.

20. Hugenholtz GG, Porte RJ, Lisman T: The platelet and platelet function testing in liver disease. *Clin Liver Dis* 13(1):11–20, 2009.

21. Kerr R, Newsome P, Germain L, et al: Effects of acute liver injury on blood coagulation. *J Thromb Haemost* 1(4):754–759, 2003.

22. Fahs SA, Hille MT, Shi Q, Weiler H, Montgomery RR: A conditional knockout mouse model reveals endothelial cells as the principal and possibly exclusive source of plasma factor VIII. *Blood* 123(24):3706–3713, 2014.

23. Blanchard RA, Furic BC, Jorgensen M, et al: Acquired vitamin K dependent carboxylation deficiency in liver disease. *N Engl J Med* 305(5):242–248, 1981.

24. Tripodi A, Mannucci PM: The coagulopathy of chronic liver disease. *N Engl J Med* 365(2):147–156, 2011.

25. de Maat MP, Nieuwenhuizen W, Knot EA, et al: Measuring plasma fibrinogen levels in patients with liver cirrhosis. The occurrence of proteolytic fibrin(ogen) degradation products and their influence on several fibrinogen assays. *Thromb Res* 78(4):353–362, 1995.

26. Francis JL, Armstrong DJ: Acquired dysfibrinogenaemia in liver disease. *J Clin Pathol* 35(6):667–672, 1982.

27. Tripodi A, Salerno F, Chantarangkul V, et al: Evidence of normal thrombin generation in cirrhosis despite abnormal conventional coagulation tests. *Hepatology* 41(3):553–558, 2005.

28. Lisman T, Bakhtiari K, Pereboom IT, et al: Normal to increased thrombin generation in patients undergoing liver transplantation despite prolonged conventional coagulation tests. *J Hepatol* 52(3):355–361, 2010.

29. Gatt A, Riddell A, Calvaruso V, et al: Enhanced thrombin generation in patients with cirrhosis-induced coagulopathy. *J Thromb Haemost* 8(9):1994–2000, 2010.

30. Potze W, Arshad F, Adelmeijer J, et al: Differential in vitro inhibition of thrombin generation by anticoagulant drugs in plasma from patients with cirrhosis. *PloS One* 9(2):e88390, 2014.

31. Lisman T, Porte RJ: Rebalanced hemostasis in patients with liver disease: Evidence and clinical consequences. *Blood* 116(6):878–885, 2010.

32. Trotter JF, Brimhall B, Arjal R, Phillips C: Specific laboratory methodologies achieve higher model for endstage liver disease (MELD) scores for patients listed for liver transplantation. *Liver Transpl* 10(8):995–1000, 2004.

33. Lisman T, van Leeuwen Y, Adelmeijer J, et al: Interlaboratory variability in assessment of the model of end-stage liver disease score. *Liver Int* 28(10):1344–1351, 2008.

34. Tripodi A, Chantarangkul V, Primignani M, et al: The international normalized ratio calibrated for cirrhosis (INR[liver]) normalizes prothrombin time results for model for end-stage liver disease calculation. *Hepatology* 46(2):520–527, 2007.

35. Bellest L, Eschwege V, Poupon R, et al: A modified international normalized ratio as an effective way of prothrombin time standardization in hepatology. *Hepatology* 46(2):528–534, 2007.

36. Leebeek FW: *Hyperfibrinolysis in Liver Disease*. CRC Press, Boca Raton, FL, 1996.

37. Leebeek FW, Kluft C, Knot EA, et al: A shift in balance between profibrinolytic and antifibrinolytic factors causes enhanced fibrinolysis in cirrhosis. *Gastroenterology* 101(5):1382–1390, 1991.

38. Lisman T, Leebeek FW, Mosnier LO, et al: Thrombin-activatable fibrinolysis inhibitor deficiency in cirrhosis is not associated with increased plasma fibrinolysis. *Gastroenterology* 121(1):131–139, 2001.

39. Stravitz RT: Potential applications of thromboelastography in patients with acute and chronic liver disease. *Nat Rev Gastroenterol Hepatol* 8(8):513–520, 2012.

40. Rijken DC, Kock EL, Guimaraes AH, et al: Evidence for an enhanced fibrinolytic capacity in cirrhosis as measured with two different global fibrinolysis tests. *J Thromb Haemost* 10(10):2116–2122, 2012.

41. Violi F, Ferro D, Basili S, et al: Association between low-grade disseminated intravascular coagulation and endotoxemia in patients with liver cirrhosis. *Gastroenterology* 109(2):531–539, 1995.

42. Francis RB Jr, Feinstein DI: Clinical significance of accelerated fibrinolysis in liver disease. *Haemostasis* 14(6):460–465, 1984.

43. Violi F, Ferro D, Basili S, et al: Hyperfibrinolysis increases the risk of gastrointestinal hemorrhage in patients with advanced cirrhosis. *Hepatology* 15(4):672–676, 1992.

44. Tripodi A, Anstee QM, Sogaard KK, et al: Hypercoagulability in cirrhosis: Causes and consequences. *J Thromb Haemost* 9(9):1713–1723, 2011.

45. Lisman T, Caldwell SH, Leebeek FW, Porte RJ: Is chronic liver disease associated with a bleeding diathesis? *J Thromb Haemost* 4(9):2059–2060, 2006.

46. Massicotte L, Lenis S, Thibeault L, et al: Effect of low central venous pressure and phlebotomy on blood product transfusion requirements during liver transplantations. *Liver Transpl* 12(1):117–123, 2006.

47. De Gottardi A, Thevenot T, Spahr L, et al: Risk of complications after abdominal paracentesis in cirrhotic patients: A prospective study. *Clin Gastroenterol Hepatol* 7(8):906–909, 2009.

48. Sogaard KK, Horvath-Puho E, Gronbaek H, et al: Risk of venous thromboembolism in patients with liver disease: A nationwide population-based case-control study. *Am J Gastroenterol* 104(1):96–101, 2009.

49. Northup PG, McMahon MM, Ruhl AP, et al: Coagulopathy does not fully protect hospitalized cirrhosis patients from peripheral venous thromboembolism. *Am J Gastroenterol* 101(7):1524–1528; quiz 1680, 2006.

50. Gulley D, Teal E, Suvannasankha A, et al: Deep vein thrombosis and pulmonary embolism in cirrhosis patients. *Dig Dis Sci* 53(11):3012–3017, 2008.

51. Vivas S, Rodriguez M, Palacio MA, et al: Presence of bacterial infection in bleeding cirrhotic patients is independently associated with early mortality and failure to control bleeding. *Dig Dis Sci* 46(12):2752–2757, 2001.

52. Munoz SJ, Rajender Reddy K, Lee W, Acute Liver Failure Study Group: The coagulopathy of acute liver failure and implications for intracranial pressure monitoring. *Neurocrit Care* 9(1):103–107, 2008.

53. Lisman T, Bakhtiari K, Adelmeijer J, et al: Intact thrombin generation and decreased fibrinolytic capacity in patients with acute liver injury or acute liver failure. *J Thromb Haemost* 10(7):1312–1319, 2012.

54. Stravitz RT, Lisman T, Luketic VA, et al: Minimal effects of acute liver injury/acute liver failure on hemostasis as assessed by thromboelastography. *J Hepatol* 56(1):129–136, 2012.

55. Hugenholtz GC, Adelmeijer J, Meijers JC, et al: An unbalance between von Willebrand factor and ADAMTS13 in acute liver failure: Implications for hemostasis and clinical outcome. *Hepatology* 58(2):752–761, 2013.

56. Pernambuco JR, Langley PG, Hughes RD, et al: Activation of the fibrinolytic system in patients with fulminant liver failure. *Hepatology* 18(6):1350–1356, 1993.

57. Stravitz RT, Bowling R, Bradford RL, et al: Role of procoagulant microparticles in mediating complications and outcome of acute liver injury/acute liver failure. *Hepatology* 58(1):304–313, 2013.

58. Munoz SJ, Stravitz RT, Gabriel DA: Coagulopathy of acute liver failure. *Clin Liver Dis* 13(1):95–107, 2009.

59. Porte RJ, Knot EA, Bontempo FA: Hemostasis in liver transplantation. *Gastroenterology* 97(2):488–501, 1989.

60. de Boer MT, Molenaar IQ, Hendriks HG, et al: Minimizing blood loss in liver transplantation: Progress through research and evolution of techniques. *Dig Surg* 22(4):265–275, 2005.

61. Massicotte L, Denault AY, Beaulieu D, et al: Transfusion rate for 500 consecutive liver transplantations: Experience of one liver transplantation center. *Transplantation* 93(12):1276–1281, 2012.

62. Kang YG, Martin DJ, Marquez J, et al: Intraoperative changes in blood coagulation and thrombelastographic monitoring in liver transplantation. *Anesth Analg* 64(9):888–896, 1985.

63. Porte RJ, Bontempo FA, Knot EA, et al: Systemic effects of tissue plasminogen activator-associated fibrinolysis and its relation to thrombin generation in orthotopic liver transplantation. *Transplantation* 47(6):978–984, 1989.

64. Sindram D, Porte RJ, Hoffman MR, et al: Platelets induce sinusoidal endothelial cell apoptosis upon reperfusion of the cold ischemic rat liver. *Gastroenterology* 118(1):183–191, 2000.

65. Agarwal S, Senzolo M, Melikian C, et al: The prevalence of a heparin-like effect shown on the thromboelastograph in patients undergoing liver transplantation. *Liver Transpl* 14(6):855–860, 2008.

66. Pereboom IT, Adelmeijer J, van Leeuwen Y, et al: Development of a severe von Willebrand factor/ADAMTS13 dysbalance during orthotopic liver transplantation. *Am J Transplant* 9(5):1189–1196, 2009.

67. Stahl RL, Duncan A, Hooks MA, et al: A hypercoagulable state follows orthotopic liver transplantation. *Hepatology* 12(3 Pt 1):553–558, 1990.

68. Boks AL, Brommer EJ, Schalm SW, Van Vliet HH: Hemostasis and fibrinolysis in severe liver failure and their relation to hemorrhage. *Hepatology* 6(1):79–86, 1986.

69. Garcia-Tsao G, Bosch J: Management of varices and variceal hemorrhage in cirrhosis. *N Engl J Med* 362(9):823–832, 2010.

70. Villanueva C, Colomo A, Bosch A, et al: Transfusion strategies for acute upper gastrointestinal bleeding. *N Engl J Med* 368(1):11–21, 2013.

71. Castaneda B, Debernardi-Venon W, Bandi JC, et al: The role of portal pressure in the severity of bleeding in portal hypertensive rats. *Hepatology* 31(3):581–586, 2000.

72. Marti-Carvajal AJ, Karakitsiou DE, Salanti G: Human recombinant activated factor VII for upper gastrointestinal bleeding in patients with liver diseases. *Cochrane Database Syst Rev* 3:CD004887, 2012.

73. Holster IL, Poley JW, Kuipers EJ, Tjwa ET: Controlling gastric variceal bleeding with endoscopically applied hemostatic powder (Hemospray). *J Hepatol* 57(6):1397–1398, 2012.

74. Sung JJ, Luo D, Wu JC, et al: Early clinical experience of the safety and effectiveness of Hemospray in achieving hemostasis in patients with acute peptic ulcer bleeding. *Endoscopy* 43(4):291–295, 2011.

75. De Gottardi A, Thevenot T, Spahr L, et al: Risk of complications after abdominal paracentesis in cirrhotic patients: A prospective study. *Clin Gastroenterol Hepatol* 7(8):906–909, 2009.

76. Piccinino F, Sagnelli E, Pasquale G, Giusti G: Complications following percutaneous liver biopsy. A multicentre retrospective study on 68,276 biopsies. *J Hepatol* 2(2):165–173, 1986.

77. Segal JB, Dzik WH, Transfusion Medicine/Hemostasis Clinical Trials Network: Paucity of studies to support that abnormal coagulation test results predict bleeding in the setting of invasive procedures: An evidence-based review. *Transfusion* 45(9):1413–1425, 2005.

78. Youssef WI, Salazar F, Dasarathy S, et al: Role of fresh frozen plasma infusion in correction of coagulopathy of chronic liver disease: A dual phase study. *Am J Gastroenterol* 98(6):1391–1394, 2003.

79. Gazzard BG, Henderson JM, Williams R: The use of fresh frozen plasma or a concentrate of factor IX as replacement therapy before liver biopsy. *Gut* 16(8):621–625, 1975.

80. Alter HJ, Klein HG: The hazards of blood transfusion in historical perspective. *Blood* 112(7):2617–2626, 2008.

81. Rockey DC, Caldwell SH, Goodman ZD, et al: American Association for the Study of Liver Diseases: Liver biopsy. *Hepatology* 49(3):1017–1044, 2009.

82. Liumbruno G, Bennardello F, Lattanzio A, et al: Recommendations for the transfusion of plasma and platelets. *Blood Transfus* 7(2):132–150, 2009.

83. Saja MF, Abdo AA, Sanai FM, et al: The coagulopathy of liver disease: Does vitamin K help? *Blood Coagul Fibrinolysis* 24(1):10–17, 2013.

84. Boberg KM, Brosstad F, Egeland T, et al: Is a prolonged bleeding time associated with an increased risk of hemorrhage after liver biopsy? *Thromb Haemost* 81(3):378–381, 1999.

85. Agnelli G, Parise P, Levi M, et al: Effects of desmopressin on hemostasis in patients with liver cirrhosis. *Haemostasis* 25(5):241–247, 1995.

86. Wong AY, Irwin MG, Hui TW, et al: Desmopressin does not decrease blood loss and transfusion requirements in patients undergoing hepatectomy. *Can J Anaesth* 50(1):14–20, 2003.

87. de Franchis R, Arcidiacono PG, Carpinelli L, et al: Randomized controlled trial of desmopressin plus terlipressin vs. terlipressin alone for the treatment of acute variceal hemorrhage in cirrhotic patients: A multicenter, double-blind study. New Italian Endoscopic Club. *Hepatology* 18(5):1102–1107, 1993.

88. Sharma P, McDonald GB, Banaji M: The risk of bleeding after percutaneous liver biopsy: Relation to platelet count. *J Clin Gastroenterol* 4(5):451–453, 1982.

89. Lisman T, Caldwell SH, Burroughs AK, et al: Hemostasis and thrombosis in patients with liver disease: The ups and downs. *J Hepatol* 53(2):362–371, 2010.

90. Violi F, Basili S, Raparelli V, et al: Patients with liver cirrhosis suffer from primary haemostatic defects? Fact or fiction? *J Hepatol* 55(6):1415–1427, 2011.

91. Slichter SJ: Evidence-based platelet transfusion guidelines. *Hematology Am Soc Hematol Educ Program* 2007:172–178.

92. Afdhal NH, Giannini EG, Tayyab G, et al: Eltrombopag before procedures in patients with cirrhosis and thrombocytopenia. *N Engl J Med* 367(8):716–724, 2012.

93. Lisman T, Porte RJ: Eltrombopag before procedures in patients with cirrhosis and thrombocytopenia. *N Engl J Med* 367(21):2055–2056, 2012.

94. de Boer MT, Boonstra EA, Lisman T, Porte RJ: Role of fibrin sealants in liver surgery. *Dig Surg* 29(1):54–61, 2012.

94a. Bakker CM, Blankensteijn JD, Schlejen P, et al: The effects of long-term graft preservation on intraoperative hemostatic changes in liver transplantation. A comparison between orthotopic and heterotopic transplantation in the pig. *HPB Surg* 7(4):265–80, 1994.

94b. de Boer MT, Westerkamp A, van den Berg AP, et al: Impact of extended criteria donor grafts on post-reperfusion transfusion requirements in liver transplantation; abstract *Liver Transpl* 15(7):S128–S129, 2009.

95. Wang SC, Shieh JF, Chang KY, et al: Thromboelastography-guided transfusion decreases intraoperative blood transfusion during orthotopic liver transplantation: Randomized clinical trial. *Transplant Proc* 42(7):2590–2593, 2010.

96. Porte RJ, Molenaar IQ, Begliomini B, et al: Aprotinin and transfusion requirements in orthotopic liver transplantation: A multicentre randomised double-blind study. EMSALT Study Group. *Lancet* 355(9212):1303–1309, 2000.

97. Boylan JF, Klinck JR, Sandler AN, et al: Tranexamic acid reduces blood loss, transfusion requirements, and coagulation factor use in primary orthotopic liver transplantation. *Anesthesiology* 85(5):1043–1048; discussion 30A–31A, 1996.

98. Fergusson DA, Hebert PC, Mazer CD, et al: A comparison of aprotinin and lysine analogues in high-risk cardiac surgery. *N Engl J Med* 358(22):2319–2331, 1996.

99. Tripodi A, Anstee QM, Sogaard KK, et al: Hypercoagulability in cirrhosis: Causes and consequences. *J Thromb Haemost* 9(9):1713–1723, 2011.

100. Northup PG, Sundaram V, Fallon MB, et al: Hypercoagulation and thrombophilia in liver disease. *J Thromb Haemost* 6(1):2–9, 2008.

101. Villa E, Camma C, Marietta M, et al: Enoxaparin prevents portal vein thrombosis and liver decompensation in patients with advanced cirrhosis. *Gastroenterology* 143(5):1253–1260, 2012.

102. Bechmann LP, Sichau M, Wichert M, et al: Low-molecular-weight heparin in patients with advanced cirrhosis. *Liver Int* 31(1):75–82, 2011.

103. Cerini F, Garcia-Pagán JC: Thromboprophylaxis with heparin in hospitalized patients with cirrhosis: Friend or foe. *Liver Int* 34(7):971–973, 2014.

104. Intagliata NM, Henry ZH, Shah N, et al: Prophylactic anticoagulation for venous thromboembolism in hospitalized cirrhosis patients is not associated with high rates of gastrointestinal bleeding. *Liver Int* 34(1):26–32, 2014.

105. Potze W, Arshad F, Adelmeijer J, et al: Routine coagulation assays underestimate levels of antithrombin-dependent drugs but not of direct anticoagulant drugs in plasma from patients with cirrhosis. *Br J Haematol* 163(5):666–673, 2013.

105a. De Gottardi A, Trebicka J, Klinger C, et al. Antithrombotic treatment with direct-acting oral anticoagulants in patients with splanchnic vein thrombosis and cirrhosis. *Liver Int.* 37(5):694–699, 2017.

106. Amitrano L, Brancaccio V, Guardascione MA, et al: Inherited coagulation disorders in cirrhotic patients with portal vein thrombosis. *Hepatology* 31(2):345–348, 2000.

107. Zocco MA, Di Stasio E, De Cristofaro R, et al: Thrombotic risk factors in patients with liver cirrhosis: Correlation with MELD scoring system and portal vein thrombosis development. *J Hepatol* 51(4):682–689, 2009.

108. Okuda K, Ohnishi K, Kimura K, et al: Incidence of portal vein thrombosis in liver cirrhosis. An angiographic study in 708 patients. *Gastroenterology* 89(2):279–286, 1985.

109. Senzolo M, Sartori T, Rossetto V, et al: Prospective evaluation of anticoagulation and transjugular intrahepatic portosystemic shunt for the management of portal vein thrombosis in cirrhosis. *Liver Int* 32(6):919–927, 2012.

110. Plessier A, Darwish-Murad S, Hernandez-Guerra M, et al: Acute portal vein thrombosis unrelated to cirrhosis: A prospective multicenter follow-up study. *Hepatology* 51(1):210–218, 2010.

111. Confer BD, Hanouneh I, Gomes M, Alraies MC: Q: Is anticoagulation appropriate for all patients with portal vein thrombosis? *Cleve Clin J Med* 80(10):611–613, 2013.

112. Intagliata N, Maitland H, Northup P, Caldwell S: Treating thrombosis in cirrhosis patients with new oral agents: Ready or not? *Hepatology* 61(2):738–739, 2015.

113. Washington K: Update on post-liver transplantation infections, malignancies, and surgical complications. *Adv Anat Pathol* 12(4):221–226, 2005.

114. Silva MA, Jambulingam PS, Gunson BK, et al: Hepatic artery thrombosis following orthotopic liver transplantation: A 10-year experience from a single centre in the United Kingdom. *Liver Transpl* 12(1):146–151, 2006.

115. Bekker J, Ploem S, de Jong KP: Early hepatic artery thrombosis after liver transplantation: A systematic review of the incidence, outcome and risk factors. *Am J Transplant* 9(4):746–757, 2009.

116. Quiroga S, Sebastia MC, Margarit C, et al: Complications of orthotopic liver transplantation: Spectrum of findings with helical CT. *Radiographics* 21(5):1085–1102, 2001.

117. Hirshfield G, Collier JD, Brown K, et al: Donor factor V Leiden mutation and vascular thrombosis following liver transplantation. *Liver Transpl Surg* 4(1):58–61, 1998.

118. Vivarelli M, La Barba G, Cucchetti A, et al: Can antiplatelet prophylaxis reduce the incidence of hepatic artery thrombosis after liver transplantation? *Liver Transpl* 13(5):651–654, 2007.

119. Warnaar N, Molenaar IQ, Colquhoun SD, et al: Intraoperative pulmonary embolism and intracardiac thrombosis complicating liver transplantation: A systematic review. *J Thromb Haemost* 6(2):297–302, 2008.

120. Jairath V, Burroughs AK: Anticoagulation in patients with liver cirrhosis: Complication or therapeutic opportunity? *Gut* 62(4):479–482, 2013.

121. Wright M, Goldin R, Hellier S, et al: Factor V Leiden polymorphism and the rate of fibrosis development in chronic hepatitis C virus infection. *Gut* 52(8):1206–1210, 2003.

122. Papatheodoridis GV, Papakonstantinou E, Andrioti E, et al: Thrombotic risk factors and extent of liver fibrosis in chronic viral hepatitis. *Gut* 52(3):404–409, 2003.

# CHAPTER 19
# DISSEMINATED INTRAVASCULAR COAGULATION

Marcel Levi and Uri Seligsohn

## SUMMARY

When procoagulants are produced or introduced into the blood and overcome the anticoagulant mechanisms of coagulation, intravascular thrombin is generated systemically, which can lead to disseminated intravascular coagulation (DIC). The clinical manifestations of intravascular coagulation include (1) multiorgan dysfunction caused by microthrombi; (2) bleeding caused by consumption of platelets, fibrinogen, and other coagulation factors; and (3) secondary fibrinolysis. Exposure of blood to tissue factor is the most common trigger. This event can occur when mononuclear cells and endothelial cells are induced to generate and express tissue factor during the systemic inflammatory response syndrome (e.g., Gram-negative and Gram-positive infections, fungemia, burns, severe trauma), or when contact is established between blood and tissue factor constitutively present on membranes of cells foreign to blood (e.g., malignant, placental, brain, adventitial cells, or traumatized tissues). Laboratory features include thrombocytopenia, reduced levels of fibrinogen and other coagulation factors (leading to prolonged partial thromboplastin, prothrombin, and thrombin times), and elevated levels of D-dimer and fibrin(ogen) degradation products. Several underlying disorders affect these hemostatic parameters and can lead to a false-positive diagnosis of DIC (e.g., liver disease–related coagulation abnormalities and thrombocytopenia) or to a false-negative diagnosis (e.g., pregnancy-related high fibrinogen levels). Reexamining these variables every 6 to 8 hours may permit a specific diagnosis. Early detection, vigorous treatment of the underlying disorder, and support of vital functions are essential for survival of affected patients. Blood component therapy is effective in patients who bleed excessively, whereas heparin administration is indicated in a limited number of circumstances. Intravascular coagulation and the underlying disorders causing it contribute to a high rate of mortality. The severity of the organ dysfunction and extent of hemostatic failure, as well as increasing patient age, have been associated with a grave prognosis.

Acronyms and Abbreviations: APACHE, Acute Physiology and Chronic Health Evaluation; APC, activated protein C; APL, acute promyelocytic leukemia; aPTT, activated partial thromboplastin time; ARDS, acute respiratory distress syndrome; AT, antithrombin; DIC, disseminated intravascular coagulation; EPCR, endothelial protein C receptor; FDP, fibrinogen degradation product; HDL, high-density lipoprotein; HELLP, hemolysis, elevated liver enzymes, low platelet count; IL, interleukin; LCAD, long-chain acyl-coenzyme A dehydrogenase; LPS, lipopolysaccharide; NET, neutrophil extracellular trap; PAI, plasminogen-activator inhibitor; PAR, protease-activated receptor; rHDL, recombinant high-density lipoprotein; TAFI, thrombin-activatable fibrinolysis inhibitor; TAT, thrombin–antithrombin; TF, tissue factor; TFPI, tissue factor pathway inhibitor; TNF, tumor necrosis factor; t-PA, tissue-type plasminogen activator.

## DEFINITION AND HISTORY

Disseminated intravascular coagulation (DIC) is a clinicopathologic syndrome in which widespread intravascular coagulation occurs as a result of exposure or production of procoagulants insufficiently balanced by natural anticoagulant mechanisms and endogenous fibrinolysis. Perturbation of the endothelium in the microcirculation, along with stimulated inflammatory cells and release of inflammatory mediators, plays a key role in this mechanism. DIC may cause tissue ischemia from occlusive microthrombi, bleeding from the consumption of platelets and coagulation factors, and, in some cases, an excessive fibrinolytic response. DIC complicates a variety of disorders, and the complexity of its pathophysiology has made it the subject of a voluminous literature.[1-7]

In 1834, Dupuy reported that injection of brain material into animals caused widespread clots in blood vessels, thus providing the first description of DIC.[8] In 1865, Trousseau described the tendency to thrombosis, sometimes disseminated, in cachectic patients with malignancies.[9] In 1873, Naunyn showed that disseminated thrombosis could be evoked by intravenous injection of dissolved red cells, and Wooldridge demonstrated that the procoagulant involved was a substance contained in the stroma of the red cells.[10-12]

In 1955, Ratnoff and associates described the hemostatic abnormalities, which we would currently classify as DIC, that occur in women with fetal death or amniotic fluid embolism.[13] The mechanism by which DIC can lead to bleeding was clarified only in 1961, when Lasch and coworkers introduced the concept of consumption coagulopathy, and McKay established that DIC is a pathogenetic feature of a variety of diseases.[1,14] Sizable series of cases were first described in the late 1960s, following the introduction of defined laboratory criteria for DIC.[15] Yet despite the vast experience that has been accumulated, DIC still constitutes a major clinicopathologic and therapeutic challenge.

## PATHOLOGY

Diffuse multiorgan bleeding, hemorrhagic necrosis, microthrombi in small blood vessels, and thrombi in medium and large blood vessels are common findings at autopsy, although patients who had unequivocal clinical and laboratory signs of DIC may not have had confirming postmortem findings.[16,17] Conversely, some patients in whom clinical and laboratory signs were not consistent with DIC had typical autopsy findings.[18,19] This occasional lack of correlation among clinical, laboratory, and pathologic findings is partly a result of extensive postmortem changes in the blood, for example, excessive fibrinolysis, but remains unexplained in most instances.[17] Organs most frequently involved by diffuse microthrombi are the lungs and kidneys, followed by the brain, heart, liver, spleen, adrenal glands, pancreas, and gut. Specific immunohistologic techniques and ultrastructural analysis have revealed that most thrombi consist of fibrin monomers or polymers in combination with platelets. In addition, involvement of activated mononuclear cells and other signs of inflammatory activation are frequently present.[20] In cases of long-lasting DIC, organization and endothelialization of the microthrombi are often observed. Acute tubular necrosis is more frequent than renal cortical necrosis.[16]

A significant proportion of patients with chronic DIC have nonbacterial thrombotic endocarditis involving mainly the mitral and aortic valves.[19] Moreover, in a retrospective pathologic study, approximately 50 percent of patients with nonbacterial thrombotic endocarditis had DIC.[18] These heart lesions can be a source of arterial embolization, leading to infarction of the brain, kidneys, and myocardium.

# ●PATHOGENESIS

## INFLAMMATION AND ENDOTHELIUM IN DISSEMINATED INTRAVASCULAR COAGULATION

Various triggers cause a hemostatic imbalance that gives rise to a procoagulant state (Fig. 19–1). The most important mediators responsible for this imbalance are cytokines.[21] There is an extensive crosstalk between coagulation and inflammatory systems, whereby inflammation leads to activation of coagulation, and coagulation stimulates inflammatory activity.[22] These interactions are highlighted in sepsis-induced systemic activation of coagulation and inflammation that lead to specific organ dysfunctions.[23] The endothelium of the capillary bed is the most important interface in which the interaction between inflammation and coagulation takes place. Endothelial cells may be a source of tissue factor and can thereby be involved in the initiation of coagulation activation. All physiologic anticoagulant systems and various adhesion molecules that may modulate both inflammation and coagulation are connected to the endothelium. In sepsis, endothelial glycosaminoglycans present in the glycocalyx are downregulated by proinflammatory cytokines, thereby impairing the functions of antithrombin (AT), tissue factor pathway inhibitor (TFPI), leukocyte adhesion, and leukocyte transmigration. Because the glycocalyx also plays a role in other endothelial functions, including maintenance of the vascular barrier function, nitric oxide–mediated vasodilation, and antioxidant activity, all these processes can be impaired in DIC (see "Role of Oxidative Stress and Vasoactive Molecules" below).[24,25] Moreover, specific disruption of the glycocalyx results in thrombin generation and platelet adhesion within a few minutes.[26,27]

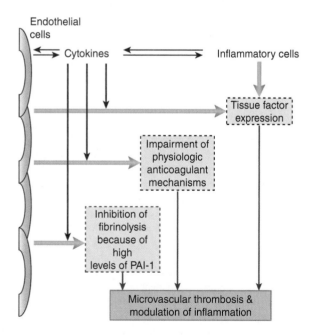

**Figure 19–1.** Schematic presentation of pathogenetic pathways involved in the activation of coagulation in disseminated intravascular coagulation (DIC). In DIC, both perturbed endothelial cells and activated mononuclear cells may produce proinflammatory cytokines that mediate coagulation activation. Activation of coagulation is initiated by tissue factor expression on activated mononuclear cells and endothelial cells. In addition, downregulation of physiologic anticoagulant mechanisms and inhibition of fibrinolysis by endothelial cells further promote intravascular fibrin deposition. PAI-1, plasminogen-activator inhibitor type 1.

Endothelial perturbation constitutes a *sine qua non* for most patients with DIC. Following injury or infection, the integrity of the endothelium is compromised, mononuclear cells are activated by cytokine and hormonal signals, additional cytokines and surface receptors are upregulated, procoagulant proteins and platelets are activated, the endothelium changes from an anticoagulant to procoagulant surface, and fibrinolysis is impeded. This sequence of events is typical for the *systemic inflammatory response syndrome* and can lead to microvascular thrombosis with ensuing multiorgan dysfunction and eventually to multiorgan failure.

## ROLE OF CYTOKINES AND TISSUE FACTOR

Tissue factor (TF) plays a central role in the initiation of inflammation-induced coagulation in DIC.[28] Blocking TF activity completely inhibits inflammation-induced thrombin generation in experimental models of endotoxemia or bacteremia.[29,30] Most cells constitutively expressing TF are found in tissues not in direct contact with blood, such as the adventitial layer of larger blood vessels. TF becomes exposed to blood upon disruption of the vascular integrity, or when cells present in the circulation, such as monocytes, are triggered to express TF. The *in vivo* expression of TF is dependent on interleukin (IL)-6 generation; inhibition of IL-6, unlike inhibition of other proinflammatory cytokines, completely abrogates TF-dependent thrombin generation in experimental endotoxemia.[21,31] In severe sepsis, monocytes, stimulated by proinflammatory cytokines, express TF, which leads to systemic activation of coagulation.[32] Even in experimental low-dose endotoxemia in healthy subjects, a 125-fold increase in TF mRNA levels in blood monocytes can be detected.[33] A potential alternative source of TF may be endothelial cells, polymorphonuclear cells, and other cell types. It is hypothesized that TF from these sources is shuttled between cells through microparticles derived from activated mononuclear cells.[34] However, it is unlikely that cells other than monocytes synthesize TF in substantial quantities.[32,35] Tumor necrosis factor (TNF)-$\alpha$ and IL-1, also generated during inflammation, impair the physiologic anticoagulant pathways.[31,36,37]

## AMPLIFYING ROLE OF THROMBIN AND PLATELETS

The TF–factor VIIa complex catalyzes the conversion of factor X to Xa, and factor Xa, in turn, forms the prothrombinase complex with factor Va, prothrombin (factor II), and calcium ions, thereby generating thrombin and converting fibrinogen into fibrin. The TF–factor VIIa complex can also activate factor IX, and factor IXa forms the tenase complex with activated factor VIII and calcium ions, generating additional factor Xa, thereby forming an essential amplification loop of thrombin generation. The assembly of the prothrombinase and tenase complexes are markedly facilitated if a suitable phospholipid surface is available, such as the membrane of activated platelets. In the setting of inflammation-induced activation of coagulation, platelets can be activated directly by endotoxin or by proinflammatory mediators, such as the membrane of platelet-activating factor. Thrombin itself is one of the strongest platelet activators (Chap. 5).

Activation of platelets may also accelerate fibrin formation by another mechanism. The expression of TF on monocytes is markedly stimulated by the presence of platelets and granulocytes in a P-selectin–dependent reaction.[38] This effect may be the result of nuclear factor kappa B (NF-$\kappa$B) activation induced by binding of activated platelets to neutrophils and mononuclear cells.[39] This cellular interaction also markedly enhances the production of IL-1$\beta$, IL-8, monocyte chemotactic protein (MCP)-1, and TNF-$\alpha$.[40]

Thrombin generated by the TF pathway amplifies both clotting and inflammation through the following activities: (1) it activates platelets, giving rise to platelet aggregation and augmenting platelet functions in coagulation; (2) it activates factors VIII, V, and XI, yielding further thrombin generation; (3) it activates proinflammatory factors via protease-activated receptors (PARs); (4) it activates factor XIII to factor XIIIa, which crosslinks fibrin clots; (5) it activates thrombin-activatable fibrinolysis inhibitor (TAFI), making clots resistant to fibrinolysis; and (6) it increases expression of adhesion molecules, such as L-selectin, thereby promoting the inflammatory effects of leukocytes.[41]

Paradoxically, at low concentrations, thrombin exhibits both anti-inflammatory and anticoagulant effects because it binds to thrombomodulin and activates protein C to the activated form, which, in turn, downregulates inflammation and serves as an "off switch" for further thrombin generation (Chap. 6).

## ROLE OF COAGULATION PROTEASES IN UPREGULATING INFLAMMATION

Coagulation proteases and protease inhibitors interact not only with coagulation proteins, but also with specific cell receptors to induce signaling pathways. In particular, protease interactions that affect inflammatory processes may be important in critically ill patients. Coagulation of whole blood *in vitro* results in a detectable expression of IL-1$\beta$ mRNA in blood cells,[42] and thrombin markedly enhances endotoxin-induced IL-1 activity in culture supernatants of guinea pig macrophages.[43] Similarly, clotted blood produces IL-8 *in vitro*.[44]

Factor Xa, thrombin, and fibrin can also activate endothelial cells, eliciting the synthesis of IL-6 and IL-8.[45,46] Coagulation proteases such as thrombin, factor Xa, and factor VIIa–TF complex induce inflammatory upregulation via leukocyte, endothelial cell, and platelet PAR-1, PAR-2, PAR-3, and PAR-4, which are located on leukocytes, endothelial cells, and platelets.[47] PARs have an extracellular domain, seven transmembrane domains, and an intracellular domain that is coupled to specific G-proteins that transmit signaling. PAR-1, PAR-3, and PAR-4 are activated by thrombin through cleavage of a specific aminoterminus bond, creating a tethered ligand that activates the receptor. PAR-2 can be cleaved by factor Xa–TF–factor VIIa complex and by other proteases.[48] Activated PARs then lead through mitogen-activated protein kinase and NF-$\kappa$B signaling pathways to cell motility, shape change, proliferation, endogenous secretagogue release, and apoptosis. The activated protein C (APC)–endothelial protein C receptor complex (see "Role of Natural Anticoagulant Pathways" below) appears to be the "off switch" for PAR activation by the proteases. These counterbalances determine the magnitude of coagulation and inflammatory upregulation by PARs. For example, factor VIIa–TF binding to PAR-2 in the lungs is proinflammatory and appears to play a role in acute respiratory distress syndrome (ARDS), raising the possibility that TFPI might be therapeutic in this circumstance.[49] This finding is consistent with data from animal studies demonstrating that TFPI can protect baboons from an LD100 of *Escherichia coli*, likely by impeding factor VIIa–TF activation of PAR-2 and thereby attenuating release of IL-6 and other proinflammatory agents.

Recent observations have pointed to an important role of extracellular DNA and DNA-binding proteins (such as histones and high mobility group box 1 protein [HMGB1]) in the pathogenesis of DIC. This cell-free DNA and DNA binding components are released from nucleosomes of degraded cells and may form a surface on which assembly of activated coagulation factor complexes may be greatly facilitated.[49a] In addition, histones activate platelets and thereby stimulate thrombin generation.[49b] Activation and binding of neutrophils by DNA components result in the formation of neutrophil extracellular traps (NETs), which have recently been identified as important contributors to vascular thrombosis and inflammation.[49c] NETs may provide the availability of inflammatory cells expressing TF.[49d] Activation of coagulation

is further enhanced by the proteolytic cleavage of physiologic anticoagulants by abundant neutrophilic elastase in NETs.[49d] NETs may also induce endothelial cell death, and detrimental inflammatory activity is an effect likely mediated by NET-associated proteases or cationic proteins, including histones.[49e,49f]

## ROLE OF FIBRINOGEN AND FIBRIN

Fibrinogen and fibrin directly influence the production of proinflammatory cytokines and chemokines (including TNF-$\alpha$, IL-1$\beta$, and MCP-1) by mononuclear cells and endothelial cells.[50] Fibrinogen-deficient mice display inhibition of macrophage adhesion and less thrombin-mediated cytokine production *in vivo*. The effects of fibrinogen on mononuclear cells seem to be mediated by toll-like receptor-4, which is also the receptor of endotoxin.

## ROLE OF NATURAL ANTICOAGULANT PATHWAYS

Procoagulant activity is regulated by three important anticoagulant pathways: AT, the protein C system, and TFPI. In DIC, the function of all three pathways can be impaired (Fig. 19–2).[51]

The serine protease inhibitor AT is the main inhibitor of thrombin and factor Xa. Without heparin, AT neutralizes coagulation enzymes in a slow, progressive manner.[52] Heparin induces conformational changes in AT that result in at least a 1000-fold enhancement of AT activity. Thus, the clinical efficacy of heparin is attributed to its interaction with AT. Endogenous glycosaminoglycans, such as heparan sulfate, also promote on the vessel wall AT-mediated inhibition of thrombin and other coagulation enzymes. During severe inflammatory responses, AT levels are markedly decreased because of impaired synthesis, degradation by elastase from activated neutrophils, and consumption as a consequence of ongoing thrombin generation.[53] Proinflammatory cytokines also cause reduced synthesis of glycosaminoglycans on the endothelial surface, thereby reducing AT function.[54]

APC appears to play a central role in the pathogenesis of sepsis and associated organ dysfunction.[55] There is ample evidence that decreased function of the protein C pathway contributes to the derangement of coagulation in sepsis.[49,56] The circulating zymogen protein C is activated by thrombin when it is bound to thrombomodulin at the endothelial cell surface.[57] APC acts with its cofactor protein S and degrades the essential cofactors Va and VIIIa, and hence, is an effective anticoagulant. The endothelial protein C receptor (EPCR) accelerates the activation of protein C several-fold, and also serves as a receptor for APC, thereby augmenting APC's anticoagulant and antiinflammatory activities.[58]

In patients with severe inflammation, the protein C pathway malfunctions at virtually all levels. Plasma levels of the zymogen protein C are decreased because of impaired synthesis, consumption, and degradation by proteolytic enzymes, such as neutrophil elastase.[59–61] Furthermore, a significant downregulation of thrombomodulin, caused by proinflammatory cytokines such as TNF-$\alpha$ and IL-1, results in diminished protein C activation.[62,63] Low levels of free protein S may further compromise the function of the protein C system. In plasma, 60 percent of protein S is complexed with a complement regulatory protein, C4b-binding protein (C4bBP), and exhibits no activity. The remaining protein S in plasma is free and functional. It was suggested that increased plasma levels of C4bBP caused by the acute-phase reaction in inflammatory diseases results in a relative protein S deficiency, which further contributes to a procoagulant state during sepsis. Indeed, infusion of C4bBP in combination with a sublethal dose of *E. coli* into baboons resulted in a lethal response with severe organ damage because of DIC.[64]

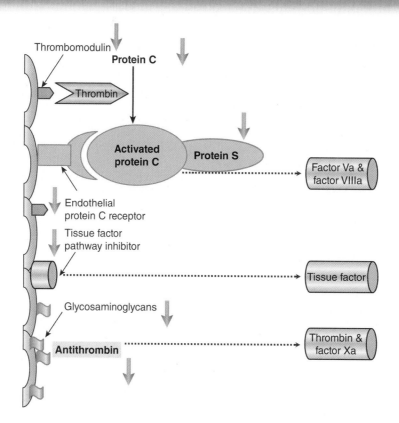

**Figure 19–2.** Schematic of the three important physiologic anticoagulant mechanisms and their point of impact in the coagulation system. In sepsis, these mechanisms are impaired by various mechanisms *(green arrows)*. The protein C system is dysfunctional as a result of low levels of zymogen protein C, downregulation of thrombomodulin and the endothelial protein C receptor, and low levels of free protein S because of acute phase–induced high levels of its binding protein (i.e., C4b-binding protein). There is a relative insufficiency of the endothelial cell–associated tissue factor pathway inhibitor. The antithrombin system is defective because of low levels of antithrombin and impaired glycosaminoglycan expression on perturbed endothelial cells.

In sepsis, the EPCR is downregulated, which further impairs the function of the protein C pathway.[65] Sepsis can also cause resistance toward APC because of a substantial increase in factor VIII levels.[66]

A third inhibitory mechanism of thrombin generation involves TFPI, the main inhibitor of the TF–factor VIIa complex and factor Xa. The role of TFPI in the regulation of inflammation-induced coagulation activation is not completely clear. Administration of recombinant TFPI blocks inflammation-induced thrombin generation in humans, and pharmacologic doses of TFPI prevent mortality during systemic infection and inflammation in experimental animals, suggesting that TFPI can modulate TF-mediated coagulation.[67,68]

## NATURAL ANTICOAGULANTS AND INFLAMMATION

AT possesses antiinflammatory properties, many of which are mediated by its actions in the coagulation cascade.[69] By inhibiting thrombin, AT blunts activation of many inflammatory mediators released by platelets and endothelial cells that recruit and activate leukocytes.[70] At high concentrations, AT also possesses potent antiinflammatory properties that are independent of its anticoagulant activity.[70] Another effect of AT is the induction of prostacyclin release from endothelial cells.[71–73] Prostacyclin inhibits platelet activation and aggregation, blocks neutrophil tethering to blood vessels, and decreases endothelial cell production of various cytokines and chemokines.[74]

AT also interacts directly with leukocytes and lymphocytes. It binds to receptors, such as syndecan-4, on the cell surfaces of neutrophils, monocytes, and lymphocytes, thereby blocking the adhesion of these cells to endothelial cells and their activation and migration. This effect, in turn, ameliorates the severity of capillary leakage and subsequent organ damage.

The protein C system also has an important function in modulating inflammation.[75,76] Blocking the protein C pathway in septic baboons exacerbates the inflammatory response, and in contrast, administration of APC ameliorates the inflammatory activation upon the intravenous infusion of *E. coli*.[77] Support for the notion that APC has antiinflammatory properties comes from *in vitro* observations demonstrating an APC binding site on monocytes that may mediate downstream inflammatory processes[78,79] and from experiments showing that APC can block NF-κB nuclear translocation, which is a prerequisite for increased proinflammatory cytokine levels and adhesion molecules.[80] These *in vitro* findings are supported by *in vivo* studies in mice with targeted disruption of the protein C gene. In these mice with genetic deficiencies of protein C, endotoxemia was associated with a more marked increase in proinflammatory cytokines and other inflammatory responses as compared with wild-type mice.[81,82]

It is likely that the antiinflammatory effects of APC are mediated by the EPCR.[75] Binding of APC to EPCR influences gene expression profiles of cells by inhibiting NF-κB nuclear translocation.[79,80] The EPCR-APC complex itself can translocate from the plasma membrane into the cell nucleus, which may be another mechanism of modulating gene expression, although the relative contribution of this nuclear translocation and cell surface signaling is uncertain.[56] Like APC, EPCR itself may have antiinflammatory properties. Blocking the EPCR with a specific monoclonal antibody aggravates both the coagulation and the inflammatory response to *E. coli* infusion.[65]

Apart from the effect on cytokine levels, APC causes diminished leukocyte chemotaxis and adhesion to the activated endothelium.[83–85] A localized antiinflammatory effect of APC has been demonstrated in the lung.[86] One mechanism for this effect may be inhibition of the expression of platelet-derived growth factor in the lung.[87] Also, APC protects against the disruption of endothelial cell barrier in sepsis.[88–90] APC also inhibits endothelial cell apoptosis by a mechanism that seems to be mediated by binding of APC to EPCR and requires PAR-1.[91,92] Signaling through this pathway can affect Bcl-2 homologue protein, which can inhibit apoptosis, and further suppresses p53, which is a proapoptotic transcription factor.[93,94]

## DYSREGULATION OF FIBRINOLYSIS

In experimental models of DIC, fibrinolysis is initially activated but subsequently inhibited, because of an increased release of plasminogen activator inhibitor-1 (PAI-1) by endothelial cells.[95] These effects are mediated by TNF-$\alpha$ and IL-1.[96,97] In a study of 69 DIC patients (31 with multiorgan failure), higher levels of tissue-type plasminogen activator (t-PA) antigen and PAI-1 with depressed levels of $\alpha_2$-antiplasmin were observed in patients with DIC and multiorgan failure compared to DIC patients without multiorgan failure.[98] This finding supports the conclusion that fibrinolysis is an important mechanism in preventing multiorgan failure.

Experiments in mice with targeted disruptions of genes encoding components of the plasminogen–plasmin system confirm that fibrinolysis plays a major role in inflammation. Mice with a deficiency of plasminogen activators have more extensive fibrin deposition in organs when challenged with endotoxin, whereas PAI-1 knockout mice, in contrast to wild-type controls, have no microvascular thrombosis upon endotoxin administration.[99]

TAFI, like PAI-1, may play a role in impeding fibrinolysis and in augmenting formation of microvascular thrombi. Studies in a DIC cohort demonstrated very low levels of TAFI proportionate to thrombin generation in such patients, particularly in those with infection-associated DIC.[100] Hence, TAFI may contribute (along with PAI-1) to microvascular thrombosis-induced ischemia in organs, resulting in multiorgan dysfunction.

## ROLE OF OXIDATIVE STRESS AND VASOACTIVE MOLECULES

Superoxides and hydroxyl radicals are generated during sepsis and other organ injury states that predispose to DIC. Each is a proinflammatory agent that may lead to recruitment of neutrophils, formation of chemotactic factors, lipid peroxidation, and stimulation of NF-$\kappa$B, which induces cytokine upregulation.[101] In addition, formation of peroxynitrite by these radicals exacerbates inflammation by (1) deactivating superoxide dismutase, which ordinarily would eliminate these superoxides and other radicals, and (2) exerting damaging effects on deoxyribonucleic acid, nicotinamide adenine dinucleotide, and ATP. For example, evidence indicates that the poor response to pressors in shock-like states associated with DIC may be directly related to their deactivation by superoxides.

Adding further insult, high levels of superoxide impair vascular response to nitrous oxide, thereby creating an imbalance in the signaling to vascular cells. Because of the strategic importance of an intact endothelium for attenuating any microangiopathic process, the most devastating effect of excessive generation of superoxides and associated free radicals may be their role in inducing endothelial apoptosis, which exacerbates capillary leak.[101]

Vasoactive substances play a critical role in the evolution of DIC. The vasodilatory agent nitric oxide (NO) and the vasoconstrictor endothelin have been measured in experimental rat models of DIC induced by both TF infusion and lipopolysaccharide (LPS) infusion.[102] LPS infusion increased both NO and endothelin remarkably, whereas TF infusion increased NO more than did LPS but did not stimulate endothelin significantly. The differential stimuli–response mechanisms may explain why LPS-induced DIC so prominently displays tissue infarction leading to multiorgan dysfunction (e.g., sepsis) compared to DIC that is predominantly induced by TF exposure (e.g., head trauma).

## METABOLIC MODULATION OF COAGULATION IN DISSEMINATED INTRAVASCULAR COAGULATION

Because there is a tight relationship between plasma lipoproteins and coagulation, it has been suggested that lipoprotein metabolism modulates coagulation in DIC.[103] *In vitro* experiments showed that plasma large very-low-density lipoprotein, small very-low-density lipoprotein, intermediate-density lipoprotein, and low-density lipoprotein stimulate activation of coagulation by supporting factor VII activation or by stimulating monocytes to express TF.[104] Lipid infusion potentiates in animals endotoxin-induced coagulation activation, as indicated by increased plasma levels of prothrombin fragments 1 and 2, thrombin–AT III complex, and PAI-1.[105] High-density lipoprotein (HDL) exerts opposite effects. Administration of recombinant HDL (rHDL) ameliorates the inflammatory response, inhibits coagulation, and augments fibrinolysis,[106] as reflected by reduced thrombin generation and increased levels of t-PA antigen following administration of endotoxin.

Endogenous lipid levels may have similar effects. Human subjects with low endogenous HDL-cholesterol plasma levels injected with small doses of endotoxin had a more pronounced increase in markers of coagulation activation in comparison with subjects with high endogenous HDL levels.[107] Also, patients heterozygous for familial hypercholesterolemia whose low-density lipoproteins level is increased were more prone to activation of coagulation upon an inflammatory stimulus.[108]

Hyperglycemia and hyperinsulinemia, as seen in type 2 diabetes mellitus and the associated metabolic syndrome, affect hemostasis.[109–111] In these circumstances, there is a marked decrease of endogenous fibrinolysis because of increased upregulation of plasma levels of PAI-1. Also, a modulatory effect of glucose/insulin on coagulation in an inflammatory setting has been described. Inflammation-induced TF gene expression was elevated in the brain, lung, kidney, heart, liver, and adipose tissues of diabetic mice compared with controls. Administration of insulin to lean mice induced enhanced inflammation-driven TF mRNA in the kidney, brain, lung, and adipose tissue.[112] In a hyperglycemic normoinsulinemic study in healthy subjects, there was an increased sensitivity toward endotoxin exhibited by upregulation of TF expression.[113] Strict glucose regulation in critically ill patients improves survival and reduces morbidity that is probably related to a better control of the derangement of coagulation and a faster resolution of coagulation abnormalities.[103]

## CONSUMPTION OF HEMOSTATIC FACTORS

The widespread generation of thrombin in DIC induces deposition of fibrin, which leads to the consumption of substantial amounts of platelets, fibrinogen, factors V and VIII, protein C, AT, and components of the fibrinolytic system. This situation results in massive depletion of these components that is further aggravated because of their decreased

**TABLE 19–1.** Clinical Conditions That May Be Complicated by Disseminated Intravascular Coagulation

Infectious diseases
    Purpura fulminans
Malignancy
    Solid tumors
    Leukemias
Trauma
    Brain injury
    Burns
Liver diseases
Heat stroke
Severe allergic/toxic reactions
    Snake bites
Vascular abnormalitles/hemanglomas
    Kasabach-Merritt syndrome
    Other vascular malformations
    Aortic aneurysms
Severe immunologic reactions (e.g., transfusion reaction)
Obstetrical conditions
    Abruptio placentae
    Amniotic fluid embolism
    Preeclampsia/eclampsia
    HELLP (hemolysis, elevated liver enzymes, and low platelet count) syndrome
    Sepsis during pregnancy
    Acute fatty liver

synthesis by the liver, which frequently is affected in DIC. Depending on the magnitude and nature of component depletion, bleeding, enhanced thrombosis, or both can result. Bleeding can be promoted by fibrinolysis-derived fibrin degradation products (FDPs) that exhibit anticoagulant and antiplatelet aggregation effects (see Fig. 19–1). Microangiopathic hemolytic anemia also occurs as a result of blood cells passing through vessels that are partially occluded by thrombi.

# CLINICAL FEATURES

Numerous disorders can provoke DIC, but only a few constitute major causes, as can be inferred from retrospective clinical studies (Table 19–1).[114] Infectious diseases and malignant disorders together account for approximately two-thirds of DIC cases in the major series (Table 19–2). Trauma was a major cause of DIC in some series, probably reflecting the specialized nature of the clinical practice in those centers.[115]

Clinical manifestations are attributable to DIC, the underlying disease, or both (Table 19–3). Bleeding manifestations were common in all series of DIC cases, but considerable variation existed in the relative frequency of shock and dysfunction of the liver, kidney, lungs, and central nervous system. These variations probably reflect the different nature of the underlying disorders in the respective series.

## BLEEDING

Acute DIC frequently is heralded by hemorrhage into the skin at multiple sites.[115] Petechiae, ecchymoses, and oozing from venipunctures, arterial lines, catheters, and injured tissues are common. Bleeding also may occur on mucosal surfaces. Hemorrhage may be life-threatening, with massive bleeding into the gastrointestinal tract, lungs, central nervous system, or orbit. Patients with chronic DIC usually exhibit only minor skin and mucosal bleeding.

## THROMBOSIS AND THROMBOEMBOLISM

Extensive organ dysfunction can result from microvascular thrombi or from venous and/or arterial thromboembolism (Table 19–4). For example, involvement of the skin can cause hemorrhagic bullae, acral necrosis, and gangrene. Thrombosis of major veins and arteries and pulmonary embolism occur but are rare. Cerebral embolism can complicate nonbacterial thrombotic endocarditis in patients with chronic DIC.

## SHOCK

Both the diseases underlying DIC and the DIC itself can cause shock. For example, septicemia and excessive blood loss because of trauma or obstetric complications by themselves can cause shock. Whatever the cause of shock, its advent in cases with DIC is a serious adverse event.

**TABLE 19–2.** Relative Frequency (%) of Major Underlying Diseases in Case Series of Patients with Disseminated Intravascular Coagulation

| Study | Number of Patients | Infectious Disease | Trauma and Major Surgery | Malignant Disease | Liver Disease | Obstetric Complications | Miscellaneous Diseases |
|---|---|---|---|---|---|---|---|
| Minna et al.[51] | 60 | 41 | 30 | 2 | 5 | 2 | 20 |
| Siegal et al.[115] | 118 | 40 | 24 | 7 | 4 | 4 | 21 |
| Spero et al.[122] | 346 | 26 | 19 | 24 | 8 | 0 | 23 |
| Matsuda et al.[52] | 503 | 15 | 2 | 61 | 6 | 4 | 12 |
| Kobayash et al.[139] | 345 | 16 | — | 55 | 4 | 5 | 20 |
| Larcan et al.[53] | 361 | 15 | 14 | 6 | 3 | 38 | 24 |

**TABLE 19–3.** Frequency (%) and Type of Organ Dysfunction or Other Clinical Manifestations in Case Series of Patients with Disseminated Intravascular Coagulation

| Study | Number of Patients | Bleeding | Thrombo-embolism | Renal Failure | Liver Failure | Respiratory Failure | CNS Manifestation | Shock | Acral Cyanosis* |
|---|---|---|---|---|---|---|---|---|---|
| Minna et al.[51] | 60 | 87 | 22 | 67 | NR | 78 | 65 | NR | 14 |
| Al-Mondhiry et al.[116] | 89 | 76 | 23 | 39 | NR | NR | 11 | NR | 0 |
| Siegal et al.[115] | 118 | 64 | 8 | 25 | 22 | 16 | 2 | 14 | 0 |
| Matsuda et al.[52] | 47 | 87 | 47 | 40 | NR | 38 | NR | NR | NR |
| Spero et al.[122] | 346 | 77 | NR | NR | NR | NR | NR | NR | NR |
| Larcan et al.[53] | 361 | 73 | 11 | 61 | 57 | 37 | 13 | 55 | 13 |

NR, not reported.

*Including necrotizing purpura and acral gangrene.

## RENAL DYSFUNCTION

Renal cortical ischemia induced by microthrombosis of afferent glomerular arterioles and acute tubular necrosis related to hypotension are the major causes of renal dysfunction in DIC. Oliguria, anuria, azotemia, and hematuria were observed in 25 to 67 percent of cases in all series (see Table 19–3).

## LIVER DYSFUNCTION

Hepatocellular dysfunction sufficient to cause jaundice has been reported in 20 to 50 percent of patients with DIC.[4,115] Infectious diseases and prolonged hypotension contribute to hepatic dysfunction.

**TABLE 19–4.** Organ Dysfunction Associated with Severe Disseminated Intravascular Coagulation

| Organ | Manifestation |
|---|---|
| Skin | Purpura, bleeding from injury sites, hemorrhagic bullae, focal necrosis, acral gangrene |
| Cardiovascular | Shock, acidosis, myocardial infarction, cerebrovascular events, thromboembolism in all types and caliber blood vessels |
| Renal | Acute renal insufficiency (acute tubular necrosis), oliguria, hematuria, renal cortical necrosis |
| Liver | Hepatic failure, jaundice |
| Lungs | Adult respiratory distress syndrome, hypoxemia, edema, hemorrhage |
| Gastrointestinal | Bleeding, mucosal necrosis and ulceration, intestinal ischemia |
| Central nervous system | Coma, convulsions, focal lesions, bleeding |
| Adrenals | Adrenal insufficiency (hemorrhagic necrosis) |

## CENTRAL NERVOUS SYSTEM DYSFUNCTION

Microthrombi, macrothrombi, emboli, and hemorrhage in the cerebral vasculature all have been held responsible for the nonspecific neurologic symptoms and signs displayed by patients with DIC.[116] These manifestations include coma, delirium, transient focal neurologic symptoms, and signs of meningeal irritation. Careful exclusion of causes other than DIC is essential.

## PULMONARY DYSFUNCTION

Symptoms and signs of respiratory dysfunction in DIC range from transient hypoxemia in mild cases to pulmonary hemorrhage and ARDS in severe cases.[117–119] Pulmonary hemorrhage is heralded by hemoptysis, dyspnea, and chest pain. Physical examination reveals rales, wheezing, and occasionally a pleural friction rub. Chest imaging shows diffuse infiltration resulting from excessive intraalveolar hemorrhage. ARDS is characterized by tachypnea, auscultatory silence, hypoxemia, low lung compliance, normal wedge pressure, and "white lungs" on chest images.[120] It stems from severe damage to the pulmonary vascular endothelium, which permits egress of blood components into the pulmonary interstitium and alveoli. This situation leads to intraalveolar hyaline membrane formation and severe respiratory insufficiency. ARDS can be caused by septic shock, severe trauma, fat embolism, amniotic fluid embolism, and heat stroke, all of which can also incite DIC. Yet only a fraction of patients with ARDS exhibit signs of DIC. When DIC and ARDS are simultaneously triggered, each aggravates the other. Regardless of the mechanism, ARDS is a serious complication in patients with DIC.

## MORTALITY

Both DIC and its underlying disorders contribute to the high mortality rate. Mortality correlates independently with the extent of organ dysfunction,[115] the degree of hemostatic failure,[121] and increasing age.[122] Mortality rates in major series of patients with DIC ranged from 31 to 86 percent,[121–124] whether or not heparin was administered. Of note, there is a clear correlation between the severity of DIC and the mortality rate.[121,123,124] In patients with sepsis, the presence of DIC is one of the strongest predictors of 28-day mortality.[124]

# LABORATORY FEATURES AND DIAGNOSIS

No single laboratory test is sensitive or specific enough to allow a definite diagnosis of DIC (Table 19–5). However, some sophisticated laboratory tests, for example, thrombin–AT complex and prothrombin fragment 1.2, are sensitive to ongoing activation of coagulation pathways. Determination of soluble fibrin in plasma is one of the best parameters for detection of ongoing DIC[125-128]; when the concentration is above a defined threshold, a diagnosis of DIC is likely.[129,130] Most of the other parameters show a sensitivity of 90 to 100 percent for the diagnosis of DIC but have a rather low specificity[131] and a wide discordance among various assays.[132] FDPs may be detected by specific enzyme-linked immunosorbent assays or by latex agglutination assays, allowing rapid and bedside determination.[133] None of the available assays discriminates between degradation products of crosslinked fibrin and fibrinogen, a situation that may cause spuriously high results.[134,135] The specificity of high levels of FDPs is therefore limited, and many other conditions, such as trauma, recent surgery, inflammation, or venous thromboembolism, are associated with elevated FDPs.

Newly developed tests are aimed at the detection of neoantigens on degraded crosslinked fibrin, one of which detects an epitope related to plasmin-degraded crosslinked γ-chain, associated with D-dimer formation. These tests better differentiate degradation of crosslinked fibrin from fibrinogen or FDPs.[136] D-dimer level is substantially elevated in patients with DIC, but this poorly distinguishes patients with DIC from patients with venous thromboembolism, recent surgery, or inflammatory conditions.[133,137]

In routine practice, simple laboratory tests in conjunction with clinical considerations are used for establishing the diagnosis of DIC. The simple tests include platelet count, prothrombin time, fibrinogen level, and fibrin-related markers, such as FDP or D-dimer. Caution should be exercised when using these laboratory parameters in the algorithms described below, because an underlying disease by itself can cause an abnormality. For example, impairment of hemostasis and/or

**TABLE 19–5.** Routine Laboratory Value Abnormalities in Disseminated Intravascular Coagulation

| Test | Abnormality | Causes Other Than DIC Contributing to Test Result |
|---|---|---|
| Platelet count | Decreased | Sepsis, impaired production, major blood loss, hypersplenism |
| Prothrombin time | Prolonged | Vitamin K deficiency, liver failure, major blood loss |
| aPTT | Prolonged | Liver failure, heparin treatment, major blood loss |
| Fibrin degradation products | Elevated | Surgery, trauma, infection, hematoma |
| Protease inhibitors (e.g., protein C, AT, protein S) | Decreased | Liver failure, capillary leakage |

aPTT, activated partial thromboplastin time, AT, antithrombin; DIC, disseminated intravascular coagulation.

**TABLE 19–6.** Diagnostic Algorithm for the Diagnosis of Overt Disseminated Intravascular Coagulation*

1. Presence of an underlying disorder known to be associated with DIC (see Table 19–2) ☐

   (no = 0, yes = 2)

2. Score global coagulation test results ☐

   Platelet count (>100 = 0; <100 = 1; <50 = 2)

   Level of fibrin markers (soluble fibrin monomers/fibrin degradation products) ☐

   (no increase: 0; moderate increase: 2; strong increase: 3)

   Prolonged prothrombin time ☐

   (<3 s = 0; >3 s but <6 s = 1; >6 s = 2)

   Fibrinogen level ☐

   (>1.0 g/L = 0; <1.0 g/L = 1)

3. Calculate score ☐

4. If ≥5: compatible with overt DIC; repeat scoring daily

   If <5: suggestive (not affirmative) for nonovert DIC; repeat next 1–2 days

DIC, disseminated intravascular coagulation.

*According to the Scientific Standardization Committee of the International Society of Thrombosis and Haemostasis.[138]

Data from Taylor FBJ, Toh CH, Hoots WK, et al: Towards definition, clinical and laboratory criteria, and a scoring system for disseminated intravascular coagulation, *Thromb Haemost.* 2001 Nov;86(5):1327–1330.

thrombocytopenia unrelated to DIC can arise from hepatic disease and from marrow involvement by leukemia. Impaired hemostasis also may occur normally in the neonatal period. Conversely, the elevated levels of some hemostatic components that are normally observed during pregnancy may obscure the presence of DIC. These limitations in laboratory diagnosis of DIC can be overcome by repeated testing, thereby following the dynamics of the process.

A scoring system utilizing the simple laboratory tests has been developed by the subcommittee on DIC of the International Society on Thrombosis and Haemostasis,[138] and Table 19–6 summarizes a five-step diagnostic algorithm to calculate a DIC score. Tentatively, a score of 5 or more is compatible with DIC, whereas a score of less than 5 may be indicative but is *not* affirmative for nonovert DIC. By using receiver-operating characteristics curves, an optimal cutoff for a quantitative D-dimer assay was determined, thereby optimizing sensitivity and the negative predictive value of the system.[131] Prospective studies show that the sensitivity of the DIC score is 93 percent, and the specificity is 98 percent.[123] The severity of DIC according to this scoring system is related to the mortality in patients with sepsis (Fig. 19–3).[124] Linking prognostic determinants from critical care measurement scores such as Acute Physiology and Chronic Health Evaluation (APACHE-II) scores to DIC scores is an important means to assess prognosis in critically ill patients. In addition, certain biochemical indicators of organ dysfunction may imply a DIC risk. For example, serial assessment of arterial lactate has proved to be a reliable prognostic indicator of DIC development among patients with the systemic inflammatory response syndrome.[139]

Criteria for less overt DIC have been more difficult to establish.[138,140] In the algorithm for nonovert DIC, the global coagulation tests are scored as with the overt DIC algorithm; however, when scoring by the algorithm

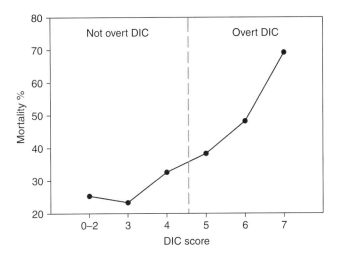

**Figure 19–3.** Number of points on the International Society of Thrombosis and Haemostasis disseminated intravascular coagulation (DIC) score and 28-day mortality in patients with severe sepsis. Data were derived from the placebo group (n = 840) in the Prowess trial on the efficacy of activated protein C in sepsis.

is being serially repeated, improvement in any laboratory test confers a negative score (rather than a zero or neutral score). This "trend" scoring allows longitudinal assessment of the patient's microangiopathy and, when therapy has been instituted, inference on whether the therapy has improved the course of the disease.[121,141] Measurements of several markers for assessing the risk of progression from nonovert to overt DIC and prediction of multiorgan dysfunction are potentially valuable and in the future can be accommodated in the nonovert DIC score. For example, impaired fibrinolysis may play a particularly important role in multiorgan dysfunction resulting from DIC of sepsis.[142] Therefore, assaying PAI-1, plasmin–antiplasmin complexes, or TAFI in septic patients may be important. Another highly sensitive early marker of impending DIC is a monoclonal antibody against APC that identifies a calcium ion–dependent epitope involved in factor Va inactivation.[143] Whether serial measurement of von Willebrand factor–cleaving protease also will identify individuals at risk early in their disease course or will help differentiate individuals with microangiopathy who are not prone to progress needs further data.[144,145]

Techniques such as rotational thrombelastography (ROTEM) enable bedside performance of this test and have again become popular in acute care settings.[146] The theoretical advantage of thrombelastography (TEG) over conventional coagulation assays is that is provides an idea of platelet function as well as fibrinolytic activity. Hyper- and hypocoagulability as demonstrated with TEG was shown to correlate with clinically relevant morbidity and mortality in several studies, although its superiority over conventional tests has not unequivocally been established.[147] Even though there are no systematic studies on the diagnostic accuracy of TEG for the diagnosis of DIC, the test may be useful for assessing the global status of the coagulation system in critically ill patients.[148]

# ● SPECIFIC UNDERLYING DISORDERS

## INFECTIOUS DISEASES

Bacterial infections are among the most common causes of DIC.[5,149] Certain patients are particularly vulnerable to infection-induced DIC,

such as immune-compromised hosts, asplenic patients whose ability to clear bacteria, particularly pneumococci and meningococci, is impaired, and newborns whose coagulation-inhibitory systems are immature. Infections are frequently superimposed on trauma and malignancies, which themselves are potential triggers of DIC. In addition, infections can aggravate bleeding and thrombosis by directly inducing thrombocytopenia, hepatic dysfunction, and shock associated with diminished blood flow in the microcirculation.[150] Clinically overt DIC may occur in 30 to 50 percent of patients with gram-negative sepsis.[151,152] DIC is similarly common in patients with gram-positive sepsis.[153,154] Extreme examples of sepsis-related DIC are as follows: (1) group A Streptococcus toxic shock syndrome, characterized by deep tissue infection, vascular collapse, vascular leakage, and multiorgan dysfunction; a streptococcal M protein forms complexes with fibrinogen, and these complexes bind to $\beta_2$ integrins of neutrophils leading to their activation[155]; and (2) meningococcemia, a fulminant gram-negative infection characterized by extensive hemorrhagic necrosis, DIC, and shock. The extent of hemostatic derangement in patients with meningococcemia correlates with prognosis.[156,157] More frequent gram-negative infections associated with DIC are caused by *Pseudomonas aeruginosa*, *E. coli*, and *Proteus vulgaris*. Patients affected by such bacteremias may have only laboratory signs of activated coagulation or may present with severe DIC, especially when shock develops.[158,159]

Severe secondary deficiency of a disintegrin-like metalloprotease with thrombospondin type 1 repeats (ADAMTS13), the von Willebrand–cleaving protease, occurs in patients with sepsis-induced DIC and is associated with a high incidence of acute renal failure.[160]

Among the gram-positive infections, *Staphylococcus aureus* bacteremia can cause DIC accompanied by renal cortical and dermal necrosis. The mechanism by which DIC is elicited may be related to an α-toxin that activates platelets and induces IL-1 secretion by macrophages.[161] *Streptococcus pneumoniae* infection is associated with the Waterhouse-Friderichsen syndrome,[162] particularly in asplenic patients. Initiation of DIC in these conditions is ascribed to the capsular antigen of the bacterium and to antigen–antibody complex formation.[163] Other gram-positive bacteria that can cause DIC are the anaerobic clostridia. Clostridial bacteremia is a highly lethal disease characterized by septic shock, DIC, renal failure, and hemolytic anemia.[164]

Activation of the coagulation system has also been documented for nonbacterial pathogens, that is, viruses (causing hemorrhagic fevers),[164,165] protozoa (malaria),[166,167] and fungi.[168] Common viral infections, such as influenza, varicella, rubella, and rubeola, rarely are associated with DIC.[169] However, purpura fulminans associated with DIC has been reported in patients with infections and either hereditary thrombophilias[170,171] or acquired antibodies to protein S.[172] Other viral infections can cause "hemorrhagic fevers" characterized by fever, hypotension, bleeding, and renal failure. Laboratory evidence of DIC can accompany Korean, Rift Valley, and dengue-related hemorrhagic fevers.[173–175] Release of TF from cells in which viruses replicate[28] and increased levels of proinflammatory cytokines have been suggested as mechanisms for initiation of the TF pathway in these conditions.[163]

## PURPURA FULMINANS

Purpura fulminans is a severe, often lethal form of DIC in which extensive areas of the skin over the extremities and buttocks undergo hemorrhagic necrosis.[176] The disease affects infants and children predominantly and occasionally adults.[177,178] Diffuse microthrombi in small blood vessels, necrosis, and occasionally vasculitis are present in biopsies of skin lesions. Onset can be within 2 to 4 weeks of a mild infection such as scarlet fever, varicella, or rubella, or can occur during an acute viral or bacterial infection in patients with acquired or hereditary thrombophilias affecting the protein C inhibitory pathway.[156,177] Homozygous protein C deficiency presents in neonates soon after birth as purpura fulminans, with or without extensive thrombosis.[179,180] Patients affected by purpura fulminans are acutely ill with fever, hypotension, and hemorrhage from multiple sites; they frequently have typical laboratory signs of DIC.[177] Excision of necrotic skin areas and grafting are indispensable at a later stage.

## SOLID TUMORS

Trousseau was the first to describe the propensity to thrombosis of patients with cancer and cachexia, and evidence for malignancy-related primary fibrinolysis and/or DIC was provided 75 years ago.[9,181,182]

In 182 patients with malignant disorders, excessive bleeding was recorded in 75 cases, venous thrombosis in 123, migratory thrombophlebitis in 96, arterial thrombosis in 45, and arterial embolism resulting from nonbacterial thrombotic endocarditis in 31.[183] Multifocal hemorrhagic infarctions of the brain, caused by fibrin microemboli and manifested as disorders of consciousness, have been described. Patients with solid tumors and DIC are more prone to thrombosis than to bleeding, whereas patients with leukemia and DIC are more prone to hemorrhage. The incidence of DIC in consecutive patients with solid tumors was 7 percent.[184]

Solid-tumor cells can express different procoagulant molecules including TF, which forms a complex with factor VII(a) to activate factors IX and X, and a cancer procoagulant, a cysteine protease with factor X–activating properties.[185,186] In breast cancer, TF is expressed by vascular endothelial cells as well as the tumor cells.[187,188] TF also appears to be involved in tumor metastasis and angiogenesis.[189–191] Cancer procoagulant is an endopeptidase that can be found in extracts of neoplastic cells but also in the plasma of patients with solid tumors.[192,193] The exact role of cancer procoagulant in the pathogenesis of cancer-related DIC is unclear.

Interactions of P- and L-selectins with mucin from mucinous adenocarcinoma can induce formation of platelet microthrombi and probably constitute a third mechanism of cancer-related thrombosis.[194] Depending on the rate and quantity of exposure or influx of shed vesicles from tumors containing TF, a nonovert or overt DIC develops.[39,195,196] For instance, a patient may be asymptomatic or present with venous thromboembolism if the tumor cells expose or release TF slowly or intermittently and the ensuing utilization of fibrinogen and platelets is compensated by increased production of these components. Conversely, massive thrombosis or severe bleeding may supervene in a patient whose circulation is deluged by TF.[184,186]

Another mechanism by which tumor cells may contribute to the pathogenesis of DIC is by expressing fibrinolytic proteins.[197,198] Despite the ability of many malignant cells to express urokinase-type plasminogen activator and t-PA, most tumors induce a hypofibrinolytic state. Because DIC is commonly characterized by a shutdown of the fibrinolytic system, mostly because of high levels of PAI-1, this may represent an alternative mechanism for the development of DIC in cancer.

Virtually all pathways that contribute to the occurrence of DIC are driven by cytokines. IL-6 has been identified as one of the most important proinflammatory cytokines that is able to induce TF expression on cells.[21,199] Indeed, inhibition of IL-6 results in an inhibition of endotoxin-stimulated activation of coagulation. In contrast, changes in fibrinolysis and microvascular physiologic anticoagulant pathways are mostly dependent on TNF-α.[200–202] Other cytokines that participate in the systemic activation of coagulation are IL-1β and IL-8, whereas antiinflammatory cytokines, such as IL-10, are able to inhibit DIC.[203–205] Because many types of tumors have the ability to synthesize and release cytokines or to stimulate other cells to activate the cytokine network,

it is likely that cytokine-dependent modulation of coagulation and fibrinolysis plays a role in cancer-related DIC.

Patients with solid tumors are vulnerable to risk factors and additional triggers of DIC that can aggravate thromboembolism and bleeding.[182] Risk factors include advanced age, stage of the disease, and use of chemotherapy or antiestrogen therapy.[197] Triggers include septicemia, immobilization, and involvement of the liver by metastases that impede the function of the liver in controlling DIC. Microangiopathic hemolytic anemia frequently is induced by DIC in patients with malignancies and is particularly severe in patients with widespread intravascular metastases of mucin-secreting adenocarcinomas.[206]

## LEUKEMIAS

Numerous reports on DIC and fibrinolysis complicating the course of acute leukemias have been published. In 161 consecutive patients who presented with acute myeloid leukemia, DIC was diagnosed in 52 (32 percent).[207] In acute lymphoblastic leukemia, DIC was diagnosed in 15 to 20 percent.[208] Some reports indicate that the incidence of DIC in acute leukemia patients might further increase during remission induction with chemotherapy.[209] In patients with acute promyelocytic leukemia (APL), DIC is present in more than 90 percent of patients at the time of diagnosis or after initiation of remission induction.[210,211]

The pathogenesis of hemostatic disturbance in APL is related to properties of the malignant cells and their interaction with the host's endothelial cells.[192,208] APL cells express TF and the cancer procoagulant that can initiate coagulation, and they release IL-1β and TNF-α, which downregulate endothelial thrombomodulin, thereby compromising the protein C anticoagulant pathway. APL cells also express increased amounts of annexin II, which mediates augmented conversion of plasminogen to plasmin (Chap. 25). The overall results of these processes are DIC and hyperfibrinolysis, followed by major bleeding that can lead to death.[212] All-trans-retinoic acid, used for induction and maintenance therapy of APL, inhibits in vitro and in vivo the deleterious effect of APL cells and has led to a reduced frequency of early hemorrhagic death; however, all-trans-retinoic acid may induce thrombotic complications.[192,213]

## TRAUMA

When DIC complicates trauma, it usually occurs in severely injured patients. Extensive exposure of TF to the blood circulation and hemorrhagic shock probably are the most immediate triggers of DIC in such instances, although direct proof of this mechanism is lacking. An alternative hypothesis is that cytokines play a pivotal role in the occurrence of DIC in trauma patients. In fact, the changes in cytokine levels are virtually identical in trauma patients and septic patients.[214] The levels of TNF-α, IL-1β, PAI-1, circulating TF, plasma elastase derived from neutrophils, and soluble thrombomodulin all can be elevated in patients with signs of DIC, predicting multiorgan dysfunction (ARDS included) and death.[215,216] Careful monitoring of laboratory signs of DIC, reduced fibrinolytic activity, and perhaps low AT levels also are useful for predicting the outcome of such patients.[217]

DIC can be aggravated in patients with severe trauma who require massive blood replacement because stored blood components are diluted and do not contain sufficient amounts of viable platelets and factors V and VIII. Moreover, in such patients, there is an activation of fibrinolysis that further aggravate bleeding in combination with acidosis and hypotension.[218–221] Infection commonly occurs in such patients and may contribute to the DIC.

The time interval between trauma and medical intervention correlates with the development and magnitude of DIC. Experience during wars proved that fast evacuation and prompt medical care reduce the risk of DIC.[222–224]

## BRAIN INJURY

Brain injury can be associated with DIC, most likely because the injury exposes the abundant TF of brain to blood. Specimens of contused brain, obtained during surgery in patients with head injury, and of liver, lungs, kidneys, and pancreas, obtained during autopsy, revealed microthrombi in arterioles and venules.[225,226] In adults and children with head injuries, a high rate of mortality occurred when DIC was present.[227] A laboratory DIC score has predictive value for prognosis in patients with head injuries, thereby supplementing the Glasgow coma score.[228] Bleeding in patients with DIC that is related to brain injury can be managed by replacement therapy.

## BURNS

TF exposed to blood at sites of burned tissue, the systemic inflammatory response syndrome induced by the burn, and the common presence of superimposed infections all can trigger DIC.[229] Bleeding, laboratory tests indicative of DIC, and vascular microthrombi in biopsies of undamaged skin have been described in patients with extensive burns.[230] Kinetic studies with labeled fibrinogen and labeled platelets disclosed that, in addition to systemic consumption of hemostatic factors, significant local consumption occurs in burned areas.[231] Laboratory signs of DIC are associated with organ failure; the extent of protein C and AT deficiencies correlates with a poor outcome.[230] A clinicopathologic study of 139 patients who died during treatment for a severe burn disclosed that 18 percent had cerebral infarctions caused by septic arterial occlusions or DIC and approximately 4 percent had intracranial hemorrhage.[232]

## LIVER DISEASES

Very complicated derangements of hemostasis occur in patients with severe liver disease and during liver transplantation (Chap. 18). Synthesis of most coagulation factors and natural anticoagulants (protein C, protein S, and AT) and of the main components of the fibrinolytic system (plasminogen, TAFI, and $\alpha_2$-antiplasmin) is reduced. The capacity of the liver to clear the circulation of activated factors IX, X, and XI, and of t-PA is decreased. Moreover, thrombocytopenia is common as a result of hypersplenism and decreased production of thrombopoietin by the liver. The similarities between the hemostatic defects observed in patients with liver disease and in patients with DIC are striking and have evoked an ongoing controversy as to whether or not DIC contributes to hemostatic derangements associated with liver disease.[233]

Several laboratory and clinical observations support the hypothesis that DIC accompanies hepatic disorders. They include a shortened half-life of radiolabeled fibrinogen and prolongation of fibrinogen half-life by administration of heparin[234,235]; failure of replacement therapy to significantly increase the levels of hemostatic factors (suggesting continuous consumption); and increased blood levels of D-dimer, thrombin–AT (TAT) complexes, and fibrinopeptide A, all consistent with ongoing thrombin generation.[236–238]

Other observations and considerations argue against the hypothesis that DIC accompanies liver diseases. They include (1) a very low incidence (2.2 percent) of microthrombosis in the tissues of patients who die of liver disease and (2) causes other than, or inconsistent with, DIC for the deranged findings in liver disease.[237] Examples of alternative explanations include the following: (1) a prolonged thrombin time may result from acquired dysfibrinogenemia[239]; (2) low levels of coagulation factors and inhibitors may result from reduced synthesis[240]; (3) increased

FDP levels may be a consequence of primary fibrinogenolysis induced by reduced synthesis of $\alpha_2$-antiplasmin and PAI-1 and by decreased clearance of t-PA; (4) factor VIII levels are commonly increased rather than decreased[241]; (5) the kinetic data show that the apparently excessive consumption of fibrinogen can be explained by loss of fibrinogen into extravascular spaces[242]; and (6) fibrinogen and plasminogen do not appear to be removed rapidly when labeled endogenously by $^{75}$Se-selenomethionine.[243]

A third hypothesis maintains that patients with liver disease usually do not present with DIC, but are extremely sensitive to the various triggers of DIC because of their impeded capacity to clear procoagulants and to synthesize essential components of the coagulation, inhibitory, and fibrinolytic systems. Patients with primary or metastatic liver disease who undergo a peritoneovenous shunt operation for severe ascites are more likely to develop DIC than are patients with ascites who undergo the same procedure because of other causes.[244]

What, then, should be the approach to patients with liver disease and bleeding without an apparent local cause? First, possible underlying causes of DIC should be considered and identified, and then a hemostatic profile should be examined at frequent intervals so as to detect any dynamic changes that may be helpful in recognizing DIC. The sensitive assays that reflect thrombin generation (TAT complex and prothrombin fragments 1.2) or concomitant thrombin and plasmin generation (D-dimer), as well as finding a normal or decreased level of factor VIII, may help establish the diagnosis of DIC in a patient with liver disease.[245]

## HEAT STROKE

In 1841, James Wellstead published his book *Travels to the City of the Caliphs* (currently known as Baghdad) and vividly described that on an extremely hot day in the Persian Gulf the decks of the ship *Liverpool* resembled a slaughterhouse, so numerous were the bleeding patients.[246] This is probably one of the first written reports on the occurrence of DIC in humans who suffer from heatstroke.[229] Heat stroke is a syndrome characterized by a rise in body temperature to higher than 42°C, which follows collapse of the thermoregulatory mechanism. The following predisposing factors have been identified: high environmental temperature, strenuous physical activity, infection, dehydration, and lack of acclimatization.[247,248] Extensive hemorrhage, unclottable blood, and venous engorgement were found as early as 1838 in postmortem examinations of patients who died of heat stroke.[246] Investigations confirm that a severe hemorrhagic diathesis and multiple organ failure often accompany heat stroke.[229,249–251] Diffuse fibrin deposition and hemorrhagic infarctions are found in fatal human cases. DIC associated with profound fibrin(ogen)olysis is evident in patients with heat stroke. The possible triggers of DIC in patients with heat stroke include endothelial cell damage and TF released from heat-damaged tissues.[249]

In a series of 18 critically ill patients from Paris with heat stroke during the 2003 heat wave in western Europe that caused numerous deaths in France alone,[251] patients had very high levels of IL-6 and IL-8. In addition, there was a striking activation of white blood cells, as demonstrated by $\beta_2$-integrin upregulation and increased production of reactive oxygen species. All patients also had evidence of a significant systemic activation of coagulation, and DIC was present in approximately 35 percent of patients. There was a marked correlation between the extent of inflammation and coagulation activation and the clinical severity of the heat stroke.

The severity of the syndrome and the stage of its development affect the type and magnitude of hemostatic alterations. Thus, in a study of 56 patients, three groups were discernible: nonbleeders, bleeders without DIC but with slight consumption of hemostatic factors, and bleeders with typical signs of DIC.[252] Prompt cooling and support of vital functions have substantially reduced the high mortality that was commonly observed in early studies.

## SNAKE BITES

Several species of snakes belonging to the Viperidae family produce venoms that have a wide range of activities affecting hemostasis. Prominent among these species are the *Vipera, Echis (E. carinatus* or *E. coloratus), Aspis, Crotalus, Bothrops,* and *Agkistrodon.* Venoms of these snakes contain enzymes or peptides that exert the following activities[253-255]: (1) thrombin-like activity, cleaving fibrinopeptide A from the Aα chain of fibrinogen *(Agkistrodon rhodostoma)*; (2) activation of prothrombin even in the absence of calcium ions *(E. carinatus)*; (3) activation of factors X and V (Russell viper venom); (4) fibrinogenolytic activity *(Agkistrodon acutus)*; (5) induction of thrombocytopenia by platelet aggregation; (6) inhibition of platelet aggregation by the low-molecular-weight arginine-glycine-aspartic acid–containing peptides from a variety of snake species; (7) activation of protein C; and (8) activities causing damage to endothelial cells, leading to bleeding, tissue ischemia, and edema. Interestingly, victims of snake bites rarely experience excessive bleeding or thromboembolism, despite the serious derangements in hemostatic tests and findings that are sometimes consistent with DIC.[256-258]

The major symptoms and signs related to envenomation are vomiting, diarrhea, apprehension, hypotension, local swelling, ischemia, and necrosis. Consequently, treatment for victims of snake bites consists of immediate immobilization, administration of antivenom and fluids, and other general measures to preserve vital functions. Local incisions, cooling, and application of tourniquet should be avoided.[253]

## HEMANGIOMAS

In 1940, Kasabach and Merritt described the association between giant hemangioma and a bleeding tendency occurring mainly in infants. The pathogenesis and management of this syndrome have been reviewed.[259] Studies using radiolabeled fibrinogen and platelets provided evidence that within the hemangioma, consumption of platelets and fibrinogen occurs because of localized intravascular clotting and excessive fibrinogenolysis.[260,261] Conceivably, concomitant local activation of the coagulation pathway and release of large amounts of t-PA by the abnormal endothelium lining the tumor vessels occur. Microangiopathic hemolytic anemia and laboratory signs of DIC and fibrinolysis have been demonstrated in patients with giant hemangiomas.[262] Accelerated growth of these hemangiomas in infants is associated with augmented consumption of hemostatic factors and can be effectively treated with glucocorticoids. Radiotherapy and interferon-α are also effective, but should only be used in life-threatening circumstances after failure of glucocorticoid therapy because of severe adverse events.[263] Spontaneous mild to moderate bleeding manifestations have been observed, but severe bleeding generally occurs only after surgery or trauma.

Extensive vascular malformation may persist and cause pain, probably resulting from thrombosis, and bleeding following trauma, which is related to the localized or generalized consumption of clotting factors and platelets and hyperfibrinolysis.[264] Graded permanent elastic compression, when possible, and low-molecular-weight heparin constitute the only effective treatment in such cases.

## AORTIC ANEURYSM

An association between aortic aneurysm and DIC is well documented.[265,266] In a series of patients with aortic aneurysm, 40 percent had elevated levels of FDPs, but only 4 percent had significant bleeding and laboratory evidence of DIC.[265] Several factors predispose patients with aortic aneurysms to the development of DIC: a large surface area, dissection, and expansion of the aneurysm.[267] Clinical and laboratory signs of DIC should be carefully sought in patients with an aortic aneurysm because bleeding may seriously complicate surgical repair of the aneurysm.[267,268] The initiation of localized and generalized intravascular coagulation can be ascribed to activation of the TF pathway by the abundant amounts of TF present in atherosclerotic plaques.[269] When patients present with significant bleeding or when surgery is planned, hemostatic defects should be sought and ongoing coagulation activation may be corrected by (low-molecular-weight) heparin.[270] Stent grafting, which is a common procedure for repair of aortic aneurysms, was complicated by DIC and death in two patients, of whom one had cirrhosis and the other underwent a lengthy procedure.[271] However, a study of 31 such patients failed to detect DIC following stent grafting of thoracic aneurysms.[272]

## TRANSFUSION REACTION

DIC accompanies incompatible blood transfusion, in which massive hemolysis is commonly associated with excessive bleeding with widespread thrombosis in fatal cases. The trigger of DIC in these cases cannot be simply ascribed to the release of red cell stroma, as patients with massive oxidative hemolysis because of glucose-6-phosphate dehydrogenase deficiency do not develop DIC.[273] Rather, extensive antigen–antibody reaction appears to cause DIC as a result of release of elastase and TNF-α from neutrophils, and activation of monocytes that release TNF-α express TF and complement, with assembly of the membrane attack complex inflicting damage to endothelial cells.[274,275]

## DISSEMINATED INTRAVASCULAR COAGULATION DURING PREGNANCY

Pregnancy predisposes patients to DIC for at least four reasons: (1) pregnancy itself produces a hypercoagulable state, manifested by evidence of low-grade thrombin generation, with elevated levels of fibrin monomer complexes and fibrinopeptide A; (2) during labor, leakage of TF from placental tissue into the maternal circulation causes a hypercoagulable state; (3) pregnancy is associated with reduced fibrinolytic activity because of increased plasma levels of PAI-1; and (4) pregnancy is associated with a decline in the plasma level of protein S. DIC may be difficult to diagnose during pregnancy because of the high initial levels of coagulation factors such as fibrinogen, factor VIII, and factor VII.[276,277] Progressive reductions in these factors, however, can confirm or exclude the diagnosis of DIC in suspected cases. Thrombocytopenia may be particularly helpful in determining whether DIC is present, provided other causes of thrombocytopenia are excluded.[278]

### Abruptio Placentae

The dramatic clinical presentation of abruptio placentae was first reported by DeLee in 1901,[279] but the immediate cause of sudden rupture of uterine spiral arteries and detachment of the placenta is still unknown. Placental abruption is a leading cause of perinatal death.[280] Older multiparous women or patients with one of the hypertensive disorders of pregnancy are thought to be at highest risk. The severe hemostatic failure accompanying abruptio placentae is the result of acute DIC emanating from the introduction of large amounts of TF into the blood circulation from the damaged placenta and uterus.[281] Amniotic fluid is able to activate coagulation *in vitro*, and the degree of placental separation correlates with the extent of DIC, suggesting that leakage of thromboplastin-like material from the placental system is responsible for the occurrence of DIC. Abruptio placentae occurs in 0.2 to 0.4 percent of pregnancies,[282] but only 10 percent of these cases are associated with DIC.[278] Different grades of severity are found among those who develop DIC, with only the more severe forms resulting in shock and fetal death. Rapid volume replenishment and evacuation of the uterus is the treatment of choice.[280] Transfusion of cryoprecipitate, fresh-frozen plasma, and platelets should be given when profuse bleeding occurs. However, in the absence of severe bleeding, administration of blood components may not be necessary because depleted coagulation factors increase rapidly following delivery. Heparin and antifibrinolytic agents are not indicated.

## Amniotic Fluid Embolism

This rare catastrophic disorder, described by Steiner and Lushbaugh in 1941, occurs only in one in 8000 to one in 80,000 deliveries.[283] A maternal mortality rate of 86 percent was reported in a 1979 review of 272 cases, but in a later population-based study, the maternal mortality (26.4 percent) was significantly lower.[284,285] Patients predisposed to amniotic fluid embolism are multiparous women whose pregnancies are postmature with large fetuses and women undergoing a tumultuous labor after pharmacologic or surgical induction. Apparently, amniotic fluid is introduced into the maternal circulation through tears in the chorioamniotic membranes, rupture of the uterus, and injury of uterine veins.[284] The trigger of DIC probably is TF present in amniotic fluid.[286,287] The mechanical obstruction of pulmonary blood vessels by fetal debris, meconium, and other particulate matter in the amniotic fluid enhances local fibrin–platelet thrombus formation and fibrinolysis. The extensive occlusion of the pulmonary arteries and an acute anaphylactoid response reminiscent of severe systemic inflammatory response syndrome provoke sudden dyspnea, cyanosis, acute cor pulmonale, left ventricular dysfunction, shock, and convulsions. These symptoms are followed within minutes to several hours by severe bleeding in 37 percent of patients.[284] Hemorrhage is particularly severe from the atonic uterus, puncture sites, gastrointestinal tract, and other organs. The best prospect for decreasing mortality lies in early termination of parturition in patients at high risk and prevention of hypertonic and tetanic uterine contractions during labor. When the syndrome is recognized, immediate termination of pregnancy under pulmonary and cardiovascular support is essential.

## Preeclampsia and Eclampsia

Thrombocytopenia described in early reports of eclampsia and widespread deposition of fibrin in blood vessels observed in fatal cases were interpreted as evidence of DIC triggered by placental TF exposure to the circulation.[1] A critical analysis of the literature concluded that the thrombocytopenia in these patients stems from endothelial injury rather than DIC.[288] However, other investigators provided evidence for significant DIC in preeclampsia and eclampsia.[289,290] Moreover, in a large series of patients, a good correlation was noted between the clinical severity and abnormalities in platelet counts and FDPs.[291] Also consistent with DIC were results of assays of sensitive parameters of thrombin generation and activation of fibrinolysis, such as TAT complexes, D-dimer, and fibrinopeptide B$\beta$1–42. Despite these observations, administration of heparin to patients with preeclampsia and eclampsia has not resulted in convincing benefits.[292]

## HELLP Syndrome

The syndrome of hemolysis (H), elevated liver enzymes (EL), low platelet count (LP), and severe epigastric pain is a complication of pregnancy-induced hypertension.[293] Seventy percent of cases occur during the third trimester of pregnancy and 30 percent occur during the postpartum period.[294] HELLP syndrome occurs more often in whites, multiparous women, and women older than 35 years.[292] Liver biopsy findings of fibrin deposition in hepatic blood vessels and laboratory

tests consistent with DIC in a significant proportion of patients imply that DIC plays a role in the pathogenesis of the syndrome.[294–296] Hepatic imaging in 33 patients revealed subcapsular hematomas in 13 and intra-parenchymal hemorrhage in six.[297] What actually triggers DIC in these cases is not known but has been related to endothelial dysfunction.[292] Multiple organ dysfunctions manifested by acute renal failure, ascites, pulmonary edema, and severe hemorrhage resulting from DIC may develop, leading to significant maternal and perinatal mortality rates. Management of patients with HELLP syndrome consists of supportive care, careful monitoring, and blood component replacement therapy. With few exceptions, immediate delivery, not necessarily by cesarean section, is indicated. HELLP syndrome tends to recur in subsequent gestations.[298]

## Sepsis During Pregnancy

Gram-negative bacteria, group A streptococci, and *Clostridium perfringens* are among the more common causes of sepsis during pregnancy. These infections are frequently associated with fulminant DIC. The pathogens gain entry into the circulation during abortion, via amnionitis that may follow invasive procedures or rupture of membranes, by endometritis developing during labor, and by way of the urinary tract. Approximately 40 percent of bacteremic patients experience shock, which is associated with significant mortality.[299] In addition, a high rate of bleeding and organ dysfunction affects the kidneys, lungs, and central nervous system.

Treatment of all cases of sepsis-related DIC should include antibiotics, support of vital functions, and surgical intervention to remove any local nidus of infection. Abortion or hysterectomy may be considered.

## Dead Fetus Syndrome

Several weeks after intrauterine fetal death, approximately one-third of patients may exhibit laboratory signs of DIC, occasionally accompanied by bleeding.[278,300] Apparently, TF from the retained dead fetus or placenta slowly enters the maternal circulation and initiates DIC, which sometimes is accompanied by significant fibrinolysis.[13] This complication currently is rarely observed because labor is induced promptly after the diagnosis of fetal death is made. However, if labor induction is unavoidably delayed, serial blood coagulation tests should be performed.

The entity of fetal death and DIC can occur following the demise of one of multiple gestations. If it occurs at term, therapy is started as discussed. If it occurs prior to fetal maturity, prolonged administration of heparin can be useful. Interestingly, when selective termination of the life of an anomalous fetus is performed in women with multiple pregnancies, hemostatic abnormalities develop in only approximately 3 percent of cases.[301]

## Acute Fatty Liver

Acute fatty liver of pregnancy is a rare disorder that occurs during the third trimester of pregnancy.[302] It can lead to hepatic failure, encephalopathy, and death of the mother and fetus.[303–306] In 15 to 20 percent of cases, acute fatty liver of pregnancy is associated with fetal homozygosity or compound heterozygosity for long-chain acyl-coenzyme A dehydrogenase (LCAD) deficiency.[307] Infants born with LCAD deficiency fail to thrive and are prone to liver failure and death. LCAD is one of four enzymes taking part in $\beta$-oxidation of fatty acids in mitochondria. When it is deficient, accumulation of medium- and long-chain fatty acid occurs. One predominant mutation (G1528C) accounts for 65 to 90 percent of cases with the deficiency. The precise mechanism by which LCAD deficiency in the fetus causes the severe liver disease in the heterozygous mother is unclear. The acute fatty liver disease of pregnancy is characterized by severe liver dysfunction, renal failure, hypertension, and signs of DIC.[304,308] The typical histologic feature is microvesicular fatty infiltration of the liver. Exceedingly low levels of AT and other laboratory signs of DIC were observed in a series of 28 patients, but no definite clinical benefit from AT concentrate infusion was achieved.[308] The primary therapy for these patients is early delivery and supportive care, which yield a maternal survival of 90 percent and perinatal survival of more than 85 percent.[304,309] Pancreatitis is a potentially lethal complication of acute fatty liver of pregnancy.[310]

## NEWBORNS

Newborns have a limited capacity to cope with triggers of DIC for several reasons: (1) their ability to clear soluble fibrin and activated factors is reduced; (2) their fibrinolytic potential is decreased because of a low plasminogen level; and (3) their capacity to synthesize coagulation factors and inhibitors is limited.[311,312] Criteria for diagnosis of DIC in newborns are different from those for diagnosis in adults.[313] Important to consider are the physiologic hemostatic findings common at this age, which include low levels of the vitamin K–dependent factors, reduced AT and protein C levels, and prolonged thrombin time. The laboratory evidence of DIC in the newborn is based on the progressive decline of hemostatic parameters, thrombocytopenia, and reduced levels of fibrinogen, factor V, and factor VIII.[311,314,315]

DIC occurs in sick neonates and particularly in those who are premature. More than one underlying cause usually can be identified in newborns with DIC. The most frequent underlying conditions are sepsis, hyaline membrane disease (respiratory distress syndrome), asphyxia, necrotizing enterocolitis, intravascular hemolysis, abruptio placentae, and eclampsia.[312,316]

Bleeding from multiple sites is the most common manifestation of DIC in newborns, with intracranial hemorrhage being the most life-threatening condition. No clinical manifestations of DIC are apparent in approximately 20 percent of neonates,[314] so a high index of suspicion in patients at risk is essential.

## ●THERAPY

Controlled studies of patients with DIC are difficult to perform in view of the variabilities in DIC triggers, clinical presentations, and grades of severity. Figure 19–4 shows general guidelines for management of patients with DIC, but decisions regarding treatment must be individualized after careful consideration of all clinically important aspects.

## TREATMENT OF UNDERLYING DISORDERS AND VITAL SUPPORT

The survival of patients with DIC depends on vigorous treatment of the underlying disorder to alleviate or remove the inciting injurious cause. For sepsis-induced DIC, treatment includes aggressive use of intravenous organism-directed antibiotics and source control (e.g., by surgery or drainage). Other examples of vigorous treatment of underlying conditions are cancer surgery or chemotherapy, uterus evacuation or even hysterectomy in patients with abruptio placentae, resection of aortic aneurysm, and debridement of crushed tissues.

Intensive support of vital functions is required. Volume replacement and correction of hypotension, acidosis, and oxygenation may improve blood flow and oxygen delivery to the microcirculation. Careful monitoring of pulmonary, cardiac, and renal function enables prompt institution of supportive measures, such as use of a respirator for respiratory support, inotropic and vasoactive drugs for improvement of organ perfusion, renal function, and maintenance of electrolyte balance.

## BLOOD COMPONENT THERAPY

Treatment of the underlying disease and vital support are necessary but usually insufficient to treat DIC or forestall progression of nonovert DIC to overt DIC. Additional supportive treatment directly aimed at the coagulation system may be required. These interventions include replacing the coagulation factors, natural anticoagulant, fibrinolytic proteins, and platelets that are actively consumed during DIC.[317]

Low levels of platelets and coagulation factors may increase the risk of bleeding. However, plasma or platelet substitution therapy should not be instituted on the basis of laboratory results alone; it is indicated only in patients with active bleeding and in those requiring an invasive procedure or who are at risk for bleeding complications.[318,319] The suggestion that administration of blood components might "add fuel to the fire" has never been proven in clinical or experimental studies. The presumed efficacy of treatment with plasma, fibrinogen concentrate, cryoprecipitate, or platelets is not based on randomized controlled trials but appears to be rational therapy in bleeding patients or in patients at risk of bleeding who have a significant depletion of these hemostatic factors.[319] One of the major challenges of infusion of fresh-frozen plasma in these dire circumstances is the propensity of the added volume, which is necessary to correct the coagulation defect, to exacerbate capillary leak. This situation can increase the risk of inducing or worsening pulmonary edema and, by extension, predispose to ARDS and induce ascites. Coagulation factor concentrates, such as prothrombin complex concentrate, may partially overcome this obstacle but do not contain essential factors, such as factor V. Moreover, caution is advocated with the use of prothrombin complex concentrates in DIC, as it may worsen the coagulopathy because of traces of activated factors that are present in these concentrates. Specific deficiencies of coagulation factors, such as fibrinogen, may be corrected by administration of purified coagulation factor concentrates.

Platelet transfusion is often required in patients with DIC to prevent bleeding into already ischemic or damaged organs (particularly the central nervous system). The threshold platelet count that should prompt transfusion is patient and disease specific. Cryoprecipitate can be used to rapidly raise the fibrinogen and factor VIII levels, particularly when bleeding is part of the DIC and fibrinogen level is less than 1 g/L. Cryoprecipitate has at least four to five times the mass of fibrinogen per milliliter of infusate compared to fresh-frozen plasma. Fresh-frozen plasma contains fibrinogen in sufficient amounts for treatment of patients with mild to moderate hypofibrinogemia.

Replacement therapy for thrombocytopenia should consist of 5 to 10 units of platelet concentrate or single-donor apheresis-derived platelets to raise the platelet count to 20 to $30 \times 10^9$/L and, in patients who need an invasive procedure, to $50 \times 10^9$/L.

## RESTORATION OF PHYSIOLOGIC ANTICOAGULANT PATHWAYS

Because the levels of the physiologic anticoagulants are reduced in patients with DIC, restoration of these inhibitors may be a rational approach.[49,320] Based on successful preclinical studies, the use of AT concentrates and heparin in patients with DIC has been examined mainly in randomized controlled trials that included patients with sepsis, septic shock, or both. All trials have shown some beneficial effect in terms of improvement of laboratory parameters, shortening of the duration of DIC, or even improvement in organ function.[6,321,322] In several small clinical trials, use of very high doses of AT concentrate showed a modest reduction in mortality, but without being statistically significant.[323-325] A large-scale, multicenter, randomized controlled trial also showed no significant reduction in mortality of

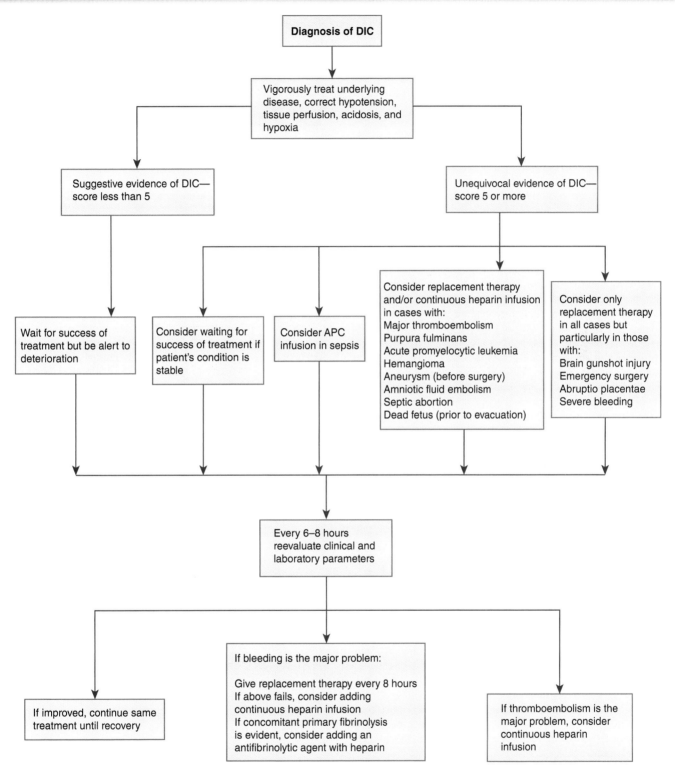

**Figure 19–4.** General guidelines for initial treatment and follow up of patients with disseminated intravascular coagulation (DIC). The success of management is related to taking rapid, vigorous measures against the underlying disease, support of vital functions, close clinical observation, thoughtful consideration in each individual patient, availability of 24-hour coagulation laboratory services, and an adequate supply of platelet concentrate, cryoprecipitate, fresh-frozen plasma, and packed red cells for replacement therapy. Heparin, when indicated, should be administered by continuous infusion. The basis and limitations of each of the outlined recommendations are detailed throughout the text. APC, activated protein C.

patients with sepsis.[326] Interestingly, *post hoc* subgroup analyses of the latter study indicated some benefit in patients who did not receive concomitant heparin, but this observation needs validation. Recent propensity-adjusted retrospective data from Japan demonstrated a significant benefit of AT-treated patients with severe infection and sepsis.[327,328] However, these observations still need prospective validation.

Adjunctive therapy with APC has also been widely studied. A phase III trial of APC concentrate in patients with sepsis was prematurely stopped because of efficacy in reducing mortality in these patients.[329] All-cause mortality at 28 days after inclusion was 24.7 percent in the APC group versus 30.8 percent in the control group (a 19.4 percent relative risk reduction). In addition, there was also an improvement of coagulation abnormalities and reduced organ failure in APC-treated patients. Of note, patients with the most severe coagulopathy benefited most from this treatment.[330] However, series of negative trials in specific populations of patients with severe sepsis led to scepticism regarding the use of APC in sepsis, and meta-analyses of published literature concluded that the basis for treatment with APC, even in patients with a high disease severity, was not very strong or even insufficient.[331] In addition, there was uncertainty regarding the bleeding risk of APC in patients with severe sepsis. The last large placebo-controlled trial in patients with severe sepsis and septic shock was prematurely stopped due to the lack of any significant benefit of APC.[332] Subsequently, the manufacturer of APC has decided to withdraw the product from the market, which has resulted in a revision of current guidelines for treatment of DIC.[333]

The most promising intervention at this moment is recombinant soluble thrombomodulin. Several preclinical studies in experimental sepsis models have shown that soluble thrombomodulin is capable of improving the derangement of coagulation and may restore organ dysfunction.[334] In phase I/II clinical studies, the pharmacokinetic profile of recombinant soluble thrombomodulin was determined.[335] In a subsequent phase III, randomized, double-blind clinical trial in patients with DIC, administration of the soluble thrombomodulin had a significantly better effect on bleeding manifestations and coagulation parameters than heparin, but the mortality rate at 28 days was similar in the two study groups.[336] When limiting these results to patients with severe infection and sepsis, DIC resolution rates were 67.5 percent in thrombomodulin-treated patients and 55.6 percent in the control group, and 28-day mortality rates were 21.4 and 31.6 percent, respectively. Subsequently, soluble thrombomodulin was evaluated in a phase II/III clinical study in 750 patients with sepsis and DIC.[337] Twenty-eight-day mortality was 17.8 percent in the thrombomodulin group and 21.6 percent in the placebo group. Markers of coagulation activation were lower in the thrombomodulin group than in the placebo group. There were no differences between groups in bleeding or thrombotic events. The promising results with recombinant soluble thrombomodulin are supported by retrospective data in large series of Japanese patients and are currently being evaluated in a large international multicenter trial.[338,339]

## HEPARIN ADMINISTRATION AND OTHER ANTICOAGULANTS

Although the question of heparin therapy in patients with DIC has been studied by several investigators, this therapy remains controversial. Experimental studies show that heparin can at least partly inhibit the activation of coagulation in DIC.[340,341] However, a beneficial effect of heparin on clinically important outcome events in patients with DIC has not been demonstrated in controlled clinical trials.[342] Also, the

safety of heparin treatment is debatable in DIC patients who are prone to bleeding. A large trial in patients with severe sepsis showed a slight, but nonsignificant benefit, of low-dose heparin on 28-day mortality in patients with severe sepsis.[343]

Notwithstanding these considerations, administration of heparin is beneficial in some categories of chronic DIC, such as metastatic carcinomas, purpura fulminans, and aortic aneurysm (prior to resection). Heparin also is indicated for treating thromboembolic complications in large vessels and before surgery in patients with chronic DIC (see Fig. 19–4). Heparin administration may be helpful in patients with acute DIC when intensive blood component replacement fails to improve excessive bleeding or when thrombosis threatens to cause irreversible tissue injury (e.g., acute cortical necrosis of the kidney or digital gangrene).

Heparin should be used cautiously in all these conditions. In patients with chronic DIC because of metastatic carcinoma or aortic aneurysm, continuous infusion of heparin 500 to 750 U/h without a bolus injection may be sufficient. If no response is obtained within 24 hours, escalating dosages can be used. In hyperacute DIC cases, such as mismatched transfusion, amniotic fluid embolism, septic abortion, and purpura fulminans, intravenous bolus injection of 5000 to 10,000 U heparin may be given simultaneously with replacement therapy with blood products. Some experts would not administer a bolus dose of heparin even under these circumstances. Continuous infusion of 500 to 1000 U/h heparin may be necessary to maintain the benefit until the underlying disease responds to treatment.[343]

Theoretically, the most logical anticoagulant agent to use in DIC is directed against TF activity. Potential agents include recombinant TFPI, inactivated factor VIIa, and recombinant nematode anticoagulant protein c2 (NAPc2), a potent and specific inhibitor of the ternary complex of TF–factor VIIa and factor Xa.[344] Phase II trials of recombinant TFPI in patients with sepsis showed promising results,[345] but a phase III trial did not show an overall survival benefit in patients who were treated with TFPI.[345,346]

Recombinant human soluble thrombomodulin binds to thrombin to form a complex that inactivates thrombin's coagulant activity and activates protein C and, thus, is a potential drug for the treatment of patients with DIC. In a phase III, randomized, double-blind clinical trial in patients with DIC, administration of the soluble thrombomodulin had a significantly better effect on bleeding manifestations and coagulation parameters than heparin.[347] Ongoing trials with soluble thrombomodulin focus on DIC, organ failure, and mortality rate.

## INHIBITORS OF FIBRINOLYSIS

Patients with DIC should not be treated with antifibrinolytic agents such as ε-aminocaproic acid or tranexamic acid because these drugs block fibrinolysis that preserves tissue perfusion in patients with DIC. Use of these agents in patients with DIC has been complicated by severe thrombosis.[348,349]

A different situation prevails in patients with DIC accompanied by primary fibrino(geno)lysis, as in some cases of APL, giant hemangioma, heat stroke, amniotic fluid embolism, some forms of liver disease, and metastatic carcinoma of the prostate. In these conditions, the use of fibrinolytic inhibitors can be considered,[350] provided (1) the patient is bleeding profusely and has not responded to replacement therapy and (2) excessive fibrino(geno)lysis is observed, that is, rapid whole blood clot lysis or a very short euglobulin lysis time. In such circumstances, use of antifibrinolytic agents should be preceded by replacement of depleted blood components and continuous heparin infusion (see Fig. 19–4).

# REFERENCES

1. McKay DG: *Disseminated Intravascular Coagulation: An Intermediary Mechanism of Disease.* Hoeber Medical, New York, 1965.
2. Mammen EF: Disseminated intravascular coagulation (DIC). *Clin Lab Sci* 13:239, 2000.
3. Colman RW, Robboy SJ, Minna JD: Disseminated intravascular coagulation: A reappraisal. *Annu Rev Med* 30:359, 1979.
4. Seligsohn U: Disseminated intravascular coagulation, in *Blood: Principles and Practice of Hematology*, edited by RI Handin, SE Lux, TP Stossel, p 1289. J.B. Lippincott, Philadelphia, 2000.
5. Levi M, ten Cate H: Disseminated intravascular coagulation. *N Engl J Med* 341:586, 1999.
6. Levi M, ten Cate H, van der Poll T: Disseminated intravascular coagulation: State of the art. *Thromb Haemost* 82:695, 1999.
7. Levi M: Disseminated intravascular coagulation. *Crit Care Med* 29:2191, 2007.
8. Dupuy M: Injections de matière cérébrale dans les veines. *Gaz Med (Paris)* 2:524, 1834.
9. Trousseau A: Phlegmasia alba dolens. *Clin Med Hotel Dieu Paris* 695, 1865.
10. Naunyn C: Untersuchungen uber Blutgerinnung im lebenden tiere und ihre Folgen. *Arch Exp Pathol Pharmacol* 1873.
11. Woolridge LC: Note on the relation of the red cell corpuscles to coagulation. *Practitioner* 187, 1886.
12. Woolridge LC: Ueber intravasculare gerinnungen. *Arch Ant Physiol Abt (Leipzig)* 397, 1886.
13. Ratnoff OD, Pritchard JA, Colopy JE: Hemorrhagic states during pregnancy. *N Engl J Med* 253:63, 1955.
14. Lasch HG, Heene DL, Huth K, et al: Pathophysiology, clinical manifestations and therapy of consumption-coagulopathy ("Verbrauchskoagulopathie"). *Am J Cardiol* 20:381, 1967.
15. Merskey C, Johnson AJ, Kleiner GJ, et al: The defibrination syndrome: Clinical features and laboratory diagnosis. *Br J Haematol* 13:528, 1967.
16. Robboy SJ, Major MC, Colman RW, et al: Pathology of disseminated intravascular coagulation (DIC). Analysis of 26 cases. *Hum Pathol* 3:327, 1972.
17. Wilde JT, Roberts KM, Greaves M, et al: Association between necropsy evidence of disseminated intravascular coagulation and coagulation variables before death in patients in intensive care units. *J Clin Pathol* 41:138, 1988.
18. Kim HS, Suzuki M, Lie JT, et al: Clinically unsuspected disseminated intravascular coagulation (DIC): An autopsy survey. *Am J Clin Pathol* 66:31, 1976.
19. Watanabe T, Imamura T, Nakagaki K, et al: Disseminated intravascular coagulation in autopsy cases. Its incidence and clinicopathologic significance. *Pathol Res Pract* 165:311, 1979.
20. Shimamura K, Oka K, Nakazawa M, et al: Distribution patterns of microthrombi in disseminated intravascular coagulation. *Arch Pathol Lab Med* 107:543, 1983.
21. Levi M, van der Poll T, ten Cate H, et al: The cytokine-mediated imbalance between coagulant and anticoagulant mechanisms in sepsis and endotoxaemia. *Eur J Clin Invest* 27:3, 1997.
22. Levi M, van der Poll T, Buller HR: The bidirectional relationship between coagulation and inflammation. *Circulation* 109:2698, 2004.
23. Aird WC: Vascular bed-specific hemostasis: Role of endothelium in sepsis pathogenesis. *Crit Care Med* 29:S28, 2001.
24. Weinbaum S, Zhang X, Han Y, et al: Mechanotransduction and flow across the endothelial glycocalyx. *Proc Natl Acad Sci U S A* 100:7988, 2003.
25. Maczewski M, Duda M, Pawlak W, et al: Endothelial protection from reperfusion injury by ischemic preconditioning and diazoxide involves a SOD-like anti-$O_2$-mechanism. *J Physiol Pharmacol* 55:537, 2004.
26. Vink H, Constantinescu AA, Spaan JA: Oxidized lipoproteins degrade the endothelial surface layer: Implications for platelet-endothelial cell adhesion. *Circulation* 101:1500, 2000.
27. Nieuwdorp M, van Haeften TW, Gouverneur MC, et al: Loss of endothelial glycocalyx during acute hyperglycemia coincides with endothelial dysfunction and coagulation activation *in vivo*. *Diabetes* 55:480, 2006.
28. Levi M, van der Poll T, ten Cate H: Tissue factor in infection and severe inflammation. *Semin Thromb Hemost* 32:33, 2006.
29. Taylor FBJ, Chang A, Ruf W, et al: Lethal *E. coli* septic shock is prevented by blocking tissue factor with monoclonal antibody. *Circ Shock* 33:127, 1991.
30. Levi M, ten Cate H, Bauer KA, et al: Inhibition of endotoxin-induced activation of coagulation and fibrinolysis by pentoxifylline or by a monoclonal anti-tissue factor antibody in chimpanzees. *J Clin Invest* 93:114, 1994.
31. van der Poll T, Levi M, Hack CE, et al: Elimination of interleukin 6 attenuates coagulation activation in experimental endotoxemia in chimpanzees. *J Exp Med* 179:1253, 1994.
32. Osterud B, Rao LV, Olsen JO: Induction of tissue factor expression in whole blood—Lack of evidence for the presence of tissue factor expression on granulocytes. *Thromb Haemost* 83:861, 2000.
33. Franco RF, de Jonge E, Dekkers PE, et al: The *in vivo* kinetics of tissue factor messenger RNA expression during human endotoxemia: Relationship with activation of coagulation. *Blood* 96:554, 2000.
34. Rauch U, Bonderman D, Bohrmann B, et al: Transfer of tissue factor from leukocytes to platelets is mediated by CD15 and tissue factor. *Blood* 96:170, 2000.
35. Osterud B, Bjorklid E: Sources of tissue factor. *Semin Thromb Hemost* 32:11, 2006.
36. van Deventer SJ, Buller HR, ten Cate JW, et al: Experimental endotoxemia in humans: Analysis of cytokine release and coagulation, fibrinolytic, and complement pathways. *Blood* 76:2520, 1990.
37. Boermeester MA, van Leeuwen P, Coyle SM, et al: Interleukin-1 blockade attenuates mediator release and dysregulation of the hemostatic mechanism during human sepsis. *Arch Surg* 130:739, 1995.
38. Osterud B: Tissue factor expression by monocytes: Regulation and pathophysiological roles. *Blood Coagul Fibrinolysis* 9(Suppl 1):S9, 1998.
39. Furie B, Furie BC: Role of platelet P-selectin and microparticle PSGL-1 in thrombus formation. *Trends Mol Med* 10:171, 2004.
40. Neumann FJ, Marx N, Gawaz M, et al: Induction of cytokine expression in leukocytes by binding of thrombin-stimulated platelets. *Circulation* 95:2387, 1997.
41. Esmon CT: Protein C anticoagulant pathway and its role in controlling microvascular thrombosis and inflammation. *Crit Care Med* 29:S48, 2001.
42. Mileno MD, Margolis NH, Clark BD, et al: Coagulation of whole blood stimulates interleukin-1 beta gene expression. *J Infect Dis* 172:308, 1995.
43. Jones A, Geczy CL: Thrombin and factor Xa enhance the production of interleukin-1. *Immunology* 71:236, 1990.
44. Johnson K, Choi Y, DeGroot E, et al: Potential mechanisms for a proinflammatory vascular cytokine response to coagulation activation. *J Immunol* 160:5130, 1998.
45. Sower LE, Froelich CJ, Carney DH, et al: Thrombin induces IL-6 production in fibroblasts and epithelial cells. Evidence for the involvement of the seven-transmembrane domain (STD) receptor for alpha-thrombin. *J Immunol* 155:895, 1995.
46. van der Poll T, de Jonge E, Levi M: Regulatory role of cytokines in disseminated intravascular coagulation. *Semin Thromb Hemost* 27:639, 2001.
47. Coughlin SR: Thrombin signalling and protease-activated receptors. *Nature* 407:258, 2000.
48. Versteeg HH, Peppelenbosch MP, Spek CA: The pleiotropic effects of tissue factor: A possible role for factor VIIa-induced intracellular signalling? *Thromb Haemost* 86:1353, 2001.
49. Levi M, de Jonge E, van der Poll T: Rationale for restoration of physiological anticoagulant pathways in patients with sepsis and disseminated intravascular coagulation. *Crit Care Med* 29:S90, 2001.
49a. Kannemeier C, Shibamiya A, Nakazawa F, et al: Extracellular RNA constitutes a natural procoagulant cofactor in blood coagulation. *Proc Natl Acad Sci U S A* 104(15):6388–6893, 2007.
49b. Semeraro F, Ammollo CT, Morrissey JH, et al: Extracellular histones promote thrombin generation through platelet-dependent mechanisms: Involvement of platelet TLR2 and TLR4. *Blood* 118(7):1952–1961, 2011.
49c. Fuchs TA, Brill A, Wagner DD: Neutrophil extracellular trap (NET) impact on deep vein thrombosis. *Arterioscler Thromb Vasc Biol* 32(8):1777–1783, 2012.
49d. von Bruhl ML, Stark K, Steinhart A, et al: Monocytes, neutrophils, and platelets cooperate to initiate and propagate venous thrombosis in mice in vivo. *J Exp Med* 209(4):819–835, 2012.
49e. Iba T, Miki T, Hashiguchi N, Tabe Y, Nagaoka I: Combination of antithrombin and recombinant thrombomodulin modulates neutrophil cell-death and decreases circulating DAMPs levels in endotoxemic rats. *Thromb Res* 134(1):169–173, 2014.
49f. Saffarzadeh M, Juenemann C, Queisser MA, et al: Neutrophil extracellular traps directly induce epithelial and endothelial cell death: A predominant role of histones. *PLoS One* 7(2):e32366, 2012.
50. Szaba FM, Smiley ST: Roles for thrombin and fibrin(ogen) in cytokine/chemokine production and macrophage adhesion *in vivo*. *Blood* 99:1053, 2002.
51. Levi M, van der Poll T: The role of natural anticoagulants in the pathogenesis and management of systemic activation of coagulation and inflammation in critically ill patients. *Semin Thromb Hemost* 34:459, 2008.
52. Levi M: Antithrombin in sepsis revisited. *Crit Care* 9:624, 2005.
53. Levi M, van der Poll T: Two-way interactions between inflammation and coagulation. *Trends Cardiovasc Med* 15:254, 2005.
54. Kobayashi M, Shimada K, Ozawa T: Human recombinant interleukin-1 beta- and tumor necrosis factor alpha-mediated suppression of heparin-like compounds on cultured porcine aortic endothelial cells. *J Cell Physiol* 144:383, 1990.
55. Levi M, van der Poll T: Recombinant human activated protein C: Current insights into its mechanism of action. *Crit Care* 11(Suppl 5):S3, 2007.
56. Esmon CT: Role of coagulation inhibitors in inflammation. *Thromb Haemost* 86:51, 2001.
57. Esmon CT: The regulation of natural anticoagulant pathways. *Science* 235:1348, 1987.
58. Esmon CT: The endothelial cell protein C receptor. *Thromb Haemost* 83:639, 2000.
59. Mesters RM, Helterbrand J, Utterback BG, et al: Prognostic value of protein C concentrations in neutropenic patients at high risk of severe septic complications. *Crit Care Med* 28:2209, 2000.
60. Vary TC, Kimball SR: Regulation of hepatic protein synthesis in chronic inflammation and sepsis. *Am J Physiol* 262:C445, 1992.
61. Eckle I, Seitz R, Egbring R, et al: Protein C degradation *in vitro* by neutrophil elastase. *Biol Chem Hoppe Seyler* 372:1007, 1991.
62. Nawroth PP, Stern DM: Modulation of endothelial cell hemostatic properties by tumor necrosis factor. *J Exp Med* 163:740, 1986.
63. Faust SN, Levin M, Harrison OB, et al: Dysfunction of endothelial protein C activation in severe meningococcal sepsis. *N Engl J Med* 345:408, 2001.
64. Taylor FB Jr, Dahlback B, Chang AC, et al: Role of free protein S and C4b binding protein in regulating the coagulant response to *Escherichia coli*. *Blood* 86:2642, 1995.
65. Taylor FB Jr, Stearns-Kurosawa DJ, Kurosawa S, et al: The endothelial cell protein C receptor aids in host defense against *Escherichia coli* sepsis. *Blood* 95:1680, 2000.

66. De Pont AC, Bakhtiari K, Hutten BA, et al: Endotoxaemia induces resistance to activated protein C in healthy humans. *Br J Haematol* 134:213, 2006.

67. de Jonge E, Dekkers PE, Creasey AA, et al: Tissue factor pathway inhibitor (TFPI) dose-dependently inhibits coagulation activation without influencing the fibrinolytic and cytokine response during human endotoxemia. *Blood* 95:1124, 2000.

68. Creasey AA, Chang AC, Feigen L, et al: Tissue factor pathway inhibitor reduces mortality from *Escherichia coli* septic shock. *J Clin Invest* 91:2850, 1993.

69. Roemisch J, Gray E, Hoffmann JN, et al: Antithrombin: A new look at the actions of a serine protease inhibitor. *Blood Coagul Fibrinolysis* 13:657, 2002.

70. Opal SM: Interactions between coagulation and inflammation. *Scand J Infect Dis* 35:545, 2003.

71. Harada N, Okajima K, Kushimoto S, et al: Antithrombin reduces ischemia/reperfusion injury of rat liver by increasing the hepatic level of prostacyclin. *Blood* 93:157, 1999.

72. Horie S, Ishii H, Kazama M: Heparin-like glycosaminoglycan is a receptor for antithrombin III-dependent but not for thrombin-dependent prostacyclin production in human endothelial cells. *Thromb Res* 59:895, 1990.

73. Mizutani A, Okajima K, Uchiba M, et al: Antithrombin reduces ischemia/reperfusion-induced renal injury in rats by inhibiting leukocyte activation through promotion of prostacyclin production. *Blood* 101:3029, 2003.

74. Uchiba M, Okajima K, Murakami K: Effects of various doses of antithrombin III on endotoxin-induced endothelial cell injury and coagulation abnormalities in rats. *Thromb Res* 89:233, 1998.

75. Esmon CT: New mechanisms for vascular control of inflammation mediated by natural anticoagulant proteins. *J Exp Med* 196:561, 2002.

76. Okajima K: Regulation of inflammatory responses by natural anticoagulants. *Immunol Rev* 184:258, 2001.

77. Taylor FB Jr, Chang A, Esmon CT, et al: Protein C prevents the coagulopathic and lethal effects of *Escherichia coli* infusion in the baboon. *J Clin Invest* 79:918, 1987.

78. Hancock WW, Tsuchida A, Hau H, et al: The anticoagulants protein C and protein S display potent antiinflammatory and immunosuppressive effects relevant to transplant biology and therapy. *Transplant Proc* 24:2302, 1992.

79. Hancock WW, Grey ST, Hau L, et al: Binding of activated protein C to a specific receptor on human mononuclear phagocytes inhibits intracellular calcium signaling and monocyte-dependent proliferative responses. *Transplantation* 60:1525, 1995.

80. White B, Schmidt M, Murphy C, et al: Activated protein C inhibits lipopolysaccharide-induced nuclear translocation of nuclear factor kappaB (NF-kappaB) and tumour necrosis factor alpha (TNF-alpha) production in the THP-1 monocytic cell line. *Br J Haematol* 110:130, 2000.

81. Levi M, Dorffler-Melly J, Reitsma PH, et al: Aggravation of endotoxin-induced disseminated intravascular coagulation and cytokine activation in heterozygous protein C deficient mice. *Blood* 101:4823, 2003.

82. Lay AJ, Donahue D, Tsai MJ, et al: Acute inflammation is exacerbated in mice genetically predisposed to a severe protein C deficiency. *Blood* 109:1984, 2007.

83. Feistritzer C, Sturn DH, Kaneider NC, et al: Endothelial protein C receptor-dependent inhibition of human eosinophil chemotaxis by protein C. *J Allergy Clin Immunol* 112:375, 2003.

84. Sturn DH, Kaneider NC, Feistritzer C, et al: Expression and function of the endothelial protein C receptor in human neutrophils. *Blood* 102:1499, 2003.

85. Hoffmann JN, Vollmar B, Laschke MW, et al: Microhemodynamic and cellular mechanisms of activated protein C action during endotoxemia. *Crit Care Med* 32:1011, 2004.

86. Nick JA, Coldren CD, Geraci MW, et al: Recombinant human activated protein C reduces human endotoxin-induced pulmonary inflammation via inhibition of neutrophil chemotaxis. *Blood* 104:3878, 2004.

87. Shimizu S, Gabazza EC, Taguchi O, et al: Activated protein C inhibits the expression of platelet-derived growth factor in the lung. *Am J Respir Crit Care Med* 167:1416, 2003.

88. Zeng W, Matter WF, Yan SB, et al: Effect of drotrecogin alfa (activated) on human endothelial cell permeability and Rho kinase signaling. *Crit Care Med* 32:S302, 2004.

89. Feistritzer C, Riewald M: Endothelial barrier protection by activated protein C through PAR1-dependent sphingosine 1-phosphate receptor-1 cross activation. *Blood* 105:3178, 2005.

90. Finigan JH, Dudek SM, Singleton PA, et al: Activated protein C mediates novel lung endothelial barrier enhancement: Role of sphingosine 1-phosphate receptor transactivation. *J Biol Chem* 280:17286, 2005.

91. Cheng T, Liu D, Griffin JH, et al: Activated protein C blocks p53-mediated apoptosis in ischemic human brain endothelium and is neuroprotective. *Nat Med* 9:338, 2003.

92. Riewald M, Petrovan RJ, Donner A, et al: Activation of endothelial cell protease activated receptor 1 by the protein C pathway. *Science* 296:1880, 2002.

93. Mosnier LO, Griffin JH: Inhibition of staurosporine-induced apoptosis of endothelial cells by activated protein C requires protease activated receptor-1 and endothelial cell protein C receptor. *Biochem J* 373:65, 2003.

94. Mosnier LO, Zlokovic BV, Griffin JH: The cytoprotective protein C pathway. *Blood* 109:3161, 2007.

95. Biemond BJ, Levi M, ten Cate H, et al: Plasminogen activator and plasminogen activator inhibitor I release during experimental endotoxaemia in chimpanzees: Effect of interventions in the cytokine and coagulation cascades. *Clin Sci* 88:587, 1995.

96. Schleef RR, Bevilacqua MP, Sawdey M, et al: Cytokine activation of vascular endothelium. Effects on tissue-type plasminogen activator and type 1 plasminogen activator inhibitor. *J Biol Chem* 263:5797, 1988.

97. van Hinsbergh VW, Kooistra T, van den Berg EA, et al: Tumor necrosis factor increases the production of plasminogen activator inhibitor in human endothelial cells *in vitro* and in rats *in vivo*. *Blood* 72:1467, 1988.

98. Asakura H, Ontachi Y, Mizutani T: An enhanced fibrinolysis prevents the development of multiple organ failure in disseminated intravascular coagulation in spite of much activation of blood coagulation. *Crit Care Med* 29:1164, 2001.

99. Yamamoto K, Loskutoff DJ: Fibrin deposition in tissues from endotoxin-treated mice correlates with decreases in the expression of urokinase-type but not tissue-type plasminogen activator. *J Clin Invest* 97:2440, 1996.

100. Nesheim M, Wang W, Boffa M, et al: Thrombin, thrombomodulin and TAFI in the molecular link between coagulation and fibrinolysis. *Thromb Haemost* 78:386, 1997.

101. Salvemini D, Cuzzocrea S: Oxidative stress in septic shock and disseminated intravascular coagulation. *Free Radic Biol Med* 33:1173, 2002.

102. Asakura H, Okudaira M, Yoshida T: Induction of vasoactive substances differs in LPS-induced and TF-induced DIC models in rats. *Thromb Haemost* 88:663, 2002.

103. Levi M, Nieuwdorp M, van der Poll T, et al: Metabolic modulation of inflammation-induced activation of coagulation. *Semin Thromb Hemost* 34:26, 2008.

104. Kjalke M, Silveira A, Hamsten A, et al: Plasma lipoproteins enhance tissue factor-independent factor VII activation. *Arterioscler Thromb Vasc Biol* 20:1835, 2000.

105. van der Poll T, Coyle SM, Levi M, et al: Fat emulsion infusion potentiates coagulation activation during human endotoxemia. *Thromb Haemost* 75:83, 1996.

106. Pajkrt D, Lerch PG, van der Poll T, et al: Differential effects of reconstituted high-density lipoprotein on coagulation, fibrinolysis and platelet activation during human endotoxemia. *Thromb Haemost* 77:303, 1997.

107. Birjmohun RS, van Leuven SI, Levels JH, et al: High-density lipoprotein attenuates inflammation and coagulation response on endotoxin challenge in humans. *Arterioscler Thromb Vasc Biol* 27:1153, 2007.

108. Bisoendial RJ, Kastelein JJ, Peters SL, et al: Effects of CRP infusion on endothelial function and coagulation in normocholesterolemic and hypercholesterolemic subjects. *J Lipid Res* 48:952, 2007.

109. Grant PJ: Diabetes mellitus as a prothrombotic condition. *J Intern Med* 262:157, 2007.

110. Juhan-Vague I, Roul C, Alessi MC, et al: Increased plasminogen activator inhibitor activity in non insulin dependent diabetic patients—Relationship with plasma insulin. *Thromb Haemost* 61:370, 1989.

111. Mansfield MW, Stickland MH, Grant PJ: PAI-1 concentrations in first-degree relatives of patients with non-insulin-dependent diabetes: Metabolic and genetic associations. *Thromb Haemost* 77:357, 1997.

112. Samad F, Pandey M, Loskutoff DJ: Regulation of tissue factor gene expression in obesity. *Blood* 98:3353, 2001.

113. Stegenga ME, van der Crabben SN, Levi M, et al: Hyperglycemia enhances coagulation and reduces neutrophil degranulation, whereas hyperinsulinemia inhibits fibrinolysis during human endotoxemia. *Blood* 112:82, 2008.

114. Levi M: Current understanding of disseminated intravascular coagulation. *Br J Haematol* 124:567, 2004.

115. Siegal T, Seligsohn U, Aghai E, et al: Clinical and laboratory aspects of disseminated intravascular coagulation (DIC): A study of 118 cases. *Thromb Haemost* 39:122, 1978.

116. Al-Mondhiry H: Disseminated intravascular coagulation: Experience in a major cancer center. *Thromb Diath Haemorrh* 34:181, 1975.

117. Hofstra JJ, Haitsma JJ, Juffermans NP, et al: Role of broncho-alveolar hemostasis in the pathogenesis of acute lung injury. *Semin Thromb Hemost* 34:475, 2008.

118. Rinaldo JE, Rogers RM: Adult respiratory distress syndrome [editorial]. *N Engl J Med* 315:578, 1986.

119. Katsumura Y, Ohtsubo K: Incidence of pulmonary thromboembolism, infarction and hemorrhage in disseminated intravascular coagulation. *Thorax* 50:160, 1995.

120. Kollef MH, Schuster DP: The acute respiratory distress syndrome. *N Engl J Med* 332:27, 1995.

121. Dhainaut JF, Shorr AF, Macias WL, et al: Dynamic evolution of coagulopathy in the first day of severe sepsis: Relationship with mortality and organ failure. *Crit Care Med* 33:341, 2005.

122. Spero JA, Lewis JH, Hasiba U: Disseminated intravascular coagulation. Findings in 346 patients. *Thromb Haemost* 43:28, 1980.

123. Bakhtiari K, Meijers JC, de Jonge E, et al: Prospective validation of the international society of thrombosis and haemostasis scoring system for disseminated intravascular coagulation. *Crit Care Med* 32:2416, 2004.

124. Dhainaut JF, Yan SB, Joyce DE, et al: Treatment effects of drotrecogin alfa (activated) in patients with severe sepsis with or without overt disseminated intravascular coagulation. *J Thromb Haemost* 2:1924, 2004.

125. Dempfle CE, Pfitzner SA, Dollman M, et al: Comparison of immunological and functional assays for measurement of soluble fibrin. *Thromb Haemost* 74:673, 1995.

126. Bredbacka S, Blomback M, Wiman B, et al: Laboratory methods for detecting disseminated intravascular coagulation (DIC): New aspects. *Acta Anaesthesiol Scand* 37:125, 1993.

127. Bredbacka S, Blomback M, Wiman B: Soluble fibrin: A predictor for the development and outcome of multiple organ failure. *Am J Hematol* 46:289, 1994.

128. McCarron BI, Marder VJ, Kanouse JJ, et al: A soluble fibrin standard: Comparable dose-response with immunologic and functional assays. *Thromb Haemost* 82:145, 1999.

129. Shorr AF, Thomas SJ, Alkins SA, et al: D-dimer correlates with proinflammatory cytokine levels and outcomes in critically ill patients. *Chest* 121:1262, 2002.

130. Dempfle CE: The use of soluble fibrin in evaluating the acute and chronic hypercoagulable state. *Thromb Haemost* 82:673, 1999.

131. Horan JT, Francis CW: Fibrin degradation products, fibrin monomer and soluble fibrin in disseminated intravascular coagulation. *Semin Thromb Hemost* 27:657, 2001.

132. McCarron BI, Marder VJ, Francis CW: Reactivity of soluble fibrin assays with plasmic degradation products of fibrin and in patients receiving fibrinolytic therapy. *Thromb Haemost* 82:1722, 1999.

133. Carr JM, McKinney M, McDonagh J: Diagnosis of disseminated intravascular coagulation. Role of D-dimer. *Am J Clin Pathol* 91:280, 1989.

134. Boisclair MD, Ireland H, Lane DA: Assessment of hypercoagulable states by measurement of activation fragments and peptides. *Blood Rev* 4:25, 1990.

135. Prisco D, Paniccia R, Bonechi F, et al: Evaluation of new methods for the selective measurement of fibrin and fibrinogen degradation products. *Thromb Res* 56:547, 1989.

136. Shorr AF, Trotta RF, Alkins SA, et al: D-dimer assay predicts mortality in critically ill patients without disseminated intravascular coagulation or venous thromboembolic disease. *Intensive Care Med* 25:207, 1999.

137. Greenberg CS, Devine DV, McCrae KM: Measurement of plasma fibrin D-dimer levels with the use of a monoclonal antibody coupled to latex beads. *Am J Clin Pathol* 87:94, 1987.

138. Taylor FB Jr, Toh CH, Hoots WK, et al: Towards definition, clinical and laboratory criteria, and a scoring system for disseminated intravascular coagulation. *Thromb Haemost* 86:1327, 2001.

139. Kobayashi S, Gando S, Morimoto Y: Serial measurement of arterial lactate concentrations as a prognostic indicator in relation to the incidence of disseminated intravascular coagulation in patients with systemic inflammatory response syndrome. *Surg Today* 31:853, 2001.

140. Wada H, Gabazza EC, Asakura H, et al: Comparison of diagnostic criteria for disseminated intravascular coagulation (DIC): Diagnostic criteria of the International Society of Thrombosis and Hemostasis and of the Japanese Ministry of Health and Welfare for overt DIC: *Am J Hematol* 74:17, 2003.

141. Kinasewitz GT, Zein JG, Lee GL, et al: Prognostic value of a simple evolving DIC score in patients with severe sepsis. *Crit Care Med* 33:2214, 2005.

142. Levi M, van der Poll T, de Jonge E, et al: Relative insufficiency of fibrinolysis in disseminated intravascular coagulation. *Sepsis* 3:103, 2000.

143. Liaw PC, Ferrell G, Esmon CT: A monoclonal antibody against activated protein C allows rapid detection of activated protein C in plasma and reveals a calcium ion dependent epitope involved in factor Va inactivation. *J Thromb Haemost* 1:662, 2003.

144. Moore JC, Hayward CP, Warkentin TE, et al: Decreased von Willebrand factor protease activity associated with thrombocytopenic disorders. *Blood* 98:1842, 2001.

145. Levi M, Lowenberg EC: Thrombocytopenia in critically ill patients. *Semin Thromb Hemost* 34:417, 2008.

146. Dempfle CE, Borggrefe M: Point of care coagulation tests in critically ill patients. *Semin Thromb Hemost* 34:445, 2008.

147. Collins PW, Macchiavello LI, Lewis SJ, et al: Global tests of haemostasis in critically ill patients with severe sepsis syndrome compared to controls. *Br J Haematol* 135:220, 2006.

148. Toh CH, Hoots WK: The scoring system of the Scientific and Standardisation Committee on Disseminated Intravascular Coagulation of the International Society on Thrombosis and Haemostasis: A 5-year overview. *J Thromb Haemost* 5:604, 2007.

149. Bone RC: Modulators of coagulation. A critical appraisal of their role in sepsis. *Arch Intern Med* 152:1381, 1992.

150. Keller TT, Mairuhu AT, de Kruif MD, et al: Infections and endothelial cells. *Cardiovasc Res* 60:40, 2003.

151. Gando S, Nanzaki S, Sasaki S, et al: Activation of the extrinsic coagulation pathway in patients with severe sepsis and septic shock. *Crit Care Med* 26:2005, 1998.

152. Wiersinga WJ, Meijers JC, Levi M, et al: Activation of coagulation with concurrent impairment of anticoagulant mechanisms correlates with a poor outcome in severe melioidosis. *J Thromb Haemost* 6:32, 2008.

153. Bone RC: Gram-positive organisms and sepsis. *Arch Intern Med* 154:26, 1994.

154. Levi M, van der Poll T: Coagulation in sepsis: All bugs bite equally. *Crit Care* 8:99, 2004.

155. Herwald H, Cramer H, Morgelin M: M-protein, a classical bacterial virulence determinant forms complexes with fibrinogen that induce vascular leakage. *Cell* 116:367, 2004.

156. Fijnvandraat K, Derkx B, Peters M, et al: Coagulation activation and tissue necrosis in meningococcal septic shock: Severely reduced protein C levels predict a high mortality. *Thromb Haemost* 73:15, 1995.

157. Hazelzet JA, Risseeuw-Appel IM, Kornelisse RF, et al: Age-related differences in outcome and severity of DIC in children with septic shock and purpura. *Thromb Haemost* 76:932, 1996.

158. Levi M, Opal SM: Coagulation abnormalities in critically ill patients. *Crit Care* 10:222, 2006.

159. Levi M: Hemostasis and thrombosis in critically ill patients. *Semin Thromb Hemost* 34:415, 2008.

160. Ono T, Mimuro J, Madoiwa S, et al: Severe secondary deficiency of von Willebrand factor-cleaving protease (ADAMTS13) in patients with sepsis-induced disseminated intravascular coagulation: Its correlation with development of renal failure. *Blood* 107:528, 2006.

161. Bhakdi S, Muhly M, Mannhardt U: Staphylococcal alpha toxin promotes blood coagulation via attack on human platelets. *J Exp Med* 168:527, 1988.

162. Ratnoff OD, Nebehay WG: Multiple coagulative defects in a patient with the Waterhouse-Friederichsen syndrome. *Ann Intern Med* 56:627, 1962.

163. van Gorp E, Suharti C, ten Cate H, et al: Review: Infectious diseases and coagulation disorders. *J Infect Dis* 180:176, 1999.

164. Levi M, Keller TT, van Gorp E, et al: Infection and inflammation and the coagulation system. *Cardiovasc Res* 60:26, 2003.

165. Heller MV, Marta RF, Sturk A, et al: Early markers of blood coagulation and fibrinolysis activation in Argentine hemorrhagic fever. *Thromb Haemost* 73:368, 1995.

166. Clemens R, Pramoolsinsap C, Lorenz R, et al: Activation of the coagulation cascade in severe falciparum malaria through the intrinsic pathway. *Br J Haematol* 87:100, 1994.

167. Mohanty D, Ghosh K, Nandwani SK, et al: Fibrinolysis, inhibitors of blood coagulation, and monocyte derived coagulant activity in acute malaria. *Am J Hematol* 54:23, 1997.

168. Fera G, Semeraro N, De MV, et al: Disseminated intravascular coagulation associated with disseminated cryptococcosis in a patient with acquired immunodeficiency syndrome. *Infection* 21:171, 1993.

169. Cosgriff TM: Viruses and haemostasis. *Rev Infect Dis* 11:672, 1989.

170. Inbal A, Kenet G, Zivelin A, et al: Purpura fulminans induced by disseminated intravascular coagulation following infection in 2 unrelated children with double heterozygosity for factor V Leiden and protein S deficiency. *Thromb Haemost* 77:1086, 1997.

171. Hofstra JJ, Schouten M, Levi M: Thrombophilia and outcome in severe infection and sepsis. *Semin Thromb Hemost* 33:604, 2007.

172. Levin M, Eley BS, Louis J: Postinfectious purpura fulminans caused by an autoantibody directed against protein S. *J Pediatr* 127:355, 1995.

173. Bhamarapravati N: Hemostatic defects in dengue hemorrhagic fever. *Rev Infect Dis* 11(Suppl 4):S826, 1989.

174. Suvatte V: Dengue hemorrhagic fever: Hematological abnormalities and pathogenesis. *J Med Assoc Thai* 61(Suppl 3):53, 1978.

175. Linder M, Muller-Berghaus G, Lasch HG, et al: Virus infection and blood coagulation. *Thromb Diath Haemorrh* 23:1, 1970.

176. Carpenter CT, Kaiser AB: Purpura fulminans in pneumococcal sepsis: Case report and review. *Scand J Infect Dis* 29:479, 1997.

177. Gerson WT, Dickerman JD, Bovill EG, et al: Severe acquired protein C deficiency in purpura fulminans associated with disseminated intravascular coagulation: Treatment with protein C concentrate. *Pediatrics* 91:418, 1993.

178. Tishler M, Abramov AL, Seligsohn U, et al: Purpura fulminans in an adult. *Isr J Med Sci* 22:820, 1986.

179. Bramson HE, Katz J, Marble R, et al: Inherited protein C deficiency and a coumarin responsive chronic relapsing purpura fulminans in a newborn infant. *Lancet* 2:1156, 1983.

180. Seligsohn U, Berger A, Abend M: Homozygous protein C deficiency manifested by massive venous thrombosis in the newborn. *N Engl J Med* 310:559, 1984.

181. Goad KE, Gralnick HR: Coagulation disorders in cancer. *Hematol Oncol Clin North Am* 10:457, 1996.

182. Levi M: Cancer and DIC: *Haemostasis* 31(Suppl 1):47, 2001.

183. Sack GH Jr, Levin J, Bell WR: Trousseau's syndrome and other manifestations of chronic disseminated coagulopathy in patients with neoplasms: Clinical, pathophysiologic, and therapeutic features. *Medicine (Baltimore)* 56:1, 1977.

184. Sallah S, Wan JY, Nguyen NP, et al: Disseminated intravascular coagulation in solid tumors: Clinical and pathological study. *Thromb Haemost* 86:828, 2001.

185. Donati MB: Cancer and thrombosis: From phlegmasia alba dolens to transgenic mice. *Thromb Haemost* 74:278, 1995.

186. Levi M: Cancer and thrombosis. *Clin Adv Hematol Oncol* 1:668, 2003.

187. Contrino J, Hair G, Kreutzer DL, et al: *In situ* detection of tissue factor in vascular endothelial cells: Correlation with the malignant phenotype of human breast disease. *Nat Med* 2:209, 1996.

188. Rickles FR, Brenner B: Tissue factor and cancer. *Semin Thromb Hemost* 34:143, 2008.

189. Bromberg ME, Konigsberg WH, Madison JF, et al: Tissue factor promotes melanoma metastasis by a pathway independent of blood coagulation. *Proc Natl Acad Sci U S A* 92:8205, 1995.

190. Zhang Y, Deng Y, Luther T, et al: Tissue factor controls the balance of angiogenic and antiangiogenic properties of tumor cells in mice. *J Clin Invest* 94:1320, 1994.

191. Nadir Y, Vlodavsky I, Brenner B: Heparanase, tissue factor, and cancer. *Semin Thromb Hemost* 34:187, 2008.

192. Falanga A, Consonni R, Marchetti M, et al: Cancer procoagulant and tissue factor are differently modulated by all-trans-retinoic acid in acute promyelocytic leukemia cells. *Blood* 92:143, 1998.

193. Levi M: Disseminated intravascular coagulation in cancer patients. *Best Pract Res Clin Haematol* 22:129, 2009.

194. Wahrenbrock M, Borsig L, Le Duc M: Selectin-mucin interactions as a probable molecular explanation for the association of Trousseau syndrome with mucinous adenocarcinoma. *J Clin Invest* 112:853, 2003.

195. Dvorak HF, Quay SC, Orenstein NS: Tumor shedding and coagulation. *Science* 212:923, 1981.

196. Zwicker JI: Tissue factor-bearing microparticles and cancer. *Semin Thromb Hemost* 34:195, 2008.

197. Nijziel MR, van OR, Hillen HF, et al: From Trousseau to angiogenesis: The link between the haemostatic system and cancer. *Neth J Med* 64:403, 2006.

198. Rickles FR, Falanga A: Molecular basis for the relationship between thrombosis and cancer. *Thromb Res* 102:V215, 2001.

199. Stouthard JM, Levi M, Hack CE, et al: Interleukin-6 stimulates coagulation, not fibrinolysis, in humans. *Thromb Haemost* 76:738, 1996.

200. van der Poll T, Coyle SM, Levi M, et al: Effect of a recombinant dimeric tumor necrosis factor receptor on inflammatory responses to intravenous endotoxin in normal humans. *Blood* 89:3727, 1997.

201. van der Poll T, Levi M, ten Cate H, et al: The role of tumor necrosis factor in systemic inflammatory responses in primate endotoxemia. *Prog Clin Biol Res* 388:425, 1994.

202. van der Poll T, Levi M, van Deventer SJ, et al: Differential effects of anti-tumor necrosis factor monoclonal antibodies on systemic inflammatory responses in experimental endotoxemia in chimpanzees. *Blood* 83:446, 1994.

203. Sewnath ME, Olszyna DP, Birjmohun R, et al: IL-10-deficient mice demonstrate multiple organ failure and increased mortality during *Escherichia coli* peritonitis despite an accelerated bacterial clearance. *J Immunol* 166:6323, 2001.

204. van der Poll T, Jansen J, Levi M, et al: Interleukin 10 release during endotoxaemia in chimpanzees: Role of platelet-activating factor and interleukin 6. *Scand J Immunol* 43:122, 1996.

205. van der Poll T, Jansen PM, Montegut WJ, et al: Effects of IL-10 on systemic inflammatory responses during sublethal primate endotoxemia. *J Immunol* 158:1971, 1997.

206. Seligsohn U, Weber H, Yoran C: Microangiopathic hemolytic anemia and defibrination syndrome in metastatic carcinoma of the stomach. *Isr J Med Sci* 4:69, 1968.

207. Uchiumi H, Matsushima T, Yamane A, et al: Prevalence and clinical characteristics of acute myeloid leukemia associated with disseminated intravascular coagulation. *Int J Hematol* 86:137, 2007.

208. Barbui T, Falanga A: Disseminated intravascular coagulation in acute leukemia. *Semin Thromb Hemost* 27:593, 2001.

209. Sarris AH, Kempin S, Berman E, et al: High incidence of disseminated intravascular coagulation during remission induction of adult patients with acute lymphoblastic leukemia. *Blood* 79:1305, 1992.

210. Avvisati G, ten Cate JW, Sturk A, et al: Acquired alpha-2-antiplasmin deficiency in acute promyelocytic leukaemia. *Br J Haematol* 70:43, 1988.

211. Falanga A: Mechanisms of hypercoagulation in malignancy and during chemotherapy. *Haemostasis* 28(Suppl 3):50, 1998.

212. Stein E, McMahon B, Kwaan H, et al: The coagulopathy of acute promyelocytic leukaemia revisited. *Best Pract Res Clin Haematol* 22:153, 2009.

213. Barbui T, Finazzi G, Falanga A: The impact of all-*trans*-retinoic acid on the coagulopathy of acute promyelocytic leukemia. *Blood* 91:3093, 1998.

214. Gando S, Nakanishi Y, Tedo I: Cytokines and plasminogen activator inhibitor-1 in posttrauma disseminated intravascular coagulation: Relationship to multiple organ dysfunction syndrome. *Crit Care Med* 23:1835, 1995.

215. Gando S: Disseminated intravascular coagulation in trauma patients. *Semin Thromb Hemost* 27:585, 2001.

216. Gando S: Tissue factor in trauma and organ dysfunction. *Semin Thromb Hemost* 32:48, 2006.

217. Owings JT, Gosselin RC, Anderson JT, et al: Practical utility of the D-dimer assay for excluding thromboembolism in severely injured trauma patients. *J Trauma* 51:425, 2001.

218. Attar S, Boyd D, Layne E, et al: Alterations in coagulation and fibrinolytic mechanisms in acute trauma. *J Trauma* 9:939, 1969.

219. Cosgriff N, Moore EE, Sauaia A, et al: Predicting life-threatening coagulopathy in the massively transfused trauma patient: Hypothermia and acidoses revisited. *J Trauma* 42:857, 1997.

220. Hess JR, Holcomb JB: Transfusion practice in military trauma. *Transfus Med* 18:143, 2008.

221. Armand R, Hess JR: Treating coagulopathy in trauma patients. *Transfus Med Rev* 17:223, 2003.

222. Simmons RL, Collins JA, Heisterkamp CA, et al: Coagulation disorders in combat casualties. I: Acute changes after wounding. II: Effects of massive transfusion. 3. Post-resuscitative changes. *Ann Surg* 169:455, 1969.

223. Gomez R, Murray CK, Hospenthal DR, et al: Causes of mortality by autopsy findings of combat casualties and civilian patients admitted to a burn unit. *J Am Coll Surg* 208:348, 2009.

224. Niles SE, McLaughlin DF, Perkins JG, et al: Increased mortality associated with the early coagulopathy of trauma in combat casualties. *J Trauma* 64:1459, 2008.

225. Kaufman HH, Hui KS, Mattson JC, et al: Clinicopathological correlations of disseminated intravascular coagulation in patients with head injury. *Neurosurgery* 15:34, 1984.

226. Stein SC, Chen XH, Sinson GP, et al: Intravascular coagulation: A major secondary insult in nonfatal traumatic brain injury. *J Neurosurg* 97:1373, 2002.

227. Olson JD, Kaufman HH, Moake J, et al: The incidence and significance of hemostatic abnormalities in patients with head injuries. *Neurosurgery* 24:825, 1989.

228. Selladurai BM, Vickneswaran M, Duraisamy S, et al: Coagulopathy in acute head injury—A study of its role as a prognostic indicator. *Br J Neurosurg* 11:398, 1997.

229. Levi M: Burning issues surrounding inflammation and coagulation in heatstroke. *Crit Care Med* 36:2455, 2008.

230. Garcia-Avello A, Lorente JA, Cesar-Perez J, et al: Degree of hypercoagulability and hyperfibrinolysis is related to organ failure and prognosis after burn trauma. *Thromb Res* 89:59, 1998.

231. Simon TL, Curreri PW, Harker LA: Kinetic characterization of hemostasis in thermal injury. *J Lab Clin Med* 89:702, 1977.

232. Winkelman MD, Galloway PG: Central nervous system complications of thermal burns. A postmortem study of 139 patients. *Medicine (Baltimore)* 71:271, 1992.

233. Carr ME Jr: Disseminated intravascular coagulation: Pathogenesis, diagnosis, and therapy. *J Emerg Med* 5:311, 1987.

234. Tytgat GN, Collen D, Verstraete M: Metabolism of fibrinogen in cirrhosis of the liver. *J Clin Invest* 50:169, 1971.

235. Coleman M, Finlayson N, Bettigole RE, et al: Fibrinogen survival in cirrhosis: Improvement by "low dose" heparin. *Ann Intern Med* 83:79, 1975.

236. Coccheri S, Mannucci PM, Palareti G, et al: Significance of plasma fibrinopeptide A and high molecular weight fibrinogen in patients with liver cirrhosis. *Br J Haematol* 52:503, 1982.

237. Oka K, Tanaka K: Intravascular coagulation in autopsy cases with liver diseases. *Thromb Haemost* 42:564, 1979.

238. Paramo JA, Rifon J, Fernandez J, et al: Thrombin activation and increased fibrinolysis in patients with chronic liver disease. *Blood Coagul Fibrinolysis* 2:227, 1991.

239. Palascak JE, Martinez J: Dysfibrinogenemia associated with liver disease. *J Clin Invest* 60:89, 1977.

240. Ben-Ari Z, Osman E, Hutton RA, et al: Disseminated intravascular coagulation in liver cirrhosis: Fact or fiction? [See comments.] *Am J Gastroenterol* 94:2977, 1999.

241. Hollestelle MJ, Geertzen HG, Straatsburg IH, et al: Factor VIII expression in liver disease. *Thromb Haemost* 91:267, 2004.

242. Straub PW: Diffuse intravascular coagulation in liver disease? *Semin Thromb Hemost* 4:29, 1977.

243. Canoso RT, Hutton RA, Deykin D: The hemostatic defect of chronic liver disease. Kinetic studies using ⁷⁵Se-selenomethionine. *Gastroenterology* 76:540, 1979.

244. Tempero MA, Davis RB, Reed E, et al: Thrombocytopenia and laboratory evidence of disseminated intravascular coagulation after shunts for ascites in malignant disease. *Cancer* 55:2718, 1985.

245. Bakker CM, Knot EA, Stibbe J, et al: Disseminated intravascular coagulation in liver cirrhosis. *J Hepatol* 15:330, 1992.

246. Wakefield FG, Hall WW: Heat injuries: A preparatory study for experimental heatstroke. *JAMA* 89:92, 1927.

247. Chao TC, Sinniah R, Pakiam JE: Acute heat stroke deaths. *Pathology* 13:145, 1981.

248. Bouchama A, Knochel JP: Heat stroke. *N Engl J Med* 346:1978, 2002.

249. Bouchama A, Hammami MM, Haq A, et al: Evidence for endothelial cell activation/injury in heatstroke. *Crit Care Med* 24:1173, 1996.

250. Gauss P, Meyer KA: Heat stroke: Report of one hundred and fifty-eight cases from Cook County Hospital, Chicago. *Am J Med Sci* 154:554, 1917.

251. Huisse MG, Pease S, Hurtado-Nedelec M, et al: Leucocyte activation: The link between inflammation and coagulation during heatstroke. A study of patients during the 2003 heat wave in Paris. *Crit Care Med* 36:2288, 2008.

252. Mustafa KY, Omer O, Khogali M, et al: Blood coagulation and fibrinolysis in heat stroke. *Br J Haematol* 61:517, 1985.

253. Seegers WH, Ouyang C: Snake venoms and blood coagulation, in *Snake Venoms*, edited by L Chen-Yuan, p 684. Springer Verlag, Berlin, 1979.

254. Huang TF, Holt JC, Lukasiewicz H, et al: Trigramin. A low molecular weight peptide inhibiting fibrinogen interaction with platelet receptors expressed on glycoprotein IIb-IIIa complex. *J Biol Chem* 262:16157, 1987.

255. Klein JD, Walker FJ: Purification of a protein C activator from the venom of the southern copperhead snake (*Agkistrodon contortrix contortrix*). *Biochemistry* 25:4175, 1986.

256. Weiss HJ, Phillips LL, Hopewell WS, et al: Heparin therapy in a patient bitten by a saw-scaled viper (*Echis carinatus*), a snake whose venom activates prothrombin. *Am J Med* 54:653, 1973.

257. Schulchynska-Castel H, Dvilansky A, Keynan A: *Echis colorata* bites: Clinical evaluation of 42 patients. A retrospective study. *Isr J Med Sci* 22:880, 1986.

258. Fainaru M, Eisenberg S, Manny N, et al: The natural course of defibrination syndrome caused by *Echis colorata* venom in man. *Thromb Diath Haemorrh* 31:420, 1974.

259. Hall GW: Kasabach-Merritt syndrome: Pathogenesis and management. *Br J Haematol* 112:851, 2001.

260. Straub PW, Kessler S, Schreiber A, et al: Chronic intravascular coagulation in Kasabach-Merritt syndrome. Preferential accumulation of fibrinogen ¹³¹I in a giant hemangioma. *Arch Intern Med* 129:475, 1972.

261. Warrell RPJ, Kempin SJ, Benua RS, et al: Intratumoral consumption of indium-111 labeled platelets in a patient with hemangiomatosis and intravascular coagulation (Kasabach-Merritt syndrome). *Cancer* 52:2256, 1983.

262. Propp RP, Scharfman WB: Hemangioma-thrombocytopenia syndrome associated with microangiopathic hemolytic anemia. *Blood* 28:623, 1966.

263. Hesselmann S, Micke O, Marquardt T, et al: Case report: Kasabach-Merritt syndrome: A review of the therapeutic options and case report of successful treatment with radiotherapy and interferon alpha. *Br J Radiol* 75:180, 2002.

264. Mazoyer E, Enjolras O, Laurian C, et al: Coagulation abnormalities associated with extensive venous malformations of the limbs: Differentiation from Kasabach-Merritt syndrome. *Clin Lab Haematol* 24:243, 2002.

265. Fisher DF Jr, Yawn DH, Crawford ES: Preoperative disseminated intravascular coagulation associated with aortic aneurysms. A prospective study of 76 cases. *Arch Surg* 118:1252, 1983.

266. Bieger R, Vreeken J, Stibbe J, et al: Arterial aneurysm as a cause of consumption coagulopathy. *N Engl J Med* 285:152, 1971.

267. ten Cate JW, Timmers H, Becker AE: Coagulopathy in ruptured or dissecting aortic aneurysms. *Am J Med* 59:171, 1975.

268. Mulcare RJ, Royster TS, Phillips LL: Intravascular coagulation in surgical procedures on the abdominal aorta. *Surg Gynecol Obstet* 143:730, 1976.

269. Wilcox JN, Smith KM, Schwartz SM, et al: Localization of tissue factor in the normal vessel wall and in the atherosclerotic plaque. *Proc Natl Acad Sci U S A* 86:2839, 1989.

270. Cummins D, Segal H, Hunt BJ, et al: Chronic disseminated intravascular coagulation after surgery for abdominal aortic aneurysm: Clinical and haemostatic response to dalteparin. *Br J Haematol* 113:658, 2001.

271. Cross KS, Bouchier-Hayes D, Leahy AL: Consumptive coagulopathy following endovascular stent repair of abdominal aortic aneurysm. *Eur J Vasc Endovasc Surg* 19:94, 2000.

272. Shimazaki T, Ishimaru S, Kawaguchi S, et al: Blood coagulation and fibrinolytic response after endovascular stent grafting of thoracic aorta. *J Vasc Surg* 37:1213, 2003.

273. Mannucci PM, Lobina GF, Caocci L, et al: Effect on blood coagulation of massive intravascular haemolysis. *Blood* 33:207, 1969.

274. Butler J, Parker D, Pillai R, et al: Systemic release of neutrophil elastase and tumour necrosis factor alpha following ABO incompatible blood transfusion. *Br J Haematol* 79:525, 1991.

275. Hamilton KK, Hattori R, Esmon CT, et al: Complement proteins C5b-9 induce vesiculation of the endothelial plasma membrane and expose catalytic surface for assembly of the prothrombinase enzyme complex. *J Biol Chem* 265:3809, 1990.

276. Weiner CP: The obstetric patient and disseminated intravascular coagulation. *Clin Perinatol* 13:705, 1986.

277. Bonnar J: Massive obstetric haemorrhage. *Best Pract Res Clin Obstet Gynaecol* 14:1, 2000.

278. Letsky EA: Disseminated intravascular coagulation. *Best Pract Res Clin Obstet Gynaecol* 15:623, 2001.

279. DeLee JB: A case of fatal hemorrhagic diathesis with premature detachment of the placenta. *Am J Obstet Gynecol* 44:785, 1901.

280. Eskes TK: Abruptio placentae. A "classic" dedicated to Elizabeth Ramsey. *Eur J Obstet Gynecol Reprod Biol* 75:63, 1997.

281. Kuczynski J, Uszynski W, Zekanowska E, et al: Tissue factor (TF) and tissue factor pathway inhibitor (TFPI) in the placenta and myometrium. *Eur J Obstet Gynecol Reprod Biol* 105:15, 2002.

282. Pritchard JA, Brekken AL: Clinical and laboratory studies on severe abruptio placentae. *Am J Obstet Gynecol* 97:681, 1967.

283. Steiner PE, Lushbaugh CC: Maternal pulmonary embolism by amniotic fluid as a cause of obstetric shock and unexpected deaths in obstetrics. *JAMA* 117:1245, 1941.

284. Morgan M: Amniotic fluid embolism. *Anaesthesia* 34:20, 1979.

285. Gilbert WM, Danielsen B: Amniotic fluid embolism: Decreased mortality in a population-based study. *Obstet Gynecol* 93:973, 1999.

286. Uszynski M, Zekanowska E, Uszynski W, et al: Tissue factor (TF) and tissue factor pathway inhibitor (TFPI) in amniotic fluid and blood plasma: Implications for the mechanism of amniotic fluid embolism. *Eur J Obstet Gynecol Reprod Biol* 95:163, 2001.

287. Boer K, den Hartog I, Meijers JC, et al: Tissue factor-dependent blood coagulation is enhanced following delivery irrespective of the mode of delivery. *J Thromb Haemost* 5:2415, 2007.

288. Gibson B, Hunter D, Neame PB, et al: Thrombocytopenia in preeclampsia and eclampsia. *Semin Thromb Hemost* 8:234, 1982.

289. O'Riordan MN, Higgins JR: Haemostasis in normal and abnormal pregnancy. *Best Pract Res Clin Obstet Gynaecol* 17:385, 2003.

290. Levi M: Disseminated intravascular coagulation (DIC) in pregnancy and the peripartum period. *Thromb Res* 123(Suppl 2):S63, 2009.

291. Giles C: Intravascular coagulation in gestational hypertension and pre-eclampsia: The value of haematological screening tests. *Clin Lab Haematol* 4:351, 1982.

292. Norwitz ER, Hsu CD, Repke JT: Acute complications of preeclampsia. *Clin Obstet Gynecol* 45:308, 2002.

293. Weinstein L: Syndrome of hemolysis, elevated liver enzymes, and low platelet count: A severe consequence of hypertension in pregnancy. *Am J Obstet Gynecol* 142:159, 1982.

294. Sibai BM, Ramadan MK, Usta I, et al: Maternal morbidity and mortality in 442 pregnancies with hemolysis, elevated liver enzymes, and low platelets (HELLP syndrome). *Am J Obstet Gynecol* 169:1000, 1993.

295. Aarnoudse JG, Houthoff HJ, Weits J, et al: A syndrome of liver damage and intravascular coagulation in the last trimester of normotensive pregnancy. A clinical and histopathological study. *Br J Obstet Gynaecol* 93:145, 1986.

296. Audibert F, Friedman SA, Frangieh AY, et al: Clinical utility of strict diagnostic criteria for the HELLP (hemolysis, elevated liver enzymes, and low platelets) syndrome. *Am J Obstet Gynecol* 175:460, 1996.

297. Barton JR, Sibai BM: Hepatic imaging in HELLP syndrome (hemolysis, elevated liver enzymes, and low platelet count. *Am J Obstet Gynecol* 174:1820, 1996.

298. Sullivan CA, Magann EF, Perry KG Jr, et al: The recurrence risk of the syndrome of hemolysis, elevated liver enzymes, and low platelets (HELLP) in subsequent gestations. *Am J Obstet Gynecol* 171:940, 1994.

299. Lee W, Clark SL, Cotton DB, et al: Septic shock during pregnancy. *Am J Obstet Gynecol* 159:410, 1988.

300. Romero R, Copel JA, Hobbins JC: Intrauterine fetal demise and hemostatic failure: The fetal death syndrome. *Clin Obstet Gynecol* 28:24, 1985.

301. Berkowitz RL, Stone JL, Eddleman KA: One hundred consecutive cases of selective termination of an abnormal fetus in a multifetal gestation. *Obstet Gynecol* 90:606, 1997.

302. Hay JE: Liver disease in pregnancy. *Hepatology* 47:1067, 2008.

303. Bacq Y, Riely CA: Acute fatty liver of pregnancy: The hepatologist's view. *Gastroenterologist* 1:257, 1993.

304. Usta IM, Barton JR, Amon EA, et al: Acute fatty liver of pregnancy: An experience in the diagnosis and management of fourteen cases. *Am J Obstet Gynecol* 171:1342, 1994.

305. Pereira SP, O'Donohue J, Wendon J, et al: Maternal and perinatal outcome in severe pregnancy-related liver disease. *Hepatology* 26:1258, 1997.

306. Rahman TM, Wendon J: Severe hepatic dysfunction in pregnancy. *Q J Med* 95:343, 2002.

307. Ibdah JA, Yang Z, Bennett MJ: Liver disease in pregnancy and fetal fatty acid oxidation defects. *Mol Genet Metab* 71:182, 2000.

308. Castro MA, Goodwin TM, Shaw KJ, et al: Disseminated intravascular coagulation and antithrombin III depression in acute fatty liver of pregnancy. *Am J Obstet Gynecol* 174:211, 1996.

309. Watson WJ, Seeds JW: Acute fatty liver of pregnancy. *Obstet Gynecol Surv* 45:585, 1990.

310. Moldenhauer JS, O'Brien JM, Barton JR, et al: Acute fatty liver of pregnancy associated with pancreatitis: A life-threatening complication. *Am J Obstet Gynecol* 190:502, 2004.

311. Hathaway WE, Mull MM, Pechet GS: Disseminated intravascular coagulation in the newborn. *Pediatrics* 43:233, 1969.

312. Corrigan JJ Jr: Activation of coagulation and disseminated intravascular coagulation in the newborn. *Am J Pediatr Hematol Oncol* 1:245, 1979.

313. Williams MD, Chalmers EA, Gibson BE: The investigation and management of neonatal haemostasis and thrombosis. *Br J Haematol* 119:295, 2002.

314. Buchanan GR: Coagulation disorders in the neonate. *Pediatr Clin North Am* 33:203, 1986.

315. Stanworth SJ, Bennett C: How to tackle bleeding and thrombosis in the newborn. *Early Hum Dev* 84:507, 2008.

316. Corrigan JJ Jr, Ray WL, May N: Changes in the blood coagulation system associated with septicemia. *N Engl J Med* 279:851, 1968.

317. Levi M, de Jonge E, van der Poll T: New treatment strategies for disseminated intravascular coagulation based on current understanding of the pathophysiology. *Ann Med* 36:41, 2004.

318. Alving BM, Spivak JL, DeLoughery TG: Consultative hematology: Hemostasis and transfusion issues in surgery and critical care medicine, in *The American Society of Hematology Education Program Book*, edited by JR McArthur, GP Schechter, SL Schrier, p 320. American Society of Hematology, Washington, DC, 1998.

319. de Jonge E, Levi M, Stoutenbeek CP, et al: Current drug treatment strategies for disseminated intravascular coagulation. *Drugs* 55:767, 1998.

320. de Jonge E, van der Poll T, Kesecioglu J, et al: Anticoagulant factor concentrates in disseminated intravascular coagulation: Rationale for use and clinical experience. *Semin Thromb Hemost* 27:667, 2001.

321. Abraham E: Coagulation abnormalities in acute lung injury and sepsis. *Am J Respir Cell Mol Biol* 22:401, 2000.

322. Levi M, Schouten M, van der Poll T: Sepsis, coagulation, and antithrombin: Old lessons and new insights. *Semin Thromb Hemost* 34:742, 2008.

323. Fourrier F, Chopin C, Huart JJ, et al: Double-blind, placebo-controlled trial of antithrombin III concentrates in septic shock with disseminated intravascular coagulation. *Chest* 104:882, 1993.

324. Eisele B, Lamy M, Thijs LG, et al: Antithrombin III in patients with severe sepsis. A randomized, placebo-controlled, double-blind multicenter trial plus a meta-analysis on all randomized, placebo-controlled, double-blind trials with antithrombin III in severe sepsis. *Intensive Care Med* 24:663, 1998.

325. Baudo F, Caimi TM, de CF, et al: Antithrombin III (ATIII) replacement therapy in patients with sepsis and/or postsurgical complications: A controlled double-blind, randomized, multicenter study. *Intensive Care Med* 24:336, 1998.

326. Warren BL, Eid A, Singer P, et al: Caring for the critically ill patient. High-dose antithrombin III in severe sepsis: A randomized controlled trial. *JAMA* 286:1869, 2001.

327. Tagami T, Matsui H, Horiguchi H, Fushimi K, Yasunaga H: Antithrombin and mortality in severe pneumonia patients with sepsis-associated disseminated intravascular coagulation: An observational nationwide study. *J Thromb Haemost* 12(9):1470–1479, 2014.

328. Iba T, Saitoh D, Wada H, Asakura H: Efficacy and bleeding risk of antithrombin supplementation in septic disseminated intravascular coagulation: A secondary survey. *Crit Care* 18(5):497, 2014.

329. Bernard GR, Vincent JL, Laterre PF, et al: Efficacy and safety of recombinant human activated protein C for severe sepsis. *N Engl J Med* 344(10):699–709, 2001.

330. Dhainaut JF, Yan SB, Joyce DE, et al: Treatment effects of drotrecogin alfa (activated) in patients with severe sepsis with or without overt disseminated intravascular coagulation. *J Thromb Haemost* 2:1924–1933, 2004.

331. Levi M: Activated protein C in sepsis: A critical review. *Curr Opin Hematol* 15(5):481–486, 2008.

332. Ranieri VM, Thompson BT, Barie PS, et al: Drotrecogin alfa (activated) in adults with septic shock. *N Engl J Med* 366(22):2055–2064, 2012.

333. Thachil J, Toh CH, Levi M, Watson HG: The withdrawal of activated protein C from the use in patients with severe sepsis and DIC [amendment to the BCSH guideline on disseminated intravascular coagulation]. *Br J Haematol* 157(4):493–494, 2012.

334. Levi M, van der Poll T: Thrombomodulin in sepsis. *Minerva Anestesiol* 79(3):294–298, 2013.

335. Tsuruta K, Yamada Y, Serada M, Tanigawara Y: Model-based analysis of covariate effects on population pharmacokinetics of thrombomodulin alfa in patients with disseminated intravascular coagulation and normal subjects. *J Clin Pharmacol* 51(9):1276–1285, 2011.

336. Saito H, Maruyama I, Shimazaki S, et al: Efficacy and safety of recombinant human soluble thrombomodulin (ART-123) in disseminated intravascular coagulation: Results of a phase III, randomized, double-blind clinical trial. *J Thromb Haemost* 5(1):31–41, 2007.

337. Vincent JL, Ramesh MK, Ernest D, et al: A randomized, double-blind, placebo-controlled, phase 2b study to evaluate the safety and efficacy of recombinant human soluble thrombomodulin, ART-123, in patients with sepsis and suspected disseminated intravascular coagulation. *Crit Care Med* 41(9):2069–2079, 2013.

338. Yamakawa K, Aihara M, Ogura H, Yuhara H, Hamasaki T, Shimazu T: Recombinant human soluble thrombomodulin in severe sepsis: A systematic review and meta-analysis. *J Thromb Haemost* 13(4):508–519, 2015.

339. Levi M: Recombinant soluble thrombomodulin: Coagulation takes another chance to reduce sepsis mortality. *J Thromb Haemost* 13(4):505–507, 2015.

340. du Toit H, Coetzee AR, Chalton DO: Heparin treatment in thrombin-induced disseminated intravascular coagulation in the baboon. *Crit Care Med* 19:1195, 1991.

341. Pernerstorfer T, Hollenstein U, Hansen JB, et al: Lepirudin blunts endotoxin-induced coagulation activation. *Blood* 95:1729, 2000.

342. Feinstein DI: Diagnosis and management of disseminated intravascular coagulation: The role of heparin therapy. *Blood* 60:284, 1982.

343. Levi M, Levy M, Williams MD, et al: Prophylactic heparin in patients with severe sepsis treated with drotrecogin alfa (activated). *Am J Respir Crit Care Med* 176:483, 2007.

344. Vlasuk GP, Bergum PW, Bradbury AE, et al: Clinical evaluation of rNAPc2, an inhibitor of the fVIIa/tissue factor coagulation complex. *Am J Cardiol* 80:66S, 1997.

345. Abraham E, Reinhart K, Svoboda P, et al: Assessment of the safety of recombinant tissue factor pathway inhibitor in patients with severe sepsis: A multicenter, randomized, placebo-controlled, single-blind, dose escalation study. *Crit Care Med* 29:2081, 2001.

346. Abraham E, Reinhart K, Opal S, et al: Efficacy and safety of tifacogin (recombinant tissue factor pathway inhibitor) in severe sepsis: A randomized controlled trial. *JAMA* 290:238, 2003.

347. Saito H, Maruyama I, Shimazaki S, et al: Efficacy and safety of recombinant human soluble thrombomodulin (ART-123) in disseminated intravascular coagulation: Results of a phase III, randomized, double-blind clinical trial. *J Thromb Haemost* 5:31, 2007.

348. Gralnick HR, Greipp P: Thrombosis with epsilon aminocaproic acid therapy. *Am J Clin Pathol* 56:151, 1971.

349. Naeye RL: Thrombotic state after a hemorrhagic diathesis, a possible complication of therapy with epsilon-aminocaproic acid. *Blood* 19:694, 1962.

350. Mannucci PM, Levi M: Prevention and treatment of major blood loss. *N Engl J Med* 356:2301, 2007.

351. Minna JD, Robboy SJ, Colman RW: *Disseminated Intravascular Coagulation in Man.* Charles C Thomas, Springfield, IL, 1974.

352. Matsuda M, Aoki N: Statistics on underlying and causative diseases of DIC in Japan, in *Disseminated Intravascular Coagulation*, edited by T Abe, M Yamanake, p 15. Karger, Basel, 1983.

353. Larcan A, Lambert H, Gerard A: *Consumption Coagulopathies.* Masson, New York, 1987.

# CHAPTER 20
# HEREDITARY THROMBOPHILIA

Saskia Middeldorp and Michiel Coppens

## SUMMARY

Thrombophilia refers to laboratory abnormalities that increase the risk of venous thromboembolism (VTE). Over the past several decades, numerous factors have been identified. The most prevalent examples of hereditary forms of thrombophilia include the factor V Leiden and prothrombin G20210A mutations; deficiencies of the natural anticoagulants antithrombin, protein C, and protein S; persistently elevated levels of coagulation factor VIII; and mild hyperhomocysteinemia. Taken together, some form of hereditary thrombophilia can be identified in more than 50 percent of patients with VTE who are without obvious reasons for VTE, such as trauma or prolonged stasis. Moreover, hereditary thrombophilia has been associated with arterial cardiovascular disease and obstetric complications such as (recurrent) pregnancy loss and preeclampsia. The high yield of thrombophilia testing has led to widespread testing for these abnormalities in patients. Nevertheless, thrombophilia testing remains a topic of ongoing debate, mostly because of the lack of evidence-based therapeutic consequences. While hereditary thrombophilia is a clear risk factor for a first VTE, the risk for recurrent episodes is only slightly increased compared with non-affected patients, and prolonged anticoagulation is probably not warranted unless VTE is recurrent. A similar lack of therapeutic consequences applies to patients with arterial cardiovascular disease and women with obstetric complications. Thrombophilia testing in asymptomatic relatives of patients with VTE may be useful in families with antithrombin, protein C, or protein S deficiency, or for siblings of patients who are homozygous for factor V Leiden, and is limited to women who intend to become pregnant or who would like to use oral contraceptives. Careful counseling with knowledge of absolute risks helps patients to make an informed decision in which their own preferences can be taken into account.

To our knowledge, the term *thrombophilia* was first used by Nygaard and Brown in 1937, when they described sudden occlusion of large arteries, sometimes with coexistent venous thrombosis.[1] In 1956, Jordan and Nandorff extensively reviewed their own and previously published cases on the familial tendency in thromboembolic disease.[2] The term *thrombophilia* was then used to describe patients with prominent manifestations of venous thromboembolism (VTE; venous thrombosis in any site or pulmonary embolism) such as recurrent spontaneous VTE, VTE at young age, a strong family history of VTE, or thrombosis in an unusual site, such as the splanchnic veins or cerebral sinuses. Currently, the term *thrombophilia* is generally used for laboratory abnormalities, usually in the coagulation system, which increase the risk of VTE. Thrombophilia can be either acquired or hereditary. An example of acquired thrombophilia is the antiphospholipid syndrome, which is characterized by a tendency toward venous or arterial thrombosis or pregnancy complications, in combination with persistent lupus anticoagulant or antibodies to cardiolipin or $\beta_2$-glycoprotein-1 (Chap. 21). Furthermore, there are many acquired and transient conditions that lead to a prothrombotic state, including cancer, surgery, strict immobilization, pregnancy and the postpartum period, and the use of estrogen-containing medication, such as oral contraceptives and hormone replacement therapy.

Patients with hereditary thrombophilia have an increased risk of developing VTE, and just like in patients without thrombophilia, approximately half of patients will develop their first episode in relation to an acquired prothrombotic risk factor. Moreover, despite young age being a criterion for thrombophilia and the mean age at time of a first thrombosis being approximately 10 years lower than in the general population, the majority of patients with thrombophilia will have the first episode later in life.[3] The theoretical concept is that patients with thrombophilia have an intrinsic prothrombotic state, which in itself is insufficient to cause thrombosis, but may lead to an event when superimposed upon (clinical) risk factors, including increasing age.[3]

The role of hereditary thrombophilia in arterial cardiovascular disease has been extensively studied.[4,5] Most of those studies did not demonstrate significant associations between hereditary thrombophilia and arterial disease, with the exception of patients with events before the age of 55 years.[5] Moreover, the relative risk increase was very modest (odds ratios [OR] of 1.1 to 1.8) in studies that did find significant associations, indicating that hereditary thrombophilia is not a major risk factor for arterial cardiovascular disease.[4]

Like the acquired antiphospholipid syndrome, most hereditary thrombophilias are also modestly associated with pregnancy-related disorders such as (recurrent) miscarriage, stillbirth, intrauterine growth retardation, preeclampsia, and the hemolysis, elevated liver enzymes, and low platelets (HELLP) syndrome of pregnancy, although for later pregnancy complications, this association is controversial.[6–8]

In the past decades, hereditary thrombophilia has evolved from a very rare genetic disorder to a prevalent trait. This evolution is a direct consequence of increasing insight into the blood coagulation system, as well as advanced genetic research tools that allowed the search for abnormalities in candidate coagulation proteins and their encoding genes. At present, some form of thrombophilia can be identified in about half of the patients presenting with VTE. Likely inspired by the high yield of thrombophilia testing, testing has increased tremendously for various indications,[9] but whether the results of such tests help in the clinical management of patients has still not been settled.[10,11] This chapter provides an overview of the most important hereditary thrombophilias and of the history of thrombophilia research. It reviews the risks associated with the most commonly tested thrombophilias and provides guidance on the indications and potential implications of the results of thrombophilia testing in various patient groups.

---

**Acronyms and Abbreviations:** APC, activated protein C; ASA, acetylsalicylic acid; CI, confidence interval; HELLP, hemolysis, elevated liver enzymes, low platelets; LMWH, low-molecular-weight heparin; MTHFR, methylenetetrahydrofolate reductase; OR, odds ratio; VKA, vitamin K antagonist; VTE, venous thromboembolism; VWF, von Willebrand factor.

# HISTORY, CLASSIFICATION, PATHOPHYSIOLOGY, AND PREVALENCE OF THROMBOPHILIA

## HISTORY OF THROMBOPHILIA RESEARCH

Research into thrombophilia began with the investigation of candidate coagulation proteins and their genes in highly thrombophilic families and linking abnormalities with the clinical phenotype within these families. As a next step, findings were confirmed in case-control studies, which yielded risk increases compared to controls, often derived from the general population. For clinicians and patients, however, absolute risk estimates were needed to guide decisions regarding prevention or treatment. These were sought again in family studies of consecutive probands with a specific thrombophilic defect. The major progress in genetic and bioinformatics techniques now allows investigation in populations of patients with VTE, as well as in thrombophilic families.[12–14]

In 1965, deficiency of the natural anticoagulant antithrombin became the first hereditary thrombophilia when Egeberg reported a Norwegian family with a remarkable tendency to VTE.[15] Deficiencies of the other anticoagulant proteins, that is, protein C and protein S, were discovered as hereditary risk factors for VTE in the early 1980s.[16,17] By that time, genes could be cloned, and numerous mutations in the genes encoding antithrombin, protein C, and protein S had been identified as underlying causes of low plasma levels of the anticoagulant proteins.[18–20] Another decade later, in 1993, Dahlbäck and colleagues described the phenomenon of activated protein C (APC) resistance, a poor anticoagulant response to APC, in a Swedish family with an increased tendency to develop VTE.[21] The genetic basis for this APC resistance was discovered independently in several laboratories in 1995 and is caused by a single point mutation in the factor V gene, which was termed *factor V Leiden*.[22–25] In 1996, genetic analysis of prothrombin revealed a G-to-A transition at position 20210 that was more common in patients with VTE and a strong family history of this disease than in healthy controls without VTE.[26] In the 1970s, it was found that individuals with non–O blood group have an increased risk of VTE.[27] Individuals with non–O blood group have higher levels of von Willebrand factor (VWF) and factor VIII than people with blood group O, which was the presumed mechanism of increased risk. In 1995, data from the Leiden Thrombophilia Study, a case-control study of patients with VTE and matched healthy controls, demonstrated that increased factor VIII (FVIII) activity, but not VWF activity, was independently associated with an increased risk of VTE.[28] Homocysteine is an intermediary amino acid formed by the conversion of methionine to cysteine. Homocystinuria or severe hyperhomocysteinemia is a rare autosomal recessive disorder characterized by severe elevations in plasma and urine homocysteine concentrations. This disease is characterized by developmental delay, osteoporosis, ocular abnormalities, and severe occlusive vascular disease. About half of the vascular complications are of venous origin.[29] Mild hyperhomocysteinemia was therefore studied as a risk factor for VTE in the 1990s, and homocysteine levels exceeding the 95th percentile of the normal population were confirmed to be a risk factor for VTE.[30]

Since then, numerous genetic variants that increase the risk of VTE to a more or lesser extent have been identified and are variably included in diagnostic panels of thrombophilia testing.[31] Essentially, the majority of hereditary thrombophilias exert their effect either by upregulation of procoagulant clotting factors or by downregulation of anticoagulant factors (Fig. 20–1). An overview of the common hereditary thrombophilias that increase the risk at least twofold and their prevalence in patients with VTE and in the general population is presented in Table 20–1. For these more common thrombophilias, a large number of clinical studies provided reliable estimates of the relative and absolute risk for VTE.

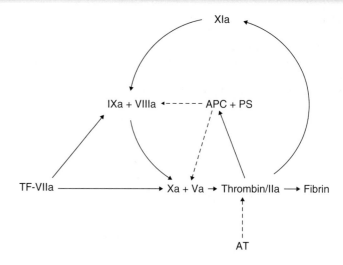

**Figure 20–1.** Regulation of blood coagulation. Coagulation is initiated by a tissue factor (TF)–factor VIIa complex that can activate factor IX or factor X. At high TF concentrations, factor X is activated primarily by the TF-VIIa complex, whereas at low TF concentrations, the contribution of the factor IXa–factor VIIIa complex to the activation of factor X becomes more pronounced. Coagulation is maintained through the activation by thrombin of factor XI. The coagulation system is regulated by the protein C pathway. Thrombin activates protein C. Together with protein S (PS), activated protein C (APC) is capable of inactivating factors Va and VIIIa, which results in a downregulation of thrombin generation and consequently in an upregulation of the fibrinolytic system. The activity of thrombin is controlled by the inhibitor antithrombin (AT). The *solid arrows* indicate activation and the *broken arrows* inhibition.

## CLASSIFICATION, PATHOPHYSIOLOGY, AND PREVALENCE OF COMMON HEREDITARY THROMBOPHILIA

### Deficiencies of the Natural Anticoagulants Antithrombin, Protein C, and Protein S

Deficiencies of the natural anticoagulants antithrombin, protein C, and protein S were among the first established hereditary thrombophilias. For antithrombin and protein C, two types of deficiencies are distinguished. In type I deficiency, levels of both antigen and activity are reduced, and in type II, antigen levels are normal, but one or more functional defects in the molecule lead to a decreased activity. Type II antithrombin

**TABLE 20–1.** Prevalence of Common Hereditary Thrombophilia

|  | General Population | Patients with VTE |
|---|---|---|
| Antithrombin, protein S, or protein C deficiency | 1%[42,43,44] | 7%[41] |
| Factor V Leiden | Whites 4–7%[46,118] Nonwhites 0–1% | 21%[22] |
| Prothrombin G20210A | Whites 2–3%[56,119] Nonwhites 0–1% | 6% |
| Elevated FVIII:c levels | 11%[28] | 25%[28] |
| Mild hyperhomocysteinemia | 5%[30] | 10%[30] |

FVIII, factor VIII; VTE, venous thromboembolism.

deficiencies are further subdivided according to the site of the defect in antithrombin. The defect is located in the thrombin binding domain (i.e., the reactive site) in type IIa deficiency and in the heparin binding domain in type IIb deficiency; type IIc deficiency comprises a pleiotropic group of mutations.[32] Interestingly, patients with type IIb deficiency seem to have a significantly lower risk of VTE than patients with other types.[32] Protein S circulates in two forms: free protein S (approximately 40 to 50 percent), which functions as a cofactor for APC, and protein S bound to complement component C4b-binding protein. In type I deficiency, total and free antigen levels and activity are all reduced; in type II deficiency, total and free antigen are normal but activity is reduced; and in type III deficiency, activity and free antigen are reduced, while total antigen is low to normal. Type I and type III are probably phenotypical variants of the same disease because family members with the same DNA mutation can present with either type I or type III deficiency.[33] Whether this classification into various subtypes is truly clinically relevant for any of the deficiencies of the natural anticoagulants is largely unknown. Moreover, most laboratory panels now only test the activity of antithrombin, protein C, or protein S, and thereby do not distinguish between different types of deficiencies. Homozygous antithrombin deficiency is extremely rare, and the only reported cases involve type IIb deficiencies.[34] Homozygous type I deficiency has never been described in humans and is believed to be incompatible with life. Complete antithrombin deficiency in knockout mice leads to embryonic death.[35] Homozygous protein C and protein S deficiencies are also very rare, and these are associated with neonatal purpura fulminans and massive thrombosis.[36,37] In a similar fashion, warfarin-induced skin necrosis has been described in patients with heterozygous protein C or S deficiencies after initiation of vitamin K antagonists (VKAs).[38,39] The concept is that after VKA initiation vitamin K–dependent protein C and S levels drop sooner than levels of factors II, IX, and X, thereby temporarily causing a paradoxical procoagulant state.[40] This is, however, a rare clinical complication, possibly resulting from concomitant treatment with (low-molecular-weight) heparin in the acute phase of VTE. Deficiencies can be caused by a large number of mutations, which are recorded in occasionally updated databases.[18-20]

Overall, deficiencies of the natural anticoagulants are rare (see Table 20–1). In cohorts of consecutive patients with VTE, the prevalence of a deficiency of one of the natural anticoagulants is below 10 percent.[41] In the general population, the prevalence of the deficiencies combined is approximately 1 percent.[42-44]

### Factor V Leiden/Factor V G1691A

In 1993, Dahlbäck and colleagues first described APC resistance in a Swedish family with a high tendency of VTE.[21] In the original paper, Dahlbäck proposed that APC resistance was best explained by a hereditary deficiency of a previously unrecognized cofactor to APC, after having ruled out several possible mechanisms, including deficiencies of protein S and protein C, or linkage with polymorphisms in the FVIII or VWF genes. He then showed that this "cofactor" was identical to coagulation factor V.[21] Soon thereafter, several laboratories reported independently from each other the underlying genetic defect, a single G-to-A substitution in the gene of factor V at nucleotide position 1691, resulting in an amino acid change from arginine (Arg) to glutamine (Gln) at position 506, the first cleavage site of factor Va for APC[22-25] (Fig. 20–2). The mutation was named factor V Leiden after the city in the Netherlands in which the group with the first publication was located.[22] The proteolytic inactivation of activated factor V (FVa) is approximately 10 times slower for Gln506-FVa compared with Arg506-FVa, which explains the partial, but not full, resistance to APC.[45] Factor V Leiden is the most common hereditary thrombophilia. In unselected consecutive patients with VTE, the prevalence is 20 to 25 percent.[22] The prevalence in the general population varies considerably between different ethnic groups. Factor V Leiden is very rare among Asians and Africans but has a high prevalence (approximately 5 percent) among whites (see Table 20–1).[46] Within Europe, the prevalence is higher in the north than in the south.[46] This implies a founder effect that suggests that the mutation occurred after the separation of non-Africans from Africans and after the divergence of whites and Asians. Studies using linkage disequilibria between factor V Leiden and specific markers indicate that the mutation occurred around 21,000 years ago.[47] The high prevalence of factor V Leiden suggests an evolutionary benefit.[48]

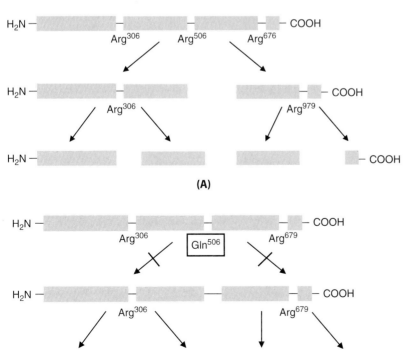

**Figure 20–2.** Pathophysiology of the factor V Leiden mutation. **A.** Activated protein C inactivates factor Va by cleaving the protein at the arginine (Arg)[506] cleavage site. **B.** In carriers of the factor V Leiden mutation, a point mutation in the gene coding for factor V causes replacement of the amino acid arginine by glutamine (Gln) at position 506 of the protein, making factor Va resistant to inactivation by activated protein C (i.e., APC resistance).

The presumed mechanism is reduced peripartum and menstrual blood loss in affected female carriers.[49,50] More recently, factor V Leiden was associated with increased sperm counts and a shorter conception time in affected male and female carriers, suggesting another evolutionary benefit.[51–53] The mechanism for this increased fertility is unknown.

### Prothrombin G20210A

The prothrombin G20210A mutation was discovered in 1996 by genetic analysis of the prothrombin gene in families with a strong tendency of VTE and confirmed in a case-control study of patients with VTE.[26] The mutation is located in the 3′-untranslated region of the prothrombin gene and augments translation and stability of prothrombin messenger RNA.[54] This leads to an average 32 percent higher blood levels of the zymogen prothrombin that is structurally identical to the protein produced by patients with the wild-type gene.[26] In unselected patients with VTE, the prevalence of prothrombin G20210A is approximately 6 percent.[55] Like factor V Leiden, the prothrombin G20210A mutation is found largely in whites, and genetic linkage disequilibrium studies date the mutation back to 24,000 years ago.[47,56] Within Europe, the prevalence of the mutation increases from 3 to 5 percent in southern Europe and the Middle East to 1 to 2 percent in northern Europe, which opposes the observed geographical gradient of factor V Leiden.[56]

### Increased Levels of Factor VIII

Most of coagulation FVIII circulates in complex with VWF. Therefore, determinants of VWF, including ABO blood group and endothelial stimulation, indirectly also determine FVIII levels.[57] Furthermore, many other factors have been associated with high FVIII levels, including increasing age, high body mass index, diabetes mellitus, and hypertriglyceridemia.[57] High FVIII levels are part of acute-phase reactions, and sustained increases are observed during pregnancy, surgery, chronic inflammation, malignancy, liver disease, hyperthyroidism, and renal disease. In most of these conditions, there is a concordant increase of FVIII and VWF levels.[57] Apart from ABO blood group, the genetic causes of high FVIII levels are largely unknown. Nevertheless, persistence over time and familial clustering of high FVIII levels in patients with VTE imply that genetic factors are prevalent. In a family study of consecutive patients with persistently elevated levels of FVIII of at least 150 percent and venous or arterial thrombosis, the prevalence of high FVIII in first-degree family members was 40 percent, which is almost in the range with what one would expect from an autosomal dominant inheritance.[58] Despite the uncertainty about the mechanisms of high FVIII levels, the association between high FVIII levels and venous thrombosis is well established. The very clear dose-dependent relationship between FVIII levels and the risk of VTE suggests that elevated FVIII is causative for thrombosis.[28] Interestingly, increased FVIII levels in patients with VTE are usually not influenced by acute-phase reactions.[57] The prevalence of elevated FVIII levels is high: 25 percent of patients with a first episode of deep vein thrombosis and 11 percent of healthy control subjects have FVIII levels of 150 percent or higher.[28] Hence, an increased level of FVIII is the most common familial, albeit not monogenetic, thrombophilia, with an estimated population attributable risk of 15 percent.[57] Whether measurement of FVIII levels should be part of a hereditary thrombophilia panel is debatable as FVIII levels may be transiently increased by a multitude of external factors including the acute VTE episode itself (Table 20–2). This leads to a significant proportion of "false-positive" test results, a necessity for repeat testing, and potentially unnecessary concern among tested patients.

### Mild Hyperhomocysteinemia

Homocysteine is an intermediate in the metabolism of the amino acids methionine and cysteine and participates in several metabolic pathways.

| **TABLE 20–2.** Acquired Conditions That Can Yield False-Positive Thrombophilia Test Results | |
|---|---|
| **Test** | **Acquired Conditions That Can Cause Abnormal Test Results** |
| Increased activated protein C (APC) resistance | Pregnancy, use of oral contraceptives, stroke, presence of lupus anticoagulant, increased factor VIII levels, autoantibodies against APC |
| Factor V Leiden | — |
| Prothrombin G20210A | — |
| Hyperhomocysteinemia | Deficiencies of folate (vitamin $B_{11}$), vitamin $B_{12}$, or vitamin $B_6$, old age, renal failure, excessive consumption of coffee, smoking |
| Increased factor VIII levels | Pregnancy, use of oral contraceptives, exercise, stress, older age, acute-phase response, liver disease, hyperthyroidism, cancer |
| Decreased level of protein C | Liver disease, use of vitamin K antagonist (VKA), vitamin K deficiency, childhood, disseminated intravascular coagulation, presence of autoantibodies against protein C |
| Decreased level of free protein S | Liver disease, use of VKA, vitamin K deficiency, pregnancy, use of oral contraceptives, nephrotic syndrome, childhood, presence of autoantibodies against protein S, disseminated intravascular coagulation |
| Decreased level of antithrombin | Use of heparin, thrombosis, disseminated intravascular coagulation, liver disease, nephrotic syndrome |

Some of the enzymes involved in homocysteine metabolism are dependent on vitamin $B_6$, folic acid, and vitamin $B_{12}$, and deficiencies lead to hyperhomocysteinemia. A polymorphism in the enzyme methylenetetrahydrofolate reductase (MTHFR), c.C677T, leads to an alanine to valine substitution at position 222, resulting in a variant enzyme with reduced activity and increased thermolability. Homozygosity for this polymorphism leads to 24 percent increased homocysteine levels and is the most common genetic cause of mild hyperhomocysteinemia.[59] The prevalence is 10 to 20 percent in whites and 10 percent in Orientals, but it is rare in Africans.[60] Many other conditions are associated with hyperhomocysteinemia, including renal failure, hypothyroidism, smoking, excessive coffee consumption, inflammatory bowel disease, psoriasis, and rheumatoid arthritis.[61] Severe hyperhomocysteinemia (plasma levels exceeding 100 $\mu$mol/L), also named homocystinuria, is a rare autosomal recessive disorder clearly associated with vascular occlusive disease.[29] Because of this association, mildly increased levels (exceeding the 95th percentile of the normal population) were studied as a risk factor for venous and arterial thrombosis. In the Leiden Thrombophilia Study, mild hyperhomocysteinemia was associated with a 2.5-fold increased risk of first VTE.[30] Interestingly, the association of homocysteine levels with VTE was stronger in men than in women and increased with age.[30] The mechanism by which hyperhomocysteinemia would lead to thrombosis is unknown. A 2005 meta-analysis that included more than 50 studies with more than 8000 cases of VTE confirmed the association of VTE with hyperhomocysteinemia and also demonstrated a 20 percent higher VTE risk in MTHFR 677TT carriers compared with 677CC carriers.[62] The association between homocysteine levels is again under scrutiny in newer studies. The single largest case-control study of more than 4000 patients with a first VTE found no association between MTHFR 677TT and VTE.[63] Furthermore, a family study of probands with mild hyperhomocysteinemia and venous or arterial thrombosis found that the association between homocysteine and VTE disappeared after adjustment for FVIII levels.[64] Finally, homocysteine lowering by B vitamins did not reduce the incidence of recurrent events both in patients with VTE as well as in patients with arterial cardiovascular disease.[65,66] As a result of these studies, homocysteine testing (either its levels or polymorphisms) as part of a thrombophilia panel has been largely abandoned.

## PITFALLS IN LABORATORY TESTING FOR HEREDITARY THROMBOPHILIA

Testing for hereditary thrombophilia is performed in many patients, or family members of patients, with various thromboembolic diseases or pregnancy complications.[9] However, it is important to realize that many acquired, often transient, conditions may affect the test results. Most known is the use of VKAs, which reduces the levels of anticoagulant factors protein C and protein S, which can thereby mimic severe deficiencies. Another example is pregnancy, which reduces free protein S levels and increases APC resistance and FVIII levels.[67] However, other factors can also affect test results and should be considered in the interpretation of results or, better yet, in the timing of testing. Table 20–2 presents an overview of acquired conditions that can yield false-positive thrombophilia tests. For deficiencies of the natural anticoagulants as well as for elevated FVIII levels, repeated testing should be performed to exclude spuriously abnormal tests. Genetic testing for deficiencies of the natural anticoagulants is not performed because of the large number of known mutations. The hereditary nature of deficiencies must be established by confirming the abnormality in a first-degree family member.

## ● HEREDITARY THROMBOPHILIA AND THE RISK OF DISEASE

### VENOUS THROMBOEMBOLISM

The relative risk of a first episode of VTE in individuals with a form of common hereditary thrombophilia ranges from 2 to 11 (Table 20–3). These figures were derived from family and population-based cohort or case-control studies.[11] Individuals homozygous for the prothrombin G20210A or factor V Leiden mutations are at higher risk for VTE than

heterozygotes. Likewise, patients with combined thrombophilic disorders have a higher risk of VTE than those with a single defect.[11] One can estimate the absolute risk of VTE by multiplying the relative risk with the absolute incidence in cohorts from the general population, in which the risk of first VTE is approximately 0.2 to 0.3 per 100 person-years.[68] However, because this may lead to imprecise estimates, it is preferable to use absolute risk estimates derived from cohort studies. Retrospective cohort studies may produce less reliable incidence estimates because retrospective studies carry the risk of (unconscious) selection of patients and data and the clinical diagnosis of VTE may not have been confirmed by objective tests. Prospective cohort studies of asymptomatic carriers of hereditary thrombophilic defects are probably better suited to estimate the true incidence of thrombosis in thrombophilic patients. It is important to note that cohort studies have been mainly performed in relatives of (consecutive) patients with a particular thrombophilic defect. Absolute risk estimates from family studies are higher than from population-based studies. Even in the absence of any hereditary thrombophilia, the risk of VTE is still two-fold increased in first-degree family members of patients with VTE.[69] This suggests cosegregation of other, unmeasured or unknown thrombophilias. Table 20–4 presents absolute risk estimates for a first-episode VTE for asymptomatic carriers with a family history of VTE. These risk estimates can be used to counsel both affected and unaffected family members about their risk of VTE. These studies also provide absolute risk estimates for VTE associated with exogenous additional risk factors such as surgery, trauma or immobilization, and pregnancy or use of hormonal contraception (Table 20–4). These incidences are derived from retrospective family studies, as prospective studies are limited by shorter follow-up duration and reduced power.

### Thrombophilia and the Risk of Recurrent Venous Thromboembolism

Regardless of thrombophilia, the absolute risk of a recurrent episode is much higher than the risk of a first episode of VTE. The most important determinant of recurrence is the presence of transient clinical risk factors during the time of the first episode.[70] After an unprovoked first episode of VTE, the risk of recurrence is approximately 10 percent in the first year after cessation of anticoagulation and approximately 5 percent per year thereafter.[70] The risk is lower after VTE that was associated with a transient risk factor, with an incidence in the first 2 years of 0.7 percent per year for surgery-provoked VTE and 4.2 percent per year for VTE provoked by estrogen use, pregnancy, temporary immobilization, or trauma.[70] Other determinants for recurrence are male sex, proximal

**TABLE 20–3.** Relative Risk Estimates for Common Hereditary Thrombophilias and Venous or Arterial Thrombosis and Pregnancy Complications

| | Relative Risk | | | |
| --- | --- | --- | --- | --- |
| | First VTE | Recurrent VTE | Arterial Thrombosis | Pregnancy Complications |
| Antithrombin deficiency | 5–10 | 1.9–2.6 | No association | 1.3–3.6 |
| Protein C deficiency | 4–6.5 | 1.4–1.8 | No consistent association | 1.3–3.6 |
| Protein S deficiency | 1–10 | 1.0–1.4 | No consistent association | 1.3–3.6 |
| Factor V Leiden | 3–5 | 1.4 | 1.3 | 1.0–2.6 |
| Prothrombin G20210A | 2–3 | 1.4 | 0.9 | 0.9–1.3 |
| Persistently elevated FVIII | 2–11 | 6–11 | – | 4.0 |
| Mild hyperhomocysteinemia | 2.5–2.6 | 2.6–3.1 | – | No consistent association |

FVIII, factor VIII; VTE, venous thromboembolism.
Risk estimated are derived from studies reviewed in detail elsewhere.[11]

**TABLE 20–4.** Absolute Incidences for a First Episode of Venous Thromboembolism in Asymptomatic Family Members of Consecutive Patients with Venous Thromboembolism

| | Incidence Any VTE (% Per Year) | Surgery, Trauma, Immobilization (% Per Episode) | Pregnancy (% Per Pregnancy Including Postpartum Period) | Oral Contraceptive Use (% Per Year of Use) |
|---|---|---|---|---|
| Antithrombin, protein C, or protein S deficiency[120] | | | | |
| Affected family members | 1.0 (0.7–1.4) | 8.1 (4.5–13.2) | 4.1 (1.7–8.3) | 4.3 (1.4–9.7) |
| Unaffected family members | 0.1 (0.0–0.2) | 0.9 (0.3–3.2) | 0.5 (0.0–2.8) | 0.7 (0.0–3.3) |
| Factor V Leiden[121] | | | | |
| Affected family members | 0.5 (0.3–0.6) | 1.8 (0.7–4.0) | 2.1 (0.7–4.9)* | 0.5 (0.1–1.4) |
| Unaffected family members | 0.1 (0.0–0.2) | 0.7 (0.1–2.7) | 0.0 (0.0–1.9)† | 0.2 (0.0–0.8) |
| Prothrombin G20210A*[122,123] | | | | |
| Affected family members | 0.4 (0.1–1.1) | 2.0 (0.8–4.2) | 2.8 (1.0–6.0) | 0.2 (0.0–0.9) |
| Unaffected family members | 0.1 (0.0–0.7) | 2.4 (1.0–4.9) | 1.2 (0.1–4.2) | 0.3 (0.0–1.1) |
| Persistently elevated FVIII[58,81] | | | | |
| Affected family members | 2.3 (1.2–4.2) | 1.2 (0.4–2.8) | 1.3 (0.4–3.4) | 0.6 (0.2–1.5) |
| Unaffected family members | 0.5 (0.1–1.2) | 1.5 (0.6–3.1) | 0.0 (0.0–1.1)† | 0.3 (0.1–0.8) |
| Mild hyperhomocysteinemia[124,125] | | | | |
| Affected family members | 0.2 (0.1–0.3) | 0.6 (0.2–2.3) | 1.9 (0.7–4.7) | 0.4 (0.1–1.0) |
| Unaffected family members | 0.1 (0.1–0.2) | 1.7 (0.8–3.5) | 0.7 (0.2–2.6) | 0.0 (0.0–0.3)† |

FVIII, factor VIII; VTE, venous thromboembolism.

*Does not apply to homozygous carriers; see Table 20–5.

†The population risk of pregnancy-related VTE is 0.2% per pregnancy.[103]

(vs. distal) deep venous thrombosis (DVT), and elevated D-dimer levels after stopping anticoagulation.[70]

Although individuals with hereditary thrombophilia have a higher risk of developing a first episode of VTE, the risk increases for recurrent events in patients with prior VTE are much lower. Numerous case-control studies in VTE patients with a specific thrombophilia with nonthrombophilic VTE patients as controls yield relative risks of 1.5 to 2.0 for most hereditary thrombophilias.[71–76] Patients develop VTE when the combination of individual susceptibility (including hereditary thrombophilia) and acquired, sometimes transient, risk factors are sufficient to cause VTE. This individual susceptibility is constant throughout life. Therefore, patients with a previous episode of VTE have proven to have sufficient individual susceptibility, irrespective of hereditary thrombophilia being part of that susceptibility. This explains why the risk for recurrence is at best only slightly increased for carriers of hereditary thrombophilia.[77]

## ARTERIAL THROMBOEMBOLIC DISEASE

The increased risk of VTE in patients with hereditary thrombophilia has led to many studies investigating the association of thrombophilia with arterial thromboembolic disease. Factor V Leiden and prothrombin G20210A are the most extensively studied as risk factors for arterial disease. The largest meta-analysis of case-control studies of patients with myocardial infarction found an OR of 1.17 (95% confidence interval [CI] 1.08 to 1.28) for factor V Leiden (60 studies with 42,390 patients) and 1.31 (95% CI 1.12 to 1.52) for prothrombin G20210A (40 studies with 26,087 patients).[4] The association between these mutations and myocardial infarction is stronger when analyses are limited to patients with myocardial infarction below the age of 55 years with ORs of 1.34

(95% CI 0.94 to 1.91) for factor V Leiden and 1.86 (95% CI 1.00 to 3.51) for prothrombin G20210A.[5] Meta-analyses of studies in patients with ischemic stroke have shown similar modest risk increases in patients with factor V Leiden or prothrombin G20210A.[78]

Deficiencies of the natural anticoagulants are less prevalent than factor V Leiden and prothrombin G20210A, and as a result, the association with arterial thromboembolic disease has not been extensively studied. Although various case reports of patients with antithrombin, protein C, or protein S deficiency have been published, most case-control studies have failed to demonstrate a significant association with myocardial infarction and ischemic stroke.[79] A retrospective cohort study of 552 first-degree family members of patients with venous or arterial thrombosis and a deficiency of either antithrombin, protein C, or protein S found no increased risk of arterial cardiovascular disease in affected family members older than age 55 years.[80] However, in persons younger than age 55 years, protein C and protein S were associated with a five- to ninefold increased risk, whereas antithrombin deficiency did not confer an increased risk.[80]

Several case-control studies have found associations with elevated FVIII levels and myocardial infarction.[57] Furthermore, prospective cohort studies of healthy individuals have demonstrated marginally increased risks of myocardial infarction and stroke in patients with elevated FVIII levels (ORs between 1.0 and 1.4).[57] In a prospective family study of asymptomatic first-degree family members of patients with elevated FVIII and either VTE or premature arterial thrombosis, the risk of arterial thromboembolism was increased 4.5-fold compared with family members with normal FVIII levels.[81] However, elevated FVIII levels are associated with several well-known risk factors for arterial cardiovascular disease, including obesity, high glucose levels, increasing age, chronic inflammatory diseases, and renal disease.[57] It is possible that studies evaluating the association between elevated FVIII and arterial thromboembolic disease have not been able to sufficiently adjust for known and unknown confounders. Moreover, acute myocardial infarction and ischemic stroke may cause acute-phase reactions that transiently increase FVIII levels, hampering interpretation of case-control or retrospective cohort studies. However, patients with hemophilia A, a genetic cause of decreased FVIII levels, have an approximate 80 percent lower risk of death from ischemic heart disease, indicating a potential causal relation between FVIII levels and arterial thrombosis.[82]

Mild hyperhomocysteinemia and MTHFR 677TT have been extensively studied in relation to arterial thromboembolic disease. A meta-analysis of studies that included more than 5000 patients with ischemic heart disease and more than 1000 patients with ischemic stroke demonstrated a significant correlation between homocysteine level and the risk of arterial thrombosis.[83] The risk increase was higher in retrospective studies than in prospective studies in which homocysteine levels are measured before the thrombotic episodes. This could, in part, be explained by the observed association between hyperhomocysteinemia and other well-known risk factors for arterial cardiovascular disease, including smoking, chronic inflammatory disorders, and renal failure.[61] As with elevated FVIII levels, it is uncertain whether studies that investigate the relation between homocysteine and arterial cardiovascular disease have been able to sufficiently adjust for confounding variables. The association between MTHFR 677TT and ischemic heart disease has shown mixed results with no association in studies in North American patients and a modest 16 percent risk increase in studies in European patients.[84] It was initially hypothesized that this difference is attributable to a lower dietary folate intake in Europe. However, this hypothesis conflicts with the results of trials in patients with vascular disease in whom homocysteine lowering with folic acid and B vitamins did not reduce the risk of recurrent episodes.[66]

## PREGNANCY COMPLICATIONS

Although many studies have observed a relationship between hereditary thrombophilia and pregnancy complications, including recurrent miscarriage, late pregnancy loss, preeclampsia, intrauterine growth restriction, and placental abruption, this should be regarded as controversial. Most associations are modest in strength and vary with type of thrombophilia and type of pregnancy complication.[8,85,86] Furthermore, the most recent and larger prospective cohort studies found lower ORs for hereditary thrombophilia than older and smaller case-control studies, which may point to a bias in the observed associations.[8,87,88] The mechanisms of how thrombophilia would lead to pregnancy complications remain largely unknown. It is unlikely that mere hypercoagulability with thrombosis of placental vasculature is the pathophysiologic substrate for an association with thrombophilia. Animal and *in vitro* studies have implicated a role for both procoagulant and inflammatory pathways in pregnancy failure and interesting effects of acetylsalicylic acid (ASA) and heparin.[89] For instance, in a murine high-risk pregnancy model, heparin rescued factor V Leiden–associated placental failure, but this was independent of anticoagulation.[90]

## ● CLINICAL IMPLICATIONS OF THROMBOPHILIA INCLUDING TESTING

### GENERAL CONSIDERATIONS OF THROMBOPHILIA TESTING

Several arguments against testing for thrombophilia should be considered.[10] First, an obvious disadvantage of testing for thrombophilia is the high cost. Although two studies concluded that testing for thrombophilia

in some scenarios could be cost-effective, the underlying assumptions from inconsistent observational studies seriously hamper their interpretation.[91,92] Second, although the psychological impact and consequences of knowing that one is a carrier of a (genetic) thrombophilic defect are considered limited, a qualitative study described several negative effects of both psychological and social origins.[93,94] Difficulties in obtaining life or disability insurance are frequently encountered by individuals who are known carriers of thrombophilia, regardless of whether they are symptomatic or asymptomatic.[93] Third, the most compelling argument against testing is the potential false reassurance that may arise from a negative thrombophilia test for individuals who come from families with a thrombotic tendency. For example, Table 20–4 indicates that, in these families, women without thrombophilia have a markedly increased risk of oral contraceptive–related VTE compared to pill users from the general population (0.7 percent in women with a natural anticoagulant deficiency versus 0.04 percent per year of use), reflecting a selection of families with a strong thrombotic tendency in which yet unknown thrombophilias have co-segregated.

The following paragraphs discuss the potential scenarios for thrombophilia testing in more detail.

## TESTING FOR THROMBOPHILIA TO MODIFY THE RISK OF A FIRST VENOUS THROMBOEMBOLISM

Having a family history of VTE is a poor predictor of the presence of thrombophilia.[69,95] Still, a potential advantage of testing patients with VTE for thrombophilia may be the identification of asymptomatic family members in order to take preventive measures if tested positive and to withhold such measures if relatives have tested negative. An important requisite is that a test result indeed dichotomizes carriers and noncarriers in terms of their risk for a first episode of VTE.

Based on the absolute risks for a first episode of VTE (see Table 20–4), it is clear that the 1 to 3 percent annual major bleeding risk associated with continuous oral anticoagulant treatment outweighs the risk of VTE.[96,97] Table 20–4 also shows that during high-risk situations such as surgery, immobilization, trauma, pregnancy, and the postpartum period, and during the use of oral contraceptives, the absolute risk is generally low, with the exception of women with a natural anticoagulant deficiency who use oral contraceptives or are pregnant.

Estimates of the effect of avoidance of oral contraceptives on the number of prevented episodes of VTE by means of thrombophilia testing can be calculated for women who have a positive first-degree relative with VTE in whom the thrombophilic defect is known.[98] To avoid one VTE event, 28 women with antithrombin, protein C, or protein S deficiency and a positive family history for VTE would need to refrain from oral contraceptives, and to identify these women, 56 female relatives would need to be tested.[98] For factor V Leiden or the prothrombin 20210A mutation, approximately 333 women would need to avoid oral contraceptives and 666 female relatives would need to be tested. Although the number of tested women for the natural deficiencies seems quite acceptable, the major argument against this scenario is that a normal level of antithrombin, protein C, or protein S in women from these families does not exclude a strongly increased risk of VTE during oral contraceptive use, as compared to the general population (see Table 20–4). The same, but to a lesser extent, is true for women from thrombophilic families who do not carry either the factor V Leiden or prothrombin mutation, but here also, the number needed to screen is unacceptably high.

Table 20–5 indicates the estimated number needed to test to initiate prophylactic measurements around pregnancy, again applicable

**TABLE 20–5.** Estimated Number of Asymptomatic Thrombophilic Women Who Should Use Low-Molecular-Weight Heparin Prophylaxis During Pregnancy and/or the Postpartum Period to Prevent Pregnancy-Related Venous Thromboembolism, and Estimated Number Needed to Test

| Thrombophilia | Risk of VTE Per Pregnancy*, % | Risk Difference Per 100 Women | Number Using Prophylaxis to Prevent 1 VTE[†] | Number of Female Relatives to Be Tested |
|---|---|---|---|---|
| Antithrombin, protein C, or protein S deficiency | | | | |
|   Deficient relatives | 4.1[‡] | 3.6 | 28 | 56 |
|   Nondeficient relatives | 0.5[‡] | | | |
| Factor V Leiden or prothrombin 20210A mutation, heterozygous | | | | |
|   Relatives with the mutation | 2.0[‡] | 1.5 | 66 | 132 |
|   Relatives without the mutation | 0.5[‡] | | | |
| Factor V Leiden or prothrombin 20210A mutation, homozygous | | | | |
|   Homozygous relatives | 16.0 | 15.5 | 6 | 24 |
|   Relatives without the mutation | 0.5[§] | | | |

VTE, venous thromboembolism.

*Antepartum and postpartum combined.

[†]These estimates apply to women with a positive family history of VTE and assume an unrealistic 100% efficacy of prophylaxis with low-molecular-weight heparin.

[‡]Based on family studies as outlined in Table 20–4.

[§]Summary estimate of the data as outlined in Table 20–4, combined for factor V Leiden and prothrombin mutation.

to women from thrombophilic families. Only for women with antithrombin, protein C, or protein S deficiency, or those who are homozygous for factor V Leiden (Table 20–5), the risks of 4 and 16 percent, respectively, during pregnancy and the postpartum period may outweigh the nuisance of daily subcutaneous low-molecular-weight heparin (LMWH) injections with frequently occurring skin reactions, and the very small risk for severe complications of anticoagulant therapy during pregnancy.[99–102] Furthermore, the numbers in Table 20–5 underestimate the number of women who need to use prophylaxis (and be tested prior to this decision) in order to avoid pregnancy-related VTE, because a 100 percent efficacy of prophylaxis is assumed in these calculations. Whether the absolute risks of pregnancy-related VTE justify prophylaxis for 8 months during pregnancy or the shorter postpartum period of 6 weeks is a matter of physicians' and patients' preference.[102] The risk of pregnancy-related VTE in women from these families who do not have the hereditary thrombophilic defect is approximately 0.5 percent, compared to 0.2 percent in the general population.[103] Hence, withholding prophylaxis from women from thrombophilic families who do not have the defect is supported by evidence from well-designed studies of individuals in the same clinical context.

## THROMBOPHILIA TESTING IN PATIENTS WITH VENOUS THROMBOEMBOLISM

Thrombophilia testing is most often considered in patients with VTE, particularly if they are young, have recurrent episodes, have thrombosis at unusual sites, or have a positive family history for the disease. However, although such a strategy may lead to an increased yield of testing, the main question is whether a positive test result should alter management. As previously discussed, thrombophilia is a poor predictor of recurrent VTE, and whether the modest risk increase warrants prolongation of the duration of anticoagulation, particularly after

provoked VTE, is a matter of debate.[70,104] Furthermore, given the rarity of homozygous or double heterozygous thrombophilias in unselected patients with VTE, the efficiency of testing is obviously very low.[10,105] A randomized controlled trial of testing for thrombophilia in patients with a first episode of VTE would provide the ultimate evidence to decide whether this is justified, but no such trials have been successfully performed.[106] To investigate whether testing for thrombophilia reduced the risk of recurrent VTE, 197 patients who had had a recurrent event were compared to 324 patients who did not have a recurrence.[107] The OR for recurrence was 1.2 (95 percent CI 0.9 to 1.8) for tested versus nontested patients, indicating that testing, with real-life clinical decisions based on the outcome of testing, did not reduce the risk of recurrent VTE in patients after a first episode.

## THROMBOPHILIA TESTING IN PATIENTS WITH ARTERIAL CARDIOVASCULAR DISEASE

The association between hereditary thrombophilia and arterial cardiovascular disease is questionable, or at least much weaker than for VTE. The association is stronger in patients with events before the age of 55 years. As a result, thrombophilia test panels are often ordered in arterial cardiovascular disease. In a survey among Dutch physicians who ordered thrombophilia tests in 2000 consecutive patients in 2003 and 2004, arterial cardiovascular disease, mainly ischemic stroke, was the indication for testing in 23 percent of patients.[9] Interestingly, only 54 percent of those patients were younger than 50 years of age. Testing for hereditary thrombophilia in patients with (premature) arterial cardiovascular disease could only be justified if the test results would mandate different secondary prevention. However, more vigorous secondary prevention such as long-term dual antiplatelet therapy or oral anticoagulation instead of ASA monotherapy is not beneficial for most patients with arterial cardiovascular events, mainly because of the increased risk of bleeding. Whether such a strategy is beneficial for patients with hereditary thrombophilia has never been tested but is very unlikely given the very modest risk increases associated with hereditary thrombophilia. Therefore, testing in this setting is not justified.

## THROMBOPHILIA TESTING IN WOMEN WITH PREGNANCY COMPLICATIONS

Thrombophilia testing in women with pregnancy complications would be indicated if a test result would alter management. However, to date, testing for hereditary thrombophilia in this setting cannot be justified[10,102] for the following reasons. For women at moderate to high risk of preeclampsia, ASA provides a modest benefit in reducing the risk of preeclampsia, but this is regardless of the presence of hereditary thrombophilia.[102,108] Whether anticoagulant treatment with heparin or LMWH improves the chance of a successful pregnancy outcome in women with pregnancy complications is presently unknown as results from randomized clinical trials are extremely inconsistent.[109–113] It is also uncertain whether presence of hereditary thrombophilia is a prerequisite for an assumed beneficial effect, if any. Only three randomized controlled trials have been exclusively dedicated to women with hereditary thrombophilia and recurrent miscarriage, a single fetal loss, or late pregnancy complications. The first trial found promising results in women with heterozygous factor V Leiden mutation, prothrombin G20210A mutation, or protein S deficiency and a single previous pregnancy loss after 10 weeks of gestation.[114] Women who were allocated to enoxaparin had a much higher chance of a livebirth than those allocated to ASA (86 percent and 29 percent, respectively; OR 15.5; 95 percent CI 7 to 34), but several methodologic issues were raised, and the results of this single study have not been confirmed by other trials.[102,115] Second, in the FRUIT trial, women with hereditary thrombophilia and a history of preeclampsia or intrauterine growth restriction requiring delivery before 34 weeks of gestation, were randomized between dalteparin with ASA and ASA alone.[116] The primary outcome (recurrence of a hypertensive disorder, e.g., preeclampsia, HELLP, or eclampsia) did not differ between the two groups, but none of the women in the LMWH/ASA group developed recurrent hypertensive disorders prior to 34 weeks of gestational age, whereas six women in the ASA-only group delivered before 34 weeks because of recurrent hypertensive disorders (risk difference 8.7 percent; 95 percent CI 1.9 to 15.5 percent). Finally, the TIPPS study included thrombophilic women at high risk for pregnancy complications or at increased risk of VTE and randomized them between dalteparin and no dalteparin.[113] The primary composite outcome (severe or early-onset preeclampsia, small-for-gestational-age infant, pregnancy loss, or VTE) did not differ between the groups. A meta-analysis limited to women with thrombophilia clearly showed no benefit of LMWH for preventing recurrent pregnancy loss,[116a] but a trial investigating this issue is still ongoing.[116b] Hence, to date, there is no evidence from sufficiently powered and adequately designed clinical trials that justify use of heparin to improve pregnancy outcome in women with hereditary thrombophilia, and heparin should only be given in the context of a clinical trial.[117]

## ● CONCLUSIONS

The knowledge about the hereditary contribution to the etiology of VTE has increased tremendously over the past decades. Still, testing for thrombophilia serves only a limited purpose and should not be performed on a routine basis. Thrombophilia testing in asymptomatic relatives may be useful in families with antithrombin, protein C, or protein S deficiency, or for siblings of patients who are homozygous for factor V Leiden, and is limited to women who intend to become pregnant or who would like to use oral contraceptives. Careful counseling with knowledge of absolute risks helps

patients make an informed decision in which their own preferences can be taken into account and in which the clinician should be cautious to not provide false reassurance in case of a negative test result. Observational studies show that patients who have had VTE and have thrombophilia are at most at a slightly increased risk for reoccurrence. Other determinants, including circumstances during the first VTE, elevated D-dimer levels, and male sex, are better predictors of recurrent VTE.[70] Furthermore, no beneficial effect on the risk of recurrent VTE was observed in patients who had been tested for inherited thrombophilia. In the absence of trials that compared routine and prolonged anticoagulant treatment in patients testing positive for thrombophilia, testing for such defects to prolong anticoagulant therapy cannot be justified. Finally, there is at present no reason to test patients with arterial cardiovascular disease or women with recurrent miscarriage or late pregnancy complications for hereditary thrombophilia, in the absence of evidence-based guidelines for changes in management.

## REFERENCES

1. Nygaard KK, Brown GE: Essential thrombophilia: Report of five cases. *Arch Intern Med* 59:82, 1937.
2. Jordan FLJ, Nandorff A: The familial tendency in thrombo-embolic disease. *Acta Med Scand* 156:267, 1956.
3. Rosendaal FR: Venous thrombosis: A multicausal disease. *Lancet* 353:1167, 1999.
4. Ye Z, Liu EH, Higgins JR, et al: Seven haemostatic gene polymorphisms in coronary disease: Meta-analysis of 66,155 cases and 91,307 controls. *Lancet* 367:651, 2006.
5. Boekholdt SM, Bijsterveld NR, Moons AH, et al: Genetic variation in coagulation and fibrinolytic proteins and their relation with acute myocardial infarction: A systematic review. *Circulation* 104:3063, 2001.
6. Lin J, August P: Genetic thrombophilias and preeclampsia: A meta-analysis. *Obstet Gynecol* 105:182, 2005.
7. Rey E, Kahn SR, David M, Shrier I: Thrombophilic disorders and fetal loss: A meta-analysis. *Lancet* 361:901, 2003.
8. Rodger MA, Walker MC, Smith GN, et al: Is thrombophilia associated with placenta-mediated pregnancy complications? A prospective cohort study. *J Thromb Haemost* 12:469, 2014.
9. Coppens M, van Mourik JA, Eckmann CM, et al: Current practice of testing for hereditary thrombophilia in The Netherlands. *J Thromb Haemost* 5:1979, 2007.
10. Baglin T, Gray E, Greaves M, et al: Clinical guidelines for testing for heritable thrombophilia. *Br J Haematol* 149:209, 2010.
11. Middeldorp S, van Hylckama Vlieg A: Does thrombophilia testing help in the clinical management of patients? *Br J Haematol* 143:321, 2008.
12. Bezemer ID, Bare LA, Doggen CJ, et al: Gene variants associated with deep vein thrombosis. *JAMA* 299:1306, 2008.
13. Gohil R, Peck G, Sharma P: The genetics of venous thromboembolism. A meta-analysis involving approximately 120,000 cases and 180,000 controls. *Thromb Haemost* 102:360, 2009.
14. Lotta LA, Wang M, Yu J, et al: Identification of genetic risk variants for deep vein thrombosis by multiplexed next-generation sequencing of 186 hemostatic/pro-inflammatory genes. *BMC Med Genomics* 5:7, 2012.
15. Egeberg O: Inherited antithrombin III deficiency causing thrombophilia. *Thromb Diath Haemorrh* 13:516, 1965.
16. Comp PC, Esmon CT: Recurrent venous thromboembolism in patients with a partial deficiency of protein S. *N Engl J Med* 311:1525, 1984.
17. Griffin JH, Evatt B, Zimmerman TS, et al: Deficiency of protein C in congenital thrombotic disease. *J Clin Invest* 68:1370, 1981.
18. Gandrille S, Borgel D, Sala N, et al: Protein S deficiency: A database of mutations—Summary of the first update. *Thromb Haemost* 84:918, 2000.
19. Lane DA, Bayston T, Olds RJ, et al: Antithrombin mutation database: 2nd (1997) update. For the Plasma Coagulation Inhibitors Subcommittee of the Scientific and Standardization Committee of the International Society on Thrombosis and Haemostasis. *Thromb Haemost* 77:197, 1997.
20. Reitsma PH, Bernardi F, Doig RG, et al: Protein C deficiency: A database of mutations, 1995 update. On behalf of the Subcommittee on Plasma Coagulation Inhibitors of the Scientific and Standardization Committee of the ISTH. *Thromb Haemost* 73:876, 1995.
21. Dahlbäck B, Carlsson M, Svensson PJ: Familial thrombophilia due to a previously unrecognized mechanism characterized by poor anticoagulant response to activated protein C: Prediction of a cofactor to activated protein C. *Proc Natl Acad Sci U S A* 90:1004, 1993.
22. Bertina RM, Koeleman BP, Koster T, et al: Mutation in blood coagulation factor V associated with resistance to activated protein C. *Nature* 369:64, 1994.
23. Greengard JS, Sun X, Xu X, et al: Activated protein C resistance caused by Arg506Gln mutation in factor Va. *Lancet* 343:1361, 1994.
24. Voorberg J, Roelse J, Koopman R, et al: Association of idiopathic venous thromboembolism with single point-mutation at Arg506 of factor V. *Lancet* 343:1535, 1994.
25. Zoller B, Dahlback B: Linkage between inherited resistance to activated protein C and factor V gene mutation in venous thrombosis. *Lancet* 343:1536, 1994.

26. Poort SR, Rosendaal FR, Reitsma PH, Bertina RM: A common genetic variation in the 3′-untranslated region of the prothrombin gene is associated with elevated plasma prothrombin levels and an increase in venous thrombosis. *Blood* 88:3698, 1996.

27. Talbot S, Wakley EJ, Ryrie D, Langman MJ: ABO blood-groups and venous thromboembolic disease. *Lancet* 1:1257, 1970.

28. Koster T, Blann AD, Briet E, et al: Role of clotting factor VIII in effect of von Willebrand factor on occurrence of deep-vein thrombosis. *Lancet* 345:152, 1995.

29. Mudd SH, Skovby F, Levy HL, et al: The natural history of homocystinuria due to cystathionine beta-synthase deficiency. *Am J Hum Genet* 37:1, 1985.

30. den Heijer M, Koster T, Blom HJ, et al: Hyperhomocysteinemia as a risk factor for deep-vein thrombosis. *N Engl J Med* 334:759, 1996.

31. Reitsma PH, Rosendaal FR: Past and future of genetic research in thrombosis. *J Thromb Haemost* 5(Suppl 1):264, 2007.

32. Finazzi G, Caccia R, Barbui T: Different prevalence of thromboembolism in the sub-types of congenital antithrombin III deficiency: Review of 404 cases. *Thromb Haemost* 58:1094, 1987.

33. Zoller B, Garcia de FP, Dahlback B: Evaluation of the relationship between protein S and C4b-binding protein isoforms in hereditary protein S deficiency demonstrating type I and type III deficiencies to be phenotypic variants of the same genetic disease. *Blood* 85:3524, 1995.

34. Okajima K, Ueyama H, Hashimoto Y, et al: Homozygous variant of antithrombin III that lacks affinity for heparin, AT III Kumamoto. *Thromb Haemost* 61:20, 1989.

35. Ishiguro K, Kojima T, Kadomatsu K, et al: Complete antithrombin deficiency in mice results in embryonic lethality. *J Clin Invest* 106:873, 2000.

36. Seligsohn U, Berger A, Abend M, et al: Homozygous protein C deficiency manifested by massive venous thrombosis in the newborn. *N Engl J Med* 310:559, 1984.

37. Mahasandana C, Suvatte V, Marlar RA, et al: Neonatal purpura fulminans associated with homozygous protein S deficiency. *Lancet* 335:61, 1990.

38. McGehee WG, Klotz TA, Epstein DJ, Rapaport SI: Coumarin necrosis associated with hereditary protein C deficiency. *Ann Intern Med* 101:59, 1984.

39. Grimaudo V, Gueissaz F, Hauert J, et al: Necrosis of skin induced by coumarin in a patient deficient in protein S. *BMJ* 298:233, 1989.

40. Weiss J, Soff GA, Halkin H, Seligsohn U: Decline of proteins C and S and factors II, VII, IX and X during the initiation of warfarin therapy. *Thromb Res* 45:783, 1987.

41. Heijboer H, Brandjes DP, Buller HR, et al: Deficiencies of coagulation-inhibiting and fibrinolytic proteins in outpatients with deep-vein thrombosis. *N Engl J Med* 323:1512, 1990.

42. Miletich J, Sherman L, Broze G Jr: Absence of thrombosis in subjects with heterozygous protein C deficiency. *N Engl J Med* 317:991, 1987.

43. Tait RC, Walker ID, Perry DJ, et al: Prevalence of antithrombin deficiency in the healthy population. *Br J Haematol* 87:106, 1994.

44. Tait RC, Walker ID, Reitsma PH, et al: Prevalence of protein C deficiency in the healthy population. *Thromb Haemost* 73:87, 1995.

45. Rosing J, Hoekema L, Nicolaes GA, et al: Effects of protein S and factor Xa on peptide bond cleavages during inactivation of factor Va and factor VaR506Q by activated protein C. *J Biol Chem* 270:27852, 1995.

46. Rees DC, Cox M, Clegg JB: World distribution of factor V Leiden. *Lancet* 346:1133, 1995.

47. Zivelin A, Mor-Cohen R, Kovalsky V, et al: Prothrombin 20210G>A is an ancestral prothrombotic mutation that occurred in whites approximately 24,000 years ago. *Blood* 107:4666, 2006.

48. Van Mens TE, Levi M, Middeldorp S: Evolution of factor V Leiden. *Thromb Haemost* 110:23, 2013.

49. Lindqvist PG, Svensson PJ, Dahlback B, Marsal K: Factor V Q506 mutation (activated protein C resistance) associated with reduced intrapartum blood loss—A possible evolutionary selection mechanism. *Thromb Haemost* 79:69, 1998.

50. Lindqvist PG, Zoller B, Dahlback B: Improved hemoglobin status and reduced menstrual blood loss among female carriers of factor V Leiden—An evolutionary advantage? *Thromb Haemost* 86:1122, 2001.

51. Cohn DM, Repping S, Buller HR, et al: Increased sperm count may account for high population frequency of factor V Leiden. *J Thromb Haemost* 8:513, 2010.

52. van Dunne FM, Doggen CJ, Heemskerk M, et al: Factor V Leiden mutation in relation to fecundity and miscarriage in women with venous thrombosis. *Hum Reprod* 20:802, 2005.

53. Kaandorp SP, Van Mens TE, Middeldorp S, et al: Time to conception and time to live birth in women with unexplained recurrent miscarriage. *Hum Reprod* 29:1146, 2014.

54. Carter AM, Sacchithananthan M, Stasinopoulos S, et al: Prothrombin G20210A is a bifunctional gene polymorphism. *Thromb Haemost* 87:846, 2002.

55. Cumming AM, Keeney S, Salden A, et al: The prothrombin gene G20210A variant: Prevalence in a U.K. anticoagulant clinic population. *Br J Haematol* 98:353, 1997.

56. Rosendaal FR, Doggen CJ, Zivelin A, et al: Geographic distribution of the 20210 G to A prothrombin variant. *Thromb Haemost* 79:706, 1998.

57. Kamphuisen PW, Eikenboom JC, Bertina RM: Elevated factor VIII levels and the risk of thrombosis. *Arterioscler Thromb Vasc Biol* 21:731, 2001.

58. Bank I, Libourel EJ, Middeldorp S, et al: Elevated levels of FVIII:c within families are associated with an increased risk for venous and arterial thrombosis. *J Thromb Haemost* 3:79, 2005.

59. Jacques PF, Bostom AG, Williams RR, et al: Relation between folate status, a common mutation in methylenetetrahydrofolate reductase, and plasma homocysteine concentrations. *Circulation* 93:7, 1996.

60. Rosenberg N, Murata M, Ikeda Y, et al: The frequent 5,10-methylenetetrahydrofolate reductase C677T polymorphism is associated with a common haplotype in whites, Japanese, and Africans. *Am J Hum Genet* 70:758, 2002.

61. Key NS, McGlennen RC: Hyperhomocyst(e)inemia and thrombophilia. *Arch Pathol Lab Med* 126:1367, 2002.

62. den Heijer M, Lewington S, Clarke R: Homocysteine, MTHFR and risk of venous thrombosis: A meta-analysis of published epidemiological studies. *J Thromb Haemost* 3:292, 2005.

63. Bezemer ID, Doggen CJ, Vos HL, Rosendaal FR: No association between the common MTHFR 677C->T polymorphism and venous thrombosis: Results from the MEGA study. *Arch Intern Med* 167:497, 2007.

64. Lijfering W, Coppens M, Veeger NJ, et al: Hyperhomocysteinemia is not a risk factor for venous and arterial thrombosis, and is associated with elevated factor VIII levels. *Thromb Res* 123:244, 2008.

65. den Heijer M, Willems HP, Blom HJ, et al: Homocysteine lowering by B vitamins and the secondary prevention of deep-vein thrombosis and pulmonary embolism. A randomized, placebo-controlled, double blind trial. *Blood* 109:139, 2007.

66. Lonn E, Yusuf S, Arnold MJ, et al: Homocysteine lowering with folic acid and B vitamins in vascular disease. *N Engl J Med* 354:1567, 2006.

67. Barco S, Nijkeuter M, Middeldorp S: Pregnancy and venous thromboembolism. *Semin Thromb Hemost* 39:549, 2013.

68. Naess IA, Christiansen SC, Romundstad P, et al: Incidence and mortality of venous thrombosis: A population-based study. *J Thromb Haemost* 5:692, 2007.

69. Bezemer ID, van der Meer FJ, Eikenboom JC, et al: The value of family history as a risk indicator for venous thrombosis. *Arch Intern Med* 169:610, 2008.

70. de Jong PG, Coppens M, Middeldorp S: Duration of anticoagulant therapy for venous thromboembolism: Balancing benefits and harms on the long term. *Br J Haematol* 158:433, 2012.

71. Baglin T, Luddington R, Brown K, Baglin C: Incidence of recurrent venous thromboembolism in relation to clinical and thrombophilic risk factors: Prospective cohort study. *Lancet* 362:523, 2003.

72. Brouwer JL, Lijfering WM, Ten Kate MK, et al: High long-term absolute risk of recurrent venous thromboembolism in patients with hereditary deficiencies of protein S, protein C or antithrombin. *Thromb Haemost* 101:93, 2009.

73. Segal JB, Brotman DJ, Necochea AJ, et al: Predictive value of factor V Leiden and prothrombin G20210A in adults with venous thromboembolism and in family members of those with a mutation: A systematic review. *JAMA* 301:2472, 2009.

74. Lijfering WM, Middeldorp S, Veeger NJ, et al: Risk of recurrent venous thrombosis in homozygous carriers, and double heterozygous carriers of factor V Leiden and prothrombin G20210A. *Circulation* 121:1706, 2010.

75. van den Belt AG, Sanson BJ, Simioni P, et al: Recurrence of venous thromboembolism in patients with familial thrombophilia. *Arch Intern Med* 157:2227, 1997.

76. Vossen CY, Walker ID, Svensson P, et al: Recurrence rate after a first venous thrombosis in patients with familial thrombophilia. *Arterioscler Thromb Vasc Biol* 25:1992, 2005.

77. Cannegieter SC, van Hylckama Vlieg A: Venous thrombosis: Understanding the paradoxes of recurrence. *J Thromb Haemost* 11(Suppl 1):161, 2013.

78. Casas JP, Hingorani AD, Bautista LE, Sharma P: Meta-analysis of genetic studies in ischemic stroke: Thirty-two genes involving approximately 18,000 cases and 58,000 controls. *Arch Neurol* 61:1652, 2004.

79. Boekholdt SM, Kramer MH: Arterial thrombosis and the role of thrombophilia. *Semin Thromb Hemost* 33:588, 2007.

80. Mahmoodi BK, Brouwer JL, Veeger NJ, van der Meer J: Hereditary deficiency of protein C or protein S confers increased risk of arterial thromboembolic events at a young age: Results from a large family cohort study. *Circulation* 118:1659, 2008.

81. Bank I, Van de Poel MH, Coppens M, et al: Absolute annual incidences of first events of venous thromboembolism and arterial vascular events in individuals with elevated FVIII:c: A prospective family cohort study. *Thromb Haemost* 98:1040, 2007.

82. Rosendaal FR, Varekamp I, Smit C, et al: Mortality and causes of death in Dutch haemophiliacs, 1973–86. *Br J Haematol* 71:71, 1989.

83. Homocysteine Studies Collaboration: Homocysteine and risk of ischemic heart disease and stroke: A meta-analysis. *JAMA* 288:2015, 2002.

84. Klerk M, Verhoef P, Clarke R, et al: MTHFR 677C—>T polymorphism and risk of coronary heart disease: A meta-analysis. *JAMA* 288:2023, 2002.

85. Robertson L, Wu O, Langhorne P, et al: Thrombophilia in pregnancy: A systematic review. *Br J Haematol* 132:171, 2006.

86. Opatrny L, David M, Kahn SR, et al: Association between antiphospholipid antibodies and recurrent fetal loss in women without autoimmune disease: A metaanalysis. *J Rheumatol* 33:2214, 2006.

87. Clark P, Walker ID, Govan L, et al: The GOAL study: A prospective examination of the impact of factor V Leiden and ABO(H) blood groups on haemorrhagic and thrombotic pregnancy outcomes. *Br J Haematol* 140:236, 2008.

88. Kahn SR, Platt R, McNamara H, et al: Inherited thrombophilia and preeclampsia within a multicenter cohort: The Montreal Preeclampsia Study. *Am J Obstet Gynecol* 200:151, 2009.

89. Bose P, Black S, Kadyrov M, et al: Heparin and aspirin attenuate placental apoptosis in vitro: Implications for early pregnancy failure. *Am J Obstet Gynecol* 192:23, 2005.

90. An J, Waitara MS, Bordas M, et al: Heparin rescues factor V Leiden-associated placental failure independent of anticoagulation in a murine high-risk pregnancy model. *Blood* 121:2127, 2013.

91. Marchetti M, Pistorio A, Barosi G: Extended anticoagulation for prevention of recurrent venous thromboembolism in carriers of factor V Leiden: Cost-effectiveness analysis. *Thromb Haemost* 84:752, 2000.

92. Wu O, Robertson L, Twaddle S, et al: Screening for thrombophilia in high-risk situations: Systematic review and cost-effectiveness analysis. The Thrombosis: Risk and Economic Assessment of Thrombophilia Screening (TREATS) study. *Health Technol Assess* 10:1, 2006.

93. Bank I, Scavenius MP, Buller HR, Middeldorp S: Social aspects of genetic testing for factor V Leiden mutation in healthy individuals and their importance for daily practice. *Thromb Res* 113:7, 2004.

94. Cohn DM, Vansenne F, Kaptein AA, et al: The psychological impact of testing for thrombophilia: A systematic review. *J Thromb Haemost* 6:1099, 2008.

95. van Sluis GL, Sohne M, El Kheir DY, et al: Family history and inherited thrombophilia. *J Thromb Haemost* 4:2182, 2006.

96. Ruff CT, Giugliano RP, Braunwald E, et al: Comparison of the efficacy and safety of new oral anticoagulants with warfarin in patients with atrial fibrillation: A meta-analysis of randomised trials. *Lancet* 383:955, 2014.

97. van Es N, Coppens M, Schulman S, et al: Direct oral anticoagulants compared with vitamin K antagonists for acute symptomatic venous thromboembolism: Evidence from phase 3 trials. *Blood* 124:1968, 2014.

98. Bleker SM, Coppens M, Middeldorp S: Sex, thrombosis and inherited thrombophilia. *Blood Rev* 28:123, 2014.

99. Bank I, Libourel EJ, Middeldorp S, et al: High rate of skin complications due to low-molecular-weight heparins in pregnant women. *J Thromb Haemost* 1:859, 2003.

100. Deruelle P, Denervaud M, Hachulla E, et al: Use of low-molecular-weight heparin from the first trimester of pregnancy: A retrospective study of 111 consecutive pregnancies. *Eur J Obstet Gynecol Reprod Biol* 127:73, 2006.

101. Schindewolf M, Gobst C, Kroll H, et al: High incidence of heparin-induced allergic delayed-type hypersensitivity reactions in pregnancy. *J Allergy Clin Immunol* 132:131, 2013.

102. Bates SM, Greer IA, Middeldorp S, et al: VTE, thrombophilia, antithrombotic therapy, and pregnancy: Antithrombotic Therapy and Prevention of Thrombosis, 9th ed: American College of Chest Physicians Evidence-Based Clinical Practice Guidelines. *Chest* 141(Suppl 2):e691S, 2012.

103. Heit JA, Kobbervig CE, James AH, et al: Trends in the incidence of venous thromboembolism during pregnancy or postpartum: A 30-year population-based study. *Ann Intern Med* 143:697, 2005.

104. Middeldorp S: Duration of anticoagulation for venous thromboembolism. *BMJ* 342:d2758, 2011.

105. Evaluation of Genomic Applications in Practice and Prevention (EGAPP) Working Group: Recommendations from the EGAPP Working Group: Routine testing for factor V Leiden (R506Q) and prothrombin (20210G>A) mutations in adults with a history of idiopathic venous thromboembolism and their adult family members. *Genet Med* 13:67, 2011.

106. Cohn DM, Vansenne F, de Borgie CA, Middeldorp S: Thrombophilia testing for prevention of recurrent venous thromboembolism. *Cochrane Database Syst Rev* 12:CD007069, 2009.

107. Coppens M, Reijnders JH, Middeldorp S, et al: Testing for inherited thrombophilia does not reduce recurrence of venous thrombosis. *J Thromb Haemost* 6:1474, 2008.

108. Henderson JT, Whitlock EP, O'Connor E, et al: Low-dose aspirin for prevention of morbidity and mortality from preeclampsia: A systematic evidence review for the U.S. Preventive Services Task Force. *Ann Intern Med* 160:695, 2014.

109. Middeldorp S: Thrombophilia and pregnancy complications: Cause or association? *J Thromb Haemost* 5:276, 2007.

110. Rodger MA, Paidas MJ, Mclintock C, et al: Inherited thrombophilia and pregnancy complications revisited: Association not proven causal and antithrombotic prophylaxis is experimental. *Obstet Gynecol* 112:320, 2008.

111. de Jong PG, Goddijn M, Middeldorp S: Antithrombotic therapy for pregnancy loss. *Hum Reprod Update* 19:674, 2013.

112. de Jong PG, Kaandorp SP, Di Nisio M, et al: Aspirin or anticoagulants for treating recurrent miscarriage in women without antiphospholipid syndrome. *Cochrane Database Syst Rev* 7:CD004734, 2014.

113. Rodger MA, Hague WM, Kingdom J, et al: Antepartum dalteparin versus no antepartum dalteparin for the prevention of pregnancy complications in pregnant women with thrombophilia (TIPPS): A multinational open-label randomised trial. *Lancet* 384:1673, 2014.

114. Gris JC, Mercier E, Quere I, et al: Low-molecular-weight heparin versus low-dose aspirin in women with one fetal loss and a constitutional thrombophilic disorder. *Blood* 103:3695, 2004.

115. Rodger M: Important publication missing key information. *Blood* 104:3413, 2004.

116. de Vries JI, van Pampus MG, Hague WM, et al: Low-molecular-weight heparin added to aspirin in the prevention of recurrent early-onset preeclampsia in women with inheritable thrombophilia: The FRUIT-RCT. *J Thromb Haemost* 10:64, 2012.

116a. Skeith L, Carrier M, Kaaja R, et al: Evidence-based focused review: A meta-analysis of low-molecular-weight heparin to prevent pregnancy loss in women with inherited thrombophilia. *Blood* 127(13):8–10, 2016.

116b. de Jong PG, Quenby S, Bloemenkamp KW, et al: ALIFE2 study: Low-molecular-weight heparin for women with recurrent miscarriage and inherited thrombophilia—Study protocol for a randomized controlled trial. *Trials* 16(1):1–10, 2015.

117. Middeldorp S: Thrombosis in women: What are the knowledge gaps in 2013? *J Thromb Haemost* 11(Suppl 1):180, 2013.

118. Ridker PM, Miletich JP, Hennekens CH, Buring JE: Ethnic distribution of factor V Leiden in 4047 men and women. Implications for venous thromboembolism screening. *JAMA* 277:1305, 1997.

119. Dilley A, Austin H, Hooper WC, et al: Prevalence of the prothrombin 20210 G-to-A variant in blacks: Infants, patients with venous thrombosis, patients with myocardial infarction, and control subjects. *J Lab Clin Med* 132:452, 1998.

120. Simioni P, Sanson BJ, Prandoni P, et al: The incidence of venous thromboembolism in families with inherited thrombophilia. *Thromb Haemost* 81:198, 1999.

121. Middeldorp S, Henkens CMA, Koopman MM, et al: The incidence of venous thromboembolism in family members of patients with factor V Leiden mutation and venous thrombosis. *Ann Intern Med* 128:15, 1998.

122. Bank I, Libourel EJ, Middeldorp S, et al: Prothrombin 20210A mutation: A mild risk factor for venous thromboembolism but not for arterial thrombotic disease and pregnancy-related complications in a family study. *Arch Intern Med* 164:1932, 2004.

123. Coppens M, van der Poel MH, Bank I, et al: A prospective cohort study on the absolute incidence of venous thromboembolism and arterial cardiovascular disease in asymptomatic carriers of the prothrombin 20210A mutation. *Blood* 108:2604, 2006.

124. Lijfering W, Coppens M, van der Poel MH, et al: The risk of venous and arterial thrombosis in hyperhomocysteinemia is low and mainly depends on concomitant thrombophilic defects. *Thromb Haemost* 98:457, 2007.

125. Van de Poel MH, Coppens M, Middeldorp S, et al: Absolute risk of venous and arterial thromboembolism associated with mild hyperhomocysteinemia. Results from a retrospective family cohort study. *J Thromb Haemost* 3(Suppl 1):P0481, 2005.

# CHAPTER 21
# THE ANTIPHOSPHOLIPID SYNDROME

Jacob H. Rand and Lucia Wolgast

## SUMMARY

The antiphospholipid (aPL) syndrome (APS) is an acquired thrombophilic disorder in which patients have vascular thrombosis and/or pregnancy complications attributable to placental insufficiency, accompanied by laboratory evidence for the presence of antiphospholipid antibodies in blood. The disorder is referred to as *primary APS* when it occurs in the absence of systemic lupus erythematosus (SLE), and *secondary APS* in its presence. Any portion of the circulatory tree can be affected, although the most frequently affected vessels are the deep veins of the lower extremities. Abnormalities that have been reported in association with the syndrome include virtually all other autoimmune disorders, immune thrombocytopenia, acquired platelet function abnormalities, hypoprothrombinemia, acquired inhibitors of coagulation factors, livedo reticularis, heart valve abnormalities, atherosclerosis, pulmonary hypertension, and migraine. Rare patients have a catastrophic form of APS (CAPS) in which there is disseminated thrombosis in large- and small-vessel thrombi, often after a triggering event such as infection or surgery and often with multiorgan ischemia and infarction.

APS is a misnomer; the main antigenic targets for thrombogenic aPL antibodies are epitopes on phospholipid-binding proteins, the most important of which appears to be $\beta_2$-glycoprotein I ($\beta_2$GPI). The syndrome is identified by persistent abnormalities of laboratory tests for antibodies against these phospholipid–protein cofactor complexes, detected by immunoassays and by coagulation assays (also known as "lupus anticoagulant assays") that, paradoxically, report the inhibition of phospholipid-dependent coagulation reactions. Long-term warfarin anticoagulant therapy is the usual treatment for thrombosis in patients with APS, although there is some controversy about whether treatment of patients with APS stroke might be better treated with aspirin. Patients with recurrent spontaneous pregnancy losses and APS generally are treated with aspirin and heparin for prophylaxis against deep vein thrombosis

**Acronyms and Abbreviations:** aCL, anticardiolipin; APC, activated protein C; aPL, antiphospholipid; APS, antiphospholipid syndrome; aPTT, activated partial thromboplastin time; ARDS, acute respiratory distress syndrome; ASIA, autoimmune/autoinflammatory syndrome induced by adjuvants; AVWS, acquired von Willebrand syndrome; BFP syphilis test, biologic false-positive serologic test for syphilis; $\beta_2$GPI, $\beta_2$-glycoprotein I; CAPS, catastrophic APS; CMV, cytomegalovirus; DOACs, direct-acting oral anticoagulants; dRVVT, dilute Russell viper venom time; ELISA, enzyme-linked immunosorbent assay; HCQ, hydroxychloroquine; Ig, immunoglobulin; IL, interleukin; LA, lupus anticoagulant; LDL, low-density lipoprotein; LMWH, low-molecular-weight heparin; MAPK, mitogen-activated protein kinase; RVV, Russell viper venom; SCR, short consensus repeat; SLE, systemic lupus erythematosus; TIA, transient ischemic attack; TLR, toll-like receptor; TM, thrombomodulin; t-PA, tissue-type plasminogen activator; UFH, unfractionated heparin; VWF, von Willebrand factor.

during their pregnancies and the postpartum period. CAPS patients have a high mortality and, in addition to anticoagulants, often require plasmapheresis and immunosuppressive agents. Patients without clinical manifestations of APS or a history of SLE should generally not undergo diagnostic screening for aPL antibodies and, if tested and found to be positive, should not be committed to antithrombotic therapy solely on the basis of laboratory abnormalities.

## ● DEFINITION AND HISTORY

The antiphospholipid (aPL) antibody syndrome (APS) is a disorder in which vascular thrombosis or pregnancy complications attributable to placental insufficiency occur in patients with laboratory evidence for antibodies directed against proteins that bind to phospholipids. The syndrome was first proposed to be a distinct entity, "the anticardiolipin (aCL) syndrome," in 1985[1] and soon was renamed APS.[2] While precise data are not available, the syndrome is thought to affect approximately 10 percent of patients with venous thrombosis[3,4] and approximately 20 percent of women with three unexplained fetal losses before 12 weeks of gestation or at least one intrauterine fetal death after 12 weeks of gestation.[5]

The term "aPL antibodies" can refer to (1) antibodies that recognize protein–phospholipid complexes as in cofactor-dependent aCL assays; (2) antibodies that recognize the proteins directly as in anti-$\beta_2$-glycoprotein I assays (anti-$\beta_2$GPI); (3) an abnormal coagulation test in several assays that report inhibition of phospholipid-dependent coagulation reactions, collectively termed as *lupus anticoagulant (LA) tests*; and (4) antibodies that recognize phospholipid directly, as in syphilis, and are not associated with the APS disease entity.

A brief review of the history of APS[6-8] helps explain the confusing terminology (Table 21–1); the reader is referred to references 6 to 8 for more detailed accounts. In retrospect, the first assay for aPL autoantibodies was Moore and Mohr's report of the "biologic false-positive" serologic tests for syphilis (BFP syphilis test) in 1952[9]; this abnormality came to be associated with systemic lupus erythematosus (SLE).[10] The contemporaneous introduction of the activated partial thromboplastin time (aPTT), which used cephalin, a phospholipid extract of animal brains, as the "partial thromboplastin" (distinct from the "complete thromboplastin," tissue factor, and phospholipid),[11] led to the recognition of a unique type of anticoagulant in patients with SLE that was frequently associated with BFP syphilis tests.[12] Because the of its initial association with SLE, this phenomenon was misnamed LA.[13] It became recognized that the LA was purely an *in vitro* phenomenon that was not limited to SLE and that was not associated with bleeding complications unless another hemostatic defect was present.[6] Furthermore, the LA came to be associated with recurrent pregnancy losses[14,15] and with thrombotic and embolic manifestations.[16] The development, in 1983, of the aCL antibody assay, which measured antibodies against the anionic phospholipid cardiolipin (diphosphatidylglycerol), the primary antigen in the syphilis test reagent,[17] was the advance that led to the identification of a new syndrome. Within a few years, it became recognized that aPL antibodies did not bind phospholipids directly but instead were directed against proteins that bound to the phospholipid, primarily $\beta_2$GPI (see "Pathogenesis" below). This information became important in helping to unravel the mechanisms for APS and in advancing diagnostic testing toward the goal of distinguishing between the syndrome and incidental false-positive tests. Table 21–2 describes the current consensus investigational criteria for diagnosing APS.[18]

Most patients with elevated aPL antibodies do not have the syndrome; elevated aPL antibody levels can occur in patients with several

**TABLE 21–1.** Paths of Development of Antiphospholipid Assays: Historical Summary

| Immunoassay Path | Coagulation Path |
|---|---|
| 1950s: Syphilis testing | 1950s: Partial thromboplastin time inhibitor |
| | 1970s: Lupus anticoagulant (LA) |
| 1980s: Antiphospholipid (aPL) antibody enzyme-linked immunosorbent assay (ELISA; e.g., anticardiolipin [aCL] immunoassays) | 1980s: Recognition that LAs are inhibitors of phospholipid-dependent coagulation reactions |
| 1990s: Anticofactor ELISA (anti-$\beta_2$-glycoprotein I [$\beta_2$GPI], antiprothrombin, etc.) | |
| 2005: Demonstration that antibodies against domain I of $\beta_2$GPI are associated with increased risk of thrombosis | 2004: Demonstration that resistance to the anticoagulant effect of annexin A5 correlates with thrombosis in antiphospholipid syndrome |

types of infections that induce formation of antibodies recognizing anionic phospholipids directly, patients taking medications such as chlorpromazine or procainamide, and even in normal healthy individuals. Testing of patients who have no clinical manifestations of the disorder or SLE for aPL antibodies should be discouraged because it incurs the risk of inappropriate diagnostic and treatment decisions.

**TABLE 21–2.** Sydney Investigational Criteria for Diagnosis of Antiphospholipid Syndrome

**Clinical**

- Vascular thrombosis (one or more episodes of arterial, venous, or small vessel thrombosis). For histopathologic diagnosis, there should <u>not</u> be evidence of inflammation in the vessel wall.

- Pregnancy morbidities attributable to placental insufficiency, including three or more otherwise unexplained recurrent spontaneous miscarriages, before 10 weeks of gestation. Also, one or more fetal losses after the 10th week of gestation, stillbirth, episode of preeclampsia, preterm labor, placental abruption, intrauterine growth restriction, or oligohydramnios that are otherwise unexplained.

**Laboratory**

- aCL or anti-$\beta_2$GPI IgG and/or IgM antibody present in medium or high titer on two or more occasions, at least 12 weeks apart, measured by standard ELISAs.

- Lupus anticoagulant in plasma, on two or more occasions, at least 12 weeks apart detected according to the guidelines of the International Society on Thrombosis and Haemostasis Scientific Standardisation Committee on Lupus Anticoagulants and Phospholipid-Dependent Antibodies.

- "Definite APS" is considered to be present if at least one of the clinical criteria and one of the laboratory criteria are met.

aCL, anticardiolipin; aPL, antiphospholipid; $\beta_2$GPI, $\beta_2$-glycoprotein I; ELISA, enzyme-linked immunosorbent assay; Ig, immunoglobulin.

Data from Miyakis S, Lockshin MD, Atsumi T, et al: International consensus statement on an update of the classification criteria for definite antiphospholipid syndrome (APS). *J Thromb Haemost* 4:295–306, 2006.

# ●ETIOLOGY AND PATHOGENESIS

## ETIOLOGY

As with most autoimmune conditions, the etiology of APS is not understood. It has been demonstrated that even normal healthy individuals have memory B cells that produce aPL antibodies. In a study of patients with infectious mononucleosis, 10 to 60 percent of immunoglobulin (Ig) M aPL-producing cells expressed CD27, the marker of memory B cells.[19] The affinity of aPL antibodies for their target becomes increased by the inclusion of amino acids lysine, arginine, and asparagine within the complementary determining regions of the heavy and light chains.[20]

Although antibodies against anionic phospholipid moieties arise during the course of infections such as syphilis and Lyme disease, those are distinct from antibodies generated by patients with the syndrome because they generally recognize phospholipid epitopes directly (also referred to as "cofactor independent") and are not associated with the clinical manifestations of the syndrome. There are intriguing hints for molecular mimicry mechanisms and that infection and vaccination-induced APS could be related to autoimmune/autoinflammatory syndrome induced by adjuvants (ASIA).[21] aPL antibodies have been reported in patients who developed thrombosis after varicella infection[8,22,23] and in patients with hepatitis C.[24,25] aPL antibodies were reported in a patient with cytomegalovirus (CMV) infection and mesenteric and femoropopliteal thrombosis.[26,27] $\beta_2$GPI cofactor–dependent antibodies against cardiolipin, phosphatidyl serine, and phosphatidyl ethanolamine have been identified in sera from patients with parvovirus B19.[28] Bacterial infections are a predisposing risk factor for the catastrophic form of APS (CAPS).[29] A high proportion of HIV-1 patients have aPL antibodies, including more than 40 percent in one study, in which 18 percent had aCL and 30 percent had anti-$\beta_2$GPI (mostly of the IgA isotype)[30]; however, positivity for these antibodies was not associated with thrombosis. A link has been proposed between the cardiac valvular disease in acute rheumatic fever and the presence of aPL antibodies.[31] aCL antibodies having $\beta_2$GPI dependence and LA activity have been generated in rabbits immunized with lipid A and lipoteichoic acid, suggesting that some bacteria can contribute to the production of pathogenic aPL antibodies.[32] It has also been proposed that cellular apoptosis, with the resulting exposure of anionic phospholipids on cell surfaces, may trigger the generation of aPL antibodies.[33–35] Molecular mimicry between $\beta_2$GPI-related synthetic peptides and structures within bacteria, viruses, and tetanus toxoid[36] has been demonstrated in an experimental model for APS.[37] Mice immunized with a CMV-derived peptide developed aPL antibodies and thrombosis and showed evidence for endothelial cell activation.[38]

Reports of familial clustering of raised aPL antibody levels[39] indicate that genetic susceptibility can play a role in their development. In one study of 84 APS patients, more than 35 percent had at least one relative and more than 20 percent had two or more relatives with evidence of at least one clinical feature of APS, such as thrombosis or recurrent fetal loss.[40]

## PATHOGENESIS

### Experimental Evidence That Antiphospholipid Antibodies Are Pathogenic

It has been clearly established in a number of experimental animal models for APS that aPL antibodies play a causal role in the development of thrombosis and pregnancy loss.[41–45] Although it is reasonable to assume that the same holds for the human disorder, the epitopic specificities of the autoantibodies that cause disease and the mechanisms by which they produce clinical manifestations require further elucidation.

## Antigenic Specificities

Antibodies against phospholipid that arise during the immunologic response to syphilis and other infections (with the notable exception of leprosy[46]) recognize anionic phospholipid epitopes directly,[47] whereas pathogenic aPL antibodies recognize phospholipid-binding proteins, primarily $\beta_2$GPI.[48,49]

$\beta_2$GPI (also named apolipoprotein H), a member of the complement control protein or short consensus repeat superfamily,[50] is a highly glycosylated single-chain plasma protein composed of 326 amino acids, with a molecular weight of approximately 50 kDa (Fig. 21-1). $\beta_2$GPI has five short consensus repeat (SCR) stretches of approximately 60 amino acids[45] (also referred to as complement control protein [CCP] repeats). Epitopic specificities for individual domains may have pathogenic and prognostic significance (see "Immunoassays" below).[51-54]

The affinity of $\beta_2$GPI for anionic phospholipids derives from cationic residues from its aminoterminus that have affinity for anionic polar heads of phospholipids and a hydrophobic loop that inserts into the lipid bilayer. $\beta_2$GPI has five domains for which antibodies have been identified. IgG antibodies against an epitope comprising Gly40-Arg43 in the domain I of $\beta_2$GPI have been reported to have a stronger correlation with thrombosis than antibodies against other epitopes.[51] Recent data support the concept that $\beta_2$GPI undergoes conformational changes that may be important for the APS disease process. By transmission electron microscopy, unbound $\beta_2$GPI appears to be in a closed conformation because of the affinity of a portion of carboxyterminal domain V for the protein's amninoterminal domain I, where the phospholipid binding site is located near the carboxy-terminus of SCR domain V (see Fig. 21-1).[55] The binding of $\beta_2$GPI to anionic phospholipid membranes requires a conformational change that exposes an epitope in domain I that had been cryptic in the unbound conformation (see Fig. 21-1).[55]

Although $\beta_2$GPI binds to phospholipids, its role in aPL-mediated cell signaling (described in the section "Proposed Pathogenic Mechanisms," below) is mediated via binding to toll-like receptors (TLRs) and not by direct binding to the lipid bilayer.

While the *in vivo* biologic function(s) of the protein has (have) not been defined, several interesting properties have been demonstrated. The molecule binds to apoptotic cells[56] and may play a role in

their phagocytosis and clearance.[57] $\beta_2$GPI binds to oxidized low-density lipoprotein (LDL) and may play a role in its clearance.[58] $\beta_2$GPI binds to lipopolysaccharide, and the scavenged complex is taken up by monocytes/macrophages.[59] $\beta_2$GPI reduces platelet adhesion to collagen in flow chambers by interfering with the platelet–von Willebrand factor (VWF) interaction by binding to its A2 domain, thereby interfering with its binding to the platelet glycoprotein Ib complex.[60] $\beta_2$GPI may also promote fibrinolysis as a cofactor for tissue-type plasminogen activator (t-PA) via its SCR domain V, which increases fibrinolytic activity.[61] The protein may have a further effect on fibrinolysis by binding to endothelial cells via annexin A2, a protein that also serves as a receptor for plasminogen and t-PA.[62] Homozygous $\beta_2$GPI-null mice have not been demonstrated to display a thrombotic phenotype.[63] However, the protein may play a role—although not a critical one—in the reproductive process, as there was a reduction in the number of viable implantation sites in $\beta_2$GPI-null mice and reduced fetal weight and fetal-to-placental weight ratio in late gestation, suggesting compromised placental function.[64]

In addition to $\beta_2$GPI, a number of other antigenic targets have been identified for aPL, including, but not limited to, prothrombin, coagulation factor V, protein C, protein S, annexin A2, annexin A5, high- and low-molecular-weight kininogens, and factors VII/VIIa and vimentin–cardiolipin complex.[65-68]

## Proposed Pathogenic Mechanisms

Table 21-3 and Fig. 21-2 summarize several of the main current hypotheses for pathogenic mechanisms in APS. The mechanisms of the human APS disease process have been difficult to elucidation, mainly for two reasons: (1) The phenotypes of vascular thrombosis and pregnancy morbidity are not unique to APS, so it is difficult to ascertain whether the candidate mechanism is playing a causal role or is incidental. (2) Antibodies isolated from APS patients recognize a multiplicity of antigenic determinants[69,70] that can have a broad range of effects, so it is difficult to determine which specificities and effects are responsible for disease manifestations in humans.

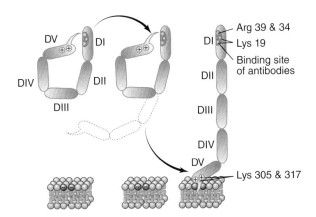

**Figure 21–1.** Schematic of the conformational states of $\beta_2$GPI. The unbound protein is in a closed conformation in which the epitope on domain I (DI) is shielded by a portion of domain V (DV). Binding to phospholipid membranes via a "barb," consisting of a hydrophobic loop formed by Ser311 to Lys317, near the carboxyterminus of DV, requires the protein to open and exposes an immunogenic epitope near the aminoterminal portion of the molecule. (*Reproduced with permission from Rand JH A snappy new concept for APS. Blood 2010 Aug 26;116(8):1193–1194.*)

**TABLE 21–3.** Proposed Pathogenic Mechanisms for Antiphospholipid Syndrome

I. Disruption of endothelial surface and annexin A5 anticoagulant shield

II. Enhanced cell signaling

   A. Mediated by antibodies against annexin A2

   B. Mediated by antibodies to ApoE2R

   C. Induction of endothelial surface proadhesive molecules

   D. Induction of tissue factor expression on monocytes and endothelial cells

   E. Complement-mediated signaling and injury

III. Impeding of fibrinolysis and endogenous anticoagulation

   A. Interference with plasminogen and tissue plasminogen activator

   B. Interference with components of the protein C activation pathway

IV. Activation of platelets

   A. Interference with $\beta_2$-glycoprotein I dampening of von Willebrand factor–mediated platelet adhesion

V. Other mechanisms

   A. Mammalian target of rapamycin complex pathway–mediated vasculopathy

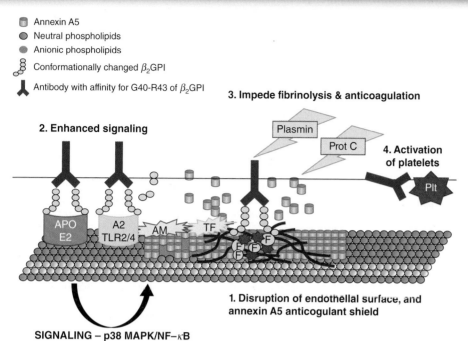

- ▢ Annexin A5
- ⬤ Neutral phospholipids
- ⬤ Anionic phospholipids
- Conformationally changed $\beta_2$GPI
- Antibody with affinity for G40-R43 of $\beta_2$GPI

**2. Enhanced signaling**

**3. Impede fibrinolysis & anticoagulation**

Plasmin

Prot C

**4. Activation of platelets**

Plt

APO E2

A2 TLR2/4

AM

TF

SIGNALING – p38 MAPK/NF–κB

**1. Disruption of endothelial surface, and annexin A5 anticogulant shield**

**Figure 21–2.** Multiple pathogenic mechanisms of aPL antibodies. (1) On a disrupted endothelial surface, anti-$\beta_2$GPI–$\beta_2$GPI complexes bind through the cationic domain V of $\beta_2$GPI to anionic structures, such as heparan sulfate, to provide a prothrombotic surface. (2) In addition, anti-$\beta_2$GPI–$\beta_2$GPI complexes activate endothelial cell receptors such as ApoE2, TLR2/TLR4, and annexin A2 to promote downstream signaling pathways involving p38 mitogen-activated protein kinase (p38 MAPK) and nuclear factor-κB (NF-κB), leading to the upregulation of tissue factor (TF) and adhesion molecules (AM) and a proinflammatory/prothrombotic phenotype. (3) Anti-$\beta_2$GPI–$\beta_2$GPI complexes also impede fibrinolysis and anticoagulation by impeding plasmin, annexin A5 anticoagulant activity, and the protein C (Prot C) pathways. (4) Anti-$\beta_2$GPI–$\beta_2$GPI complexes bind to directly to activate platelets (Plt) and promote aggregation.

**Disruption of the Endothelial Surface and Annexin A5 Anticoagulant Shield** Annexin A5 is a potent anticoagulant protein with high affinity for phospholipid membranes that contain anionic phospholipids, specifically phosphatidyl serine.[71] Annexin A5 forms two-dimensional crystals over the phospholipid bilayers that shield them from binding coagulation factors,[72] and it has been proposed that the protein may play a thrombomodulatory role on the surfaces of cells lining the placental and systemic vasculatures. Annexin A5 is highly expressed on the apical membranes of placental syncytiotrophoblasts, the location where maternal blood interfaces with fetal cells.[73] Pregnant annexin A5–null mice develop placental infarctions of fetuses and yield reduced litter sizes.[74] Pregnant mice treated with anti–annexin A5 antibodies developed placental necrosis, fibrosis, and pregnancy loss.[75] Dissociation of annexin A5 from the surface of human placental trophoblasts and human umbilical vein endothelial cells accelerates the coagulation of plasma exposed to those cells.[76] Annexin A5 binds to the surfaces of endothelial cells and inhibits thrombin formation.[77]

aPL antibody–antigen complexes disrupt the crystallization of annexin A5 and displace the protein from phospholipid membrane surfaces (Fig. 21–3).[78–81] In contrast to the LA phenomenon, aPL antibodies accelerate coagulation reactions in systems that include annexin A5.[78,82–85] IgG fractions from APS patients reduce the quantity of annexin A5 on cultured placental trophoblasts[76,86] and endothelial cells[76,87] and accelerate the coagulation of plasma exposed to these cells.[76] This effect of aPL antibodies on annexin A5 binding has been correlated with IgG antibodies that recognize a specific epitope—domain I of $\beta_2$GPI in patients with APS who have thrombosis[52] and spontaneous pregnancy losses. Figure 21–2 includes a model for this mechanism.

**Binding to Endothelial Surface Receptors Enhances Cell Signaling** aPL antibodies can bind, injure, and activate cultured vascular endothelial cells.[88–91] Cultured endothelial cells incubated with aPL antibodies with specificity for cell surface $\beta_2$GPI express increased levels of cell adhesion molecules[92] triggered by their binding to cell surface $\beta_2$GPI.[93] Annexin A2 serves as a receptor for $\beta_2$GPI,[62] and anti-$\beta_2$GPI antibodies may thereby stimulate expression of tissue factor on endothelial cells.[94] In animal models, the signaling effects of aPL antibodies were significantly reduced in mice treated with an anti–annexin A2 monoclonal antibody and also in annexin A2–null transgenic mice.[95] These effects of the aPL antibodies may be mediated by TLR-4 of the innate immunity system,[96,97] although there are data indicating participation of

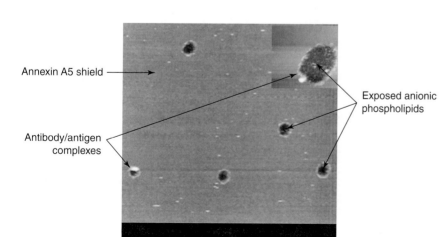

Annexin A5 shield

Exposed anionic phospholipids

Antibody/antigen complexes

**Figure 21–3.** Disruption of annexin A5 shield by monoclonal antiphospholipid antibodies and $\beta_2$-glycoprotein I ($\beta_2$GPI). Atomic force microscopy picture showing the effect of a monoclonal aPL antibody on a preformed annexin A5 crystal. The figure demonstrates the smooth lipid bilayer covered by the annexin A5 crystals, disrupted by antibody–$\beta_2$GPI complexes (*white circles*) and exposing anionic phospholipids (*black holes*) to coagulation factors and accelerated coagulation. (*Modifed with permission from Rand JH, Wu XX, Quinn AS, et al. Human monoclonal antiphospholipid antibodies disrupt the annexin A5 anticoagulant crystal shield on phospholipid bilayers: evidence from atomic force microscopy and functional assay. Am J Pathol 2003 Sep; 163(3):1193–1200.*)

other TLRs, particularly TLR-2.[98] This binding results in downstream signaling that involves TRAF6 (tumor necrosis factor receptor-associated factor 6) and MyD88 (myeloid differentiation factor 88).[99] Increased expression of tissue factor is mediated by p38 mitogen-activated protein kinase (MAPK).[100]

Binding of autoantibodies to annexin A2 may also promote thrombosis by inhibiting fibrinolysis. APS patients have increased titers of antibodies against annexin A2, an endothelial surface receptor for t-PA, and plasminogen.[101] The blocking of annexin A2 by aPL antibodies impedes plasmin generation in a t-PA–dependent generation assay and inhibits cell surface plasmin generation on human umbilical vein endothelial cells.[94] Several additional mechanisms have been identified by which aPL antibodies can interfere with fibrinolysis. $\beta_2$GPI is a cofactor for t-PA–mediated activation of plasminogen, and aPL antibodies against $\beta_2$GPI interfere with its binding to t-PA, thereby downregulating plasminogen activation.[61] Finally, fibrinolysis may also be impaired by autoantibodies directed against the catalytic site of plasmin or t-PA,[102,103] by an increased level of plasminogen activator inhibitor-1,[104] and by inhibition of autoactivation of factor XII with ensuing reductions of kallikrein and urokinase.[105]

Apolipoprotein E receptor 2 (apoER2), a member of the LDL-receptor family, is found on endothelial surfaces,[106] monocytes,[107] and platelets, and may also serve as receptor for anti-$\beta_2$GPI–$\beta_2$GPI complexes where it can also trigger the phosphatidylinositol 3′-kinase (PI3K)/Akt pathway[108] and increase tissue factor and cell adhesion molecule expression. IgG-mediated dimerization of $\beta_2$GPI and binding to ApoER2′ increase the sensitivity of platelets to agonists of aggregation.[109]

**Complement-Mediated Injury** Complement activation may play a role in the APS disease process. The IgG$_2$ subtype of aPL most closely correlates with thrombosis.[110,111] Blockade of complement activation using a C3 convertase inhibitor or genetic deletion of C3 protected mice from pregnancy complications induced by aPL antibodies.[112–114] These effects involve the aPL-stimulated expression of tissue factor by myeloid cells[115] and proteinase-activated G-protein–coupled receptor (PAR)-2 signaling,[116] indicating that complement activation can be pathogenic via both direct injury and downstream signaling.

**Induction of Tissue Factor Activity in Leukocytes** aPL antibodies can promote tissue factor expression by leukocytes.[115,117–119] The specific binding site on these cells has not been elucidated.

**Inhibition of Fibrinolysis and Endogenous Anticoagulation** aPL antibodies can interfere with fibrinolysis in several ways. Antibodies against annexin A2, an endothelial surface receptor for t-PA and plasminogen, can interfere with binding of plasminogen and t-PA and thereby reduce plasmin formation and fibrinolysis.[94,101,103] Monoclonal aPL antibodies derived from APS patients can directly inhibit plasmin's enzymatic activity.[102] $\beta_2$GPI is a cofactor for t-PA–mediated activation of plasminogen,[120] and anti-$\beta_2$GPI can interfere with this activity. Also, it has been reported that women with APS have significantly increased levels of circulating plasminogen activator inhibitor-1 (PAI-1), implying impaired fibrinolysis.[104]

**Interference with Components of the Protein C Activation Pathway** The protein C pathway (Chap. 4) is initiated by thrombin binding to thrombomodulin (TM), which activates protein C bound to the endothelial protein C receptor (EPCR). Activated protein C (APC), together with free protein S, then proteolyses coagulation factors Va and VIIIa. APC also modulates signaling events by interfering with PAR-1 signalling.[121,122] aPL antibodies can interfere with the activation of protein C by TM–thrombin and with the activity of APC, as well as protect factors Va and VIIIa from proteolysis by APC.[65] Acquired APC resistance has been described in APS plasmas[123] and has been correlated with anti-$\beta_2$GPI domain I antibodies,[124] a risk factor for thrombosis. The presence of antibodies against EPCR in APS patients was proposed to be a risk factor for fetal death.[125]

**Antiphospholipid Antibodies Activate Platelets** An experimental animal model that includes *in vivo* imaging has provided data indicating that aPL-induced thrombosis is a consequence of platelet activation that then promotes endothelial activation and fibrin formation.[126] aPL antibodies can induce platelet aggregation,[127] an effect that might be promoted via signaling through apoER2 receptors; the $\beta_2$GPI binding site for apoER2 on platelets was localized to its domain V.[128] As described above (see "Antigenic Specificities"), $\beta_2$GPI also has a dampening effect on platelet adhesion by interfering with the platelet–VWF interaction, and consequently, aPL antibodies, by interfering with this $\beta_2$GPI-mediated dampening, can increase platelet adhesion in flow systems.[60]

**Other Mechanisms** APS patients have been shown to have autoantibodies against tissue factor pathway inhibitor.[129] Some aPL antibodies cross-react with heparin and heparinoid molecules, which are highly polyanionic, and hence, inhibit their contribution to antithrombin activity.[69] aPL antibodies show cross-reactivity against oxidized LDL[130] and are associated with an increased risk of atherosclerosis.[131] Antibodies against $\beta_2$GPI-oxidized LDL complexes have been proposed to be atherogenic by reducing their clearance.[132] Finally, in addition to promoting thrombosis, aPL antibodies may contribute to other vascular lesions by stimulating the mammalian target of rapamycin complex (mTORC) pathway (Fig. 21–4).[133]

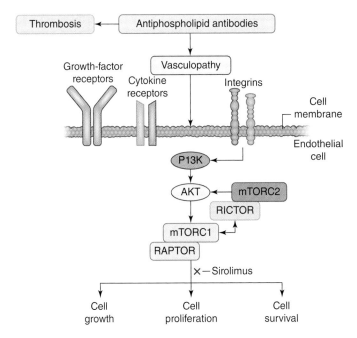

**Figure 21–4.** Pathogenesis of vasculopathy in the antiphospholipid syndrome. In addition to promoting thrombosis, antiphospholipid antibodies also trigger vasculopathy by binding to vascular endothelial cells and activating the mammalian target of rapamycin (mTOR) signaling pathway. Extracellular and intracellular signals through the phosphatidylinositide 3′-kinase (PI3K)-AKT pathway activate the mTOR pathway, which regulates cell growth, proliferation, and survival. The mTOR enzyme is a component of two complexes, mammalian target of rapamycin complex (mTORC) 1 and mTORC2. The activity of mTORC1 is regulated by a subunit of the regulatory-associated protein of mTORC1 (RAPTOR), whereas the activity of mTORC2 is regulated by a subunit of the rapamycin-insensitive companion of mTOR (RICTOR). *(Modified with permission from Eikelbloom JW, Weitz JI. The mTORC pathway in the antiphospholipid syndrome, N Engl J Med 2014 Jul 24;371(4):369–371.)*

# ●CLINICAL FEATURES

Table 21–4 summarizes the clinical features of APS. Patients generally present with thrombotic manifestations, that is, evidence for vasoocclusion or end-organ ischemia or infarction, and/or pregnancy losses and complications attributable to placental insufficiency. The usual age at presentation with thrombosis is approximately 35 to 45 years. Except for patients with SLE, men and women are equally susceptible to thrombotic manifestations. No differences have been observed between the arterial and venous distributions of thromboses of primary and secondary APS patients.[134]

## SYSTEMIC VASCULAR THROMBOSIS

Patients can present with spontaneous venous and/or arterial thrombosis or embolism in any site; however, about half of all patients have deep vein thrombosis of the lower extremities.[135,136] Other sites of venous thromboembolic events include pulmonary embolism, thoracic veins (superior vena cava, subclavian vein, or jugular vein), and abdominal or pelvic veins.[136] Approximately one-fourth of patients present with arterial thromboses; the remainder present with concurrent arterial and venous thrombosis.[136] Patients may also present with stroke, cerebral venous thrombosis, upper-extremity venous thrombosis,[135] myocardial infarction, adrenal infarction, acalculous gallbladder infarction, aortic thrombosis with renal infarction,[120] and mesenteric artery thrombosis.[137,138] Thrombosis may occur spontaneously or in the presence of some other risk factor such as estrogen replacement therapy, oral contraceptives,[134,139] vascular stasis, surgery, or trauma. Women are at particularly high risk for venous thrombosis during pregnancy and in the postpartum period.[134] Some APS patients with venous thrombosis have concurrent genetic thrombophilic conditions such as the factor V Leiden variant, and it has been postulated that this may increase the risk of thrombosis.[140-143] Concurrent positivity for all three aPL antibody assays—that is, the aCL

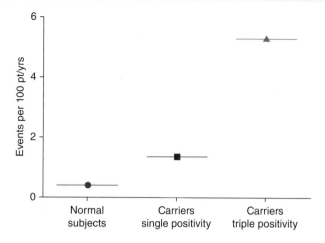

**Figure 21–5.** Average annual rates of first cardiovascular events (including venous thromboembolism) among antiphospholipid (aPL) antibody–negative and aPL antibody–positive populations. Concurrent positivity for all three aPL antibody assays—that is, "triple positivity" for the aCL antibody assay, anti-$\beta_2$GPI antibody assay, and the lupus anticoagulant assay—is a highly significant risk factor for a first thrombotic event. (Modified with permission from Pengo V, Ruffatti A, Legnani C et al. Incidence of a first thromboembolic event in asymptomatic carriers of high-risk antiphospholipid antibody profile: a multicenter prospective study, Blood 2011 Oct 27; 118(17):4714–4718.)

antibody assay, anti-$\beta_2$GPI antibody assay, and the LA assay—appears to be a highly significant risk factor for having an initial thrombotic event (Fig. 21–5).[144] If this finding is confirmed, it could identify a group of patients who might warrant consideration for prophylactic treatment. A history of having had a thromboembolic event is probably the most significant risk factor for recurrence of venous thromboembolism in APS, with a reported frequency that reached approximately 30 percent in patients followed for 4 years after the first episode.[145] The risk of recurrent thromboembolism correlates with the titer of antibodies[145,146] and with the presence of LA. In addition, it appears that the presence of anti-$\beta_2$GPI domain I antibodies significantly increases the risk of thrombosis, compared to patients who have antibodies that are not domain I dependent and LA that is not domain I dependent.[51]

## SYSTEMIC LUPUS ERYTHEMATOSUS AND OTHER AUTOIMMUNE CONDITIONS

APS patients frequently present with other autoimmune conditions. A significant proportion of SLE patients have elevated aPL antibodies, with estimates ranging between 12 and 30 percent for aCL antibodies and 15 and 34 percent for LA antibodies.[147] APS has been associated with the concurrence of other autoimmune conditions including, but not limited to, rheumatoid arthritis,[148] Sjögren syndrome,[149] myasthenia gravis,[150] Budd-Chiari syndrome in the setting of SLE,[151] Graves disease,[152] autoimmune hemolytic anemia, progressive systemic sclerosis,[153] Evans syndrome,[154] Takayasu arteritis,[155] polyarteritis nodosa,[156] and immune thrombocytopenia (see section "Thrombocytopenia" below and also Chap. 7).

## STROKE AND OTHER NEUROLOGIC CONDITIONS

The most common neurologic manifestations of APS are stroke or transient ischemic attacks (TIAs), which were the initial presentation of up to 30 percent of adults with APS in a large European cohort.[157] In the European Catastrophic Antiphospholipid Antibody Syndrome (CAPS)

---

**TABLE 21–4.** Clinical Manifestations Associated with APS

- Venous and arterial thromboembolism*
- Pregnancy complications attributable to placental insufficiency, including spontaneous pregnancy losses as detailed in Table 21–2, intrauterine growth restriction, preeclampsia, preterm labor, and placental abruption*
- Thrombocytopenia
- Thrombotic and embolic stroke*
- Cerebral vein thrombosis*
- Livedo reticularis, necrotizing skin vasculitis
- Coronary artery disease
- Valvular heart disease
- Kidney disease
- Pulmonary hypertension
- Acute respiratory distress syndrome
- Atherosclerosis and peripheral artery disease
- Nonthrombotic retinal disease
- Adrenal failure, hemorrhagic adrenal infarction*
- Budd-Chiari syndrome, mesenteric and portal vein obstructions, hepatic infarction, esophageal necrosis, gastric and colonic ulceration, gallbladder necrosis*
- Catastrophic antiphospholipid syndrome with thrombotic microangiopathy*

*Manifestations that qualify as consensus criteria for diagnosis of antiphospholipid syndrome.[18]

Registry, cerebral manifestations occurred in 62 percent of patients and caused 13 percent of deaths.[158] Recurrent strokes are more likely in patients with APS and other risk factors for cerebrovascular disease, such as cigarette smoking, hypertension hyperlipidemia, oral contraceptive use, and SLE.[159,160]

Most APS patients with stroke have arterial thromboembolic occlusive events that are clinically indistinguishable from the more common arteriosclerotic strokes. APS should be suspected in young patients with TIAs or stroke, particularly when the more typical risk factors for cerebrovascular disease are absent.[161] Cerebral venous thrombosis is less common in APS patients, presents at a younger age, and is more extensive than in non-APS patients with the disorder.[162] In one series of 40 cases of cerebral venous thrombosis, three patients (8 percent) had elevated aPL antibody levels.[163] Superior sagittal sinus thrombosis has been reported with primary APS.[164]

There is controversy about whether migraines in patients with aPL antibodies should be regarded as thromboocclusive events.[165] Other neurologic abnormalities reported to be associated with aPL antibodies include seizures/epilepsy,[166] chorea, Guillain-Barré syndrome, transient global amnesia, dementia, diabetic peripheral neuropathy, and orthostatic hypotension.[167] Recurrent acute transverse myelopathy has been described with APS.[168–172] However, in one study of 315 SLE patients, including 10 with a history of transverse myelopathy, that disorder was not associated with aPL antibodies.[173] Multiple sclerosis patients have a high incidence of elevated aCL antibody levels (in one series, 9 percent had IgG antibodies and 44 percent had IgM antibodies)[174]; however, no clinical distinctions were found between aPL-positive and aPL-negative patients, and the antibodies do not appear to be associated with thrombosis. Patients with psychotic disorders have an increased prevalence of LA and aCL antibodies, even in the absence of treatment with antipsychotic drugs.[175]

## CATASTROPHIC ANTIPHOSPHOLIPID SYNDROME

CAPS is a relatively infrequent but devastating presentation of APS and is characterized by severe widespread vascular occlusions.[176] Diagnostic criteria for CAPS include evidence of involvement of at least three organs, systems, and/or tissues; development of manifestations simultaneously or in less than 1 week; histopathologic confirmation of small-vessel occlusion; and laboratory confirmation of the presence of aPL antibodies.[177] According to the CAPS Registry, a web-based database of 433 patients with CAPS (https://ontocrf.costaisa.com/en/web/caps/), the majority of CAPS patients are female (69 percent) and in their late thirties (mean age of 38.5 years), but the condition can present at any age (range: 0 to 85 years). In half of the CAPS cases, the patients' catastrophic event was their first APS manifestation. Precipitating factors of CAPS include infections, drugs (sulfur-containing diuretics, captopril, and oral contraceptives), surgical procedures, and cessation of prior anticoagulant therapy. In 26.9 percent of cases, the patients also had SLE. The most frequently affected organ was the kidney (73 percent of episodes), followed by lungs (58.9 percent), the brain (55.9 percent), the heart (49.7 percent), and the skin (45.4 percent). Other organs were also affected, including the peripheral vessels, intestines, spleen, adrenal glands, pancreas, retina, and marrow. Patients present with evidence for severe multiorgan ischemia/infarction, often with concurrent disseminated microvascular thrombosis. Patients with CAPS can present with renal insufficiency; respiratory failure resulting from acute respiratory distress syndrome (ARDS) and pulmonary emboli; cerebral manifestations such as encephalopathy, stroke, and seizures; cardiac problems such as heart failure, myocardial infarction, and valvular defects; and skin complications such as livedo reticularis and skin necrosis.[178] Most patients show histologic evidence of microangiopathy mainly affecting small vessels of the kidneys, lungs, brain, heart, and liver. Only a minority of patients experience large-vessel occlusions. Laboratory evidence for disseminated intravascular coagulation is frequently present. An LA is present in 81.7 percent of patients, and the aCL IgG is the most common positive aPL antibody.[178] Improved treatment has reduced mortality from approximately 50 percent to approximately 20 percent.[176] Relapse is rare in survivors. The only identified predictive factor for adverse outcome is underlying SLE.[179]

## PREGNANCY LOSSES, OBSTETRIC COMPLICATIONS, AND INFERTILITY

At this time, aPL screening of otherwise asymptomatic obstetrical patients with no history of prior complications is not warranted because of the high frequency of false-positive tests; most studies have estimated the prevalence of aPL antibodies among general obstetric populations to be approximately 5 percent or less, and most of these aPL-positive patients are not clinically affected.[180]

Among obstetric patients with recurrent fetal losses, approximately 16 to 38 percent have aPL antibodies. In addition, pregnant women with elevated aPL antibodies had significantly more obstetric complications, including preeclampsia, abruption placentae, miscarriage, prematurity, intrauterine fetal demise, intrauterine growth restriction, and oligohydramnios, than aPL antibody–negative pregnant women.[181–183] In approximately half of patients, the pregnancy losses occur in the first trimester. Other patients present with later losses, most in the second trimester, but some occur even later, including stillbirth. Pregnancy complications attributable to APS include three or more recurrent spontaneous first-trimester miscarriages, one or more fetal losses during the second trimester, stillbirth, episode of preeclampsia, preterm labor, placental abruption, intrauterine growth restriction, and oligohydramnion.[184–186] Pregnant patients with APS are also more prone to developing deep vein thrombosis during pregnancy or the puerperium. Rarely, pregnant patients develop CAPS.[187,188] The best predictor for pregnancy loss in a patient who tests positive for aPL antibodies has been demonstrated to simply be a previous history of pregnancy loss, complications, or thrombosis.[146,189] A recent study reported that aPL antibody–positive women with an unexplained early loss prior to 10 weeks have a higher risk of complications in their second pregnancy,[190] but the degree of laboratory abnormalities was not associated with increased risk. Positivity by more than one assay appears to correlate with increased pregnancy morbidities.[182,191] Histologic abnormalities were found in many, but not all, placentas of aPL patients.[192] Studies of placental pathology in patients with aPL antibodies, but without a prior history of fetal loss, showed that approximately half had evidence of uteroplacental vascular pathology, approximately half had evidence of thrombotic occlusion, and approximately one-third had chronic villitis and/or decidual plasma cell infiltrates.[193,194]

Overall, it appears that the presence of aPL antibodies does not affect the success rate of implantation. Although one group has reported data that indicated that women with recurrent implantation failure were more likely to have positive assays for aPL antibodies compared to fertile negative controls,[195] a review of 29 studies showed mixed results.[196] Many of the studies were noted to have limitations, including problems with study design and statistical power. The current consensus is that aPL antibodies are not a cause of infertility.[197] Recently, the 14th International Congress on Antiphospholipid Antibodies Task Force also concluded that "there are no data to support the inclusion of infertility as criteria for APS and investigation of APS in patients with infertility should not be done in routine clinical practice, being reserved only for research purposes."[196]

## CUTANEOUS MANIFESTATIONS

The cutaneous manifestations of APS may compose the first signs of APS in some patients.[198,199] Livedo reticularis is relatively common, occurring in 24 percent of a series of 1000 aPL patients,[200] and occasionally presents in a necrosing form.[201] Noninflammatory vascular thrombosis is the most frequent histopathologic feature. Necrotizing vasculitis, livedoid vasculitis, thrombophlebitis, cutaneous ulceration and necrosis, erythematous macules, purpura, ecchymoses, painful skin nodules, subungual splinter hemorrhages, anetoderma (macular atrophy), discoid lupus erythematosus, and cutaneous T-cell lymphoma have all been reported.

## CORONARY ARTERY DISEASE

aPL antibodies are associated with increased susceptibility to coronary artery disease,[202] particularly premature atherosclerosis.[203,204] APS should be considered in patients who lack the usual risk factors for coronary artery disease and in patients with evidence for thrombotic or embolic coronary artery occlusion who lack angiographic evidence of atherosclerotic disease. aPL antibodies appear to be a risk factor for adverse outcomes following all coronary revascularization procedures[202] and for restenosis after percutaneous transluminal coronary angioplasty.[205,206] An ultrasound study of carotid arteries provided evidence supporting an association of aPL antibodies with premature atherosclerosis; relatively young primary APS patients (mean age: 37 ± 11 years) had significantly increased intimal medial thickness compared to control non-APS groups.[207]

## VALVULAR HEART DISEASE

Approximately 35 percent of patients with primary APS have cardiac valvular abnormalities detected by echocardiography.[208] In one study, approximately 20 percent of cardiac patients with valvular heart disease had evidence for aPL antibodies compared with approximately 10 percent of matched control subjects.[209] Valvulopathy includes leaflet thickening, vegetations, regurgitation, and stenosis.[210] The mitral valve is mainly affected, followed by the aortic valve.[211] Histologically, APS valvular lesions consist mainly of superficial or intravalvular fibrin deposits in association with variable degrees of vascular proliferation, fibroblast influx, fibrosis, and calcification. These can result in valve thickening, fusion, and rigidity, nd can lead to functional abnormalities.[212] Deposits of immunoglobulins, including aCL antibodies, and of complement components are commonly found in the affected valves.[213]

## PERIPHERAL VASCULAR DISEASE

Approximately one-third of patients with peripheral arterial disease undergoing bypass grafting procedures had elevated aPL antibody levels (mostly aCL antibodies).[214] Intraarterial thromboembolic events are common at presentation of these patients and may complicate surgical management. However, these patients did not have an increased risk for reocclusion, a finding that was attributable to the use of anticoagulant therapy.

## PULMONARY MANIFESTATIONS

Patients with APS may present with in situ thrombosis in pulmonary vessels. aPL antibodies are associated with pulmonary hypertension.[215] In one prospective trial of 38 consecutive patients with precapillary pulmonary hypertension, approximately 30 percent had aPL antibodies with various phospholipid specificities.[216] An interinstitutional study of 687 patients with chronic thromboembolic pulmonary hypertension reported that aPL antibodies were a significant risk factor.[217] The majority

of patients with CAPS (see "Catastrophic Antiphospholipid Syndrome" above) have dyspnea, and most of these individuals have ARDS.[218]

## ABDOMINAL MANIFESTATIONS

The liver is the most frequently affected abdominal organ in APS, with occlusion of hepatic vessels, including those supplying the biliary tree.[219] aPL antibody levels frequently are elevated in patients with chronic liver disease of various causes. In one prospective study of patients with liver disease, approximately half of patients with alcoholic liver disease and one-third of patients with chronic hepatitis C virus had elevated aPL antibody levels. The frequency was even higher in patients with more severe cirrhosis.[220] A review reported that approximately 20 percent of patients with chronic hepatitis B and hepatitis C had aPL antibodies, most of which were cofactor independent.[221] Some patients with hepatitis C present with true autoimmune aPL antibodies, the most common features reported being intraabdominal thrombosis and myocardial infarction.[222]

Reported gastrointestinal manifestations of APS also include esophageal necrosis with perforation, intestinal ischemia and infarction, pancreatitis, and colonic ulceration. Primary biliary cirrhosis,[223] acute acalculous cholecystitis with gallbladder necrosis,[224,225] and giant gastric ulceration are associated with APS.[226] APS has been reported in patients with mesenteric inflammatory venoocclusive disease[227] and in patients with mesenteric and portal venous obstruction.[228]

## THROMBOCYTOPENIA

Approximately 20 to 40 percent of patients with APS have varying degrees of thrombocytopenia. The decrease in platelet count is generally mild or moderate and is rarely significant enough to cause bleeding complications or affect anticoagulant therapy.[229,230] The majority of patients with APS and thrombocytopenia have antibodies against $\alpha_{IIb}\beta_3$ integrin and/or glycoprotein Ib–IX complex.[231] Patients presenting with immune thrombocytopenic purpura frequently have elevated aPL antibodies, and these patients are more prone to thrombosis.[232] aPL antibodies and antibodies against platelet membrane glycoprotein were present simultaneously in approximately 70 percent of patients with immune-mediated thrombocytopenia.[233] Thrombocytopenia itself is not protective against thrombosis in these patients. In a prospective cohort study, 5-year thrombosis-free survival rates of aPL-positive and aPL-negative immune thrombocytopenic purpura patients were 39 percent and 98 percent, respectively.[234]

## BLEEDING

The presence of a concurrent hemostasis defect needs to be considered when patients with APS exhibit a bleeding tendency (Table 21–5). Acquired hypoprothrombinemia with severe bleeding has been reported.[235,236] This diagnosis may be missed when coagulation abnormalities are attributed only to the LA effect, so a specific assay for prothrombin should be performed when the prothrombin time is prolonged.

**TABLE 21–5.** Causes of Bleeding in Antiphospholipid Syndrome

- Hypoprothrombinemia
- Thrombocytopenia
- Acquired platelet function abnormality
- Acquired inhibitor to specific coagulation factor, e.g., factor VIII
- Acquired von Willebrand syndrome

Other causes of bleeding in APS include acquired thrombocytopathies, thrombocytopenia (see "Thrombocytopenia," above), acquired inhibitors against specific coagulation factors, such as factor VIII, and the acquired von Willebrand syndrome (AVWS).

## RETINAL ABNORMALITIES

The diagnosis of aPL antibody retinopathy should be suspected in patients with diffuse retinal vasoocclusion, particularly when characterized by involvement of arteries and veins, neovascularization at presentation, and symptoms of systemic rheumatologic disease.[237] aPL antibodies were present in 5 to 33 percent of patients with retinal vein occlusion.[238,239] Cilioretinal artery occlusion,[240] optic neuropathy,[241] and severe vasoocclusive retinopathy[242] have been described with APS.

## KIDNEY DISEASES

APS may affect the renal system. Patients may present with renal artery stenosis and/or thrombosis, renal infarction, renal vein thrombosis, and glomerulonephritis that is distinct from vasoocclusive disease.[200,243] An entity named "APS nephropathy" has been described, which consists of a vasoocclusive disease of small-size intrarenal vessels.[244] This nephropathy features fibrous intimal hyperplasia, focal cortical atrophy, and thrombotic microangiopathy. A review of 29 consecutive renal biopsies from patients with primary APS, performed at two institutions over 22 years, described 20 cases of APS nephropathy and nine cases with other distinct pathologic features.[243] These features included membranous nephropathy, minimal change disease/focal segmental glomerulonephritis, mesangial C3 nephropathy, and pauci-immune crescentic glomerulonephritis.

## ANTIPHOSPHOLIPID SYNDROME AND AIDS

Although patients with HIV-1 infection frequently have elevated aPL antibody levels, they do not often have thrombotic manifestations. A review indicated that approximately 50 percent of HIV-1 patients test positive for aPL antibodies, most of which are not cofactor dependent.[221] HIV-infected patients with manifestations of APS have also presented with avascular bone and cutaneous necrosis.[222]

## ANTIPHOSPHOLIPID SYNDROME IN CHILDREN

Increasingly, APS has become recognized in children,[245] in whom diverse clinical features are common. The results of a European registry have been reported.[246] Review of 121 cases indicated that although the thrombotic manifestations were similar to adults with APS, there was a difference between children with primary APS and secondary APS; the children with primary APS were younger and had a higher frequency of arterial thrombotic events, whereas the children with secondary APS had a higher frequency of venous thrombotic events associated with hematologic and skin manifestations. CAPS has been reported in children but is rare.[247,248]

Thrombosis is rare in newborns delivered from mothers with APS, and only a few cases are reported, mostly associated with other prothrombotic factors.[249] aPL antibodies have been found in up to 30 percent of offspring of mothers with APS.[250]

In a recent European prospective study, 17 percent of neonates born to APS mothers were premature; however, no specific complications were found during the 5-year follow-up.[251] The study did show a higher rate of neurodevelopmental abnormalities with learning disabilities similar to two retrospective reports where learning disabilities without other neurodevelopmental abnormalities were present in 15 to 20 percent of cases.[252,253]

## OTHER MANIFESTATIONS

Acute adrenal failure secondary to bilateral infarction of the adrenal glands has been reported as the first manifestation of primary APS.[254] Adrenal hemorrhage has been reported.[255] aPL antibodies have been associated with marrow necrosis.[256]

## ●LABORATORY FEATURES

Diagnosis of APS requires the demonstration of antibodies against phospholipids and/or relevant protein cofactors (Table 21–6). The current tests for APS recommended by the most recent consensus on investigational criteria[18] and the Scientific Standardisation Committee of the International Society on Thrombosis and Haemostasis are aCL, anti-$\beta_2$GPI (IgG and IgM), and LA.[257] The laboratory diagnosis of APS is frequently problematic, with limitations that have been detailed.[258,259] aCL IgG and IgM assays are the most sensitive but the least specific. Anti-$\beta_2$GPI IgG and IgM assays are more specific but less sensitive. LA assays, of which the dilute Russell viper venom time (dRVVT) is the most common, generally tend to be the least sensitive but the most specific. The current recommended tests are less than ideal because they are empirically derived tests and do not yet measure antibodies directed against disease-specific epitopes or functional parameters that correlate with disease mechanisms. Despite these limitations, positivity for all three criteria assays ("triple positivity") has been correlated with an increased risk for a future thrombotic event (see Fig. 21–5).[144]

**TABLE 21–6.** Diagnostic Tests for Antiphospholipid Syndrome

**Immunoassays**

Anticardiolipin IgG and IgM antibodies*

Anti-$\beta_2$GPI IgG and IgM antibodies*

Serologic test for syphilis ("biologic false-positive")

Antiphosphatidyl serine antibodies

Antiprothrombin antibodies

**Coagulation Tests†**

Dilute Russell viper venom time with mixing incubations and neutralization with excess phospholipid

aPTT with mixing incubation and neutralization with excess phospholipids

aPL-sensitive and -insensitive reagents and platelet neutralization procedure

Kaolin clotting time

Dilute prothrombin time (a.k.a. tissue thromboplastin inhibition test)

Hexagonal phase array test

Textarin/ecarin test

---

aPL, antiphospholipid; APS, antiphospholipid syndrome; aPTT, activated partial thromboplastin time; $\beta_2$GPI, $\beta_2$-glycoprotein I; Ig, immunoglobulin; LA, lupus anticoagulant.

*Recommended by the International Society on Thrombosis and Haemostasis (ISTH) Scientific and Standardisation Committee (SSC) Subcommittee on Lupus Anticoagulants and Antiphospholipid Antibodies.[258]

†The committee recommended that two coagulation assays be performed if LA or APS is suspected, preferably the dilute Russell viper venom time (dRVVT) and aPTT.

Investigational criteria have been developed to identify patients with "definite" autoimmune APS (see Table 21–3).[18] Because no single test is sufficient for diagnosing the disorder, a panel of tests, including antibodies against cardiolipin and $\beta_2$GPI and coagulation tests for LA, should be performed when APS is suspected.[257] The investigational criteria require that positive results have to be obtained on two or more occasions at least 12 weeks apart to qualify for diagnosis.

## IMMUNOASSAYS

### Anticardiolipin Antibody Assays

Most patients with APS are identified by elevated levels of aCL antibodies, a test with high sensitivity but poor specificity. The prevalence of positive tests in the asymptomatic healthy population has generally ranged from approximately 3 to 10 percent. In a prospective study of 2132 consecutive Spanish patients with venous thromboembolism, 4.1 percent had elevated levels of aCL antibodies (i.e., about the same prevalence as in the asymptomatic healthy population),[260] but in a group of healthy young women in another study, the prevalence of elevated levels of aCL was 18.2 percent.[261] Many individuals have antibody levels that are elevated in response to infections that are not associated with thrombotic complications. Patients with syphilis, Lyme disease, and other infections may be misdiagnosed with APS based on elevated aCL antibody levels when concurrent stroke or arterial thrombosis is present, so these conditions must always be ruled out in susceptible patients. In a systematic literature review, 15 of 28 studies showed significant associations between aCL antibodies and thrombosis.[262] In all cases, a correlation existed between high antibody titers and a high risk of thrombosis. Elevated levels of aCL antibodies, whether high or low titer, were significantly associated with both myocardial infarction and cerebral stroke. Only high-titer aCL antibodies significantly increased the risk of deep vein thrombosis. During a 10-year follow-up of patients with elevated levels of aCL antibodies, approximately 50 percent of patients who presented with the antibodies but without clinical manifestations of the syndrome subsequently developed the APS.[263] The presence of elevated titers of aCL antibodies 6 months after an episode of venous thromboembolism is a predictor for increased risk of recurrence and of death.[145] Women with aCL IgM antibodies or with an aCL IgG antibody titer less than 20 IgG-binding units and without a positive LA do not appear to be at risk for APS.[264] In contrast, women with an aCL IgG titer greater than 20 binding units or a positive LA were more likely to develop complications.[264] With respect to pregnancy losses, a meta-analysis of 25 studies on aPL antibodies in women with recurrent fetal losses showed a significant correlation with increased aCL IgG and particularly with LA.[262]

With respect to stroke, elevated levels of aCL antibodies of IgG or IgM isotype were reported to be significant risk factors.[265] aPL antibodies also are an independent risk factor for stroke in young women.[266]

Approximately 20 percent of patients taking procainamide have moderate to high levels of aCL antibodies.[267] In these patients, the antibodies are associated with anti-$\beta_2$GPI specificity. There have been case reports of associated thrombosis.[268] Treatment with chlorpromazine has been associated with the development of aCL antibodies,[269] although more recent data indicate that aPL antibodies are frequently elevated in patients with severe psychiatric disorders whether or not they are treated with antipsychotic medications.[270]

### Anti-$\beta_2$-Glycoprotein I Antibody Assays

$\beta_2$GPI is believed to be the major protein cofactor for aPL antibodies. Enzyme-linked immunosorbent assays (ELISAs) for anti-$\beta_2$GPI antibodies are considered to be more specific but less sensitive to APS than to aCL assays.[271] In a systematic literature review, 34 of 60 studies showed significant associations between anti-$\beta_2$GPI antibodies and thrombosis.[262] None of the studies were prospective. Of the 10 studies that included multivariate analysis, only two confirmed that anti-$\beta_2$GPI IgG antibodies were independent risk factors for venous thrombosis. Anti-$\beta_2$GPI antibodies were more often associated with venous than arterial thrombosis. Anti-$\beta_2$GPI IgA antibodies were significantly associated with thrombosis.

Although these antibodies usually are present in conjunction with abnormal aCL and antiphosphatidyl serine antibodies, some patients with APS present solely with antibodies to $\beta_2$GPI.[272,273] Despite their higher specificity for APS (98 percent), $\beta_2$GPI antibodies alone cannot be relied upon for the diagnosis because of their low sensitivity (40 to 50 percent).[274,275] Also, interlaboratory variability is a significant problem with anti-$\beta_2$GPI antibody assays.[276]

Epitope-specific anti-$\beta_2$GPI antibodies, not yet in general use, may offer a better predictive value for diagnosis and prognosis of APS. A recent analysis of 198 samples from patients with a variety of auto-immune conditions revealed that the 52 patients with anti-$\beta_2$GPI IgG antibodies could be divided into those that recognize domain I alone and those with reactivity for all domains[51]; the former were positive for LA and were associated with an increased risk for thrombosis. As mentioned earlier, positivity for this assay has been correlated with positivity for a functional coagulation assay that measures resistance to annexin A5 anticoagulant activity.[52]

### Assays for Antibodies Against Prothrombin and Phosphatidyl Serine

Prothrombin is considered the second major cofactor for aPL antibodies. In a systematic literature review, 17 of 46 studies showed significant associations between antiprothrombin antibodies and thrombosis.[262] Of the eight studies that included multivariate analysis, two confirmed that antiprothrombin antibodies were independent risk factors for thrombosis, and three other studies showed that antiprothrombin antibodies added to the risk borne by LA or aCL antibodies. A recent study indicated that the sensitivity of antiprothrombin immunoassays in the primary aPL syndrome is too low to warrant inclusion in recommendations for APS testing.[277]

Tests for antibodies against phosphatidyl serine have been hypothesized to be more relevant than antibodies against cardiolipin, because the latter are present in intracellular membranes, whereas phosphatidyl serine is exposed on syncytialized cells, on apoptotic cells, and on activated platelets. Antibodies against phosphatidyl serine were reported to correlate more specifically with APS than aCL antibodies, particularly in arterial thrombosis.[278,279] However, antiphosphatidyl serine antibody tests are not included as an international consensus criterion.[257]

Newer studies indicate that assays for detecting autoantibodies that recognize prothrombin complexed to the anionic phospholipid, phosphatidyl serine, may have improved utility for diagnosing APS by identifying patients suspected for the disorder but with negative results in the conventional assays; in one series of 728 patients who were suspected of having APS but tested negative by conventional assays, 41 were found to be positive for anti–prothrombin/phosphatidyl serine.[280] It has also been suggested that positivity for these assays may correlate with positivity for LA assays.[281]

### Assays for Antibodies Against Other Phospholipids

Some investigators have advocated testing for antibodies against a panel of phospholipids other than cardiolipin,[282–285] but others have disagreed.[286] Although one review has indicated that measurement for antiphosphatidyl ethanolamine antibodies may identify some patients whose conventional tests are negative for aPL antibodies,[287] the current consensus holds that no benefit has been demonstrated for tests for antibodies against panels of different phospholipids.[257]

# COAGULATION TESTS

## Lupus Anticoagulants

One of the most intriguing aspects of APS is the LA phenomenon.[288,289] The various LA tests all report the inhibition of phospholipid-dependent blood coagulation reactions,[6] but by different detection methods. These include modifications of the aPTT test with LA-sensitive and LA-insensitive reagents, the kaolin clotting time, the dRVVT, the tissue thromboplastin inhibition time, the hexagonal phase array test, and the platelet neutralization procedure. Readers who are interested in the latest consensus recommendations on details of the procedures are directed to reference 257.

The results of LA tests can be so variable that even specialized laboratories will disagree as to the results of LA tests. For example, three surveys in the United Kingdom have shown that although most laboratories agreed on identification of plasmas containing strong positive LA activity, they frequently have disagreed about samples with a weak LA activity.[286]

Despite these limitations, the presence of a positive LA appears to be the strongest predictive diagnostic test for future thrombosis. In a meta-analysis of the risk for aPL-associated venous thromboembolism in individuals with aPL antibodies without an underlying autoimmune disease or previous thrombosis, the mean odds ratios were 1.6 for aCL antibodies, 3.2 for high titers of aCL, and 11.0 for LA.[290] In a systematic literature review, 12 of 12 studies showed significant associations between LA and thrombosis, with odds ratios from 5.7 to 9.4.[262] LA increased the risks of arterial and venous events to the same extent. Positivity for both LA and aCL, but not for aCL alone, predicted a higher risk of recurrent thromboocclusive events in patients with first ischemic stroke.[135] In a prospective study of pregnant women, the PROMISSE study (Predictors of Pregnancy Outcome: Biomarkers in Antiphospholipid Antibody Syndrome and Systemic Lupus Erythematosus study), LA was the primary predictor of adverse pregnancy outcome after 12 weeks of gestation in aPL-associated pregnancies; aCL antibody and anti-$\beta_2$GPI did not predict adverse pregnancy outcome if LA was not also present.[291]

In patients with SLE as well, the presence of LA activity is more predictive and more specific for the occurrence of thrombosis or pregnancy loss than aCL assays.[292] This was also found in a meta-analysis of women without autoimmune conditions who had recurrent pregnancy losses.[293]

## Dilute Russell Viper Venom Time

dRVVT is considered to be one of the most sensitive of the LA tests. The assay uses Russell viper venom (RVV) in a system containing limiting quantities of diluted rabbit brain phospholipid. RVV directly activates coagulation factor X, leading to formation of fibrin clot. LA prolongs dRVVT by interfering with assembly of the prothrombinase complex; however, the prolongation is reversed by adding excess phospholipid to the reaction (sometimes referred to a "confirmatory test"). To ensure that prolongation of the clotting time is not a result of a factor deficiency, the procedure includes mixture of patient and control plasmas. Anticoagulant therapy with heparin, warfarin, or direct thrombin inhibitors can yield falsely abnormal test results.

## Activated Partial Thromboplastin Time Tests

Prolongation of the aPTT detects some LAs, and prolonged aPTTs in otherwise healthy individuals are most frequently caused by LAs.[294] The various commercial aPTT reagents vary widely with regard to sensitivity to LA, so it is important to know the characteristics of the particular reagent(s) that is (are) being used. When the aPTT of a particular plasma sample is prolonged and not correctable by immediate mixture

with normal plasma, the presence of an LA should be suspected, especially if the patient does not have bleeding symptoms. The LA needs to be differentiated from inhibitors of specific coagulation factors and from anticoagulants such as heparin. Besides specific assays to exclude the latter two possibilities, the clinician should check whether the aPTT normalizes when an LA-insensitive aPTT reagent is used or when the assay is performed using frozen washed platelets as the source of phospholipid, a procedure referred to as the platelet neutralization procedure. The effects of incubation with normal plasma may be helpful in differentiating LAs from coagulation factor inhibitors. aPTTs performed on mixtures of normal plasma and plasma containing a factor VIII inhibitor usually show no prolongation immediately after mixing but marked prolongation following incubation for 1 to 2 hours at 37°C, whereas LA-containing plasmas usually prolong the aPTT immediately after mixing with normal plasma and show no further prolongation with incubation. The clinician should be aware that both types of anticoagulants, LA and specific coagulation factor inhibitors, may coexist in rare patients and yield confusing laboratory results. Specific coagulation factor inhibitor assays and using an aPTT reagent that is insensitive to LA are helpful for clarifying most of these cases. LAs may result in artifactual decreases in contact activation pathway coagulation factor assays, because these assays are based on aPTT. Consequently, these patients are sometimes misdiagnosed as having multiple coagulation factor deficiencies. This problem can be handled by repeating the coagulation factor assays following dilution of the plasma samples; this usually results in complete or partial normalization of coagulation factor levels with progressive dilution. The use of an aPTT reagent that is insensitive to LA for specific factor assays is another way to solve this problem.

## Other Methods for Detecting Lupus Anticoagulant

The dilute prothrombin time (dPT) (also known as the tissue thromboplastin inhibition test [TTIT]) is essentially a prothrombin time assay done with diluted tissue factor–phospholipid complex. It can be performed with standard or recombinant tissue factor.[295,296] The results are expressed as a ratio of the patient-to-control clotting times.

The kaolin clotting time (KCT) depends on the ability of aPL antibodies to block the coagulant activity of trace amounts of phospholipid present in centrifuged plasma. Some authors maintain that the KCT–LA test reflects dependence on prothrombin as a cofactor and is less likely to be associated with thrombosis than the dRVVT, which appears to be more dependent on $\beta_2$GPI.[297,298] The hexagonal phase array test is based on a prior idea that aPL antibodies recognize phosphatidyl ethanolamine directly in the hexagonal phase array configuration but not in the lamellar phase. Although this assay remains in use, the correction of the prolonged clotting time with hexagonal phase phosphatidyl ethanolamine is probably similar to the confirmatory step used in the other LA assays, that is, a result of the excess of phospholipid in the reaction.

The textarin/ecarin test depends on the difference in phospholipid dependence of coagulation mechanisms triggered by two snake venoms: textarin, which activates prothrombin via a phospholipid-dependent pathway, and ecarin, which activates prothrombin directly without phospholipid.[296]

## Annexin A5 Resistance Assay

In addition to the various LA tests, there is a coagulation test that reports on a thrombogenic mechanism—resistance to annexin A5 anticoagulant activity.[80] This test is an immunoassay for IgG antibodies against domain I of $\beta_2$GPI.[52] The assay has two stages: a first, in which a tissue factor–phospholipid suspension is exposed to test plasma, and a second, in which the washed suspension is used to coagulate pooled normal plasma in the presence and absence of annexin A5. This assay has been correlated with significantly increased risk for thrombosis in patients with antiphospholipid antibodies. Patients with annexin A5 resistance show a less-than-expected annexin A5 anticoagulant effect, reported as a reduction in the annexin A5 anticoagulant ratio. In contrast to the lupus "anticoagulant" effect, this assay measures and reports a procoagulant effect for the antibodies.[70] (*Disclosure: One of the authors [J.H.R.] is the inventor of this assay, U.S. Patents #6284475 and #7252959.*)

# DIFFERENTIAL DIAGNOSIS

Chapters 23 and 24 address the general subject of vascular thrombosis and its differential diagnosis. When vascular occlusion occurs in the setting of a known autoimmune disorder such as SLE, the possibility of a vasculitis, rather than a thrombotic condition, should be considered. Patients with CAPS may, at first, appear to have other multisystem vasoocclusive disorders, such as thrombotic thrombocytopenic purpura or disseminated vasculitis, and may also manifest laboratory findings of disseminated intravascular coagulation.

The differential diagnosis of a prolonged aPTT includes hereditary and acquired coagulation factor deficiencies, inhibitors to coagulation proteins (e.g., acquired hemophilia A; Chap. 18), and the presence, or use, of anticoagulants. The diagnosis of LA is substantiated through plasma mixing studies and specific factor assays. A positive immunoassay for aPL—that is, aCL and/or anti-$\beta_2$GPI antibodies—helps confirm the diagnosis.

When an elevated aPL antibody level is detected, the clinician must exclude the possibility of an infectious etiology for the antibodies; these occur frequently in syphilis, Lyme disease, HIV-1, and hepatitis C. Occasional patients may have artifactually elevated antibodies from increased polyclonal immunoglobulin levels.[299] In such cases, diagnosis is aided by specific tests for suspected infection, quantitative measurement of serum immunoglobulins, and subtraction of background controls using uncoated microtiter wells. Antipsychotic or other medications should be excluded as causative agents.

## PREGNANCY COMPLICATIONS

A systematic review of treatments given to maintain pregnancy in women with prior miscarriages and APS concluded that combined unfractionated heparin and aspirin may reduce pregnancy loss by 54 percent compared to aspirin alone.[300] Three trials of aspirin alone showed no significant reduction in pregnancy loss[300]; intravenous immunoglobulin, whether or not in combination with unfractionated heparin (UFH) and aspirin, was associated with an increased risk of pregnancy loss or premature birth when compared to UFH or low-molecular-weight heparin (LMWH) combined with aspirin.

Taking together the available data, women with a history of three or more spontaneous pregnancy losses and evidence of aPL antibodies should be treated with a combination of low-dose aspirin (75 to 81 mg/d) and prophylactic doses of UFH (i.e., 5000 U every 12 hours subcutaneously). Treatment should be started as soon as pregnancy is documented and continued until delivery so as to reduce the rate of late complications.[183,301] In especially high-risk situations, induction of early delivery may be necessary. Unfractionated heparin at the prophylactic dosage of 5000 U every 12 hours subcutaneously should be started approximately 4 to 6 hours after delivery, if significant bleeding has ceased, and continued at least until the patient is fully ambulatory. Many physicians recommend continuing prophylactic therapy for 6 weeks after delivery even if the patients have not experienced thrombosis. For patients who experienced thromboembolism, prophylaxis by heparin or oral anticoagulant therapy is warranted for at least 6 weeks after delivery.

Although treatment with LMWH has become widely used for recurrent fetal loss as a replacement for prophylactic dose UFH, a prospective randomized controlled trial has questioned the benefit of LMWH treatment versus aspirin therapy. In the LMWH/aspirin group 35 of 47 patients (77.8 percent) had a live birth, and in the aspirin group, 34 of 43 patients (79.1 percent) had a live birth (p = 0.7).[302]

The presence of positive aPL laboratory assays alone is not an indication for treatment in pregnant women without a history of spontaneous pregnancy losses, other attributable pregnancy complications, thrombosis, or SLE. Therefore, the inclusion of aPL tests in routine prenatal testing panels should be discouraged.

Although prednisone was reported to possibly improve the outcome of pregnancy in women with APS, those benefits are associated with significant toxicity.[303] Glucocorticoids or intravenous IgG should be considered only for patients who are refractory to anticoagulant therapy, who have a severe immune thrombocytopenia, or who have a significant contraindication to heparin therapy. Treatment with the combination of prednisone and heparin is associated with an increased risk of osteopenia and vertebral fractures.[304]

# THERAPY, COURSE, AND PROGNOSIS

There is general agreement that APS patients with recurrent spontaneous thrombosis require long-term, and perhaps lifelong, anticoagulant therapy and APS patients with recurrent spontaneous pregnancy losses require antithrombotic therapy for most of the gestational period. There are differences of opinion among experts regarding the approaches to treatment of patients with a single thrombotic event, patients with a history of thrombotic events in the distant past (>5 years), patients with stroke, and patients with thrombotic events that were associated with a provocative factor such as trauma, surgery, stasis, pregnancy, and estrogens.

## THROMBOSIS

The accumulated evidence from randomized controlled trials indicates that patients with APS and thrombosis should be treated with warfarin for the long-term and maintained at a therapeutic international normalized ratio (INR) of 2.0 to 3.0.[305] Patients with arterial thrombosis may require a higher anticoagulant intensity as a retrospective study showed that a higher intensity (INR >3.0) was necessary for preventing recurrences in this group of patients, but this issue is controversial.[306] Two other studies reported no benefit for high-intensity warfarin, but the number of patients with arterial thrombosis was not high.[299,305] The issue of appropriate antithrombotic treatment of aPL-associated stroke is even more controversial. One major study concluded that there was no benefit for warfarin anticoagulation compared to aspirin therapy.[307]

For patients treated acutely with intravenous UFH, care must be taken to determine whether the patient has a preexisting LA that can interfere with aPTT monitoring of heparin levels. This problem can be circumvented by using an LA-insensitive aPTT reagent or be avoided by treatment, where appropriate, with an LMWH.

An important practical consequence of the LA effect is that prothrombin time and INR results can be artifactually elevated in some patients with APS and LAs treated with warfarin anticoagulant therapy.[308] A multicenter study reported that all but one of the commercial thromboplastins in use at nine centers provided acceptable INR values for APS patients with LA.[309] New thromboplastins should be checked for their responsiveness to LA prior to their use in monitoring oral anticoagulant treatment in patients with APS. Chromogenic factor X (CFX) assays can be used as an alternative to INR for APS patients, especially in patients with a prolonged baseline prothrombin time prior to initiating warfarin therapy, those who are persistently positive for LA, and those who continue to have recurrent venous thromboembolism (VTE).[310] Therapeutic CFX values range from 20 to 40 percent; thus, a

CFX of 40 percent would approximate an INR of 2.0, and a CFX of 20 percent would approximate an INR of 3.0.

Direct-acting oral anticoagulants (DOACs), either direct factor Xa or thrombin inhibitors, are effective for treatment of VTE.[311] However, their use specifically in APS patients has not been thoroughly evaluated. In two recent case studies, DOACs failed to prevent thrombosis in APS patients. Of six APS patients studied, five suffered recurrent VTE and one suffered a recurrent TIA after transitioning to DOACs.[312,313]

At the time of writing, there have been two prospective randomized controlled trials comparing warfarin to rivaroxaban in patients with thrombotic APS. The first, named RAPS (Rivaroxaban in Antiphospholipid Syndrome) (study ISRCTN68222801), was recently completed.[313a] Of the 116 patients who were recruited and randomized to either drug, no thrombosis or major bleeding was seen. A second trial, named TRAPS (Rivaroxaban in Thrombotic APS) (ClinicalTrials.gov identifier: NCT02157272), is expected to be completed in December 2020. At present, DOACs may be considered for selected APS patients, particularly those who have difficulty with warfarin anticoagulation. Nevertheless, the results of additional confirmatory trials are awaited.

Fibrinolytic treatment has been reported for patients with primary APS and extensive thrombosis of the common femoral and iliac veins extending to the lower vena cava,[314] acute ischemic stroke,[315] and acute myocardial infarction.[316]

The antimalarial drug hydroxychloroquine (HCQ) is associated with reduced risk of thrombosis in patients with APS[271–273,317–319] and SLE.[319–321] The potential effectiveness of this treatment has been supported by an animal model for aPL thrombosis[322] and by a recent report that HCQ directly disrupts aPL IgG–$\beta_2$GPI complexes[323] and also reverses the aPL antibody-mediated disruption of annexin A5 binding on phospholipid bilayers[324] and on human placental syncitiotrophoblasts.[325] In a longitudinal cohort study consisting of 272 patients with APS and 152 taking HCQ (17 of 272 patients on warfarin, 203 on prednisolone, 112 on azathioprine, 38 on aspirin), investigators found fewer thrombotic complications for patients on HCQ (odds ratio [OR] 0.17, 95% confidence interval 0.07 to 0.44; p <0.0001).[326] In asymptomatic aPL antibody–positive patients with SLE, primary prophylaxis with aspirin and HCQ appeared to reduce the frequency of thrombotic events.[327] A published prospective, nonrandomized study compared oral anticoagulant plus HCQ versus oral anticoagulant alone. In this study, 30 percent (6/20) of patients had a thrombotic event if they were on oral anticoagulant alone, despite therapeutic range INR, versus no thrombotic events in the oral anticoagulant plus HCQ group (0/20). However, this study was limited given the small number of patients studied and short follow-up.[328] Recently, the natural 4-aminoquinolone, quinine, was shown *in vitro* to disrupt the immune complexes bound to phospholipid layers.[329] However, both HCQ and quinine will require clinical testing in appropriately designed clinical trials. A prospective randomized controlled trial comparing HCQ to placebo in aPL-positive patients without a prior history for thrombosis was recently discontinued because of difficulty in reaching the recruitment targets.

Other proposed treatments for APS include statins, rituximab, and vitamin D. Statins have immunomodulatory, anti-inflammatory, and antithrombotic properties that may benefit APS patients. In recent studies, APS patients treated with statins demonstrated downregulation of tissue factor and reduced proinflammatory/prothrombotic markers such as interleukin-1$\beta$, vascular endothelial growth factor, tumor necrosis factor $\alpha$, interferon-inducible protein 10, and soluble CD40L.[330,331] It has been suggested that a B-cell inhibitor such as rituximab may be useful in reducing aPL antibody titers in APS patients. The Rituximab in Antiphospholipid Syndrome (RITAPS) trial did not show reduction in aPL antibody profiles by rituximab; however, rituximab may be effective in controlling noncriteria manifestations of APS.[332] Because low

vitamin D levels correlate with arterial and venous thrombosis as well as noncriteria APS manifestations,[333–335] it is recommended that vitamin D deficiency (<10 to 20 ng/mL) and insufficiency (<30 ng/mL) be corrected in aPL antibody–positive patients.[336]

Conventional anticoagulant therapy is usually not sufficient for treatment of CAPS; these patients require aggressive treatment because of the high mortality.[176] Treatment for CAPS is directed toward the thrombotic events and suppression of the cytokine cascade. This includes anticoagulation with heparin and immunosuppressive therapy in the form of high-dose glucocorticoids. A triple therapy strategy of anticoagulation, glucocorticoids, and either intravenous immunoglobulin or plasma exchange or both has improved outcomes. Cyclophosphamide is recommended for patients with CAPS and inflammatory features of SLE or high-titer aPL antibodies. Rituximab may be useful in refractory or relapsing cases of CAPS.[178]

## PREGNANCY COMPLICATIONS

The current approach to treating pregnant women with APS and recurrent pregnancy losses or the other aPL antibody–associated complications of pregnancy includes daily low-dose aspirin (75 to 81 mg/d) and either UFH or LMWH.[300,337,338] Although clinical studies have shown efficacy with UFH, most clinicians treat with LMWH because it has a better pharmacokinetic profile and a lower risk of heparin-induced thrombocytopenia and osteopenia. Heparin is then withheld when labor begins or 24 hours prior to a cesarean section. Anticoagulation is resumed 6 weeks postpartum because of the increased risk of VTE in this time period.[301] Interestingly, the current standard of care for pregnant APS patients is based on two randomized controlled trials conducted prior to 2000 that included only 150 patients. Newer trials show conflicting results, with some showing no difference in prevention of pregnancy loss in APS patients receiving aspirin alone versus aspirin and LMWH,[302] and others showing a small benefit.[339] With this management, the likelihood of a good pregnancy outcome in women with APS has been estimated to be approximately 75 to 80 percent.

Other treatment modalities such as glucocorticoids or intravenous IgG (IVIG) should be considered only for patients who are refractory to anticoagulant therapy, who have a severe immune thrombocytopenia, or who have a significant contraindication to heparin therapy. The addition of glucocorticoids has shown no clear benefits and has been associated with premature rupture of membranes or preeclampsia; however, a newer study showed that for patients with refractory APS, the addition of low-dose prednisolone (10 mg) from the time of a positive pregnancy test up to 14 weeks of gestation may help to increase live birth rates.[340] Although the addition of IVIG has not been shown to be superior to heparin and aspirin in large multicenter clinical trials,[341] it has shown some efficacy in patients with refractory APS in small case studies.[342,343]

## REFERENCES

1. Hughes GR: The anticardiolipin syndrome. *Clin Exp Rheumatol* 3:285–286, 1985.
2. Harris EN, Hughes GRV, Gharavi AE: The antiphospholipid antibody syndrome. *J Rheumatol Suppl* 13:210, 1987.
3. Simioni P, Prandoni P, Zanon E, et al: Deep venous thrombosis and lupus anticoagulant. A case-control study. *Thromb Haemost* 76:187–189, 1996.
4. Ginsberg JS, Wells PS, Brill-Edwards P, et al: Antiphospholipid antibodies and venous thromboembolism. *Blood* 86:3685–3691, 1995.
5. Out HJ, Bruinse HW, Christiaens GC, et al: Prevalence of antiphospholipid antibodies in patients with fetal loss. *Ann Rheum Dis* 50:553–557, 1991.
6. Shapiro SS, Thiagarajan P: Lupus anticoagulants. *Prog Hemost Thromb* 6:263–285, 1982.
7. Shapiro SS: Lupus anticoagulants and anticardiolipin antibodies: Personal reminiscences, a little history, and some random thoughts. *J Thromb Haemost* 3:831–833, 2005.
8. Asherson RA: The primary, secondary, catastrophic, and seronegative variants of the antiphospholipid syndrome: A personal history long in the making. *Semin Thromb Hemost* 34:227–235, 2008.

9. Moore JE, Mohr CF: Biologically false positive serological tests for syphilis: Type, incidence, and cause. *JAMA* 150:467–473, 1952.

10. Moore JE, Lutz WB: Natural history of systemic lupus erythematosus: Approach to its study through chronic biologic false positive reactors. *J Chronic Dis* 1:297–316, 1955.

11. Bell WN, Alton HG: A brain extract as a substitute for platelet suspensions in the thromboplastin generation test. *Nature* 174:880–881, 1955.

12. Conley CL, Hartmann RC: A hemorrhagic disorder caused by circulating anticoagulant in patients with disseminated lupus erythematosus. *J Clin Invest* 31:621, 1952.

13. Feinstein DI, Rapaport SI: Acquired inhibitors of blood coagulation, in *Progress in Hemostasis and Thrombosis*, edited by TH Spaet, pp 75–95. Grune & Stratton, New York, 1972.

14. Beaumont JL: Acquired hemorrhagic syndrome caused by a circulating anticoagulant; inhibition of the thromboplastic function of the blood platelets; description of a specific test. *Sang* 25:1–15, 1954.

15. Nilsson IM, Astedt B, Hedner U, Berezin D: Intrauterine death and circulating anticoagulant ("antithromboplastin"). *Acta Med Scand* 197:153–159, 1975.

16. Bowie EJ, Thompson JH Jr, Pascuzzi CA, Owen GA Jr: Thrombosis in systemic erythematosus despite circulating anticoagulants. *J Clin Invest* 62:416–430, 1963.

17. Harris EN, Gharavi AE, Boey ML, et al: Anticardiolipin antibodies: Detection by radioimmunoassay and association with thrombosis in systemic lupus erythematosus. *Lancet* 2:1211–1214, 1983.

18. Miyakis S, Lockshin MD, Atsumi T, et al: International consensus statement on an update of the classification criteria for definite antiphospholipid syndrome (APS). *J Thromb Haemost* 4:295–306, 2006.

19. Lieby P, Soley A, Knapp AM, et al: Memory B cells producing somatically mutated antiphospholipid antibodies are present in healthy individuals. *Blood* 102:2459–2465, 2003.

20. Giles I, Lambrianides A, Rahman A: Examining the non-linear relationship between monoclonal antiphospholipid antibody sequence, structure and function. *Lupus* 17:895–903, 2008.

21. Cruz-Tapias P, Blank M, Anaya JM, Shoenfeld Y: Infections and vaccines in the etiology of antiphospholipid syndrome. *Curr Opin Rheumatol* 24:389–393, 2012.

22. Barcat D, Constans J, Seigneur M, et al: Deep venous thrombosis in an adult with varicella. *Rev Med Interne* 19:509–511, 1998.

23. Peyton BD, Cutler BS, Stewart FM: Spontaneous tibial artery thrombosis associated with varicella pneumonia and free protein S deficiency. *J Vasc Surg* 27:563–567, 1998.

24. Prieto J, Yuste JR, Beloqui O, et al: Anticardiolipin antibodies in chronic hepatitis C: Implication of hepatitis C virus as the cause of the antiphospholipid syndrome [see comments]. *Hepatology* 23:199–204, 1996.

25. Cojocaru IM, Cojocaru M, Iacob SA: High prevalence of anticardiolipin antibodies in patients with asymptomatic hepatitis C virus infection associated acute ischemic stroke. *Rom J Intern Med* 43:89–95, 2005.

26. Labarca JA, Rabagliati RM, Radrigan FJ, et al: Antiphospholipid syndrome associated with cytomegalovirus infection: Case report and review. *Clin Infect Dis* 24:197–200, 1997.

27. Delbos V, Abgueguen P, Chennebault JM, et al: Acute cytomegalovirus infection and venous thrombosis: Role of antiphospholipid antibodies. *J Infect* 54:e47–e50, 2007.

28. Loizou S, Cazabon JK, Walport MJ, et al: Similarities of specificity and cofactor dependence in serum antiphospholipid antibodies from patients with human parvovirus B19 infection and from those with systemic lupus erythematosus. *Arthritis Rheum* 40:103–108, 1997.

29. Martin E, Winn R, Nugent K: Catastrophic antiphospholipid syndrome in a community-acquired methicillin-resistant *Staphylococcus aureus* infection: A review of pathogenesis with a case for molecular mimicry. *Autoimmun Rev* 10:181–188, 2011.

30. Galrao L, Brites C, Atta ML, et al: Antiphospholipid antibodies in HIV-positive patients. *Clin Rheumatol* 26:1825–1830, 2007.

31. Blank M, Aron-Maor A, Shoenfeld Y: From rheumatic fever to Libman-Sacks endocarditis: Is there any possible pathogenetic link? *Lupus* 14:697–701, 2005.

32. Gotoh M, Matsuda J: Induction of anticardiolipin antibody and/or lupus anticoagulant in rabbits by immunization with lipoteichoic acid, lipopolysaccharide and lipid A. *Lupus* 5:593–597, 1996.

33. Eschwege V, Freyssinet JM: The possible contribution of cell apoptosis and necrosis to the generation of phospholipid-binding antibodies. *Ann Med Interne (Paris)* 147(Suppl 1):33–35, 1996.

34. Price BE, Rauch J, Shia MA, et al: Anti-phospholipid autoantibodies bind to apoptotic, but not viable, thymocytes in a beta 2-glycoprotein I-dependent manner. *J Immunol* 157:2201–2208, 1996.

35. Pittoni V, Isenberg D: Apoptosis and antiphospholipid antibodies. *Semin Arthritis Rheum* 28:163–178, 1998.

36. Inic-Kanada A, Stojanovic M, Zivkovic I, et al: Murine monoclonal antibody 26 raised against tetanus toxoid cross-reacts with beta2-glycoprotein I: Its characteristics and role in molecular mimicry. *Am J Reprod Immunol* 61:39–51, 2009.

37. Blank M, Asherson RA, Cervera R, Shoenfeld Y: Antiphospholipid syndrome infectious origin. *J Clin Immunol* 24:12–23, 2004.

38. Gharavi AE, Pierangeli SS, Espinola RG, et al: Antiphospholipid antibodies induced in mice by immunization with a cytomegalovirus-derived peptide cause thrombosis and activation of endothelial cells in vivo. *Arthritis Rheum* 46:545–552, 2002.

39. Hellan M, Kuhnel E, Speiser W, et al: Familial lupus anticoagulant: A case report and review of the literature. *Blood Coagul Fibrinolysis* 9:195–200, 1998.

40. Weber M, Hayem G, DeBandt M, et al: The family history of patients with primary or secondary antiphospholipid syndrome (APS). *Lupus* 9:258–263, 2000.

41. Garcia CO, Kanbour-Shakir A, Tang H, et al: Induction of experimental antiphospholipid antibody syndrome in PL/J mice following immunization with beta 2 GPI. *Am J Reprod Immunol* 37:118–124, 1997.

42. Holers VM, Girardi G, Mo L, et al: Complement C3 activation is required for antiphospholipid antibody-induced fetal loss. *J Exp Med* 195:211–220, 2002.

43. Pierangeli SS, Liu X, Espinola R, et al: Functional analyses of patient-derived IgG monoclonal anticardiolipin antibodies using in vivo thrombosis and in vivo microcirculation models. *Thromb Haemost* 84:388–395, 2000.

44. Jankowski M, Vreys I, Wittevrongel C, et al: Thrombogenicity of beta 2-glycoprotein I-dependent antiphospholipid antibodies in a photochemically induced thrombosis model in the hamster. *Blood* 101:157–162, 2003.

45. Arad A, Proulle V, Furie RA, et al: Beta(2)-glycoprotein-1 autoantibodies from patients with antiphospholipid syndrome are sufficient to potentiate arterial thrombus formation in a mouse model. *Blood* 117:3453–3459, 2011.

46. Loizou S, Singh S, Wypkema E, Asherson RA: Anticardiolipin, anti-beta(2)-glycoprotein I and antiprothrombin antibodies in black South African patients with infectious disease. *Ann Rheum Dis* 62:1106–1111, 2003.

47. Roubey RA, Pratt CW, Buyon JP, Winfield JB: Lupus anticoagulant activity of autoimmune antiphospholipid antibodies is dependent upon beta 2-glycoprotein I. *J Clin Invest* 90:1100–1104, 1992.

48. Galli M, Comfurius P, Maassen C, et al: Anticardiolipin antibodies (ACA) directed not to cardiolipin but to a plasma protein cofactor. *Lancet* 335:1544–1547, 1990.

49. McNeil HP, Simpson RJ, Chesterman CN, Krilis SA: Anti-phospholipid antibodies are directed against a complex antigen that includes a lipid-binding inhibitor of coagulation: Beta 2-glycoprotein I (apolipoprotein H). *Proc Natl Acad Sci U S A* 87:4120–4124, 1990.

50. Goldsmith GH, Pierangeli SS, Branch DW, et al: Inhibition of prothrombin activation by antiphospholipid antibodies and beta 2-glycoprotein 1. *Br J Haematol* 87:548–554, 1994.

51. de Laat HB, Derksen RH, Urbanus RT, de Groot PG: IgG antibodies that recognize epitope Gly40-Arg43 in domain I of beta 2-glycoprotein I cause LAC, and their presence correlates strongly with thrombosis. *Blood* 105:1540–1545, 2005.

52. de Laat B, Wu XX, van Lummel M, et al: Correlation between antiphospholipid antibodies that recognize domain i of $\beta_2$-glycoprotein I and a reduction in the anticoagulant activity of annexin A5. *Blood* 109:1490–1494, 2007.

53. Hunt BJ, Wu XX, de Laat B, et al: Association of anti-$\beta_2$GPI domain I IgG and resistance to annexin A5 with obstetrical antiphospholipid syndrome: Evidence for a specific mechanism in a patient subset. *Blood* 112(abstr):3821, 2008.

54. Hunt BJ, Wu XX, de Laat B, et al: Resistance to annexin A5 anticoagulant activity in women with histories for obstetric antiphospholipid syndrome. *Am J Obstet Gynecol* 205:485.e17–485.e23, 2011.

55. Agar C, van Os GM, Mörgelin M, et al: Beta-2-glycoprotein I can exist in 2 conformations: Implications for our understanding of the antiphospholipid syndrome. *Blood* 116:1336–1343, 2010.

56. Balasubramanian K, Maiti SN, Schroit AJ: Recruitment of beta-2-glycoprotein 1 to cell surfaces in extrinsic and intrinsic apoptosis. *Apoptosis* 10:439–446, 2005.

57. Maiti SN, Balasubramanian K, Ramoth JA, Schroit AJ: Beta-2-glycoprotein 1-dependent macrophage uptake of apoptotic cells. Binding to lipoprotein receptor-related protein receptor family members. *J Biol Chem* 283:3761–3766, 2008.

58. Matsuura E, Kobayashi K, Matsunami Y, Lopez LR: The immunology of atherothrombosis in the antiphospholipid syndrome: Antigen presentation and lipid intracellular accumulation. *Autoimmun Rev* 8:500–505, 2009.

59. Agar C, de Groot PG, Morgelin M, et al: Beta2-glycoprotein I: A novel component of innate immunity. *Blood* 117:6939–6947, 2011.

60. Hulstein JJ, Lenting PJ, de Laat B, et al: Beta2-glycoprotein I inhibits von Willebrand factor dependent platelet adhesion and aggregation. *Blood* 110:1483–1491, 2007.

61. Bu C, Gao L, Xie W, et al: Beta2-glycoprotein I is a cofactor for tissue plasminogen activator-mediated plasminogen activation. *Arthritis Rheum* 60:559–568, 2009.

62. Ma K, Simantov R, Zhang JC, et al: High affinity binding of beta 2-glycoprotein I to human endothelial cells is mediated by annexin II. *J Biol Chem* 275:15541–15548, 2000.

63. Sheng Y, Reddel SW, Herzog H, et al: Impaired thrombin generation in beta 2-glycoprotein I null mice. *J Biol Chem* 276:13817–13821, 2001.

64. Robertson SA, Roberts CT, van Beijering E, et al: Effect of beta2-glycoprotein I null mutation on reproduction outcome and antiphospholipid antibody mediated pregnancy pathology in mice. *Mol Hum Reprod* 10:409–416, 2004.

65. de-Groot PG, Horbach DA, Derksen RH: Protein C and other cofactors involved in the binding of antiphospholipid antibodies: Relation to the pathogenesis of thrombosis. *Lupus* 5:488–493, 1996.

66. Atsumi T, Khamashta MA, Amengual O, et al: Binding of anticardiolipin antibodies to protein C via beta2-glycoprotein I (beta2-GPI): A possible mechanism in the inhibitory effect of antiphospholipid antibodies on the protein C system. *Clin Exp Immunol* 112:325–333, 1998.

67. Bidot CJ, Jy W, Horstman LL, et al: Factor VII/VIIa: A new antigen in the anti-phospholipid antibody syndrome. *Br J Haematol* 120:618–626, 2003.

68. Ortona E, Capozzi A, Colasanti T, et al: Vimentin/cardiolipin complex as a new antigenic target of the antiphospholipid syndrome. *Blood* 116:2960–2967, 2010.

69. Shibata S, Harpel PC, Gharavi A, et al: Autoantibodies to heparin from patients with antiphospholipid antibody syndrome inhibit formation of antithrombin III-thrombin complexes. *Blood* 83:2532–2540, 1994.

70. Lieby P, Soley A, Levallois H, et al: The clonal analysis of anticardiolipin antibodies in a single patient with primary antiphospholipid syndrome reveals an extreme antibody heterogeneity. *Blood* 97:3820–3828, 2001.

71. Andree HAM, Hermens WT, Hemker HC, Willems GM: Displacement of factor Va by annexin V, in *Phospholipid Binding and Anticoagulant Action of Annexin V*, edited by HAM Andree, pp 73–85. Universitaire Pers Maastricht, Maastricht, The Netherlands, 1992.

72. Reviakine I, Bergsma-Schutter W, Brisson A: Growth of protein 2-D crystals on supported planar lipid bilayers imaged in situ by AFM. *J Struct Biol* 121:356–361, 1998.

73. Krikun G, Lockwood CJ, Wu XX, et al: The expression of the placental anticoagulant protein, annexin V, by villous trophoblasts: Immunolocalization and in vitro regulation. *Placenta* 15:601–612, 1994.

74. Ueki H, Mizushina T, Laoharatchatathanin T, et al: Loss of maternal annexin A5 increases the likelihood of placental platelet thrombosis and foetal loss. *Sci Rep* 2:827, 2012.

75. Wang X, Campos B, Kaetzel MA, Dedman JR: Annexin V is critical in the maintenance of murine placental integrity. *Am J Obstet Gynecol* 180:1008–1016, 1999.

76. Rand JH, Wu XX, Andree HA, et al: Pregnancy loss in the antiphospholipid-antibody syndrome—A possible thrombogenic mechanism. *N Engl J Med* 337:154–160, 1997.

77. van Heerde WL, Poort S, van't Veer C, et al: Binding of recombinant annexin V to endothelial cells: Effect of annexin V binding on endothelial-cell-mediated thrombin formation. *Biochem J* 302:305–312, 1994.

78. Rand JH, Wu XX, Andree HAM, et al: Antiphospholipid antibodies accelerate plasma coagulation by inhibiting annexin-V binding to phospholipids: A "lupus procoagulant" phenomenon. *Blood* 92:1652–1660, 1998.

79. Rand JH, Wu XX, Quinn AS, et al: Human monoclonal antiphospholipid antibodies disrupt the annexin A5 anticoagulant crystal shield on phospholipid bilayers: Evidence from atomic force microscopy and functional assay. *Am J Pathol* 163:1193–1200, 2003.

80. Wolgast LR, Arslan AA, Wu XX, et al: Reduction of annexin A5 anticoagulant ratio identifies antiphospholipid antibody-positive patients with adverse clinical outcomes. *J Thromb Haemost* 15(7):1412-1421, 2017.

81. Wu XX, Pierangeli SS, Rand JH: Resistance to annexin A5 binding and anticoagulant activity in plasmas from patients with the antiphospholipid syndrome but not with syphilis. *J Thromb Haemost* 4:271–273, 2006.

82. Hanly JG, Smith SA: Anti-beta2-glycoprotein I (GPI) autoantibodies, annexin V binding and the anti-phospholipid syndrome. *Clin Exp Immunol* 120:537–543, 2000.

83. Tomer A: Antiphospholipid antibody syndrome: Rapid, sensitive, and specific flow cytometric assay for determination of anti-platelet phospholipid autoantibodies. *J Lab Clin Med* 139:147–154, 2002.

84. Tomer A, Bar-Lev S, Fleisher S, et al: Antiphospholipid antibody syndrome: The flow cytometric annexin A5 competition assay as a diagnostic tool. *Br J Haematol* 139:113–120, 2007.

85. Gaspersic N, Ambrozic A, Bozic B, et al: Annexin A5 binding to giant phospholipid vesicles is differentially affected by anti-beta2-glycoprotein I and anti-annexin A5 antibodies. *Rheumatology* 46:81–86, 2007.

86. Rand JH, Wu XX, Guller S, et al: Reduction of annexin-V (placental anticoagulant protein-I) on placental villi of women with antiphospholipid antibodies and recurrent spontaneous abortion. *Am J Obstet Gynecol* 171:1566–1572, 1994.

87. Cederholm A, Svenungsson E, Jensen-Urstad K, et al: Decreased binding of annexin V to endothelial cells: A potential mechanism in atherothrombosis of patients with systemic lupus erythematosus. *Arterioscler Thromb Vasc Biol* 25:198–203, 2005.

88. Dueymes M, Levy Y, Ziporen L, et al: Do some antiphospholipid antibodies target endothelial cells? *Ann Med Interne (Paris)* 147(Suppl 1):22–23, 1996.

89. Del-Papa N, Raschi E, Catelli L, et al: Endothelial cells as a target for antiphospholipid antibodies: Role of anti-beta 2 glycoprotein I antibodies. *Am J Reprod Immunol* 38:212–217, 1997.

90. Matsuda J, Gotoh M, Gohchi K, et al: Anti-endothelial cell antibodies to the endothelial hybridoma cell line (EAhy926) in systemic lupus erythematosus patients with antiphospholipid antibodies. *Br J Haematol* 97:227–232, 1997.

91. Navarro M, Cervera R, Teixido M, et al: Antibodies to endothelial cells and to beta 2-glycoprotein I in the antiphospholipid syndrome: Prevalence and isotype distribution. *Br J Rheumatol* 35:523–528, 1996.

92. Simantov R, Lo SK, Gharavi A, et al: Antiphospholipid antibodies activate vascular endothelial cells. *Lupus* 5:440–441, 1996.

93. Meroni PL, Papa ND, Beltrami B, et al: Modulation of endothelial cell function by antiphospholipid antibodies. *Lupus* 5:448–450, 1996.

94. Cockrell E, Espinola RG, McCrae KR: Annexin A2: Biology and relevance to the antiphospholipid syndrome. *Lupus* 17:943–951, 2008.

95. Romay-Penabad Z, Montiel-Manzano MG, Shilagard T, et al: Annexin A2 is involved in antiphospholipid antibody-mediated pathogenic effects in vitro and in vivo. *Blood* 114:3074–3083, 2009.

96. Raschi E, Borghi MO, Grossi C, et al: Toll-like receptors: Another player in the pathogenesis of the anti-phospholipid syndrome. *Lupus* 17:937–942, 2008.

97. Xie H, Sheng L, Zhou H, Yan J: The role of TLR4 in pathophysiology of antiphospholipid syndrome-associated thrombosis and pregnancy morbidity. *Br J Haematol* 164:165–176, 2014.

98. Brandt KJ, Fickentscher C, Boehlen F, et al: NF-kappaB is activated from endosomal compartments in antiphospholipid antibodies-treated human monocytes. *J Thromb Haemost* 12:779–791, 2014.

99. Raschi E, Testoni C, Bosisio D, et al: Role of the MyD88 transduction signaling pathway in endothelial activation by antiphospholipid antibodies. *Blood* 101:3495–3500, 2003.

100. Vega-Ostertag ME, Ferrara DE, Romay-Penabad Z, et al: Role of p38 mitogen-activated protein kinase in antiphospholipid antibody-mediated thrombosis and endothelial cell activation. *J Thromb Haemost* 5:1828–1834, 2007.

101. Cesarman-Maus G, Rios-Luna NP, Deora AB, et al: Autoantibodies against the fibrinolytic receptor, annexin 2, in antiphospholipid syndrome. *Blood* 107:4375–4382, 2006.

102. Chen PP, Yang CD, Ede K, et al: Some antiphospholipid antibodies bind to hemostasis and fibrinolysis proteases and promote thrombosis. *Lupus* 17:916–921, 2008.

103. Cugno M, Cabibbe M, Galli M, et al: Antibodies to tissue-type plasminogen activator (tPA) in patients with antiphospholipid syndrome: Evidence of interaction between the antibodies and the catalytic domain of tPA in 2 patients. *Blood* 103:2121–2126, 2004.

104. Ames PR, Tommasino C, Iannaccone L, et al: Coagulation activation and fibrinolytic imbalance in subjects with idiopathic antiphospholipid antibodies—A crucial role for acquired free protein S deficiency. *Thromb Haemost* 76:190–194, 1996.

105. Schousboe I, Rasmussen MS: Synchronized inhibition of the phospholipid mediated autoactivation of factor XII in plasma by beta 2-glycoprotein I and anti-beta 2-glycoprotein I. *Thromb Haemost* 73:798–804, 1995.

106. Sacre SM, Stannard AK, Owen JS: Apolipoprotein E (apoE) isoforms differentially induce nitric oxide production in endothelial cells. *FEBS Lett* 540:181–187, 2003.

107. Yang XV, Banerjee Y, Fernandez JA, et al: Activated protein C ligation of ApoER2 (LRP8) causes Dab1-dependent signaling in U937 cells. *Proc Natl Acad Sci U S A* 106:274–279, 2009.

108. Shi T, Giannakopoulos B, Yan X, et al: Anti-beta2-glycoprotein I antibodies in complex with beta2-glycoprotein I can activate platelets in a dysregulated manner via glycoprotein Ib-IX-V. *Arthritis Rheum* 54:2558–2567, 2006.

109. Lutters BC, Derksen RH, Tekelenburg WL, et al: Dimers of beta 2-glycoprotein I increase platelet deposition to collagen via interaction with phospholipids and the apolipoprotein E receptor 2′. *J Biol Chem* 278:33831–33838, 2003.

110. Graham A, Ford I, Morrison R, et al: Anti-endothelial antibodies interfere in apoptotic cell clearance and promote thrombosis in patients with antiphospholipid syndrome. *J Immunol* 182:1756–1762, 2009.

111. Sammaritano LR: Significance of aPL IgG subclasses. *Lupus* 5:436–439, 1996.

112. Salmon JE, Girardi G, Holers VM: Complement activation as a mediator of antiphospholipid antibody induced pregnancy loss and thrombosis. *Ann Rheum Dis* 61(Suppl 2):ii46–ii50, 2002.

113. Salmon JE, Girardi G: The role of complement in the antiphospholipid syndrome. *Curr Dir Autoimmun* 7:133–148, 2004.

114. Girardi G, Redecha P, Salmon JE: Heparin prevents antiphospholipid antibody-induced fetal loss by inhibiting complement activation. *Nat Med* 10:1222–1226, 2004.

115. Redecha P, Tilley R, Tencati M, et al: Tissue factor: A link between C5a and neutrophil activation in antiphospholipid antibody induced fetal injury. *Blood* 110:2423–2431, 2007.

116. Redecha P, Franzke CW, Ruf W, et al: Neutrophil activation by the tissue factor/Factor VIIa/PAR2 axis mediates fetal death in a mouse model of antiphospholipid syndrome. *J Clin Invest* 118:3453–3461, 2008.

117. Zhou H, Wolberg AS, Roubey RA: Characterization of monocyte tissue factor activity induced by IgG antiphospholipid antibodies and inhibition by dilazep. *Blood* 104:2353–2358, 2004.

118. Roubey RA: New approaches to prevention of thrombosis in the antiphospholipid syndrome: Hopes, trials, and tribulations. *Arthritis Rheum* 48:3004–3008, 2003.

119. Martini F, Farsi A, Gori AM, et al: Antiphospholipid antibodies (aPL) increase the potential monocyte procoagulant activity in patients with systemic lupus erythematosus. *Lupus* 5:206–211, 1996.

120. Bu C, Gao L, Xie W, et al: Beta2-glycoprotein i is a cofactor for tissue plasminogen activator-mediated plasminogen activation. *Arthritis Rheum* 60:559–568, 2009.

121. Riewald M, Ruf W: Protease-activated receptor-1 signaling by activated protein C in cytokine-perturbed endothelial cells is distinct from thrombin signaling. *J Biol Chem* 280:19808–19814, 2005.

122. Niessen F, Furlan-Freguia C, Fernandez JA, et al: Endogenous EPCR/aPC-PAR1 signaling prevents inflammation-induced vascular leakage and lethality. *Blood* 113:2859–2866, 2009.

123. Nojima J, Kuratsune H, Suehisa E, et al: Acquired activated protein C resistance associated with IgG antibodies against beta2-glycoprotein I and prothrombin as a strong risk factor for venous thromboembolism. *Clin Chem* 51:545–552, 2005.

124. de Laat B, Eckmann CM, van SM, et al: Correlation between the potency of a beta2-glycoprotein I-dependent lupus anticoagulant and the level of resistance to activated protein C. *Blood Coagul Fibrinolysis* 19:757–764, 2008.

125. Hurtado V, Montes R, Gris JC, et al: Autoantibodies against EPCR are found in antiphospholipid syndrome and are a risk factor for fetal death. *Blood* 104:1369–1374, 2004.

126. Proulle V, Furie RA, Merrill-Skoloff G, Furie BC: Platelets are required for enhanced activation of the endothelium and fibrinogen in a mouse thrombosis model of APS. *Blood* 124:611–622, 2014.

127. Lin YL, Wang CT: Activation of human platelets by the rabbit anticardiolipin antibodies. *Blood* 80:3135–3143, 1992.

128. van Lummel M, Pennings MT, Derksen RH, et al: The binding site in (beta)2-glycoprotein I for ApoER2′ on platelets is located in domain V. *J Biol Chem* 280:36729–36736, 2005.

129. Forastiero RR, Martinuzzo ME, Broze GJ: High titers of autoantibodies to tissue factor pathway inhibitor are associated with the antiphospholipid syndrome. *J Thromb Haemost* 1:718–724, 2003.

130. Witztum JL, Horkko S: The role of oxidized LDL in atherogenesis: Immunological response and anti-phospholipid antibodies. *Ann N Y Acad Sci* 811:88–96, 1997.

131. Vaarala O: Antiphospholipid antibodies and atherosclerosis. *Lupus* 5:442–447, 1996.

132. Lopez LR, Kobayashi K, Matsunami Y, Matsuura E: Immunogenic oxidized low-density lipoprotein/beta2-glycoprotein I complexes in the diagnostic management of atherosclerosis. *Clin Rev Allergy Immunol* 37:12–19, 2009.

133. Canaud G, Bienaime F, Tabarin F, et al: Inhibition of the mTORC pathway in the antiphospholipid syndrome. *N Engl J Med* 371:303–312, 2014.

134. Krnic BS, O'Connor CR, Looney SW, et al: A retrospective review of 61 patients with antiphospholipid syndrome. Analysis of factors influencing recurrent thrombosis. *Arch Intern Med* 157:2101–2108, 1997.

135. Martinelli I, Cattaneo M, Panzeri D, et al: Risk factors for deep venous thrombosis of the upper extremities. *Ann Intern Med* 126:707–711, 1997.

136. Provenzale JM, Ortel TL, Allen NB: Systemic thrombosis in patients with antiphospholipid antibodies: Lesion distribution and imaging findings. *AJR Am J Roentgenol* 170:285–290, 1998.

137. Poux JM, Boudet R, Lacroix P, et al: Renal infarction and thrombosis of the infrarenal aorta in a 35-year-old man with primary antiphospholipid syndrome. *Am J Kidney Dis* 27:721–725, 1996.

138. Kojima E, Naito K, Iwai M, et al: Antiphospholipid syndrome complicated by thrombosis of the superior mesenteric artery, co-existence of smooth muscle hyperplasia. *Intern Med* 36:528–531, 1997.

139. Girolami A, Zanon E, Zanardi S, et al: Thromboembolic disease developing during oral contraceptive therapy in young females with antiphospholipid antibodies. *Blood Coagul Fibrinolysis* 7:497–501, 1996.

140. Montaruli B, Borchiellini A, Tamponi G, et al: Factor V Arg506–>Gln mutation in patients with antiphospholipid antibodies. *Lupus* 5:303–306, 1996.

141. Simantov R, Lo SK, Salmon JE, et al: Factor V Leiden increases the risk of thrombosis in patients with antiphospholipid antibodies. *Thromb Res* 84:361–365, 1996.

142. Schutt M, Kluter H, Hagedorn GM, et al: Familial coexistence of primary antiphospholipid syndrome and factor V Leiden. *Lupus* 7:176–182, 1998.

143. Brenner B, Vulfsons SL, Lanir N, Nahir M: Coexistence of familial antiphospholipid syndrome and factor V Leiden: Impact on thrombotic diathesis. *Br J Haematol* 94:166–167, 1996.

144. Pengo V, Ruffatti A, Legnani C, et al: Incidence of a first thromboembolic event in asymptomatic carriers of high-risk antiphospholipid antibody profile: A multicenter prospective study. *Blood* 118:4714–4718, 2011.

145. Schulman S, Svenungsson E, Granqvist S: Anticardiolipin antibodies predict early recurrence of thromboembolism and death among patients with venous thromboembolism following anticoagulant therapy. Duration of Anticoagulation Study Group. *Am J Med* 104:332–338, 1998.

146. Finazzi G, Brancaccio V, Moia M, et al: Natural history and risk factors for thrombosis in 360 patients with antiphospholipid antibodies: A four-year prospective study from the Italian Registry. *Am J Med* 100:530–536, 1996.

147. Gezer S: Antiphospholipid syndrome. *Dis Mon* 49:696–741, 2003.

148. Gladd DA, Olech E: Antiphospholipid antibodies in rheumatoid arthritis: Identifying the dominoes. *Curr Rheumatol Rep* 11:43–51, 2009.

149. Fauchais AL, Lambert M, Launay D, et al: Antiphospholipid antibodies in primary Sjogren's syndrome: Prevalence and clinical significance in a series of 74 patients. *Lupus* 13:245–248, 2004.

150. Shoenfeld Y, Meroni PL: The beta-2-glycoprotein I and antiphospholipid antibodies. *Clin Exp Rheumatol* 10:205–209, 1992.

151. Yun YY, Yoh KA, Yang HI, et al: A case of Budd-Chiari syndrome with high antiphospholipid antibody in a patient with systemic lupus erythematosus. *Korean J Intern Med* 11:82–86, 1996.

152. Hofbauer LC, Spitzweg C, Heufelder AE: Graves' disease associated with the primary antiphospholipid syndrome. *J Rheumatol* 23:1435–1437, 1996.

153. Chun WH, Bang D, Lee SK: Antiphospholipid syndrome associated with progressive systemic sclerosis. *J Dermatol* 23:347–351, 1996.

154. Frolow M, Jankowski M, Swadzba J, Musial J: Evan's syndrome with antiphospholipid-protein antibodies. *Pol Merkur Lekarski* 1:344–345, 1996.

155. Yokoi K, Hosoi E, Akaike M, et al: Takayasu's arteritis associated with antiphospholipid antibodies. Report of two cases. *Angiology* 47:315–319, 1996.

156. Dasgupta B, Almond MK, Tanqueray A: Polyarteritis nodosa and the antiphospholipid syndrome. *Br J Rheumatol* 36:1210–1212, 1997.

157. Cervera R, Boffa MC, Khamashta MA, Hughes GR: The Euro-Phospholipid project: Epidemiology of the antiphospholipid syndrome in Europe. *Lupus* 18:889–893, 2009.

158. Bucciarelli S, Espinosa G, Cervera R: The CAPS Registry: Morbidity and mortality of the catastrophic antiphospholipid syndrome. *Lupus* 18:905–912, 2009.

159. Urbanus RT, Siegerink B, Roest M, et al: Antiphospholipid antibodies and risk of myocardial infarction and ischaemic stroke in young women in the RATIO study: A case-control study. *Lancet Neurol* 8:998–1005, 2009.

160. Levine SR, Deegan MJ, Futrell N, Welch KM: Cerebrovascular and neurologic disease associated with antiphospholipid antibodies: 48 cases. *Neurology* 40:1181–1189, 1990.

161. Weingarten K, Filippi C, Barbut D, Zimmerman RD: The neuroimaging features of the cardiolipin antibody syndrome. *Clin Imaging* 21:6–12, 1997.

162. Carhuapoma JR, Mitsias P, Levine SR: Cerebral venous thrombosis and anticardiolipin antibodies. *Stroke* 28:2363–2369, 1997.

163. Deschiens MA, Conard J, Horellou MH, et al: Coagulation studies, factor V Leiden, and anticardiolipin antibodies in 40 cases of cerebral venous thrombosis. *Stroke* 27:1724–1730, 1996.

164. Nagai S, Horie Y, Akai T, et al: Superior sagittal sinus thrombosis associated with primary antiphospholipid syndrome—Case report. *Neurol Med Chir (Tokyo)* 38:34–39, 1998.

165. Tanasescu R, Nicolau A, Caraiola S, et al: Antiphospholipid antibodies and migraine: A retrospective study of 428 patients with inflammatory connective tissue diseases. *Rom J Intern Med* 45:355–363, 2007.

166. Ong MS, Kohane IS, Cai T, et al: Population-level evidence for an autoimmune etiology of epilepsy. *JAMA Neurol* 71:569–574, 2014.

167. Brey RL, Escalante A: Neurological manifestations of antiphospholipid antibody syndrome. *Lupus* 7(Suppl 2):S67–S74, 1998.

168. Matsushita T, Kanda F, Yamada H, Chihara K: Recurrent acute transverse myelopathy: An 83-year-old man with antiphospholipid syndrome. *Rinsho Shinkeigaku* 37:987–991, 1997.

169. Ruiz AG, Guzman RJ, Flores FJ, Garay MJ: Refractory hiccough heralding transverse myelitis in the primary antiphospholipid syndrome. *Lupus* 7:49–50, 1998.

170. Takamura Y, Morimoto S, Tanooka A, Yoshikawa J: Transverse myelitis in a patient with primary antiphospholipid syndrome—A case report. *No To Shinkei* 48:851–855, 1996.

171. Campi A, Filippi M, Comi G, Scotti G: Recurrent acute transverse myelopathy associated with anticardiolipin antibodies. *AJNR Am J Neuroradiol* 19:781–786, 1998.

172. Smyth AE, Bruce IN, McMillan SA, Bell AL: Transverse myelitis: A complication of systemic lupus erythematosus that is associated with the antiphospholipid syndrome. *Ulster Med J* 65:91–94, 1996.

173. Mok CC, Lau CS, Chan EY, Wong RW: Acute transverse myelopathy in systemic lupus erythematosus: Clinical presentation, treatment, and outcome. *J Rheumatol* 25:467–473, 1998.

174. Sugiyama Y, Yamamoto T: Characterization of serum anti-phospholipid antibodies in patients with multiple sclerosis. *Tohoku J Exp Med* 178:203–215, 1996.

175. Schwartz M, Rochas M, Weller B, et al: High association of anticardiolipin antibodies with psychosis. *J Clin Psychiatry* 59:20–23, 1998.

176. Espinosa G, Bucciarelli S, Asherson RA, Cervera R: Morbidity and mortality in the catastrophic antiphospholipid syndrome: Pathophysiology, causes of death, and prognostic factors. *Semin Thromb Hemost* 34:290–294, 2008.

177. Erkan D, Cervera R, Asherson RA: Catastrophic antiphospholipid syndrome: Where do we stand? *Arthritis Rheum* 48:3320–3327, 2003.

178. Cervera R, Rodriguez-Pinto I, Colafrancesco S, et al: 14th International Congress on Antiphospholipid Antibodies Task Force report on catastrophic antiphospholipid syndrome. *Autoimmun Rev* 13:699–707, 2014.

179. Bucciarelli S, Espinosa G, Cervera R, et al: Mortality in the catastrophic antiphospholipid syndrome: Causes of death and prognostic factors in a series of 250 patients. *Arthritis Rheum* 54:2568–2576, 2006.

180. Lockshin MD: Pregnancy loss and antiphospholipid antibodies. *Lupus* 7(Suppl 2):S86–S89, 1998.

181. Saha SP, Bhattacharjee N, Ganguli RP, et al: Prevalence and significance of antiphospholipid antibodies in selected at-risk obstetrics cases: A comparative prospective study. *J Obstet Gynaecol* 29:614–618, 2009.

182. Ruffatti A, Calligaro A, Hoxha A, et al: Laboratory and clinical features of pregnant women with antiphospholipid syndrome and neonatal outcome. *Arthritis Care Res (Hoboken)* 62:302–307, 2010.

183. Rai R: Obstetric management of antiphospholipid syndrome. *J Autoimmun* 15:203–207, 2000.

184. Rai R, Regan L: Obstetric complications of antiphospholipid antibodies. *Curr Opin Obstet Gynecol* 9:387–390, 1997.

185. Saha SP, Bhattacharjee N, Ganguli RP, et al: Prevalence and significance of anti-phospholipid antibodies in selected at-risk obstetrics cases: A comparative prospective study. *J Obstet Gynaecol* 29:614–618, 2009.

186. Ruffatti A, Calligaro A, Hoxha A, et al: Laboratory and clinical features of pregnant women with antiphospholipid syndrome and neonatal outcome. *Arthritis Care Res (Hoboken)* 62:302–307, 2010.

187. Ornstein MH, Rand JH: An association between refractory HELLP syndrome and antiphospholipid antibodies during pregnancy; a report of 2 cases. *J Rheumatol* 21:1360–1364, 1994.

188. Neuwelt CM, Daikh DI, Linfoot JA, et al: Catastrophic antiphospholipid syndrome: Response to repeated plasmapheresis over three years. *Arthritis Rheum* 40:1534–1539, 1997.

189. Ramsey-Goldman R, Kutzer JE, Kuller LH, et al: Pregnancy outcome and anti-cardiolipin antibody in women with systemic lupus erythematosus. *Am J Epidemiol* 138:1057–1069, 1993.

190. Chauleur C, Galanaud JP, Alonso S, et al: Observational study of pregnant women with a previous spontaneous abortion before the 10th gestation week with and without antiphospholipid antibodies. *J Thromb Haemost* 8:699–706, 2010.

191. Bergrem A, Jacobsen EM, Skjeldestad FE, et al: The association of antiphospholipid antibodies with pregnancy-related first time venous thrombosis—A population-based case-control study. *Thromb Res* 125:e222–e227, 2010.

192. Locatelli A, Patane L, Ghidini A, et al: Pathology findings in preterm placentas of women with autoantibodies: A case-control study. *J Matern Fetal Neonatal Med* 11:339–344, 2002.

193. Salafia CM, Cowchock FS: Placental pathology and antiphospholipid antibodies: A descriptive study. *Am J Perinatol* 14:435–441, 1997.

194. Salafia CM, Parke AL: Placental pathology in systemic lupus erythematosus and phospholipid antibody syndrome. *Rheum Dis Clin North Am* 23:85–97, 1997.

195. Sauer R, Roussev R, Jeyendran RS, Coulam CB: Prevalence of antiphospholipid antibodies among women experiencing unexplained infertility and recurrent implantation failure. *Fertil Steril* 93:2441–2443, 2010.

196. de Jesus GR, Rodrigues G, de Jesus NR, Levy RA: Pregnancy morbidity in antiphospholipid syndrome: What is the impact of treatment? *Curr Rheumatol Rep* 16:403, 2014.

197. Practice Committee of American Society for Reproductive Medicine: Anti-phospholipid antibodies do not affect IVF success. *Fertil Steril* 90(5 Suppl):S172–S173, 2008.

198. Kriseman YL, Nash JW, Hsu S: Criteria for the diagnosis of antiphospholipid syndrome in patients presenting with dermatologic symptoms. *J Am Acad Dermatol* 57:112–115, 2007.

199. Gibson GE, Su WP, Pittelkow MR: Antiphospholipid syndrome and the skin. *J Am Acad Dermatol* 36:970–982, 1997.

200. Asherson RA, Cervera R: The antiphospholipid syndrome: Multiple faces beyond the classical presentation. *Autoimmun Rev* 2:140–151, 2003.

201. Aronoff DM, Callen JP: Necrosing livedo reticularis in a patient with recurrent pulmonary hemorrhage. *J Am Acad Dermatol* 37:300–302, 1997.

202. Greco TP, Conti-Kelly AM, Matsuura E, et al: Antiphospholipid antibodies in patients with coronary artery disease: New cardiac risk factors? *Ann N Y Acad Sci* 1108:466–474, 2007.

203. Vaarala O: Antiphospholipid antibodies and myocardial infarction. *Lupus* 7(Suppl 2):S132–S134, 1998.

204. Sherer Y, Shoenfeld Y: Antiphospholipid antibodies: Are they pro-atherogenic or an epiphenomenon of atherosclerosis? *Immunobiology* 207:13–16, 2003.

205. Ludia C, Domenico P, Monia C, et al: Antiphospholipid antibodies: A new risk factor for restenosis after percutaneous transluminal coronary angioplasty? *Autoimmunity* 27:141–148, 1998.

206. Chambers-JD J, Haire HD, Deligonul U: Multiple early percutaneous transluminal coronary angioplasty failures related to lupus anticoagulant. *Am Heart J* 132:189–190, 1996.

207. Ames PR, Antinolfi I, Scenna G, et al: Atherosclerosis in thrombotic primary antiphospholipid syndrome. *J Thromb Haemost* 7:537–542, 2009.

208. Niaz A, Butany J: Antiphospholipid antibody syndrome with involvement of a bioprosthetic heart valve. *Can J Cardiol* 14:951–954, 1998.

209. Bouillanne O, Millaire A, de Groote P, et al: Prevalence and clinical significance of antiphospholipid antibodies in heart valve disease: A case-control study. *Am Heart J* 132:790–795, 1996.

210. Nesher G, Ilany J, Rosenmann D, Abraham AS: Valvular dysfunction in antiphospholipid syndrome: Prevalence, clinical features, and treatment. *Semin Arthritis Rheum* 27:27–35, 1997.

211. Hojnik M, George J, Ziporen L, Shoenfeld Y: Heart valve involvement (Libman-Sacks endocarditis) in the antiphospholipid syndrome. *Circulation* 93:1579–1587, 1996.

212. Bulckaen HG, Puisieux FL, Bulckaen ED, et al: Antiphospholipid antibodies and the risk of thromboembolic events in valvular heart disease. *Mayo Clin Proc* 78:294–298, 2003.

213. Ziporen L, Goldberg I, Arad M, et al: Libman-Sacks endocarditis in the antiphospholipid syndrome: Immunopathologic findings in deformed heart valves. *Lupus* 5:196–205, 1996.

214. Lee RW, Taylor LM Jr, Landry GJ, et al: Prospective comparison of infrainguinal bypass grafting in patients with and without antiphospholipid antibodies. *J Vasc Surg* 24:524–531, 1996.

215. Porres-Aguilar M, Pena-Ruiz MA, Burgos JD, et al: Chronic thromboembolic pulmonary hypertension as an uncommon presentation of primary antiphospholipid syndrome. *J Natl Med Assoc* 100:734–736, 2008.

216. Karmochkine M, Cacoub P, Dorent R, et al: High prevalence of antiphospholipid antibodies in precapillary pulmonary hypertension. *J Rheumatol* 23:286–290, 1996.

217. Bonderman D, Wilkens H, Wakounig S, et al: Risk factors for chronic thromboembolic pulmonary hypertension. *Eur Respir J* 33:325–331, 2009.

218. Asherson RA: The catastrophic antiphospholipid syndrome, 1998. A review of the clinical features, possible pathogenesis and treatment. *Lupus* 7(Suppl 2):S55–S62, 1998.

219. Uthman I, Khamashta M: The abdominal manifestations of the antiphospholipid syndrome. *Rheumatology (Oxford)* 46:1641–1647, 2007.

220. Biron C, Andreani H, Blanc P, et al: Prevalence of antiphospholipid antibodies in patients with chronic liver disease related to alcohol or hepatitis C virus: Correlation with liver injury. *J Lab Clin Med* 131:243–250, 1998.

221. Sene D, Piette JC, Cacoub P: Antiphospholipid antibodies, antiphospholipid syndrome and infections. *Autoimmun Rev* 7:272–277, 2008.

222. Ramos-Casals M, Cervera R, Lagrutta M, et al: Clinical features related to antiphospholipid syndrome in patients with chronic viral infections (hepatitis C virus/HIV infection): Description of 82 cases. *Clin Infect Dis* 38:1009–1016, 2004.

223. Hoffman M, Burke M, Fried M, et al: Primary biliary cirrhosis associated with antiphospholipid syndrome. *Isr J Med Sci* 33:681–686, 1997.

224. Date K, Shirai Y, Hatakeyama K: Antiphospholipid antibody syndrome presenting as acute acalculous cholecystitis. *Am J Gastroenterol* 92:2127–2128, 1997.

225. Dessailloud R, Papo T, Vaneecloo S, et al: Acalculous ischemic gallbladder necrosis in the catastrophic antiphospholipid syndrome. *Arthritis Rheum* 41:1318–1320, 1998.

226. Kalman DR, Khan A, Romain PL, Nompleggi DJ: Giant gastric ulceration associated with antiphospholipid antibody syndrome. *Am J Gastroenterol* 91:1244–1247, 1996.

227. Gul A, Inanc M, Ocal L, et al: Primary antiphospholipid syndrome associated with mesenteric inflammatory veno-occlusive disease. *Clin Rheumatol* 15:207–210, 1996.

228. Lee HJ, Park JW, Chang JC: Mesenteric and portal venous obstruction associated with primary antiphospholipid antibody syndrome. *J Gastroenterol Hepatol* 12:822–826, 1997.

229. Galli M, Finazzi G, Barbui T: Thrombocytopenia in the antiphospholipid syndrome. *Br J Haematol* 93:1–5, 1996.

230. Cuadrado MJ, Mujic F, Munoz E, Khamashta MA, Hughes GR: Thrombocytopenia in the antiphospholipid syndrome. *Ann Rheum Dis* 56:194–196, 1997.

231. Macchi L, Rispal P, Clofent SG, et al: Anti-platelet antibodies in patients with systemic lupus erythematosus and the primary antiphospholipid antibody syndrome: Their relationship with the observed thrombocytopenia. *Br J Haematol* 98:336–341, 1997.

232. Pierrot-Deseilligny DC, Michel M, Khellaf M, et al: Antiphospholipid antibodies in adults with immune thrombocytopenic purpura. *Br J Haematol* 142:638–643, 2008.

233. Lipp E, von-Felten A, Sax H, Muller D, Berchtold P: Antibodies against platelet glycoproteins and antiphospholipid antibodies in autoimmune thrombocytopenia. *Eur J Haematol* 60:283–288, 1998.

234. Diz-Kucukkaya R, Hacihanefioglu A, Yenerel M, et al: Antiphospholipid antibodies and antiphospholipid syndrome in patients presenting with immune thrombocytopenic purpura: A prospective cohort study. *Blood* 98:1760–1764, 2001.

235. Vivaldi P, Rossetti G, Galli M, Finazzi G: Severe bleeding due to acquired hypoprothrombinemia-lupus anticoagulant syndrome. Case report and review of literature. *Haematologica* 82:345–347, 1997.

236. Hudson N, Duffy CM, Rauch J, Paquin JD, Esdaile JM: Catastrophic haemorrhage in a case of paediatric primary antiphospholipid syndrome and factor II deficiency. *Lupus* 6:68–71, 1997.

237. Dunn JP, Noorily SW, Petri M, et al: Antiphospholipid antibodies and retinal vascular disease. *Lupus* 5:313–322, 1996.

238. Coniglio M, Platania A, Di Nucci GD, et al: Antiphospholipid-protein antibodies are not an uncommon feature in retinal venous occlusions. *Thromb Res* 83:183–188, 1996.

239. Glacet BA, Bayani N, Chretien P, et al: Antiphospholipid antibodies in retinal vascular occlusions. A prospective study of 75 patients. *Arch Ophthalmol* 112:790–795, 1994.

240. Dori D, Gelfand YA, Brenner B, Miller B: Cilioretinal artery occlusion: An ocular complication of primary antiphospholipid syndrome. *Retina* 17:555–557, 1997.

241. Reino S, Munoz RF, Cervera R, et al: Optic neuropathy in the "primary" antiphospholipid syndrome: Report of a case and review of the literature. *Clin Rheumatol* 16: 629–631, 1997.

242. Au A, O'Day J: Review of severe vaso-occlusive retinopathy in systemic lupus erythematosus and the antiphospholipid syndrome: Associations, visual outcomes, complications and treatment. *Clin Experiment Ophthalmol* 32:87–100, 2004.

243. Fakhouri F, Noel LH, Zuber J, et al: The expanding spectrum of renal diseases associated with antiphospholipid syndrome. *Am J Kidney Dis* 41:1205–1211, 2003.

244. Nochy D, Daugas E, Droz D, et al: The intrarenal vascular lesions associated with primary antiphospholipid syndrome. *J Am Soc Nephrol* 10:507–518, 1999.

245. Breda L, Nozzi M, De SS, Chiarelli F: Laboratory tests in the diagnosis and follow-up of pediatric rheumatic diseases: An update. *Semin Arthritis Rheum* 40:53–72, 2010.

246. Avcin T, Cimaz R, Silverman ED, et al: Pediatric antiphospholipid syndrome: Clinical and immunologic features of 121 patients in an international registry. *Pediatrics* 122: e1100–e1107, 2008.

247. Falcini F, Taccetti G, Ermini M, Trapani S, Matucci CM: Catastrophic antiphospholipid antibody syndrome in pediatric systemic lupus erythematosus. *J Rheumatol* 24: 389–392, 1997.

248. Ol'binskaia LI, Poptsov VN, Gofman AM: [Hemodynamic changes in patients with myocardial infarct complicated by acute left ventricular failure during combined nitroglycerin and dobutamine therapy] [in Russian]. *Kardiologiia* 31:49–51, 1991.

249. Boffa MC, Lachassine E: Infant perinatal thrombosis and antiphospholipid antibodies: A review. *Lupus* 16:634–641, 2007.

250. Motta M, Chirico G, Rebaioli CB, et al: Anticardiolipin and anti-beta2 glycoprotein I antibodies in infants born to mothers with antiphospholipid antibody-positive autoimmune disease: A follow-up study. *Am J Perinatol* 23:247–251, 2006.

251. Mekinian A, Lachassinne E, Nicaise-Roland P, et al: European registry of babies born to mothers with antiphospholipid syndrome. *Ann Rheum Dis* 72:217–222, 2013.

252. Brewster JA, Shaw NJ, Farquharson RG: Neonatal and pediatric outcome of infants born to mothers with antiphospholipid syndrome. *J Perinat Med* 27:183–187, 1999.

253. Nacinovich R, Galli J, Bomba M, et al: Neuropsychological development of children born to patients with antiphospholipid syndrome. *Arthritis Rheum* 59:345–351, 2008.

254. Marie I, Levesque H, Heron F, et al: Acute adrenal failure secondary to bilateral infarction of the adrenal glands as the first manifestation of primary antiphospholipid antibody syndrome. *Ann Rheum Dis* 56:567–568, 1997.

255. Espinosa G, Santos E, Cervera R, et al: Adrenal involvement in the antiphospholipid syndrome: Clinical and immunologic characteristics of 86 patients. *Medicine (Baltimore)* 82:106–118, 2003.

256. Paydas S, Kocak R, Zorludemir S, Baslamisli F: Bone marrow necrosis in antiphospholipid syndrome. *J Clin Pathol* 50:261–262, 1997.

257. Pengo V, Tripodi A, Reber G, et al: Update of the guidelines for measuring the presence of Lupus Anticoagulant. *J Thromb Haemost* 7:1737–1740, 2009.

258. de Groot PG, Derksen RH, de Laat B: Twenty-two years of failure to set up undisputed assays to detect patients with the antiphospholipid syndrome. *Semin Thromb Hemost* 34:347–355, 2008.

259. Favaloro EJ: Variability and diagnostic utility of antiphospholipid antibodies including lupus anticoagulants. *Int J Lab Hematol* 35:269–274, 2013.

260. Mateo J, Oliver A, Borrell M, et al: Laboratory evaluation and clinical characteristics of 2,132 consecutive unselected patients with venous thromboembolism—Results of the Spanish Multicentric Study on Thrombophilia (EMET-Study). *Thromb Haemost* 77:444–451, 1997.

261. Naarendorp M, Spiera H: Sudden sensorineural hearing loss in patients with systemic lupus erythematosus or lupus-like syndromes and antiphospholipid antibodies. *J Rheumatol* 25:589–592, 1998.

262. Galli M, Luciani D, Bertolini G, Barbui T: Anti-beta 2-glycoprotein I, antiprothrombin antibodies, and the risk of thrombosis in the antiphospholipid syndrome. *Blood* 102:2717–2723, 2003.

263. Shah NM, Khamashta MA, Atsumi T, Hughes GR: Outcome of patients with anti-cardiolipin antibodies: A 10 year follow-up of 52 patients. *Lupus* 7:3–6, 1998.

264. Silver RM, Porter TF, van Leeuwen I, et al: Anticardiolipin antibodies: Clinical consequences of "low titers." *Obstet Gynecol* 87:494–500, 1996.

265. Tuhrim S, Rand JH, Wu XX, et al: Elevated anticardiolipin antibody titer is a stroke risk factor in a multiethnic population independent of isotype or degree of positivity. *Stroke* 30:1561–1565, 1999.

266. Brey RL, Stallworth CL, McGlasson DL, et al: Antiphospholipid antibodies and stroke in young women. *Stroke* 33:2396–2400, 2002.

267. Merrill JT, Shen C, Gugnani M, et al: High prevalence of antiphospholipid antibodies in patients taking procainamide. *J Rheumatol* 24:1083–1088, 1997.

268. El-Rayes BF, Edelstein M: Unusual case of antiphospholipid antibody syndrome presenting with extensive cutaneous infarcts in a patient on long-term procainamide therapy. *Am J Hematol* 72:154, 2003.

269. Karmochkine M, Piette JC, Mazoyer E, et al: Antiphospholipid antibodies: Cause of thrombosis or an epiphenomenon? *Presse Med* 24:267–270, 1995.

270. Delluc A, Rousseau A, Le GM, et al: Prevalence of antiphospholipid antibodies in psychiatric patients users and non-users of antipsychotics. *Br J Haematol* 164:272–279, 2014.

271. Amengual O, Atsumi T, Khamashta MA, et al: Specificity of ELISA for antibody to beta 2-glycoprotein I in patients with antiphospholipid syndrome. *Br J Rheumatol* 35:1239–1243, 1996.

272. Alarcon-Segovia D, Mestanza M, Cabiedes J, Cabral AR: The antiphospholipid/cofactor syndromes. II. A variant in patients with systemic lupus erythematosus with antibodies to beta 2-glycoprotein I but no antibodies detectable in standard antiphospholipid assays. *J Rheumatol* 24:1545–1551, 1997.

273. Cabral AR, Amigo MC, Cabiedes J, Alarcon-Segovia D: A primary variant with antibodies to beta 2-glycoprotein-I but no antibodies detectable in standard antiphospholipid assays. *Am J Med* 101:472–481, 1996.

274. Sanmarco M, Soler C, Christides C, et al: Prevalence and clinical significance of IgG isotype anti-beta 2-glycoprotein I antibodies in antiphospholipid syndrome: A comparative study with anticardiolipin antibodies. *J Lab Clin Med* 129:499–506, 1997.

275. Day HM, Thiagarajan P, Ahn C, et al: Autoantibodies to beta2-glycoprotein I in systemic lupus erythematosus and primary antiphospholipid antibody syndrome: Clinical correlations in comparison with other antiphospholipid antibody tests. *J Rheumatol* 25:667–674, 1998.

276. Reber G, Schousboe I, Tincani A, et al: Inter-laboratory variability of anti-beta2-glycoprotein I measurement. A collaborative study in the frame of the European Forum on Antiphospholipid Antibodies Standardization Group. *Thromb Haemost* 88:66–73, 2002.

277. Hoxha A, Ruffatti A, Pittoni M, et al: The clinical significance of autoantibodies directed against prothrombin in primary antiphospholipid syndrome. *Clin Chim Acta* 413:911–913, 2012.

278. Lopez LR, Dier KJ, Lopez D, et al: Anti-beta 2-glycoprotein I and antiphosphatidylserine antibodies are predictors of arterial thrombosis in patients with antiphospholipid syndrome. *Am J Clin Pathol* 121:142–149, 2004.

279. Audrain MA, El-Kouri D, Hamidou MA, et al: Value of autoantibodies to beta(2)-glycoprotein 1 in the diagnosis of antiphospholipid syndrome. *Rheumatology (Oxford)* 41:550–553, 2002.

280. Sanfelippo MJ, Joshi A, Schwartz S, et al: Antibodies to phosphatidylserine/prothrombin complex in suspected antiphospholipid syndrome in the absence of antibodies to cardiolipin or beta-2-glycoprotein I. *Lupus* 22:1349–1352, 2013.

281. Sciascia S, Khamashta MA, Bertolaccini ML: New tests to detect antiphospholipid antibodies: Antiprothrombin (aPT) and anti-phosphatidylserine/prothrombin (aPS/PT) antibodies. *Curr Rheumatol Rep* 16:415, 2014.

282. Berard M, Chantome R, Marcelli A, Boffa MC: Antiphosphatidylethanolamine antibodies as the only antiphospholipid antibodies. I. Association with thrombosis and vascular cutaneous diseases. *J Rheumatol* 23:1369–1374, 1996.

283. Rauch J, Janoff AS: Antibodies against phospholipids other than cardiolipin: Potential roles for both phospholipid and protein. *Lupus* 5:498–502, 1996.

284. Yetman DL, Kutteh WH: Antiphospholipid antibody panels and recurrent pregnancy loss: Prevalence of anticardiolipin antibodies compared with other antiphospholipid antibodies. *Fertil Steril* 66:540–546, 1996.

285. de Maistre E, Gobert B, Bene MC, et al: Comparative assessment of phospholipid-binding antibodies indicates limited overlapping. *J Clin Lab Anal* 10:6–12, 1996.

286. Branch DW, Silver R, Pierangeli S, et al: Antiphospholipid antibodies other than lupus anticoagulant and anticardiolipin antibodies in women with recurrent pregnancy loss, fertile controls, and antiphospholipid syndrome. *Obstet Gynecol* 89:549–555, 1997.

287. Staub HL, Bertolaccini ML, Khamashta MA: Anti-phosphatidylethanolamine antibody, thromboembolic events and the antiphospholipid syndrome. *Autoimmun Rev* 12:230–234, 2012.

288. Shapiro SS: The lupus anticoagulant/antiphospholipid syndrome. *Annu Rev Med* 47:533–553, 1996.

289. Triplett DA: Antiphospholipid-protein antibodies: Clinical use of laboratory test results (identification, predictive value, treatment). *Haemostasis* 26(Suppl 4):358–367, 1996.

290. Nojima J, Suehisa E, Akita N, et al: Risk of arterial thrombosis in patients with anticardiolipin antibodies and lupus anticoagulant. *Br J Haematol* 96:447–450, 1997.

291. Lockshin MD, Kim M, Laskin CA, et al: Prediction of adverse pregnancy outcome by the presence of lupus anticoagulant, but not anticardiolipin antibody, in patients with antiphospholipid antibodies. *Arthritis Rheum* 64:2311–2318, 2012.

292. Somers E, Magder LS, Petri M: Antiphospholipid antibodies and incidence of venous thrombosis in a cohort of patients with systemic lupus erythematosus. *J Rheumatol* 29:2531–2536, 2002.

293. Opatrny L, David M, Kahn SR, Shrier I, Rey E: Association between antiphospholipid antibodies and recurrent fetal loss in women without autoimmune disease: A metaanalysis. *J Rheumatol* 33:2214–2221, 2006.

294. Kitchens CS: Prolonged activated partial thromboplastin time of unknown etiology: A prospective study of 100 consecutive cases referred for consultation. *Am J Hematol* 27:38–45, 1988.

295. Liu HW, Wong KL, Lin CK, et al: The reappraisal of dilute tissue thromboplastin inhibition test in the diagnosis of lupus anticoagulant. *Br J Haematol* 72:229–234, 1989.

296. Forastiero RR, Cerrato GS, Carreras LO: Evaluation of recently described tests for detection of the lupus anticoagulant. *Thromb Haemost* 72:728–733, 1994.

297. Galli M, Barbui T: Prothrombin as cofactor for antiphospholipids. *Lupus* 7(Suppl 2):S37–S40, 1998.

298. Galli M, Finazzi G, Bevers EM, Barbui T: Kaolin clotting time and dilute Russell's viper venom time distinguish between prothrombin-dependent and beta 2-glycoprotein I-dependent antiphospholipid antibodies. *Blood* 86:617–623, 1995.

299. Lenzi R, Rand JH, Spiera H: Anticardiolipin antibodies in pregnant patients with systemic lupus erythematosus. *N Engl J Med* 314:1392–1393, 1986.

300. Empson M, Lassere M, Craig J, Scott J: Prevention of recurrent miscarriage for women with antiphospholipid antibody or lupus anticoagulant. *Cochrane Database Syst Rev* 2:CD002859, 2005.

301. Galli M, Barbui T: Antiphospholipid antibodies and pregnancy. *Best Pract Res Clin Haematol* 16:211–225, 2003.

302. Laskin CA, Spitzer KA, Clark CA, et al: Low molecular weight heparin and aspirin for recurrent pregnancy loss: Results from the randomized, controlled HepASA trial. *J Rheumatol* 36:279–287, 2009.

303. Cowchock S, Reece EA: Do low-risk pregnant women with antiphospholipid antibodies need to be treated? Organizing Group of the Antiphospholipid Antibody Treatment Trial. *Am J Obstet Gynecol* 176:1099–1100, 1997.

304. Cowchock S: Treatment of antiphospholipid syndrome in pregnancy. *Lupus* 7(Suppl 2):S95–S97, 1998.

305. Lim W, Crowther MA, Eikelboom JW: Management of antiphospholipid antibody syndrome: A systematic review. *JAMA* 295:1050–1057, 2006.

306. Khamashta MA, Cuadrado MJ, Mujic F, et al: The management of thrombosis in the antiphospholipid-antibody syndrome. *N Engl J Med* 332:993–997, 1995.

307. Levine SR, Brey RL, Tilley BC, et al: Antiphospholipid antibodies and subsequent thrombo-occlusive events in patients with ischemic stroke. *JAMA* 291:576–584, 2004.

308. Moll S, Ortel TL: Monitoring warfarin therapy in patients with lupus anticoagulants. *Ann Intern Med* 127:177–185, 1997.

309. Tripodi A, Chantarangkul V, Clerici M, et al: Laboratory control of oral anticoagulant treatment by the INR system in patients with the antiphospholipid syndrome and lupus anticoagulant. Results of a collaborative study involving nine commercial thromboplastins. *Br J Haematol* 115:672–678, 2001.

310. Crowl A, Schullo-Feulner A, Moon JY: A review of warfarin monitoring in antiphospholipid syndrome and lupus anticoagulant. *Ann Pharmacother* 48:1479–1483, 2014.

311. Agnelli G, Becattini C, Franco L: New oral anticoagulants for the treatment of venous thromboembolism. *Best Pract Res Clin Haematol* 26:151–161, 2013.

312. Schaefer JK, McBane RD, Black DF, et al: Failure of dabigatran and rivaroxaban to prevent thromboembolism in antiphospholipid syndrome: A case series of three patients. *Thromb Haemost* 112:947–950, 2014.

313. Win K, Rodgers GM: New oral anticoagulants may not be effective to prevent venous thromboembolism in patients with antiphospholipid syndrome. *Am J Hematol* 89:1017, 2014.

313a. Cohen H, Hunt BJ, Efthymiou M, et al: Rivaroxaban versus warfarin to treat patients with thrombotic antiphospholipid syndrome, with or without systemic lupus erythematosus (RAPS): A randomised, controlled, open-label, phase 2/3, non-inferiority trial. *Lancet Haematol* 3(9):e426–436, 2016.

314. Camps GM, Guil M, Sanchez LJ, et al: Fibrinolytic treatment in primary antiphospholipid syndrome. *Lupus* 5:627–629, 1996.

315. Julkunen H, Hedman C, Kauppi M: Thrombolysis for acute ischemic stroke in the primary antiphospholipid syndrome. *J Rheumatol* 24:181–183, 1997.

316. Ho YL, Chen MF, Wu CC, et al: Successful treatment of acute myocardial infarction by thrombolytic therapy in a patient with primary antiphospholipid antibody syndrome. *Cardiology* 87:354–357, 1996.

317. Wallace DJ: The use of chloroquine and hydroxychloroquine for non-infectious conditions other than rheumatoid arthritis or lupus: A critical review. *Lupus* 5(Suppl 1): S59–S64, 1996.

318. Erkan D, Yazici Y, Peterson MG, Sammaritano L, Lockshin MD: A cross-sectional study of clinical thrombotic risk factors and preventive treatments in antiphospholipid syndrome. *Rheumatology (Oxford)* 41:924–929, 2002.

319. Tektonidou MG, Laskari K, Panagiotakos DB, Moutsopoulos HM: Risk factors for thrombosis and primary thrombosis prevention in patients with systemic lupus erythematosus with or without antiphospholipid antibodies. *Arthritis Rheum* 61:29–36, 2009.

320. Petri M: Thrombosis and systemic lupus erythematosus: The Hopkins Lupus Cohort perspective. *Scand J Rheumatol* 25:191–193, 1996.

321. Kaiser R, Cleveland CM, Criswell LA: Risk and protective factors for thrombosis in systemic lupus erythematosus: Results from a large, multi-ethnic cohort. *Ann Rheum Dis* 68:238–241, 2009.

322. Edwards MH, Pierangeli S, Liu X, et al: Hydroxychloroquine reverses thrombogenic properties of antiphospholipid antibodies in mice. *Circulation* 96:4380–4384, 1997.

323. Rand JH, Wu XX, Quinn AS, et al: Hydroxychloroquine directly reduces the binding of antiphospholipid antibody-beta2-glycoprotein I complexes to phospholipid bilayers. *Blood* 112:1687–1695, 2008.

324. Rand JH, Wu XX, Quinn AS, et al: Hydroxychloroquine reverses a procoagulant mechanism for antiphospholipid syndrome: Evidence for a novel effect for an old antimalarial drug. *Blood* 115:2292–2299, 2010.

325. Wu XX, Guller S, Rand JH: Hydroxychloroquine reduces binding of antiphospholipid antibodies to syncytiotrophoblasts and restores annexin A5 expression. *Am J Obstet Gynecol* 205:576.e7–576.e14, 2011.

326. Mok MY, Chan EY, Fong DY, et al: Antiphospholipid antibody profiles and their clinical associations in Chinese patients with systemic lupus erythematosus. *J Rheumatol* 32:622–628, 2005.

327. Wahl DG, Bounameaux H, de MP, Sarasin FP: Prophylactic antithrombotic therapy for patients with systemic lupus erythematosus with or without antiphospholipid antibodies: Do the benefits outweigh the risks? A decision analysis. *Arch Intern Med* 160:2042–2048, 2000.

328. Schmidt-Tanguy A, Voswinkel J, Henrion D, et al: Antithrombotic effects of hydroxychloroquine in primary antiphospholipid syndrome patients. *J Thromb Haemost* 11: 1927–1929, 2013.

329. Bezati E, Wu XX, Quinn A, et al: A new trick for an ancient drug: Quinine dissociates antiphospholipid immune complexes. *Lupus* 24:32–41, 2014.

330. Lopez-Pedrera C, Ruiz-Limon P, Aguirre MA, et al: Global effects of fluvastatin on the prothrombotic status of patients with antiphopholipid syndrome. *Ann Rheum Dis* 70:675–682, 2011.

331. Erkan D, Willis R, Murthy VL, et al: A prospective open-label pilot study of fluvastatin on proinflammatory and prothrombotic biomarkers in antiphospholipid antibody positive patients. *Ann Rheum Dis* 73:1176–1180, 2014.

332. Erkan D, Vega J, Ramon G, et al: A pilot open-label phase II trial of rituximab for non-criteria manifestations of antiphospholipid syndrome. *Arthritis Rheum* 65:464–471, 2013.

333. Agmon-Levin N, Blank M, Zandman-Goddard G, et al: Vitamin D: An instrumental factor in the anti-phospolipid syndrome by inhibition of tissue factor expression. *Ann Rheum Dis* 70:145–150, 2011.

334. Andreoli L, Piantoni S, Dall'Ara F, et al: Vitamin D and antiphospholipid syndrome. *Lupus* 21:736–740, 2012.

335. Piantoni S, Andreoli L, Allegri F, et al: Low levels of vitamin D are common in primary antiphospholipid syndrome with thrombotic disease. *Reumatismo* 64:307–313, 2012.

336. Erkan D, Aguiar CL, Andrade D, et al: 14th International Congress on Antiphospholipid Antibodies: Task force report on antiphospholipid syndrome treatment trends. *Autoimmun Rev* 13:685–696, 2014.

337. Kutteh WH: Antiphospholipid antibody-associated recurrent pregnancy loss: Treatment with heparin and low-dose aspirin is superior to low-dose aspirin alone. *Am J Obstet Gynecol* 174:1584–1589, 1996.

338. Rai R, Cohen H, Dave M, Regan L: Randomised controlled trial of aspirin and aspirin plus heparin in pregnant women with recurrent miscarriage associated with phospholipid antibodies (or antiphospholipid antibodies) [see comments]. *BMJ* 314:253–257, 1997.

339. Cohn DM, Goddijn M, Middeldorp S, et al: Recurrent miscarriage and antiphospholipid antibodies: Prognosis of subsequent pregnancy. *J Thromb Haemost* 8:2208–2213, 2010.

340. Bramham K, Thomas M, Nelson-Piercy C, et al: First trimester low-dose prednisolone in refractory antiphospholipid antibody-related pregnancy loss. *Blood* 117:6948–6951, 2011.

341. Dendrinos S, Sakkas E, Makrakis E: Low-molecular-weight heparin versus intravenous immunoglobulin for recurrent abortion associated with antiphospholipid antibody syndrome. *Int J Gynaecol Obstet* 104:223–225, 2009.

342. Sherer Y, Levy Y, Shoenfeld Y: Intravenous immunoglobulin therapy of antiphospholipid syndrome. *Rheumatology* 39:421–426, 2000.

343. Branch DW, Peaceman AM, Druzin M, et al: A multicenter, placebo-controlled pilot study of intravenous immune globulin treatment of antiphospholipid syndrome during pregnancy. The Pregnancy Loss Study Group. *Am J Obstet Gynecol* 182:122–127, 2000.

# CHAPTER 22
# THROMBOTIC MICROANGIOPATHIES

J. Evan Sadler

## SUMMARY

*Thrombotic microangiopathy* is a general term for the combination of micro-angiopathic hemolytic anemia and thrombocytopenia, often accompanied by signs and symptoms consistent with disseminated microvascular thrombosis. Thrombotic thrombocytopenic purpura (TTP) refers to thrombotic micro-angiopathy, without an obvious predisposing condition, and without oliguric renal failure. TTP is caused by autoantibodies to ADAMTS13 (a disintegrin and metalloprotease with a thrombospondin type 1 motif member 13), a plasma metalloprotease that normally cleaves von Willebrand factor (VWF) and regu-lates VWF-dependent platelet aggregation. Inherited deficiency of ADAMTS13 causes congenital TTP, which typically responds to plasma infusion. Most patients with acquired TTP respond to plasma exchange, although many have relapsing disease. Hemolytic uremic syndrome (HUS) refers to thrombotic microangiopathy that usually causes oliguric or anuric renal failure. Ingestion of *Shiga* toxin–producing *Escherichia coli* can cause the most common or "typical" form of HUS that is usually preceded by bloody diarrhea. Inherited or acquired defects in the regulation of the alternative complement pathway cause HUS referred to as "atypical" because it occurs without a prodrome of bloody diar-rhea. Secondary thrombotic microangiopathy can occur in association with metastatic cancer, infections, organ transplantation, and certain drugs. These variants of thrombotic microangiopathy differ in pathogenesis and prognosis but can be difficult to distinguish because their clinical features often overlap.

## ● THROMBOTIC THROMBOCYTOPENIC PURPURA

### DEFINITION AND HISTORY

Thrombotic thrombocytopenic purpura (TTP) refers to thrombotic microangiopathy without another apparent cause and without acute renal failure, although mild or modest renal insufficiency may be seen.

Acronyms and Abbreviations: ADAMTS, a disintegrin and metalloprotease with thrombospondin repeats; aHUS, atypical hemolytic uremic syndrome; ANA, anti-nuclear antibody; APS, antiphospholipid syndrome; aPTT, activated partial throm-boplastin time; CFH, complement factor H; CFHR, complement factor H-related protein; DDAVP, desmopressin; DGKE, diacylglycerol kinase ε ; Gb3, globotriaos-ylceramide 3; HELLP, hemolysis, elevated liver enzymes, low platelet count; HIT, heparin-induced thrombocytopenia; HUS, hemolytic uremic syndrome; LDH, lactate dehydrogenase; MCP, membrane cofactor protein; MMACHC, methylmalonic aciduria and homocystinuria type C protein; PT, prothrombin time; SLE, systemic lupus ery-thematosus; STEC, *Shiga* toxin–producing *Escherichia coli*; Stx, *Shiga* toxin; TM, thrombomodulin (gene name *THBD*); TTP, thrombotic thrombocytopenic pur-pura; VEGF, vascular endothelial growth factor; VWF, von Willebrand factor.

Tissue injury can affect almost any organ but often results in neuro-logic damage. TTP is associated with autoantibodies against the plasma metalloprotease ADAMTS13 (a member of the "a disintegrin and metalloprotease with thrombospondin repeats" family) that reduce plasma ADAMTS13 activity to less than 10 percent of normal.

Eli Moschcowitz reported the first detailed description of TTP in 1924.[1] The patient was a 16-year-old girl with fever, severe anemia, leukocytosis, petechiae, and hemiparesis. Her renal function was not impaired, but the urine contained albumin, hyaline casts, and granular casts. She became comatose and died 2 weeks after her first symptoms. At autopsy, hyaline thrombi were found diffusely in terminal arterioles and capillaries, particularly of the heart and kidney. For many years, patients with similar findings were said to have Moschcowitz disease. The name *TTP* was proposed in 1947[2] and widely adopted thereafter.

In 1966, a review of 272 published cases defined the major clinical features of TTP.[3] Most patients were females between the ages of 10 and 39 years. The symptoms and physical findings included thrombocytope-nia, hemolytic anemia with numerous fragmented red cells or schisto-cytes, neurologic findings, renal damage, and fever. Mortality exceeded 90 percent; the average hospital stay was only 14 days before death, and 80 percent of patients lived fewer than 90 days after the onset of symp-toms. However, dramatic recoveries occurred in some cases following splenectomy.

This grim prognosis was recorded before a report in 1976 that whole blood exchange transfusions induced prompt remissions in eight of 14 patients.[4] Similar responses were described after plasmapher-esis with plasma replacement.[5] One remarkable case report showed that plasmapheresis was effective if the replacement fluid was plasma or cryoprecipitate-depleted plasma, but ineffective if the replacement fluid contained just albumin.[6] Furthermore, simple plasma infusions without plasmapheresis could induce sustained remissions, suggesting that replacement of a missing plasma factor sometimes was sufficient to ameliorate TTP.[6]

These reports led to the widespread adoption of plasma therapy for TTP, and two studies published in 1991 provided compelling evidence for its efficacy. Plasma infusion was associated with 91 percent survival in 108 patients, an impressive improvement over historical experi-ence.[7] The same year, a prospective randomized comparison of plasma exchange and plasma infusion in 102 patients with TTP was reported.[8] Long-term survival was 78 percent for the plasma exchange group and 63 percent for the plasma infusion group, a significant difference in favor of plasma exchange.

A link between TTP and von Willebrand factor (VWF) was pro-posed in 1982, based on studies of four patients with chronic relapsing TTP.[9] Their plasma VWF multimers were much larger than those of healthy controls and similar in size to the VWF multimers secreted by endothelial cells. Patients with TTP were proposed to lack a depoly-merase activity, perhaps a protease or a reductase, that shortens newly secreted VWF multimers *in vivo* and produces the multimer distribu-tion of normal plasma. The absence of this depolymerase would cause the persistence of "unusually large" VWF, which promotes intravascular platelet aggregation, thrombocytopenia, and microvascular thrombosis. Plasma exchange therapy could provide the missing depolymerase activity or remove other factors that provoke clinical relapses.

A candidate depolymerase was identified in 1996, when a metal-loprotease in plasma was shown to cleave VWF multimers subjected to high fluid shear stress or to mild protein denaturants.[10,11] Soon thereafter, children with congenital TTP were shown to have inherited deficiency of this metalloprotease,[12] and adults with acquired TTP were shown to have autoantibody inhibitors of the enzyme.[13,14] The VWF cleaving protease was purified,[15,16] cloned,[17,18] and named ADAMTS13, a new member of the ADAMTS family of metalloproteases. Simultaneously, the *ADAMTS13* locus was identified by linkage analysis in families affected by congenital TTP, and causative *ADAMTS13* mutations were characterized.[19]

## ETIOLOGY AND PATHOGENESIS

TTP is caused by unregulated VWF-dependent platelet thrombosis. Large VWF multimers mediate platelet adhesion at sites of vascular injury by binding to connective tissue and to glycoprotein Ib (GPIb) on the platelet surface (Chap. 10). The VWF subunit from which multimers are constructed has a modular structure consisting of five types of conserved structural motifs (Fig. 22–1). VWF multimers bind to collagen through domain A3 and to platelet GPIb through domain A1. When platelets bind to VWF under conditions of high fluid shear stress, the VWF multimer is stretched and the $Tyr^{1605}$-$Met^{1606}$ bond within domain A2 becomes accessible to ADAMTS13, which cleaves it and thereby can release any adherent platelets. ADAMTS13 deficiency prevents this feedback inhibition of platelet adhesion and leads to widespread microvascular thrombosis. ADAMTS13 levels greater than 10 percent appear sufficient to prevent thrombotic microangiopathy.

ADAMTS13 deficiency in TTP is caused by polyclonal autoantibodies against ADAMTS13, usually immunoglobulin (Ig) G but occasionally IgA or IgM.[13,14] These antibodies almost always bind the ADAMTS13 spacer domain, and often bind to the CUB domains and first thrombospondin-1 repeat; they bind less frequently to other thrombospondin-1 repeats, the metalloprotease domain, or the propeptide.[20-22] Most patients have autoantibodies that inhibit ADAMTS13 activity. The rest have noninhibitory antibodies that are likely to mediate clearance of ADAMTS13 from the circulation.[23]

## EPIDEMIOLOGY

The annual incidence of TTP reportedly is two to six per million population in the United States and approximately 2.2 per million in the United Kingdom.[24,25] Seasonal or geographical trends have not been observed consistently. The demographics of TTP are similar to those of systemic lupus erythematosus (SLE). TTP is relatively uncommon before age 20 years, with a peak incidence between ages 30 and 50 years.[24,25] Across many reports, the female-to-male ratio averages approximately 2:1, but female preponderance is more pronounced below age 50 years and the ratio approaches equality above age 60 years.[24,25] Other risk factors for TTP include African ancestry[26,27] and obesity.[27,28] Women have a tendency to present during late pregnancy or peripartum (reviewed in Refs. 29 and 30). HLA-DRB1*11 is overrepresented severalfold in whites with TTP.[31,32]

## CLINICAL FEATURES

The onset of TTP can be dramatically acute or insidious, developing over weeks. Approximately one-third of patients have symptoms of hemolytic anemia.[3,29] Thrombocytopenia typically causes petechiae or purpura; oral, gastrointestinal, or genitourinary bleeding is less common but can be severe. Many patients describe an antecedent upper respiratory tract infection or flu-like illness. Abdominal pain and tenderness are common. Nausea, vomiting, and diarrhea may occur, but bloody diarrhea is uncommon.

Systemic microvascular thrombosis typically affects the kidney, heart, brain, pancreas, adrenals, skin, spleen, marrow, and most other tissues except the lungs, which are spared. Renal involvement is common, but acute renal failure occurs in fewer than 10 percent of cases.[26,27,29] Neurologic findings can be transient or persistent and may include headache, visual disturbances, vertigo, personality change, confusion, lethargy, syncope, coma, seizures, aphasia, hemiparesis, and other focal sensory or motor deficits.[3,29] The frequency of neurologic findings or fever has decreased from more than 90 percent to approximately 50 percent over the past 40 years,[3,8,26,27,29] probably because these features no longer are recognized as necessary to diagnose TTP.

The symptoms of TTP sometimes can be quite atypical, either at first presentation or upon relapse. Thrombocytopenia without hemolytic anemia may herald the onset of disease. In rare instances, visual disturbances, pancreatitis, stroke, or other thrombosis may

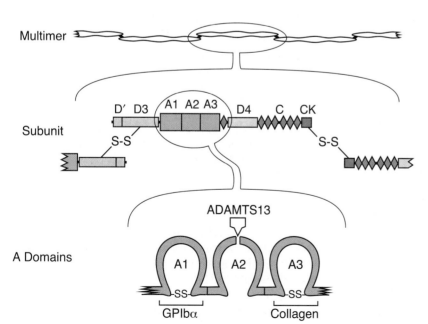

**Figure 22–1.** Structure of von Willebrand factor (VWF). Multimeric VWF *(top)* is composed of identical subunits with four kinds of structural motifs, including three A domains, six C domains and a homologous D4N domain, two complete and one partial D domains, and a cystine knot (CK) domain. Subunits *(middle)* are linked into multimers by disulfide bonds between C-terminal CK domains and N-terminal D3 domains. Domain A1 *(bottom)* binds platelet glycoprotein Ibα (GPIbα), domain A3 binds collagen in extracellular matrix, and domain A2 contains a Tyr-Met bond that is susceptible to cleavage by ADAMTS13 (a disintegrin and metalloprotease with a thrombospondin type 1 motif member 13).

precede overt thrombotic microangiopathy by days to months.[33–36] Macrovascular venous or arterial thrombosis occurs in up to one-half of patients.[37]

Cardiac involvement may cause chest pain, myocardial infarction, congestive heart failure, or arrhythmias.[29,38,39] Direct pulmonary involvement is uncommon, but severe acute respiratory distress syndrome may occur, possibly secondary to cardiac failure.[29] Gastrointestinal symptoms are common and can include abdominal pain, nausea, vomiting, and diarrhea.[3,29] Physical examination may suggest acute pancreatitis or mesenteric ischemia. Infrequent findings include Raynaud phenomenon, arthralgia, myalgia, and retinal hemorrhage or detachment.[3,29]

## LABORATORY FEATURES

The symptoms and signs of TTP are nonspecific. The diagnosis depends on laboratory testing to document microangiopathic hemolytic anemia and thrombocytopenia, without another predisposing cause. Anemia is almost universal, with a mean hemoglobin of approximately 8 g/dL.[27,40] Thrombocytopenia typically is severe, with a mean platelet count of approximately $20 \times 10^9$/L.[26,27,40] Hemolysis is indicated by an elevated reticulocyte count and serum lactate dehydrogenase (LDH), undetectable serum haptoglobin, and increased total and unconjugated bilirubin. Coombs test is almost always negative.[7,8] Renal microvascular injury is common with microhematuria, granular or red cell casts, and proteinuria, but the serum creatinine is often normal and seldom greater than 2 mg/dL.[7,8,27,40] Approximately 50 percent of patients have a positive antinuclear antibody (ANA) test.[40]

Almost all patients have normal values for plasma fibrinogen, prothrombin time (PT), and activated partial thromboplastin time (aPTT),[7,8] reflecting a minor role of blood coagulation in TTP. Evidence of myocardial damage is common, with elevated troponin levels.[38,39]

The characteristic morphologic feature of TTP on the blood film is a marked increase in schistocytes. Schistocytes are helmet cells, or small irregular triangular or crescent-shaped cells with pointed projections, that lack central pallor.[41] Patients with TTP often have markedly increased schistocytes; in a study of six patients, schistocytes composed a mean of 8.3 percent of all red cells, with a range of 1 percent to 18.4 percent.[42] Spherocytes also may be seen.

ADAMTS13 activity is characteristically less than 10 percent, and this degree of acquired ADAMTS13 deficiency appears to be specific for TTP.[13,14,43,44] If adult patients with thrombotic microangiopathy are selected with no plausible secondary cause, no diarrheal prodrome, and no features suggestive of hemolytic uremic syndrome (HUS) (e.g., oliguria, severe hypertension, dialysis, serum creatinine >3.5 mg/dL), then at least 80 percent of those selected have ADAMTS13 activity less than 10 percent of normal. The majority of patients with severe ADAMTS13 deficiency have autoantibody inhibitors,[13,14,26,45] and almost all patients have autoantibodies that bind ADAMTS13 by enzyme-linked immunosorbent assay (ELISA).

Depending on the clinical context, laboratory tests should be considered to detect conditions that may cause thrombotic microangiopathy by mechanisms other than ADAMTS13 deficiency such as pregnancy, cobalamin deficiency, SLE and other autoimmune diseases, antiphospholipid syndrome (APS), HIV, and *Shiga* toxin–producing organisms.

The histologic appearance of microvascular lesions in TTP is consistent with a pathophysiologic role of VWF-dependent platelet thrombosis. Amorphous thrombi and subendothelial hyaline deposits may be found in the small arterioles and capillaries of any organ, but are particularly common (in order of decreasing severity) in the myocardium, pancreas, kidney, adrenal gland, and brain. The liver and lung are relatively spared. The lesions consist mainly of platelets and VWF, with little fibrin and few inflammatory cells. They often include focal endothelial cell proliferation.[46,47]

## DIFFERENTIAL DIAGNOSIS

The diagnosis of TTP should be entertained for any patient with microangiopathic hemolytic anemia and thrombocytopenia, without evidence for disseminated intravascular coagulation, and without features associated with *Shiga* toxin–producing *Escherichia coli* (STEC)-HUS such as a prodromal diarrheal illness and acute oliguric or anuric renal failure. These criteria can only be approximate, however, because many diseases associated with secondary thrombotic microangiopathy can produce overlapping clinical and laboratory findings. As a consequence, making a diagnosis of TTP can be a challenge, and a wide differential diagnosis often must be considered (Table 22–1).

Schistocytes occur in a variety of conditions besides TTP, although the level seldom enters the 1 to 18 percent range typical of TTP. For example, schistocytes were seen in the blood film of 58 percent of healthy controls, with a mean of 0.05 percent and a range of 0 to 0.27 percent of all red cells.[42] Up to 0.6 percent schistocytes were observed in patients with chronic renal failure, preeclampsia, or properly functioning prosthetic heart valves.[42] Severe hemolysis and marked schistocytosis occur in patients with defective mechanical heart valves. Patients receiving marrow allografts or autografts

**TABLE 22–1.** Classification and Differential Diagnosis of Thrombotic Microangiopathy

| |
|---|
| **Thrombotic Thrombocytopenic Purpura (TTP)** |
|   Autoimmune, with antibodies against ADAMTS13 |
| **Congenital Thrombotic Thrombocytopenic Purpura (Upshaw-Schulman Syndrome)** |
|   Inherited ADAMTS13 deficiency, with mutations in *ADAMTS13* |
| ***Shiga* Toxin–Producing *Escherichia Coli* Hemolytic Uremic Syndrome (STEC-HUS)** |
| **Atypical Hemolytic Uremic Syndrome (aHUS)** |
|   Alternative complement pathway defects |
|   Diacylglycerol kinase ε (DGKE) defects |
| **Secondary Thrombotic Microangiopathy** |
|   Disseminated intravascular coagulation |
|   Infections (viral, bacterial, fungal) |
|     *Streptococcus pneumoniae* |
|   Tissue transplant-associated |
|     Chemotherapy or radiation injury |
|     Tissue rejection |
|     Graft-versus-host disease |
|   Cancer |
|   Pregnancy associated (preeclampsia, eclampsia, HELLP [hemolysis, elevated liver enzymes, low platelet count] syndrome) |
|   Autoimmune disorders |
|     Systemic lupus erythematosus and other vasculitides |
|     Antiphospholipid syndrome |
|   Drugs (commonly implicated) |
|     Immune (quinine, ticlopidine) |
|     Toxic (cyclosporine, tacrolimus, mitomycin C, gemcitabine) |
|   Cobalamin metabolic defects |
|   Malignant hypertension |
|   Mechanical hemolysis (e.g., malfunctioning aortic or mitral valve prosthesis) |

for a variety of indications had a mean of 0.7 percent schistocytes 6 weeks after transplantation, with a range of 0 to approximately 4 percent schistocytes.[48,49] Approximately 10 percent of patients had at least 1.3 percent schistocytes, placing them at risk for a diagnosis of thrombotic microangiopathy.[49]

ADAMTS13 levels are normal to moderately decreased in newborns, during pregnancy, after surgery, and in chronic liver cirrhosis, chronic renal insufficiency, acute inflammatory states, and a variety of thrombocytopenic disorders other than TTP.[44,50] Severe sepsis may sometimes cause acquired severe ADAMTS13 deficiency, although the incidence and clinical significance of the finding remain uncertain.[51] Some patients with acute viral hepatitis, severe liver cirrhosis,[52] or venoocclusive disease after stem cell transplantation[53] have had severe ADAMTS13 deficiency (<10 percent) at least transiently, which is consistent with the synthesis of ADAMTS13 in liver.[17-19]

## THERAPY

### Plasma Exchange

The mainstay of therapy for TTP is plasma exchange, which removes antibody inhibitors of ADAMTS13 and replenishes the enzyme. After diagnosing TTP, or determining that the diagnosis is sufficiently likely to justify treatment, plasma exchange therapy should be started as soon as feasible. Studies establishing the value of plasma therapy have excluded secondary thrombotic microangiopathy,[7,8] so the efficacy of plasma exchange has been demonstrated directly only for TTP. The optimal dose of plasma is not known, but a common practice is to perform plasma exchange once daily at a volume of 40 or 60 mL/kg, equivalent to 1.0 or 1.5 plasma volumes. Most centers will start with 1.5× plasma volume exchange for the initial procedures followed by 1.0× plasma volume thereafter. For refractory disease, the intensity of plasma exchange can be increased to 1 plasma volume twice daily.[54] Prompt treatment is important, and if plasma exchange must be delayed more than a few hours, plasma should be given by simple infusion at 20 to 40 mL/kg total dose per day, consistent with the patient's ability to tolerate the fluid load.[55]

The replacement fluid should contain ADAMTS13. Satisfactory results have been obtained with fresh-frozen plasma,[7,8] plasma cryosupernatant,[56-58] and various pathogen-inactivated plasma products, which are considered equivalent.[59] The incidence of allergic reactions and transfusion-associated lung injury may be lower with solvent/detergent-treated plasma than with fresh-frozen plasma,[60] but the incidence of thrombosis may be increased with some preparations.[59,61] Cryosupernatant is depleted in the largest VWF multimers but has normal ADAMTS13 levels,[62] which could make cryosupernatant particularly suitable for the treatment of TTP. Nevertheless, small randomized trials suggest that cryosupernatant is not superior to fresh-frozen plasma for the initial treatment of TTP.[56,57] Methylene blue–treated plasma may be less effective than fresh-frozen plasma,[59,63] despite having a similar concentration of ADAMTS13.[59]

Plasma exchange should be continued daily until the patient has a treatment response as shown by a platelet count greater than $150 \times 10^9$/L for at least 2 days.[55] Whether plasma exchange then should be simply stopped or tapered is not known. A typical strategy is to reduce the frequency of plasma exchange to every other day (or twice per week) for several days. If the disease remains quiescent, then treatment can be stopped and the patient monitored closely for recurrence. Alternatively, plasma exchange can be stopped abruptly with monitoring for recurrent thrombocytopenia over several days.

### Glucocorticoids

TTP is an autoimmune disease, and the use of glucocorticoids is logical, although a beneficial effect has not been demonstrated conclusively.

Common practice is to give prednisone or equivalent at a total daily dose of 1 mg/kg, in one or two doses, for the duration of plasma exchange, followed by tapering. An alternative regimen is methylprednisolone 1 g intravenously daily for 3 days.[55] High-dose methylprednisolone (10 mg/kg/d for 3 days followed by 2.5 mg/kg/d) was more effective than standard-dose methylprednisolone (1 mg/kg/d) in a small randomized trial.[63a]

### Antiplatelet Agents

The use of antiplatelet agents in TTP is controversial. Aspirin and dipyridamole often are combined with plasma exchange but have not been shown conclusively to modify the course of TTP.[8,64] Low-dose aspirin (e.g., 80 mg/d) has been suggested for thromboprophylaxis, once the platelet count exceeds $50 \times 10^9$/L.[55]

### Platelet Transfusion

Transfusion of platelets may correlate with acute deterioration and death in TTP.[7,29,65,66] Therefore, platelet transfusions are relatively contraindicated and should be reserved for the treatment of life-threatening hemorrhage, preferably after plasma exchange treatment has been initiated. Platelets generally need not be given prophylactically before establishing venous access for plasma exchange.[67,68] Platelets have been transfused before emergency surgery, immediately after preparation by intensive plasma exchange.[65]

### Rituximab

TTP that is refractory to plasma exchange usually responds to rituximab (e.g., 375 mg/m² weekly for 4 doses). Almost 90 percent of patients have complete responses within 1 to 3 weeks of starting treatment,[69] including a normal ADAMTS13 level and disappearance of anti-ADAMTS13 antibodies (if present). Relapses occur in a minority of patients after successful treatment, usually after intervals of 6 months to 4 years, and most such patients respond to retreatment.

Acute reactions to rituximab are controlled by premedication with glucocorticoids, antihistamines, and analgesics. Because rituximab is removed by plasma exchange, it should be administered immediately after plasma exchange to maximize the interval until the next plasma exchange.

Rituximab has been given together with plasma exchange at the time of initial diagnosis, which may shorten the time to treatment response and reduce the incidence of relapse.[55,69,70] Rituximab also has been administered preemptively to patients with persistent or recurrent severe ADAMTS13 deficiency after achieving remission of TTP, and this approach may prevent subsequent relapses.[70,71,71a]

In some settings, rare but serious complications associated with rituximab have included bronchospasm, hypotension, serum sickness, susceptibility to infections, and progressive multifocal leukoencephalopathy.[72] Such events have been very rare for patients with autoimmune diseases like TTP.[73,74]

Patients who have not been vaccinated for hepatitis B should be screened for hepatitis B infection before receiving rituximab. Those with evidence of past infection should be considered for antiviral prophylaxis as well as monitoring for hepatic injury and viral reactivation for 6 to 12 months after treatment.[74]

### Splenectomy

Splenectomy can result in lasting remissions or reduce the frequency of relapses for some patients with TTP that is refractory to plasma exchange or immunosuppressive therapy, presumably by removing a major site of anti-ADAMTS13 antibody production.[75,76] Laparoscopic splenectomy can be performed safely in most patients regardless of platelet count.[77]

### Other Treatments

Anecdotal experience suggests that vincristine may be beneficial for refractory TTP, although its efficacy is difficult to assess. Dosing schedules have included 2 mg intravenously on day 1 followed by 1 mg on days 4 and 7,[78] or 2 mg intravenously per week for 2 to 14 weeks.[79] Prostacyclin analogues[80,81] and high-dose intravenous immunoglobulins[82,83] have been used without convincing evidence of efficacy.

Although cyclosporine can cause secondary thrombotic microangiopathy, apparent responses, with normalization of ADAMTS13 activity, have been observed with cyclosporine 2 to 3 mg/kg daily in two divided doses as an adjunct to plasma exchange.[84]

Other treatments have included oral or intravenous cyclophosphamide, oral azathioprine,[55] bortezomib,[85] mycophenolate,[86] N-acetylcysteine,[87] combination chemotherapy with cyclophosphamide, doxorubicin, vincristine, and prednisone,[88] and autologous stem cell transplantation.[89] Agents that prevent the binding of VWF to platelets are under development and may prove useful for the treatment of TTP.[90,91]

### Supportive Therapy

Daily laboratory monitoring should include complete blood count with platelet count, LDH, electrolytes, blood urea nitrogen, and creatinine. Because of the high incidence of cardiac damage,[29] continuous electrocardiographic monitoring and periodic assessment of cardiac enzymes should be considered. Patients should receive supplemental folic acid and vaccination for hepatitis B.[55] Allergic reactions, metabolic alkalosis, and hypocalcemia associated with plasma exchange should be prevented or treated by appropriate adjustments in therapy.

After the platelet count increases to above $50 \times 10^9$/L, prophylaxis for venous thromboembolism may be instituted with low-molecular-weight heparin[61] and low-dose aspirin.[55]

## COURSE AND PROGNOSIS

The platelet count normalizes after a median of 11 plasma exchanges, with a wide range of four to 55 sessions.[92] Normalization of serum LDH lags behind the platelet count by approximately 9 days, and persistent elevation of LDH does not correlate with the risk of exacerbation or relapse.[93]

Exacerbations are defined as TTP recurring within 30 days after a treatment response, and 25 to 50 percent of patients have an acute exacerbation within 2 weeks that requires further treatment with plasma exchange. Some have repeated exacerbations over several months.[94] A durable treatment response, lasting more than 30 days, is achieved eventually in approximately 80 percent of patients.[92]

Relapses, defined as recurrences more than 30 days after a complete response, occur in up to one-third of patients within 2 years after treatment with plasma exchange and glucocorticoids alone. Most relapses occur during the first year, but have occurred 13 years or more after diagnosis.[26,94] Evaluation for relapsing TTP should be considered for any symptom compatible with thrombotic microangiopathy, especially in association with a common trigger of relapse such as infection, surgery, or pregnancy.[34,95] Relapsing patients typically respond to plasma exchange. Relapses in TTP are associated with severe ADAMTS13 deficiency and detectable ADAMTS13 autoantibody inhibitors. Conversely, patients without severe ADAMTS13 deficiency at diagnosis rarely relapse (approximately 9 percent across several studies) (reviewed in Ref. 96).

Serious catheter-related complications of plasma exchange therapy occur in approximately 26 percent of patients with TTP and include pneumothorax and hemorrhage, cardiac perforation, venous thrombosis, catheter thrombosis, and bacterial or fungal infections.[97]

Hives or pruritic reactions to fresh-frozen plasma occur in one-to two-thirds of patients but usually can be managed by premedication with antihistamines. High-volume plasma exchange causes metabolic alkalosis and hypocalcemia and may cause unintentional platelet removal. Serious complications attributable to plasma are less common, occurring in approximately 4 percent of patients, and include bronchospasm, anaphylaxis, hypotension, hypoxia, and serum sickness.[97]

The mortality rate for TTP treated with plasma exchange ranges from 10 to 20 percent. Most deaths occur within a few days after presentation, and almost all occur within the first month.[7,8,26,94]

Late sequelae of TTP may include long-term deficits in quality of life and cognition in many patients,[98,99] severe persistent neurologic deficits in 5 to 13 percent,[100] chronic renal insufficiency in up to 25 percent,[100] and dialysis-dependent renal failure in 3 to 8 percent of patients.[100,101]

## ● CONGENITAL THROMBOTIC THROMBOCYTOPENIC PURPURA

### DEFINITION AND HISTORY

Congenital TTP, or Upshaw-Schulman syndrome, refers to TTP that is caused by inherited deficiency of ADAMTS13.

Schulman and colleagues[102] and Upshaw[103] first described a congenital disorder resembling TTP characterized by autosomal recessive inheritance and chronic relapsing thrombotic microangiopathy from infancy. Congenital TTP, or Upshaw-Schulman syndrome, shared many features with acquired TTP in adults, including the consistent response to plasma.[103]

### ETIOLOGY AND PATHOGENESIS

Congenital TTP is caused by homozygosity or compound heterozygosity for inactivating mutations in the *ADAMTS13* gene[19] on chromosome 9q34 (reviewed in Ref. 104). The mutations usually impair the synthesis or secretion of ADAMTS13. As yet no evidence convincingly indicates locus heterogeneity in congenital TTP.

### EPIDEMIOLOGY

Congenital TTP is autosomal recessive and affects the genders almost equally.[105] The prevalence of congenital TTP is approximately one per million population in Japan[106] and appears to be similar elsewhere. Congenital TTP accounts for a small percentage of patients presenting with TTP.

### CLINICAL FEATURES

The clinical features of congenital TTP are similar to those of acquired TTP, except for age of onset. Most children with congenital ADAMTS13 deficiency have neonatal jaundice and hemolysis but no evidence of ABO blood group or Rh incompatibility. Approximately half of the children continue to have a chronic relapsing course from infancy. The remaining children usually develop symptoms in their late teens or early twenties. In either case, acute exacerbations often are triggered by infections, otitis media, surgery, or other inflammatory stress.[105,107] Patients may suffer an acute attack after receiving desmopressin (DDAVP), which stimulates the release of VWF from endothelial cell stores; one such patient was receiving a low dose of intranasal DDAVP for enuresis.[108] As in acquired TTP, most patients with congenital TTP have some renal involvement with proteinuria, hematuria, or a mildly elevated serum creatinine during acute attacks. Chronic renal failure can occur, usually after a prolonged course of relapsing disease.[107]

Females often present during their first pregnancy, possibly because VWF levels are increased late in pregnancy. If untreated, pregnancies usually end in spontaneous abortion, stillbirth, or premature delivery.

TTP usually occurs in the third trimester or postpartum, whereas fetal loss is most common in the second trimester.[109]

## LABORATORY FEATURES

Severe congenital ADAMTS13 deficiency (<5 percent) is characteristic of congenital TTP. Alloantibodies to ADAMTS13 as a consequence of treatment with plasma are extremely rare in congenital TTP; only one such patient has been reported.[110] Other laboratory findings in congenital TTP are similar to those in acquired TTP. The histologic features of congenital TTP are similar to those of acquired TTP.[111]

## DIFFERENTIAL DIAGNOSIS

For patients presenting during early childhood, other causes of thrombotic microangiopathy to consider include STEC-HUS, atypical HUS, and secondary thrombotic microangiopathy associated with disorders that are characteristic of childhood. For adolescents and adults, the differential diagnosis is the same as for acquired TTP (see Table 22–1).

Testing of stool and urine for STEC should be considered for all patients with thrombotic microangiopathy because a significant fraction of patients with STEC infection never have bloody diarrhea.

## THERAPY

Congenital TTP can be treated with periodic infusions of fresh-frozen plasma or an equivalent virucidally treated product, if available. The half-life of ADAMTS13 is 2 to 3 days,[112] and the level of ADAMTS13 required to avoid symptoms is approximately 5 percent of normal; 5 to 20 mL/kg of plasma every 2 to 3 weeks usually is sufficient to maintain ADAMTS13 at a greater than 5 percent level and prevent symptoms.[105,107] Patients with severe allergic reactions to plasma have been treated successfully with plasma-derived factor VIII/VWF concentrates that contain significant amounts of ADAMTS13.[55]

### Pregnancy Management

Fetal loss and premature birth can be prevented by plasma infusions of 10 mL/kg every 2 weeks beginning at 8 weeks of gestation, increasing to weekly in the second trimester. Any sign of thrombotic microangiopathy is an indication to increase the volume or frequency of plasma infusion. Plasma exchange may be necessary to avoid fluid overload.[55,109]

## COURSE AND PROGNOSIS

The severity of congenital TTP varies considerably and correlates to some extent with the underlying genotype and residual plasma ADAMTS13 activity. Patients with ADAMTS13 activity of less than 2.5 percent of normal tend to have their first TTP episode in childhood, have more than one episode of TTP per year, and require regular plasma prophylaxis. Conversely, patients with ADAMTS13 activity of 2.5 to 6.0 percent tend to present in adulthood and have infrequent episodes of disease.[113,114] Some of these patients have prolonged symptom-free intervals and can be treated on demand. However, inadequately treated patients are at risk for developing chronic renal failure and stroke.[55]

## ● *SHIGA* TOXIN *ESCHERICHIA COLI*– ASSOCIATED HEMOLYTIC UREMIC SYNDROME

### DEFINITION AND HISTORY

HUS refers to thrombotic microangiopathy that mainly affects the kidney and usually causes oliguric or anuric renal failure. Ingestion of STEC causes HUS (STEC-HUS) that is usually is associated with a prodrome of diarrhea. Other names in the literature for STEC-HUS include diarrhea-associated HUS (D+HUS) and "typical" HUS.

In 1955, the term *HUS* was proposed for thrombotic microangiopathy occurring in children and associated with acute anuric renal failure, which is uncommon in TTP.[115] HUS was often preceded by a diarrheal illness, and unlike TTP in adults, the prognosis was relatively favorable. Most patients survived and recovered normal renal function with only supportive care.[116] Although cases were known to cluster in endemic areas, the cause of HUS was unknown until 1983, when *E. coli* O157:H7 was shown to express a *Shiga*-like toxin and cause epidemic hemorrhagic colitis that could evolve into HUS.[117-119]

## ETIOLOGY AND PATHOGENESIS

STEC may make two types of *Shiga* toxin (Stx) that are similar in structure and function to ricin. Stx1 is identical to *Shigella dysenteriae* serotype 1 toxin. Stx2 is approximately 50 percent identical in sequence to Stx1 and occurs in several closely related forms. Both toxins consist of pentameric B subunits that bind globotriaosylceramide (Gb3) on cell surfaces and a single A subunit that is responsible for cytotoxicity. Pathogenic *E. coli* almost always express a variant of Stx2, and approximately two-thirds express Stx1.[120]

When STEC colonize the gut, they damage the epithelium and secrete Stx that is delivered to target organs through the blood, probably by neutrophils. Stx bound to Gb3 on cell surfaces is endocytosed and transported in a retrograde fashion through the secretory pathway to the endoplasmic reticulum, where the A subunit is translocated into the cytoplasm. The A subunit is an *N*-glycosidase that removes a specific base from the large ribosomal subunit, which inhibits protein synthesis and activates a response pathway that leads to apoptosis. The observed predilection for renal injury is a result of the relatively high expression of Gb3 on renal tubular epithelial, mesangial, and glomerular endothelial cells.

## EPIDEMIOLOGY

STEC-HUS can occur at any age but affects mainly children younger than age 5 years and is rare before age 6 months. The disease occurs sporadically and in epidemics, associated with ingestion of foods or other materials contaminated with Stx-producing bacteria. *E. coli* O157:H7 accounts for at least 80 percent of cases in many series, but STEC-HUS can be caused by other toxin-bearing *E. coli* serotypes[121,122] or by *S. dysenteriae* type 1. Most cases occur in summer and autumn in rural environments. The incidence is approximately 10 to 30 per million children per year but depends on the risk of exposure, which varies considerably with the time of year, location, and other factors. STEC-HUS is a common cause of chronic renal failure in children.[120]

## CLINICAL FEATURES

Patients develop abdominal pain, tenderness, and diarrhea between 2 and 12 days after ingesting STEC, with a mean incubation period of 3 to 7 days and a median of 3 days. The diarrhea usually becomes bloody within 1 to 3 days, at which time patients are typically afebrile. Nausea and vomiting are common. The abdominal pain is greater than is typical for other causes of gastroenteritis, and defecation is often painful. Most patients recover spontaneously within a few days. Of children younger than 10 years of age with bloody diarrhea and *E. coli* O157:H7 infection, approximately 15 percent will develop STEC-HUS with the acute onset of microangiopathic hemolytic anemia, thrombocytopenia, and renal injury an average of 7 days (range: 5 to 13 days) after the start of diarrhea.[120]

## LABORATORY FEATURES

Aside from signs of dehydration or electrolyte imbalances from diarrhea or vomiting, laboratory testing may be unremarkable before bloody diarrhea develops. Thrombocytopenia and hemolysis with associated laboratory abnormalities develop after bloody diarrhea and usually before renal failure. The platelet count falls to an average of $40 \times 10^9/L$. Renal signs may include a rising creatinine, proteinuria, hematuria, hypertension, and oliguria or anuria. Usually the PT and aPTT are normal or minimally prolonged, plasma fibrinogen is normal or elevated, and fibrin degradation products may be moderately elevated.[120,123] ADAMTS13 levels are normal.[124,125]

Stool should be cultured on selective media for *E. coli* O157:H7 and tested for Stxs to detect non-O157 strains. STEC in the stool are found in at least 90 percent of patients during the first 6 days but in less than 30 percent of patients at later times. Fecal leukocytes are not always present and generally are not abundant.[120]

Serologic testing for antibodies to STEC surface antigens at diagnosis and after 2 weeks can facilitate the diagnosis of STEC-HUS if stool cultures are not informative. Titers rise after infection and persist for 8 to 12 weeks.

STEC-HUS mainly affects the renal cortex, which often shows extensive necrosis. Lesions occur less frequently in the pancreas, brain, adrenal glands, and myocardium. The thrombi of HUS typically involve glomerular capillaries and arterioles and are composed mainly of fibrin and red cells with few platelets.[47,126]

## DIFFERENTIAL DIAGNOSIS

Unlike STEC-HUS, bloody diarrhea caused by *Salmonella*, *Shigella*, or *Clostridium difficile* is likely to be accompanied by fever and prostration. Coinfection with STEC and *C. difficile* can occur. Otherwise the differential diagnosis of apparent STEC-HUS includes unusual presentations of other causes of thrombotic microangiopathy (see Table 22–1).

## THERAPY

Patients with acute bloody diarrhea should be admitted to the hospital for diagnosis and management of presumed STEC infection as well as infection control. Early intravenous hydration to maintain renal perfusion protects against the development of HUS.[120] Most patients require red cell transfusions. Daily monitoring of hemoglobin, platelet count, electrolytes, blood urea nitrogen (BUN), and creatinine is important.

The risks and benefits of antibiotic use in STEC-HUS may depend on the stage of illness. Antibiotics should not be used early in the course of acute diarrheal illness caused by *E. coli* O157:H7 because antibiotics increase the risk of HUS.[127] However, retrospective analysis of a 2011 outbreak of *E. coli* O104:H4 infection suggests that treatment with multiple antibiotics after the development of HUS may have reduced the incidence of seizures and death.[128]

Antimotility agents and narcotics increase the risk of HUS and neurologic complications. Nonsteroidal antiinflammatory drugs and antihypertensives that reduce renal perfusion such as angiotensin-converting enzyme inhibitors and angiotensin receptor blockers should be avoided. No convincing data indicate that antiplatelet agents, anticoagulants, plasma exchange, glucocorticoids, rituximab, or an inhibitor of the terminal components of complement, eculizumab, add benefit to supportive therapy and dialysis, for children or adults.[58,120,128]

## COURSE AND PROGNOSIS

Patients often have a degree of diffuse vascular injury and may become edematous with intravenous hydration. Consequently, more sodium than expected may be required for adequate volume replacement, and monitoring for fluid overload and hypertension is essential. A rising platelet count signals the end of the period of risk for developing HUS. For patients with HUS, hemolysis can persist as the HUS resolves and require additional red cell transfusions.

Extrarenal involvement is common, although the incidence of specific complications varies widely. Depending on the outbreak, central nervous system involvement (seizures, coma, or stroke) occurs in 10 to 65 percent of cases and is more common in older patients. Cardiac dysfunction is associated with ischemia or congestive heart failure. Patients may require mechanical ventilation for seizures, coma, pulmonary edema, or pneumonia. Gastrointestinal involvement can include hemorrhagic colitis, necrosis, perforation, peritonitis, pancreatitis, diabetes mellitus, and rectal prolapse.[120,128,129]

The incidence of death and end-stage renal failure also varies widely, but correlates with the need for initial dialysis and central nervous system involvement. In a meta-analysis of more than 3400 patients with STEC-HUS, an average of 9 percent died and 3 percent developed permanent end-stage renal failure 1 or more years later. Another 25 percent had persistent hypertension, proteinuria, or chronic renal insufficiency.[130]

Inability to detect STEC may not strongly affect the clinical course. In a study of 268 patients with HUS, 59 percent had prodromal diarrhea plus bacteriologic or serologic evidence of infection by STEC; 21 percent had only diarrhea, and 10 percent had only positive bacteriologic or serologic studies. All three groups had similar outcomes: approximately 1 percent died and 73 percent recovered normal renal function. In contrast, the 11 percent of patients with neither diarrhea nor documented STEC infection had a significantly worse outcome; 10 percent died and only 34 percent recovered normal renal function.[121] Most of these latter patients probably had "atypical hemolytic uremic syndrome (aHUS)," which has a distinct cause and prognosis.

# ● ATYPICAL HEMOLYTIC UREMIC SYNDROME

### DEFINITION AND HISTORY

*Diarrhea-negative HUS*, or *aHUS*, is not associated with diarrhea or Stx-producing organisms and occurs in patients without an obvious predisposing condition.

Reporting on patients seen in southern Africa in 1965, Barnard and Kibel first distinguished typical diarrhea-associated HUS from "atypical" patients who did not have diarrhea.[131] In the 1970s, Kaplan proposed that recurrent familial cases of HUS represented a distinct genetic illness.[132,133] By 1993, aHUS was an accepted diagnosis of uncertain cause,[134] although increased consumption of complement C3 and deficiency of factor H had been described in some patients.[135] In 1998, Warwicker and colleagues showed that mutations in complement factor H (CFH) caused familial HUS,[136] and mutations in other proteins of the alternative complement pathway quickly followed. These results provided a rationale for treating aHUS with inhibitors of complement activation, which has proved very effective.[137]

### ETIOLOGY AND PATHOGENESIS

The alternative complement pathway drives the pathogenesis of aHUS. Complement component C3 is spontaneously converted to C3b at a low rate and deposited on cell surfaces. Under normal circumstances, this C3b is promptly cleaved and inactivated by the serine protease factor I, and this reaction is accelerated by factor H or membrane cofactor protein

**TABLE 22–2.** Complement Defects in Atypical Hemolytic Uremic Syndrome

| Gene or Subgroup | Prevalence in aHUS | Low C3 | Progression to End-Stage Renal Disease | Death |
|---|---|---|---|---|
| *CFH* | 25–30% | 50–60% | 50–60% | 5–20% |
| *CFI* | 4–10% | 20–50% | ~60% | 0–10% |
| *MCP* | 7–10% | 6–30% | 6–35% | 0% |
| *CFB* | <1.5% | ≤100% | ~50% | 0% |
| *C3* | 4–8% | 70–80% | 55–70% | 0% |
| *THBD* (TM)* | <5% | ~50% | ~50% | ~30% |
| Anti–complement factor H antibody | 3–7% | ~40% | 30–60% | 0% |
| No mutation | 30–50% | ~20% | ~40% | 3–7% |

Based on outcomes after 5 years from the International Registry of Recurrent and Familial HUS/TTP[138] and after 3 years from the French Study Group for aHUS.[139]

*THBD* is the gene for thrombomodulin.

(MCP, CD46). These cofactors are structurally and functionally similar, but factor H is a plasma protein, whereas MCP is a transmembrane protein found on the surface of almost all cells. If not restrained by these inhibitors, C3b interacts with factor B to form a potent C3 convertase that amplifies the deposition of C3b, which attracts phagocytes and promotes membrane attack complex formation on renal glomerular and arteriolar endothelium and basement membrane. The resultant vascular damage causes thrombotic microangiopathy.

Heterozygous mutations in alternative complement pathway proteins have been identified in 60 to 70 percent of patients with aHUS (Table 22–2). These include loss-of-function mutations in factor H, MCP, factor I, complement factor H–related proteins 1 and 3 (CFHR1, CFHR3), thrombomodulin (TM), and gain-of-function mutations in factor B and C3. In addition, autoantibodies to factor H have been identified in some patients with aHUS, often in association with mutations in CFHR1 and CFHR3. Patients sometimes have mutations at more than one locus or a combination of autoantibodies to CFH and mutations.[138,139]

Homozygous or compound heterozygous mutations in diacylglycerol kinase ε (DGKE) cause aHUS with high penetrance that presents before 1 year of age with hypertension, hematuria, and proteinuria. How DGKE mutations cause aHUS is not established. DGKE mutations may account for a small percentage of aHUS.[140]

## EPIDEMIOLOGY

Atypical HUS affects approximately 5 percent as many children as develop STEC-HUS, with an estimated incidence of two per million population per year.[141] Approximately one-half of patients are younger than age 18 years. Approximately 60 percent of affected children have their first episode of aHUS before age 2 years, and 25 percent before age 6 months. In contrast, STEC-HUS is rare before age 6 months. Most adults have their first episode of aHUS between ages 20 and 40 years. Childhood aHUS affects males and females equally, whereas onset in adults disproportionately affects females mainly because of disease triggered by pregnancy. Analysis of relatives of probands shows that the penetrance of aHUS may be approximately 50 percent for mutations in any of the predisposing genes.[138,139]

## CLINICAL FEATURES

Approximately 20 percent of patients have a subacute or chronic course of mild anemia, variable thrombocytopenia, and relatively normal renal function. However, patients usually present acutely with thrombotic microangiopathy and renal failure, sometimes with progressive hypertension. Most patients report a possible triggering event such as a viral or bacterial upper respiratory infection, gastroenteritis, or pregnancy. aHUS is not classically preceded by bloody or painful diarrhea.[138,139]

Women with pregnancy-associated aHUS usually present postpartum. Most of the rest develop symptoms in the third trimester, sometimes complicated by fetal loss and preeclampsia.[142]

Extrarenal symptoms occur in 10 to 20 percent of patients. Central nervous system involvement is most common. Myocardial infarction, pancreatitis, and necrosis of skin or digits have been reported. Extrarenal involvement is relatively uncommon for aHUS caused by MCP mutations.[138,139]

## LABORATORY FEATURES

Patients have the laboratory findings characteristic of microangiopathic hemolysis, as observed for TTP and STEC-HUS. The mean platelet count in aHUS is $40 \times 10^9$/L, typically higher than in TTP. Serum creatinine can be markedly elevated, with microhematuria and proteinuria if the patient is not anuric.

Complement C4 is usually normal and C3 may be low, consistent with activation of the alternative complement pathway, but the likelihood of a low C3 level varies considerably and depends on the involved locus (see Table 22–2). Approximately 3 to 7 percent of patients have autoantibodies against CFH that can be detected by ELISA. In favorable cases, flow cytometry on peripheral blood leukocytes can identify cell-surface MCP deficiency for patients with *MCP* mutations. Assays of CFH and CFI may be useful to identify specific deficiencies, but patients are usually heterozygous and mutations at these loci may not clearly decrease the factor levels.[138,139]

DNA sequencing should be considered to detect mutations in *CFH, CFI, MCP, C3, CFB,* and *TM* before renal transplantation because the risk of relapse and need for subsequent prophylaxis depends on the affected locus. Candidate mutations in one of these loci or antibodies to CFH can be found in approximately 70 percent of patients with aHUS. Sequencing of *DGKE* should be considered for patients presenting before age 1 year.

As in STEC-HUS, renal lesions in aHUS are rich in fibrin but poor in platelets or VWF.

## DIFFERENTIAL DIAGNOSIS

Signs and symptoms consistent with aHUS may occur in TTP or STEC-HUS, and distinguishing among these entities is important because they are treated differently. Correct diagnosis is not always straightforward. For example, MCP mutations may cause thrombotic microangiopathy without renal insufficiency that resolves coincidentally during a course of plasma exchange and therefore resembles TTP except for normal ADAMTS13 activity.[143] Infection with STEC may be difficult to document, and some patients with STEC-HUS do not have a diarrheal prodrome.[121]

Secondary causes of thrombotic microangiopathy should be considered (see Table 22–1). For children, conditions that usually present in that age group deserve special attention such as *Streptococcus pneumoniae* infections and inherited cobalamin defects.

## THERAPY

### Plasma Exchange

For patients without a previous diagnosis of aHUS, plasma exchange should be started at 1 to 2 volumes daily for adults or 50 to 100 mL/kg for children.[141] Plasma exchange can induce responses, at least transiently, for patients with deficiency of plasma complement proteins or autoantibodies to CFH but not for deficiency of the membrane protein MCP. If an isolated *MCP* mutation is identified, plasma exchange can be stopped.

### Eculizumab

After excluding severe ADAMTS13 deficiency, STEC, and secondary causes of thrombotic microangiopathy, plasma exchange can be stopped and eculizumab started for presumptive aHUS at 900 mg intravenously every week for 4 weeks, followed by 1200 mg in week 5 and every other week thereafter, in many cases indefinitely. For patients younger than 18 years of age, doses are adjusted based on body weight. Supplementary doses are recommended during plasma exchange or infusion,[137] but concurrent plasma exchange and eculizumab are not beneficial and should be avoided.

Adverse reactions to eculizumab during the treatment of aHUS have included infections, fever, hypertension, headache, diarrhea, abdominal pain, nausea, and vomiting. Adverse reactions are common but seldom require discontinuation of therapy.

Ideally, patients should be vaccinated against *Neisseria meningitides* at least 2 weeks before treatment. If timely vaccination is not possible or the available vaccine does not cover prevalent strains, then antibiotic prophylaxis should be considered. Children also should be vaccinated for *S. pneumoniae* and *Haemophilus influenzae* type b.

### Rituximab

Rituximab and glucocorticoids can be added to eculizumab for treatment of aHUS caused by autoantibodies to CFH. If the autoantibodies are eradicated, then eculizumab can be discontinued.

### Renal Transplantation

Patients with end-stage renal disease that does not improve on eculizumab may be treated by renal transplantation. Living related donors generally are not used because the donated kidney may be at risk for aHUS and the donor may have the same risk factors as the recipient and develop aHUS after donation.

Mutation screening should be performed before transplantation to guide subsequent therapy. Unless patients are treated preemptively with eculizumab, aHUS recurs predictably in transplanted kidneys. Isolated MCP deficiency is an exception because normal membrane-bound MCP in the transplanted kidney protects it from complement attack. HUS has not recurred after renal transplantation in children with *DGKE* mutations.[141,144]

Liver transplantation or combined liver-kidney transplantation can cure aHUS caused by deficiency of plasma complement proteins that are synthesized in the liver. However, the risk and complications of liver transplantation can be avoided by prophylactic treatment with eculizumab after renal transplantation.[141,144]

## COURSE AND PROGNOSIS

Treatment of aHUS with just plasma exchange and supportive care is associated with up to 8 percent mortality during the first episode of disease and rapid progression to end-stage renal failure in many survivors. Mortality at 1 year appears substantially higher for children, but progression to end-stage renal failure is more common for adults. MCP mutations are associated with a less aggressive clinical course: patients may improve during plasma exchange but have similar outcomes

without plasma exchange, with 90 percent alive and dialysis free after several years (see Table 22–2).[138,139]

Treatment with eculizumab is associated with sustained resolution of thrombotic microangiopathy, improvement in renal function, and prevention of relapses. The platelet count normalizes in approximately 50 percent of patients by day 7 and in 80 to 90 percent of patients by week 26. Earlier initiation of eculizumab is associated with greater improvement in renal function.[137]

Most patients are likely to need lifelong treatment to prevent recurrent thrombotic microangiopathy and progressive renal failure. Some patients with aHUS and no remaining renal function may still benefit from eculizumab to prevent the progression of neurologic or other extrarenal injury. Patients with MCP mutations can have a relatively mild course with normal renal function and long intervals between exacerbations; they may not need chronic prophylaxis with eculizumab.[138,139]

*DGKE* mutations are associated with the development of nephrotic syndrome,[140] which is otherwise uncommon in aHUS. Case reports suggest that aHUS caused by *DGKE* mutations is associated with complement activation and can respond to plasma therapy.[145,146] The efficacy of eculizumab is not known. HUS has not recurred after renal transplantation in children with *DGKE* mutations.[140,145,146]

## ● SECONDARY THROMBOTIC MICROANGIOPATHY

Secondary thrombotic microangiopathy occurs in patients with predisposing medical conditions such as metastatic cancer, malignant hypertension, systemic infection, solid-organ or hematopoietic stem cell transplantation, vasculitis, catastrophic APS, radiation exposure, chemotherapy, certain other drugs, inherited or acquired metabolic disorders, and various causes of disseminated intravascular coagulation. Endothelial injury may be a common cause, although the mechanism of disease varies and in most cases is not understood.

The clinical features of secondary thrombotic microangiopathy usually are dominated by the predisposing illness, and the most important clinical intervention is correcting the underlying "primary" condition. The clinical history and laboratory testing can identify most causes of secondary thrombotic microangiopathy. Severe ADAMTS13 deficiency almost never occurs in secondary thrombotic microangiopathy, and treatment with plasma exchange, rituximab, or eculizumab is not known to be beneficial.

## DISSEMINATED INTRAVASCULAR COAGULATION

Conditions resulting in disseminated intravascular coagulation sometimes cause microangiopathic changes and thrombocytopenia with little change in blood coagulation tests, which can suggest a diagnosis of TTP.

## INFECTIONS

Infections may trigger disease in patients with severe ADAMTS13 deficiency, but infections typically cause secondary thrombotic microangiopathy by other mechanisms. Secondary thrombotic microangiopathy caused by infections may respond to antimicrobial or antiviral therapy, but not to plasma exchange.

Thrombotic microangiopathy, often with acute renal failure, is a rare complication of invasive infections with *S. pneumoniae* in children. A surveillance study in Atlanta, Georgia, identified HUS in 0.6 percent of pneumococcal infections in children younger than 2 years of age.[147]

Patients usually have complicated pneumococcal pneumonia or meningitis, with normal plasma fibrinogen and normal or minimally prolonged PT and aPTT. The pathophysiology is thought to involve bacterial neuraminidase, made by *S. pneumoniae* and some other organisms, which removes sialic acid residues from cell surface glycoproteins and exposes Thomsen-Friedenreich antigen (T antigen). T antigen is recognized by naturally occurring antibodies that fix complement, causing hemolysis and damaging the renal microvasculature. Because donor blood usually contains high levels of antibodies against T antigen, red cells and platelets should be washed before transfusion, and plasma should not be used as a replacement fluid. Exchange transfusion has been proposed to stop hemolysis by replacing T-antigen–bearing red blood cells and removing circulating neuraminidase, but the efficacy of this treatment is uncertain.[148]

## TISSUE TRANSPLANTS

Recipients of solid-organ transplants can develop thrombotic microangiopathy, often dominated by renal involvement associated with immunosuppression by cyclosporine or tacrolimus.[149] These drugs appear to damage renal endothelial cells directly and can cause neurotoxicity, adding another feature suggestive of TTP. Similarly, hematopoietic stem cell transplant recipients may develop thrombotic microangiopathy associated with high-dose chemotherapy or radiation, immunosuppressive drugs, graft-versus-host disease, or infections. ADAMTS13 levels are normal,[150] and plasma therapy is ineffective.[151]

## CANCER

Thrombotic microangiopathy occurs in a small fraction of patients with cancer, most commonly with adenocarcinoma of the pancreas, lung, prostate, stomach, colon, ovary, breast, or unknown primary site that usually is widely metastatic. These cancers also are associated with Trousseau syndrome or paraneoplastic hypercoagulability and thrombosis. Patients often have variable prolongation of the PT and aPTT and increased fibrin degradation products. The thrombosis of Trousseau syndrome may respond to anticoagulation with heparin but not warfarin.[152,153] Abundant schistocytes also have been described in acute erythroleukemia.[154] Plasma exchange is ineffective.[26,27,153]

## PREGNANCY-ASSOCIATED THROMBOTIC MICROANGIOPATHY

The differential diagnosis of thrombotic microangiopathy in pregnancy includes preeclampsia, eclampsia, HELLP syndrome (hemolysis, elevated liver enzymes, low platelet count), acute fatty liver of pregnancy, abruptio placenta, amniotic fluid embolism, and retained products of conception (Chap. 19). Severe ADAMTS13 deficiency has not been observed in these conditions.[155] Pregnancy also can trigger disease in patients with congenital or acquired ADAMTS13 deficiency or defects in the alternative complement pathway.

## AUTOIMMUNE DISORDERS

Autoimmune thrombocytopenia may be confused with TTP if other causes of microangiopathic hemolytic anemia are present. Asymptomatic thrombocytopenia also may sometimes be the only finding in TTP. Patients have been described in whom TTP and autoimmune thrombocytopenia appeared to occur simultaneously or sequentially.[156] Evan syndrome (autoimmune hemolytic anemia with autoimmune thrombocytopenia) usually can be distinguished from TTP by a positive Coombs test and the prominence of spherocytes relative to schistocytes in the blood film. Heparin-induced thrombocytopenia (HIT) may sometimes resemble TTP (Chap. 8).

SLE can cause autoimmune hemolysis and thrombocytopenia, and lupus vasculitis can cause microangiopathic changes, renal insufficiency, and neurologic defects consistent with TTP. Vasculitis associated with other autoimmune disorders can pose a similar diagnostic problem. Although ADAMTS13 deficiency is uncommon among patients with SLE,[157] in rare cases, they develop autoimmune ADAMTS13 deficiency and TTP that responds to plasma exchange.[158] Conversely, patients with TTP and autoantibodies against ADAMTS13 may have other markers of autoimmune disease, including ANA or anti-DNA antibodies, polyarthritis, discoid lupus, or ulcerative colitis.[101,159]

Thrombotic microangiopathy can develop in patients with APS, with or without concurrent SLE.

Thrombotic microangiopathy occurs in patients with progressive systemic sclerosis, particularly in association with acute scleroderma renal crisis and malignant hypertension. Treatment with angiotensin-converting enzyme inhibitors may be effective.[160]

## DRUG-INDUCED THROMBOTIC MICROANGIOPATHY

Nearly 80 drugs are associated with thrombotic microangiopathy, and evidence supports a definite or probable causal association for approximately 44 of them. Three drugs (quinine, cyclosporine, tacrolimus) account for 60 percent of the patient reports with definite evidence.[161] Some agents cause disease by an immune mechanism and others by direct toxicity; a few drugs reportedly act by either mechanism. With the exception of ticlopidine-induced disease, plasma exchange appears to be ineffective or possibly harmful for drug-induced thrombotic microangiopathy.[162]

### Immune Mechanisms

Quinine is the most common cause of drug-induced thrombotic microangiopathy. Most patients are women. Severe thrombotic microangiopathy occurs suddenly within several hours after ingestion of a quinine tablet or a beverage containing it, such as tonic water, with fever, abdominal and back pain, nausea, vomiting, diarrhea, rash, and oliguric renal failure. Neurologic changes are common.[163] ADAMTS13 levels are normal.[164] The mechanism involves a broad range of quinine-dependent antibodies against platelets, endothelium, and other cells. Most patients recover with normal renal function over several weeks, although some develop end-stage renal disease.

The antiplatelet drug ticlopidine is unusual because it induces autoantibody inhibitors of ADAMTS13, effectively causing TTP that responds to plasma exchange.[165] The related thienopyridine drugs clopidogrel, prasugrel, and ticagrelor do not appear to cause thrombotic microangiopathy by this mechanism.

### Direct Toxicity

Cyclosporine and tacrolimus are structurally distinct immunosuppressive drugs that indirectly inhibit calcineurin and suppress T-cell activation. Both agents cause dose-dependent nephrotoxicity, neurotoxicity, and thrombotic microangiopathy.[166–168] The renal damage is thought to involve toxic effects on endothelium.[166] Thrombotic microangiopathy can develop during the first few weeks of treatment, although graft rejection, graft-versus-host disease, or systemic infections can cause similar microangiopathic changes. The thrombotic microangiopathy often remits with dose reduction or substitution of other immunosuppressive drugs and may not recur if therapy with cyclosporine or tacrolimus is reinstituted.

Mitomycin C is an alkylating agent that is used for anal carcinoma and for some adenocarcinomas. It appears to cause dose-dependent nephrotoxicity, with renal failure occurring in approximately 16 percent of patients who receive a cumulative dose of at least 50 mg.[169] About half of the patients with renal toxicity also develop thrombotic microangiopathy, usually 4 to 8 weeks after the latest dose. Mitomycin C–induced thrombotic microangiopathy does not respond to plasma exchange and has a high mortality rate of approximately 70 percent within 4 months of onset.[170]

Gemcitabine is a nucleoside analogue often used for carcinoma of the pancreas, bladder, or lung. Thrombotic microangiopathy with renal failure occurs with an incidence of approximately 0.3 percent.[171] The median time to develop thrombotic microangiopathy is 7 months with a median cumulative dose of 22 g/m², although the range of doses is broad, and very low doses have been associated with thrombotic microangiopathy.[172] Death or disability usually results from cancer progression or renal failure, not from extrarenal manifestations of thrombotic microangiopathy.

Drugs that inhibit vascular endothelial growth factor (VEGF) signaling like sunitinib and bevacizumab are associated with proteinuria, hypertension, and mild thrombotic microangiopathy that usually improve when the drug is discontinued. Inhibition of VEGF produced within the kidney appears to damage glomerular endothelium.[173] In some cases, disease has responded to an angiotensin receptor blocker, allowing continued treatment with the VEGF inhibitor.[174]

## COBALAMIN METABOLIC DEFECTS

Cobalamin C deficiency is a rare autosomal recessive condition caused by mutations in the *MMACHC* (methylmalonic aciduria and homocystinuria type C protein) gene. Clinical features may include developmental delay, ataxia, seizures, cognitive impairment, pulmonary hypertension, thrombotic microangiopathy, and renal failure. Symptoms usually appear during infancy but can occur later in childhood or rarely in adulthood. Laboratory studies show elevated plasma methylmalonic acid and homocysteine, low plasma methionine, and normal or elevated plasma vitamin B₁₂. Treatment with high-dose hydroxycobalamin and betaine may reverse or prevent HUS.[175]

The abnormal red cell and platelet morphology in adults with severe vitamin B₁₂ deficiency rarely may suggest thrombotic microangiopathy.

## MALIGNANT HYPERTENSION

Malignant hypertension is associated with microangiopathic hemolytic anemia, thrombocytopenia, neurologic symptoms, and renal insufficiency.[176]

## MECHANICAL HEMOLYSIS

A malfunctioning aortic or mitral valve prosthesis may sufficiently increase the fluid shear stress experienced by the blood to cause significant hemolysis, with schistocytes and thrombocytopenia, suggesting a diagnosis of thrombotic microangiopathy.[41,42] Such patients also are likely to have acquired von Willebrand syndrome.

## REFERENCES

1. Moschcowitz E: Hyaline thrombosis of the terminal arterioles and capillaries: A hitherto undescribed disease. *Proc N Y Pathol Soc* 24:21, 1924.
2. Singer K, Bornstein FP, Wile SA: Thrombotic thrombocytopenic purpura. Hemorrhagic diathesis with generalized platelet thromboses. *Blood* 2:542, 1947.
3. Amorosi EL, Ultmann JE: Thrombotic thrombocytopenic purpura: Report of 16 cases and review of the literature. *Medicine (Baltimore)* 45:139, 1966.
4. Bukowski RM, Hewlett JS, Harris JW, et al: Exchange transfusions in the treatment of thrombotic thrombocytopenic purpura. *Semin Hematol* 13:219, 1976.
5. Bukowski RM, King JW, Hewlett JS: Plasmapheresis in the treatment of thrombotic thrombocytopenic purpura. *Blood* 50:413, 1977.
6. Byrnes JJ, Khurana M: Treatment of thrombotic thrombocytopenic purpura with plasma. *N Engl J Med* 297:1386, 1977.
7. Bell WR, Braine HG, Ness PM, Kickler TS: Improved survival in thrombotic thrombocytopenic purpura-hemolytic uremic syndrome. Clinical experience in 108 patients. *N Engl J Med* 325:398, 1991.
8. Rock GA, Shumak KH, Buskard NA, et al: Comparison of plasma exchange with plasma infusion in the treatment of thrombotic thrombocytopenic purpura. Canadian Apheresis Study Group. *N Engl J Med* 325:393, 1991.
9. Moake JL, Rudy CK, Troll JH, et al: Unusually large plasma factor VIII:von Willebrand factor multimers in chronic relapsing thrombotic thrombocytopenic purpura. *N Engl J Med* 307:1432, 1982.
10. Furlan M, Robles R, Lämmle B: Partial purification and characterization of a protease from human plasma cleaving von Willebrand factor to fragments produced by *in vivo* proteolysis. *Blood* 87:4223, 1996.
11. Tsai H-M: Physiologic cleavage of von Willebrand factor by a plasma protease is dependent on its conformation and requires calcium ion. *Blood* 87:4235, 1996.
12. Furlan M, Robles R, Solenthaler M, et al: Deficient activity of von Willebrand factor-cleaving protease in chronic relapsing thrombotic thrombocytopenic purpura. *Blood* 89:3097, 1997.
13. Furlan M, Robles R, Galbusera M, et al: Von Willebrand factor-cleaving protease in thrombotic thrombocytopenic purpura and the hemolytic-uremic syndrome. *N Engl J Med* 339:1578, 1998.
14. Tsai HM, Lian EC: Antibodies to von Willebrand factor-cleaving protease in acute thrombotic thrombocytopenic purpura. *N Engl J Med* 339:1585, 1998.
15. Fujikawa K, Suzuki H, McMullen B, Chung D: Purification of human von Willebrand factor-cleaving protease and its identification as a new member of the metalloproteinase family. *Blood* 98:1662, 2001.
16. Gerritsen HE, Robles R, Lammle B, Furlan M: Partial amino acid sequence of purified von Willebrand factor-cleaving protease. *Blood* 98:1654, 2001.
17. Zheng X, Chung D, Takayama TK, et al: Structure of von Willebrand factor-cleaving protease (ADAMTS13), a metalloprotease involved in thrombotic thrombocytopenic purpura. *J Biol Chem* 276:41059, 2001.
18. Soejima K, Mimura N, Hirashima M, et al: A novel human metalloprotease synthesized in the liver and secreted into the blood: Possibly, the von Willebrand factor-cleaving protease? *J Biochem* 130:475, 2001.
19. Levy GG, Nichols WC, Lian EC, et al: Mutations in a member of the ADAMTS gene family cause thrombotic thrombocytopenic purpura. *Nature* 413:488, 2001.
20. Klaus C, Plaimauer B, Studt JD, et al: Epitope mapping of ADAMTS13 autoantibodies in acquired thrombotic thrombocytopenic purpura. *Blood* 103:4514, 2004.
21. Luken BM, Turenhout EA, Hulstein JJ, et al: The spacer domain of ADAMTS13 contains a major binding site for antibodies in patients with thrombotic thrombocytopenic purpura. *Thromb Haemost* 93:267, 2005.
22. Zheng XL, Wu HM, Shang D, et al: Multiple domains of ADAMTS13 are targeted by autoantibodies against ADAMTS13 in patients with acquired idiopathic thrombotic thrombocytopenic purpura. *Haematologica* 95:1555, 2010.
23. Scheiflinger F, Knobl P, Trattner B, et al: Nonneutralizing IgM and IgG antibodies to von Willebrand factor-cleaving protease (ADAMTS-13) in a patient with thrombotic thrombocytopenic purpura. *Blood* 102:3241, 2003.
24. Miller DP, Kaye JA, Shea K, et al: Incidence of thrombotic thrombocytopenic purpura/hemolytic uremic syndrome. *Epidemiology* 15:208, 2004.
25. Terrell DR, Williams LA, Vesely SK, et al: The incidence of thrombotic thrombocytopenic purpura-hemolytic uremic syndrome: All patients, idiopathic patients, and patients with severe ADAMTS-13 deficiency. *J Thromb Haemost* 3:1432, 2005.
26. Zheng XL, Kaufman RM, Goodnough LT, Sadler JE: Effect of plasma exchange on plasma ADAMTS13 metalloprotease activity, inhibitor level, and clinical outcome in patients with idiopathic and nonidiopathic thrombotic thrombocytopenic purpura. *Blood* 103:4043, 2004.
27. Kremer Hovinga JA, Vesely SK, Terrell DR, et al: Survival and relapse in patients with thrombotic thrombocytopenic purpura. *Blood* 115:1500, 2010.
28. Nicol KK, Shelton BJ, Knovich MA, Owen J: Overweight individuals are at increased risk for thrombotic thrombocytopenic purpura. *Am J Hematol* 74:170, 2003.
29. Ridolfi RL, Bell WR: Thrombotic thrombocytopenic purpura. Report of 25 cases and review of the literature. *Medicine (Baltimore)* 60:413, 1981.
30. McMinn JR, George JN: Evaluation of women with clinically suspected thrombotic thrombocytopenic purpura-hemolytic uremic syndrome during pregnancy. *J Clin Apher* 16:202, 2001.
31. Coppo P, Busson M, Veyradier A, et al: HLA-DRB1*11: A strong risk factor for acquired severe ADAMTS13 deficiency-related idiopathic thrombotic thrombocytopenic purpura in Caucasians. *J Thromb Haemost* 8:856, 2010.
32. Scully M, Brown J, Patel R, et al: Human leukocyte antigen association in idiopathic thrombotic thrombocytopenic purpura: Evidence for an immunogenetic link. *J Thromb Haemost* 8:257, 2010.
33. O'Brien TE, Crum ED: Atypical presentations of thrombotic thrombocytopenic purpura. *Int J Hematol* 76:471, 2002.
34. Sarode R: Atypical presentations of thrombotic thrombocytopenic purpura: A review. *J Clin Apher* 24:47, 2009.
35. Imanirad I, Rajasekhar A, Zumberg M: A case series of atypical presentations of thrombotic thrombocytopenic purpura. *J Clin Apher* 27:221, 2012.
36. Htun KT, Davis AK: Neurological symptoms as the sole presentation of relapsed thrombotic thrombocytopenic purpura without microangiopathic haemolytic anaemia. *Thromb Haemost* 112:838, 2014.

37. Camous L, Veyradier A, Darmon M, et al: Macrovascular thrombosis in critically ill patients with thrombotic micro-angiopathies. *Intern Emerg Med* 9:267, 2014.

38. Hawkins BM, Abu-Fadel M, Vesely SK, George JN: Clinical cardiac involvement in thrombotic thrombocytopenic purpura: A systematic review. *Transfusion* 48:382, 2008.

39. Hughes C, McEwan JR, Longair I, et al: Cardiac involvement in acute thrombotic thrombocytopenic purpura: Association with troponin T and IgG antibodies to ADAMTS 13. *J Thromb Haemost* 7:529, 2009.

40. Benhamou Y, Assie C, Boelle PY, et al: Development and validation of a predictive model for death in acquired severe ADAMTS13 deficiency-associated idiopathic thrombotic thrombocytopenic purpura: The French TMA Reference Center experience. *Haematologica* 97:1181, 2012.

41. Zini G, d'Onofrio G, Briggs C, et al: ICSH recommendations for identification, diagnostic value, and quantitation of schistocytes. *Int J Lab Hematol* 34:107, 2012.

42. Burns ER, Lou Y, Pathak A: Morphologic diagnosis of thrombotic thrombocytopenic purpura. *Am J Hematol* 75:18, 2004.

43. Veyradier A, Obert B, Houllier A, et al: Specific von Willebrand factor-cleaving protease in thrombotic microangiopathies: A study of 111 cases. *Blood* 98:1765, 2001.

44. Bianchi V, Robles R, Alberio L, et al: Von Willebrand factor-cleaving protease (ADAMTS13) in thrombocytopenic disorders: A severely deficient activity is specific for thrombotic thrombocytopenic purpura. *Blood* 100:710, 2002.

45. Tsai HM: Is severe deficiency of ADAMTS-13 specific for thrombotic thrombocytopenic purpura? Yes. *J Thromb Haemost* 1:625, 2003.

46. Asada Y, Sumiyoshi A, Hayashi T, et al: Immunohistochemistry of vascular lesion in thrombotic thrombocytopenic purpura, with special reference to factor VIII related antigen. *Thromb Res* 38:469, 1985.

47. Hosler GA, Cusumano AM, Hutchins GM: Thrombotic thrombocytopenic purpura and hemolytic uremic syndrome are distinct pathologic entities. A review of 56 autopsy cases. *Arch Pathol Lab Med* 127:834, 2003.

48. Zomas A, Saso R, Powles R, et al: Red cell fragmentation (schistocytosis) after bone marrow transplantation. *Bone Marrow Transplant* 22:777, 1998.

49. Kanamori H, Takaishi Y, Takabayashi M, et al: Clinical significance of fragmented red cells after allogeneic bone marrow transplantation. *Int J Hematol* 77:180, 2003.

50. Mannucci PM, Canciani MT, Forza I, et al: Changes in health and disease of the metalloprotease that cleaves von Willebrand factor. *Blood* 98:2730, 2001.

51. Kremer Hovinga JA, Zeerleder S, Kessler P, et al: ADAMTS-13, von Willebrand factor and related parameters in severe sepsis and septic shock. *J Thromb Haemost* 5:2284, 2007.

52. Uemura M, Fujimura Y, Matsumoto M, et al: Comprehensive analysis of ADAMTS13 in patients with liver cirrhosis. *Thromb Haemost* 99:1019, 2008.

53. Park YD, Yoshioka A, Kawa K, et al: Impaired activity of plasma von Willebrand factor-cleaving protease may predict the occurrence of hepatic veno-occlusive disease after stem cell transplantation. *Bone Marrow Transplant* 29:789, 2002.

54. Nguyen L, Li X, Duvall D, et al: Twice-daily plasma exchange for patients with refractory thrombotic thrombocytopenic purpura: The experience of the Oklahoma Registry, 1989 through 2006. *Transfusion* 48:349, 2008.

55. Scully M, Hunt BJ, Benjamin S, et al: Guidelines on the diagnosis and management of thrombotic thrombocytopenic purpura and other thrombotic microangiopathies. *Br J Haematol* 158:323, 2012.

56. Zeigler ZR, Shadduck RK, Gryn JF, et al: Cryoprecipitate poor plasma does not improve early response in primary adult thrombotic thrombocytopenic purpura (TTP). *J Clin Apher* 16:19, 2001.

57. Rock G, Anderson D, Clark W, et al: Does cryosupernatant plasma improve outcome in thrombotic thrombocytopenic purpura? No answer yet. *Br J Haematol* 129:79, 2005.

58. Michael M, Elliott EJ, Craig JC, et al: Interventions for hemolytic uremic syndrome and thrombotic thrombocytopenic purpura: A systematic review of randomized controlled trials. *Am J Kidney Dis* 53:259, 2009.

59. Prowse C: Properties of pathogen-inactivated plasma components. *Transfus Med Rev* 23:124, 2009.

60. McCarthy LJ: Evidence-based medicine for apheresis: An ongoing challenge. *Ther Apher Dial* 8:112, 2004.

61. Yarranton H, Cohen H, Pavord SR, et al: Venous thromboembolism associated with the management of acute thrombotic thrombocytopenic purpura. *Br J Haematol* 121:778, 2003.

62. Allford SL, Harrison P, Lawrie AS, et al: Von Willebrand factor—Cleaving protease activity in congenital thrombotic thrombocytopenic purpura. *Br J Haematol* 111:1215, 2000.

63. del Rio-Garma J, Alvarez-Larran A, Martinez C, et al: Methylene blue-photoinactivated plasma versus quarantine fresh frozen plasma in thrombotic thrombocytopenic purpura: A multicentric, prospective cohort study. *Br J Haematol* 143:39, 2008.

63a. Balduini CL, Gugliotta L, Luppi M, et al: High versus standard dose methylprednisolone in the acute phase of idiopathic thrombotic thrombocytopenic purpura. *Ann Hematol* 89:591–596, 2010.

64. Bobbio-Pallavicini E, Gugliotta L, Centurioni R, et al: Antiplatelet agents in thrombotic thrombocytopenic purpura (TTP). Results of a randomized multicenter trial by the Italian Cooperative Group for TTP. *Haematologica* 82:429, 1997.

65. Coppo P, Lassoued K, Mariette X, et al: Effectiveness of platelet transfusions after plasma exchange in adult thrombotic thrombocytopenic purpura: A report of two cases. *Am J Hematol* 68:198, 2001.

66. Goel R, Ness PM, Takemoto CM, et al: Platelet transfusions in platelet consumptive disorders are associated with arterial thrombosis and in-hospital mortality. *Blood* 125:1470, 2015.

67. Doerfler ME, Kaufman B, Goldenberg AS: Central venous catheter placement in patients with disorders of hemostasis. *Chest* 110:185, 1996.

68. Rizvi MA, Vesely SK, George JN, et al: Complications of plasma exchange in 71 consecutive patients treated for clinically suspected thrombotic thrombocytopenic purpura-hemolytic-uremic syndrome. *Transfusion* 40:896, 2000.

69. Lim W, Vesely SK, George JN: The role of rituximab in the management of patients with acquired thrombotic thrombocytopenic purpura. *Blood* 125:1526, 2015.

70. Westwood JP, Webster H, McGuckin S, et al: Rituximab for thrombotic thrombocytopenic purpura: Benefit of early administration during acute episodes and use of prophylaxis to prevent relapse. *J Thromb Haemost* 11:481, 2013.

71. Hie M, Gay J, Galicier L, et al: Preemptive rituximab infusions after remission efficiently prevent relapses in acquired thrombotic thrombocytopenic purpura. *Blood* 124:204, 2014.

71a. Cuker A: Adjuvant rituximab to prevent TTP relapse. *Blood* 127:2952–2953, 2016.

72. Carson KR, Evens AM, Richey EA, et al: Progressive multifocal leukoencephalopathy after rituximab therapy in HIV-negative patients: A report of 57 cases from the Research on Adverse Drug Event and Reports project. *Blood* 113:4834, 2009.

73. Bharat A, Xie F, Baddley JW, et al: Incidence and risk factors for progressive multifocal leukoencephalopathy among patients with selected rheumatic diseases. *Arthritis Care Res (Hoboken)* 64:612, 2012.

74. Lunel-Fabiani F, Masson C, Ducancelle A: Systemic diseases and biotherapies: Understanding, evaluating, and preventing the risk of hepatitis B reactivation. *Joint Bone Spine* 81:478, 2014.

75. Aqui NA, Stein SH, Konkle BA, et al: Role of splenectomy in patients with refractory or relapsed thrombotic thrombocytopenic purpura. *J Clin Apher* 18:51, 2003.

76. Kappers-Klunne MC, Wijermans P, Fijnheer R, et al: Splenectomy for the treatment of thrombotic thrombocytopenic purpura. *Br J Haematol* 130:768, 2005.

77. Katkhouda N, Hurwitz MB, Rivera RT, et al: Laparoscopic splenectomy: Outcome and efficacy in 103 consecutive patients. *Ann Surg* 228:568, 1998.

78. Ferrara F, Annunziata M, Pollio F, et al: Vincristine as treatment for recurrent episodes of thrombotic thrombocytopenic purpura. *Ann Hematol* 81:7, 2002.

79. Bobbio-Pallavicini E, Porta C, Centurioni R, et al: Vincristine sulfate for the treatment of thrombotic thrombocytopenic purpura refractory to plasma-exchange. The Italian Cooperative Group for TTP. *Eur J Haematol* 52:222, 1994.

80. Bobbio-Pallavicini E, Porta C, Tacconi F, et al: Intravenous prostacyclin (as epoprostenol) infusion in thrombotic thrombocytopenic purpura. Four case reports and review of the literature. Italian Cooperative Group for Thrombotic Thrombocytopenic Purpura. *Haematologica* 79:429, 1994.

81. Sagripanti A, Carpi A, Rosaia B, et al: Iloprost in the treatment of thrombotic microangiopathy: Report of thirteen cases. *Biomed Pharmacother* 50:350, 1996.

82. Dervenoulas J, Tsirigotis P, Bollas G, et al: Efficacy of intravenous immunoglobulin in the treatment of thrombotic thrombocytopaenic purpura. A study of 44 cases. *Acta Haematol* 105:204, 2001.

83. Anderson D, Ali K, Blanchette V, et al: Guidelines on the use of intravenous immune globulin for hematologic conditions. *Transfus Med Rev* 21:S9, 2007.

84. Cataland SR, Jin M, Lin S, et al: Cyclosporin and plasma exchange in thrombotic thrombocytopenic purpura: Long-term follow-up with serial analysis of ADAMTS13 activity. *Br J Haematol* 139:486, 2007.

85. Shortt J, Oh DH, Opat SS: ADAMTS13 antibody depletion by bortezomib in thrombotic thrombocytopenic purpura. *N Engl J Med* 368:90, 2013.

86. Ahmad HN, Thomas-Dewing RR, Hunt BJ: Mycophenolate mofetil in a case of relapsed, refractory thrombotic thrombocytopenic purpura. *Eur J Haematol* 78:449, 2007.

87. Li GW, Rambally S, Kamboj J, et al: Treatment of refractory thrombotic thrombocytopenic purpura with N-acetylcysteine: A case report. *Transfusion* 54:1221, 2014.

88. Spiekermann K, Wormann B, Rumpf KW, Hiddemann W: Combination chemotherapy with CHOP for recurrent thrombotic thrombocytopenic purpura. *Br J Haematol* 97:544, 1997.

89. Passweg JR, Rabusin M, Musso M, et al: Haematopoetic stem cell transplantation for refractory autoimmune cytopenia. *Br J Haematol* 125:749, 2004.

90. Callewaert F, Roodt J, Ulrichts H, et al: Evaluation of efficacy and safety of the anti-VWF Nanobody ALX-0681 in a preclinical baboon model of acquired thrombotic thrombocytopenic purpura. *Blood* 120:3603, 2012.

91. Cataland SR, Peyvandi F, Mannucci PM, et al: Initial experience from a double-blind, placebo-controlled, clinical outcome study of ARC1779 in patients with thrombotic thrombocytopenic purpura. *Am J Hematol* 87:430, 2012.

92. O'Brien KL, Price TH, Howell C, Delaney M: The use of 50% albumin/plasma replacement fluid in therapeutic plasma exchange for thrombotic thrombocytopenic purpura. *J Clin Apher* 28:416, 2013.

93. Zhan H, Streiff MB, King KE, Segal JB: Thrombotic thrombocytopenic purpura at the Johns Hopkins Hospital from 1992 to 2008: Clinical outcomes and risk factors for relapse. *Transfusion* 50:868, 2010.

94. Bandarenko N, Brecher ME: United States Thrombotic Thrombocytopenic Purpura Apheresis Study Group (US TTP ASG): Multicenter survey and retrospective analysis of current efficacy of therapeutic plasma exchange. *J Clin Apher* 13:133, 1998.

95. Tsai H-M, Shulman K: Rituximab induces remission of cerebral ischemia caused by thrombotic thrombocytopenic purpura. *Eur J Haematol* 70:183, 2003.

96. Sadler JE: Von Willebrand factor, ADAMTS13, and thrombotic thrombocytopenic purpura. *Blood* 112:11, 2008.

97. McClain RS, Terrell DR, Vesely SK, George JN: Plasma exchange complications in patients treated for thrombotic thrombocytopenia purpura-hemolytic uremic syndrome: 2011 to 2014. *Transfusion* 54:3257, 2014.

98. Kennedy AS, Lewis QF, Scott JG, et al: Cognitive deficits after recovery from thrombotic thrombocytopenic purpura. *Transfusion* 49:1092, 2009.

99. Lewis QF, Lanneau MS, Mathias SD, et al: Long-term deficits in health-related quality of life after recovery from thrombotic thrombocytopenic purpura. *Transfusion* 49:118, 2009.

100. Hayward CP, Sutton DM, Carter WH Jr, et al: Treatment outcomes in patients with adult thrombotic thrombocytopenic purpura-hemolytic uremic syndrome. *Arch Intern Med* 154:982, 1994.

101. Coppo P, Bengoufa D, Veyradier A, et al: Severe ADAMTS13 deficiency in adult idiopathic thrombotic microangiopathies defines a subset of patients characterized by various autoimmune manifestations, lower platelet count, and mild renal involvement. *Medicine (Baltimore)* 83:233, 2004.

102. Schulman I, Pierce M, Lukens A, Currimbhoy Z: Studies on thrombopoiesis. I. A factor in normal human plasma required for platelet production; chronic thrombocytopenia due to its deficiency. *Blood* 16:943, 1960.

103. Upshaw JD Jr: Congenital deficiency of a factor in normal plasma that reverses microangiopathic hemolysis and thrombocytopenia. *N Engl J Med* 298:1350, 1978.

104. Zheng XL, Sadler JE: Pathogenesis of thrombotic microangiopathies. *Annu Rev Pathol* 3:249, 2008.

105. Furlan M, Lämmle B: Aetiology and pathogenesis of thrombotic thrombocytopenic purpura and haemolytic uraemic syndrome: The role of von Willebrand factor-cleaving protease. *Best Pract Res Clin Haematol* 14:437, 2001.

106. Miyata T, Kokame K, Matsumoto M, Fujimura Y: ADAMTS13 activity and genetic mutations in Japan. *Hamostaseologie* 33:131, 2013.

107. Loirat C, Girma JP, Desconclois C, et al: Thrombotic thrombocytopenic purpura related to severe ADAMTS13 deficiency in children. *Pediatr Nephrol* 24:19, 2009.

108. Veyradier A, Meyer D, Loirat C: Desmopressin, an unexpected link between nocturnal enuresis and inherited thrombotic thrombocytopenic purpura (Upshaw-Schulman syndrome). *J Thromb Haemost* 4:700, 2006.

109. Scully M, Thomas M, Underwood M, et al: Thrombotic thrombocytopenic purpura and pregnancy: Presentation, management, and subsequent pregnancy outcomes. *Blood* 124:211, 2014.

110. Raval JS, Padmanabhan A, Kremer Hovinga JA, Kiss JE: Development of a clinically significant ADAMTS13 inhibitor in a patient with hereditary thrombotic thrombocytopenic purpura. *Am J Hematol* 90:E22, 2015.

111. Wallace DC, Lovric A, Clubb JS, Carseldine DB: Thrombotic thrombocytopenic purpura in four siblings. *Am J Med* 58:724, 1975.

112. Furlan M, Robles R, Morselli B, et al: Recovery and half-life of von Willebrand factor-cleaving protease after plasma therapy in patients with thrombotic thrombocytopenic purpura. *Thromb Haemost* 81:8, 1999.

113. Lotta LA, Wu HM, Mackie IJ, et al: Residual plasmatic activity of ADAMTS13 is correlated with phenotype severity in congenital thrombotic thrombocytopenic purpura. *Blood* 120:440, 2012.

114. Camilleri RS, Scully M, Thomas M, et al: A phenotype-genotype correlation of ADAMTS13 mutations in congenital thrombotic thrombocytopenic purpura patients treated in the United Kingdom. *J Thromb Haemost* 10:1792, 2012.

115. Gasser C, Gautier E, Steck A, et al: Hämolytisch-urämische Syndrome: Bilaterale Nierenrindennekrosen bei akuten erworbenen hämolytischen Anämien. *Schweiz Med Wochenschr* 85:905, 1955.

116. Kibel MA, Barnard PJ: The haemolytic-uraemic syndrome: A survey in Southern Africa. *S Afr Med J* 42:692, 1968.

117. Karmali MA, Steele BT, Petric M, Lim C: Sporadic cases of haemolytic-uraemic syndrome associated with faecal cytotoxin and cytotoxin-producing *Escherichia coli* in stools. *Lancet* 1:619, 1983.

118. O'Brien AO, Lively TA, Chen ME, et al: *Escherichia coli* O157:H7 strains associated with haemorrhagic colitis in the United States produce a Shigella dysenteriae 1 (SHIGA) like cytotoxin. *Lancet* 1:702, 1983.

119. Riley LW, Remis RS, Helgerson SD, et al: Hemorrhagic colitis associated with a rare *Escherichia coli* serotype. *N Engl J Med* 308:681, 1983.

120. Tarr PI, Gordon CA, Chandler WL: Shiga-toxin-producing *Escherichia coli* and haemolytic uraemic syndrome. *Lancet* 365:1073, 2005.

121. Gianviti A, Tozzi AE, De Petris L, et al: Risk factors for poor renal prognosis in children with hemolytic uremic syndrome. *Pediatr Nephrol* 18:1229, 2003.

122. Frank C, Werber D, Cramer JP, et al: Epidemic profile of Shiga-toxin-producing *Escherichia coli* O104:H4 outbreak in Germany. *N Engl J Med* 365:1771, 2011.

123. Proesmans W: The role of coagulation and fibrinolysis in the pathogenesis of diarrhea-associated hemolytic uremic syndrome. *Semin Thromb Hemost* 27:201, 2001.

124. Tsai HM, Chandler WL, Sarode R, et al: Von Willebrand factor and von Willebrand factor-cleaving metalloprotease activity in *Escherichia coli* O157:H7-associated hemolytic uremic syndrome. *Pediatr Res* 49:653, 2001.

125. Hunt BJ, Lämmle B, Nevard CH, et al: Von Willebrand factor-cleaving protease in childhood diarrhoea-associated haemolytic uraemic syndrome. *Thromb Haemost* 85: 975, 2001.

126. Inward CD, Howie AJ, Fitzpatrick MM, et al: Renal histopathology in fatal cases of diarrhoea-associated haemolytic uraemic syndrome. British Association for Paediatric Nephrology. *Pediatr Nephrol* 11:556, 1997.

127. Wong CS, Mooney JC, Brandt JR, et al: Risk factors for the hemolytic uremic syndrome in children infected with *Escherichia coli* O157:H7: A multivariable analysis. *Clin Infect Dis* 55:33, 2012.

128. Menne J, Nitschke M, Stingele R, et al: Validation of treatment strategies for enterohaemorrhagic *Escherichia coli* O104:H4 induced haemolytic uraemic syndrome: Case-control study. *BMJ* 345:e4565, 2012.

129. Braune SA, Wichmann D, von Heinz MC, et al: Clinical features of critically ill patients with Shiga toxin-induced hemolytic uremic syndrome. *Crit Care Med* 41:1702, 2013.

130. Garg AX, Suri RS, Barrowman N, et al: Long-term renal prognosis of diarrhea-associated hemolytic uremic syndrome: A systematic review, meta-analysis, and meta-regression. *JAMA* 290:1360, 2003.

131. Barnard PJ, Kibel M: The haemolytic-uraemic syndrome of infancy and childhood. A report of eleven cases. *Cent Afr J Med* 11:31, 1965.

132. Kaplan BS, Chesney RW, Drummond KN: Hemolytic uremic syndrome in families. *N Engl J Med* 292:1090, 1975.

133. Kaplan BS: Hemolytic uremic syndrome with recurrent episodes: An important subset. *Clin Nephrol* 8:495, 1977.

134. Fitzpatrick MM, Walters MD, Trompeter RS, et al: Atypical (non-diarrhea-associated) hemolytic-uremic syndrome in childhood. *J Pediatr* 122:532, 1993.

135. Thompson RA, Winterborn MH: Hypocomplementaemia due to a genetic deficiency of beta 1H globulin. *Clin Exp Immunol* 46:110, 1981.

136. Warwicker P, Goodship TH, Donne RL, et al: Genetic studies into inherited and sporadic hemolytic uremic syndrome. *Kidney Int* 53:836, 1998.

137. Legendre CM, Licht C, Muus P, et al: Terminal complement inhibitor eculizumab in atypical hemolytic-uremic syndrome. *N Engl J Med* 368:2169, 2013.

138. Noris M, Caprioli J, Bresin E, et al: Relative role of genetic complement abnormalities in sporadic and familial aHUS and their impact on clinical phenotype. *Clin J Am Soc Nephrol* 5:1844, 2010.

139. Fremeaux-Bacchi V, Fakhouri F, Garnier A, et al: Genetics and outcome of atypical hemolytic uremic syndrome: A nationwide French series comparing children and adults. *Clin J Am Soc Nephrol* 8:554, 2013.

140. Lemaire M, Fremeaux-Bacchi V, Schaefer F, et al: Recessive mutations in DGKE cause atypical hemolytic-uremic syndrome. *Nat Genet* 45:531, 2013.

141. Taylor CM, Machin S, Wigmore SJ, et al: Clinical practice guidelines for the management of atypical haemolytic uraemic syndrome in the United Kingdom. *Br J Haematol* 148:37, 2010.

142. Fakhouri F, Roumenina L, Provot F, et al: Pregnancy-associated hemolytic uremic syndrome revisited in the era of complement gene mutations. *J Am Soc Nephrol* 21:859, 2010.

143. Rossio R, Lotta LA, Pontiggia S, et al: A novel CD46 mutation in a patient with microangiopathy clinically resembling thrombotic thrombocytopenic purpura and normal ADAMTS13 activity. *Haematologica* 100:e87, 2015.

144. Noris M, Remuzzi G: Managing and preventing atypical hemolytic uremic syndrome recurrence after kidney transplantation. *Curr Opin Nephrol Hypertens* 22:704, 2013.

145. Sanchez Chinchilla D, Pinto S, Hoppe B, et al: Complement mutations in diacylglycerol kinase-epsilon-associated atypical hemolytic uremic syndrome. *Clin J Am Soc Nephrol* 9:1611, 2014.

146. Westland R, Bodria M, Carrea A, et al: Phenotypic expansion of DGKE-associated diseases. *J Am Soc Nephrol* 25:1408, 2014.

147. Cabrera GR, Fortenberry JD, Warshaw BL, et al: Hemolytic uremic syndrome associated with invasive Streptococcus pneumoniae infection. *Pediatrics* 101:699, 1998.

148. Copelovitch L, Kaplan BS: Streptococcus pneumoniae-associated hemolytic uremic syndrome. *Pediatr Nephrol* 23:1951, 2008.

149. Singh N, Gayowski T, Marino IR: Hemolytic uremic syndrome in solid-organ transplant recipients. *Transpl Int* 9:68, 1996.

150. Arai S, Allan C, Streiff M, et al: Von Willebrand factor-cleaving protease activity and proteolysis of von Willebrand factor in bone marrow transplant-associated thrombotic microangiopathy. *Hematol J* 2:292, 2001.

151. Ho VT, Cutler C, Carter S, et al: Blood and marrow transplant clinical trials network toxicity committee consensus summary: Thrombotic microangiopathy after hematopoietic stem cell transplantation. *Biol Blood Marrow Transplant* 11:571, 2005.

152. Sack GH Jr, Levin J, Bell WR: Trousseau's syndrome and other manifestations of chronic disseminated coagulopathy in patients with neoplasms: Clinical, pathophysiologic, and therapeutic features. *Medicine (Baltimore)* 56:1, 1977.

153. Elliott MA, Letendre L, Gastineau DA, et al: Cancer-associated microangiopathic hemolytic anemia with thrombocytopenia: An important diagnostic consideration. *Eur J Haematol* 85:43, 2010.

154. Domingo-Claros A, Larriba I, Rozman M, et al: Acute erythroid neoplastic proliferations. A biological study based on 62 patients. *Haematologica* 87:148, 2002.

155. Lattuada A, Rossi E, Calzarossa C, et al: Mild to moderate reduction of a von Willebrand factor cleaving protease (ADAMTS-13) in pregnant women with HELLP microangiopathic syndrome. *Haematologica* 88:1029, 2003.

156. Baron BW, Martin MS, Sucharetza BS, et al: Four patients with both thrombotic thrombocytopenic purpura and autoimmune thrombocytopenic purpura: The concept of a mixed immune thrombocytopenia syndrome and indications for plasma exchange. *J Clin Apher* 16:179, 2001.

157. Mannucci PM, Vanoli M, Forza I, et al: Von Willebrand factor cleaving protease (ADAMTS-13) in 123 patients with connective tissue diseases (systemic lupus erythematosus and systemic sclerosis). *Haematologica* 88:914, 2003.

158. Güngör T, Furlan M, Lämmle B, et al: Acquired deficiency of von Willebrand factor-cleaving protease in a patient suffering from acute systemic lupus erythematosus. *Rheumatology (Oxford)* 40:940, 2001.

159. Ahmed S, Siddiqui AK, Chandrasekaran V: Correlation of thrombotic thrombocytopenic purpura disease activity with von Willebrand factor-cleaving protease level in ulcerative colitis. *Am J Med* 116:786, 2004.

160. Steen VD: Scleroderma renal crisis. *Rheum Dis Clin North Am* 29:315, 2003.

161. Al-Nouri ZL, Reese JA, Terrell DR, et al: Drug-induced thrombotic microangiopathy: A systematic review of published reports. *Blood* 125:616, 2015.

162. Schwartz J, Winters JL, Padmanabhan A, et al: Guidelines on the use of therapeutic apheresis in clinical practice-evidence-based approach from the Writing Committee of the American Society for Apheresis: The sixth special issue. *J Clin Apher* 28:145, 2013.

163. Kojouri K, Vesely SK, George JN: Quinine-associated thrombotic thrombocytopenic purpura-hemolytic uremic syndrome: Frequency, clinical features, and long-term outcomes. *Ann Intern Med* 135:1047, 2001.

164. Dlott JS, Danielson CF, Blue-Hnidy DE, McCarthy LJ: Drug-induced thrombotic thrombocytopenic purpura/hemolytic uremic syndrome: A concise review. *Ther Apher Dial* 8:102, 2004.

165. Bennett CL, Kim B, Zakarija A, et al: Two mechanistic pathways for thienopyridine-associated thrombotic thrombocytopenic purpura: A report from the SERF-TTP Research Group and the RADAR Project. *J Am Coll Cardiol* 50:1138, 2007.

166. Remuzzi G, Bertani T: Renal vascular and thrombotic effects of cyclosporine. *Am J Kidney Dis* 13:261, 1989.

167. Bechstein WO: Neurotoxicity of calcineurin inhibitors: Impact and clinical management. *Transpl Int* 13:313, 2000.

168. Scott LJ, McKeage K, Keam SJ, Plosker GL: Tacrolimus: A further update of its use in the management of organ transplantation. *Drugs* 63:1247, 2003.

169. Valavaara R, Nordman E: Renal complications of mitomycin C therapy with special reference to the total dose. *Cancer* 55:47, 1985.

170. Lesesne JB, Rothschild N, Erickson B, et al: Cancer-associated hemolytic-uremic syndrome: Analysis of 85 cases from a national registry. *J Clin Oncol* 7:781, 1989.

171. Humphreys BD, Sharman JP, Henderson JM, et al: Gemcitabine-associated thrombotic microangiopathy. *Cancer* 100:2664, 2004.

172. Glezerman I, Kris MG, Miller V, et al: Gemcitabine nephrotoxicity and hemolytic uremic syndrome: Report of 29 cases from a single institution. *Clin Nephrol* 71:130, 2009.

173. Eremina V, Jefferson JA, Kowalewska J, et al: VEGF inhibition and renal thrombotic microangiopathy. *N Engl J Med* 358:1129, 2008.

174. Bollee G, Patey N, Cazajous G, et al: Thrombotic microangiopathy secondary to VEGF pathway inhibition by sunitinib. *Nephrol Dial Transplant* 24:682, 2009.

175. Carrillo-Carrasco N, Chandler RJ, Venditti CP: Combined methylmalonic acidemia and homocystinuria, cblC type. I. Clinical presentations, diagnosis and management. *J Inherit Metab Dis* 35:91, 2012.

176. van den Born BJ, van der Hoeven NV, Groot E, et al: Association between thrombotic microangiopathy and reduced ADAMTS13 activity in malignant hypertension. *Hypertension* 51:862, 2008.

# CHAPTER 23
# VENOUS THROMBOSIS

Gary E. Raskob, Russell D. Hull, and Harry R. Buller

## SUMMARY

Venous thromboembolism, consisting of deep vein thrombosis and/or pulmonary embolism, is a common disorder with an estimated 900,000 patients each year in the United States and more than 1 million each year in the European Union. Approximately one-third of these cases are fatal pulmonary emboli, and the remaining two-thirds are nonfatal episodes of symptomatic deep vein thrombosis or pulmonary embolism. The majority of fatal events occur as sudden death, underscoring the importance of prevention as the critical strategy for reducing death from pulmonary embolism. Of the nonfatal cases, approximately 60 percent present clinically as deep vein thrombosis and 40 percent present as pulmonary embolism. Most clinically important pulmonary emboli arise from proximal deep vein thrombosis of the leg (popliteal, femoral, or iliac vein thrombosis). Upper-extremity deep vein thrombosis also may lead to clinically important pulmonary emboli. The clinical features of deep vein thrombosis and pulmonary embolism are nonspecific. Objective diagnostic testing is required to confirm or exclude the presence of venous thromboembolism. A validated assay for plasma D-dimer, if available, provides a simple, rapid, and cost-effective first-line exclusion test in patients with low, unlikely, or intermediate clinical probability. Compression ultrasonography is highly sensitive and specific for clinically important deep vein thrombosis and is the primary imaging test for symptomatic patients. Compression ultrasonography of the proximal veins performed at presentation, and if normal, repeated once 5 to 7 days later can safely exclude clinically important deep vein thrombosis. In centers with the expertise, a single comprehensive evaluation of the proximal and calf veins with duplex ultrasonography is sufficient. In patients with suspected pulmonary embolism, computed tomographic angiography, with or without additional testing using computed tomographic venography or compression ultrasonography of the legs, provides a definitive basis to give or withhold antithrombotic therapy in 90 percent of patients. Anticoagulant therapy is the preferred treatment for most patients with acute venous thromboembolism. Initial treatment with heparin or low-molecular-weight heparin, followed by long-term treatment with an oral vitamin K antagonist such as warfarin, is highly effective for preventing recurrent venous thromboembolism and has been the traditional standard of care. More recently, the direct oral anticoagulants, including the thrombin inhibitor dabigatran and the factor Xa inhibitors rivaroxaban, apixaban, and edoxaban, have been established to be as effective as and safer than traditional standard anticoagulant therapy. Rivaroxaban and apixaban can be used as a single-drug approach. Dabigatran and edoxaban are preceded by at least 5 days of heparin or low-molecular-weight heparin treatment. The direct oral anticoagulants are preferred over the vitamin K antagonists in most new patients commencing anticoagulant therapy. In cancer patients with venous thromboembolism, treatment with low-molecular-weight heparin for at least 6 months is the recommended approach. Thrombolytic therapy is indicated for patients with pulmonary embolism who present with hypotension or shock and in selected patients who have impaired right ventricular function who are at high risk of hemodynamic collapse. Insertion of a vena cava filter is indicated for patients who have an absolute contraindication to anticoagulant therapy or who have recurrent venous thromboembolism despite adequate anticoagulant treatment. Anticoagulant treatment should be continued for at least 3 months in all patients, and treatment duration of 3 months is sufficient for patients with first episode of venous thromboembolism secondary to a reversible risk factor. Indefinite anticoagulant therapy should be considered for patients with unprovoked (idiopathic) venous thromboembolism and those with recurrent venous thromboembolism.

Acronyms and Abbreviations: aPTT, activated partial thromboplastin time; CDT, catheter-directed thrombolysis; CI, confidence interval; CT, computed tomography; CTA, computed tomographic angiography; CTV, computed tomographic venography; DOAC, direct-acting oral anticoagulant; DVT, deep vein thrombosis; ELISA, enzyme-linked immunosorbent assay; INR, international normalized ratio; LMW, low molecular weight; PCDT, pharmacomechanical catheter-directed thrombolysis; PE, pulmonary embolism; PIOPED, Prospective Investigation of Pulmonary Embolism Diagnosis; VTE, venous thromboembolism.

## ● DEFINITION AND EPIDEMIOLOGY

Venous thrombosis commonly develops in the deep veins of the leg or the arm or in the superficial veins of these extremities. Venous thrombosis of superficial veins is a relatively benign disorder unless extension into the deep venous system occurs. Confusingly, one of the major deep veins in the leg is called the superficial femoral vein. Thrombosis involving the deep veins of the leg is divided into two prognostic categories: (1) calf vein thrombosis, in which thrombi remain confined to the deep calf veins, and (2) proximal vein thrombosis, in which thrombosis involves the popliteal, femoral, or iliac veins.[1]

Pulmonary emboli originate from thrombi in the deep veins of the leg in 90 percent or more of patients. Other less common sources of pulmonary embolism (PE) include the deep pelvic veins, renal veins, inferior vena cava, right side of the heart, and axillary veins. Most clinically important PE arise from proximal deep vein thrombosis (DVT) of the leg. Upper-extremity DVT also may lead to important PE.[2] DVT and/or PE are referred to collectively as *venous thromboembolism (VTE)*.

VTE is a common disorder.[3] The estimated annual incidence of clinically evident VTE ranges between 0.75 and 2.7 per 1000 population based on studies done in North America, Western Europe, Australia, and Argentina.[3] The literature indicates a strong and consistent association of increasing incidence of VTE with increasing age. The annual incidence increased to between two and seven per 1000 population among those 70 years of age and to between three and 12 per 1000 population among those 80 years of age or older.[3] Although the incidence is lower in individuals of Chinese and Korean ethnicity,[3] their disease burden is not low because of population aging. The high incidence of VTE in the elderly likely reflects the high prevalence of comorbid acquired risk factors in these patients, especially malignancy, heart failure, and surgery or hospitalization for medical illness, which account for the majority of the population-attributable risk of VTE in older individuals.

VTE causes a major burden of disease across low-, middle-, and high-income countries. VTE associated with hospitalization was the leading cause of premature death and years lived with disability in low- and middle-income countries and the second-highest cause in high-income countries and is responsible for more premature death and disability than nosocomial pneumonia, catheter-related bloodstream infections, and adverse drug events.[3]

The direct ascertainment of deaths from VTE is difficult because of the low rate of autopsy in most countries and because autopsy studies have consistently demonstrated that PE is often not diagnosed antemortem. The strongest evidence comes from the study by Cohen and colleagues, who used an incidence-based model in six European countries to estimate that there were 534,454 deaths related to VTE across the European Union in 2004.[4] A similar approach applied to the data from the United States suggested approximately 300,000 deaths from VTE each year.[5] The majority of deaths from VTE occur as sudden death, underscoring the critical role of prevention for reducing death from VTE.

Effective prophylaxis against VTE is available for most high-risk patients. Use of prophylaxis is more effective for preventing death and morbidity from VTE than is treatment of the established disease. Evidence-based recommendations for prevention are available.[6-9] Multifaceted interventions with alerts, such as computerized reminders or stickers on patient charts, are effective for increasing the prescription of appropriate thromboprophylaxis in hospitalized adult medical or surgical patients.[10] There is also evidence that inclusion of VTE risk assessment at the time of hospital admission and the provision of appropriate prophylaxis are effective for reducing VTE-related death and readmission with nonfatal VTE.[11,12] All hospitals should routinely assess the risk of VTE in all patients at the time of admission and provide thromboprophylaxis appropriate for the patient's risk.[12a] Historically, the majority of the disease burden from VTE occurred in hospitalized patients. The burden of illness from VTE has shifted to the community setting such that most patients now present as outpatients to their primary care physician or to the emergency department. The main reason for this shift is the greatly reduced length of hospital stay for most surgical procedures or medical conditions, such that patients are discharged from the hospital before the period of risk of VTE has ended or patients are discharged who have subclinical venous thrombi that subsequently evolve to symptomatic DVT or PE. The shift in burden of illness from the hospital to the community setting has led to an emphasis on effective and safe methods for outpatient prophylaxis, diagnosis, and treatment.

The recently completed APEX trial[12b] is an important advance toward reducing the community burden of VTE. This randomized trial evaluated extended thromboprophylaxis (35 to 45 days) using the oral factor Xa inhibitor betrixaban with the current standard practice of prophylaxis with low-molecular-weight heparin given for 10 to 14 days among 7513 patients who were hospitalized for acute medical illness and who were at high risk for VTE based on the presence of multiple clinical risk factors or an elevated plasma D-dimer level. Extended thromboprophylaxis resulted in a 24 percent relative risk reduction, from 7.0 percent to 5.3 percent (p = 0.006), in the composite outcome of asymptomatic proximal vein thrombosis, symptomatic DVT or PE, or VTE-related death.[12b] Symptomatic VTE was reduced from 1.5 percent to 0.9 percent (relative risk reduction 36 percent, p = 0.04) by extended thromboprophylaxis. Major bleeding was not increased with the use of extended thromboprophylaxis compared to prophylaxis given for 10 to 14 days (rates of 0.6 percent and 0.7 percent, respectively). Fatal bleeding was rare and occurred in only one patient of 3716 in each group, whereas VTE-related death occurred in 26 patients (0.7 percent) in the 10- to 14-day prophylaxis group and in 15 patients (0.4 percent) in the extended prophylaxis group. Thus, VTE is a much more common cause of mortality in this population than bleeding. Extended thromboprophylaxis with betrixaban was safe and resulted in an important reduction in clinically important VTE from both an individual patient perspective and from a population health perspective (number needed to treat of 59 to prevent one event of proximal vein thrombosis, symptomatic VTE, or VTE-related death). Given the many millions of patients admitted to hospital each year for acute medical conditions, extended thromboprophylaxis in this population can produce an important reduction in the burden of disease from VTE.

# ETIOLOGY AND PATHOGENESIS

Venous thrombi are composed mainly of fibrin and red blood cells, with variable numbers of platelets and leukocytes. The formation, growth, and breakdown of venous thromboemboli reflect a balance between thrombogenic stimuli and protective mechanisms. The thrombogenic stimuli first identified by Virchow in the 19th century are (1) venous stasis, (2) activation of blood coagulation, and (3) vascular damage. The protective mechanisms are (1) inactivation of activated coagulation factors by circulating inhibitors (e.g., antithrombin and activated protein C), (2) clearance of activated coagulation factors and soluble fibrin polymer complexes by mononuclear phagocytes and the liver, and (3) lysis of fibrin by fibrinolytic enzymes derived from plasma and endothelial cells.

PE occurs in at least 50 percent of patients with documented proximal vein thrombosis.[1] Many of these emboli are asymptomatic. The clinical importance of PE depends on the size of the embolus and the patient's cardiorespiratory reserve. Usually only part of the thrombus embolizes, and 30 to 70 percent of patients with PE detected by angiography also have identifiable DVT of the legs.[13,14] DVT and PE are not separate disorders but a continuous syndrome of VTE in which the initial clinical presentation may be symptoms of either DVT or PE. Therefore, strategies for diagnosis of VTE include both tests for detection of PE (e.g., computed tomography [CT] or lung scanning)[13-16] and tests for DVT of the legs (e.g., ultrasonography)[17-19] (see "Objective Testing for Pulmonary Embolism" and "Objective Testing for Deep Vein Thrombosis" below).

Acquired and inherited risk factors for VTE have been identified[20-23] and are shown in Table 23–1 (Chap. 20). Aging is the dominant risk factor for VTE (population attributable risk >90 percent).[23] Comorbidities, such as malignancy and heart failure, contribute to a higher population-attributable risk in older patients (≥65 years).[23] The risk of VTE increases when more than one risk factor is present.[24]

Activated protein C resistance is the most common hereditary abnormality predisposing to VTE. The defect results from substitution

**TABLE 23–1.** Risk Factors for Thromboembolism*

| Acquired | Hereditary Thrombophilias* |
|---|---|
| Advancing age (age >40 years) | Activated protein C resistance |
| History of prior thromboembolic event | Prothrombin G20210A mutation |
| Recent surgery | Antithrombin deficiency |
| Recent trauma | Protein C deficiency |
| Prolonged immobilization | Protein S deficiency |
| Certain forms of cancer | Dysfibrinogenemia |
| Congestive heart failure | |
| Recent myocardial infarction | |
| Paralysis of legs | |
| Use of female hormones | |
| Pregnancy or postpartum period | |
| Varicose veins | |
| Obesity | |
| Antiphospholipid antibody syndrome** | |
| Hyperhomocysteinemia | |

*See also Chap. 20
**See also Chap. 21

of glutamine for arginine at residue 506 in the factor V molecule, making factor Va resistant to proteolysis by activated protein C. The gene mutation is commonly designated *factor V Leiden* and follows autosomal dominant inheritance. Patients who are homozygous for the factor V Leiden mutation have a markedly increased risk of VTE and present with clinical thromboembolism at a younger age (median age: 31 years) than those who are heterozygous (median age: 46 years).[20,22] Factor V Leiden is present in approximately 5 percent of the normal population of European descent, 16 percent of patients with a first episode of DVT, and up to 35 percent of patients with unprovoked (idiopathic) DVT.[20,22,25] Prothrombin G20210A is another common gene mutation that predisposes to VTE. It is present in approximately 2 to 3 percent of apparently healthy individuals and in 7 percent of those with DVT.[22] An inherited abnormality cannot be detected in up to 40 to 50 percent of patients with unprovoked DVT, suggesting that as yet undefined gene mutations are present that have an etiologic role (Chap. 20).

# CLINICAL FEATURES

## VENOUS THROMBOSIS

The clinical features of DVT include leg pain, tenderness, and swelling, a palpable cord representing a thrombosed vessel, discoloration, venous distention, prominence of the superficial veins, and cyanosis. The clinical diagnosis of DVT is highly nonspecific because each of the symptoms or signs can be caused by nonthrombotic disorders. The rare exception is the patient with phlegmasia cerulea dolens (occlusion of the whole venous circulation, extreme swelling of the leg, and compromised arterial flow), in whom the diagnosis of massive iliofemoral thrombosis is obvious. This syndrome occurs in less than 1 percent of patients with symptomatic venous thrombosis. In most patients, the symptoms and signs are nonspecific. In 50 to 85 percent of patients, the clinical suspicion of DVT is not confirmed by objective testing.[17-19] Patients with minor symptoms and signs may have extensive DVT. Conversely, patients with florid leg pain and swelling, suggesting extensive DVT, may have negative results by objective testing.

Although the clinical diagnosis is nonspecific, prospective studies have established that patients can be categorized as low, moderate, or high probability for DVT using a clinical prediction rule that incorporates signs, symptoms, and risk factors. A systematic review[26] of the studies found that the prevalence of DVT in the low, moderate, and high probability categories, respectively, was 5 percent (95 percent confidence interval [95% CI]: 4 to 8 percent), 17 percent (95% CI: 13 to 23 percent), and 53 percent (95% CI: 44 to 61 percent). The prevalence in the pretest category of "low probability" is not sufficiently low to withhold further diagnostic testing and treatment, and the prevalence in the "high probability" category is not sufficiently high to give anticoagulant therapy without performing further diagnostic testing. Consequently, the key role for clinical pretest categorization is for use within integrated diagnostic strategies employing measurement of D-dimer and venous imaging.

## PULMONARY EMBOLISM

The clinical features of acute PE include the following symptoms and signs that may overlap: (1) transient dyspnea and tachypnea in the absence of other clinical features; (2) pleuritic chest pain, cough, hemoptysis, pleural effusion, and pulmonary infiltrates noted on chest radiogram caused by pulmonary infarction or congestive atelectasis (also known as *ischemic pneumonitis* or *incomplete infarction*); (3) severe dyspnea and tachypnea and right-sided heart failure; (4) cardiovascular collapse with hypotension, syncope, and coma (usually associated with massive PE); and (5) several less common and nonspecific clinical presentations,

including unexplained tachycardia or arrhythmia, resistant cardiac failure, wheezing, cough, fever, anxiety/apprehension, and confusion. All of these clinical features are nonspecific and can be caused by a variety of cardiorespiratory disorders. Patients can be assigned to categories of pretest probability using implicit clinical judgement or clinical decision rules such as the Geneva score or Wells approach.[27-30] However, the prevalences of PE in these categories are not sufficiently low or high to withhold further investigation altogether, and the measurement of D-dimer and/or diagnostic imaging is mandatory to exclude or confirm the presence of PE. The assessment of clinical pretest probability is an important first step in integrated diagnostic strategies that employ, for example, D-dimer, computed tomographic angiography (CTA), and objective testing for DVT.[27-30]

# LABORATORY FEATURES

VTE is associated with nonspecific laboratory changes that constitute the acute-phase response to tissue injury. This response includes elevated levels of fibrinogen and factor VIII, increases in leukocyte and platelet counts, and systemic activation of blood coagulation, fibrin formation, and fibrin breakdown, with increases in plasma concentrations of prothrombin fragment 1.2, fibrinopeptide A, complexes of thrombin–antithrombin, and fibrin degradation products. All of these changes are nonspecific and may occur as a result of surgery, trauma, infection, inflammation, or infarction. None of the above reported laboratory changes can be used to establish the diagnosis of VTE or predict its development with high probability. The fibrin breakdown fragment D-dimer can be measured by an enzyme-linked immunosorbent assay (ELISA) or by a latex agglutination assay. Some of these assays have a rapid turnaround time, and some are quantitative. A negative D-dimer result is useful for excluding the diagnosis in many patients with suspected DVT or suspected PE (see "Objective Testing for Deep Vein Thrombosis" and "Objective Testing for Pulmonary Embolism" below).[16,27,28,31] A positive result is highly nonspecific.

# DIFFERENTIAL DIAGNOSIS OF DEEP VEIN THROMBOSIS

The differential diagnosis in patients with clinically suspected DVT includes muscle strain or tear, direct twisting injury to the leg, lymphangitis or lymphatic obstruction, venous reflux, popliteal cyst, cellulitis, leg swelling in a paralyzed limb, and abnormality of the knee joint. An alternate diagnosis frequently is not evident at presentation, so excluding DVT is not possible without objective testing. The cause of symptoms often can be determined by careful follow-up once DVT has been excluded by objective testing. In approximately 25 percent of patients, however, the cause of pain, tenderness, and swelling remains uncertain even after careful follow-up.[19]

# OBJECTIVE TESTING FOR DEEP VEIN THROMBOSIS

## D-DIMER ASSAY

Measurement of plasma D-dimer has been extensively evaluated as an exclusion test in patients with clinically suspected DVT.[31] The different D-dimer assays (ELISA, quantitative rapid ELISA, latex agglutination, and whole-blood agglutination) have different sensitivities, specificities, and likelihood ratios for DVT. ELISA and quantitative rapid ELISA have high sensitivity (96 percent) and negative likelihood ratios of approximately 0.10 for DVT in symptomatic patients. Thus, for excluding DVT in symptomatic patients with a low or intermediate clinical pretest probability, a negative D-dimer result by a quantitative rapid ELISA technique is as diagnostically useful as a negative result by duplex ultrasonography.[31] Measurement of D-dimer using an appropriate assay method can also be combined with ultrasonography imaging. If the two tests are negative at presentation, repeat ultrasonography imaging is unecessary.[32] Use of the D-dimer test for patient care decisions depends on the local availability of an appropriate assay that has high sensitivity and has been validated by clinical outcome studies. The use of age-adjusted D-dimer cut-off levels for a negative result enhances the clinical utility of the test. Figure 23–1 shows a practical approach for the diagnosis of suspected DVT.

## IMAGING TESTS

The objective diagnostic imaging tests that have a role in patients with clinically suspected DVT are ultrasonography and venography. Both of these tests have been validated by properly designed clinical trials, including prospective studies with long-term follow-up that have established the safety of withholding anticoagulant treatment in patients with negative test results.[17–19,33] Ultrasonography is the preferred imaging test for most patients. The role of venography is for selected patients, such as those in whom ultrasonography is unavailable or inconclusive. Ultrasonography using vein compression is effective for identifying patients with proximal vein thrombosis. Compression ultrasonography of the proximal veins performed at presentation (and, if normal, repeated once 5 to 7 days later) is a safe approach in symptomatic patients.[17] In centers with experienced ultrasonography staff, a single comprehensive evaluation of the proximal and calf veins with duplex ultrasonography is sufficient, and if negative, a repeat test is not required.[18] A randomized trial supports the equivalence of a comprehensive whole-leg color-coded Doppler ultrasonography approach to that of an approach using

combined D-dimer testing and repeated ultrasonography for the management of suspected DVT.[34]

The positive predictive value of a positive ultrasonography result isolated to the calf veins may vary among centers based on expertise and thrombosis prevalence. Therefore, the number of repeat ultrasonography evaluations avoided by evaluating the calf veins may be partially offset by an increased number of patients with positive ultrasonography results confined to the calf, for whom additional diagnostic testing and/or anticoagulant treatment is required. Most patients with a negative ultrasonographic result at presentation require a follow-up visit to establish the alternate diagnosis and to guide further care, so the return visit for repeat ultrasonography at 5 to 7 days may have added practical value.[17]

Diagnosis of acute recurrent DVT is particularly challenging because recurrent symptoms such as pain and swelling are common in patients with DVT despite adequate anticoagulant therapy and because both ultrasonography and venography have limitations for excluding the presence of acute recurrent DVT.[35] Compression ultrasonography may remain abnormal for 1 year in 50 percent of patients, and for even longer in some patients,[36] because of persistent noncompressibility of the vein caused by fibrous organization of the original thrombus. Venography is of limited value for excluding the diagnosis of recurrent DVT because of obliteration or recanalization of the previously affected venous segments or nonfilled venous segments. Thus, measurement of plasma D-dimer may be particularly useful as an exclusion test in patients with suspected acute recurrent DVT. However, use of D-dimer must be evaluated separately in this patient group because many patients with a past history of VTE are receiving long-term oral anticoagulant therapy, which has the potential to cause a false-negative D-dimer result. Promising initial results were obtained in one study,[37] but further studies in larger numbers of patients are needed before using a negative D-dimer alone to exclude acute recurrent DVT can be routinely recommended.

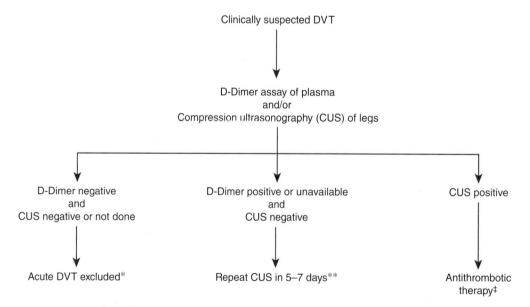

**Figure 23–1.** Diagnosis of patients with suspected first episode of deep vein thrombosis (DVT). *Negative D-dimer can be used to exclude acute DVT, without the need for further diagnostic testing with compression ultrasonography (CUS), if the patient has low, unlikely, moderate, or intermediate clinical probability.[26,31] Ultrasonography should be performed in patients with a high clinical probability. A negative D-dimer can also be used with a negative CUS at presentation to exclude acute DVT without the need for a repeat CUS.[32,34] **CUS is performed with imaging of the common femoral vein in the groin and of the popliteal vein in the popliteal fossa extending distally 10 cm from midpatella. A repeat CUS is required in 5 to 7 days to detect extending calf vein thrombi.[17] In centers with the expertise, a single negative result of full-leg duplex ultrasonography (CUS plus flow evaluation) is sufficient to exclude acute DVT.[18,34] ‡CUS that indicates noncompressibility of deep vein segments is highly predictive of DVT (>95 percent) and provides an indication for antithrombotic therapy in most patients. If CUS is positive at a single site isolated in the groin, additional testing with venography, computed tomography, or magnetic resonance imaging should be performed because of the potential for false-positive CUS results from disorders producing vein compression in the groin (e.g., tumor mass).

# DIFFERENTIAL DIAGNOSIS OF PULMONARY EMBOLISM

The differential diagnosis in patients with suspected PE includes cardiopulmonary disorders for each of the modes of presentation (see "Pulmonary Embolism" above). For the presentation of dyspnea and tachypnea, they include atelectasis, pneumonia, pleuritis, pneumothorax, acute pulmonary edema, bronchitis, bronchiolitis, and acute bronchial obstruction. For pulmonary infarction exhibited by pleuritic chest pain or hemoptysis, they include pneumonia, pneumothorax, pericarditis, pulmonary or bronchial neoplasm, bronchiectasis, acute bronchitis, tuberculosis, diaphragmatic inflammation, myositis, muscle strain, and rib fracture. For the clinical presentation of right-sided heart failure, they include myocardial infarction, myocarditis, and cardiac tamponade. For cardiovascular collapse, they include myocardial infarction, acute massive hemorrhage, gram-negative septicemia, cardiac tamponade, and spontaneous pneumothorax.

# OBJECTIVE TESTING FOR PULMONARY EMBOLISM

The objective diagnostic imaging tests include CT, CTA, radionuclide lung scanning, selective pulmonary arteriography, and objective testing for DVT. Measurement of plasma D-dimer is useful as an exclusion test in patients with an unlikely or intermediate clinical probability.

## D-DIMER ASSAY

The assay for plasma D-dimer is useful as an exclusion test, provided an appropriately validated test is available. A negative result by the rapid quantitative ELISA for D-dimer has a negative likelihood ratio similar to that of a normal perfusion scan.[31] A positive D-dimer result is not useful diagnostically. Several management studies have found that PE can be excluded without performing imaging studies in patients with a low, intermediate, or unlikely clinical probability.[38] When combined with pretest clinical probability assessment, the use of an age-adjusted D-dimer cutoff value, instead of a fixed D-dimer cutoff of 500 mcg/mL, improves the utility of the test, and enables more patients to have the diagnosis of PE safely excluded.[39]

## COMPUTED TOMOGRAPHY IMAGING AND ANGIOGRAPHY

CT imaging is the primary imaging test for the diagnosis of PE in most centers. Single-detector spiral CT is highly sensitive for large emboli (segmental or larger arteries) but is much less sensitive for emboli in subsegmental pulmonary arteries[16,40]; such emboli may be clinically important in patients with severely impaired cardiorespiratory reserve. Therefore, a negative result by single-detector spiral CT should not be used alone to exclude the diagnosis of PE. A filling defect of a segmental or larger artery on single-detector spiral CT is associated with a high probability (>90 percent) of PE.[40]

The development of multidetector row CT, together with the use of contrast enhancement, has established CT as the preferred diagnostic imaging test in most patients.[41–43] Contrast-enhanced CTA has the advantage of providing clear results (positive or negative), with a low rate of nondiagnostic test results, good characterization of nonvascular structures for alternate or associated diagnoses, and the ability to simultaneously evaluate the deep venous system of the legs (computed tomographic venography [CTV]).

The accuracy and clinical utility of multidetector CTA and combined CTA-CTV were evaluated in the Prospective Investigation of Pulmonary Embolism Diagnosis (PIOPED) II study.[43] Among 824 patients with a reference diagnosis and a completed CT study, CTA was inconclusive in 51 (6 percent) because of poor image quality. The sensitivity of CTA was 83 percent and the specificity was 96 percent. CTA-CTV was inconclusive in 87 (11 percent) of 824 patients because the image quality of either CTA or CTV was poor. Multidetector CTA-CTV had a higher sensitivity (90 percent) than CTA alone (83 percent), with similar specificity (~95 percent for both testing techniques). Positive results on CTA in combination with a high probability or intermediate probability of PE by the clinical assessment or normal findings on CTA with a low clinical probability had a predictive value (positive or negative) of 92 to 96 percent.[43] Such values are consistent with those generally considered adequate to confirm or rule out the diagnosis of PE. Additional testing is necessary when the clinical probability is discordant with CTA or CTA-CTV imaging results.[43]

Figure 23-2 summarizes the approach to diagnosis of suspected PE using CTA or CTA-CTV as the primary imaging test. A high-quality image by CTA is sufficient to establish or exclude the diagnosis of PE with high predictive value in most patients, and withholding anticoagulant therapy based on a negative CTA alone is associated with a low rate of subsequent VTE on follow-up.[44] Objective testing for DVT is useful in patients in whom the CTA image is of poor quality or inconclusive and in patients who also have symptoms suggesting DVT. CTV has the advantage of being easily performed at the time of CTA, but incurs the risk of added radiation exposure for the patient. Compression ultrasonography can also be used and avoids added radiation exposure and can be performed serially if needed.

## RADIONUCLIDE LUNG SCANNING

Radionuclide lung scanning continues to have a role in the diagnosis of suspected PE. A normal perfusion lung scan excludes the diagnosis of clinically important PE.[15,45] A normal perfusion lung scan is found in approximately 10 percent of all patients with suspected PE seen at academic health centers or tertiary referral centers. A high-probability lung scan result (i.e., large perfusion defects with ventilation mismatch) has a positive predictive value for PE of 85 percent and provides a diagnostic end point to give antithrombotic treatment in most patients.[15,46,47] A high-probability lung scan is found in approximately 10 to 15 percent of symptomatic patients. For patients with a history of PE, careful comparison of the lung scan results to the most recent lung scan is required to ensure the perfusion defects are new. Further diagnostic testing is indicated for patients with a high-probability lung scan who have a "low" pretest clinical suspicion, and in those who are at high risk for major bleeding, to reduce the likelihood of a false-positive diagnosis.

The major limitation of lung scanning is that the results are inconclusive in most patients, even when considered together with the pretest clinical probability.[15] The nondiagnostic lung scan patterns are found in approximately 70 percent of all patients with suspected PE.[13,15,47] These lung scan results have historically been called "low probability" (matching ventilation–perfusion abnormalities or small perfusion defects), "intermediate probability," or "indeterminate" (because the perfusion defects correspond to an area of abnormality on chest radiograph). Further diagnostic testing is required in most of these patients because, regardless of the pretest clinical suspicion, the posttest probabilities of PE associated with these lung scan results are neither sufficiently high to give antithrombotic treatment nor sufficiently low to withhold therapy. The uncommon exception is the patient with a low clinical suspicion and a so-called low-probability lung scan result. However, even in these patients, objective testing for DVT with ultrasonography and/or

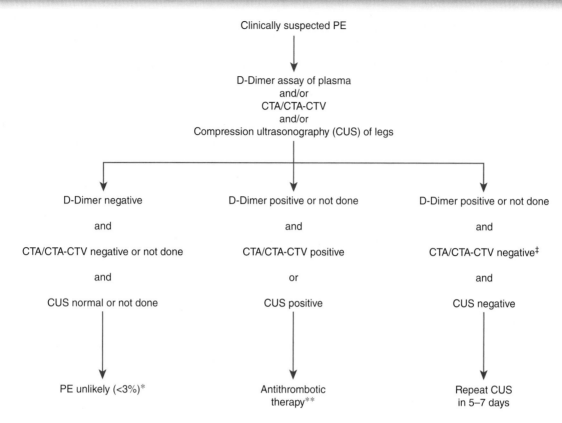

**Figure 23–2.** Integrated strategy for diagnosis of patients with suspected pulmonary embolism (PE) using computed tomographic angiography (CTA) as the primary imaging test. *Negative D-dimer alone can be used as an exclusion test with high negative predictive value (>96 percent) in patients with low or moderate probability by the clinical assessment.[27,30,31] Patients with a high clinical probability should undergo imaging with CTA or combined CTA-computed tomographic venography (CTV). **Positive results on CTA or combined CTA-CTV, in patients with a high or moderate probability of pulmonary embolism by the clinical assessment, have positive predictive value of 90% or more for venous thromboembolism. Similarly, abnormal results by compression ultrasonography (CUS) of the proximal deep veins of the legs have high positive predictive value for proximal vein thrombosis and provide an indication to give antithrombotic therapy. If the patient has a low probability by the clinical assessment, positive results by CTA or CTA-CTV in the main or lobar pulmonary arteries are still highly predictive (97 percent) for the presence of pulmonary embolism[43]; further testing is recommended for patients with low clinical probability and positive CTA results only of segmental or subsegmental arteries, and the options include pulmonary arteriography or serial CUS. ‡Negative results by CTA or by combined CTA-CTV have high negative predictive value (96 percent) in patients with low probability by the clinical assessment.[43] For patients with moderate clinical probability, the negative predictive value for combined CTA-CTV is also high (92 percent), but slightly lower for CTA alone (89 percent)[43]; in CTA-alone group and in patients with a high probability by the clinical assessment, serial CUS and pulmonary arteriography are recommended options.

measurement of plasma D-dimer is without risk for the patient and may provide added diagnostic value (see "Objective Testing for Deep Vein Thrombosis" below). A randomized trial has established that CTA is not inferior to using ventilation–perfusion lung scanning for excluding the diagnosis of PE when either test is used in an algorithm together with venous ultrasonography of the legs.[48]

In centers where CTA is available, the major role for lung scanning is in select patients; for example, in younger women to reduce radiation exposure to the breast. Lung scanning can be useful in such patients who are less likely to have comorbid cardiorespiratory disorders and therefore a higher proportion of diagnostic scan results (normal or high probability).

## MAGNETIC RESONANCE ANGIOGRAPHY

The accuracy of magnetic resonance angiography for diagnosing PE, with or without the addition of magnetic resonance venography, was evaluated in the PIOPED III study.[49] This was a prospective study of 371 adults with suspected PE recruited from seven hospitals and their emergency services. Magnetic resonance angiography was technically inadequate in 25 percent of patients (92 of 371); this rate ranged from

11 percent to 52 percent among the centers. If a technically adequate image was obtained, magnetic resonance angiography had a sensitivity of 78 percent and a specificity of 99 percent, and combined magnetic resonance angiography and venography had a sensitivity of 92 percent and a specificity of 96 percent. However, 52 percent of patients (194 of 370) had technically inadequate results with the combined approach.[49] Based on these findings, magnetic resonance angiography has a very limited role in the diagnosis of PE. In centers that routinely perform it well with a high rate of technically adequate images, magnetic resonance angiography and venography may be useful for patients in whom CTA or lung scanning is contraindicated.

## PULMONARY ANGIOGRAPHY

Pulmonary angiography using selective catheterization of the pulmonary arteries is a relatively safe technique for patients who do not have pulmonary hypertension or cardiac failure.[13,15] If the expertise is available, pulmonary angiography should be used when other approaches are inconclusive and when definitive knowledge about the presence or absence of PE is required, because the risk of angiography in properly selected patients is less than the risk of unnecessary anticoagulant therapy.

## OBJECTIVE TESTING FOR DEEP VEIN THROMBOSIS

Objective testing for DVT is useful in patients with suspected PE, particularly those with nondiagnostic lung scan results[33,47] or inconclusive CT results.[50] Detection of proximal vein thrombosis by objective testing provides an indication for anticoagulant treatment, regardless of the presence or absence of PE, and prevents the need for further testing. However, a negative result by objective testing for DVT does not exclude the presence of PE.[13,14] If the patient has adequate cardiorespiratory reserve, then serial ultrasonography testing for proximal vein thrombosis can be used as an alternative to pulmonary angiography in patients with nondiagnostic lung scan or inconclusive CT results, and withholding anticoagulant therapy is safe if repeated ultrasonography testing of the legs is negative.[33,47,50] The rationale is that the clinical objective in such patients is to prevent recurrent PE, which is unlikely in the absence of proximal vein thrombosis. Selective pulmonary angiography should be done among patients with features suggesting a possible alternate source of embolism to proximal DVT of the leg (e.g., upper-extremity thrombosis, renal vein thrombosis, pelvic vein thrombosis, or right-heart thrombus).

## ●THERAPY, COURSE, AND PROGNOSIS

### CLINICAL COURSE OF VENOUS THROMBOEMBOLISM

#### Proximal Vein Thrombosis

Proximal vein thrombosis is a serious and potentially lethal condition. Untreated proximal vein thrombosis is associated with a 10 percent rate of fatal PE. Inadequately treated proximal vein thrombosis results in a 20 to 50 percent risk of recurrent VTE events.[51] Prospective studies of patients with clinically suspected DVT or PE indicate that new VTE events on follow-up are uncommon (≤2 percent) among patients in whom proximal vein thrombosis is absent by objective testing.[17,32,33,47,50] The aggregate data from diagnostic and treatment studies indicate that the presence of proximal vein thrombosis is the key prognostic marker for recurrent VTE.

#### Calf Vein Thrombosis

Thrombosis that remains confined to the calf veins is associated with low risk (≤1 percent) of clinically important PE. Extension of thrombosis into the popliteal vein or more proximally occurs in 15 to 25 percent of patients with untreated calf vein thrombosis.[1] Patients with documented calf vein thrombosis should either receive anticoagulant treatment to prevent extension or undergo monitoring for proximal extension using serial ultrasonography.

#### Postthrombotic Syndrome

The postthrombotic syndrome is a frequent complication of DVT.[52] Patients with the postthrombotic syndrome complain of pain, heaviness, swelling, cramps, and itching or tingling of the affected leg. Ulceration may occur. The symptoms usually are aggravated by standing or walking and improve with rest and elevation of the leg. A prospective study documented a 25 percent incidence of moderate-to-severe postthrombotic symptoms 2 years after the initial diagnosis of proximal vein thrombosis in patients who were treated with initial heparin and oral anticoagulants for 3 months.[53] The study also demonstrated that ipsilateral recurrent venous thrombosis is strongly associated with subsequent development of moderate or severe postthrombotic symptoms. Thus, prevention of ipsilateral recurrent DVT likely reduces the incidence of the postthrombotic syndrome. Application of a properly fitted graded compression stocking, as soon after diagnosis as the patient's symptoms will allow, can improve edema and pain in the acute stage of DVT and may also help control or relieve symptoms in patients who develop the postthrombotic syndrome. Conflicting findings have been found in randomized trials of graded compression stockings for preventing the development of the postthrombotic syndrome.[54,55]

#### Chronic Thromboembolic Pulmonary Hypertension

Chronic thromboembolic pulmonary hypertension is a serious complication of PE. Historically, thromboembolic pulmonary hypertension was believed to be relatively rare and to occur only several years after the diagnosis of PE. A prospective cohort study provides important information on the incidence and timing of thromboembolic pulmonary hypertension.[56] The results indicate that thromboembolic pulmonary hypertension is more common and occurs earlier than previously thought. On prospective follow-up of 223 patients with documented PE, the cumulative incidence of chronic thromboembolic pulmonary hypertension was 3.8 percent at 2 years after diagnosis, despite state-of-the-art treatment for PE. The strongest independent risk factors were a history of PE (odds ratio 19) and idiopathic PE at presentation (odds ratio 5.7).[56]

## OBJECTIVES AND PRINCIPLES OF ANTITHROMBOTIC TREATMENT

The objectives of treatment in patients with established VTE are to (1) prevent death from PE, and (2) prevent morbidity from recurrent DVT or PE, especially the postthrombotic syndrome and chronic pulmonary hypertension.

For most patients, these objectives are achieved by providing adequate anticoagulant treatment. Thrombolytic therapy is indicated in selected patients (see "Thrombolytic Therapy" below). Use of an inferior vena cava filter is indicated to prevent death from PE in patients in whom anticoagulant treatment is absolutely contraindicated and in other selected patients (see "Anticoagulant Therapy" below). These recommendations and those below are linked to the strength of the evidence from clinical trials and evidence-based guidelines.[9,30,57,58,58a]

## ANTICOAGULANT THERAPY

Anticoagulant therapy is the treatment of choice for most patients with proximal vein thrombosis or PE.[9,57,58,58a] Patients with proximal DVT require both adequate initial anticoagulant treatment with heparin or low-molecular-weight (LMW) heparin and adequate long-term anticoagulant therapy to prevent recurrent VTE.[51,59,60] Anticoagulant therapy for at least 3 months is required to prevent a high frequency (15 to 25 percent) of symptomatic extension of thrombosis and/or recurrent venous thromboembolic events.[51,60,61] Adequate anticoagulant treatment reduces the incidence of recurrence during the first 3 months after diagnosis to 5 percent or less.[51,59–61]

The absolute contraindications to anticoagulant treatment include intracranial bleeding, severe active bleeding, recent brain, eye, or spinal cord surgery, and malignant hypertension. Relative contraindications include recent major surgery, recent cerebrovascular accident, active gastrointestinal tract bleeding, severe hypertension, severe renal or hepatic failure, and severe thrombocytopenia (platelets $<50 \times 10^9$/L).

### Parenteral Anticoagulants

**Heparin and Low-Molecular-Weight Heparin** Initial therapy with continuous intravenous heparin was the standard approach to treatment of VTE during the 1970s and 1980s. During the 1990s, LMW heparin given by subcutaneous injection once or twice daily was evaluated by clinical trials and shown to be as effective and safe as continuous intravenous heparin for the initial treatment of patients with proximal

DVT and submassive PE.[57,58,62] The advantage of LMW heparin is that it does not require anticoagulant monitoring. LMW heparin given subcutaneously once or twice daily is preferred over intravenous unfractionated heparin for the initial treatment of most patients with either DVT or PE.[57,58] LMW heparin enables outpatient therapy for many patients with uncomplicated DVT and selected patients with PE. Intravenous unfractionated heparin remains a useful approach for initial anticoagulant therapy in patients with severe renal failure. Initial treatment with LMW heparin or unfractionated heparin should be continued for at least 5 days. Table 23–2 lists the specific LMW heparin regimens for the treatment of VTE.

If unfractionated heparin is used for initial therapy, it is important to achieve an adequate anticoagulant effect, defined as an activated partial thromboplastin time (aPTT) above the lower limit of therapeutic range within the first 24 hours.[63,64] Failure to achieve an adequate aPTT effect early during therapy is associated with a high incidence (25 percent) of recurrent VTE.[63] Two-thirds of the recurrent events

occur between 2 and 12 weeks after the initial diagnosis despite treatment with oral anticoagulants, and the initial management with either unfractionated heparin or LMW heparin is critical to the patient's long-term outcome.[63,64]

**Fondaparinux** The synthetic pentasaccharide fondaparinux, which is an indirect inhibitor of factor Xa, has been evaluated by large randomized clinical trials.[65,66] These studies indicate fondaparinux is as effective and safe as LMW heparin for treatment of established DVT and as effective and safe as intravenous heparin for treatment of symptomatic PE. Fondaparinux is given subcutaneously once daily at a dose of 7.5 mg for patients weighing between 50 and 100 kg (85 percent of all patients evaluated in the clinical trials), 5 mg for patients weighing less than 50 kg, and 10 mg for patients weighing more than 100 kg.[65,66]

## Oral Anticoagulants

**Vitamin K Antagonists** Oral anticoagulant treatment using a vitamin K antagonist (e.g., sodium warfarin) has been the standard approach for long-term treatment in most patients for more than 60 years. Treatment with a vitamin K antagonist is started with initial heparin or LMW heparin therapy and overlapped for 4 to 5 days.

The preferred intensity of the anticoagulant effect of treatment with a vitamin K antagonist has been established by clinical trials.[67–70] The dose of vitamin K antagonist should be adjusted to maintain the international normalized ratio (INR) between 2.0 and 3.0. High-intensity vitamin K antagonist treatment (INR 3.0 to 4.0) should not be used because it has not improved effectiveness in patients with the antiphospholipid syndrome and recurrent thrombosis[69] and has caused more bleeding.[70] Low-intensity therapy (INR 1.5 to 1.9) is not recommended because it is less effective than standard-intensity treatment (INR 2.0 to 3.0) and does not reduce bleeding complications.[68]

Long-term treatment with LMW heparin is indicated for select patients in whom vitamin K antagonists are contraindicated (e.g., pregnant women) and in patients with concurrent cancer for whom LMW heparin regimens are more effective.[71,72]

**Direct Oral Anticoagulants** Oral anticoagulants that bind directly to the target coagulation enzyme of either thrombin or factor Xa have been evaluated in phase III clinical trials for the treatment of patients with VTE.[73–78] The advantages of these drugs are: (1) they can be administered orally once or twice daily without the need for anticoagulant monitoring and dose titration; (2) they have fewer clinically relevant drug interactions; (3) because of a fast onset of anticoagulant action, similar to that of LMW heparin, they can simplify treatment for many patients by replacing the standard approach of a parenteral drug (heparin, LMW heparin, or fondaparinux) followed by an oral vitamin K antagonist with a single drug given for both initial and long-term therapy; and (4) they result in less clinically important bleeding. Table 23-2 lists the direct-acting oral anticoagulant (DOAC) regimens that have been evaluated by clinical trials for the treatment of established VTE.

Six phase III clinical trials evaluating the DOACs for the treatment of acute VTE have been completed and published.[73–78] Table 23–3 outlines the design features of these trials and the efficacy and bleeding results. Each of these trials met the prespecified criteria for noninferiority of the efficacy of the DOAC for preventing recurrent VTE.

The six trials included more than 27,000 patients with acute VTE, and meta-analyses of these studies have been done.[79] The meta-analyses provide added clinically useful information regarding specific major bleeding outcomes (intracranial bleeding and fatal bleeding) and regarding the risk-to-benefit profile in key patient subgroups commonly encountered by the clinician. These subgroups are patients

---

**TABLE 23–2.** Anticoagulant Drug Regimens for Treatment of Venous Thromboembolism

| Drug | Regimen |
|---|---|
| **Low-Molecular-Weight Heparins** | |
| Enoxaparin | 1.0 mg/kg BID* |
| Dalteparin | 200 IU/kg once daily† |
| Tinzaparin | 175 IU/kg once daily‡ |
| Nadroparin | 6150 IU BID for 50–70 kg |
| | 4100 IU BID if patient weighs <50 kg |
| | 9200 IU BID if patient weighs >70 kg |
| Reviparin | 4200 IU BID for 46–60 kg |
| | 3500 IU BID if patient weighs 35–45 kg |
| | 6300 IU BID if patient weighs >60 kg |
| **Indirect Factor Xa Inhibitor** | |
| Fondaparinux | 7.5 mg once daily if patient weighs 50–100 kg |
| | 5.0 mg once daily if patient weighs <50 kg |
| | 10.0 mg once daily if patient weighs >100 kg |
| **Direct Oral Anticoagulants** | |
| Dabigatran | 150 mg BID after 5 days of parenteral low-molecular-weight heparin or heparin |
| Rivaroxaban | 15 mg BID for 21 days, then 20 mg once daily Taken with food |
| Apixaban | 10 mg BID for 7 days, then 5 mg BID After 6 months, 2.5 mg BID for extended therapy |
| Edoxaban | 60 mg once daily after 5 days of parenteral low-molecular-weight heparin or heparin§ |

*A once-daily regimen of 1.5 mg/kg can be used but probably is less effective in patients with cancer.

†After 1 month, can be followed by 150 IU/kg once daily as an alternative to an oral vitamin K antagonist for long-term treatment.

‡This regimen can also be used for long-term treatment as an alternative to an oral vitamin K antagonist.

§30 mg once daily if patient's creatinine clearance is 30–50 mL/min or weight is ≤60 kg or if patient is taking strong P-glycoprotein inhibitor drugs.

**TABLE 23-3.** Clinical Trials of Direct Oral Anticoagulants for Treatment of Venous Thromboembolism

|  | Hokusai-VTE[78] | AMPLIFY[77] | EINSTEIN-DVT[75] | EINSTEIN-PE[76] | RE-COVER II[74] | RE-COVER I[73] |
|---|---|---|---|---|---|---|
| Drug | Edoxaban | Apixaban | Rivaroxaban | Rivaroxaban | Dabigatran | Dabigatran |
| Study design | Double-blind | Double-blind | Open label | Open label | Double-blind | Double-blind |
| Heparin lead-in | At least 5 days | None | None | None | At least 5 days | At least 5 days |
| Regimen | 60 mg QD<br><br>30 mg QD if CrCl 30–50 mL/min, bw ≤60 kg or P-gp inhibitors | 10 mg BID × 7 days then 5 mg BID | 15 mg BID × 21 days then 20 mg QD | 15 mg BID × 21 days then 20 mg QD | 150 mg BID | 150 mg BID |
| Sample size | 8292 | 5400 | 3449 | 4832 | 2568 | 2564 |
| Treatment duration | Flexible: 3–12 months | 6 months | Prespecified: 3, 6, or 12 months | Prespecified: 3, 6, or 12 months | 6 months | 6 months |
| Recurrent VTE | Edoxaban 3.2%*<br><br>(LMW) Hep/ warfarin 3.5%*<br><br>$p < 0.001$ noninferiority | Apixaban 2.3%<br><br>Enoxaparin/ warfarin 2.7%<br><br>$p < 0.001$ noninferiority | Rivaroxaban 2.1%<br><br>Enoxaparin/VKA 3.0%**<br><br>$p < 0.001$ noninferiority | Rivaroxaban 2.1%<br><br>Enoxaparin/VKA 1.8%<br><br>$p = 0.003$ noninferiority | Dabigatran 2.4%<br><br>Warfarin 2.1%<br><br>$p < 0.001$ noninferiority | Dabigatran 2.3%<br><br>Warfarin 2.2%<br><br>$p < 0.001$ noninferiority |
| Major bleeding | Edoxaban 1.4%<br><br>(LMW) Hep/ warfarin 1.6% | Apixaban 0.6%<br><br>Enoxaparin/ warfarin 1.8%<br><br>$p < 0.001$ superiority | Rivaroxaban 0.8%<br><br>Enoxaparin/VKA 1.2% | Rivaroxaban 1.1%<br><br>Enoxaparin/VKA 2.2%<br><br>$p = 0.003$ superiority | Dabigatran 1.6%<br><br>Warfarizn 1.9% | Dabigatran 1.2%<br><br>Warfarin 1.7% |
| CRNM bleeding | Edoxaban 7.2%<br><br>(LMW) Hep/ warfarin 8.9%<br><br>$p = 0.004$ superiority | Apixaban 3.8%<br><br>Enoxaparin/ warfarin 8.0%<br><br>$p < 0.001$ superiority | Rivaroxaban 7.3%<br><br>Enoxaparin/VKA 7.0% | Rivaroxaban 9.5%<br><br>Enoxaparin/VKA 9.8% | Dabigatran 5.6%§<br><br>Warfarin 8.8%§<br><br>$p = 0.002$ superiority | Dabigatran 5.0%§<br><br>Warfarin 7.9%§<br><br>$p < 0.05$ superiority |

bw, body weight; CrCl, creatinine clearance; CRNM, clinically relevant non major bleeding; Hep, heparin; LMW, low molecular weight; P-gp, P glycoprotein; VKA, vitamin K antagonist; VTE, venous thromboembolism.

*During overall study period. On-treatment rates were 1.6% for edoxaban and 1.9% for heparin/warfarin. The analysis for all the other studies used rates on treatment.

**Either warfarin or acenocoumarol was used for the vitamin K antagonist therapy.

§Rates are for the composite of major and clinically relevant nonmajor bleeding.

Adapted with permission from Raskob G, Büller H, Prins M, et al: Edoxaban for the long-term treatment of venous thromboembolism: rationale and design of the Hokusai-venous thromboembolism study—methodological implications for clinical trials, *J Thromb Haemost* 2013 Jul;11(7):1287–1294.

presenting with symptomatic PE or symptomatic DVT, the elderly (age ≥75 years), the obese, patients with moderate renal impairment (creatinine clearance 30 to 49 mL/min), and patients with cancer. The DOACs were associated with clinically important reductions in major bleeding (relative risk [RR] 0.61), intracranial bleeding (RR 0.37), and fatal bleeding (RR 0.36).[79] For each of these outcomes, the results are consistent among the trials; none of the trials have a point estimate for these outcomes in favor of the vitamin K antagonists (supplementary data online[79]). The number of patients who would need to be treated with a DOAC rather than a vitamin K antagonist to avoid one event of intracranial bleeding is 588, and for fatal bleeding, it is 1250. In view of the large number of VTE patients each year and the devastating nature of these bleeding events, these are important impacts on population health. The results of cost-effectiveness studies have shown the DOACs to be cost-effective.

Regarding the key patient subgroups evaluated, the noninferior efficacy of the DOACs was consistent across all subgroups, with possibly superior efficacy in the elderly and in cancer patients.[79] The safety advantage of reduced major bleeding was also consistent across the subgroups, except possibly in cancer patients, in whom the pooled estimate of a 33 percent risk reduction did not achieve statistical significance.

The DOACs are preferred over vitamin K antagonists in most new patients commencing anticoagulant treatment for VTE. The exceptions are patients with severe renal impairment (creatinine clearance <30 mL/min), because they were not included in the clinical trials, and cancer patients, because only relatively small numbers of selected cancer patients were included, and because clinical trials comparing DOACs to the currently recommended standard therapy with LMW heparin have not been performed. For patients already taking long-term vitamin K antagonist therapy who are well controlled with a high proportion of time in therapeutic range and for whom regular anticoagulant monitoring is not a burden, switching treatment to a DOAC is not indicated unless a clinical reason develops.

Some practical issues remain incompletely resolved. Rivaroxaban and apixaban can be used as a single-drug approach, whereas dabigatran and edoxaban are preceded by at least 5 days of heparin or LMW heparin treatment. Whether DOAC monotherapy is sufficient for the full spectrum of VTE severity or whether "lead-in" heparin treatment is preferred in some patients, such as those with PE who have right ventricular dysfunction,[78] remains uncertain. A specific reversal is available for dabigatran,[79a] but the oral factor Xa inhibitors continue to lack a specific reversal agent. In general, this should not be a reason to withhold from most patients the benefit of significantly reduced risks of major bleeding, intracranial bleeding, and fatal bleeding with the DOACs. Dabigatran may be the preferred DOAC in patients in whom prompt and measurable reversal of the anticoagulant effect will be required because of planned surgery or invasive procedures. Because the DOACs do not require laboratory monitoring, patients receiving DOACs may have less frequent contact with their physician or anticoagulation clinic, and nonadherence to the prescribed therapy may not be detected as readily. Physicians and health systems should employ evidence-based strategies to enhance adherence and should evaluate patients at intervals to assess if ongoing anticoagulant therapy is appropriate and adhered to. The effectiveness and safety of the DOACs compared with LMW heparin treatment in cancer patients with VTE have not been evaluated by direct comparison in randomized trials, and LMW heparin remains indicated for these patients.

### Duration of Anticoagulant Therapy

Anticoagulant treatment should be continued for at least 3 months in all patients with VTE.[9,57,58,80] Stopping treatment at 4 to 6 weeks resulted in an increased incidence of recurrent VTE during the following 6 months (absolute risk increase 8 percent).[57,80–82] In contrast, treatment for 3 to 6 months resulted in a low rate of recurrence during the following 1 to 2 years (annual incidence 3 percent).[80–82]

The decision to stop anticoagulant therapy or continue treatment after 3 months is influenced mainly by the patient's clinical presentation of thromboembolism as either "provoked," which refers to VTE occurring in association with known risk factors, or "unprovoked," in which identifiable risk factors for VTE are absent. Approximately 20 to 40 percent of all symptomatic patients present as unprovoked VTE.

In patients with a first episode of DVT or PE provoked by a reversible risk factor (e.g., surgery), treatment for 3 months is usually sufficient if the risk factor(s) is no longer present. If the risk factor(s) persists, for example, prolonged immobility or cancer, treatment should be continued until the risk factor is reversed. It has been a customary practice to treat patients with PE for 6 months rather than 3 months, but clinical trials indicate there is little to no added benefit of doing so, with a small but additional risk of bleeding.[80] Thus, for patients with DVT or PE provoked by a risk factor that has reversed, 3 months is sufficient and recommended over longer therapy.[57]

Patients with a first episode of unprovoked VTE should be considered for indefinite anticoagulant therapy.[57,58] The term "indefinite" refers to continued treatment without a scheduled stopping date; treatment may be stopped in the future if the patient's risk-to-benefit profile or preference for continued treatment changes. The decision to stop or continue anticoagulation after 3 months in patients with a first episode of unprovoked VTE should take into consideration the risk of recurrent VTE, the risk of bleeding, and patient preference. If indefinite anticoagulant treatment is chosen, the risks and benefits of continuing such treatment should be reassessed at periodic intervals.[57]

There has been significant research to develop strategies to aid the clinician in assessing the risk of recurrent VTE in patients with unprovoked VTE. The presence of residual DVT assessed by compression ultrasonography,[83] elevated levels of plasma D-dimer after discontinuing anticoagulant treatment,[84] and male gender[85] are associated with an increased incidence of recurrent thromboembolism. The challenge,

however, has been to identify the subgroup of patients with a sufficiently low annual risk of recurrence to warrant stopping anticoagulant therapy. Palaretti and colleagues evaluated an approach for patients with a first episode of unprovoked VTE or VTE associated with a minor risk factor (e.g., estrogens, pregnancy, or travel-related thrombosis) that combined evaluation of the presence or absence of residual thrombosis by ultrasonography with serial D-dimer measurement to guide the decision to stop or continue anticoagulant therapy.[86] Patients in whom residual vein thrombosis was absent after 3 months of treatment or patients with residual vein thrombosis who had been treated for at least 1 year, and who had serially negative D-dimer measurements for 3 months after stopping vitamin K antagonist treatment, had an annual rate of recurrent VTE of 3 percent during follow-up off anticoagulant therapy; this compared to 0.7 percent per year in 373 patients who resumed anticoagulation because of an elevated D-dimer measurement, and 8.8 percent per year among the 109 patients with elevated D-dimer who did not continue anticoagulant therapy.[86] An annual risk of recurrent VTE of 3 percent may be low enough to discontinue therapy in patients in whom the annual risk of bleeding, especially major bleeding, is similar or higher. However, if the risk of major bleeding is low, for example, 1 percent per year or lower, then the annual risk of recurrent VTE of 3 percent may not be sufficiently low to stop anticoagulation, especially if the patient's preference is on avoiding further recurrent VTE events.

A variety of thrombophilic conditions have been identified and can be evaluated in the laboratory. These include deficiencies of the naturally occurring inhibitors of coagulation such as antithrombin, protein C, and protein S; specific gene mutations including factor V Leiden and prothrombin 20210A; elevated levels of coagulation factor VIII; and the presence of antiphospholipid antibodies (Chap. 21). The role of the presence or absence of thrombophilia in guiding decisions about duration of therapy has been controversial and is incompletely resolved. Indefinite anticoagulant treatment should be considered in patients with a first episode of VTE and antiphospholipid antibodies or the presence of one or a combination of the more potent thrombophilias (deficiency of antithrombin, protein C or protein S, homozygous factor V Leiden, or prothrombin 20210A gene mutation, or one of these with a family history of VTE). Again, patient preference is important to the decision.

The DOACs have been evaluated by randomized trials for the extended treatment of patients with VTE who have completed an initial course of 6 months of anticoagulant therapy.[75,87–89] Most of the patients in these trials had unprovoked VTE at their initial presentation, and all had clinical equipoise about the benefit-to-risk trade-off of receiving extended anticoagulant therapy. The results of the trials are consistent. The DOACs produced 80 percent or greater reductions in the annual incidence of recurrent VTE of 7 to 9 percent per year in patients receiving placebo to approximately 2 percent per year in those given DOACs.[75,87–89] The rates of major bleeding were 0.1 to 0.7 percent. Clinically relevant nonmajor bleeding occurred in 3 to 4 percent of patients.[75,87–89] In the AMPLIFY Extension trial,[89] the rate of major bleeding for the 2.5-mg apixaban regimen was 0.2 percent per year, compared with 0.5 percent for placebo. The low rates of major bleeding, coupled with the advantage of not requiring laboratory monitoring of the anticoagulant effect, will likely tip the balance in favor of extended treatment for more patients with unprovoked VTE.

Aspirin has also been evaluated for the extended treatment of patients with a first episode of unprovoked VTE who have received a course of 6 months or more of anticoagulant therapy.[90,91] Aspirin produced a statistically significant 42 percent RR reduction in recurrent VTE in one study (from 11.2 percent to 6.6 percent per year),[90] and a nonsignificant ($p = 0.09$) 26 percent RR reduction in the second study (from 6.5 percent to 4.8 percent per year).[91] The rates of major bleeding for aspirin (0.5 to 0.6 percent per year) were similar to placebo. The relative efficacy and safety of the DOAC rivaroxaban compared with aspirin for the extended treatment of VTE have been evaluated recently in the EINSTEIN CHOICE trial.[91a] A total of 3396 patients with VTE who had received 6 to 12 months of anticoagulant therapy were randomly assigned to one of three regimens for extended treatment: rivaroxaban 20 mg once daily, rivaroxaban 10 mg once daily, or aspirin 100 mg daily. The study treatment was given for up to 12 months. Recurrent VTE occurred in 17 of 1107 patients (1.5 percent) given rivaroxaban 20 mg and in 13 of 1127 patients (1.2 percent) given rivaroxaban 10 mg, as compared with 50 of 1131 patients (4.4 percent) given aspirin (p <0.001 for both comparisons of rivaroxaban to aspirin).[91a] The rates of major bleeding were 0.5 percent in the group given rivaroxaban 20 mg, 0.4 percent in the group given rivaroxaban 10 mg, and 0.3 percent in the aspirin group.[91a] These results have three important implications for practice. First, anticoagulant therapy using a DOAC is more effective than aspirin and produces a clinically important reduction in recurrent VTE (absolute risk difference about 3 percent during the year). Second, aspirin had no safety advantage over the regimens of rivaroxaban. Taken together with the results of the AMPLIFY Extension trial,[89] which showed that 2.5 mg of apixaban daily did not increase major bleeding compared to placebo, the findings indicate that if extended antithrombotic treatment of VTE is indicated and/or preferred, a DOAC is preferred over aspirin. Aspirin should now have a very limited, if any, role for extended treatment of VTE. Third, two studies using DOACs now indicate that, after an initial 6 to 12 months of anticoagulant treatment, the daily maintenance dose of either apixaban or rivaroxaban can be reduced by 50 percent without loss of efficacy for preventing recurrent VTE. Unfortunately, neither the EINSTEIN CHOICE trial nor the AMPLIFY Extension trial had sufficient statistical power to determine whether the reduced dose of DOAC achieves an important reduction in nonmajor clinically important bleeding.

Oral anticoagulant treatment should be given indefinitely for most patients with a second episode of unprovoked VTE,[57,58,92] because stopping treatment at 3 to 6 months in these patients results in a high incidence (21 percent) of recurrent VTE during the following 4 years.[92] The risk of recurrent thromboembolism during the 4-year follow-up was reduced by 87 percent (from 21 percent to 3 percent) by continuing anticoagulant treatment[92]; this benefit is partially offset by the risk of bleeding.

### Anticoagulant Therapy of Venous Thromboembolism in Cancer Patients

Use of LMW heparin for long-term treatment of VTE has been evaluated in clinical trials.[71,72,93] The studies indicate that long-term treatment with subcutaneous LMW heparin for 3 to 6 months is at least as effective as, and in cancer patients is more effective than, an oral vitamin K antagonist adjusted to maintain the INR between 2.0 and 3.0. Therefore, patients with VTE associated with concurrent cancer should be treated with LMW heparin for the first 3 to 6 months of long-term treatment.[9,57,58] The patients then should receive anticoagulation indefinitely or until the cancer resolves. The regimens of LMW heparin that are established as effective for long-term treatment are dalteparin 200 U/kg once daily for 1 month, followed by 150 U/kg daily thereafter, or tinzaparin 175 U/kg once daily.

### Anticoagulant Therapy During Pregnancy

LMW heparin and adjusted-dose subcutaneous heparin are the options for anticoagulant therapy of pregnant patients with VTE.[94–96] LMW heparin is preferred because it has the safety advantages of causing less thrombocytopenia and probably less osteoporosis than unfractionated heparin. An additional advantage is that LMW heparin is effective when

given once daily, whereas unfractionated heparin requires twice-daily injection. A study indicates no major change in the peak anti–factor Xa levels over the course of pregnancy in most patients treated with a once-daily therapeutic LMW heparin regimen (tinzaparin 175 U/kg).[96] Measurement of the anti–factor Xa level may provide reassurance that major drug accumulation is not occurring. However, the appropriate dose adjustments in response to a decreased anti–factor Xa level are uncertain. The DOACs have not been evaluated in pregnant patients. Evidence-based guidelines for antithrombotic therapy during pregnancy are available.[94]

### Side Effects of Anticoagulant Therapy

**Bleeding** Bleeding is the most common side effect of anticoagulant therapy. Bleeding can be classified as major or clinically relevant nonmajor according to standardized international criteria. *Major bleeding* is defined as clinically overt bleeding resulting in a decline of hemoglobin of at least 2 g/dL, transfusion of at least 2 U of packed red cells, or bleeding that is retroperitoneal or intracranial or occurs into other critical spaces. The rates of major bleeding in contemporary clinical trials of initial therapy with intravenous heparin, LMW heparin, or fondaparinux are 1 to 2 percent.[65,66,73–78] Patients at increased risk of major bleeding are those who have undergone surgery or experienced trauma within the previous 14 days; those with a history of gastrointestinal or intracranial bleeding, peptic ulcer disease, or genitourinary bleeding; and those with miscellaneous conditions predisposing to bleeding, such as thrombocytopenia, liver disease, and multiple invasive lines.

Major bleeding occurs in approximately 1 to 2 percent of patients during the first 3 months of oral anticoagulant treatment using a vitamin K antagonist and in 1 to 3 percent per year of treatment thereafter.[97] A meta-analysis suggests the clinical impact of major bleeding during long-term oral vitamin K antagonist treatment is greater than widely appreciated.[97] The estimated case fatality rate for this major bleeding is 13 percent, and the rate of intracranial bleeding was 1.15 per 100 patient-years. These risks are important considerations in the decision about extended or indefinite anticoagulant therapy in patients with VTE. As noted above, clinical trials of the DOACs and meta-analysis indicate clinically important lower rates of bleeding, including major, intracranial, and fatal bleeding, than the vitamin K antagonists.[73–79]

**Heparin-Induced Thrombocytopenia** (See also Chap. 8.) Heparin or LMW heparin may cause thrombocytopenia. In large clinical studies of acute VTE treatment, thrombocytopenia occurred in less than 1 percent of more than 2000 patients treated with unfractionated heparin or LMW heparin.[66] Nevertheless, heparin-induced thrombocytopenia can be a serious complication when accompanied by extension or recurrence of VTE or the development of arterial thrombosis. Such complications may precede or coincide with the fall in platelet count and are associated with a high rate of limb loss and a high mortality. Heparin in all forms should be discontinued when the diagnosis of heparin-induced thrombocytopenia is made on clinical grounds, and treatment with an alternative anticoagulant, such as danaparoid, bivalirudin, or argatroban, should be initiated. The DOACs have potential to be useful for anticoagulant therapy in patients with heparin-induced thrombocytopenia, but their use has not been evaluated by clinical trials in this patient group.

**Heparin-Induced Osteoporosis** Osteoporosis may occur as a result of long-term treatment with heparin or LMW heparin (usually after more than 3 months). The earliest clinical manifestation of heparin-associated osteoporosis usually is nonspecific low back pain primarily involving the vertebrae or the ribs. Patients also may present with spontaneous fractures. Up to one-third of patients treated with long-term heparin may have subclinical reduction in bone density. Whether these patients are predisposed to future fractures is not known. The incidence of symptomatic osteoporosis in clinical trials of LMW heparin treatment for 3 to 6 months was very low and was not increased compared to warfarin treatment. Patients with osteoporosis or fractures often had other risk factors such as bone metastases.

**Other Side Effects of Heparin** Heparin or LMW heparin may cause elevated liver transaminase levels. These elevations are of unknown clinical significance and usually return to normal after the heparin or LMW heparin is discontinued. Awareness of this biochemical effect is important so as to avoid unnecessary interruption of heparin therapy and unnecessary liver biopsies in patients who may develop elevated transaminase levels during heparin or LMW heparin therapy. Additional rare side effects of heparin include hypersensitivity and skin reactions, such as skin necrosis, alopecia, and hyperkalemia occurring as a result of hypoaldosteronism.

## THROMBOLYTIC THERAPY

Thrombolytic therapy is indicated for patients with PE who present with hypotension or shock and for select patients with PE who have evidence of right ventricular dysfunction and are at high risk of hemodynamic collapse.[30] Thrombolytic therapy provides more rapid lysis of pulmonary emboli and more rapid restoration of right ventricular function and pulmonary perfusion than does anticoagulant treatment.[30,98,99] Effective regimens are 100 mg of recombinant tissue plasminogen activator by intravenous infusion over 2 hours (50 mg/h) or 30 to 50 mg (depending on body weight) of tenecteplase given as a single bolus injection.[98,99] Heparin then is given by continuous infusion once the thrombin time or aPTT is less than twice the control value.[98,99] The starting infusion dose is 1000 U/h. Chapter 25 provides further details of thrombolytic therapy.

The recently reported PEITHO trial[99] evaluated the effectiveness and safety of thrombolysis with tenecteplase followed by anticoagulant therapy compared with anticoagulant therapy alone in 1006 patients with PE and evidence of both right ventricular dysfunction by echocardiography or CT scan and evidence of myocardial injury by the results of troponin I or troponin T measurement. The primary outcome of death or hemodynamic compensation (or collapse) within 7 days occurred in 13 of 506 patients (2.6 percent) given thrombolysis, compared with 28 of 499 (5.6 percent) receiving anticoagulant therapy alone (p = 0.02).[99] Stroke occurred in 12 patients (2.4 percent) in the thrombolysis group, compared with one patient (0.2 percent) in the anticoagulant alone group (p = 0.003). Extracranial bleeding occurred in 32 patients (6.3 percent) given thrombolysis and in six patients (1.2 percent) receiving anticoagulant therapy alone (p <0.001). At day 7, death had occurred in six patients (1.2 percent) given thrombolysis and in nine patients (1.8 percent) given anticoagulant therapy alone; the corresponding rates at day 30 were 2.4 percent and 3.2 percent, respectively.[99] The findings indicate thrombolytic therapy prevented hemodynamic decompensation, but increased the risk of major bleeding and stroke. The study was not large enough to resolve the key question of whether thrombolysis will improve survival. At present, the risk of thrombolysis outweighs the benefit for most patients with PE who do not have hypotension but who do have evidence of right ventricular dysfunction. Further trials are needed in this group of patients.

The role of thrombolytic therapy in patients with DVT is limited. Thrombolytic therapy may be indicated in patients with acute massive proximal vein thrombosis (phlegmasia cerulea dolens with impending venous gangrene) or in occasional patients with extensive iliofemoral vein thrombosis who have severe symptoms because of venous outflow obstruction. Thrombolytic therapy can be given by systemic infusion or catheter-directed infusion. Catheter-directed thrombolysis (CDT) may be effective for reducing the incidence or severity of the postthrombotic syndrome.[100] Although it was hoped that the catheter-directed approach might be associated with a lower risk of major bleeding, particularly intracranial bleeding, than systemic injection, comparative effectiveness research data suggest the risks of bleeding still outweigh the benefits of this approach.[101] From a national database of more than 90,000 patients with a principal diagnosis of proximal DVT or thrombosis involving the vena cava, the outcomes of the 3600 patients who received CDT with a similar number of propensity-matched patients treated with anticoagulation alone were compared. The CDT patients were more likely to have intracranial bleeding (0.9 percent vs. 0.3 percent) and transfusion (11.1 percent vs. 6.5 percent) and more likely to have filter placement (34.8 percent vs. 15.6 percent) and to experience PE (17.9 percent vs. 11.4 percent).[101] The important message from this analysis of CDT use in practice is that the rate of intracranial bleeding is appreciable (0.9 percent) and not sufficiently low to recommend the routine use of CDT for DVT.

The effectiveness and safety of pharmacomechanical catheter-directed thrombolysis (PCDT) was evaluated in a recently reported randomized trial.[101a] The ATTRACT study compared the use of PCDT in addition to standard therapy (anticoagulation and compression) with standard therapy alone in 692 patients with proximal DVT. The primary outcome was the cumulative incidence of the postthrombotic syndrome between 6 and 24 months after randomization. The incidence of this outcome was 46.7 percent in the 337 patients who received PCDT and 48.2 percent in the 335 patients in the standard therapy group. The respective incidences of moderate to severe postthrombotic syndrome were 17.9 percent and 23.7 percent (p = 0.035); this difference was confined to the patients who entered the study with iliofemoral DVT. There was a trend toward more recurrent VTE in the PCDT group (12.5 percent) compared with the standard therapy group (8.5 percent; p = 0.09). Major bleeding within 10 days occurred in 1.7 percent of patients in the PCDT group and in 0.3 percent of patients in the standard therapy group (p = 0.049); none of these major bleeds were intracranial or fatal.[101a] Leg pain and leg swelling at 10 days and 30 days were significantly improved in the PCDT group.[101a] The ATTRACT study findings indicate that PCDT does not prevent the occurrence of the postthrombotic syndrome, but does reduce early DVT symptoms of pain and swelling and the severity of the postthrombotic syndrome in patients with iliofemoral DVT. This benefit is significantly offset by an increased risk of major bleeding, consistent with the findings of data from routine clinical practice,[101] and probably also by an increased risk of recurrent VTE.

In conclusion, the available evidence indicates that PCDT should have a limited role in the care of patients with DVT, such as the occasional patient with iliofemoral DVT and persistent venous outflow obstruction in whom limb viability is threatened or in whom leg symptoms persist or worsen.

## INFERIOR VENA CAVA FILTER

Insertion of an inferior vena cava filter is indicated for patients with acute VTE and an absolute contraindication to anticoagulant therapy and also indicated for the rare patients who have objectively documented recurrent VTE during adequate anticoagulant therapy.

Insertion of a vena cava filter is effective for preventing PE. However, use of a permanent filter results in an increased incidence of recurrent DVT 1 to 2 years after insertion (increase in cumulative incidence at 2 years increases from 12 percent to 21 percent).[102] Therefore, if the indication for filter placement is transient, such as a contraindication to anticoagulation as the result of a temporary high risk of bleeding, a retrievable vena cava filter should be used. A retrievable filter can then be removed in the several weeks to months later, once the filter is no longer required. If a permanent filter is placed, long-term anticoagulant treatment should be given as soon as safely possible to prevent morbidity from recurrent DVT.

# REFERENCES

1. Moser KM, Lemoine JR: Is embolic risk conditioned by localization of deep venous thrombosis? *Ann Intern Med* 94:439, 1981.

2. Prandoni P, Polistena P, Bernardi E, et al: Upper-extremity deep vein thrombosis. Risk factors, diagnosis, and complications. *Arch Intern Med* 157:57, 1997.

3. ISTH Steering Committee for World Thrombosis Day: Thrombosis: A major contributor to the global disease burden. *J Thromb Haemost* 12:1580, 2014.

4. Cohen AT, Agnelli G, Anderson FA, et al: VTE Impact Assessment Group in Europe (VITAE): Venous thromboembolism (VTE) in Europe. The number of VTE events and associated morbidity and mortality. *Thromb Haemost* 98:756, 2007.

5. Heit J, Cohen A, Anderson FJ: Estimated annual number of incident and recurrent, fatal and non-fatal venous thromboembolism (VTE) events in the US. *Blood* 106:267A, 2005.

6. Kahn S, Lim W, Dunn AS, et al: American College of Chest Physicians: Prevention of VTE in nonsurgical patients: Antithrombotic Therapy and Prevention of Thrombosis, 9th ed: American College of Chest Physicians Evidence-Based Clinical Practice Guidelines. *Chest* 141(2 Suppl):e195S, 2012.

7. Gould MK, Garcia DA, Wren SM, et al: American College of Chest Physicians: Prevention of VTE in nonorthopedic surgical patients: Antithrombotic Therapy and Prevention of Thrombosis, 9th ed: American College of Chest Physicians Evidence-Based Clinical Practice Guidelines. *Chest* 141(2 Suppl):e227S, 2012.

8. Falck-Yitter Y, Francis CW, Johanson NA, et al: American College of Chest Physicians. Prevention of VTE in orthopedic surgery patients: Antithrombotic Therapy and Prevention of Thrombosis, 9th ed: American College of Chest Physicians Evidence-Based Clinical Practice Guidelines. *Chest* 141(2 Suppl):e278S, 2012.

9. Nicolaides AN, Fareed J, Kakkar AK, et al: Prevention and treatment of venous thromboembolism—International consensus statement. *Int Angiol* 32:111, 2013.

10. Kahn SR, Morrison DR, Cohen JM, et al: Interventions for implementation of thromboprophylaxis in hospitalized medical and surgical patients at risk for venous thromboembolism. *Cochrane Database Syst Rev* 7:CD008201, 2013.

11. Lester W, Freemantle N, Begaj I, et al: Fatal venous thromboembolism associated with hospital admission: A cohort study to assess the impact of a national risk assessment target. *Heart* 99:1734, 2013.

12. Catterick D, Hunt BJ: Impact of the national venous thromboembolism risk assessment tool in secondary care in England: Retrospective population-based database study. *Blood Coagul Fibrinolysis* 25:571, 2014.

12a. ISTH Steering Committee for World Thrombosis Day: Venous thromboembolism: A call for risk assessment in all hospitalized patients. *Thromb Haemost* 116:777–779, 2016.

12b. Cohen A, Harrington R, Goldhaber S, et al: Extended thromboprophylaxis with betrixaban in acutely ill medical patients. *N Engl J Med* 375:534–544, 2016.

13. Hull R, Hirsh J, Carter C, et al: Diagnostic value of ventilation-perfusion lung scanning in patients with suspected pulmonary embolism. *Chest* 88:819, 1985.

14. Turkstra F, Kuijer P, van Beck EJ, et al: Diagnostic utility of ultrasonography of leg veins in patients suspected of having pulmonary embolism. *Ann Intern Med* 126:775, 1997.

15. PIOPED Investigators: Value of the ventilation/perfusion scan in acute pulmonary embolism: Results of the Prospective Investigation of Pulmonary Embolism Diagnosis (PIOPED). *JAMA* 263:2753, 1990.

16. Kruip M, Leclercq M, van der Heul C, et al: Diagnostic strategies for excluding pulmonary embolism in clinical outcome studies. A systematic review. *Ann Intern Med* 138:941, 2003.

17. Birdwell BG, Raskob GE, Whitsett TL, et al: The clinical validity of normal compression ultrasonography in outpatients suspected of having deep venous thrombosis. *Ann Intern Med* 128:1, 1998.

18. Stevens S, Elliott CG, Chan K, et al: Withholding anticoagulation after a negative result on Duplex ultrasonography for suspected symptomatic deep venous thrombosis. *Ann Intern Med* 140:985, 2004.

19. Hull R, Hirsh J, Sackett DL, et al: Clinical validity of a negative venogram in patients with clinically suspected venous thrombosis. *Circulation* 64:622, 1981.

20. Rosendaal FR: Risk factors for venous thrombosis: Prevalence, risk and interaction. *Semin Hematol* 34:171, 1997.

21. Heit JA, O'Fallon WM, Peterson TM, et al: Relative impact of risk factors for deep vein thrombosis and pulmonary embolism: A population-based study. *Arch Intern Med* 162:1245, 2002.

22. Bezemer ID, Bare LA, Doggen CJ, et al: Gene variants associated with deep vein thrombosis. *JAMA* 299:1306, 2008.

23. Engbers MJ, Van Hylckama Vlieg A, Rosendaal F: Venous thrombosis in the elderly: Incidence, risk factors, and risk groups. *J Thromb Haemost* 8:2105, 2010.

24. Hull R, Merali T, Mills A, et al: Venous thromboembolism in elderly high-risk medical patients: Time course of events and influence of risk factors. *Clin Appl Thromb Hemost* 19:357, 2013.

25. Simioni P, Prandoni P, Lensing AW, et al: The risk of recurrent venous thromboembolism in patients with an Arg506Gln mutation in the gene for factor V (factor V Leiden). *N Engl J Med* 336:399, 1997.

26. Wells PS, Owen C, Doucette S, et al: Does this patient have deep vein thrombosis? *JAMA* 295:199, 2006.

27. Stein PD, Woodard PK, Weg JG, et al: Diagnostic pathways in acute pulmonary embolism: Recommendations of the PIOPED II Investigators. *Am J Med* 119:1048, 2006.

28. Qaseem A, Snow V, Barry P, et al: Current diagnosis of venous thromboembolism in primary care: A clinical practice guideline from the American Academy of Family Physicians and the American College of Physicians. *Ann Fam Med* 5:57, 2007.

29. Mos IC, Douma RA, Erkens PM, et al: Diagnostic outcome management study in patients with clinically suspected recurrent pulmonary embolism with a structured algorithm. *Thromb Res* 133:1039, 2014.

30. Konstantinides SV, Torbicki A, Agnelli G, et al: Task Force for the Diagnosis and Management of Acute Pulmonary Embolism of the European Society of Cardiology (ESC) endorsed by the European respiratory Society (ERS): 2014 ESC Guidelines on the diagnosis and management of acute pulmonary embolism. *Eur Heart J* 35:3033, 2014.

31. Stein P, Hull RD, Patel K, et al: D-dimer for the exclusion of acute venous thrombosis and pulmonary embolism. A systematic review. *Ann Intern Med* 140:589, 2004.

32. Bernardi E, Prandoni P, Lensing AW, et al: D-dimer testing as an adjunct to ultrasonography in patients with clinically suspected deep-vein thrombosis: Prospective cohort study. *BMJ* 317:1037, 1998.

33. Kearon C, Ginsberg J, Hirsh J: The role of venous ultrasonography in the diagnosis of suspected deep vein thrombosis and pulmonary embolism. *Ann Intern Med* 129:1044, 1998.

34. Bernardi E, Camporese G, Buller HR, et al: Serial 2-point ultrasonography plus D-dimer vs whole-leg color-coded Doppler ultrasonography for diagnosing suspected symptomatic deep vein thrombosis: A randomized controlled trial. *JAMA* 300:1653, 2008.

35. Hull RD, Carter CJ, Jay RM, et al: The diagnosis of acute, recurrent deep-vein thrombosis: A diagnostic challenge. *Circulation* 67:901, 1983.

36. Prandoni P, Cogo A, Bernardi E, et al: A simple ultrasound approach for detection of recurrent proximal-vein thrombosis vein diameter. *Circulation* 88:1730, 1993.

37. Rathbun S, Whitsett T, Raskob G: Negative D-dimer to exclude recurrent deep-vein thrombosis in symptomatic patients. *Ann Intern Med* 141:839, 2004.

38. Ten Cate-Hoek AJ, Prins MH: Management studies using a combination of D-dimer test result and clinical probability to rule out venous thromboembolism: A systematic review. *J Thromb Haemost* 3:2465, 2005.

39. Righini M, Van Es J, Den Exter PL, et al: Age-adjusted D-dimer cutoff levels to rule out pulmonary embolism: The ADJUST-PE study. *JAMA* 311:1117, 2014.

40. Rathbun S, Whitsett T, Raskob G: Sensitivity and specificity of helical computed tomography in the diagnosis of pulmonary embolism: A systematic review. *Ann Intern Med* 132:227, 2000.

41. Patel S, Kazerooni EA, Cascade PN: Pulmonary embolism: Optimization of small pulmonary artery visualization at multi-detector row CT. *Radiology* 227:455, 2003.

42. Perrier A, Roy PM, Sanchez O, et al: Multi-detector row computed tomography in suspected pulmonary embolism. *N Engl J Med* 352:1760, 2005.

43. Stein PD, Fowler SE, Goodman LR, et al: Multi-detector computed tomography for acute pulmonary embolism. *N Engl J Med* 354:2317, 2006.

44. van Belle A, Büller HR, Huisman MV, et al: Effectiveness of managing suspected pulmonary embolism using an algorithm combining clinical probability, D-dimer testing, and computed tomography. *JAMA* 295:172, 2006.

45. Hull R, Raskob G, Coates G, Panju A: Clinical validity of a normal perfusion lung scan in patients with suspected pulmonary embolism. *Chest* 97:23, 1990.

46. Miniati M, Prediletto R, Fornichi B, et al: Accuracy of clinical assessment in the diagnosis of pulmonary embolism. *Am J Respir Crit Care Med* 159:864, 1999.

47. Hull RD, Raskob GE, Ginsberg JS, et al: A noninvasive strategy for the treatment of patients with suspected pulmonary embolism. *Arch Intern Med* 154:289, 1994.

48. Anderson DR, Kahn SR, Rodger MA, et al: Computed tomographic pulmonary angiography vs ventilation-perfusion lung scanning in patients with suspected pulmonary embolism: A randomized controlled trial. *JAMA* 298:2743, 2007.

49. Stein PD, Chenevert TL, Fowler SE, et al: Gadolinium-enhanced magnetic resonance angiography for pulmonary embolism: A multicenter prospective study (PIOPED III). *Ann Intern Med* 152:434, 2010.

50. van Strijen M, de Monye W, Schiereck J, et al: Single-detector helical computed tomography as the primary diagnostic test in suspected pulmonary embolism: A multicenter clinical management study of 510 patients. *Ann Intern Med* 138:307, 2003.

51. Hull R, Delmore T, Genton E, et al: Warfarin sodium versus low-dose heparin in the long-term treatment of venous thrombosis. *N Engl J Med* 301:855, 1979.

52. Prandoni P, Kahn S: Post-thrombotic syndrome: Prevalence, prognostication and need for progress. *Br J Haematol* 145:286, 2009.

53. Prandoni P, Lensing AWA, Cogo A, et al: The long-term clinical course of acute deep venous thrombosis. *Ann Intern Med* 125:1, 1996.

54. Prandoni P, Lensing AW, Prins MH, et al: Below knee elastic compression stockings to prevent the post-thrombotic syndrome: A randomized controlled trial. *Ann Intern Med* 141:249, 2004.

55. Kahn SR, Shapiro S, Wells PS, et al: SOX Trial Investigators: Compression stockings to prevent post-thrombotic syndrome: A randomized placebo-controlled trial. *Lancet* 383:880, 2014.

56. Pengo V, Lensing A, Prins M, et al: Incidence of chronic thromboembolic pulmonary hypertension after pulmonary embolism. *N Engl J Med* 350:2257, 2004.

57. Kearon C, Akl EA, Comerota A, et al: Antithrombotic therapy for VTE disease. Antithrombotic Therapy and Prevention of Thrombosis, 9th ed: American College of Chest Physicians Evidence-based Clinical Practice Guidelines. *Chest* 141(2 Suppl):E419S, 2012.

58. Wells PS, Forgie MA, Rodger MA: Treatment of venous thromboembolism. *JAMA* 311:717, 2014.

58a. Kearon C, Akl E, Ornelas J, et al: Antithrombotic therapy for VTE Disease. CHEST Guideline and Expert Panel Report. *Chest* 149:315–352, 2016.

59. Hull R, Raskob G, Hirsh J, et al: Continuous intravenous heparin compared with intermittent subcutaneous heparin in the initial treatment of proximal vein thrombosis. *N Engl J Med* 315:1109, 1986.

60. Brandjes D, Heijboer H, Buller H, et al: Acenocoumarol and heparin compared with acenocoumarol alone in the initial treatment of proximal-vein thrombosis. *N Engl J Med* 327:1485, 1992.

61. Lagerstedt C, Olsson C, Fagher B, et al: Need for long-term anticoagulant treatment in symptomatic calf-vein thrombosis. *Lancet* 2:515, 1986.

62. Quinlan D, McQuillan A, Eikelboom J: Low-molecular-weight heparin compared with intravenous unfractionated heparin for treatment of pulmonary embolism. *Ann Intern Med* 140:175, 2004.

63. Hull RD, Raskob GE, Brant RF, et al: Relation between the time to achieve the lower limit of the APTT therapeutic range and recurrent venous thromboembolism during heparin treatment for deep vein thrombosis. *Arch Intern Med* 157:2562, 1997.

64. Hull RD, Raskob GE, Brant RF, et al: The importance of initial heparin treatment on long-term clinical outcomes of antithrombotic therapy: The emerging theme of delayed recurrence. *Arch Intern Med* 157:2317, 1997.

65. Buller H, Davidson B, Decousus H, et al: Fondaparinux or enoxaparin for the initial treatment of symptomatic deep venous thrombosis. A randomized trial. *Ann Intern Med* 140:867, 2004.

66. Matisse Investigators: Subcutaneous fondaparinux versus intravenous unfractionated heparin in the initial treatment of pulmonary embolism. *N Engl J Med* 349:1695, 2003.

67. Ridker P, Goldhaber S, Danielson E, et al: Long-term low-intensity warfarin therapy for the prevention of recurrent venous thromboembolism. *N Engl J Med* 348:1425, 2003.

68. Kearon C, Ginsberg J, Kovacs M, et al: Comparison of low-intensity warfarin therapy with conventional intensity warfarin therapy for long-term prevention of recurrent venous thromboembolism. *N Engl J Med* 349:631, 2003.

69. Crowther M, Ginsberg J, Julian J, et al: A comparison of two intensities of warfarin for the prevention of recurrent thrombosis in patients with the antiphospholipid antibody syndrome. *N Engl J Med* 349:1133, 2003.

70. Hull R, Hirsh J, Jay R, et al: Different intensities of oral anticoagulant therapy in the treatment of proximal-vein thrombosis. *N Engl J Med* 307:1676, 1982.

71. Lee A, Levine M, Baker R, et al: Low-molecular-weight heparin versus Coumadin for the prevention of recurrent venous thromboembolism in patients with cancer. *N Engl J Med* 349:146, 2003.

72. Hull R, Pineo G, Brant R, et al: Long-term low-molecular-weight heparin versus usual care in proximal-vein thrombosis patients with cancer. *Am J Med* 119:1062, 2006.

73. Schulman S, Kearon C, Kakkar A, et al: Dabigatran versus warfarin in the treatment of acute venous thromboembolism. *N Engl J Med* 361:2342, 2009.

74. Schulman S, Kakkar AK, Goldhaber SZ, et al: Treatment of acute venous thromboembolism with dabigatran or warfarin and pooled analysis. *Circulation* 129:764, 2014.

75. EINSTEIN Investigators, Bauersachs R, Berkowitz SD, et al: Oral rivaroxaban for symptomatic venous thromboembolism. *N Engl J Med* 363:2499, 2010.

76. EINSTEIN-PE Investigators, Büller HR, Prins MH, et al: Oral rivaroxaban for the treatment of symptomatic pulmonary embolism. *N Engl J Med* 366:1287, 2012.

77. Agnelli G, Buller H, Cohen A, et al: Oral apixaban for the treatment of acute venous thromboembolism. *N Engl J Med* 369:799, 2013.

78. Hokusai-VTE Investigators, Büller HR, Décousus H, et al: Edoxaban versus warfarin for the treatment of symptomatic venous thromboembolism. *N Engl J Med* 369:1406, 2013.

79. van Es N, Coppens M, Schulman S, et al: Direct oral anticoagulants compared with vitamin K antagonists for acute symptomatic venous thromboembolism: Evidence from phase 3 trials. *Blood* 124:1968, 2014.

79a. Pollack C, Reilly P, Eikelboom J, et al: Idarucizumab for dabigatran reversal. *N Engl J Med* 373:511–520, 2015.

80. Kearon C, Akl E: Duration of anticoagulant therapy for deep vein thrombosis and pulmonary embolism. *Blood* 123:1794, 2014.

81. Schulman S, Rhedin A-S, Lindmarker P, et al: A comparison of six weeks with six months of oral anticoagulant therapy after a first episode of venous thromboembolism. *N Engl J Med* 332:1661, 1995.

82. Levine M, Hirsh J, Gent M, et al: Optimal duration of oral anticoagulant therapy: A randomized trial comparing four weeks with three months of warfarin in patients with proximal deep-vein thrombosis. *Thromb Haemost* 74:606, 1995.

83. Prandoni P, Lensing A, Prins M, et al: Residual venous thrombosis as a predictive factor of recurrent venous thromboembolism. *Ann Intern Med* 137:955, 2002.

84. Palareti G, Cosmi B, Vigano D'Angelo S, et al: D-dimer testing to determine the duration of anticoagulant therapy. *N Engl J Med* 355:1780, 2006.

85. Kyrle P, Minar E, Bialonczyk, et al: The risk of recurrent venous thromboembolism in men and women. *N Engl J Med* 350:2558, 2004.

86. Palareti G, Cosmi B, Legnani C et al: D-dimer to guide the duration of anticoagulation in patients with venous thromboembolism: A management study. *Blood* 124:196, 2014.

87. Connors JM. Extended treatment of venous thromboembolism. *N Engl J Med* 368:767–769, 2013.

88. Schulman S, Kearon C, Kakkar A, et al: Extended use of dabigatran, warfarin, or placebo in venous thromboembolism. *N Engl J Med* 368:709, 2013.

89. Agnelli G, Buller H, Cohen A, et al: Apixaban for extended treatment of venous thromboembolism. *N Engl J Med* 368:699, 2013.

90. Becattini C, Agnelli G, Schenone A, et al: Aspirin for preventing the recurrence of venous thromboembolism. *N Engl J Med* 366:1959, 2012.

91. Brighton T, Eikelboom J, Mann K, et al: Low-dose aspirin for preventing recurrent venous thromboembolism. *N Engl J Med* 367:1979, 2012.

91a. Weitz J, Lensing A, Prins M, et al: Rivaroxaban or aspirin for extended treatment of venous thromboembolism. *N Engl J Med* 376:1211–1222, 2017.

92. Schulman S, Granqvist S, Holmström M, et al: The duration of oral anticoagulant therapy after a second episode of venous thromboembolism. *N Engl J Med* 336:393, 1997.

93. Hull R, Pineo G, Brant R, et al: Self-managed long-term low-molecular-weight heparin therapy: The balance of benefits and harms. *Am J Med* 120:72, 2007.

94. Bates S, Greer IA, Middledorp S, et al: VTE, thrombophilia, antithrombotic therapy, and pregnancy: Antithrombotic Therapy and Prevention of Thrombosis, 9th ed: American College of Chest Physicians Evidence-Based Clinical Practice Guidelines. *Chest* 141(2 Suppl):E691S, 2012.

95. Pettila V, Kaaja R, Leinonen P, et al: Thromboprophylaxis with low molecular weight heparin (dalteparin) in pregnancy. *Thromb Res* 96:275, 1999.

96. Smith M, Norris L, Steer P, et al: Tinzaparin sodium for thrombosis treatment and prevention during pregnancy. *Am J Obstet Gynecol* 190:495, 2004.

97. Linkins L, Choi P, Douketis J: Clinical impact of bleeding in patients taking oral anticoagulant therapy for venous thromboembolism. A meta-analysis. *Ann Intern Med* 139:893, 2003.

98. Goldhaber SZ, Haire WD, Feldstein ML, et al: Alteplase versus heparin in acute pulmonary embolism: Randomized trial assessing right-ventricular function and pulmonary perfusion. *Lancet* 341:507, 1993.

99. Meyer G, Vicaut E, Danays T, et al: Fibrinolysis for patients with intermediate-risk pulmonary embolism. *N Engl J Med* 370:1402, 2014.

100. Enden T, Haig Y, Klow NE, et al: CaVenT Study Group: Long-term outcome after additional catheter-directed thrombolysis versus standard treatment for acute iliofemoral deep vein thrombosis (the CaVenT study): A randomized controlled trial. *Lancet* 379:31, 2012.

101. Bashir R, Zack CJ, Zhao H, et al: Comparative outcomes of catheter-directed thrombolysis plus anticoagulation vs anticoagulation alone to treat lower-extremity proximal deep vein thrombosis. *JAMA Intern Med* 174:1494, 2014.

101a. Endovascular Today: 2-Year ATTRACT data: Anticoagulation alone best for most DVT; PCDT benefits seen in certain iliofemoral DVT patients. available at: http://evtoday.com/2017/02/2-year-attract-data-anticoagulation-alone-best-for-most-dvt-pcdt-benefits-seen-in-certain-iliofemoral-patients/

102. Decousus H, Leizorovicz A, Parent F, et al: A clinical trial of vena caval filters in the prevention of pulmonary embolism in patients with proximal deep-vein thrombosis. *N Engl J Med* 338:409, 1998.

# CHAPTER 24

# ATHEROTHROMBOSIS: DISEASE INITIATION, PROGRESSION, AND TREATMENT

Emile R. Mohler III and Andrew I. Schafer

## SUMMARY

The consequences of atherosclerotic vascular disease are the leading cause of morbidity and mortality in the developed countries of the world and are rapidly approaching that status in the developing world. This chapter reviews the pathologic mechanisms of atherosclerotic disease development and progression and details the interaction of these processes with the coagulation system. The earliest morphologically visible lesion of arterial atherosclerosis, the fatty streak, already is an advanced metabolic and immunologic locus that manifests as abnormalities of vascular tone, inflammation, cellular growth, and endothelial cell dysfunction. After years to decades, the lesions advance to form plaques that grow and eventually either impinge on the arterial lumen or rupture. Rupture of a vulnerable plaque is a catastrophic event that, through activation of both platelets and the coagulation cascade, triggers thrombosis, which leads to complete occlusion, and unless collateral circulation has already been established, results in tissue ischemia. Based on an increased understanding of the pathogenesis and consequences of atheromatous plaque development and progression, medical management of atherothrombotic syndromes has improved and is reviewed for the coronary, cerebrovascular, and peripheral arteries.

**Acronyms and Abbreviations:** ACC, American College of Cardiology; ACCF, American College of Cardiology Foundation; ACCP, American College of Chest Physicians; ACS, acute coronary syndrome; AHA, American Heart Association; apo, apolipoprotein; aPTT, activated partial thromboplastin time; CABG, coronary artery bypass graft; CAD, coronary artery disease; CAPRIE, Clopidogrel Versus Aspirin in Patients at Risk of Ischaemic Events; CCL, CC chemokine ligand; CK, creatine kinase; CVD, cardiovascular disease; DAPT, dual antiplatelet therapy; ECG, electrocardiogram; eNOS, endothelial nitric oxide synthase; EPC, endothelial progenitor cell; EV, extracellular vesicle; GP, glycoprotein; HAART, highly active antiretroviral therapy; HDL, high-density lipoprotein; hsCRP, high-sensitivity C-reactive protein; IFN, interferon; Ig, immunoglobulin; IL, interleukin; LDL, low-density lipoprotein; Lp-PLA$_2$, lipoprotein phospholipase A$_2$; MCP, monocyte chemoattractant protein; MHC, major histocompatibility complex; MI, myocardial infarction; NO, nitric oxide; NOX, nicotinamide adenine dinucleotide phosphate oxidase; NSTEMI, non–ST-segment elevation myocardial infarction; PAD, peripheral arterial disease; PAI, plasminogen-activator inhibitor; PCI, percutaneous coronary intervention; RBC, red blood cell; SLE, systemic lupus erythematosus; SNP, single nucleotide polymorphisms; STEMI, ST-segment elevation myocardial infarction; TF, tissue factor; TFPI, tissue factor pathway inhibitor; TGF, transforming growth factor; Th, T helper; t-PA, tissue-type plasminogen activator; VCAM, vascular cell adhesion molecule; VLDL, very-low-density lipoprotein; VWF, von Willebrand factor.

## ● ATHEROSCLEROSIS

Atherothrombosis describes a disease process that begins with atherosclerosis and predisposes to thrombosis in the artery. In the 1850s, Virchow[1] described atherosclerosis as an inflammatory and prothrombotic process. Rokitansky, and later Duguid, posited that atherosclerotic lesions are initiated by incorporation of platelet lipids into the vessel wall ("encrustation") following thrombosis. It was subsequently demonstrated that insudation of plasma lipoproteins is responsible for most of the lipid content of the atherosclerotic lesions. In 1913, Anitschkow noted atherosclerosis developing in rabbits fed a relatively high cholesterol diet. Although the involvement of inflammation in atherosclerosis has been known for more than 100 years, the molecular mechanisms of atherosclerotic disease initiation and progression have become clearer only in the recent past.[2] It is now understood that the classical disagreement between the "lipid" hypothesis and the "inflammation" hypothesis of atherogenesis can be reconciled because there is direct linkage between cholesterol deposition and arterial inflammation in the process.[3,4]

Lipid accumulation in the arterial intima, termed a *fatty streak*, can occur in adolescents and may progress in paroxysmal fashion to a hemodynamically significant lesion causing arterial insufficiency. Autopsy studies of young soldiers and young trauma victims indicated that occult coronary atherosclerotic plaques are commonly present in healthy individuals in their teens and twenties.[5,6] In addition, intracoronary ultrasonography studies demonstrated the presence of coronary atherosclerosis in 37 percent of healthy heart donors age 20 to 29 years, 60 percent of those age 30 to 39 years, and 85 percent of those older than age 50 years.[7] Several theories are espoused for this propitious condition. One well-recognized theory is the *response to injury hypothesis* whereby the inciting event that predisposes to atherosclerosis is injury to the endothelial lining of the artery. This hypothesis was formulated in animal studies that showed vessel narrowing and intimal thickening after endothelial denudation with angioplasty.[8,9] However, human pathologic studies of early atherosclerotic plaques indicate that endothelium is structurally present but is dysfunctional.[9a] The dysfunctional state of endothelium induces abnormalities in vascular tone, inflammation, growth, and thrombosis. Atherosclerotic risk factors contribute to endothelial dysfunction and promote atherosclerosis. This section describes the mechanisms responsible for endothelial dysfunction and the impact of atherosclerotic risk factors.

### ATHEROSCLEROTIC RISK FACTORS

Increasing age, male gender, and heredity are the major atherosclerotic cardiovascular disease risk factors that cannot be modified (Table 24–1). Abnormal lipids, smoking, improperly controlled hypertension, improperly controlled diabetes mellitus, abdominal obesity, physical inactivity, and psychosocial factors are established risk factors that can be modified, accounting for most of the risk of myocardial infarction worldwide in both sexes and at all ages.[10]

In addition to these traditional risk factors, newer risk factors have been recognized.[11] With the use of highly active antiretroviral therapy (HAART), HIV-infected patients have demonstrated a dramatic overall increase in life expectancy.[12] At the same time, HAART-treated HIV patients also have an increased risk of developing premature cardiovascular disease over time. Both HIV viral proteins and the antiretroviral drugs themselves cause endothelial dysfunction. They activate cell signaling cascades, induce oxidative stress, disturb mitochondrial function, alter gene expression, and impair lipid metabolism in vascular cells, macrophages, and adipocytes.[13,14]

Cardiovascular morbidity and mortality are also recognized to be exceedingly high in patients with chronic renal failure.[15,16] Increased

**TABLE 24–1.** Cardiovascular Risk Factors That Cause Impaired Endothelium-Dependent Vasodilation

Smoking

Dyslipidemia

Hypertension

Diabetes mellitus

Hyperhomocysteinemia

risk of premature atherosclerotic cardiovascular disease in patients on chronic hemodialysis has been known for many years, but recent studies point to an increased risk even at early stages of chronic kidney diseases. Low glomerular filtration rates and/or proteinuria are independently associated with increased rates of cardiovascular disease.[17] Other factors, such as sympathetic overactivity,[18] are likely to contribute to the pathophysiology of cardiac risk in these patients. Among other emerging risk factors is obstructive sleep apnea, in which treatment may improve cardiovascular outcomes.[19] The Framingham Study and others have shown that individuals with higher levels of hemoglobin and hematocrit are at increased risk of cardiovascular disease. Red blood cells (RBCs) promote arterial thrombosis by enhancing platelet accumulation at the site of vascular intimal injury.[19a] In addition to their metabolic effects on enhancing platelet activation (see section on "Platelet Activation" below), RBCs are principal determinants of whole blood viscosity and rheologically narrow the RBC-free zone of flowing blood along the intimal surface, thereby enhancing platelet contact with an injured vessel wall and the growing thrombus at those sites.

## ENDOTHELIAL DYSFUNCTION

Cardiovascular risk factors and abnormal blood rheology are thought to result in endothelial dysfunction that predisposes the aorta and arteries to atherosclerotic plaque development, sparing the arterioles and capillaries (Fig. 24–1). *Endothelial dysfunction* is a term that encompasses perturbations in the diverse physiologic functions of normal arteries, including regulation of vascular tone, inflammation, growth, and preservation of blood fluidity. Lipid accumulation[20] and endothelial dysfunction are intimately connected and seminal to the initiation and progression of atherosclerosis. Endothelial dysfunction occurs early in the development of plaque and is systemic in nature, afflicting vessels throughout the arterial circulation without gross evidence of atherosclerotic plaque formation. Emerging data indicate that proatherosclerotic genes are upregulated and antiatherosclerotic genes are downregulated in areas of turbulent blood flow, as seen at branch points of arteries,[21] resulting in vascular adhesion molecule expression and recruitment of monocytes.[22] The atherosclerotic plaque initially may expand outward rather than inward into the vessel wall, making some significant lesions difficult to visualize by angiography. The components of the mature atherosclerotic lesion include smooth muscle cells, macrophages, T lymphocytes, and calcification, in addition to accumulation of lipoproteins.[23] Neutrophils and mast cells also are implicated in the atherosclerotic process.[22] Later in the process, increased activity of matrix metalloproteinases in the atherosclerotic cap predisposes to plaque rupture or ulceration, resulting in tissue factor (TF) exposure and platelet adhesion, culminating in thrombus formation.[24] The thrombus may undergo endogenous fibrinolysis with plaque healing or become occlusive and produce organ damage (e.g., myocardial infarction [MI]). In severe lesions, lamellar bone, presumably from endochondral

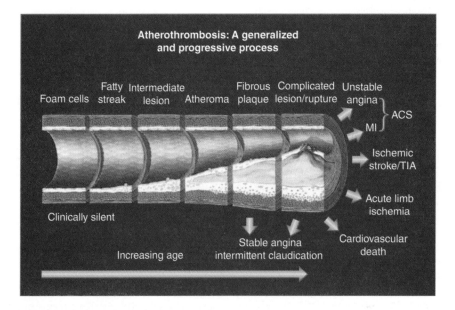

**Figure 24–1.** Schematic showing the life span of the atherosclerotic plaque, beginning with the fatty streak and resulting in a thrombotic event. Cardiovascular risk factors and disturbed blood flow at branch points of vessels are thought to cause endothelial dysfunction that results in atherosclerotic plaque development in the aorta and conduit arteries. Early lipid accumulation in the intimal layer is called the *fatty streak*. A series of stimuli, including lipid peroxidation, are thought to signal adhesion molecule expression on the endothelium, which results in monocyte adhesion and diapedesis into the intimal space. The monocytes develop into macrophages and become sessile with accumulation of lipid (foam cells). Smooth muscle cells, primarily from the media, enter the plaque and participate in cap formation. The plaque accumulates hydroxyapatite mineral and forms calcific deposits. Matrix metalloproteinases also accumulate in the lesion and may predispose to plaque rupture or ulceration, resulting in tissue factor exposure and thrombus formation. Risk factor modification favors a more stable plaque, which may have relatively less lipid accumulation and more sclerotic tissue than an unstable plaque. Severe lesions may even develop lamellar bone. ACS, acute coronary syndrome; MI, myocardial infarction; TIA, transient ischemic attack.

calcification, may appear.[25] There is evolving evidence that extracellular vesicles (EVs), also known as microparticles, are involved in the atherosclerotic process.[26] The following sections describe in detail the major manifestations of endothelial dysfunction that occur early in the atherosclerotic process.

## Abnormal Vascular Tone

The importance of the endothelium in maintaining vascular tone was first recognized when endothelial cells of rabbit aorta were inadvertently removed and resulted in paradoxical vasoconstriction after administration of acetylcholine.[27] The major endothelium-dependent vasodilator normally produced was found to be nitric oxide (NO), a free radical gas with multiple physiologic properties,[28] including inhibition of platelet aggregation and inflammation and stimulation of angiogenesis. Numerous studies indicate that the endothelium does not vasodilate appropriately in the setting of traditional and emerging cardiovascular risk factors. Cardiovascular risk factors are thought to reduce NO availability through a variety of mechanisms, including increased oxidative stress, through generation of reactive oxygen species, and in so doing create an environment conducive to development of atherosclerosis.[29] Major sources of reactive oxygen species are nicotinamide adenine dinucleotide phosphate (NADPH) oxidases (NOXs). The catalytic subunits of the NOXs are the NOX proteins and are found in atherosclerotic lesions.[30] A reduction in NO synthesis is thought to occur because of decreased availability of tetrahydrobiopterin, an essential cofactor for synthesis of NO.[31] Administration of sepiapterin, a substrate for tetrahydrobiopterin, improves endothelial dysfunction.[32] Also, recent evidence indicates that the transcription factor p53 and the adaptor protein Shc both play essential roles in impairing endothelium-dependent vascular relaxation.[33] High cholesterol levels are thought to produce oxygen free radicals that may inactivate NO. NO synthases are the enzymes responsible for converting L-arginine to NO (Fig. 24–2) (Chap. 5). The enzyme may be perturbed by modified low-density lipoprotein (LDL), resulting in decreased NO production. Supplementation of the diet with L-arginine leads to improvement in endothelial-dependent vasodilation.[34] Elevated levels of asymmetric dimethylarginine, an endogenous competitive inhibitor of NO synthase, found in patients with hypercholesterolemia and diabetes, also may result in decreased NO availability.[35] Oxidized LDL is thought to increase the elaboration of asymmetric dimethylarginine by endothelial cells and decrease its degradation by the enzyme dimethylarginine dimethylaminohydrolase.[36] Administration of acetylcholine to patients with elevated serum LDL[37] and relatively low high-density lipoprotein (HDL)[38] may result in abnormal vasoconstriction, which can be reversed with nitroglycerin (an endothelium-independent vasodilator).[39] Intravenous infusion of HDL improves endothelial-mediated vasodilation through improved NO availability.[40] The decreased vasodilatory capacity because of dyslipidemia may facilitate the development of coronary ischemia.

Impaired endothelial vasodilation is noted with advanced aging,[41] when the hands are exposed acutely to cold, and during mental stress. The impairment may be mediated by increased production of endothelin, a potent vasoconstrictor.[42] Sex differences are also seen in endothelial function as women in middle age tend to have more endothelial vasodilation than men at any age.[43] Proinflammatory cytokines may induce formation of endothelial-derived EVs, making them a surrogate marker for endothelial dysfunction[44] and a biomarker for cardiovascular events.[45] Infection with concomitant inflammation is associated with impaired endothelial vasodilation. For example, repeated infection with *Chlamydia pneumoniae* results in endothelial dysfunction via impaired NO availability.[46] The combination of coronary artery disease and elevated serum levels of high-sensitivity C-reactive protein (hsCRP) is an independent predictor of abnormal endothelial vasoreactivity.[47] External radiation therapy also results in endothelial dysfunction and may explain the increased risk of atherosclerosis in patients receiving mantle irradiation for Hodgkin lymphoma.[48]

## Endothelial Inflammation

The endothelium does not routinely interact with inflammatory cells but is poised to express adhesion molecules after stimulation with inflammatory mediators. An inflammatory response is thought to begin in the vessel wall after "invasion" of pathogenic lipoproteins.[49] The presence of lipoproteins, especially oxidized LDL, results in expression of adhesion molecules such as vascular cell adhesion molecule (VCAM)-1 on the luminal surface of endothelial cells, leading to adherence of monocytes (Fig. 24–3).[50] Endothelial cell expression of adhesion molecules and accumulation of monocytes can be regarded as endothelial dysfunction because these events may occur in the absence of morphologic changes in the vessel wall. Inflammation may develop without the demonstrable presence of an external microbial pathogen. It is now recognized that diseases with inflammatory component such as psoriasis and systemic lupus erythematosus (SLE) confer an increased risk for atherosclerosis and MI.[51] The complex interactions of inflammation and the endothelium on the initiation and progression of atherosclerosis are reviewed in more detail in "Inflammation and Atherosclerosis" below.

## Abnormal Control of Vascular Growth: Smooth Muscle Cells and Extracellular Matrix

Normal endothelium inhibits vascular smooth muscle cell proliferation.[52] The specific function of vascular smooth muscle cells in atherosclerosis is unclear. However, evidence indicates that, in early atherosclerosis, vascular smooth muscle cells contribute to the development of atheroma through production of proinflammatory mediators such as CC chemokine ligand (CCL) 2 (previously termed *monocyte chemoattractant protein*, or MCP-1) and VCAMs. Although smooth muscle cells primarily play a

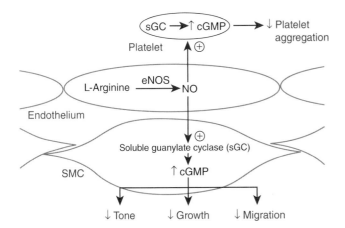

**Figure 24–2.** Vascular tone depends on endothelial production and release of various vasoconstricting and vasodilating substances. The endothelial-derived vasodilators include nitric oxide (NO) and prostacyclin. NO is generated from the amino acid L-arginine by constitutive endothelial NO synthase (eNOS, or NOSIII). The enzyme is stimulated by blood flow across the endothelial surface (shear stress) or by chemical mediators, such as acetylcholine, which stimulate receptors on the endothelial surface. NO diffuses to the underlying smooth muscle cells (SMCs), where it stimulates guanylate cyclase to generate cyclic guanosine V monophosphate (cGMP), which causes smooth muscle relaxation and vasodilation. It also diffuses into blood, where it increases intraplatelet cGMP and thereby inhibits platelet adhesion and aggregation.

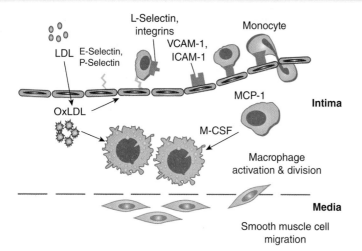

**Figure 24–3.** Atherosclerotic lesion initiation is stimulated by oxidized low-density lipoprotein (OxLDL). Induction of inflammatory gene products in vascular cells is activated by the transcription factor nuclear factor-κB, which results in increased expression of cellular adhesion molecules. The adhesion molecules have specific functions for endothelial leuko-cyte interaction. The selectins tether and trap monocytes and other leukocytes. Vascular cell adhesion molecule-1 (VCAM-1) and intracel-lular adhesion molecule-1 (ICAM-1) mediate firm attachment of these leukocytes to the endothelial layer. OxLDL also augments expression of monocyte chemoattractant protein-1 (MCP-1 or CCL2) and macro-phage colony-stimulating factor (M-CSF). MCP-1 mediates the attrac-tion of monocytes and leukocytes and facilitates diapedesis through the endothelium into the intima. M-CSF is an important cytokine for the transformation of monocytes to macrophage foam cells. Macrophages express scavenger receptors and internalize oxidized low-density lipo-protein (LDL) during their transformation into foam cells. Smooth mus-cle cells migrate from the media into the intima and participate in the formation of a fibrous atheroma. *(Adapted with permission from Kinlay S, Selwyn AP, Libby P: Inflammation, the endothelium, and the acute coronary syndromes, J Cardiovasc Pharmacol 1998;32 Suppl 3:S62–S66.)*

role in modulating vascular tone, they also are involved in the control of extracellular matrix formation and degradation through matrix modula-tors such as proteases, protease inhibitors, matrix proteins, and integrins (Fig. 24–4).

The importance of vascular smooth muscle cells in controlling the synthesis of matrix molecules is evident at the clinical level. They pro-vide a thick, fibrous cap that promotes stability and inhibits plaque rup-ture and ulceration. Factor VII–activating protease, thought to play a role in coagulation and fibrinolysis, is also a potent inhibitor of vascular smooth muscle cell proliferation and migration *in vitro*, and local appli-cation of factor VII–activating protease (but not Marburg I variant) in animal models reduces neointima formation.[53] Furthermore, it has been localized to unstable atherosclerotic plaques and may contribute to plaque instability.

Evidence indicates that vascular smooth muscle cells that undergo apoptosis, especially at the shoulder region of the plaque, may create a more unstable cap.[54] Both intact vascular smooth muscle cells and fibroblasts are thought to stabilize plaques through modulation of extra-cellular calcification and formation of a fibrocalcific plaque.

Vascular smooth muscle cells arise primarily from the medial layer and are considered monoclonal in origin.[55] Evidence also indicates that vascular smooth muscle cells may originate from the adventitia.[56] The rate and timing of smooth muscle cell replication are unclear. It may occur at a constant low rate throughout the development of the

atherosclerotic lesion or episodically at a higher rate. Animal studies indicate that new intimal cells may originate from outside the vessel wall from subpopulations of marrow- and non–marrow-derived circu-lating cells.[57] Smooth muscle progenitor cells circulating in blood may contribute to the arterial remodeling that occurs after angioplasty and after bypass graft surgery.[58]

Vascular proliferation and inflammation are linked processes. Inflammation-induced impaired NO bioactivity contributes to vascular smooth muscle proliferation.[2] Overexpression of NO synthase results in reduction of atherosclerotic or restenotic lesion formation in rabbits through both inhibition of vascular smooth muscle cell proliferation and inhibition of adhesion and chemoattractant molecule expression, with subsequent reduction of vascular mononuclear cell infiltration.[59] Thus, the vascular smooth muscle cell participates in the atherosclerotic process by affecting lipoprotein retention, modulating inflammation, and controlling plaque stability through formation of the fibrous cap. Several vascular disorders involve vascular smooth muscle proliferation as the primary pathophysiologic mechanism, including in-stent rest-enosis, transplant vasculopathy, and vein bypass graft failure.[60] The con-trol of smooth muscle proliferation is thought to involve NR4A nuclear receptors that are expressed in atherosclerotic lesion macrophages, smooth muscle cells, and endothelial cells, and are induced by athero-genic stimuli. Inhibition of the transcriptional activity of the NR4A nuclear receptors results in enhanced smooth muscle proliferation.[61] The NR4A nuclear receptors are also expressed in vein segments exposed to arterial pressure, and it is postulated that they are responsible for an inhibitory feedback mechanism that occurs in activated vascular cells. Drug-eluting vascular stents that release agents such as sirolimus and paclitaxel interfere with the cell cycle and inhibit restenosis in part via decreased smooth muscle cell proliferation.[62]

### Abnormal Endothelial Control of Blood Fluidity

Endothelial cells normally elaborate a number of antithrombotic sub-stances. Some of these substances are released into blood, whereas others are properties of the unactivated endothelial cell surface. These antiplate-let, anticoagulant, and profibrinolytic activities of endothelium, some of which also possess vasodilatory properties (e.g., prostacyclin, NO), act in concert to promote blood fluidity under normal circumstances. Acute activation or chronic dysfunction of endothelial cells alters the hemo-static balance, transforming them from predominantly antithrombotic to prothrombotic cells.[63]

To this end, endothelial cells modulate the activities of thrombin in health and disease. In the presence of intact and normally func-tioning endothelium, the prothrombotic actions of thrombin are quenched and the antithrombotic actions of the enzyme predominate. Thrombin binds to thrombomodulin, an integral membrane protein expressed by endothelial cells, and activates protein C (accelerated in the presence of endothelial protein C receptor, another endothelial cell protein) (Chap. 6). Activated protein C, in concert with its cofactor, protein S, has anticoagulant and profibrinolytic actions. It degrades by proteolytic digestion factors Va and VIIIa and inactivates plasminogen-activator inhibitor (PAI)-1. Simultaneously, by binding to thrombo-modulin, enzymatically active procoagulant thrombin is removed from the circulation, thereby limiting its availability to catalyze fibrin forma-tion. Endothelial dysfunction causes loss of thrombomodulin activity from the vascular surface. In fact, increased circulating plasma levels of free (truncated) thrombomodulin represent a marker of endothe-lial damage. In addition to the role of thrombomodulin in clearance of circulating thrombin, the procoagulant activity of thrombin is nor-mally blocked by endothelial cells through the action of antithrombin, which binds to heparin-like glycosaminoglycans on their luminal sur-face, thereby catalyzing the inactivation of thrombin by antithrombin.

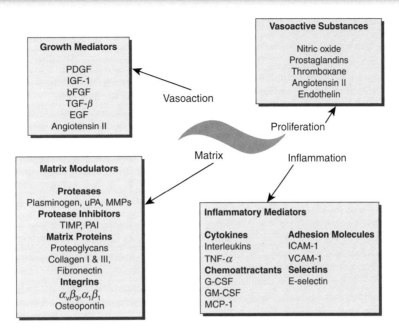

**Figure 24–4.** Vascular smooth muscle cells mediate vascular proliferation, inflammation, matrix composition, and contraction. Many of these mediators have multiple functions. For example, angiotensin is a vasoconstrictor, but it also stimulates proliferation and inflammation. This is only a partial list of mediators secreted by vascular smooth muscle cells. bFGF, basic fibroblast growth factor; EGF, epidermal growth factor; G-CSF, granulocyte colony-stimulating factor; GM-CSF, granulocyte-monocyte colony-stimulating factor; ICAM, intracellular adhesion molecule; IGF, insulin-like growth factor; MCP, monocyte chemoattractant protein; MMPs, matrix metalloproteinases; PAI, plasminogen-activator inhibitor; PDGF, platelet-derived growth factor; TGF-β, transforming growth factor-β; TIMP, tissue inhibitor of metalloproteinases; TNF, tumor necrosis factor; uPA, urokinase-type plasminogen activator; VCAM, vascular cell adhesion molecule. *(Adapted with permission from Dzau VJ, Braun-Dullaeus RC, Sedding DG. Vascular proliferation and atherosclerosis: new perspectives and therapeutic strategies,* Nat Med *2002 Nov;8(11):1249–1256.)*

Like thrombomodulin, this thrombin-neutralizing action of endothelial heparan sulfate glycosaminoglycans is lost with endothelial dysfunction.

Endothelial cells do not normally express TF, but they do so upon activation by inflammatory cytokines or exposure to endothelium-activating levels of homocysteine or free thrombin. The procoagulant effects of expression of TF by dysfunctional endothelial cells are potentially compounded by the loss of TF pathway inhibitor (TFPI), which normally is synthesized by endothelial cells. Studies show that monocyte-derived EVs (or microparticles) express TF and platelet-derived EVs express phosphatidylserine and thus support coagulation complex formation.[64] There is also evidence that P-selectin on platelets binds to P-selection protein ligand-1 on EVs.[65]

Normal endothelium is profibrinolytic. It synthesizes and releases tissue-type plasminogen activator (t-PA); it possesses binding sites for t-PA and plasminogen to provide a surface for the concentrated assembly of the fibrinolytic complex and thereby enhance local plasmin generation; and it fails to produce significant amounts of PAI-1. This profibrinolytic state is converted to an antifibrinolytic state in the presence of endothelial dysfunction. In activated or dysfunctional endothelium, PAI-1 gene expression and PAI-1 secretion are induced; simultaneously, the profibrinolytic properties of normal endothelium are lost (Chap. 25).

The antithrombotic profile of normal endothelium also manifests through the elaboration of several antiplatelet substances. NO is constitutively released into blood by normal endothelial cells and inhibits platelet adhesion and aggregation by stimulating platelet soluble guanylyl cyclase and raising intraplatelet levels of cyclic guanosine monophosphate (see Fig. 24–2).[66] Physiologic flow and shear forces maintain the activity of endothelial (endothelium-derived) NO synthase (eNOS)[67] under normal circumstances. Vascular cell-derived carbon monoxide, a

product of heme catabolism by heme oxygenase, may have similar antiplatelet activity.[68,69] Prostacyclin (prostaglandin I$_2$) likewise is released basally by normal endothelial cells and inhibits platelet aggregation by inducing platelet adenylyl cyclase and raising intraplatelet levels of cyclic adenosine monophosphate.[70]

NO, carbon monoxide, and prostaglandin I$_2$ are labile autacoids, acting only in the immediate vicinity of their release into blood from endothelial cells. An endothelial surface ecto-adenosine diphosphatase (CD39) also blocks platelet activity by metabolizing and disposing of platelet agonist adenosine diphosphate (ADP).[71] In endothelial dysfunction, these various antiplatelet activities are lost, and endothelial release of von Willebrand factor (VWF) is increased, which promotes platelet adhesion. In the case of NO, oxidative stress in the microenvironment of endothelial dysfunction actually "uncouples" eNOS activity[68,72] to preferentially generate superoxide over NO. Oxygen free radicals bind any remaining available NO to produce the toxic product peroxynitrite. Bioactive NO is further reduced in endothelial dysfunction by the presence of asymmetric dimethylarginine, which competes to block eNOS and limit NO production.[67,73]

### Progenitor Cells and Atherosclerosis

Endothelial progenitor cells (EPCs) are heterogenous in origin and participate in endothelial cell regeneration and neovascularization of ischemic tissue. The mobilization of EPCs from the marrow is stimulated by hypoxia, cytokines such as vascular endothelial growth factor, hormones such as erythropoietin, and statin drugs, whereas mobilization is inhibited in the diabetic state.[74] The role of EPCs in atherosclerosis is unclear as there are conflicting data.[22] A study in apolipoprotein (apo) E–/– mice showed that there is rapid turnover of endothelial cells in atherosclerosis-prone areas and marrow-derived EPCs are recruited to sites of atheroprogression.[75]

## INFLAMMATION AND ATHEROSCLEROSIS

### Innate Immunity and Atherosclerosis

The endothelial response to injury manifests as a chronic inflammatory response that involves both innate and adaptive immunity.[76] Innate immunity provides the first line of defense for the host and involves several cell types, most importantly macrophages and dendritic cells, which express a limited number of highly conserved sensing molecules such as scavenger receptors and toll-like receptors.[76,77] Microbial infection can be detected by pathogen-associated molecular patterns, which are present in bacteria, viruses, and yeasts, but not in mammalian cells, and are recognized by the toll-like receptors.[78] Ligation of a pathogen or other substances containing pathogen-associated molecular patterns (such as lipopolysaccharides, aldehyde-derivatized proteins, mannans, teichoic acids) elicits endocytosis or activation of endothelial cells (e.g., through nuclear factor-$\kappa$B) that results in an inflammatory response.[77,79] Proinflammatory cytokines, such as tumor necrosis factor, nuclear factor-$\kappa$B, and interleukin (IL)-1, magnify the innate inflammatory response.

Innate defense involves soluble factors, such as complement, which is involved in atherosclerotic lesion formation. hsCRP has been found to be an important and independent predictor for cardiovascular events.[80] Natural antibodies that are generated in the absence of known antigen stimulation, mainly immunoglobulin (Ig) M, provide an immediate response against bacteria and viruses but also may be involved in atherosclerosis. For example, innate B lymphocytes, the so-called B1 cells, express a restricted set of germline–encoded antigen receptors that may bind oxidized LDL.

### Adaptive Immunity and Atherosclerosis

Compared to innate immunity, adaptive immunity is slower but more precise.[76] T cells can be activated by dendritic cells and macrophages, whereas most antigens cannot stimulate B cells without assistance from CD4+ T cells, which recognize the peptide–major histocompatibility complex (MHC) complexes on B cells. By genetic recombination, the number of T-cell and B-cell receptors that can be formed is almost unlimited and far exceeds the number of pattern recognition receptors used by the innate immune system. Most CD4+ cells are cytokine-secreting T-helper (Th) cells and express $\alpha\beta$–T-cell receptors, which interact with MHC class II molecules. A smaller number of Th cells express $\gamma\delta$–T-cell receptors, which interact with the nonpolymorphic, nonclassic MHC molecules, CD1, which present certain antigens (particularly lipids and glycolipids). Th cells are classified according to the cytokines they secrete. Th1 cells secrete interferon (IFN)-$\gamma$ and IL-2 and promote cell-mediated immunity. Th2 cells secrete IL-4, IL-5, IL-10, and IL-13, and help B cells produce antibodies. CD8+ T cells are primarily cytotoxic killer cells, although they can secrete cytokines, such as tumor necrosis factor-$\alpha$, IFN-$\gamma$, and lymphotoxin. Some thymus-independent antigens can activate these cells without the help of T cells. Oxidized LDL is considered such an antigen because it expresses multiple copies of oxidation-specific epitopes on a single LDL particle.

### Adhesion Molecules and Atherosclerosis

Monocyte recruitment to inflammatory foci initially involves the expression of endothelial cell selectins, which mediate monocyte rolling on the endothelium (see Fig. 24–3). The rolling phenomenon is followed by a firmer attachment to endothelial cells mediated by integrins. Perhaps the most important of these is VCAM-1, which is upregulated in cultured endothelial cells in the presence of oxidized LDL. The appearance of this molecule before the development of grossly visible atherosclerotic lesions supports oxidized LDL as an initial recruiter of macrophages. The finding of reduced atherosclerosis in VCAM-1–deficient mice further supports the important role of macrophages and VCAM-1 in the pathogenesis of atherosclerosis.[81,82] Other adhesion molecules, such as P-selectin and intracellular cell adhesion molecule-1, also may be involved in monocyte adhesion at sites of lesion formation.[83] The entry of monocytes into the vascular intima leads to their differentiation into resident macrophages. Here they take up cholesterol that has also accumulated in the vascular intima, thereby becoming cholesterol-engorged foam cells.[84] It has been demonstrated that the accumulation of macrophage foam cells in established atherosclerotic lesions actually originates mainly from the proliferation of macrophages within the lesion rather than from the recruitment of circulating monocytes.[85] Platelet-derived EVs contain and deliver the chemokine "regulated upon activation, normal T-cell expressed and secreted" (RANTES) to activate endothelium in atherosclerosis to promote attraction of monocytes.[86]

### Lipoprotein Phospholipase A$_2$ and Atherosclerosis

Lipoprotein phospholipase A$_2$ (Lp-PLA$_2$) is an inflammatory enzyme belonging to the large family of phospholipases that are capable of hydrolyzing the sn-2 ester bond of phospholipids of cell membranes and lipoproteins.[87] This enzyme, produced by macrophages, circulates bound to LDL and in the intimal space of the artery can produce oxidized fatty acids and lysophosphatidyl choline. These molecules have a range of potentially atherogenic effects, including chemoattraction of monocytes, increased expression of adhesion molecules, and inhibition of endothelial NO production.[88] Although originally designated as platelet-activating factor acetylhydrolase because of its ability to degrade platelet-activating factor, the clinical importance of this effect is not thought significant. Numerous epidemiologic studies show that Lp-PLA$_2$ is a significant biomarker associated with cardiovascular events. The selective inhibition of Lp-PLA$_2$ with the drug darapladib reduced development of advanced coronary atherosclerosis in diabetic and hypercholesterolemic swine.[89] A phase II clinical study of patients with cardiovascular disease showed that sustained inhibition of plasma Lp-PLA$_2$ activity with background of intensive atorvastatin therapy resulted in reduction in IL-6 and hsCRP after 12 weeks of darapladib 160 mg, suggesting a possible reduction in inflammatory burden.[90] However, in a prospective double-blind phase III trial of 15,828 patients, darapladib did not reduce the composite end point of cardiovascular death, MI, or stroke. There was a significant reduction in major coronary events and total coronary events.[91]

### Immune Cells and Atherosclerosis

Macrophages are essential for the clearance of modified lipoproteins and the efflux of lipoprotein-derived cholesterol to HDL receptors for reverse cholesterol transport, the process by which HDL removes cholesterol from cells. Multiple lines of evidence indicate that macrophages promote lesion initiation and progression. For example, hypercholesterolemic mice become markedly resistant to atherosclerosis if they are bred to macrophage-deficient animals.[92]

The earliest grossly visible sign of atherosclerosis is the fatty streak, which is composed mainly of macrophage foam cells containing relatively large amounts of cholesterol. Foam cells also can derive from smooth muscle cells, as these cells can express scavenger receptors when appropriately activated.[93,94] Formation of the fatty streak is thought to begin with adherence of circulating monocytes to activated endothelial cells at sites in the arterial system prone to atherosclerotic disease, such as at branch points in vessels. Multiple chemoattractant molecules have been identified in these nascent lesions, which recruit monocytes and induce their diapedesis into the subendothelial space where they further differentiate into macrophages. As noted above, however, more recent evidence indicates that microenvironment-supported macrophage proliferation *in situ* within the atherosclerotic lesion is likewise a key event in atherogenesis.[84]

The chemoattractant CCL2 (MCP-1) facilitates recruitment of monocytes to atherosclerotic lesions, as noted in studies of mouse models of atherosclerosis, such as apoE–/– or LDL receptor (LDLR–/–)–deficient mice fed a Western-style diet. When these mice are crossed to the model lacking CCL2, or its receptor CCR-2, lesion development decreases significantly.[95–97]

Macrophages and T cells were once thought to be the only inflammatory cells to significantly promote angiogenesis. More recent data showing that neutrophils are found at sites of plaque rupture or erosion and in thrombus from patients with acute coronary artery syndromes indicate that they also have an important role in atherothrombosis.[18] Mast cells have been found in the adventitia of lesions and in areas of plaque hemorrhage; they have been implicated in macrophage apoptosis, increased vascular permeability, degradation of HDL, and reduced cholesterol efflux.[22] Neutrophils and mast cells are recruited to atherosclerotic lesions in response to CXC-chemokine receptor 2 (CXCR2) signals. The mobilization of neutrophils to atherosclerotic lesions is inhibited by CXC-chemokine receptor 4 (CXCR4) and its ligand CXC-chemokine ligand 12 (CXCRL12; also known as stromal-derived factor [SDF] 1). A subset of CD31+ T cells, so called T$_{ang}$ cells, was shown to promote endothelial repair and revascularization and to be inversely correlated with age and cardiovascular disease (CVD) risk in patients undergoing coronary angiography.[98]

### Lipid Peroxidation and Atherosclerosis

Macrophages control the amount of cholesterol loading by down-regulating the native LDL receptor. Therefore, knowing how cholesterol is taken up into macrophages is important. Cell culture experiments revealed a "foam cell paradox," in which macrophages engulf only modified lipids. Treatment of native LDL with copper or acetic anhydride (causing acetylation) led to increased LDL uptake through use of the scavenger receptor, leading to the formation of lipid-laden macrophages. These experiments led to the peroxidation theory of atherosclerosis,[94] whereby LDL modification is an essential step in the development of foam cells. Although the precise mechanisms responsible for LDL oxidation remain unclear, enzymes including myeloperoxidase, inducible NO synthase, and NADPH oxidases are involved in the process.[99,100] Of note, macrophages express each of these enzymes, which normally are used as antimicrobial reactive oxygen species essential for innate immunity.[101] Thus, accumulation of cholesterol in the macrophage occurs via scavenger (not LDL) receptors of oxidized (and not native) LDL. Myeloperoxidase is an enzyme thought to cause lipid peroxidation in the intimal space, and circulating levels are associated with adverse clinical outcomes in the setting of acute coronary syndromes and predictive of major adverse cardiovascular events.[99]

### Scavenger Receptors and Atherosclerosis

Conserved pattern recognition receptors expressed by macrophages include scavenger receptors A and B1 and CD36, all of which internalize oxidized LDL.[102,103] Macrophages express various genes in response to oxidized LDL, including peroxisome proliferator-activated receptor-γ and adenosine triphosphate–binding cassette transporter A1, which profoundly influence macrophage-mediated inflammation and atherosclerotic activity.

Cell culture studies indicate that scavenger receptor A recognizes acetylated LDL but, unlike the LDL receptor, is not downregulated in response to increased cholesterol content and thus likely accounts for foam cell formation.[104] However, no evidence indicates that acetyl LDL is generated *in vivo*, indicating other modifications of LDL, such as oxidation, may be required for foam cell formation.[105,106] Another scavenger receptor presumed to be involved in the atherosclerotic process is CD36, a receptor that avidly binds oxidized LDL.

Circulating IgG and IgM antibodies against products of lipid peroxidation are present in the plasma of animals and humans.[107] These antibodies closely correlate with measures of lipid peroxidation and with atherosclerotic progression and regression in murine models.[108] Immunization of hypercholesterolemic rabbits and mice with products of oxidized LDL, such as malonyldialdehyde LDL or copper-oxidized LDL, inhibits the progression of atherosclerotic lesion formation.[109–112] These experiments have been interpreted to indicate that an immunologic response to oxidized LDL components can alter the atherosclerotic process.

Leukocyte-derived 5-lipoxygenase also contributes to atherosclerosis susceptibility in mice.[113] Animal studies indicate the importance of lipoxygenases in atherosclerosis as disruption of the 12,15-lipoxygenase gene diminishes atherosclerosis in apoE-deficient mice, and overexpression of 15-lipoxygenase in vascular endothelium accelerates early atherosclerosis in LDL receptor–deficient mice.[114,115] This enzyme is under study as a potential target to inhibit the atherosclerotic process.[116]

**Gut Microbiome** There are newer data indicating that intestinal microbes are involved in cardiometabolic diseases.[117,117a] Systemic inflammation is activated in the setting of chronic bacterial translocation (secondary to increased intestinal permeability), leading to macrophage influx into adipose tissue and resulting in insulin resistance and nonalcoholic fatty liver disease. The increased inflammation may also be secondary to trimethylamine-*N*-oxide via influx of macrophages and cholesterol accumulation via upregulation of macrophage scavenger receptors and reduction in reverse cholesterol transport. Thus, gut microbiota may accelerate atherosclerosis risk.[117b]

### Accumulation of Low-Density Lipoprotein in the Vascular Wall

Three potential factors lead to accumulation of LDL in the vascular wall: increased permeability of the endothelium, prolonged retention of lipoproteins in the intima, and slow removal of lipoproteins from the vessel wall.[118] Rabbits fed a high-cholesterol diet develop aortic wall lesions at specific lesion-susceptible sites; however, endothelial permeability is not increased at those sites, indicating that LDL is selectively retained in these regions.[119,120] Retention of LDL molecules likely results from their adherence to proteoglycans in the vessel wall.[121] LDL genetically engineered to not bind to proteoglycans is hypothesized to be less atherogenic than native LDL.[20]

Oxidized LDL and its products, oxidized phospholipids and oxysterols, have other properties that make them potentially proatherogenic.[122] These properties include proinflammatory characteristics, such as chemotactic signaling for monocytes, smooth muscle cells, and T lymphocytes (but not for B lymphocytes or neutrophils, neither of which is found in lesions), and increased expression of VCAM-1 on, and stimulation of CCL2 release from, endothelial cells.[123] Oxidized LDL also may contribute to instability of the atherosclerotic plaque via induction of type 1 metalloproteinase expression and increase in TF activity.[124] For oxidized LDL to be a ligand for the scavenger receptor, extensive degradation of the polyunsaturated fatty acid in the sn-2 position of phospholipids by oxidation is essential.

To test the oxidized LDL hypothesis, several clinical studies have been conducted using antioxidant vitamins, most commonly vitamin E; however, most of the completed studies gave negative results.[125,126] At the present time, treatment with vitamin E does not appear to be beneficial in preventing cardiovascular events.

### High-Density Lipoprotein and Atherosclerosis

A low level of HDL cholesterol is a strong predictor of adverse cardiovascular events, presumably because the low level is associated with insufficient reverse cholesterol transport. Animal studies using liver-directed gene transfer of human apoA–apoI resulted in significant promotion of reverse cholesterol transport and regression of preexisting atherosclerotic lesions in LDL receptor–deficient mice.[127,128] The HDL level may not be as important as amount of reverse cholesterol transport. For example, the capacity of HDL to accept cholesterol from macrophages is predictive of atherosclerotic burden.[129] However, HDL has additional antiatherogenic properties that may confer protection against atherosclerosis.[130] For example, HDL is protective against oxidation of LDL, at least in part because of paraoxonase, an enzyme physically associated with HDL that degrades organophosphates.[131] Paraoxonase polymorphisms are associated with increased risk of CVD, also indicating that oxidized LDL is an important factor in atherosclerotic development.[132]

Research studies currently are evaluating novel ways to increase HDL levels or to use apoA–apoI variants and mimetics that hopefully will cause regression of atherosclerosis. So far, initial clinical studies were not successful. Cholesteryl ester transfer protein promotes the transfer of cholesteryl esters from antiatherogenic HDLs to proatherogenic apoB-containing lipoproteins, including very-low-density lipoproteins (VLDLs), VLDL remnants, intermediate-density lipoproteins, and LDLs. A deficiency of this molecule results in increased HDL levels and decreased LDL levels, a lipid profile that is antiatherogenic. A large clinical study in humans showed that inhibition of the transfer protein with torcetrapib increased HDL levels but was associated with increased mortality and hypertension.[133] It is supposed that the increase in mortality was a result of an off-target effect of the drug increasing blood pressure and not because of cholesterol ester transfer protein inhibition. Clinical trials evaluating the effect of other inhibitors of cholesteryl ester transfer protein on atherosclerosis and cardiovascular events have not shown clinical efficacy thus far. Along similar lines, delivery of a mutant form of apoA1 (apoA1 Milano) resulted in regression of plaque size as measured by intravascular ultrasound in a small phase II clinical trial.[134] However, studies evaluating the effect of apoA1 mimetics on atherosclerosis also are have not shown compelling data regarding reducing plaque size or cardiovascular events.[135]

### CD40, CD40 Ligand, and Atherosclerosis

Studies indicate that human atherosclerotic lesions express the immune mediator CD40 and its soluble ligand, sCD40L. Increasing evidence indicates that the CD40–sCD40L signaling pathway plays a central role in several inflammatory processes, including atherosclerosis and graft rejection following transplantation.[136] Interruption of CD40 signaling in hyperlipidemic mice reduces the size of aortic atherosclerotic lesions and their lipid, macrophage, and T-lymphocyte content.[137] Atorvastatin, lovastatin, pravastatin, and simvastatin reduce IFN-γ–induced CD40 expression in a dose-dependent manner. Activation of atheroma-associated cells with human recombinant sCD40L is reduced when cells are treated with statins. In addition, retrospective ex vivo immunostaining of human carotid atherosclerotic lesions of patients treated with simvastatin for more than 3 months revealed less CD40 expression and atheroma-associated cells compared with patients who were not treated with the drug. A reduction in sCD40L is associated with pravastatin or cerivastatin therapy.[138] These findings support the notion that statins are antiinflammatory, in addition to their cholesterol-lowering effects.

### Transforming Growth Factor-β and Atherosclerosis

Transforming growth factor (TGF)-β is a cytokine secreted by macrophages, smooth muscle cells, and the Th3 subset of Th cells that has multiple regulatory functions. TGF-β is speculated to contribute to plaque stabilization because it stimulates collagen synthesis and is fibrogenic. One study found that inhibition of TGF-β signaling by neutralizing antibodies led to a larger plaque size with an unstable phenotype.[139] Further studies are needed to clarify the role of TGF-β in atherosclerotic plaque initiation and growth.

**ABO Blood Type and Cardiovascular Risk** The ABO blood group is determined from presence of A and B antigens on the surface of the red blood cells and is thought to confer cardiovascular risk.[140] These antigens are also expressed on the surface of platelets and the endothelium and consist of terminal carbohydrate molecules, which are synthesized by the sequential action of the ABO glycosyltransferases. Genetic studies showed that carriers of single nucleotide polymorphisms (SNPs) that mark non-O blood group types have higher levels of plasma VWF when compared to O individuals. Epidemiologic and genetic studies show that the non-O blood group is associated with adverse cardiovascular events. One study demonstrated that the SNP rs514659 was associated with coronary artery diseases (CADs) when complicated by MI but not with CAD without MI, suggesting that the primary relationship of ABO to clinical CAD is through modulation of coronary thrombosis or plaque rupture in patients with established coronary atherosclerosis rather than through primary promotion of atherosclerosis per se.

### Infection and Atherosclerosis

Several infectious agents have been implicated as pathogens in atherosclerosis.[141] A well-studied infectious pathogen is C. pneumoniae. Animals infected with this agent develop atherosclerosis, and patients with CVD have higher titers of antibodies against this pathogen. Viruses, such as herpes simplex and cytomegalovirus, also are implicated in human atherosclerotic lesion formation. Gingivitis as a consequence of poor dental hygiene or smoking may lead to cellular immune activation and provoke atherosclerosis by cytokines or antibodies.[142] Endogenous proteins, such as heat shock proteins, also are implicated in atherosclerosis. One study showed that progression of carotid disease correlated with antibodies against heat shock proteins 65 and 60.[143]

### Splenectomy and Atherosclerosis

The relationship between the immune system and atherosclerosis is complex, as evident from an animal study that showed that splenectomy of cholesterol-fed apoE–/– mice led to significantly increased atherosclerosis.[144] This proatherogenic effect was rescued by transfer of either purified B cells or T cells from the spleens of atherosclerotic apoE–/– donors. A long-term study of soldiers who underwent splenectomy after trauma found the soldiers had a twofold increased incidence of CAD, providing evidence that the spleen has antiatherogenic activity.[145] Further studies are needed to determine if splenectomy significantly impacts the atherosclerotic process, and if so, by what mechanism.

### Genetics and Myocardial Infarction

Atherosclerotic disease is a complex human trait involving multiple genes and environmental factors. Through the study of linkage analysis of families and sibling pairs as well as candidate genes and genome-wide association studies, the genetic predisposition to MI is starting to be understood.[146] The clinical importance of this knowledge is the potential identification of markers of disease for risk prediction and potential intervention to lower the risk of atherosclerotic-based cardiovascular events.

The use of genome-wide linkage analyses of families or sib-pairs has identified chromosomal loci linked to or genetic variations in the arachidonic 5-lipoxygenase-activating protein gene (ALOX5AP)[147] and leukotriene A4 hydrolase gene (LTA4H).[148] The genes are both involved in inflammation-related pathway of leukotriene B4 production. Interestingly, a small-molecule inhibitor of ALOX5AP was shown to reduce leukotriene production and plasma levels of C-reactive protein.

Several association studies of unrelated individuals have identified genetic variations that confer susceptibility to atherosclerotic disease and cardiovascular events. Studies using genome-wide linkage analysis identified four SNPs on chromosome 9p21.3 that were associated with MI in white cohorts.[146,149] Other genetic polymorphisms also contribute to increased risk of CVD through a variety of mechanisms.[150]

## ATHEROSCLEROTIC PLAQUE

### Plaque Classification

The American Heart Association classification of atherosclerotic plaques into types I through VIII is based on lesion composition and structure (Fig. 24–5).[23] Types I through III atherosclerotic plaques have foam cells organized in a fatty streak, ranging from those not visible on close examination (type I) to those that are apparent on examination (type III). Types I through III lesions are small and clinically silent, whereas types IV through VI lesions may obstruct the lumen and produce a clinical event. Type IV lesions contain a confluent pool of lipid and in most patients do not cause anginal symptoms because of the ability of the artery to remodel outward. Type V lesions contain a fibromuscular cap resulting from replacement of tissue disrupted by accumulated lipid and hematoma or organized thrombotic deposits. Type VI lesions involve thrombosis that may be either mural or obstructive. Of note, a type IV lesion may develop type VI changes without ever passing through a type V change and accumulating significant fibrous tissue. Plaques that are complex and primarily composed of calcium are type VII lesions or, if fibrous tissue predominates, are type VIII lesions.

### Vulnerable Plaque and the Vulnerable Patient

The pathologic mechanisms responsible for converting chronic coronary atherosclerosis to an acute coronary event result, in part, from *plaque disruption*, a term that was synonymously used with *plaque rupture*.[151,152] The term *vulnerable plaque* was used by Muller and colleagues[153,154] to describe rupture-prone plaques as the underlying cause of most clinical coronary events. The current definition for "vulnerable plaque" includes all thrombosis-prone plaques and those with a high probability of undergoing rapid progression, thus becoming culprit plaques (Fig. 24–6).[155,155a] Criteria for development of the vulnerable plaque have been proposed based on histopathologic study of culprit plaques (Table 24–2).[155] The major criteria involve the presence of active inflammation, a thin cap with large lipid core, endothelial denudation with superficial platelet aggregation, a fissured plaque, and stenosis greater than 90 percent. The minor criteria for a vulnerable plaque include superficial calcified nodule, glistening yellow plaque, intraplaque hemorrhage, endothelial

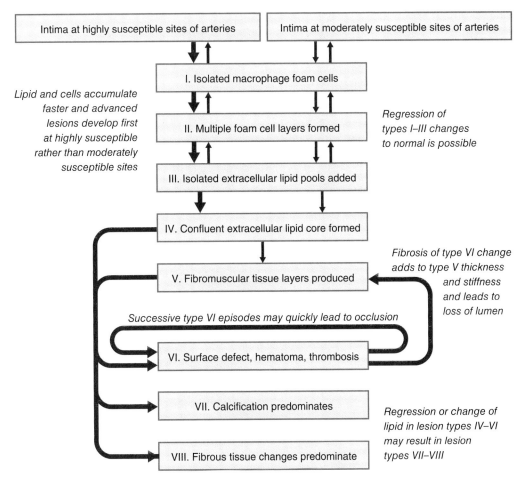

**Figure 24–5.** Flow diagram in *center column* indicates pathways in evolution and progression of human atherosclerotic lesions. *Roman numerals* indicate histologically characteristic types of lesions. The direction of *arrows* indicates sequence in which characteristic morphologies may change. From type I to type IV, changes in lesion morphology occur primarily because of increasing accumulation of lipid. The *loop* between types V and VI illustrates how lesions increase in surfaces. Thrombotic deposits may develop repeatedly over varied time spans in the same location and may be the principal mechanism for gradual occlusion of medium-sized arteries.

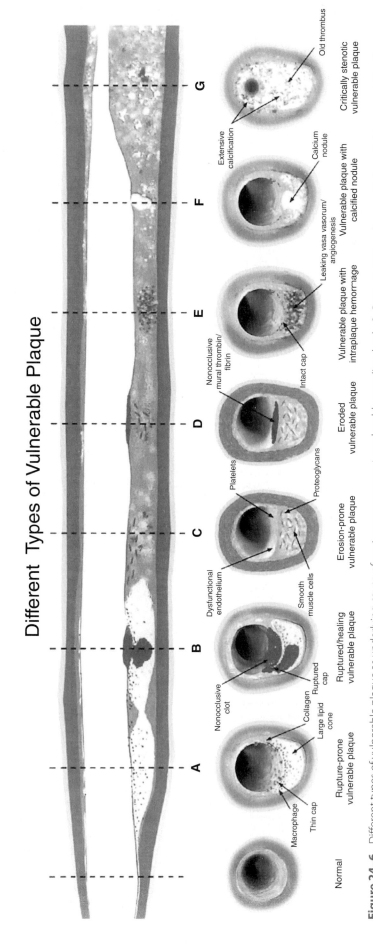

## Different Types of Vulnerable Plaque

**Figure 24–6.** Different types of vulnerable plaque as underlying cause of acute coronary events and sudden cardiac death. **A.** Rupture-prone plaque with large lipid core and thin fibrous cap infiltrated by macrophages. **B.** Ruptured plaque with subocclusive thrombus and early organization. **C.** Erosion-prone plaque with proteoglycan matrix in a smooth muscle cell–rich plaque. **D.** Eroded plaque with subocclusive thrombus. **E.** Intraplaque hemorrhage secondary to leaking vasa vasorum. **F.** Calcific nodule protruding into the vessel lumen. **G.** Chronically stenotic plaque with severe calcification, old thrombus, and eccentric lumen. *(Reproduced with permission from Naghavi M, Libby P, Falk E et al. From vulnerable plaque to vulnerable patient: a call for new definitions and risk assessment strategies: Part I, Circulation 2003 Oct 7;108(14):1664–1672.)*

**TABLE 24–2.** Criteria for Defining the Vulnerable Plaque, Based on the Study of Culprit Plaques

| Major Criteria |
| --- |
| Active inflammation (monocyte/macrophage and sometimes T-cell infiltration) |
| Thin cap with large lipid core |
| Endothelial denudation with superficial platelet aggregation |
| Fissured plaque |
| Stenosis >90% |

| Minor Criteria |
| --- |
| Superficial calcified nodule |
| Glistening yellow |
| Intraplaque hemorrhage |
| Endothelial dysfunction |
| Outward (positive) remodeling |

Reproduced with permission from Naghavi M, Libby P, Falk E et al. From vulnerable plaque to vulnerable patient: a call for new definitions and risk assessment strategies: Part I, *Circulation* 2003 Oct 7; 108(14):1664–1672.

**TABLE 24–3.** Blood Hypercoagulability Factors That May Contribute to Patient Vulnerability to Coronary Heart Disease Events

1. Markers of blood hypercoagulability

   Decreased anticoagulation factors (e.g., proteins C and S and antithrombin)

   Prothrombotic gene polymorphisms (e.g., factor V Leiden, G20210A prothrombin mutation)

   Increased coagulation factors (e.g., fibrinogen, factor VII, factor VIII, von Willebrand factor)

2. Increased platelet activation (e.g., gene polymorphisms of platelet integrin $\alpha_{IIb}\beta_3$, integrin $\alpha_2\beta_1$, glycoprotein Ib/IX)

3. Decreased endogenous fibrinolysis activity (e.g., reduced tissue-type plasminogen activator, increased plasminogen-activator inhibitor [PAI]-1, certain PAI-1 polymorphisms)

4. Other thrombogenic factors (e.g., anticardiolipin antibodies, thrombocytosis, sickle cell disease, polycythemia, diabetes mellitus, hyperhomocysteinemia, hypercholesterolemia)

5. Increased viscosity

6. Transient hypercoagulability (e.g., smoking, dehydration, infection, adrenergic surge, cocaine, estrogens, postprandial)

Data from Naghavi M, Libby P, Falk E et al. From vulnerable plaque to vulnerable patient: a call for new definitions and risk assessment strategies: Part I, *Circulation* 2003 Oct 7;108(14):1664–1672.

dysfunction, and outward (positive) remodeling. Some studies indicate plaques that are heavily calcified and without a significant lipid core are more stable.[25,48]

An important concept concerning plaque remodeling is that atherosclerotic plaques commonly grow outward (positive remodeling) before a luminal stenosis occurs. Therefore, a contrast dye coronary angiogram may underestimate the plaque burden in the vessel. Arterial thrombosis may result from plaque hemorrhage (majority of events) or occur in an area of endothelial denudation (30 to 40 percent) without breach of the intimal space.[156] Thrombosis has also been reported in plaques that have a superficial calcified nodule protruding into the lumen.[156] Most atherosclerotic plaques that underlie a fatal or non-fatal MI are, as shown by angiography, less than 70 percent stenosed.[157] Some patients have more than one vulnerable plaque, which underscores the importance of medical therapy in addition to coronary revascularization.[158] Several technologies are currently being tested to identify the location of the vulnerable plaque.[159] Hopefully these developing technologies will shed more light on the natural history of the vulnerable plaque and afford the ability to conduct studies using local or regional antiatherosclerotic therapy.

Because of the dynamic interaction of atherosclerotic plaque with circulating blood, the term *cardiovascular vulnerable patient* has been proposed to define subjects susceptible to an acute coronary syndrome (ACS) or sudden cardiac death based on atherosclerotic plaque or blood or myocardial vulnerability.[160] The vulnerable (thrombogenic) blood includes serum markers of atherosclerosis and inflammation, such as hsCRP, inflammatory cytokines (e.g., IL-6, sCD40L), EVs, and hypercoagulable factors. The blood markers of vulnerability that reflect the hypercoagulable state include those of the fibrinolytic system and platelets (Table 24–3).[161] Patients may have an MI because of a nonfatal or fatal arrhythmia as a result of coronary atherosclerosis or other non-atherosclerotic disease, such as hypertrophic cardiomyopathy or right ventricular dysplasia. Thus, a vulnerable patient should be considered from the standpoint of the combined presence of a vulnerable atherosclerotic plaque, vulnerable blood (prone to thrombosis), and/or vulnerable myocardium (prone to life-threatening arrhythmia).

## Arterial Thrombosis

*Atherothrombosis* refers to the occurrence of thrombosis upon atherosclerotic lesions,[161] the typical setting for arterial thrombosis. It represents the acute event that converts chronic atherosclerosis—a silent, asymptomatic, progressive disease—into symptomatic, life-threatening clinical complications, including acute MI, stroke, and critical limb ischemia. The previous section described in detail the current concepts of the consecutive stages of atherosclerotic lesion development.

However, thrombosis is not simply the final occlusive event. It also contributes to atherosclerosis lesion development. Intraplaque hemorrhage and *in situ* thrombosis localize thrombin activity within plaques. Thus, atheroma evolution is not only a proliferative process but also involves thrombosis.[162]

## Pathobiology of Arterial Thrombi

Fundamental pathologic and pathophysiologic distinctions exist between arterial and venous thrombi (Table 24–4). Arterial thrombi usually are occlusive in smaller arteries and arterioles. Nonocclusive mural thrombi often occur in the lumina of the heart chambers and large arteries, such as the aorta and the iliac and common carotid arteries. In any arterial vessel, however, thrombi develop almost invariably upon preexisting abnormal intimal surfaces, which typically are atherosclerotic lesions. Less commonly, arterial thrombosis is superimposed on other forms of vascular disease, such as vasculitis or traumatic injury.[163] Thus, in the high-flow and high-pressure arterial system, thrombi form in response to increased local shear forces and exposure of thrombogenic substances on damaged vascular surfaces. Arterial thrombi, referred to as *white thrombi*, are composed mainly of platelets and relatively little fibrin or red cells. Leukocytes are likewise actively recruited into growing, platelet-rich arterial thrombi.[164]

Thus, at sites of atherosclerotic plaque rupture, circulating platelets are activated not only by thrombogenic substances exposed to them by a disrupted plaque but also directly by the locally increased shear forces the platelets encounter.[85] At any given point in the circulation, shear

**TABLE 24–4.** Pathophysiologic Differences Between Arterial and Venous Thrombi

| | Arterial Thrombosis | Venous Thrombosis |
|---|---|---|
| Underlying vasculature | Abnormal<br>• Atherosclerosis<br>• Vasculitis<br>• Trauma | Normal |
| Thrombus pathology | Occlusive or nonocclusive (mural thrombi in large arteries) | Occlusive |
| | "White thrombus" composed mainly of platelets | "Red thrombus" composed mainly of fibrin, red cells |
| Pathophysiology | Local shear stress and thrombogenic vascular surface | Stasis and hypercoagulability |

rates are maximal adjacent to the vessel wall (measured as "wall shear rates"), and they are minimal in the center of the vessel lumen where velocity of flowing blood is the greatest. Normally, wall shear rates are in the range of 300 to 800 $s^{-1}$ in large arteries, and they increase to about 500 to 1600 $s^{-1}$ in arterioles of the microcirculation. However, in pathologically stenotic vessels, the wall shear rates can reach 10,000 $s^{-1}$ or even higher. Increased shear stress in the microenvironment of an atherosclerotic plaque is usually compounded by turbulent blood flow. These locally abnormal hemodynamic forces can directly activate platelets as they pass through the region. Disturbed flow can simultaneously cause localized endothelial dysfunction.[165]

High shear stresses, especially in the presence of marked shear gradients around stenotic sites, are sufficient to cause the release of VWF from endothelial cells and promote the unfolding and binding of VWF to its receptors on platelet surface glycoprotein (GP) Ib–V–IX. This interaction, which does not occur in the normal circulation, mediates the adhesion of platelets to the intimal surface and triggers GPIb–V–IX–dependent platelet thrombus formation. The mechanisms of arterial thrombogenesis are further elaborated below in the section titled "Platelet Activation."

In contrast, wall shear rates are much lower in the venous circulation where the hemodynamic forces are insufficient to directly activate platelets.[166] Venous thrombi are almost always occlusive and may form virtual casts of the vessel in which they arise. Unlike the setting for arterial thrombi, gross vascular damage generally is not found at sites of venous thrombosis. Any ultrastructural abnormalities of adjacent endothelium likely are the consequences rather than the causes of thrombus formation. Therefore, in the low-flow and low-pressure venous system, reduced blood flow (stasis) and systemic activation of the coagulation cascade play the primary pathophysiologic roles. Venous thrombi are composed predominantly of red cells enmeshed in fibrin and contain relatively few platelets; hence, they have been described pathologically as *red thrombi*.

The generalizations described are consistent with the following clinical observations: (1) hereditary hypercoagulable states (also called "thrombophilias"), characterized by chronic hyperactivity of the coagulation system, are primarily associated with venous rather than arterial thrombosis; and (2) anticoagulants that prevent fibrin formation (e.g., heparin, warfarin) are generally used to prevent venous thrombosis, whereas antiplatelet agents (e.g., aspirin) are more effective in preventing arterial thrombosis. The differences between arterial and venous thrombosis are not, however, absolute because both types of thrombi are composed of different amounts of platelets, fibrin, and leukocytes. In addition, all thrombi continually undergo propagation, organization, embolization, lysis, and rethrombosis, and this dynamic remodeling results in their constantly changing compositions.

### Site-Specific Arterial Thrombosis

The model of atherothrombosis described is best characterized in coronary arteries. This pathophysiology may not be entirely applicable to arterial thrombosis at other sites. It cannot be assumed that the local determinants of thrombosis that are operative in the coronary arteries are identical to those encountered in the cerebrovascular and peripheral arterial circulations. Basic regional differences may involve (1) distribution and composition of atherosclerotic lesions, (2) variable local rheology, and (3) underlying vascular cell heterogeneity.

Atherosclerosis is highly localized within the systemic vasculature. Lesion formation particularly affects the carotid artery bifurcation, coronary arteries (especially the left coronary artery bifurcation), abdominal aorta (especially its posterior wall downstream of the renal arteries, but with little disease usually present in the upstream thoracic aorta), and profunda femoral arteries. These lesion-prone sites in the arterial circulation correspond to regions where wall shear stress is very low and may even oscillate between positive and negative directions (i.e., reversal of flow) during the cardiac cycle. A strong correlation exists between local hemodynamic conditions of low shear stress and the development of atherosclerotic plaque formation and intimal thickening.[167–169] However, as arteries become progressively diseased and as stenoses develop at these sites, local hemodynamics change. Stenotic flows are characterized by sharp increases in shear rate that achieve their peak just upstream of the stenosis throat, with development of intensive turbulence downstream of the stenosis. The mechanisms of platelet activation and accumulation that initiate arterial thrombosis at these high-shear sites are further described in "Platelet Activation" below.

Striking heterogeneity is seen in the composition of atherothrombotic plaques, even within the same individual. In addition to plaque composition, the basic structural differences between specific arteries contribute to differences in thrombogenic substrates that are exposed upon arterial injury. For example, carotid and iliac arteries contain relatively more elastic fibers and proportionately fewer smooth muscle cells than coronary arteries.[170] Furthermore, ACSs typically result from disruption of only modestly stenotic, lipid-rich plaques, whereas disruption-prone, high-risk plaques in the carotid arteries usually are severely stenotic. Thus, a proposed more appropriate term is *high-risk plaque* rather than *vulnerable plaque* (which connotes its composition) to define a disruption-prone or thrombosis-prone plaque in different parts of the circulation.[171]

The pathophysiology of arterial thrombosis at different sites in the circulation may also be determined in part by vascular bed-specific heterogeneity of endothelial and smooth muscle cells. Endothelial cell–derived anticoagulant and procoagulant activities are differentially expressed throughout the vascular tree. Endothelial cell heterogeneity throughout the circulation is a function of varying organ- and tissue-specific microenvironments, hemodynamic forces, and site-specific changes in epigenetic footprinting. The heterogeneity of endothelial cells and the vascular bed-specific signaling pathways that control endothelial gene expression have been considered to play an important role in the localization of arterial thrombosis.[172] Heterogeneity of vascular smooth muscle cells likewise exists throughout the arterial tree. They vary in embryonic origin, sources of progenitors, and lineage. With subsequent development, they acquire various phenotypes that can be traced to preferential sites within vessel walls.[173]

Less is known about the pathophysiology of cerebrovascular thrombosis, and even less about peripheral arterial thrombosis, than about coronary artery thrombosis. Future research in these areas should permit the development of more rational antithrombotic strategies in noncoronary artery thrombosis.

### Overview of Arterial Thrombotic Process

Arterial thrombosis typically occurs in the presence of underlying atherosclerosis (hence the term "atherothrombosis"). Less frequently, however, it may also occur in nonatherosclerotic arteries, such as in the setting of vasculitis.

**Atherothrombosis** Disruption of an atherosclerotic plaque triggers an explosive cascade of events that results in the formation of a platelet-rich thrombus at the site of arterial injury.[57] Focal loss of the antithrombotic and the vasodilatory properties of endothelium is compounded by plaque rupture or erosion. These events induce the local activation of platelets and the coagulation system by exposure of blood to previously encrypted thrombogenic substances (e.g., subendothelial cells, such as smooth muscle cells and fibroblasts; subendothelial structures, such as collagen; and subendothelial prothrombotic substances, such as TF, from all of which flowing blood is normally insulated by the barrier of a healthy endothelial monolayer). The local milieu for thrombus formation is aggravated by focal vasoconstriction, rapidly increased shear forces, and platelet-mediated recruitment of leukocytes. Platelet and coagulation activation are inseparable, reciprocally self-amplifying processes. Activation of platelets generates procoagulant properties on their cell surfaces. Combined with non–platelet-dependent local activators of the coagulation cascade, platelet activation culminates in the formation of thrombin, which itself is a potent stimulus for further platelet activation. Superimposed on these local determinants of arterial thrombosis, the thrombotic process may be modulated by systemic, circulating factors. The factors include the systemic state of activation of platelets and coagulation, which may be governed by acquired or genetic factors and by hormonal influences (e.g., adrenergic state).

Arterial thrombi generally are localized to the site of acute vascular injury. They are prevented from extending beyond this site by the restoration of hemostatic balance that promotes blood fluidity along healthy endothelial surfaces immediately adjacent to the site of injury. Thrombus propagation may occur, however, through a bloodborne pool of thrombogenic substances that originate at the site of vascular injury and thrombosis. These substances can be in the form of platelets, leukocytes, red cells, sloughed endothelial cells, other cellular microparticles, and circulating active TF derived from leukocytes activated within the thrombus.[174,175] In fact, cellular microparticles[176] constitute the main reservoir of bloodborne TF, the principal initiator of coagulation.

Thrombus persistence within an artery depends on the local balance between prothrombotic, antithrombotic, and fibrinolytic factors. Ulcerated and thrombotic atherosclerotic plaques, particularly in the aorta, tend to persist or recur.[177] Atherosclerotic plaques of the aortic arch have been detected in almost one-third of patients with cryptogenic stroke. Although aortic arch atheroma are more frequent and more severe causes of cryptogenic stroke in individuals older than 55 years of age, patent foramen ovale (and presumably paradoxical embolism) are more strongly associated with cryptogenic stroke in those younger than 55 years of age.[178]

Advances in the development of coronary stents have created a new form of arterial thrombosis that usually can only be prevented by administration of two different platelet inhibitors (e.g., aspirin in combination with a thienopyridine derivative, such as clopidogrel or prasugrel). Although drug-eluting stents that deliver sirolimus or paclitaxel have been successful in reducing the problem of restenosis that is caused by smooth muscle cell proliferation and intimal hyperplasia following the coronary intervention, they have actually increased the occurrence of "late stent thrombosis" compared to bare metal stents. This form of arterial thrombosis, which typically occurs after discontinuation of (dual) antiplatelet therapy, is probably caused by eluting drugs interfering with endothelialization of the stent surface.[179]

**Thrombosis in Nonatherosclerotic Arteries** Thrombosis may occur in arteries that are affected by vasculitis.[180] As both SLE and atherosclerosis are immune-driven processes, it is to be expected that some patients with active SLE are more susceptible to accelerated atherosclerosis (and related atherothrombosis) resulting from autoantibody-mediated proatherogenic mechanisms.[181,182] However, even in the absence of underlying atherosclerosis, various types of arterial thrombosis can complicate active vasculitis. For example, patients with SLE may have MI with angiographically normal coronary arteries. Giant cell arteritis, which characteristically targets the extracranial carotid and vertebral arteries, leads to inflammation and necrosis of the arterial wall and subsequent arterial occlusions in a distribution that is quite different from that of atherosclerosis. Takayasu arteritis has an unusual predilection for the aortic arch and its branches, leading to panarteritis, medial layer enlargement with luminal narrowing, and sometimes thrombotic occlusion. Other types of vasculitis and autoimmune processes that may cause arterial thrombosis include polyarteritis nodosa, Behçet disease, and antiphospholipid antibody syndrome.

Arterial thrombosis in the absence of atherosclerosis is also seen with immune- and nonimmune disorders of platelets and/or the vascular endothelium, such as heparin-induced thrombocytopenia (with arterial thrombosis most commonly occurring in the aorta, iliofemoral arteries, as well as in cerebral and coronary arteries),[183] and in the myeloproliferative neoplasms (e.g., essential thrombocythemia, polycythemia vera).[184-186]

### Platelet Activation

Disruption of an advanced atherosclerotic plaque results in abrupt exposure of highly thrombogenic material to flowing blood. This process leads locally to both thrombin generation and platelet activation, which operate simultaneously in a mutually self-amplifying process. As noted above in the section on "Pathobiology of Arterial Thrombi," plaque rupture and the development of new intimal surface irregularities also suddenly alter local rheologic characteristics, increasing local shear rates. Increased shear stress resulting from sudden changes in degree of stenosis following rupture is compounded by increased focal vasoconstriction induced by thrombin, thromboxane $A_2$, and other vasoactive substances released in the milieu of acute injury.

At high shear rates ($>1000$ s$^{-1}$), platelets must be initially tethered to the vascular surface through a shear-activated interaction between the platelet membrane GPIb$\alpha$ (of the GPIb–IX–V complex) and its adhesive ligand, VWF.[187-189] Platelet adhesion also involves collagen binding to platelet collagen receptors (integrin $\alpha_2\beta_1$ and GPVI). Other matrix constituents that become exposed to platelets and serve as adhesive ligands include fibronectin, laminin, fibrinogen, and fibrin. These initial adhesive interactions induce intracellular signaling pathways that activate platelets. High shear stress also activates platelets both directly,[190] as noted previously, and by lowering the threshold of platelet activation by chemical agonists to which platelets are simultaneously exposed in the microenvironment of the arterial thrombus.[191] Thus, following adhesion, platelets are explosively activated by several interacting pathways: (1) intracellular signaling initiated by the adhesion event itself, (2) direct action of locally increased shear stress, and (3) agonists released (e.g., ADP, thromboxane $A_2$) and generated (e.g., thrombin) at the site of vascular injury.

Finally, the occlusive arterial platelet thrombus is created by the aggregation of platelets. This process is mediated by several alternative ligands (VWF, fibrinogen, fibronectin) that bind to their activated receptors in the platelet integrin $\alpha_{IIb}\beta_3$ complex. Stability of the platelet aggregate is conferred by additional ligand–receptor interactions, including CD40L binding to integrin $\alpha_{IIb}\beta_3$.[192] Platelet thrombus stabilization is designed to counteract shear forces that promote not only the formation of arterial thrombi but also their embolization.

The importance of the inflammatory component of arterial thrombosis,[164] which is characterized by complex interactions among leukocytes, endothelial cells, and platelets, is increasingly being recognized. Activated platelets recruit leukocytes to the site of vascular damage, promoting their adhesion to endothelium and their activation on endothelium-bound chemokines. In fact, the presence of leukocytosis in myeloproliferative neoplasms is a better predictor of pathologic thrombosis than the platelet count.

### Tissue Factor and Phospholipids

TF is a cell-surface–bound transmembrane protein that normally is not exposed to circulating blood. When expressed, TF initiates coagulation by binding to factor VIIa and activates factors IX and X, thereby triggering the common pathway of coagulation and the formation of thrombin. Strong evidence indicates that TF is the principal thrombogenic factor in the lipid-rich core of atherosclerotic plaques. While much of this TF is associated with monocytes/macrophages and vascular smooth muscle cells, more recent studies suggest that TF-positive microparticles are the most abundant sources of TF in atherosclerotic plaques. The main inhibitor of TF-mediated coagulation is TFPI. In atherosclerotic plaques, TFPI colocalizes with TF and therefore may play an atheroprotective role.[162,193]

Upon rupture of the atherosclerotic plaque, exposure of vascular TF to flowing blood initiates the coagulation cascade. Coagulation reactions are accelerated on the surfaces of activated platelets, microparticles, and on other activated cells in the microenvironment of vascular injury. The surfaces of these activated cells express anionic phospholipids, particularly phosphatidylserine. Apoptotic cells, with which advanced lesions are enriched, likewise translocate phospholipids from the inner to the outer leaflet of the cell membrane.[194] Plasma lipoproteins can provide a phospholipid surface for the assembly of enzymatic complexes of the coagulation cascade; in particular, oxidized LDL, LDL, and VLDL have procoagulant effects.[195,196] In contrast, HDL has multiple antithrombotic actions, including suppression of the coagulation cascade, stimulation of fibrinolysis, and stimulation of endothelial cell release of prostacyclin and NO, which are inhibitors of platelet activation.[197]

Arterial thrombosis is triggered by the acute exposure of circulating blood to TF and anionic phospholipids, leading to explosive thrombin formation. Thrombin, a potent platelet agonist, further fuels the platelet activation process described in the previous section. These reactions create a self-amplifying process that is tightly localized to the site of vascular injury. The arterial thrombus is further contained to this site by the restoration of normal, antithrombotic endothelium in adjacent areas of the vessel wall.

### Systemic Factors

As described above in "Overview of Arterial Thrombotic Process," the pathophysiology of arterial thrombosis is primarily determined by local, "solid-state" factors that operate in concert in the immediate microenvironment of acute vascular injury, typically disruption of an atherosclerotic plaque. However, interindividual differences in systemic, circulating factors can modify susceptibility to the focal formation of an arterial thrombus.[198] Systemic determinants of blood thrombogenicity (i.e., hypercoagulability) can enhance the local risk of arterial thrombosis. There is increasing evidence for an association between venous

and arterial thrombosis, with several studies now showing that patients with venous thromboembolism (deep vein thrombosis and/or pulmonary embolism) are at increased risk of having coexisting asymptomatic atherosclerosis or subsequent symptomatic atherothrombotic events. Conversely, patients with clinically overt atherosclerotic CVD are at increased risk of venous thromboembolism.[199–201] In addition to certain thrombophilic abnormalities, such as antiphospholipid antibody syndrome, hyperhomocysteinemia, and the myeloproliferative neoplasms, which are known to predispose individuals to both venous and arterial thromboembolism, some traditional cardiovascular risk factors (e.g., advanced age, obesity, metabolic syndrome, abnormal lipid profiles, immobility, estrogens) also appear to be independent risk factors for venous thromboembolism.[39,202–204]

Genetic determinants of the coagulation system may exert modifying effects on susceptibility to arterial thrombosis. The known hypercoagulable states that predispose to venous thrombosis (e.g., factor V Leiden, prothrombin gene mutation, antithrombin deficiency, protein C and protein S deficiencies) generally are weakly[205] or not at all associated with increased risk of arterial thrombosis. However, decreased mortality from ischemic heart disease has been noted in patients with hemophilia A or B and even in carriers of hemophilia.[206] This finding most likely results from reduced arterial thrombotic tendency in these individuals because early atherogenesis itself does not appear to be significantly affected by the coexistence of hemophilia.[207] Conversely, some epidemiologic studies have correlated elevated levels of fibrinogen and some other coagulation factors with both subclinical atherosclerosis and clinical cardiovascular events,[208,209] although cause-and-effect relationships between elevated levels of hemostatic factors and cardiovascular risk have not been established.

Several lines of evidence suggest that genetic determinants of increased platelet reactivity likewise enhance focal determinants of arterial thrombosis. Animal models of atherosclerosis in pigs and mice with von Willebrand disease suggest that an extremely low or absent VWF level exerts a protective effect on the development and distribution of atherosclerotic lesions,[210,211] although these observations are inconclusive. Whether or not von Willebrand disease protects against development of human atherosclerosis remains in dispute.

Platelet membrane glycoproteins are highly polymorphic and can be recognized as alloantigens or autoantigens. Polymorphisms in platelet membrane glycoprotein receptors have been considered to increase platelet reactivity, thereby potentially contributing to susceptibility to arterial thrombosis.[212,213] The first such genetic variation reported involves the HPA-1a/HPA-1b polymorphism, which results in a Leu33Pro substitution in the $\beta_3$ subunit of the platelet integrin $\alpha_{IIb}\beta_3$ complex. The 33Pro (HPA-1b) allele was found to be associated with risk of MI in young individuals.[214] Most, but not all, subsequent studies have agreed that the HPA-1b allele represents an inherited risk factor for ACS.[213] Other platelet receptor polymorphisms that have been inconclusively linked to risk of CVD include three different polymorphisms of the integrin $\alpha_{IIb}$ (HPA-3), GPIb gene, and a polymorphism of the collagen receptor integrin $\alpha_2\beta_1$. However, as is the case for the soluble hemostatic factors, lack of a clear relationship among genotype, phenotype, and clinical manifestations has failed to establish convincing cause-and-effect relationships for any of these genetic variations.

Although none of these individual hemostatic proteins or platelet polymorphisms plays a clear, dominant role in the pathophysiology of arterial thrombosis, future application of platelet proteomics[215] and genomics is likely to reveal new disorders of platelet activation associated with arterial thrombosis.

High blood levels of catecholamines likely contribute systemically to localized arterial thrombus formation. Catecholamines may be increased by physical or emotional stress or by cigarette smoking, thereby triggering acute cardiovascular events in these settings. In addition to their vasoactive actions, catecholamines are direct platelet agonists and enhance shear stress–induced platelet activation.[191,216]

Changes in lipid metabolism may exert systemic prothrombotic actions. The thrombogenicity of lipoprotein(a) has been attributed to its structural similarity to plasminogen, leading to reduced plasmin formation and impaired thrombolysis.[163] Elevated LDL cholesterol can contribute to blood hypercoagulability.[217] The prothrombotic state of diabetes involves multiple mechanisms, including platelet hyperreactivity and increased leukocyte procoagulant activity.[177]

# ● ISCHEMIC VASCULAR DISEASE

## MYOCARDIAL INFARCTION

MI is a term that reflects necrosis of cardiac myocytes caused by prolonged ischemia. In the past, MI was defined by the combination of two of three characteristics: typical symptoms (i.e., chest discomfort), a rise in serum enzymatic markers derived from myocardial cells, and a typical electrocardiographic pattern involving the development of Q waves. The advent of sensitive and specific serologic biomarkers and precise imaging techniques has led to the development of revised criteria for MI.[218] For example, patients can be diagnosed with an "ST-segment elevation MI"[219] or "non–Q-wave or non–ST-segment elevation" MI (NSTEMI)[220] if certain criteria are met. The criteria agreed upon by the American College of Cardiology (ACC) for acute, evolving, or recent MI[218] are as follows:

1. Typical rise and gradual fall (troponin) or more rapid rise and fall (creatinine kinase-MB isoform) or biochemical markers of myocardial necrosis with at least one of the following: (A) ischemic symptoms; (B) development of pathologic Q waves on the electrocardiogram (ECG); (C) electrocardiographic changes indicative of ischemia (ST-segment elevation or depression); or (D) coronary artery intervention (e.g., coronary angioplasty).
2. Pathologic findings of an acute MI.

The criteria for established MI[218] (i.e., event that occurred in the past) is any one of the following:

1. Development of new pathologic Q waves on serial ECGs. The patient may or may not remember previous symptoms. Biochemical markers of myocardial necrosis may have normalized, depending on the length of time since the infarct developed.
2. Pathologic findings of a healed or healing MI.

### Clinical Features of Acute Coronary Syndromes

*Stable angina pectoris* is ischemic discomfort symptomatology caused by a narrowed coronary artery that does not allow sufficient oxygen delivery to meet the metabolic demands of the myocardium. *Unstable angina* is defined clinically as a change in the pattern of stable angina to more frequent or more severe symptoms, uninterrupted angina symptoms for 20 minutes or more, or the development of angina at rest. The term *acute coronary syndrome* has evolved as a useful description of the spectrum of patients presenting with angina pectoris caused by unstable angina through MI.[220] The underlying pathologic mechanism for the development of ACS is usually a vulnerable atherosclerotic plaque with either plaque rupture or plaque ulceration leading to thrombosis. Unstable angina and NSTEMI are differentiated by pathologic elevation in the levels of cardiac biomarkers that confirm MI.

Angina pectoris can be associated with other symptoms, such as diaphoresis, dizziness, nausea, clamminess, and fatigue. Some patients with ACS present with atypical symptoms rather than chest pain. The presentation may be dyspnea alone, nausea and/or vomiting, palpitations/syncope, or cardiac arrest. Rarely, patients with diabetes mellitus and other patients have a "silent MI" diagnosed incidentally on ECG or cardiac imaging study.

The initial ECG is often not diagnostic in patients with ACS. In one clinical study, the ECG was not diagnostic in approximately 45 percent and was normal in 20 percent of patients who subsequently were shown to have experienced an acute MI.[221] ST-segment elevation and Q waves are consistent with ST-segment elevation myocardial infarction (STEMI), but other conditions, such as acute pericarditis with early repolarization variant and hypertrophic cardiomyopathy with Q waves, may mimic the ECG manifestations of STEMI.

### Laboratory Features of Acute Myocardial Infarction

A variety of serum biomarkers are used to evaluate patients with suspected acute MI. The three most commonly used tests are (1) troponin I and troponin T, (2) creatine kinase (CK) and its isoform CK-myocardial band (MB), and (3) myoglobin. An elevated serum concentration of one or more of the three biomarkers is seen in almost all patients with acute MI. The preferred biomarkers are the troponins because the troponin assays are more specific than the other tests.

### Therapy for Acute Coronary Syndromes

**Therapy for Acute Myocardial Infarction** The initial management of patients with STEMI depends on prompt recognition and therapy to reduce morbidity and mortality. A carefully coordinated plan of care is essential for optimal results in patients with STEMI, given that multiple therapies usually are initiated simultaneously. The goals of therapy are to reduce ischemic pain, stabilize hemodynamic status, and quickly establish myocardial reperfusion. The ACC Foundation (ACCF)/American Heart Association (AHA) guidelines for management of patients with acute MI were published in 2013.[222] They include specific guidelines for management of STEMI at percutaneous coronary intervention (PCI)-capable as well as non–PCI-capable hospitals.

**Antiplatelet Agents** Unless contraindicated, all patients with acute MI should be given antiplatelet therapy. The Antiplatelet Trialists' Collaboration indicated a 30 percent reduction in vascular events with an absolute benefit of 38 vascular events prevented per 1000 patients at 1 month with antiplatelet therapy.[220] Non–enteric-coated aspirin at a dose of 162 to 325 mg/d or a P2Y$_{12}$ receptor antagonist is commonly used in the setting of MI. The initial dose of aspirin is followed by an indefinite duration daily maintenance dose of 81 to 325 mg.[222,223] The addition of an oral P2Y$_{12}$ inhibitor (clopidogrel, prasugrel, or ticagrelor) to aspirin is recommended for all higher-risk patients. The ACCF/AHA guidelines recommend giving aspirin to patients with STEMI at a dose of 162 to 325 mg before PCI, with continuation of aspirin indefinitely after PCI. In addition, a loading dose of a P2Y$_{12}$ receptor inhibitor should be given as early as possible or at the time of PCI and continued at maintenance doses (clopidogrel 75 mg daily, prasugrel 10 mg daily, or ticagrelor 90 mg twice daily) for 1 year to patients with STEMI who are stented (with a bare metal stent or a drug-eluting stent) during primary PCI. With newer generation drug-eluting stents, more recent evidence suggests that the risk of major hemorrhage with prolonged dual antiplatelet therapy (DAPT) may outweigh its benefits in reducing stent thrombosis,[224] leading to recommendations to individualize the duration of DAPT.[225] Vorapaxar, a protease-activated receptor-1 (PAR-1) antagonist, is indicated for the reduction of thrombotic events in patients with a history of MI or with peripheral artery disease (PAD).[226] Contraindications to antiplatelet therapy include active bleeding, coagulopathy, and severe, untreated hypertension (a relative contraindication). The combination of dipyridamole and aspirin has not been proven to provide incremental clinical benefit over aspirin alone.

Intravenously administered platelet GPIIb/IIIa inhibitors (abciximab, eptifibatide, tirofiban) provide rapid onset of antiplatelet activity in the treatment of ACSs, before PCI, or for management of periprocedural thrombotic complications. However, their antithrombotic effectiveness can be offset by their bleeding risks, so there has been a decline in routine GPIIb/IIIa inhibitor use and an increase in their use as provisional or "bailout" therapy. Meta-analysis of 41 randomized clinical trials of PCI showed that antithrombotic therapy with routine platelet GPIIb/IIIa inhibitor administration was associated with reductions in recurrent MI and major adverse cardiovascular events, but also significantly increased risk of bleeding compared with either heparin or bivalirudin using a provisional GPIIb/IIIa inhibitor strategy. Among the different GPIIb/IIIa inhibitors, high-dose bolus tirofiban was more effective in reducing all-cause mortality and was superior to heparin and eptifibatide.[227]

**β-Adrenergic Blockade**  The control of heart rate with β-adrenergic blocker agents has been efficacious in the setting of acute MI or unstable angina.[222] According to guidelines, oral β-blocker should be initiated during the first 24 hours of care of STEMI. Intravenous administration of β-blockers should be given only to selected, hemodynamically stable patients according to guidelines.

**Management of Chest Pain**  A cornerstone of ischemic pain management has been intravenous nitroglycerin (beginning at 5 to 10 mcg/min) in combination with morphine sulfate if necessary. Nitroglycerin also may improve hypertension and symptoms of heart failure, if present. Intravenous nitroglycerin therapy has not been proven to improve mortality and usually is discontinued within 24 to 48 hours of presentation.[222] Patients who have taken drugs (e.g., sildenafil) for erectile dysfunction within the preceding 24 hours are at increased risk for vasodilation and hypotension, so caution is advised in these patients when intravenous nitroglycerin is given.

**Reperfusion Therapy**  The overriding goal of treatment of STEMI is restoration of myocardial blood flow and salvage of myocardial tissue. Emergency reperfusion of ischemic myocardium that is in the process of becoming infarcted is the primary therapeutic goal.[228] A decision should be made immediately whether the patient will undergo a primary (direct) PCI or receive a fibrinolytic agent. The currently preferred approach is PCI, but the relative advantages and limitations of each therapy should be considered. The most important factor to consider is whether PCI is immediately available. Several randomized trials indicate enhanced survival with PCI compared to fibrinolysis, with a lower rate of early death, intracranial hemorrhage, and recurrent MI.[229,230] Transfer to a center that can provide PCI, if necessary, should be accomplished in less than 2 hours.[231]

At PCI-capable hospitals, patients seen within 12 hours of onset of symptoms of STEMI should undergo prompt primary PCI (angioplasty and stenting), with a goal of revascularization <90 minutes from the time of first medical contact. There has been progressive improvement in outcomes with the evolution of stents from bare metal stents to first-generation and then second-generation drug-eluting stents,[228] with cobalt chromium everolimus-eluting stents currently having the most favorable safety and efficacy profile.[232] To reduce the problem of bleeding at the access site with the traditional transfemoral artery approach to coronary angiography and PCI, radial artery access is being increasingly used.[233] Although it slightly prolongs the procedure time, radial artery access is associated with decreases in major bleeding events and even deaths compared with femoral artery access.[234]

Fibrinolytic therapy should be given immediately if PCI cannot be performed promptly.[219] Prior to fibrinolysis, the patient should be initially assessed for possible contraindications, which include active bleeding, history of cerebrovascular disease, intracranial neoplasm, drug allergy, and trauma. A systolic blood pressure greater than 175 torr

is a relative contraindication but should not prohibit therapy, especially if the pressure can be rapidly controlled. Many different fibrinolytic regimens with different dosing schemes are available. Streptokinase was the first thrombolytic agent tested but has proved less effective than alteplase.[235] In addition, streptokinase is antigenic and can cause an allergic reaction, particularly with repeat administration. Other thrombolytic agents, such as tenecteplase and reteplase, have reportedly similar results compared to alteplase.[236] Tenecteplase is popular on hospital formularies because of its relatively easy single-bolus administration and reported lower rate of noncerebral bleeding.[237]

**Anticoagulation**  Heparin, both unfractionated and low molecular weight, is commonly used in patients with STEMI.[219] The exact role of heparin therapy with different fibrinolytic agents is evolving. Patients who undergo primary PCI usually are given unfractionated heparin 7500 U subcutaneously twice daily or low-molecular-weight heparin, for example, enoxaparin 1 mg/kg twice daily, unless contraindications are evident. For patients receiving intravenous unfractionated heparin, the recommended dose is an initial 60 to 70 U/kg bolus (maximum: 5000 U) followed by 12 to 15 U/kg per hour (maximum: 1000 U/h) as continuous infusion with monitoring of the activated partial thromboplastin time (aPTT) measured at 6 hours. The heparin dose is adjusted to maintain an aPTT between 50 and 75 seconds.

Current guidelines recommend maintaining the aPTT at 50 to 75 seconds for short-term use. Heparin should be continued beyond this period only in the case of high risk of systemic or venous thromboembolism. Patients can be switched to a subcutaneously administered heparin or converted to oral warfarin during the high-risk period. The anticoagulant drugs unfractionated heparin, enoxaparin, fondaparinux, and bivalirudin are all excreted by the kidneys; consequently, although the first dose is usually safe, longer-term therapy should be guided by assessment of creatinine clearance.[223] The Coumadin-Aspirin Reinfarction Study (CARS) did not show a significant benefit with the combination of low-dose warfarin (1 or 3 mg) and aspirin 80 mg daily compared to aspirin 160 mg daily monotherapy on cardiovascular morbidity in patients who had an MI.[238] Subsequent studies have suggested that long-term anticoagulant therapy decreases the risk of cardiovascular events, but it does so at the cost of increased risk of bleeding. At this time, the FDA has not approved the use of novel anticoagulants, such as rivaroxaban, apixaban, or dabigatran, in the treatment of coronary artery disease.[239]

**Statins**  All patients with MI should be started on a 3-hydroxy-3-methylglutaryl-coenzyme A reductase inhibitor (statin) unless the MI was caused by a nonatherosclerotic process such as coronary vasospasm, vasculitis, or embolus. Numerous studies indicate that statins reduce the risk of subsequent MI by approximately 30 to 50 percent.[240] Current evidence suggests that a serum LDL level less than 80 mg/dL with statin treatment is more efficacious in retarding atherosclerotic disease progression than a serum LDL level of 100 mg/dL or above.[241] Other nonstatin drugs, such as ezetimibe, PCSK9 inhibitors, and microsomal triglyceride transfer protein inhibitors, also reduce cholesterol levels but relative reduction in cardiovascular events compared to statins is not yet clear.

**Therapy for Unstable Angina Pectoris and Non–ST-Elevation Myocardial Infarction**  The distinction between unstable angina and NSTEMI initially may be difficult because levels of troponins and/or CK-MB may not be elevated until hours after presentation. Similar to STEMI, the initial treatment of unstable angina and NSTEMI includes supplemental oxygen, pain control, and bed rest.[223] Nitrates, given either intravenously or subcutaneously, are the treatment of choice for angina pectoris. Oral β-blockers also are routinely given to patients with unstable angina to relieve symptoms of angina and to reduce the risk of progression to MI.

Treatment of unstable angina and NSTEMI involves administration of an antiplatelet agent and anticoagulation.[223] For patients with acute coronary syndrome without ST-segment elevation, the urgency and approach to revascularization differ from those of STEMI.[228] Fibrinolytic therapy is not beneficial in these patients, and its use is associated with unacceptably high bleeding risk. Therefore, these patients are triaged to either an invasive strategy or an ischemia-guided strategy.[223] An invasive strategy is favored for most patients because of improved outcomes. However, an ischemia-guided medical strategy is used for patients, especially women, who are at low risk for recurrent ischemia, patients for whom PCI carries excessive risk, or in hospitals where PCI is not available.[226]

Antiplatelet treatment, most commonly aspirin at a dose of 325 mg daily, was shown in the Antithrombotic Trialists' Collaboration study to reduce the combined end point of subsequent nonfatal MI, nonfatal stroke, or vascular death (8.0 percent vs. 13.3 percent) in patients with non–ST-segment elevation ACS.[242] Clinical trials involving patients with non–ST-segment elevation ACS have demonstrated significantly reduced cardiovascular events and mortality with aspirin administration, mostly at a lower dose of 80 to 100 mg orally once per day.[243-245] Some patients do not benefit from aspirin, and this finding has generated an interest as to whether these patients are "aspirin resistant." Nonrandomized studies indicate that aspirin resistance may occur, but because of the limitations of these studies, the definition and prognostic significance of this phenomenon are uncertain.[246]

The thienopyridine clopidogrel (75 mg/d) is effective in reducing the risk of MI and mortality in patients with unstable angina.[220] The combination of aspirin and clopidogrel has been tested in patients with NSTEMI and unstable angina. The combination of these antiplatelet agents resulted in improved survival and decreased progression to MI.[247] The patients with non–ST-segment elevation ACS who underwent PCI benefited the most from the combination of aspirin and clopidogrel.[248] However, the combination was associated with an increase in major bleeding and reoperation for bleeding in patients who underwent coronary artery bypass grafting (CABG). Therefore, a 5-day, but preferably a 7-day, period off clopidogrel is recommended before CABG.[249]

A meta-analysis of randomized clinical trials found that intravenous platelet integrin IIb/IIIa inhibitors substantially benefited patients with non–ST-segment elevation ACS undergoing coronary intervention.[250] The integrin $\alpha_{IIb}\beta_{IIIa}$ receptor antagonist abciximab (ReoPro) is a monoclonal antibody fragment that reduces short-term and long-term clinical events in patients with ACS undergoing angioplasty with or without stent placement. Other platelet integrin $\alpha_{IIb}\beta_{IIIa}$ antagonists, such as tirofiban and eptifibatide, also are effective and safe in treating unstable angina when combined with heparin anticoagulation.[251] Guidelines from an ACC/AHA task force recommend administration of an integrin $\alpha_{IIb}\beta_{IIIa}$ inhibitor, in addition to aspirin and heparin, for patients with unstable angina/NSTEMI undergoing planned PCI.[220]

Unfractionated heparin reduces the rate of MI and death and relieves anginal pain when used in combination with an antiplatelet agent.[220] Intravenous heparin usually is given as a 5000-U bolus followed by continuous infusion. Low-molecular-weight heparins can be substituted for unfractionated heparin. Some studies have shown superior efficacy of low-molecular-weight heparins, but other studies have not indicated a significant difference. Direct thrombin inhibitors, such as hirudin and bivalirudin, have been shown to reduce the rate of death, nonfatal MI, and refractory angina compared to heparin.[252,253] The American College of Chest Physicians (ACCP) recommends lepirudin (recombinant hirudin), argatroban, bivalirudin, or danaproid in patients with a history of heparin-associated thrombocytopenia,[254] although some of these agents are no longer available in the United States.

**Therapy for Stable Angina Pectoris** Patients with stable angina pectoris can be treated with either medical management or revascularization.[255] Limited clinical trial data comparing revascularization, either percutaneous or surgical, to medical therapy are available. The older trials evaluating percutaneous and surgical revascularization were limited by several factors: antiplatelet treatment, angiotensin-converting enzyme inhibitors, and aggressive lipid lowering with statins were not given as background medical therapy of angina. Given these limitations, determining whether revascularization is better than medical management for long-term care of patients with stable angina in modern practice is difficult.

Both PCI and coronary bypass surgery significantly reduce angina. The Coronary Artery Surgery Study (CASS) showed more patients remained symptom-free after CABG compared to medical therapy 5 years after the procedure.[256] At 10 years, however, no significant difference in symptoms was observed. Clinical trials showed significant improvement in angina with PCI compared to medical therapy; however, patients who underwent the former had similar rates of death and MI as those undergoing medical therapy and were less likely to have angina and more likely to have undergone a coronary bypass graft.[257]

Restenosis is a complex process involving inflammation, cellular proliferation, thrombosis, and matrix deposition. Restenosis occurring after PCI may result in flow-limiting luminal narrowing in 20 to 30 percent of therapeutically dilated vessels.[258] Numerous pharmacologic agents, including heparin,[259] have been given in an attempt to reduce the restenosis rate but have met with limited or no success. Intraarterial radiation (brachytherapy) reduces the restenosis rate but is cumbersome to perform because of radiation safety issues and has fallen out of favor. Drug-eluting arterial stents, including the immunosuppressive macrocyclic lactone rapamycin (sirolimus)[260] and the chemotherapeutic agent paclitaxel (Taxol),[261] significantly reduce the rate of restenosis. Because drug-eluting stents were not available at the time of the previous clinical trials, extrapolating the benefits of PCI versus CABG or over medical therapy is difficult. The medical management of patients with stable angina pectoris should include antiplatelet therapy, statin drug treatment, a $\beta$-blocker, an angiotensin-converting enzyme inhibitor, and a long-acting nitrate.

# PERIPHERAL ARTERY DISEASE

PAD is a term that encompasses any arterial disease of the lower extremities, upper extremities, and iliac vessels. It most commonly results from atherosclerosis.[262] Patients who have atherosclerotic disease that compromises blood flow to the extremities may present with exertional pain in a muscle group, called *claudication* (derived from the Latin *claudicare* meaning "to limp"). Claudication is an intermittent but reproducible discomfort of a defined group of muscles that is induced by exercise and relieved with rest.[263] Acute limb ischemia[264] is a relatively rare problem in patients with PAD. In general, it is caused by *in situ* thrombosis or an embolic event from arrhythmias, such as atrial fibrillation, or after manipulation of an artery or aorta with a catheter. Only a minority of patients with claudication (estimated at <10 percent to 15 percent over 5 years or longer) progress to *critical limb ischemia*,[265] which is defined as rest pain and/or foot ulceration that heralds impending tissue loss.

The 5-year mortality rate is estimated to be 30 percent in patients with lower-extremity PAD.[266] Approximately 75 percent of mortality results from a cardiovascular event, such as MI or stroke.[266] The ankle-brachial index is a noninvasive measure of limb vascular pressure in the lower extremities and has been noted in several studies to be predictive of cardiovascular events.[263] However, a decreased index is not just a predictor; it also is a physical finding that indicates significant atherosclerotic plaque burden is present. Other noninvasive imaging studies for PAD include the combination of segmental pressures and pulse volume recordings, duplex Doppler ultrasound, computed tomographic angiography, and magnetic resonance imaging.[267,268]

Medical therapy for patients with PAD includes risk factor modification, antiplatelet therapy, and treatment of claudication symptoms with exercise rehabilitation and possible pharmacologic agents.[269] The risk factors for development of peripheral atherosclerosis include cigarette smoking, diabetes mellitus, hypertension, and dyslipidemia.[270] Aggressive management of risk factors for PAD is recommended to prevent disease progression.[271] Treatment with antiplatelet agents reduces the risk of cardiovascular events, such as MI and stroke, in patients with PAD.[266] The Antithrombotic Trialists' Collaboration evaluated 9214 patients with PAD enrolled in 42 trials and found that use of antiplatelet drugs, such as aspirin 75 to 325 mg/d, resulted in a proportional reduction of 23 percent in serious vascular events.[242] Evaluation of patients with PAD in the Physicians' Health Study found that aspirin 325 mg every other day decreased the need for peripheral artery surgery.[272] However, no difference between the aspirin and placebo groups with regard to development of claudication was observed. Several studies have evaluated the ADP receptor blockers ticlopidine and clopidogrel. Clopidogrel was evaluated in 19,185 patients in the Clopidogrel Versus Aspirin in Patients at Risk of Ischaemic Events (CAPRIE) study.[273] A dose of clopidogrel 75 mg/d had a modest but significant advantage over aspirin 325 mg/d in preventing stroke, MI, and peripheral vascular disease. Subgroup analysis revealed that the patients with PAD benefited the most with clopidogrel treatment. One study evaluating the effect of aspirin, 100 mg, compared to placebo in asymptomatic patients with diabetes mellitus and PAD found no benefit in reducing cardiovascular events.[274] The PAR-1 antagonist, vorapaxar, is approved to prevent cardiovascular events in patients with PAD.[226] The clinical consensus is that antiplatelet therapy should be offered to all patients with PAD unless contraindicated by allergy or comorbidities.[275]

The options for treating claudication symptoms include exercise rehabilitation, pharmacologic agents, and a revascularization procedure. Several studies indicate exercise rehabilitation improves the symptoms of claudication, and a supervised program is better than an unstructured program, and comparable to percutaneous revascularization.[276,277] Two drugs are approved by the FDA for treatment of claudication symptoms: pentoxifylline, a methylxanthine derivative that may improve abnormal red cell deformability and reduce blood viscosity, and cilostazol, a type III phosphodiesterase inhibitor with antiplatelet and vasodilating properties. Cilostazol is generally considered more effective than pentoxifylline for improving walking distance in patients with claudication.[278] However, side effects, including headache, diarrhea, dizziness, and palpitations, can be severe enough to require discontinuation of cilostazol in up to 20 percent of patients.[269] The addition of cilostazol to either aspirin or clopidogrel does not increase the bleeding risk.[279]

A revascularization procedure in patients with stable, intermittent claudication generally is reserved for those with severe lifestyle-limiting symptoms or manifestation of critical limb ischemia despite guideline-directed management and therapy.[269] Revascularization can be performed by either (1) endovascular methods (e.g., angioplasty, stents, and atherectomy), or (2) surgical approaches (e.g., femoral-popliteal bypass). Randomized, controlled trials are ongoing to compare contemporary endovascular and surgical treatments.[269,280]

## CEREBROVASCULAR DISEASE

The etiology of ischemic stroke is multifactorial and can be categorized into embolic, small-vessel disease, large-vessel disease, and cryptogenic. Carotid artery disease accounts for approximately 30 percent of strokes. The distinction between stroke and transient ischemic attack (TIA) has become less important in recent years because many of the preventive approaches are applicable to both and they share pathophysiologic mechanisms.[281] Furthermore, the advent of contemporary imaging modalities has required a revision of the strictly duration-based definition of TIA (i.e., focal neurologic symptoms lasting <24 hours). Imaging now shows that up to one-third of such patients already have an infarction by that time. Major risk factors for developing carotid artery atherosclerosis are hypertension, diabetes, smoking, and dyslipidemia.[282] Emerging risk factors for stroke include hyperhomocysteinemia and an elevated plasma level of lipoprotein(a). An elevated hsCRP level is a risk factor associated with ischemic stroke in both men and women.[283] However, at this time, hsCRP is not routinely measured as an additional marker for increased risk of stroke. A large body of evidence supports a link between migraine and ischemic stroke. However, there is no indication that prevention of migraine reduces stroke risk.[284] Similar to CAD and PAD, control of atherosclerotic risk factors is essential in the primary prevention of stroke in patients with evidence of carotid atherosclerosis and for those who have undergone carotid endarterectomy.

Assessment of eligibility for reperfusion therapy is a critical component of the initial evaluation of acute ischemic stroke.[285] Intravenous thrombolysis with alteplase (tissue plasminogen activator) within 4.5 hours of symptom onset improves patient outcome at 3 to 6 months. More recently, several multicenter, open-label, randomized clinical trials have shown that early intra-arterial treatment with mechanical thrombectomy for large anterior circulation occlusions is superior to intravenous thrombolysis alone in terms of functional neurologic outcomes.[286–290]

Carotid revascularization with endarterectomy or with angioplasty and stenting are established treatments for patients with symptomatic carotid stenosis of >70 percent.[291] However, guidelines for carotid revascularization for asymptomatic carotid stenosis are being reassessed in view of more recent advances in both medical and interventional therapies.[291] Current guidelines acknowledge that the effectiveness of carotid endarterectomy in asymptomatic patients with >70 percent stenosis, compared with best medical management, is not well established, but recommend that it be considered in these individuals if the risk of periprocedural stroke, MI, and death is <3 percent.[292] Over 10 years of follow-up, no significant difference has been found between patients who underwent stenting and those who underwent endarterectomy with respect to the risk of periprocedural stroke, MI, subsequent ipsilateral stroke, and death.[293] Carotid stents with embolic protection[294] and mesh-covered stents[295] are under development for the treatment of carotid atherosclerosis in selective patients.

Two antiplatelet drug regimens are approved for prevention of stroke: clopidogrel (Plavix) and the combination of aspirin 25 mg and dipyridamole 200 mg daily. Approval of clopidogrel is based on the CAPRIE study, which showed a reduction in the combined end point of stroke, MI, and death in patients treated with clopidogrel 75 mg/d compared to those treated with aspirin 325 mg/d.[273] The FDA indication for dipyridamole/aspirin is primarily based on the European Stroke Protection Study 2, which noted a reduction in stroke with the combination of dipyridamole 200 mg and aspirin 25 mg given together (Aggrenox) twice per day.[296] The Prevention Regimen for Effectively Avoiding Second Strokes (PRoFESS) trial was a secondary stroke–prevention trial comparing the combination of aspirin and extended-release dipyridamole (Aggrenox) versus clopidogrel (Plavix) in preventing stroke recurrence after a first event. The difference between the agents was not statistically significant for the primary outcome of recurrent stroke.[297] Fish oil (omega-3 fatty acids) lowers triglycerides and VLDLs and may reduce serum viscosity by lowering fibrinogen. Some studies suggest that fish oil consumption lowers the risk of ischemic stroke. The effect of fish oils on carotid atherosclerosis is unknown.[298]

Warfarin anticoagulation is used instead of antiplatelet agents for the prevention of cardioembolic stroke. The newer direct oral anticoagulants include dabigatran, a direct thrombin inhibitor, and rivaroxaban, apixaban, and edoxaban, direct factor Xa inhibitors. Clinical use of direct oral anticoagulants has provided a promising alternative to warfarin therapy. The direct oral anticoagulants offer a major advantage over warfarin therapy in cardioembolic stroke prevention not only by obviating the need for dose adjustments via blood monitoring and dietary control, but also by decreasing the risk of intracranial hemorrhage.[299]

# ● ATHEROEMBOLISM

*Atheromatous embolism* refers to the dislodgment into the bloodstream of arterial plaque material, including cholesterol crystals ("cholesterol embolism") from ulcerated vascular plaques. The cholesterol embolization syndrome involves systemic microembolism to the end arteries of almost any circulatory bed. Atheroembolism most characteristically originates from lesions in the abdominal aorta and ileofemoral arteries. Cholesterol emboli that lodge in an arteriole incite an acute inflammatory response, followed by a foreign-body reaction, intravascular thrombus formation, endothelial proliferation, and eventually fibrosis. These processes generally result in ischemia that sometimes leads to infarction and necrosis.[300] Mortality rate of clinically diagnosed atheroembolism can be as high as 80 percent, depending on the anatomic location and size of the vascular beds involved.[301]

Patients with atheroembolism, including the cholesterol embolization syndrome, generally have advanced atherosclerosis, often complicated by a history of hypertension, diabetes mellitus, renal failure, or aortic aneurysms. Atherosclerotic plaques can disrupt and embolize spontaneously; however, the clinical syndrome typically is triggered by vascular intervention, including vascular surgery, catheterization, angioplasty, endarterectomy, or angiography. Anticoagulation or thrombolytic therapy may be risk factors with atheroembolism.[301] Clinical presentation depends on the sites of embolization. When these sites involve the distal extremity microcirculation, the "blue toe syndrome" may develop. The syndrome presents with the acute appearance of painful and tender discoloration or mottled blue and patchy appearance of one or more toes that may progress to ulceration and gangrene. Other common cutaneous manifestations are livedo reticularis involving the legs, buttocks, or abdomen, painful nodules, and purpura. Cerebrovascular embolism can cause transient neurologic abnormalities. Cholesterol emboli lodged in retinal arterial bifurcations can be visualized by ophthalmoscopy as bright, refractile, yellow rectangular crystals. Visceral organs most commonly affected by atheroembolism include the kidneys, sometimes causing renal failure, and the gastrointestinal tract, where abdominal pain, ischemic colitis, and bleeding may ensue.

Diagnosis is based on clinical presentation associated with imaging evidence of atherosclerosis of the arterial supply of affected organs.[301] Transient eosinophilia occurs in most cases.[302] Treatment of atheroembolism should include surgical removal or bypass of the source of emboli. No medical treatment modalities have been established to be effective. Anticoagulation or fibrinolytic therapy may increase the risk of further atheroembolism.

# REFERENCES

1. Virchow R: *Cellular Pathology: As Based upon Physiological and Pathological Histology.* Dover, New York, 1863.
2. Ross R: Atherosclerosis-an inflammatory disease. *N Engl J Med* 340:115–126, 1999.
3. Ridker PM: Inflammation, C-reactive protein, and cardiovascular disease: Moving past the marker versus mediator debate. *Circ Res* 114:594–595, 2014.
4. Duewell P, Kono H, Rayner KJ, et al: NLRP3 inflammasomes are required for atherogenesis and activated by cholesterol crystals. *Nature* 464:1357–1361, 2010.
5. Enos WF, Holmes RH, Beyer J: Coronary disease among United States soldiers killed in action in Korea; preliminary report. *J Am Med Assoc* 152:1090–1093, 1953.
6. Joseph A, Ackerman D, Talley JD, et al: Manifestations of coronary atherosclerosis in young trauma victims—An autopsy study. *J Am Coll Cardiol* 22:459–467, 1993.
7. Tuzcu EM, Kapadia SR, Tutar E, et al: High prevalence of coronary atherosclerosis in asymptomatic teenagers and young adults: Evidence from intravascular ultrasound. *Circulation* 103:2705–2710, 2001.
8. Ross R, Glomset JA: The pathogenesis of atherosclerosis (first of two parts). *N Engl J Med* 295:369–377, 1976.
9. Ross R, Glomset JA: The pathogenesis of atherosclerosis (second of two parts). *N Engl J Med* 295:420–425, 1976.
10. Yusuf S, Hawken S, Ounpuu S, et al: Effect of potentially modifiable risk factors associated with myocardial infarction in 52 countries (the INTERHEART study): Case-control study. *Lancet* 364:937–952, 2004.
11. Mallika V, Goswami B, Rajappa M: Atherosclerosis pathophysiology and the role of novel risk factors: A clinicobiochemical perspective. *Angiology* 58:513–522, 2007.
12. Hemkens LG, Bucher HC: HIV infection and cardiovascular disease. *Eur Heart J* 35:1373–1381, 2014.
13. Kline ER, Sutliff RL: The roles of HIV-1 proteins and antiretroviral drug therapy in HIV-1-associated endothelial dysfunction. *J Investig Med* 56:752–769, 2008.
14. Calza L, Manfredi R, Pocaterra D, Chiodo F: Risk of premature atherosclerosis and ischemic heart disease associated with HIV infection and antiretroviral therapy. *J Infect* 57:16–32, 2008.
15. de Zeeuw D: Renal disease: A common and a silent killer. *Nat Clin Pract Cardiovasc Med* 5(Suppl 1):S27–S35, 2008.
16. Budoff MJ, Rader DJ, Reilly MP, et al: Relationship of estimated GFR and coronary artery calcification in the CRIC (Chronic Renal Insufficiency Cohort) Study. *Am J Kidney Dis* 58:519–526, 2011.
17. Said S, Hernandez GT: The link between chronic kidney disease and cardiovascular disease. *J Nephropathol* 3:99–104, 2014.
18. Vonend O, Rump LC, Ritz E: Sympathetic overactivity—The Cinderella of cardiovascular risk factors in dialysis patients. *Semin Dial* 21:326–330, 2008.
19. Bradley TD, Floras JS: Obstructive sleep apnoea and its cardiovascular consequences. *Lancet* 373:82–93, 2009.
19a. Walton BL, Lehmann M, Skorczewski T, et al: Elevated hematocrit enhances platelet accumulation following vascular injury. *Blood* 129:2537–2546, 2017.
20. Skalen K, Gustafsson M, Rydberg EK, et al: Subendothelial retention of atherogenic lipoproteins in early atherosclerosis. *Nature* 417:750–754, 2002.
21. Passerini AG, Polacek DC, Shi C, et al: Coexisting proinflammatory and antioxidative endothelial transcription profiles in a disturbed flow region of the adult porcine aorta. *Proc Natl Acad Sci U S A* 101:2482–2487, 2004.
22. Weber C, Zernecke A, Libby P: The multifaceted contributions of leukocyte subsets to atherosclerosis: Lessons from mouse models. *Nat Rev Immunol* 8:802–815, 2008.
23. Stary HC, Chandler AB, Dinsmore RE, et al: A definition of advanced types of atherosclerotic lesions and a histological classification of atherosclerosis. A report from the Committee on Vascular Lesions of the Council on Arteriosclerosis, American Heart Association. *Circulation* 92:1355–1374, 1995.
24. Johnson JL: Matrix metalloproteinases: Influence on smooth muscle cells and atherosclerotic plaque stability. *Expert Rev Cardiovasc Ther* 5:265–282, 2007.
25. Hunt JL, Fairman R, Mitchell ME, et al: Bone formation in carotid plaques: A clinicopathological study. *Stroke* 33:1214–1219, 2002.
26. Curtis AM, Edelberg J, Jonas R, et al: Endothelial microparticles: Sophisticated vesicles modulating vascular function. *Vasc Med* 18:204–214, 2013.
27. Furchgott RF, Zawadzki JV: The obligatory role of endothelial cells in the relaxation of arterial smooth muscle by acetylcholine. *Nature* 288:373–376, 1980.
28. Loscalzo J: The identification of nitric oxide as endothelium-derived relaxing factor. *Circ Res* 113:100–103, 2013.
29. Lubos E, Handy DE, Loscalzo J: Role of oxidative stress and nitric oxide in atherothrombosis. *Front Biosci* 13:5323–5344, 2008.
30. Guzik TJ, Chen W, Gongora MC, et al: Calcium-dependent NOX5 nicotinamide adenine dinucleotide phosphate oxidase contributes to vascular oxidative stress in human coronary artery disease. *J Am Coll Cardiol* 52:1803–1809, 2008.
31. De Pascali F, Hemann C, Samons K, et al: Hypoxia and reoxygenation induce endothelial nitric oxide uncoupling in endothelial cells through tetrahydrobiopterin depletion and S-glutathionylation. *Biochemistry* 53:3679–3688, 2014.
32. Tiefenbacher CP, Bleeke T, Vahl C, et al: Endothelial dysfunction of coronary resistance arteries is improved by tetrahydrobiopterin in atherosclerosis. *Circulation* 102:2172–2179, 2000.
33. Kim CS, Jung SB, Naqvi A, et al: P53 impairs endothelium-dependent vasomotor function through transcriptional upregulation of p66shc. *Circ Res* 103:1441–1450, 2008.
34. Creager MA, Gallagher SJ, Girerd XJ, et al: L-Arginine improves endothelium-dependent vasodilation in hypercholesterolemic humans. *J Clin Invest* 90:1248–1253, 1992.
35. Chen S, Li N, Deb-Chatterji M, et al: Asymmetric dimethylarginine as marker and mediator in ischemic stroke. *Int J Mol Sci* 13:15983–16004, 2012.
36. Niu PP, Cao Y, Gong T, et al: Hypermethylation of DDAH2 promoter contributes to the dysfunction of endothelial progenitor cells in coronary artery disease patients. *J Transl Med* 12:170, 2014.
37. Ludmer PL, Selwyn AP, Shook TL, et al: Paradoxical vasoconstriction induced by acetylcholine in atherosclerotic coronary arteries. *N Engl J Med* 315:1046–1051, 1986.

38. Kuhn FE, Mohler ER, Satler LF, et al: Effects of high-density lipoprotein on acetylcholine-induced coronary vasoreactivity. *Am J Cardiol* 68:1425–1430, 1991.

39. Kuhn FE, Mohler ER 3rd, Rackley CE: Cholesterol and lipoproteins: Beyond atherogenesis. *Clin Cardiol* 15:883–890, 1992.

40. Luscher TF, Landmesser U, von Eckardstein A, Fogelman AM: High-density lipoprotein: Vascular protective effects, dysfunction, and potential as therapeutic target. *Circ Res* 114:171–182, 2014.

41. Oakley R, Tharakan B: Vascular hyperpermeability and aging. *Aging Dis* 5:114–125, 2014.

42. van den Heuvel M, Sorop O, Koopmans SJ, et al: Coronary microvascular dysfunction in a porcine model of early atherosclerosis and diabetes. *Am J Physiol Heart Circ Physiol* 302:H85–H94, 2012.

43. Mohler ER 3rd, O'Hare K, Darze ES, et al: Cardiovascular function in normotensive offspring of persons with essential hypertension and black race. *J Clin Hypertens (Greenwich)* 9:506–512, 2007.

44. Yong PJ, Koh CH, Shim WS: Endothelial microparticles: Missing link in endothelial dysfunction? *Eur J Prev Cardiol* 20:496–512, 2013.

45. Nozaki T, Sugiyama S, Koga H, et al: Significance of a multiple biomarkers strategy including endothelial dysfunction to improve risk stratification for cardiovascular events in patients at high risk for coronary heart disease. *J Am Coll Cardiol* 54:601–608, 2009.

46. Liuba P, Karnani P, Pesonen E, et al: Endothelial dysfunction after repeated *Chlamydia pneumoniae* infection in apolipoprotein E-knockout mice. *Circulation* 102:1039–1044, 2000.

47. Fichtlscherer S, Rosenberger G, Walter DH, et al: Elevated C-reactive protein levels and impaired endothelial vasoreactivity in patients with coronary artery disease. *Circulation* 102:1000–1006, 2000.

48. Beckman JA, Ganz J, Creager MA, et al: Relationship of clinical presentation and calcification of culprit coronary artery stenoses. *Arterioscler Thromb Vasc Biol* 21:1618–1622, 2001.

49. Libby P, Ridker PM, Maseri A: Inflammation and atherosclerosis. *Circulation* 105:1135–1143, 2002.

50. Moore KJ, Sheedy FJ, Fisher EA: Macrophages in atherosclerosis: A dynamic balance. *Nat Rev Immunol* 13:709–721, 2013.

51. Takeshita J, Mohler ER, Krishnamoorthy P, et al: Endothelial cell-, platelet-, and monocyte/macrophage-derived microparticles are elevated in psoriasis beyond cardiometabolic risk factors. *J Am Heart Assoc* 3:e000507, 2014.

52. Lim S, Park S: Role of vascular smooth muscle cell in the inflammation of atherosclerosis. *BMB Rep* 47:1–7, 2014.

53. Kanse SM, Parahuleva M, Muhl L, et al: Factor VII-activating protease (FSAP): Vascular functions and role in atherosclerosis. *Thromb Haemost* 99:286–289, 2008.

54. Fuster V: Lewis A. Conner Memorial Lecture. Mechanisms leading to myocardial infarction: Insights from studies of vascular biology. *Circulation* 90:2126–2146, 1994.

55. Schwartz SM, Murry CE: Proliferation and the monoclonal origins of atherosclerotic lesions. *Annu Rev Med* 49:437–460, 1998.

56. Scott NA, Cipolla GD, Ross CE, et al: Identification of a potential role for the adventitia in vascular lesion formation after balloon overstretch injury of porcine coronary arteries. *Circulation* 93:2178–2187, 1996.

57. Sakakura K, Nakano M, Otsuka F, et al: Pathophysiology of atherosclerosis plaque progression. *Heart Lung Circ* 22:399–411, 2013.

58. Majesky MW, Dong XR, Regan JN, Hoglund VJ: Vascular smooth muscle progenitor cells: Building and repairing blood vessels. *Circ Res* 108:365–377, 2011.

59. Der Leyen HE, Gibbons GH, Morishita R, et al: Gene therapy inhibiting neointimal vascular lesion: In vivo transfer of endothelial cell nitric oxide synthase gene. *Proc Natl Acad Sci U S A* 92:1137–1141, 1995.

60. Dzau VJ, Braun-Dullaeus RC, Sedding DG: Vascular proliferation and atherosclerosis: New perspectives and therapeutic strategies. *Nat Med* 8:1249–1256, 2002.

61. Bonta PI, Pols TW, de Vries CJ: NR4A nuclear receptors in atherosclerosis and vein-graft disease. *Trends Cardiovasc Med* 17:105–111, 2007.

62. Lemos PA, Lee CH, Degertekin M, et al: Early outcome after sirolimus-eluting stent implantation in patients with acute coronary syndromes: Insights from the Rapamycin-Eluting Stent Evaluated at Rotterdam Cardiology Hospital (RESEARCH) registry. *J Am Coll Cardiol* 41:2093–2099, 2003.

63. Sagripanti A, Carpi A: Antithrombotic and prothrombotic activities of the vascular endothelium. *Biomed Pharmacother* 54:107–111, 2000.

64. van Der Meijden PE, van Schilfgaarde M, van Oerle R, Renne T, et al: Platelet- and erythrocyte-derived microparticles trigger thrombin generation via factor XIIa. *J Thromb Haemost* 10:1355–1362, 2012.

65. Falati S, Liu Q, Gross P, et al: Accumulation of tissue factor into developing thrombi in vivo is dependent upon microparticle P-selectin glycoprotein ligand 1 and platelet P-selectin. *J Exp Med* 197:1585–1598, 2003.

66. Feil R, Lohmann SM, de Jonge H, et al: Cyclic GMP-dependent protein kinases and the cardiovascular system: Insights from genetically modified mice. *Circ Res* 93:907–916, 2003.

67. Gonzalez MA, Selwyn AP: Endothelial function, inflammation, and prognosis in cardiovascular disease. *Am J Med* 115(Suppl 8A):99S–106S, 2003.

68. Anderson TJ: Nitric oxide, atherosclerosis and the clinical relevance of endothelial dysfunction. *Heart Fail Rev* 8:71–86, 2003.

69. Tulis DA, Durante W, Liu X, et al: Adenovirus-mediated heme oxygenase-1 gene delivery inhibits injury-induced vascular neointima formation. *Circulation* 104:2710–2715, 2001.

70. Sachais BS: Platelet-endothelial interactions in atherosclerosis. *Curr Atheroscler Rep* 3:412–416, 2001.

71. Marcus AJ, Broekman MJ, Drosopoulos JH, et al: Metabolic control of excessive extracellular nucleotide accumulation by CD39/ecto-nucleotidase-1: Implications for ischemic vascular diseases. *J Pharmacol Exp Ther* 305:9–16, 2003.

72. Landmesser U, Merten R, Spiekermann S, et al: Vascular extracellular superoxide dismutase activity in patients with coronary artery disease: Relation to endothelium-dependent vasodilation. *Circulation* 101:2264–2270, 2000.

73. Cooke JP: Does ADMA cause endothelial dysfunction? *Arterioscler Thromb Vasc Biol* 20:2032–2037, 2000.

74. Mohler ER 3rd, Shi Y, Moore J, et al: Diabetes reduces bone marrow and circulating porcine endothelial progenitor cells, an effect ameliorated by atorvastatin and independent of cholesterol. *Cytometry A* 75:75–82, 2009.

75. Foteinos G, Hu Y, Xiao Q, et al: Rapid endothelial turnover in atherosclerosis-prone areas coincides with stem cell repair in apolipoprotein E-deficient mice. *Circulation* 117:1856–1863, 2008.

76. Binder CJ, Chang MK, Shaw PX, et al: Innate and acquired immunity in atherogenesis. *Nat Med* 8:1218–1226, 2002.

77. Medzhitov R: Toll-like receptors and innate immunity. *Nat Rev Immunol* 1:135–145, 2001.

78. Erridge C: The roles of pathogen-associated molecular patterns in atherosclerosis. *Trends Cardiovasc Med* 18:52–56, 2008.

79. Medzhitov R, Janeway CA Jr: Decoding the patterns of self and nonself by the innate immune system. *Science* 296:298–300, 2002.

80. Ridker PM: Clinical application of C-reactive protein for cardiovascular disease detection and prevention. *Circulation* 107:363–369, 2003.

81. Dansky HM, Barlow CB, Lominska C, et al: Adhesion of monocytes to arterial endothelium and initiation of atherosclerosis are critically dependent on vascular cell adhesion molecule-1 gene dosage. *Arterioscler Thromb Vasc Biol* 21:1662–1667, 2001.

82. Cybulsky MI, Iiyama K, Li H, et al: A major role for VCAM-1, but not ICAM-1, in early atherosclerosis. *J Clin Invest* 107:1255–1262, 2001.

83. Collins RG, Velji R, Guevara NV, et al: P-Selectin or intercellular adhesion molecule (ICAM)-1 deficiency substantially protects against atherosclerosis in apolipoprotein E-deficient mice. *J Exp Med* 191:189–194, 2000.

84. Parks BW, Lusis AJ: Macrophage accumulation in atherosclerosis. *N Engl J Med* 369:2352–2353, 2013.

85. Robbins CS, Hilgendorf I, Weber GF, et al: Local proliferation dominates lesional macrophage accumulation in atherosclerosis. *Nat Med* 19:1166–1172, 2013.

86. Weber C, Noels H: Atherosclerosis: Current pathogenesis and therapeutic options. *Nat Med* 17:1410–1422, 2011.

87. Zalewski A, Macphee C, Nelson JJ: Lipoprotein-associated phospholipase A2: A potential therapeutic target for atherosclerosis. *Curr Drug Targets Cardiovasc Haematol Disord* 5:527–532, 2005.

88. Shi Y, Zhang P, Zhang L, et al: Role of lipoprotein-associated phospholipase A(2) in leukocyte activation and inflammatory responses. *Atherosclerosis* 191:54–62, 2006.

89. Wilensky RL, Shi Y, Mohler ER 3rd, et al: Inhibition of lipoprotein-associated phospholipase A2 reduces complex coronary atherosclerotic plaque development. *Nat Med* 14:1059–1066, 2008.

90. Mohler ER 3rd, Ballantyne CM, Davidson MH, et al: The effect of darapladib on plasma lipoprotein-associated phospholipase A2 activity and cardiovascular biomarkers in patients with stable coronary heart disease or coronary heart disease risk equivalent: The results of a multicenter, randomized, double-blind, placebo-controlled study. *J Am Coll Cardiol* 51:1632–1641, 2008.

91. Investigators S, White HD, Held C, et al: Darapladib for preventing ischemic events in stable coronary heart disease. *N Engl J Med* 370:1702–1711, 2014.

92. Smith JD, Trogan E, Ginsberg M, et al: Decreased atherosclerosis in mice deficient in both macrophage colony-stimulating factor (op) and apolipoprotein E. *Proc Natl Acad Sci U S A* 92:8264–8268, 1995.

93. Endemann G, Stanton LW, Madden KS, et al: CD36 is a receptor for oxidized low density lipoprotein. *J Biol Chem* 268:11811–11816, 1993.

94. Steinberg D, Parthasarathy S, Carew TE, et al: Beyond cholesterol: Modifications of low-density lipoprotein that increase its atherogenicity. *N Engl J Med* 320:915–924, 1989.

95. Boring L, Gosling J, Cleary M, Charo IF: Decreased lesion formation in CCR2−/− mice reveals a role for chemokines in the initiation of atherosclerosis. *Nature* 394:894–897, 1998.

96. Gu L, Okada Y, Clinton SK, et al: Absence of monocyte chemoattractant protein-1 reduces atherosclerosis in low density lipoprotein receptor-deficient mice. *Mol Cell* 2:275–281, 1998.

97. Gosling J, Slaymaker S, Gu L, et al: MCP-1 deficiency reduces susceptibility to atherosclerosis in mice that overexpress human apolipoprotein B. *J Clin Invest* 103:773–778, 1999.

98. Hur J, Yang HM, Yoon CH, et al: Identification of a novel role of T cells in postnatal vasculogenesis: Characterization of endothelial progenitor cell colonies. *Circulation* 116:1671–1682, 2007.

99. Tang WH, Wu Y, Nicholls SJ, Hazen SL: Plasma myeloperoxidase predicts incident cardiovascular risks in stable patients undergoing medical management for coronary artery disease. *Clin Chem* 57:33–39, 2011.

100. Sugiyama S, Okada Y, Sukhova GK, et al: Macrophage myeloperoxidase regulation by granulocyte macrophage colony-stimulating factor in human atherosclerosis and implications in acute coronary syndromes. *Am J Pathol* 158:879–891, 2001.

101. Babior BM: Phagocytes and oxidative stress. *Am J Med* 109:33–44, 2000.

102. Suzuki H, Kurihara Y, Takeya M, et al: A role for macrophage scavenger receptors in atherosclerosis and susceptibility to infection. *Nature* 386:292–296, 1997.

103. Febbraio M, Podrez EA, Smith JD, et al: Targeted disruption of the class B scavenger receptor CD36 protects against atherosclerotic lesion development in mice. *J Clin Invest* 105:1049–1056, 2000.

104. Kodama T, Reddy P, Kishimoto C, Krieger M: Purification and characterization of a bovine acetyl low density lipoprotein receptor. *Proc Natl Acad Sci U S A* 85:9238–9242, 1988.

105. Henriksen T, Mahoney EM, Steinberg D: Enhanced macrophage degradation of low density lipoprotein previously incubated with cultured endothelial cells: Recognition by receptors for acetylated low density lipoproteins. *Proc Natl Acad Sci U S A* 78:6499–6503, 1981.

106. Steinbrecher UP, Parthasarathy S, Leake DS, Witztum JL, Steinberg D: Modification of low density lipoprotein by endothelial cells involves lipid peroxidation and degradation of low density lipoprotein phospholipids. *Proc Natl Acad Sci U S A* 81:3883–3887, 1984.

107. Shaw PX, Horkko S, Chang MK, et al: Natural antibodies with the T15 idiotype may act in atherosclerosis, apoptotic clearance, and protective immunity. *J Clin Invest* 105:1731–1740, 2000.

108. Tsimikas S, Palinski W, Witztum JL: Circulating autoantibodies to oxidized LDL correlate with arterial accumulation and depletion of oxidized LDL in LDL receptor-deficient mice. *Arterioscler Thromb Vasc Biol* 21:95–100, 2001.

109. Palinski W, Ord VA, Plump AS, et al: ApoE-deficient mice are a model of lipoprotein oxidation in atherogenesis. Demonstration of oxidation-specific epitopes in lesions and high titers of autoantibodies to malondialdehyde-lysine in serum. *Arterioscler Thromb* 14:605–616, 1994.

110. Ameli S, Hultgardh-Nilsson A, Regnstrom J, et al: Effect of immunization with homologous LDL and oxidized LDL on early atherosclerosis in hypercholesterolemic rabbits. *Arterioscler Thromb Vasc Biol* 16:1074–1079, 1996.

111. Freigang S, Horkko S, Miller E, et al: Immunization of LDL receptor-deficient mice with homologous malondialdehyde-modified and native LDL reduces progression of atherosclerosis by mechanisms other than induction of high titers of antibodies to oxidative neoepitopes. *Arterioscler Thromb Vasc Biol* 18:1972–1982, 1998.

112. Zhou X, Caligiuri G, Hamsten A, et al: LDL immunization induces T-cell-dependent antibody formation and protection against atherosclerosis. *Arterioscler Thromb Vasc Biol* 21:108–114, 2001.

113. Mehrabian M, Allayee H, Wong J, et al: Identification of 5-lipoxygenase as a major gene contributing to atherosclerosis susceptibility in mice. *Circ Res* 91:120–126, 2002.

114. Cyrus T, Witztum JL, Rader DJ, et al: Disruption of the 12/15-lipoxygenase gene diminishes atherosclerosis in apo E-deficient mice. *J Clin Invest* 103:1597–1604, 1999.

115. Harats D, Shaish A, George J, et al: Overexpression of 15-lipoxygenase in vascular endothelium accelerates early atherosclerosis in LDL receptor-deficient mice. *Arterioscler Thromb Vasc Biol* 20:2100–2105, 2000.

116. Whatling C, McPheat W, Herslof M: The potential link between atherosclerosis and the 5-lipoxygenase pathway: Investigational agents with new implications for the cardiovascular field. *Expert Opin Investig Drugs* 16:1879–1893, 2007.

117. Vinje S, Stroes E, Nieuwdorp M, Hazen SL: The gut microbiome as novel cardiometabolic target: The time has come! *Eur Heart J* 35:883–887, 2014.

117a. Tang WH, Kitai T, Hazen SL: Gut microbiota in cardiovascular health and disease. *Circ Res* 120:1183–1196, 2017.

117b. Jonsson AL, Bäckhed F: Role of the gut microbiota in atherosclerosis. *Nat Rev Cardiol* 14:79–87, 2017.

118. Williams KJ, Feig JE, Fisher EA: Cellular and molecular mechanisms for rapid regression of atherosclerosis: From bench top to potentially achievable clinical goal. *Curr Opin Lipidol* 18:443–450, 2007.

119. Schwenke DC: Comparison of aorta and pulmonary artery: I. Early cholesterol accumulation and relative susceptibility to atheromatous lesions. *Circ Res* 81:338–345, 1997.

120. Schwenke DC: Comparison of aorta and pulmonary artery: II. LDL transport and metabolism correlate with susceptibility to atherosclerosis. *Circ Res* 81:346–354, 1997.

121. Camejo G, Hurt-Camejo E, Wiklund O, Bondjers G: Association of apo B lipoproteins with arterial proteoglycans: Pathological significance and molecular basis. *Atherosclerosis* 139:205–222, 1998.

122. Navab M, Hama SY, Reddy ST, et al: Oxidized lipids as mediators of coronary heart disease. *Curr Opin Lipidol* 13:363–372, 2002.

123. Rajavashisth TB, Andalibi A, Territo MC, et al: Induction of endothelial cell expression of granulocyte and macrophage colony-stimulating factors by modified low-density lipoproteins. *Nature* 344:254–257, 1990.

124. Steinberg D: Atherogenesis in perspective: Hypercholesterolemia and inflammation as partners in crime. *Nat Med* 8:1211–1217, 2002.

125. MRC/BHF Heart Protection Study of antioxidant vitamin supplementation in 20,536 high-risk individuals: A randomised placebo-controlled trial. *Lancet* 360:23–33, 2002.

126. Brown BG, Zhao XQ, Chait A, et al: Simvastatin and niacin, antioxidant vitamins, or the combination for the prevention of coronary disease. *N Engl J Med* 345:1583–1592, 2001.

127. Tangirala RK, Tsukamoto K, Chun SH, et al: Regression of atherosclerosis induced by liver-directed gene transfer of apolipoprotein A-I in mice. *Circulation* 100:1816–1822, 1999.

128. Zhang Y, Zanotti I, Reilly MP, et al: Overexpression of apolipoprotein A-I promotes reverse transport of cholesterol from macrophages to feces in vivo. *Circulation* 108:661–663, 2003.

129. Khera AV, Cuchel M, de la Llera-Moya M, et al: Cholesterol efflux capacity, high-density lipoprotein function, and atherosclerosis. *N Engl J Med* 364:127–135, 2011.

130. Mineo C, Deguchi H, Griffin JH, Shaul PW: Endothelial and antithrombotic actions of HDL. *Circ Res* 98:1352–1364, 2006.

131. Shih DM, Gu L, Xia YR, et al: Mice lacking serum paraoxonase are susceptible to organophosphate toxicity and atherosclerosis. *Nature* 394:284–287, 1998.

132. Haraguchi Y, Toh R, Hasokawa M, et al: Serum myeloperoxidase/paraoxonase 1 ratio as potential indicator of dysfunctional high-density lipoprotein and risk stratification in coronary artery disease. *Atherosclerosis* 234:288–294, 2014.

133. Barter PJ, Caulfield M, Eriksson M, et al: Effects of torcetrapib in patients at high risk for coronary events. *N Engl J Med* 357:2109–2122, 2007.

134. Nissen SE, Tsunoda T, Tuzcu EM, et al: Effect of recombinant ApoA-I Milano on coronary atherosclerosis in patients with acute coronary syndromes: A randomized controlled trial. *JAMA* 290:2292–2300, 2003.

135. Van Lenten BJ, Navab M, Anantharamaiah GM, et al: Multiple indications for anti-inflammatory apolipoprotein mimetic peptides. *Curr Opin Investig Drugs* 9:1157–1162, 2008.

136. Rizvi M, Pathak D, Freedman JE, Chakrabarti S: CD40-CD40 ligand interactions in oxidative stress, inflammation and vascular disease. *Trends Mol Med* 14:530–538, 2008.

137. Zhang B, Wu T, Chen M, et al: The CD40/CD40L system: A new therapeutic target for disease. *Immunol Lett* 153:58–61, 2013.

138. Cipollone F, Mezzetti A, Porreca E, et al: Association between enhanced soluble CD40L and prothrombotic state in hypercholesterolemia effects of statin therapy. *Circulation* 106:399–402, 2002.

139. Mallat Z, Gojova A, Marchiol-Fournigault C, et al: Inhibition of transforming growth factor-beta signaling accelerates atherosclerosis and induces an unstable plaque phenotype in mice. *Circ Res* 89:930–934, 2001.

140. Zhang H, Mooney CJ, Reilly MP: ABO blood groups and cardiovascular diseases. *Int J Vasc Med* 2012:641917, 2012.

141. Gurfinkel E, Lernoud V: The role of infection and immunity in atherosclerosis. *Expert Rev Cardiovasc Ther* 4:131–137, 2006.

142. Ford PJ, Yamazaki K, Seymour GJ: Cardiovascular and oral disease interactions: What is the evidence? *Prim Dent Care* 14:59–66, 2007.

143. Mayr M, Kiechl S, Willeit J, et al: Infections, immunity, and atherosclerosis: Associations of antibodies to *Chlamydia pneumoniae*, *Helicobacter pylori*, and cytomegalovirus with immune reactions to heat-shock protein 60 and carotid or femoral atherosclerosis. *Circulation* 102:833–839, 2000.

144. Caligiuri G, Nicoletti A, Poirier B, Hansson GK: Protective immunity against atherosclerosis carried by B cells of hypercholesterolemic mice. *J Clin Invest* 109:745–753, 2002.

145. Robinette CD, Fraumeni JF Jr: Splenectomy and subsequent mortality in veterans of the 1939–45 war. *Lancet* 2:127–129, 1977.

146. Yamada Y, Ichihara S, Nishida T: Molecular genetics of myocardial infarction. *Genomic Med* 2:7–22, 2008.

147. Helgadottir A, Manolescu A, Thorleifsson G, et al: The gene encoding 5-lipoxygenase activating protein confers risk of myocardial infarction and stroke. *Nat Genet* 36:233–239, 2004.

148. Topol EJ, Smith J, Plow EF, Wang QK: Genetic susceptibility to myocardial infarction and coronary artery disease. *Hum Mol Genet* 15(Spec No 2):R117–R123, 2006.

149. Helgadottir A, Thorleifsson G, Manolescu A, et al: A common variant on chromosome 9p21 affects the risk of myocardial infarction. *Science* 316:1491–1493, 2007.

150. Roberts R: Genetics of coronary artery disease. *Circ Res* 114:1890–1903, 2014.

151. Falk E: Plaque rupture with severe pre-existing stenosis precipitating coronary thrombosis. Characteristics of coronary atherosclerotic plaques underlying fatal occlusive thrombi. *Br Heart J* 50:127–134, 1983.

152. Davies MJ, Thomas AC: Plaque fissuring—The cause of acute myocardial infarction, sudden ischaemic death, and crescendo angina. *Br Heart J* 53:363–373, 1985.

153. Muller JE: Circadian variation and triggering of acute coronary events. *Am Heart J* 137:S1–S8.

154. Muller JE, Abela GS, Nesto RW, Tofler GH: Triggers, acute risk factors and vulnerable plaques: The lexicon of a new frontier. *J Am Coll Cardiol* 23:809–813, 1994.

155. Naghavi M, Libby P, Falk E, et al: From vulnerable plaque to vulnerable patient: A call for new definitions and risk assessment strategies: Part I. *Circulation* 108:1664–1672, 2003.

155a. Stefanadis C, Antoniou CK, Tsiachris D, Pietri P: Coronary atherosclerotic vulnerable plaque: Current perspectives. *J Am Heart Assoc* 6(3):pii:e005543, 2017.

156. Virmani R, Kolodgie FD, Burke AP, et al: Lessons from sudden coronary death: A comprehensive morphological classification scheme for atherosclerotic lesions. *Arterioscler Thromb Vasc Biol* 20:1262–1275, 2000.

157. Casscells W, Naghavi M, Willerson JT: Vulnerable atherosclerotic plaque: A multifocal disease. *Circulation* 107:2072–2075, 2003.

158. Uchida Y, Nakamura F, Tomaru T, et al: Prediction of acute coronary syndromes by percutaneous coronary angioscopy in patients with stable angina. *Am Heart J* 130:195–203, 1995.

159. Ambrose JA: In search of the "vulnerable plaque": Can it be localized and will focal regional therapy ever be an option for cardiac prevention? *J Am Coll Cardiol* 51:1539–1542, 2008.

160. Naghavi M, Libby P, Falk E, et al: From vulnerable plaque to vulnerable patient: A call for new definitions and risk assessment strategies: Part II. *Circulation* 108:1772–1778, 2003.

161. Davi G, Patrono C: Platelet activation and atherothrombosis. *N Engl J Med* 357:2482–2494, 2007.

162. Owens AP 3rd, Mackman N: Role of tissue factor in atherothrombosis. *Curr Atheroscler Rep* 14:394–401, 2012.

163. Frostegard J: Systemic lupus erythematosus and cardiovascular disease. *Lupus* 17:364–367, 2008.

164. Rohla M, Weiss TW: Metabolic syndrome, inflammation and atherothrombosis. *Hamostaseologie* 33:283–294, 2013.

165. Heo KS, Fujiwara K, Abe J: Shear stress and atherosclerosis. *Mol Cells* 37:435–440, 2014.

166. Cosemans JM, Angelillo-Scherrer A, Mattheij NJ, Heemskerk JW: The effects of arterial flow on platelet activation, thrombus growth, and stabilization. *Cardiovasc Res* 99:342–352, 2013.

167. Aird WC: Vascular bed-specific thrombosis. *J Thromb Haemost* 5(Suppl 1):283–291, 2007.

168. Chien S: Effects of disturbed flow on endothelial cells. *Ann Biomed Eng* 36:554–562, 2008.

169. Helderman F, Segers D, de Crom R, et al: Effect of shear stress on vascular inflammation and plaque development. *Curr Opin Lipidol* 18:527–533, 2007.

170. Badimon JJ, Ortiz AF, Meyer B, et al: Different response to balloon angioplasty of carotid and coronary arteries: Effects on acute platelet deposition and intimal thickening. *Atherosclerosis* 140:307–314, 1998.

171. Halvorsen B, Otterdal K, Dahl TB, et al: Atherosclerotic plaque stability—What determines the fate of a plaque? *Prog Cardiovasc Dis* 51:183–194, 2008.

172. Regan ER, Aird WC: Dynamical systems approach to endothelial heterogeneity. *Circ Res* 111:110–130, 2012.

173. Cheung C, Bernardo AS, Pedersen RA, Sinha S: Directed differentiation of embryonic origin-specific vascular smooth muscle subtypes from human pluripotent stem cells. *Nat Protoc* 9:929–938, 2014.

174. Lechner D, Weltermann A: Circulating tissue factor-exposing microparticles. *Thromb Res* 122(Suppl 1):S47–S54, 2008.

175. George FD: Microparticles in vascular diseases. *Thromb Res* 122(Suppl 1):S55–S59, 2008.

176. Lacroix R, Dubois C, Leroyer AS, et al: Revisited role of microparticles in arterial and venous thrombosis. *J Thromb Haemost* 11(Suppl 1):24–35, 2013.

177. Rauch U, Osende JI, Fuster V, et al: Thrombus formation on atherosclerotic plaques: Pathogenesis and clinical consequences. *Ann Intern Med* 134:224–238, 2001.

178. Ma B, Liu G, Chen X, et al: Risk of stroke in patients with patent foramen ovale: An updated meta-analysis of observational studies. *J Stroke Cerebrovasc Dis* 23:1207–1215, 2014.

179. Nallu K, Yang DC, Swaminathan RV, et al: Innovations in drug-eluting stents. *Panminerva Med* 55:345–352, 2013.

180. Springer J, Villa-Forte A: Thrombosis in vasculitis. *Curr Opin Rheumatol* 25:19–25, 2013.

181. Matsuura E, Kobayashi K, Lopez LR: Preventing autoimmune and infection triggered atherosclerosis for an enduring healthful lifestyle. *Autoimmun Rev* 7:214–222, 2008.

182. Mok CC: Accelerated atherosclerosis, arterial thromboembolism, and preventive strategies in systemic lupus erythematosus. *Scand J Rheumatol* 35:85–95, 2006.

183. Dasararaju R, Singh N, Mehta A: Heparin induced thrombocytopenia: Review. *Expert Rev Hematol* 6:419–428, 2013.

184. Barbui T, Finazzi G, Falanga A: Myeloproliferative neoplasms and thrombosis. *Blood* 122:2176–2184, 2013.

185. Casini A, Fontana P, Lecompte TP: Thrombotic complications of myeloproliferative neoplasms: Risk assessment and risk-guided management. *J Thromb Haemost* 11:1215–1227, 2013.

186. Finazzi G, De Stefano V, Barbui T: Are MPNs vascular diseases? *Curr Hematol Malig Rep* 8:307–316, 2013.

187. De Ceunynck K, De Meyer SF, Vanhoorelbeke K: Unwinding the von Willebrand factor strings puzzle. *Blood* 121:270–277, 2013.

188. Nightingale T, Cutler D: The secretion of von Willebrand factor from endothelial cells; an increasingly complicated story. *J Thromb Haemost* 11(Suppl 1):192–201, 2013.

189. Wong AK: Platelet biology: The role of shear. *Expert Rev Hematol* 6:205–212, 2013.

190. Kulkarni S, Dopheide SM, Yap CL, et al: A revised model of platelet aggregation. *J Clin Invest* 105:783–791, 2000.

191. Wagner CT, Kroll MH, Chow TW, et al: Epinephrine and shear stress synergistically induce platelet aggregation via a mechanism that partially bypasses VWF-GP IB interactions. *Biorheology* 33:209–229, 1996.

192. Andre P, Prasad KS, Denis CV, et al: CD40L stabilizes arterial thrombi by a beta3 integrin-dependent mechanism. *Nat Med* 8:247–252, 2002.

193. Winckers K, ten Cate H, Hackeng TM: The role of tissue factor pathway inhibitor in atherosclerosis and arterial thrombosis. *Blood Rev* 27:119–132, 2013.

194. Tedgui A, Mallat Z: Apoptosis as a determinant of atherothrombosis. *Thromb Haemost* 86:420–426, 2001.

195. Shah PK: Inflammation and plaque vulnerability. *Cardiovasc Drugs Ther* 23:31–40, 2009.

196. Kuge Y, Kume N, Ishino S, et al: Prominent lectin-like oxidized low density lipoprotein (LDL) receptor-1 (LOX-1) expression in atherosclerotic lesions is associated with tissue factor expression and apoptosis in hypercholesterolemic rabbits. *Biol Pharm Bull* 31:1475–1482, 2008.

197. van der Stoep M, Korporaal SJ, Van Eck M: High-density lipoprotein as a modulator of platelet and coagulation responses. *Cardiovasc Res* 103:362–371, 2014.

198. Endler G, Mannhalter C: Polymorphisms in coagulation factor genes and their impact on arterial and venous thrombosis. *Clin Chim Acta* 330:31–55, 2003.

199. Prandoni P, Bilora F, Marchiori A, et al: An association between atherosclerosis and venous thrombosis. *N Engl J Med* 348:1435–1441, 2003.

200. Franchini M, Mannucci PM: Association between venous and arterial thrombosis: Clinical implications. *Eur J Intern Med* 23:333–337, 2012.

201. Lind C, Flinterman LE, Enga KF, et al: Impact of incident venous thromboembolism on risk of arterial thrombotic diseases. *Circulation* 129:855–863, 2014.

202. Celermajer DS, Sorensen KE, Spiegelhalter DJ, et al: Aging is associated with endothelial dysfunction in healthy men years before the age-related decline in women. *J Am Coll Cardiol* 24:471–476, 1994.

203. Franchini M, Targher G, Montagnana M, Lippi G: The metabolic syndrome and the risk of arterial and venous thrombosis. *Thromb Res* 122:727–735, 2008.

204. Lowe GD: Common risk factors for both arterial and venous thrombosis. *Br J Haematol* 140:488–495, 2008.

205. Ye Z, Liu EH, Higgins JP, et al: Seven haemostatic gene polymorphisms in coronary disease: Meta-analysis of 66,155 cases and 91,307 controls. *Lancet* 367:651–658, 2006.

206. Kamphuisen PW, ten Cate H: Cardiovascular risk in patients with hemophilia. *Blood* 123:1297–1301, 2014.

207. Sramek A, Reiber JH, Gerrits WB, Rosendaal FR: Decreased coagulability has no clinically relevant effect on atherogenesis: Observations in individuals with a hereditary bleeding tendency. *Circulation* 104:762–767, 2001.

208. Haverkate F: Levels of haemostatic factors, arteriosclerosis and cardiovascular disease. *Vascul Pharmacol* 39:109–112, 2002.

209. Kannel WB: Overview of hemostatic factors involved in atherosclerotic cardiovascular disease. *Lipids* 40:1215–1220, 2005.

210. Montoro-Garcia S, Shantsila E, Lip GY: Potential value of targeting von Willebrand factor in atherosclerotic cardiovascular disease. *Expert Opin Ther Targets* 18:43–53, 2014.

211. van Galen KP, Tuinenburg A, Smeets EM, Schutgens RE: Von Willebrand factor deficiency and atherosclerosis. *Blood Rev* 26:189–196, 2012.

212. Williams MS, Bray PF: Genetics of arterial prothrombotic risk states. *Exp Biol Med (Maywood)* 226:409–419, 2001.

213. Lekakis J, Bisti S, Tsougos E, et al: Platelet glycoprotein IIb HPA-3 polymorphism and acute coronary syndromes. *Int J Cardiol* 127:46–50, 2008.

214. Weiss EJ, Bray PF, Tayback M, et al: A polymorphism in a platelet glycoprotein receptor as an inherited risk factor for coronary thrombosis. *N Engl J Med* 334:1090–1094, 1996.

215. Burkhart JM, Gambaryan S, Watson SP, et al: What can proteomics tell us about platelets? *Circ Res* 114:1204–1219, 2014.

216. Berger JS, Becker RC, Kuhn C, et al: Hyperreactive platelet phenotypes: Relationship to altered serotonin transporter number, transport kinetics and intrinsic response to adrenergic co-stimulation. *Thromb Haemost* 109:85–92, 2013.

217. Rauch U, Osende JI, Chesebro JH, et al: Statins and cardiovascular diseases: The multiple effects of lipid-lowering therapy by statins. *Atherosclerosis* 153:181–189, 2000.

218. Alpert JS, Thygesen K, Antman E, Bassand JP: Myocardial infarction redefined—A consensus document of the Joint European Society of Cardiology/American College of Cardiology Committee for the redefinition of myocardial infarction. *J Am Coll Cardiol* 36:959–969, 2000.

219. O'Gara PT, Kushner FG, Ascheim DD, et al: 2013 ACCF/AHA guideline for the management of ST-elevation myocardial infarction: Executive summary: A report of the American College of Cardiology Foundation/American Heart Association Task Force on Practice Guidelines: Developed in collaboration with the American College of Emergency Physicians and Society for Cardiovascular Angiography and Interventions. *Catheter Cardiovasc Interv* 82:E1–E27, 2013.

220. Wright RS, Anderson JL, Adams CD, et al: 2011 ACCF/AHA focused update incorporated into the ACC/AHA 2007 Guidelines for the Management of Patients with Unstable Angina/Non-ST-Elevation Myocardial Infarction: A report of the American College of Cardiology Foundation/American Heart Association Task Force on Practice Guidelines developed in collaboration with the American Academy of Family Physicians, Society for Cardiovascular Angiography and Interventions, and the Society of Thoracic Surgeons. *J Am Coll Cardiol* 57:e215–e367, 2011.

221. Pope JH, Ruthazer R, Beshansky JR, et al: Clinical features of emergency department patients presenting with symptoms suggestive of acute cardiac ischemia: A multicenter study. *J Thromb Thrombolysis* 6:63–74, 1998.

222. American College of Emergency Physicians, Society for Cardiovascular Angiography and Interventions, O'Gara PT, et al: 2013 ACCF/AHA guideline for the management of ST-elevation myocardial infarction: A report of the American College of Cardiology Foundation/American Heart Association Task Force on Practice Guidelines. *J Am Coll Cardiol* 61:e78–e140, 2013.

223. Amsterdam EA, Wenger NK, Brindis RG, et al: 2014 AHA/ACC guideline for the management of patients with non-ST-elevation acute coronary syndromes: Executive summary. *Circulation* 130:2354–2394, 2014.

224. Bittl JA, Baber U, Bradley SM, Wijeysundera DN: Duration of dual antiplatelet therapy: A systematic review for the 2016 ACC/AHA guideline focused update on duration of dual antiplatelet therapy in patients with coronary artery disease. *Circulation* 134:e156–e178, 2016.

225. Moseley AD, Collado FM, Volgman AS, et al: Duration of dual antiplatelet therapy in coronary artery disease: A review article. *Curr Atheroscler Rep* 18:45, 2016.

226. Morrow DA, Braunwald E, Bonaca MP, et al: Vorapaxar in the secondary prevention of atherothrombotic events. *N Engl J Med* 366:1404–1413, 2012.

227. Lipinski MJ, Lee RC, Gaglia MA Jr, et al: Comparison of heparin, bivalirudin, and different glycoprotein IIb/IIIa inhibitor regimens for anticoagulation during percutaneous coronary intervention: A network meta-analysis. *Cardiovas Revasc Med* 17:535–545, 2016.

228. Anderson JL, Morrow DA: Acute myocardial infarction. *N Engl J Med* 376:2053–2064, 2017.

229. Grines CL, Browne KF, Marco J, et al: A comparison of immediate angioplasty with thrombolytic therapy for acute myocardial infarction. The Primary Angioplasty in Myocardial Infarction Study Group. *N Engl J Med* 328:673–679, 1993.

230. Le May MR, Davies RF, Labinaz M, et al: Hospitalization costs of primary stenting versus thrombolysis in acute myocardial infarction: Cost analysis of the Canadian STAT Study. *Circulation* 108:2624–2630, 2003.

231. Pollack CV Jr, Braunwald E: 2007 Update to the ACC/AHA guidelines for the management of patients with unstable angina and non-ST-segment elevation myocardial infarction: Implications for emergency department practice. *Ann Emerg Med* 51:591–606, 2008.

232. Palmerini T, Biondi-Zoccai G, Della Riva D, et al: Clinical outcomes with drug-eluting and bare-metal stents in patients with ST-segment elevation myocardial infarction: Evidence from a comprehensive network meta-analysis. *J Am Coll Cardiol* 62:496–504, 2013.

233. Hinohara TT, Rao SV: Current state of radial artery catheterization in ST-elevation myocardial infarction. *Prog Cardiovasc Dis* 58:241–246, 2015.

234. Valgimigli M, Gagnor A, Calabró P, et al: Radial versus femoral access in patients with acute coronary syndromes undergoing invasive management: A randomised, multicenter trial. *Lancet* 385:2465–2476, 2015.

235. Califf RM, White HD, Van de Werf F, et al: One-year results from the Global Utilization of Streptokinase and TPA for Occluded Coronary Arteries (GUSTO-I) trial. GUSTO-I Investigators. *Circulation* 94:1233–1238, 1996.

236. Llevadot J, Giugliano RP, Antman EM: Bolus fibrinolytic therapy in acute myocardial infarction. *JAMA* 286:442–449, 2001.

237. Brieger DB, Mak KH, White HD, et al: Benefit of early sustained reperfusion in patients with prior myocardial infarction (the GUSTO-I trial). Global Utilization of Streptokinase and TPA for occluded arteries. *Am J Cardiol* 81:282–287, 1998.

238. Coumadin Aspirin Reinfarction Study (CARS) Investigators: Randomised double-blind trial of fixed low-dose warfarin with aspirin after myocardial infarction. *Lancet* 350:389–396, 1997.

239. McMahon SR, Brummel-Ziedins K, Schneider DJ: Novel oral anticoagulants in the management of coronary artery disease. *Coron Artery Dis* 27:412–419, 2016.

240. Stone NJ, Robinson JG, Lichtenstein AH, et al: 2013 ACC/AHA guideline on the treatment of blood cholesterol to reduce atherosclerotic cardiovascular risk in adults: A report of the American College of Cardiology/American Heart Association Task Force on Practice Guidelines. *J Am Coll Cardiol* 63:2889–2934, 2014.

241. Cannon CP, Murphy SA, Braunwald E: Intensive lipid lowering with atorvastatin in coronary disease. *N Engl J Med* 353:93–96; author reply 93–96, 2005.

242. Antithrombotic Trialists' Collaboration: Collaborative meta-analysis of randomised trials of antiplatelet therapy for prevention of death, myocardial infarction, and stroke in high risk patients. *BMJ* 324:71–86, 2002.

243. Lewis HD Jr, Davis JW, Archibald DG, et al: Protective effects of aspirin against acute myocardial infarction and death in men with unstable angina. Results of a Veterans Administration Cooperative Study. *N Engl J Med* 309:396–403, 1983.

244. Cairns JA, Gent M, Singer J, et al: Aspirin, sulfinpyrazone, or both in unstable angina. Results of a Canadian multicenter trial. *N Engl J Med* 313:1369–1375, 1985.

245. Boersma E, Harrington RA, Moliterno DJ, et al: Platelet glycoprotein IIb/IIIa inhibitors in acute coronary syndromes. *Lancet* 360:342–343, 2002.

246. Gaglia MA Jr, Clavijo L: Cardiovascular pharmacology core reviews: Aspirin. *J Cardiovasc Pharmacol Ther* 18:505–513, 2013.

247. Yusuf S, Zhao F, Mehta SR, et al: Effects of clopidogrel in addition to aspirin in patients with acute coronary syndromes without ST-segment elevation. *N Engl J Med* 345:494–502, 2001.

248. Mehta SR: Aspirin and clopidogrel in patients with ACS undergoing PCI: CURE and PCI-CURE. *J Invasive Cardiol* 15(Suppl B):17B–20B, 2003.

249. Hongo RH, Ley J, Dick SE, Yee RR: The effect of clopidogrel in combination with aspirin when given before coronary artery bypass grafting. *J Am Coll Cardiol* 40:231–237, 2002.

250. Antoniucci D, Migliorini A, Parodi G, et al: Abciximab-supported infarct artery stent implantation for acute myocardial infarction and long-term survival: A prospective, multicenter, randomized trial comparing infarct artery stenting plus abciximab with stenting alone. *Circulation* 109:1704–1706, 2004.

251. Nguyen CM, Harrington RA: Glycoprotein IIb/IIIa receptor antagonists: A comparative review of their use in percutaneous coronary intervention. *Am J Cardiovasc Drugs* 3:423–436, 2003.

252. Direct thrombin inhibitors in acute coronary syndromes: Principal results of a meta-analysis based on individual patients' data. *Lancet* 359:294–302, 2002.

253. Lincoff AM, Kleiman NS, Kereiakes DJ, et al: Long-term efficacy of bivalirudin and provisional glycoprotein IIb/IIIa blockade vs heparin and planned glycoprotein IIb/IIIa blockade during percutaneous coronary revascularization: REPLACE-2 randomized trial. *JAMA* 292:696–703, 2004.

254. Linkins LA, Dans AL, Moores LK, et al: Treatment and prevention of heparin-induced thrombocytopenia: Antithrombotic Therapy and Prevention of Thrombosis, 9th ed: American College of Chest Physicians Evidence-Based Clinical Practice Guidelines. *Chest* 141:e495S–530S, 2012.

255. Fraker TD Jr, Fihn SD, Chronic Stable Angina Writing Committee, et al: 2007 chronic angina focused update of the ACC/AHA 2002 guidelines for the management of patients with chronic stable angina: A report of the American College of Cardiology/American Heart Association Task Force on Practice Guidelines Writing Group to develop the focused update of the 2002 guidelines for the management of patients with chronic stable angina. *J Am Coll Cardiol* 50:2264–2274, 2007.

256. Kaiser GC, Davis KB, Fisher LD, et al: Survival following coronary artery bypass grafting in patients with severe angina pectoris (CASS). An observational study. *J Thorac Cardiovasc Surg* 89:513–524, 1985.

257. Shaw LJ, Berman DS, Maron DJ, et al: Optimal medical therapy with or without percutaneous coronary intervention to reduce ischemic burden: Results from the Clinical Outcomes Utilizing Revascularization and Aggressive Drug Evaluation (COURAGE) trial nuclear substudy. *Circulation* 117:1283–1291, 2008.

258. Mintz GS, Kimura T, Nobuyoshi M, Leon MB: Intravascular ultrasound assessment of the relation between early and late changes in arterial area and neointimal hyperplasia after percutaneous transluminal coronary angioplasty and directional coronary atherectomy. *Am J Cardiol* 83:1518–1523, 1999.

259. Wilensky RL, Tanguay JF, Ito S, et al: Heparin Infusion Prior to Stenting (HIPS) trial: Final results of a prospective, randomized, controlled trial evaluating the effects of local vascular delivery on intimal hyperplasia. *Am Heart J* 139:1061–1070, 2000.

260. Morice MC, Serruys PW, Sousa JE, et al: A randomized comparison of a sirolimus-eluting stent with a standard stent for coronary revascularization. *N Engl J Med* 346:1773–1780, 2002.

261. Simonton CA, Brodie B, Cheek B, et al: Comparative clinical outcomes of paclitaxel- and sirolimus-eluting stents: Results from a large prospective multicenter registry—STENT Group. *J Am Coll Cardiol* 50:1214–1222, 2007.

262. Kullo IJ, Rooke TW: Peripheral artery disease. *N Engl J Med* 374:861–871, 2016.

263. Mohler ER 3rd: Peripheral arterial disease: Identification and implications. *Arch Intern Med* 163:2306–2314, 2003.

264. Lukasiewicz A: Treatment of acute lower limb ischaemia. *Vasa* 45:213–221, 2016.

265. Shishehbor MH, White CJ, Gray BH, et al: Critical limb ischemia: An expert statement. *J Am Coll Cardiol* 68:2002–2015, 2016.

266. Rooke TW, Hirsch AT, Misra S, et al: 2011 ACCF/AHA focused update of the guideline for the management of patients with peripheral artery disease (updating the 2005 guideline): A report of the American College of Cardiology Foundation/American Heart Association Task Force on Practice Guidelines. *J Am Coll Cardiol* 58:2020–2045, 2011.

267. Norgren L, Hiatt WR, Dormandy JA, et al: Inter-Society Consensus for the Management of Peripheral Arterial Disease (TASC II). *Eur J Vasc Endovasc Surg* 33(Suppl 1):S1–S75, 2007.

268. Goyen M, Edelman M, Perreault P, et al: MR angiography of aortoiliac occlusive disease: A phase III study of the safety and effectiveness of the blood-pool contrast agent MS-325. *Radiology* 236:825–833, 2005.

269. Gerhard-Herman MD, Gornik HL, et al: 2016 AHA/ACC guideline on the management of patients with lower extremity peripheral artery disease: executive summary. *J Am Coll Cardiol* 69:1465–1508, 2017.

270. Mohler ER 3rd: Therapy insight: Peripheral arterial disease and diabetes—From pathogenesis to treatment guidelines. *Nat Clin Pract Cardiovasc Med* 4:151–162, 2007.

271. Mohler ER, Jaff MR: *Peripheral Arterial Disease*. American College of Physicians, Philadelphia, 2008.

272. Goldhaber SZ, Manson JE, Stampfer MJ, et al: Low-dose aspirin and subsequent peripheral arterial surgery in the Physicians' Health Study. *Lancet* 340:143–145, 1992.

273. CAPRIE Steering Committee: A randomised, blinded, trial of clopidogrel versus aspirin in patients at risk of ischaemic events (CAPRIE). *Lancet* 348:1329–1339, 1996.

274. Belch J, MacCuish A, Campbell I, et al: The prevention of progression of arterial disease and diabetes (POPADAD) trial: Factorial randomised placebo controlled trial of aspirin and antioxidants in patients with diabetes and asymptomatic peripheral arterial disease. *BMJ* 337:a1840, 2008.

275. Mohler E 3rd, Giri J: Management of peripheral arterial disease patients: Comparing the ACC/AHA and TASC-II guidelines. *Curr Med Res Opin* 24:2509–2522, 2008.

276. Gardner AW, Poehlman ET: Exercise rehabilitation programs for the treatment of claudication pain. A meta-analysis. *JAMA* 274:975–980, 1995.

277. Murphy TP, Cutlip DE, Regensteiner JG, et al: Supervised exercise versus primary stenting for claudication resulting from aortoiliac peripheral artery disease: Six-month outcomes from the claudication: Exercise versus endoluminal revascularization (CLEVER) study. *Circulation* 125:130–139, 2012.

278. Reilly MP, Mohler ER 3rd: Cilostazol: Treatment of intermittent claudication. *Ann Pharmacother* 35:48–56, 2001.

279. Wilhite DB, Comerota AJ, Schmieder FA, et al: Managing PAD with multiple platelet inhibitors: The effect of combination therapy on bleeding time. *J Vasc Surg* 38: 710–713, 2003.

280. Popplewell MA, Davies H, Jarrett H, et al: Bypass versus angioplasty in severe ischaemia of the leg-2 (BASIL-2) trial: Study protocol for a randomised controlled trial. *Trials* 17:11, 2016.

281. Kernan WN, Ovbiagele B, Black HR, et al: Guidelines for the prevention of stroke in patients with stroke and transient ischemic attack. A guideline for healthcare professionals from the American Heart Association/American Stroke Association. *Stroke* 45:2160–2236, 2014.

282. Bogousslavsky J, Kaste M, Skyhoj OT, et al: Risk factors and stroke prevention. European Stroke Initiative (EUSI). *Cerebrovasc Dis* 10(Suppl 3):12–21, 2000.

283. Zhang YB, Yin Z, Han X, et al: Association of circulating high-sensitivity C-reactive protein with late recurrence after ischemic stroke. *Neuroreport* 28:598–603, 2017.

284. Gryglas A, Smigiel R: Migraine and stroke: What's the link? What to do? *Curr Neurol Neurosci Rep* 17:22, 2017.

285. Christophe BR, Mehta SH, Garton ALA, et al: Current and future perspectives on the treatment of cerebral ischemia. *Expert Opin Pharmacother* 18:573–580, 2017.

286. Berkhemer OA, Fransen PSS, Beumer D, et al: A randomized trial of intraarterial treatment for acute ischemic stroke. *N Engl J Med* 372:11–20, 2015.

287. Goyal M, Demchuck AM, Menon BK, et al: Randomized assessment of rapid endovascular treatment of ischemic stroke. *N Engl I Med* 372:1019–1030, 2015.

288. Saver JL, Goyal M, Bonafe A, et al: Stent-retriever thrombectomy after intravenous t-PA vs, t-PA alone in stroke. *N Engl J Med* 372:2285–2295, 2015.

289. Campbell BC, Mitchell PJ, Kleinig TJ, et al: Endovascular therapy for ischemic stroke with perfusion-imaging selection. *N Engl J Med* 372:1009–1018, 2015.

290. Jovin TG, Chamorro A, Cobo E, et al: Thrombectomy within 8 hours after symptom onset in ischemic stroke. *N Engl J Med* 372:2296–2306, 2015.

291. Barrett KM, Brott TG: Stroke caused by extracranial disease. *Circ Res* 120:496–501, 2017.

292. Meschia JF, Bushnell C, Boden-Albala B, et al: Guidelines for the primary prevention of stroke: A statement for healthcare professionals from the American Heart Association/American Stroke Association. *Stroke* 45:3754–3832, 2014.

293. Brott TG, Howard G, Roubin GS, et al: Long-term results of stenting versus endarterectomy for carotid-artery stenosis. *N Engl J Med* 374:1021–1031, 2016.

294. Giri J, Parikh SA, Kennedy KF, et al: Proximal versus distal embolic protection for carotid artery stenting: A national cardiovascular data registry analysis. *JACC Cardiovasc Interv* 8:609–615, 2015,

295. Schofer J, Musialek P, Bijuklic K, et al: A prospective, multicenter study of a novel mesh-covered carotid stent: The CGuard CARENET Trial (Carotid Embolic Protection Using MicroNET). *JACC Cardiovasc Interv* 8:1129–1134, 2015.

296. Diener HC, Cunha L, Forbes C, et al: European Stroke Prevention Study. 2. Dipyridamole and acetylsalicylic acid in the secondary prevention of stroke. *J Neurol Sci* 143:1–13, 1996.

297. Sacco RL, Diener HC, Yusuf S, et al: Aspirin and extended-release dipyridamole versus clopidogrel for recurrent stroke. *N Engl J Med* 359:1238–1251, 2008.

298. Chowdhury R, Stevens S, Gorman D, et al: Association between fish consumption, long chain omega 3 fatty acids, and risk of cerebrovascular disease: Systematic review and meta-analysis. *BMJ* 345:e6698.

299. Kapil N, Datta YH, Alakbarova N, et al: Antiplatelet and anticoagulant therapies for prevention of ischemic stroke. *Clin Appl Thromb Hemost* 23:301–318, 2017.

300. Li X, Bayliss G, Zhuang S: Cholesterol crystal embolism and chronic kidney disease. *Int J Mol Sci* 18:pii:E1120.doi: 10.3390/ijms18061120, 2017.

301. Voetsch B, Afshar-Kharghan V, Loscalzo J, Schafer AI: Less common thrombotic and embolic disorders, in *Thrombosis and Hemorrhage*, edited by J Loscalzo AI Schafer, pp 707–762. Lippincott Williams & Wilkins, Philadelphia, 2003.

302. Quinones A, Saric M: The cholesterol emboli syndrome in atherosclerosis. *Curr Atheroscler Rep* 15:315, 2013.

# CHAPTER 25
# FIBRINOLYSIS AND THROMBOLYSIS

Katherine A. Hajjar and Jia Ruan

## SUMMARY

Improved understanding of the molecular mechanisms of fibrinolysis has led to major advances in fibrinolytic and antifibrinolytic therapy. Characterization of the genes for all the major fibrinolytic proteins has revealed the structure of the relevant serine proteases, their inhibitors, and their receptors. The development of genetically engineered animals deficient in one or more fibrinolytic protein(s) has revealed both expected and unexpected functions. In addition, we now have a catalog of acquired and inherited disorders reflective of either fibrinolytic deficiency with thrombosis or fibrinolytic excess with hemorrhage. These advances have led to development of more effective and safer protocols for both pro- and antifibrinolytic therapy in a variety of circumstances.

## ● BASIC CONCEPTS OF FIBRINOLYSIS

In response to vascular injury, fibrin, the insoluble end product of the action of thrombin on fibrinogen, is deposited in blood vessels, thus stemming the flow of blood. Once the vessel has healed, the fibrinolytic system is activated, converting fibrin to its soluble degradation products through the action of the serine protease, plasmin (Fig. 25–1A). Fibrinolysis is subject to precise control because of the actions of multiple activators, inhibitors, and cofactors.[1] In addition, receptors expressed by endothelial, monocytoid, and myeloid cells provide specialized, protected environments where plasmin can be generated without compromise by circulating inhibitors (Fig. 25–1B).[2,3] Beyond its more traditional role in fibrin degradation, the fibrinolytic system also supports a variety of tissue remodeling mechanisms. This chapter reviews the fundamental features of plasmin generation, considers the major clinical syndromes resulting from abnormalities in fibrinolysis, and discusses approaches to fibrinolytic and antifibrinolytic therapy.

## ● COMPONENTS OF THE FIBRINOLYTIC SYSTEM

### PLASMINOGEN

Synthesized primarily in the liver,[4,5] plasminogen is a Mr approximately 92,000 single-chain proenzyme that circulates in plasma at a

Acronyms and Abbreviations: $\alpha_2$-PI, alpha-2 plasmin inhibitor; APL, acute promyelocytic leukemia; CI, confidence interval; CT, computed tomography; DIC, disseminated intravascular coagulation; HC, homocysteine; IL, interleukin; LDL, low-density lipoprotein; MMP, matrix metalloproteinase; MRI, magnetic resonance imaging; Plg, plasminogen; PAI, plasminogen activator inhibitor; TAFI, thrombin-activatable fibrinolysis inhibitor; TGF-$\beta$, transforming growth factor beta; t-PA, tissue-type plasminogen activator; u-PA, urokinase-type plasminogen activator; uPAR, urokinase-type plasminogen activator receptor.

concentration of approximately 1.5 $\mu$M[6] (Table 25–1). The plasma half-life of plasminogen in adults is approximately 2 days.[7] Its 791 amino acids are crosslinked by 24 disulfide bridges, 16 of which give rise to five homologous triple loop structures called "kringles" (Fig. 25–2).[8] The first (K1) and fourth (K4) of these 80-amino-acid, Mr approximately 10,000 structures impart high- and low-affinity lysine binding, respectively.[9] The lysine-binding domains of plasminogen appear to mediate its specific interactions with fibrin, cell surface receptors, and other proteins, including its circulating inhibitor $\alpha_2$-plasmin inhibitor ($\alpha_2$-PI).[10–14]

Posttranslational modification of plasminogen results in two glycosylation variants (forms 1 and 2; see Table 25–1).[15–17] O-linked oligosaccharide, consisting of sialic acid, galactose, and galactosamine resident on Thr345, is common to both forms. Only form 2, however, contains N-linked oligosaccharide on Asn 288 that is comprised of sialic acid, galactose, glucosamine, and mannose. The carbohydrate portion of plasminogen appears to regulate its affinity for cellular receptors and may also specify its physiologic degradation pathway.

Activation of plasminogen results from cleavage of a single Arg–Val peptide bond at position 560–561,[6] giving rise to the active protease, plasmin (see Table 25–1). Plasmin contains a typical serine protease catalytic triad (His 602, Asp 645, and Ser 740), but exhibits broad substrate specificity when compared to other proteases of this class.[18] The circulating form of plasminogen, aminoterminal glutamic acid plasminogen (Glu–Plg), can be converted by limited proteolysis to several modified forms known collectively as Lys–Plg.[19,20] Hydrolysis of the Lys77–Lys78 peptide bond gives rise to a conformationally modified form of the zymogen that more readily binds fibrin, displays two- to threefold higher avidity for cellular receptors, and is activated 10 to 20 times more rapidly than Glu–Plg.[11,21,22] Lys–Plg does not normally circulate in plasma[21] but has been identified on cell surfaces.[23,24]

Spanning 52.5 kb of DNA on chromosome 6q26–27, the Plg gene consists of 19 exons[25,26] and directs expression of a 2.7-kb mRNA[8] (see Fig. 25–2). The 5′ upstream region of the Plg gene contains two regulatory elements common to genes for acute-phase reactants (CTGGGA) and six interleukin (IL)-6 response elements.[26] Plg gene activity, moreover, is stimulated by the acute-phase-mediator IL-6 both in vitro and in vivo.[27] The gene is closely linked and structurally related to that of apolipoprotein(a), an apoprotein associated with the highly atherogenic low-density lipoprotein–like particle lipoprotein(a),[28] and more distantly related to other kringle-containing proteins such as tissue-type plasminogen activator (t-PA), urokinase-type plasminogen activator (u-PA), macrophage-stimulating protein, and hepatocyte growth factor.[29–34]

### The Physiologic Functions of Plasmin(ogen)

Mice made completely deficient in Plg through gene targeting undergo normal embryogenesis and development, are fertile, and survive to adulthood (Table 25–2).[35,36] These animals display runting and ligneous conjunctivitis,[37] and harbor spontaneous thrombi in the liver, stomach, colon, rectum, lung, and pancreas, as well as fibrin deposition in the liver and ulcerative lesions in the gastrointestinal tract and rectum. These results suggested that Plg is not strictly required for normal development, but does play a central role in fibrin homeostasis. In humans, Plg deficiency presents most often with ligneous mucositis as a result of fibrin deposition and is rarely a cause of macrovascular thrombosis (see "Fibrinolytic Deficiency and Thrombosis" below).

### PLASMINOGEN ACTIVATORS

#### Tissue-Type Plasminogen Activator

One of two major endogenous Plg activators, t-PA consists of 527 amino acids comprising a glycoprotein of Mr approximately 72,000 (see Table 25–1).[38] t-PA contains five structural domains including a

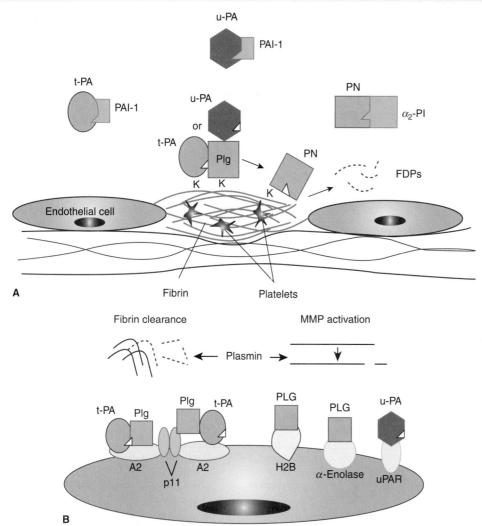

**Figure 25–1.** Overview of the fibrinolytic system. **A.** Fibrin-based plasminogen activation. The zymogen plasminogen (Plg) is converted to the active serine protease, plasmin (PN), through the action of tissue-type plasminogen activator (t-PA) or urokinase-type plasminogen activator (u-PA). The activity of t-PA is greatly enhanced by its assembly with Plg through lysine residues (K) on a fibrin-containing thrombus. u-PA acts independently of fibrin. Both t-PA and u-PA can be inhibited by plasminogen activator inhibitor-1 (PAI-1), the main physiologic regulator of plasminogen activator activity. By binding to fibrin, PN is protected from its major inhibitor, $a_2$-plasmin inhibitor ($a_2$–PI). Fibrin-bound plasmin degrades crosslinked fibrin, giving rise to soluble fibrin degradation products (FDPs). **B.** Cell surface plasminogen activation. Although many cell types express receptors for Plg, urokinase, and t-PA, only the endothelial cell is depicted here. The annexin A2 heterotetramer, consisting of two copies each of annexin A2 (A2) and protein p11 (p11), binds both t-PA and Plg, thereby augmenting the efficiency of plasmin generation on endothelial cells. Plg may also bind to other endothelial cell receptors, including histone H2B (H2B) and $a$-enolase, and may be activated by u-PA bound to its receptor, uPAR, to effect plasmin generation.

**TABLE 25–1.** Fibrinolytic Proteins

**A. Major Proteases**

| Property | Plasminogen | t-PA | u-PA |
|---|---|---|---|
| Molecular mass | 92,000 | 72,000 | 54,000 |
| Amino acids | 791 | 527 | 411 |
| Chromosome | 6 | 8 | 10 |
| Site of synthesis | Liver | Endothelium | Endothelium, kidney |
| Plasma concentration | | | |
| nM | 1500 | 0.075 | 0.150 |
| mcg/mL | 140 | 0.005 | 0.008 |
| Plasma half-life | 48 h | 5 min | 8 min |
| N-Glycosylation (%) | 2 | 13 | 7 |
| Form 1 | – | Asn117, Asn184, Asn448 | Asn302 |
| Form 2 | Asn288 | Asn117, –, Asn448 | – |
| O-Glycosylation | | | |
| $a$-Fucose | – | Thr61 | Thr18 |
| Complex | Thr345 | – | – |

(continued)

**TABLE 25–1.** Fibrinolytic Proteins *(Continued)*

| Two-chain cleavage site | Arg560-Val561 | Arg275-Ile276 | Lys158-Ile159 |
|---|---|---|---|
| Heavy-chain domains | | | |
| Finger | No | Yes | No |
| Growth factor | No | Yes | Yes |
| Kringles (no.) | 5 | 2 | 1 |
| Light-chain catalytic triad | His602, Asp645, Ser740 | His322, Asp371, Ser478 | His204, Asp255, Ser356 |

**B. Major Serpin Inhibitors**

| Property | $\alpha_2$-PI | PAI-1 | PAI-2 |
|---|---|---|---|
| Molecular mass | 70,000 | 52,000 | 60,000 (glycosylated) 47,000 (nonglycosylated) |
| Amino acids | 452 | 402 | 393 |
| Chromosome | 18 | 7 | 18 |
| Sites of synthesis | Kidney, liver | Endothelium Monocytes/macrophages Hepatocytes Adipocytes | Placenta Monocytes/macrophages Tumor cells |
| Plasma concentration | | | |
| nM | 900 | 0.1–0.4 | ND |
| mcg/mL | 50 | 0.02 | ND |
| Serpin reactive site | Arg364–Met365 | Arg346–Met347 | Arg358–Thr359 |
| Specificity | Plasmin | u-PA = t-PA | u-PA > t-PA |

**C. Major Activation Receptors**

| Property | uPAR | Annexin A2 | p11 | Plg-R$_{KT}$ | Histone 2B |
|---|---|---|---|---|---|
| Molecular mass | 55,000–60,000 | 36,000 | 11,000 | 17,000 | 17,000 |
| Amino acids | 313 | 339 | 4544 | 147 | 126 |
| Chromosome | 19 | 15 | 12 | 9 | 6 |
| Source | Endothelial cells | Endothelial cells | Endothelial cells | – | Endothelial cells |
| | Monocytes | Monocytes | Monocytes | Monocytes | Monocytes |
| | Macrophages | Macrophages | Macrophages | Macrophages | Macrophages |
| | Fibroblasts | Myeloid cells | Myeloid cells | Myeloid cells | Neutrophils |
| | Tumor cells | Tumor cells | Tumor cells | Tumor cells | |
| Ligand(s) | u-PA | t-PA, Plg | Plg | Plg | |

$\alpha_2$-PI, $\alpha_2$-plasmin inhibitor; ND, not determined; PAI-1, plasminogen activator inhibitor type 1; PAI-2, plasminogen activator inhibitor type 2; Plg, plasminogen; Plg-R$_{KT}$, plasminogen receptor with terminal lysine; PN, plasmin; t-PA, tissue-type plasminogen activator; u-PA, urokinase-type plasminogen activator; uPAR, urokinase plasminogen activator receptor.

fibronectin-like "finger," an epidermal growth factor–like domain, two "kringle" structures homologous to those of Plg, and a serine protease domain (see Fig. 25–2). Cleavage of the Arg275–Ile276 peptide bond by plasmin converts t-PA to a disulfide-linked, two-chain form.[38] Although single-chain t-PA is less active than two-chain t-PA in the fluid phase, both forms demonstrate equivalent activity when fibrin bound.[39]

The two glycosylation forms of t-PA are distinguishable by the presence (type 1) or absence (type 2) of a complex N-linked oligosaccharide moiety on Asn184 (see Table 25–1).[40,41] Both types, however, contain high mannose carbohydrate on Asn 117, complex oligosaccharide on

Asn448, and an O-linked $\alpha$-fucose residue on Thr61.[42] The carbohydrate moieties of t-PA may modulate its functional activity, regulate its binding to cell surface receptors, and specify its degradation pathways.

Located on chromosome 8p12–q11.2, the gene for human t-PA is encoded by 14 exons spanning a total of 36.6 kb (see Fig. 25–2).[43–45] Although exon 1 encodes a 58-nucleotide mRNA leader sequence, each of the structural domains of t-PA is encoded by one or two of the remaining 13 exons. This arrangement suggests that the t-PA gene arose by an evolutionary process called "exon shuffling," whereby functionally related genes evolved through rearrangement of exons

Plasminogen

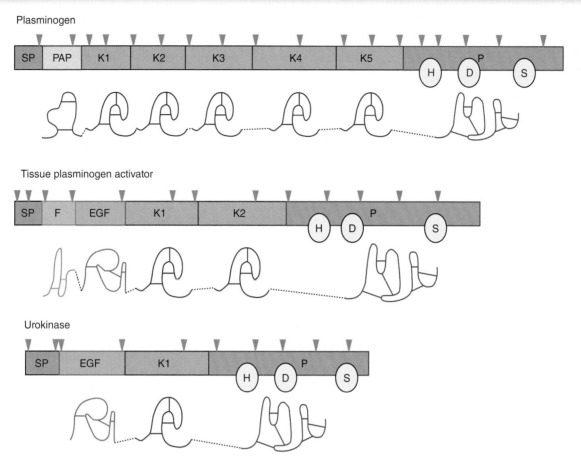

**Figure 25–2.** Alignment of the intron–exon structure of plasminogen, tissue plasminogen activator, and urokinase genes showing functional protein domains. Protein domains are labeled signal peptide (SP), preactivation peptide (PAP), "kringle" domains (K), fibronectin-like "finger" (F), epidermal growth factor–like domain (EGF), and protease (P). The positions of the catalytic triad amino acids histidine (H), aspartic acid (D), and serine (S) are shown within individual protease domains. The positions of individual introns relative to amino acid encoding exons are indicated with inverted triangles.

encoding autonomous domains. Consistent with this hypothesis, deletion of exons encoding the fibronectin-like finger or kringle 2, but not kringle 1, domains of t-PA results in expression of mutants resistant to the cofactor activity of fibrin, while catalytic activity in the absence of fibrin remains intact.[46]

The proximal promoter of the human t-PA gene contains binding sequences for potentially important transcription factors including AP1, NF1, SP1, and AP2,[47,48] as well as a potential cyclic adenosine monophosphate (cAMP)–responsive element (CRE).[49] In vitro, many agents have been shown to exert small effects on the expression of t-PA mRNA, but relatively few enhance t-PA synthesis without augmenting plasminogen activator inhibitor (PAI)-1 synthesis as well. Agents that regulate t-PA gene expression independently of PAI-1 include histamine, butyrate, retinoids, arterial levels of shear stress, and dexamethasone.[50-55] Forskolin, which increases intracellular cAMP levels, has been reported to decrease synthesis of both t-PA and PAI-1.[48,56]

In the vascular system, t-PA is synthesized and secreted primarily by endothelial cells belonging to a restricted set of blood vessels. In rodents, t-PA expression appears in 7- to 30-$\mu$m diameter precapillary arterioles in the lung, postcapillary venules, and vasa vasorum; much less expression is seen in endothelial cells of the femoral artery, femoral vein, carotid artery, or aorta.[57] In the mouse lung, bronchial arteriolar endothelial cells express t-PA antigen, especially at branch points, while pulmonary blood vessels are uniformly negative.[51,58-60] t-PA has also been

detected in sympathetic neurons associated with the blood vessel wall.[61] Release of t-PA is governed by a variety of stimuli such as thrombin, histamine, bradykinin, epinephrine, acetylcholine, arginine vasopressin, gonadotropins, exercise, venous occlusion, and shear stress.[50,51,62,63] Its circulating half-life is exceedingly short (~5 minutes). Alone, t-PA is actually a poor activator of Plg, but, in the presence of fibrin, the catalytic efficiency of t-PA–dependent plasmin generation ($k_{cat}/K_m$) increases by at least two orders of magnitude.[22] This is the result of a dramatic increase in affinity (decreased $K_m$) between t-PA and its substrate Plg in the presence of fibrin. Although it is also expressed by extravascular cells, t-PA appears to represent the major intravascular activator of Plg.[18]

## Urokinase

The second endogenous Plg activator, single-chain u-PA or prourokinase, is an Mr approximately 54,000 glycoprotein consisting of 411 amino acids (see Table 25–1). u-PA possesses an epidermal growth factor–like domain, a single Plg-like "kringle," and a classical catalytic triad (His204, Asp255, Ser356) within its serine protease domain (see Fig. 25–2).[64] Cleavage of the Lys158–Ile159 peptide bond by plasmin or kallikrein converts single-chain u-PA to a disulfide-linked two-chain derivative.[65] Located on chromosome 10, the human u-PA gene is encoded by 11 exons spanning 6.4 kb and expressed by activated endothelial cells, macrophages, renal epithelial cells, and some tumor cells.[66,67] Its intron–exon structure is closely related to that of the t-PA gene.

**TABLE 25–2.** Mouse Gene Deletion Models Relevant to Fibrinolysis

| Genotype | Some Phenotypic Features | References |
|---|---|---|
| **Plasminogen** | | |
| Plg–/– | Spontaneous thrombosis, runting, premature death | 35, 36 |
| | Fibrin in liver, lungs, stomach; gastric ulcers | 35, 36 |
| | Impaired wound healing | 243, 244 |
| | Ligneous mucositis | 37 |
| | Impaired monocyte recruitment | 245 |
| | Impaired neointima formation after electrical injury | 246 |
| | Impaired dissemination of *Borrelia burgdorferi* | 247 |
| **Plasminogen Activators** | | |
| t-PA–/– | Reduced lysis of fibrin clot | 84 |
| | Increased endotoxin-induced thrombosis | 84 |
| u-PA–/– | Occasional fibrin in liver/intestine | 84 |
| | Rectal prolapse, ulcers of eyelids, face, ears | 84 |
| | Reduced macrophage degradation of fibrin | 84 |
| | Increased endotoxin-induced thrombosis | 84 |
| u-PA–/– t-PA–/– | Reduced growth, fertility, and life span; cachexia | 84 |
| | Fibrin deposits in liver, gonads, lungs | 84 |
| | Ulcers in intestine, skin, ears; rectal prolapse | 84 |
| | Impaired clot lysis | 84 |
| **Inhibitors** | | |
| $\alpha_2$PI–/– | Reduced fibrin deposition following endotoxin | 90 |
| | Enhanced lysis of injected plasma clots | 90 |
| PAI-1–/– | Mildly increased lysis of fibrin clot | 123 |
| | Resistance to endotoxin-induced thrombosis | 124 |
| TAFI–/– | Increased clot lysis | 140, 142 |
| | Reduced injury-related venous thrombosis | 141 |
| **Receptors** | | |
| uPAR–/– | Normal development and fertility | 163 |
| | Normal clot lysis | 164 |
| Annexin A2–/– | Fibrin deposition in microvasculature | 205 |
| | Impaired clearance of arterial thrombi | 205 |
| | Impaired postnatal neoangiogenesis | 198, 205, 270 |
| S100A10–/– | Reduced baseline fibrin deposition | 199 |

u-PA expression appears to be induced during neoplastic transformation, possibly through the action of transcription factors AP1 and AP2.[68] Other *in vitro* u-PA inducers include hormones, angiogenic growth factors, and cAMP,[55] as well as tumor necrosis factor and transforming growth factor-$\beta$ (TGF-$\beta$).[69–71]

Two-chain u-PA occurs in both high- (Mr 54,000) and low-molecular-weight (Mr 33,000) forms that differ by the presence or absence, respectively, of a 135-residue aminoterminal fragment released by plasmin cleavage between Lys135 and Lys136.[72,73] Although both forms are capable of activating Plg, only the high-molecular-weight form binds to the u-PA receptor (see "Urokinase Plasminogen Activator Receptors" below). u-PA has much lower affinity for fibrin than t-PA and is an effective Plg activator both in the presence and in the absence of fibrin.[74,75]

### Accessory Plasminogen Activators and Fibrinolysins

Under certain conditions, proteases traditionally classified within the intrinsic arm of the coagulation cascade have been shown to be capable of activating Plg directly. These include kallikrein, factor XIa, and factor XIIa.[76–78] These proteases, however, normally account for no more than 15 percent of total plasmin-generating activity in plasma.[79] In addition, the membrane type 1 matrix metalloproteinase (MT1-MMP) appears to exert fibrinolytic activity in the absence of Plg and may explain the unexpectedly mild phenotype observed in Plg-deficient mice.[80]

### Physiologic Function of the Plasminogen Activators

Because there are no clinical examples of complete deficiency of t-PA or u-PA in humans, except for patients with deficient release in the setting of chronic renal disease and hypertension,[81–83] the most compelling data regarding the physiologic functions of t-PA and u-PA come from gene disruption analysis in mice.[84] Both u-PA– and t-PA–null deletion mice exhibit normal fertility and embryonic development. However, u-PA–/– mice develop rectal prolapse, nonhealing ulcerations of the face and eyelids, and occasional fibrin deposition in tissues. Although they show normal lysis rates of pulmonary clots injected via the jugular vein, endotoxin-induced microvascular thrombus formation is significantly enhanced. t-PA–deficient mice also display a normal spontaneous phenotype but have a decreased rate of lysis of artificially induced pulmonary thrombi, as well as enhanced thrombus formation, in response to injection of endotoxin. Like Plg–/– mice, mice doubly deficient in t-PA and u-PA (t-PA–/–; u-PA–/–) exhibit rectal prolapse, nonhealing ulceration, runting, and cachexia, with extensive fibrin deposition in liver, intestine, gonads, and lung. Not surprisingly, clot lysis is also markedly impaired.

## INHIBITORS OF FIBRINOLYSIS

### Plasmin Inhibitors

The action of plasmin is negatively modulated by a family of serine protease inhibitors, called serpins (see Table 25–1).[85] Serpins form an irreversible complex with the active site serine of their target protease following proteolytic cleavage of the inhibitor by the target protease. Within such a complex, both protease and inhibitor lose their activity.

A single-chain glycoprotein of Mr approximately 70,000, $\alpha_2$-PI is synthesized primarily in the liver, circulates in plasma at relatively high concentrations (~0.9 $\mu$M), and enjoys a plasma half-life of 2.4 days (see Table 25–1).[86] This serpin contains approximately 13 percent carbohydrate by mass and consists of 452 amino acids with two disulfide bridges.[87] In humans, the gene is located on chromosome 18 and contains 10 exons distributed over 16 kb of DNA.[88] The promoter region of the $\alpha_2$-PI gene contains a hepatitis B–like enhancer element that directs tissue-specific expression in the liver.[87] $\alpha_2$-PI is also a constituent of platelet $\alpha$ granules.[89] Plasmin released into flowing blood or in the vicinity of a platelet-rich thrombus is immediately neutralized upon forming an irreversible 1:1 stoichiometric, lysine-binding site–dependent complex with $\alpha_2$-PI. Interaction with plasmin is accompanied by cleavage of the Arg364–Met365 peptide bond, and the resulting covalent complexes are cleared in the liver. Mice globally deficient in $\alpha_2$-PI display reduced fibrin deposition following treatment with endotoxin and enhanced lysis of injected plasma clots, but no spontaneous bleeding (see Table 25–2).[90]

Several additional proteins can act as plasmin inhibitors (see Table 25–1). $\alpha_2$-Macroglobulin is an Mr 725,000 dimeric protein synthesized by endothelial cells and macrophages and found in platelet $\alpha$ granules. This nonserpin inhibits plasmin with approximately 10 percent of the efficiency exhibited by $\alpha_2$-PI by forming noncovalent complexes with several distinct serine proteases.[91] $C_1$-esterase inhibitor can inhibit t-PA in plasma,[92] and protease nexin may function as a noncirculating cell surface inhibitor of trypsin, thrombin, factor Xa, urokinase, or plasmin, resulting in protease–inhibitor complexes that are endocytosed via a specific nexin receptor.[93,94] The purpose of these multiple plasmin inhibitors is to guard against premature plasmin activation and subsequent degradation of fibrinogen, until intravascular fibrin begins to appear.

### Plasminogen Activator Inhibitors

**Plasminogen Activator Inhibitor-1** Of the two major Plg activator inhibitors, PAI-1 is the most ubiquitous (see Table 25–1).[95] This Mr approximately 52,000 single-chain, cysteine-less glycoprotein is released by endothelial cells, monocytes, macrophages, hepatocytes, adipocytes, and platelets.[96-98] Release of PAI-1 is stimulated by many cytokines, growth factors, and lipoproteins common to the global inflammatory response.[69,70,99,100,101] The PAI-1 gene consists of nine exons, spanning 12.2 kb on chromosome 7q21.3–q22.[102] The serpin-reactive site is located at Arg346–Met347, and activity of this labile serpin is stabilized upon complex formation with vitronectin, a component of plasma and pericellular matrix.[103-105]

Regulation of PAI-1 gene expression is complex.[106,107] The upstream regulatory region of the human PAI-1 gene contains a strong endothelial cell/fibroblast-specific element,[108,109] a glucocorticoid-responsive enhancer,[109] and TGF-$\beta$ responsive elements.[110] TGF-$\beta$ is known to stimulate fos and jun, the two components of the AP1 complex, and an AP1 binding site (GGAGTCA) is located upstream of the PAI-1 cap site.[111] Agents shown to enhance expression of PAI-1 at the message level, the protein level, or both, without affecting t-PA synthesis, include the inflammatory cytokines lipopolysaccharide, IL-1, tumor necrosis factor-$\alpha$,[69,70,99,112,113] TGF-$\beta$ and basic fibroblast growth factor,[71,99,110,114] very-low-density lipoprotein and lipoprotein(a),[115,116] angiotensin II,[117] thrombin,[118,119] and phorbol esters.[120] In addition, endothelial cell PAI-1 is downregulated by forskolin[56] and by endothelial cell growth factor in the presence of heparin.[121]

PAI-1 is the most important and rapidly acting physiologic inhibitor of both t-PA and u-PA. Transgenic mice that overexpress PAI-1 exhibit thrombotic occlusion of tail veins and swelling of hind limbs within 2 weeks of birth.[122] Mice deficient in PAI-1, on the other hand, exhibit normal fertility, viability, tissue histology, and development, and are resistant to endotoxin-induced thrombosis, but show no evidence of overt hemorrhage (see Table 25–2).[123,124] These observations contrast with the moderately severe bleeding disorder observed in a human patient with complete PAI-1 deficiency.[125]

**Plasminogen Activator Inhibitor-2** Originally purified from human placenta, PAI-2 is a 393-amino-acid member of the serpin family whose reactive site is the Arg358–Thr359 peptide bond[126] (see Table 25–1). The gene encoding PAI-2 is located on chromosome 18q21–23, spans 16.5 kb, and contains eight exons.[127] PAI-2 exists as both an Mr 47,000 nonglycosylated intracellular form and an Mr 60,000 glycosylated form secreted by leukocytes and fibrosarcoma cells. Functionally, PAI-2

inhibits both two-chain t-PA and two-chain u-PA with comparable efficiency (second order rate constants $10^5$ $M^{-1}s^{-1}$). However, it is less effective toward single-chain t-PA (second order rate constant $10^3$ $M^{-1}s^{-1}$) and does not inhibit prourokinase.

Significant levels of PAI-2 are found in human plasma primarily during pregnancy. The gene's 5′-untranslated region contains a potent silencer, the PAUSE-1 element, which may be responsible for its low level of expression in nonpregnant individuals.[127,128] The 3′-downstream sequences include the TTATTTAT motif, which has been identified with inflammatory mediators.[129,130] In macrophages in vitro, secretion of PAI-2 is enhanced by endotoxin and phorbol esters,[130,131] and dexamethasone decreases PAI-2 expression in HT-1080 cells.[55]

### Thrombin-Activatable Fibrinolysis Inhibitor

Thrombin-activatable fibrinolysis inhibitor (TAFI) is a plasma carboxypeptidase with specificity for carboxy terminal arginine and lysine residues.[132] The action of TAFI eliminates binding sites for Plg and t-PA on fibrin.[133] This single-chain Mr 60,000 polypeptide circulates in plasma at concentrations of approximately 75 nM, and undergoes limited proteolysis in the presence of thrombin, which leads to its activation.[134-136] The profibrinolytic effect of activated protein C in plasma is a result of its ability to inactivate coagulation factors Va and VIIIa, which reduces activation of thrombin, the primary activator of TAFI.[132] The profibrinolytic effect of activated protein C in an in vitro plasma-based system was TAFI-dependent,[137] and in a system of purified components, TAFI has been shown to downregulate t-PA–induced fibrinolysis half-maximally at a concentration of approximately 1 nM, which is 2 percent of its concentration in plasma.[138] Inhibition of either the intrinsic pathway of coagulation or TAFI itself results in a doubling of endogenous clot lysis in an in vivo rabbit jugular vein model of thrombolysis.[139,140] TAFI-deficient mice display increased lysis of plasma clots and reduced injury-induced venous thrombosis (see Table 25–2).[141,142] In plasma, TAFI may regulate Plg binding to both cell surface receptors and to fibrin.[143]

## CELLULAR RECEPTORS

A large number of structurally diverse fibrinolytic "activation" and "clearance" receptors have been described. Here, we focus on endothelial cell activation receptors that are likely to contribute to homeostatic control of plasmin activity (see Table 25–1).[2] Clearance receptors eliminate plasmin and Plg activators from the blood or focal microenvironments.

### Activation Receptors

**Plasminogen Receptors** Proposed Plg receptors include $\alpha$-enolase, glycoprotein IIb/IIIa complex, the Heymann nephritis antigen, amphoterin, the annexin A2/S100A10 complex, histone H2B, and plasminogen receptor-KT (Plg-$R_{KT}$)[2,3]; these are expressed on a wide spectrum of cells, including monocytoid cells, platelets, renal epithelial cells, neuroblastoma cells, endothelial cells, and tumor cells.[144-151] Typically, Plg receptors interact with the kringle structures of Plg through carboxyl-terminal lysine residues that are either present on the native protein or generated by limited proteolysis.[144]

**Urokinase Plasminogen Activator Receptor** The u-PA receptor (uPAR) is expressed on monocytes, macrophages, fibroblasts, endothelial cells, and many tumor cells (see Table 25–1).[152,153] uPAR complementary DNA (cDNA) was cloned and sequenced from a human fibroblast cDNA library[154] and encodes a protein of 313 amino acids with a 21-residue signal peptide. The gene consists of seven exons distributed over 23 kb of genomic DNA and places this glycoprotein within the Ly-1/elapid venom toxin superfamily of cysteine-rich proteins.[155,156] uPAR is anchored to the plasma membrane through glycosylphosphatidylinositol linkages.[157] u-PA bound to its receptor maintains its activity and susceptibility to the physiologic inhibitor, PAI-1.[158] Formation of u-PA–PAI-1 complexes hastens clearance of u-PA by hepatic or monocytoid cells.[158-161]

Although originally thought to function only as a means of localizing Plg activation to the cell surface, uPAR now appears to play a central role in cellular signaling and adhesion events.[152,162] The uPAR-deficient mouse has normal development and fertility and unimpaired fibrin clot lysis (see Table 25–2).[163,164] uPAR binds the adhesive glycoprotein vitronectin at a site distinct from the u-PA binding domain,[165,166] and u-PA transfected renal epithelial cells acquire enhanced adhesion to vitronectin while they lose their adhesion to fibronectin.[167] uPAR, furthermore, colocalizes with integrins in focal contacts and at the leading edge of migrating cells,[168] and also associates with caveolin, a major component of caveolae, structures abundant in endothelial cells and thought to participate in signaling events.[169-171] In addition, cleaved and soluble forms of uPAR have recently been detected in the sera of patients with cancer, and these modified forms are thought to regulate the activity of several receptors involved in inflammatory and angiogenic responses.[153]

**The Annexin A2–S100A10 System** Annexin A2, an Mr 36,000, 339-amino-acid member of the annexin superfamily of calcium-dependent, phospholipid-binding proteins, forms a heterotetramer with the S100 family protein, S100A10 (see Table 25–1).[172-174] It is highly conserved and abundantly expressed on endothelial cells,[175-178] monocyte/macrophages,[179,180] early myeloid cells,[181] developing neuronal cells,[182] and some tumor cells.[183-185] All of the more than 60 annexin family members have in common a conserved membrane-binding C-terminal "core" region and a more variable N-terminal "tail."[186] The human annexin A2 gene consists of 13 exons distributed over 40 kb of genomic DNA on chromosome 15 (15q21).[187]

Annexin A2 is unique among fibrinolytic receptors in that it possesses binding affinity for both Plg (Kd 114 nM)[148] and t-PA (Kd 30 nM), but not u-PA.[149] In a fluid phase system of purified proteins, native human annexin A2 stimulates the catalytic efficiency of t-PA–dependent Plg activation by 60-fold.[188] This effect is completely inhibited in the presence of lysine analogues or upon treatment of annexin A2 with carboxypeptidase B, an agent that removes basic carboxyl-terminal amino acids. Although it lacks a classical signal peptide, annexin A2 is constitutively translocated to the endothelial cell surface within 16 hours of its biosynthesis. This translocation event can be stimulated either by thrombin or by heat stress, in a process that requires phosphorylation of annexin A2 at Tyr23, the action of a Src family kinase, and the presence of the annexin A2 binding protein p11 (S100A10).[189]

At the cell surface, A2 binds phospholipid via core repeat 2, which contains the linear amino acid sequence KGLGT and downstream aspartate residue (Asp 161); together these moieties constitute a classical "annexin" motif.[190] The annexin A2 heterotetramer, which consists of two A2 monomers and two protein p11 subunits and constitutes the cell surface form of A2, appears to have even greater stimulatory effects on t-PA–dependent plasmin generation.[177] Interestingly, A2 regulates endogenous levels of protein p11 in the endothelial cell by masking a polyubiquitination site on p11, which otherwise directs p11 to the proteasome where it is rapidly degraded.[191]

Plg and t-PA appear to bind to distinct domains. Lys307 appears to be crucial for the effective interaction of Plg with annexin A2 and may be revealed upon limited proteolysis of the parent protein.[188] The atherogenic low-density lipoprotein (LDL)-like particle, lipoprotein(a), competes with Plg for binding to annexin A2 *in vitro*,[192] thereby reducing cell surface plasmin generation. t-PA binding to annexin A2 requires a domain consisting of residues 8 to 13 (LCKLSL) within the receptor's amino terminal "tail" domain.[193] This region is a target for homocysteine (HC), a thiol-containing amino acid that accumulates in association with nutritional deficiencies of vitamin $B_6$, vitamin $B_{12}$, or folic acid,

or in inherited abnormalities of cystathionine $\beta$-synthase, methylenetetrahydrofolate reductase, or methionine synthase,[194] and is associated with atherothrombotic disease.[195,196] *In vitro*, HC impairs t-PA–dependent plasmin generation at the endothelial cell surface by approximately 50 percent[197] by forming a covalent derivative with Cys,[197] and mice with diet-induced hyperhomocysteinemia have deficient annexin A2 function[198] The half-maximal dose of HC for inhibition of t-PA binding to annexin A2 is approximately 11 $\mu$M HC, a value close to the upper limit of normal for HC in plasma (12 $\mu$M).

The important role of S100A10 in fibrin balance has recently been underscored. S100A10–/– mice display increased deposition of fibrin in the vasculature and reduced clearance of batroxobin-induced vascular thrombi, and S100A10-deficient endothelial cells demonstrate a 40 percent reduction in Plg binding and plasmin generation *in vitro* (see Table 25–2).[199] S100A10 also appears to contribute to Plg-dependent macrophage invasion *in vitro* by enhancing plasmin-dependent activation of matrix metalloporetinase-9.[200]

Several studies suggest a physiologic role for the annexin A2 system in fibrin homeostasis. First, blast cells from human patients with acute promyelocytic leukemia overexpress annexin A2 in proportion to their degree of hyperfibrinolytic coagulopathy[181]; S100A10 also appears to be upregulated by the PML-RAR-$\alpha$ oncoprotein,[201] and both annexin A2 and S100A10 are downregulated by treatment with all-*trans*-retinoic acid. Second, in rats, arterial thrombosis can be significantly attenuated by pretreatment with intravenous annexin A2.[202] Third, the prevalence of high-titer anti–annexin A2 antibodies correlates with a history of severe thrombosis in humans with antiphospholipid syndrome and in a cohort of individuals with cerebral venous thrombosis.[203,204] Finally, mice with total deficiency of annexin A2 display impaired clearance of artificial arterial thrombi, fibrin deposition in the microvasculature, and angiogenic defects in a variety of tissues (see Table 25–2).[205]

### Clearance Receptors

Clearance of serpin–enzyme complexes, such as t-PA–PAI-1 and u-PA–PAI-1, occurs mainly in the liver and is mediated by a large two-chain receptor called the LDL receptor–related protein 1 (LRP1).[206,207] LRP1 binds a large number of serpin–protease complexes and other ligands, indicating a multifunctional role in mammalian physiology. An additional Mr 39,000 "receptor-associated protein" copurifies with LRP1 and appears to regulate the binding and uptake of LRP1 ligands.[208] Interestingly, LRP1 "knockout" embryos undergo developmental arrest by 13.5 days after conception, suggesting that regulation of serine protease activity may be crucial for early embryogenesis.[209,210] Although PAI-1–independent clearance pathways for t-PA have been proposed involving the mannose receptor[211] or an $\alpha$-fucose–specific receptor,[212] *in vivo* studies in mice suggest that LRP1 and the mannose receptor play a dominant role in t-PA clearance.[213]

## THE FIBRINOLYTIC ACTIONS OF PLASMIN

### DEGRADATION OF FIBRINOGEN AND FIBRIN

#### Fibrinogen

Plasmin releases carboxyl-terminal A$\alpha$ and N-terminal fibrinopeptide B moieties from fibrinogen (Fig. 25–5). This reaction is distinct from the proteolytic cleavage of fibrinogen by thrombin, which releases fibrinopeptide A, exposing the Gly–Pro–Arg tripeptide sequence and allowing fibrinogen to polymerize and form insoluble fibrin.[214] Plasmin cleavage of fibrinogen (Mr 340,000) initially produces carboxyl-terminal fragments from the $\alpha$ chain within the D domain of

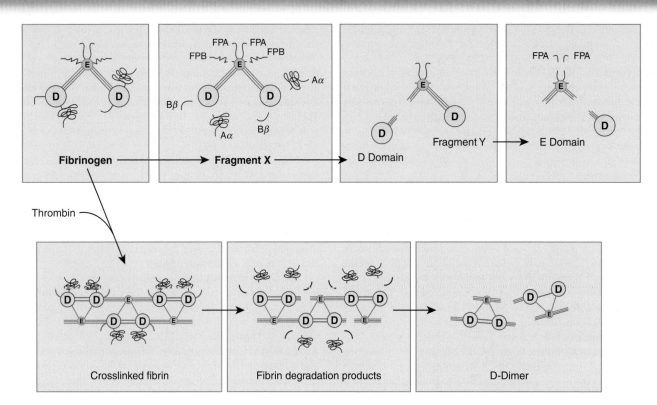

**Figure 25–3.** Degradation of fibrinogen and crosslinked fibrin by plasmin. **Top panel:** On fibrinogen, plasmin initially cleaves the C-terminal regions of the α and β chains within the D domain, releasing the Aα and Bβ fragments. In addition, a fragment containing fibrinopeptide B (FPB) from the N-terminal region of the β chain is released giving rise to the intermediate fragment known as "fragment X." Subsequently, plasmin cleaves the three connecting polypeptide chains connecting D and E domains, giving rise to fragments D, E, and Y. **Bottom panel:** Upon polymerization by thrombin, fibrinogen forms fibrin. When degrading crosslinked fibrin, plasmin initially cleaves the C-terminal region of the α and β chains within the D domain. Subsequently, some of the connecting regions between the D and E domains are severed. Fibrin is ultimately solubilized upon hydrolysis of additional peptide bonds within the central portions of the coiled–coil connectors, giving rise to fibrin degradation products such as D-dimer. (*Reproduced with permission Nathan DG, Orkin SH, Ginsburg D, et al: Hematology of Infancy and Childhood, 6th ed. WB Saunders, Philadelphia, 2003.*)

fibrinogen (Aα fragment).[205–208,215–218] Simultaneously, but more slowly, the N–terminal segments of the β chains are cleaved, releasing a peptide containing fibrinopeptide B. The resulting Mr approximately 250,000 molecule is termed fragment X and represents a clottable form of fibrinogen. Additional cleavage events may release the Bβ fragment from the β chain's carboxyl-terminus, and in a series of subsequent reactions, plasmin cleaves the three polypeptide chains that connect the D and E domains giving rise to free D domain (Mr ~100,000) plus the binodular D–E fragment known as fragment Y (Mr ~150,000). Finally, domains D and E are separated from each other, and some of the N-terminal fibrinopeptide A sites on domain E are also modified. Although fragment X can be converted to fibrin by thrombin, the fragments Y, D, and E are all nonclottable and, in fact, may inhibit polymerization of fibrinogen.[219]

### Fibrin

Plasmin degradation of fibrin leads to a distinct set of molecular products (see Fig. 25–3).[220] Species similar to fragments Y, D, and E, but lacking fibrinopeptide sites, are released from noncrosslinked fibrin. If fibrin has been extensively crosslinked by factor XIII, however, the resulting D fragments are crosslinked to an E domain fragment. Assay of crosslinked D-dimer fragments is employed clinically to identify disseminated intravascular coagulation–like states associated with excessive plasmin-mediated fibrinolysis. Several biologic activities, including inhibition of platelet function,[221] potentiation of the hypotensive effects

of bradykinin,[222] chemotaxis,[223] and immune modulation,[224] have been ascribed to fibrin breakdown products.

## TISSUE-TYPE PLASMINOGEN ACTIVATOR–MEDIATED PLASMINOGEN ACTIVATION

With or without fibrin, t-PA–mediated activation of Plg follows Michaelis–Menten kinetics.[22] In the absence of fibrin, t-PA is a weak activator of Plg. However, in the presence of fibrin, the catalytic efficiency ($k_{cat}/K_m$) of t-PA–dependent Plg activation is enhanced by approximately 500-fold. This is the basis for its specificity as a lytic agent in the treatment of thrombosis. The affinity between t-PA and Plg in the absence of fibrin is low ($K_m$ 65 μM), but increases significantly in its presence ($K_m$ 0.16 μM), even though the catalytic rate constant remains essentially unchanged ($k_{cat}$ ~0.05 s$^{-1}$). When plasmin forms on the fibrin surface, both its lysine binding sites and its active site are occupied. Thus, it is relatively protected from its physiologic inhibitor, $\alpha_2$-PI.[225]

The interaction of t-PA with fibrin is probably initiated by its "finger" domain. However, once fibrin is modified by plasmin, carboxy-terminal lysine residues are generated, and these become binding sites for "kringle" 2 of t-PA and "kringles" 1 and 4 of Plg.[226] Therefore, fibrin accelerates its own destruction by (1) enhancing the catalytic efficiency of plasmin formation by t-PA, (2) protecting plasmin from its physiologic inhibitor, $\alpha_2$-PI, and (3) providing new binding sites for Plg and t-PA once its degradation has begun.

## UROKINASE-TYPE PLASMINOGEN ACTIVATOR–MEDIATED PLASMIN GENERATION

For the activation of Glu–Plg by u-PA in a fibrin-free system, reported Michaelis constants ($K_m$) vary from 1.4 to 200 $\mu$M, while catalytic rate constants ($k_{cat}$) range from 0.26 to 1.48 s$^{-1}$.[1] Interestingly, activation of Glu–Plg by two-chain u-PA is increased in the presence of fibrin by approximately 10-fold even though u-PA does not bind to fibrin.[227] In contrast, single-chain u-PA has considerable fibrin specificity. This may reflect neutralization by fibrin of components in plasma that impair Plg[74] and also reflect a conformational change in Plg upon binding to fibrin.[228] It is important to recognize, however, that the intrinsic Plg activating potential of single-chain u-PA is less than 1 percent of that of two-chain u-PA. Two-chain u-PA has been used effectively as a thrombolytic agent for many years.[229]

## ● THE NONFIBRINOLYTIC ACTIONS OF PLASMIN

### PLASMIN AS A TISSUE REMODELER

A large number of *in vitro* studies suggest a role for plasmin in tissue remodeling. Basement membrane proteins such as thrombospondin,[230] laminin,[231] fibronectin,[232] and fibrinogen,[233] are readily degraded by plasmin *in vitro,* suggesting possible roles in inflammation,[234] tumor cell invasion,[235] embryogenesis,[236] ovulation,[237] neurodevelopment,[238,239] and prohormone activation.[240,241] Plasmin also activates MMPs 3 and 13 in the mouse, thereby facilitating the degradation of matrix proteins such as the collagens, laminin, fibronectin, vitronectin, elastin, aggrecan, and tenascin C.[242] On the other hand, activation of other MMPs apparently proceeds in the absence of Plg, possibly providing the basis for the mild phenotype observed in Plg-null homozygote animals.[80]

Roles for plasmin in tissue remodeling and host defense mechanisms are further supported by *in vivo* observations in Plg-deficient mice (see Table 25–2). Impaired wound healing is observed in the Plg "knockout"[243] and is reversed upon simultaneous deletion of fibrinogen.[244] Plg-deficient mice also display diminished recruitment of monocytes in response to intraperitoneal thioglycolate[245] and impaired neointima formation following electrical injury to blood vessels.[246] In studies involving *Borrelia burgdorferi*, the agent of Lyme disease, dissemination of the spirochete within its arthropod vector *Ixodes dammini* is absolutely dependent upon host Plg even though the deer tick contains no fibrin.[247] Furthermore, kainate-induced excitotoxicity and attendant neuronal cell dropout in the hippocampus is not observed in Plg knockout mice but does occur in fibrinogen-deficient animals.[248] The latter two studies may define new roles for plasmin, which appear to be unrelated to degradation of fibrin.

In the lung, the fibrinolytic system mediates lung matrix remodeling through mechanisms that appear to be independent of fibrin degradation.[249] In mice, deficiency of fibrinogen has no effect on the development of bleomycin-induced pulmonary fibrosis.[250] Mice lacking either PAI-1 or TAFI are protected from lung fibrosis in the same model,[251–253] whereas inducible expression of u-PA within alveoli abrogates the fibrotic response.[254]

Plasmin may play a role in the activation of growth factors. TGF-$\beta$ is an Mr 25,000 homodimeric polypeptide that regulates vascular cell responses and epithelial–mesenchymal transformation in development and in tissue fibrosis.[255,256] In culture, cell-associated plasmin appears to convert latent TGF-$\beta$ to its physiologically relevant active state. Inhibition of wound healing in this system was dependent upon active TGF-$\beta$, and activation of this agent could be blocked in the presence of plasmin inhibitors such as aprotinin or $\alpha_2$-PI. Activation of TGF-$\beta$ by plasmin may reflect alteration of its tertiary structure upon cleavage of an aminoterminal glycopeptide.[257] Once activated by plasmin, TGF-$\beta$ can stimulate production of PAI-1, thus impairing further activation of Plg.

The role of the fibrinolytic system in vascular remodeling during atherosclerosis appears to be complex.[258] In the evolution of an injury to the endothelial cell lining of blood vessels, deposition of intravascular fibrin and organization of a thrombus occur.[259] As the injury resolves, fibrin participates in plaque growth and luminal narrowing. Evidence of the importance of fibrinolytic balance in this process is that, in the absence of PAI-1, there is less neointima formation and reduced luminal stenosis, possibly because of more rapid resolution of fibrin.[260] In areas of the vasculature where injury is not associated with fibrin deposition, however, absence of PAI-1 may lead to enhanced lesion formation, as cells that invade the developing plaque may require plasmin activity for their directed migration.[261]

## FIBRINOLYSIS AND ANGIOGENESIS

Although the fibrinolytic system has generally been assumed to be proangiogenic by virtue of its ability to promote "tunneling" of endothelial cells through fibrin-containing matrices, its effect, in actuality, appears to be context specific.[262,263] PAI-1 deficiency in mice, for example, seems to prevent tumor vascularization in a malignant keratinocyte model.[264] The same mice are also resistant to laser-induced neovascularization of the choroid.[265,266] The paradoxical proangiogenic effect of PAI-1 in some settings may relate to its ability to protect endothelial cells from apoptosis mediated by FasL, which is activated by plasmin.[267]

In the mouse cornea, absence of t-PA, u-PA, or TAFI, had no effect on neovascularization, whereas loss of Plg, PAI-1, or annexin A2 significantly diminished this response.[205,268] Within the atherosclerotic plaque, moreover, expression of a truncated form of PAI-1 (rPAI-1$_{23}$) was antiangiogenic, inhibiting the proliferation of vasa vasorum and reducing overall plaque area and plaque cholesterol in the descending aorta.[269] As a gene product that is transcriptionally upregulated by hypoxia, annexin A2 is required for the normal corneal angiogenic response to growth factor stimulation and also for hypoxia-induced retinal angiogenesis.[198,205,270]

## ● DISORDERS OF PLASMIN GENERATION

### FIBRINOLYTIC DEFICIENCY AND THROMBOSIS

Although partial human Plg deficiency was first described in a young man with a history of venous thrombosis and pulmonary embolism,[271] there is currently little evidence that hypoplasminogenemia alone is a significant cause of deep venous thrombosis.[272] In a study of 23 consecutive patients with thrombophilia, the prevalence of Plg deficiency was only 1.9 percent.[273] Approximately half of these individuals had other risk factors such as deficiency of antithrombin, protein C, or protein S, or resistance to activated protein C. Among 93 patients with type I Plg deficiency, the prevalence of thrombosis was 24 percent, or 9 percent when the propositi were excluded.[274] Two additional epidemiologic studies concluded, moreover, that isolated hypoplasminogenemia is not a risk factor for thrombosis.[275,276]

Although there are no reported cases of complete absence of Plg in humans, a large number of Plg polymorphisms and dysplasminogenemias have been reported.[272] Congenital Plg deficiency has been classified into two types: in type I, the concentration of immunoreactive Plg is reduced in parallel with functional activity,[277] whereas in type II (dysplasminogenemia), immunoreactive protein is normal while functional activity is reduced.[278] Patients with type I Plg deficiency are most likely to present with ligneous conjunctivitis, which resolves completely upon infusion of Lys–Plg.[279,280] In a study of a Japanese cohort, approximately 27 percent of individuals with type II deficiency had a clinical history of thrombosis, but it is not clear whether there were other explanations for thrombophilia in these individuals.[281] Acquired Plg deficiency may occur in liver disease, sepsis, and Argentine hemorrhagic fever due to decreased synthesis and/or increased catabolism,[282] but associated thrombosis may be due to abnormalities in other hemostatic factors in these very ill patients. Similarly, there are no reported cases of complete t-PA or u-PA deficiency in humans, and no mutations or polymorphisms in these genes have so far been clinically linked to thrombophilia. Defects in Plg activator release, as well as increased inhibition of t-PA by PAI-1, have been reported in associated with thrombosis[283,284] and with chronic renal disease and hypertension.[81,83]

Global deficiency in fibrinolytic function, moreover, is associated with increased risk for venous thrombosis, as well as first myocardial infarction in young men.[285,286] Increased circulating PAI-1 appears to represent an independent risk factor for vascular reocclusion in young survivors of myocardial infarction.[287] In addition, increased levels of PAI-1 have been associated with deep vein thrombosis in patients undergoing hip replacement surgery[288] and in individuals with insulin resistance.[289] Although a 4G versus 5G polymorphism in the PAI-1 promoter has been reported, with the 4G form being associated with higher PAI-1 plasma levels, it is not yet established as to whether this allele correlates with elevated thrombotic risk.[290,291] With regard to such studies, one should bear in mind that PAI-1 is itself an acute-phase reactant and thus may not be directly responsible for the observed prothrombotic tendency.[292]

## ENHANCED FIBRINOLYSIS AND BLEEDING

Enhanced fibrinolysis resulting from congenital or acquired loss of fibrinolytic inhibitor activity may be associated with a bleeding diathesis.[293] Patients with congenital deficiency of $\alpha_2$-PI may present with a severe hemorrhagic disorder as a result of impaired inactivation of plasmin and premature lysis of the hemostatic plug.[294] Acquired $\alpha_2$-PI deficiency may be seen in patients with severe liver disease from decreased synthesis, disseminated intravascular coagulation from consumption, nephrotic syndrome from urinary losses, or during thrombolytic therapy, which induces excessive utilization of the inhibitor.[294] TAFI levels are markedly reduced in liver cirrhosis, correlating with enhanced plasma fibrinolysis and serving as an independent predictor of mortality.[295]

Patients with acute promyelocytic leukemia demonstrate excessive expression of annexin A2 on their developmentally arrested promyelocytes. Bleeding in this disorder is accompanied by evidence of high levels of plasmin generation and depletion of $\alpha_2$-PI. Bleeding resolves upon initiation of all-*trans*-retinoic acid therapy, which eliminates expression of promyelocyte annexin A2, probably through a transcriptional mechanism.[181] In this setting, A2 acts most likely in concert with S100A10, which is also upregulated in an acute promyelocytic leukemia (APL) cell line.[201,296]

Complete loss of PAI-1 expression resulting in hemorrhage in a 9-year-old child was associated with severe hemorrhage in the setting of trauma or surgery.[297] This autosomal recessive trait reflected a frameshift mutation within exon 4 that induced a premature stop codon. This case demonstrates that PAI-1 is a central regulator of fibrinolysis in humans.

## DEVELOPMENTAL REGULATION OF THE FIBRINOLYTIC SYSTEM

In the resting, nonstressed state, the plasmin-generating potential in the newborn is significantly less than that of the adult.[298,299] Although the amino acid composition and apparent molecular mass of neonatal Plg are indistinguishable from those of the adult protein,[300,301] plasma concentrations of Plg in the neonate are approximately 50 to 75 percent of those observed in adults.[300,302,303] On the other hand, levels of histidine-rich glycoprotein, a carrier protein that may limit Plg's interaction with fibrin, are also reduced by 50 to 80 percent in healthy, term newborns.[304] Neonatal Plg is heavily glycosylated, less readily activated by t-PA, and only weakly bound to the endothelial cell surface.[301] Throughout childhood, global plasma fibrinolytic activity and plasmin generation are decreased in comparison to adults, and this relative deficiency may contribute to the high frequency of thrombosis associated with central venous line placement, Kawasaki disease, and Henoch-Schönlein purpura in this age group.[305]

Although t-PA antigen and activity levels are reduced by 50 to 75 percent compared with adult values throughout childhood,[303] stressed infants, such as those with severe congenital heart disease or respiratory distress syndrome, may have t-PA antigen levels that are increased by up to eightfold because of the t-PA release response.[306,307] In contrast, the principal plasmin inhibitors undergo only minimal change from birth to adulthood.[302,308–310] Thus, reduced fibrinolytic activity may contribute to the thrombogenic state commonly observed in the newborn,[311] but this predilection may be reversed under conditions of physiologic stress.

## FIBRINOLYTIC ACTIVITY DURING PREGNANCY AND PUERPERIUM

Pregnancy is a hypofibrinolytic state.[312–314] Both Plg and fibrinogen levels in plasma increase by 50 to 60 percent in the third trimester. However, overall fibrinolytic activity, as reflected in euglobulin lysis activity, is reduced, and increased fibrin deposition is suggested by increasing D-dimer levels throughout pregnancy.[315] Between the 20th week of pregnancy and term, PAI-1 levels increase to three times their normal level, while PAI-2 levels rise to 25 times their level in early pregnancy.[312] Less dramatic increases in both u-PA and t-PA levels are also observed. Within 1 hour of delivery, however, concentrations of both PAI-1 and PAI-2 begin to decrease and return to normal within 3 to 5 days.[312]

In preeclampsia, the hemostatic and fibrinolytic imbalances seen in pregnancy are further exaggerated.[316] Circulating PAI-1 levels exceed those in normal pregnancy, and fibrin deposition is seen in the glomerular capillaries and spiral arteries of the placenta. Interestingly, levels of PAI-2, a marker of placental function, are reduced during preeclampsia compared with normal pregnancy, and this decrease correlates with intrauterine growth retardation of the fetus. Elevated TAFI levels may be a cause of fibrin deposition and occlusion of placental vessels in preeclampsia.[317]

## ● FIBRINOLYTIC THERAPY

The goal of thrombolytic therapy is rapid restoration of flow to an occluded vessel achieved by accelerating fibrinolytic proteolysis of the thrombus.[318] The fibrinolytic system functions physiologically to remove fibrin deposits through the action of plasmin, but this is often too slow to prevent tissue injury following acute vascular occlusion. Because arterial thrombosis immediately renders distal tissue ischemic with rapid onset of dysfunction and necrosis, a critical problem is minimizing time to restoration of flow. Thrombolytic therapy should be viewed as one part of an overall antithrombotic plan that frequently includes anticoagulants, antiplatelet agents, and mechanical approaches, all designed to rapidly restore flow, prevent reocclusion, and promote healing. Here we review thrombolytic approaches to stroke and peripheral vascular disease. Thrombolytic therapy for deep vein thrombosis, pulmonary embolism, and myocardial infarction are discussed elsewhere.

## PRINCIPLES OF THERAPY

The basic principle of all fibrinolytic therapy is administration of sufficient Plg activator to achieve a high local concentration at the site of the thrombus, thereby accelerating conversion of Plg to plasmin and increasing the rate of fibrin dissolution. However, if large amounts of Plg activator overwhelm the natural regulatory systems, plasmin may be formed in the blood, resulting in degradation of susceptible proteins, the "lytic state."[319] In addition, if high concentrations of activator reach fibrin deposits at sites of injury, bleeding, often exacerbated by plasmic proteolysis of other proteins in the blood, may ensue.

Several therapeutic agents, from both recombinant and natural sources, are available and approved for thrombolytic use (Table 25–3). The degree of "fibrin specificity" is critical in determining the intensity of action at the site of a thrombus. The plasma half-life of most agents is short, ranging, for example, from 5 to 70 minutes for t-PA and anistreplase, respectively. Decisions to administer by bolus versus continuous infusion, as well as the duration of therapy, are determined by the agent's half-life and the condition being treated. Regarding site of delivery, systemic therapy via peripheral vein is simpler and does not require specialized facilities but results in greater systemic complications. Regional delivery with a catheter placed close to the proximal end of the thrombus can provide a high local concentration with a smaller total dose, thereby increasing the local effect and limiting systemic exposure. Fibrinolytic therapy is often administered in combination with an anticoagulant to block fibrin formation and with an antiplatelet agent to limit continued platelet deposition. Anticoagulant therapy is routinely continued after completion of fibrinolytic therapy to prevent reocclusion. In addition, mechanical approaches such as percutaneous coronary intervention often play a vital role in removing the underlying cause of thrombosis.

The activation of plasmin has effects beyond the thrombus, including a reduction in fibrinogen, increase in fibrinogen degradation products, and depletion of Plg and $\alpha_2$-plasmin inhibitor. Screening coagulation tests, including the activated partial thromboplastin time (aPTT), prothrombin time (PT), and thrombin clotting time, will be prolonged depending on the intensity of the lytic state. Tests reflecting Plg activation, such as the euglobulin clot lysis time, will be abnormal. Platelet membrane proteins may also be degraded, resulting in abnormal platelet function.[320-322] Overall, these effects contribute to a hypocoagulable lytic state that may be beneficial for vessel patency, but may also exacerbate a bleeding complication. High doses of a nonspecific activator, such as streptokinase, will cause a more marked lytic state, compared to that seen with a fibrin-specific agent such as reteplase.

Patient selection for fibrinolytic therapy depends on careful consideration of risks and benefits (Table 25–4). For patients with acute myocardial infarction or stroke, there is a higher tolerance of bleeding complications, because lytic therapy can be life-saving and limit disability. Timing of treatment is also critical, with greater benefit achieved with earlier administration. Whereas fibrinolytic therapy for acute pulmonary embolism may be life-saving, the potential benefits for venous disease are less clear and more likely to be associated with bleeding problems.

## THROMBOLYTIC THERAPY FOR STROKE

Stroke is the third leading cause of death and the leading cause of serious disability in the United States.[323] Its incidence has been declining in

---

**TABLE 25–3.** Comparison of Plasminogen Activators

| Agent (Regimen) | Source (Approved) | Antigenic | Half-Life (min) |
|---|---|---|---|
| Streptokinase (infusion) | *Streptococcus* (Y) | Yes | 20 |
| Urokinase (infusion) | Cell culture; recombinant (Y) | No | 15 |
| Alteplase (t-PA) (infusion) | Recombinant (Y) | No | 5 |
| Anistreplase (bolus) | *Streptococcus* + plasma product (Y) | No | 70 |
| Reteplase (double bolus) | Recombinant (Y) | No | 15 |
| Saruplase (scu-PA) (infusion) | Recombinant (N) | No | 5 |
| Staphylokinase (infusion) | Recombinant (N) | Yes | |
| Tenecteplase (bolus) | Recombinant (Y) | No | 15 |

N, no; scu-PA, single chain urokinase-type plasminogen activator; t-PA, tissue-type plasminogen activator; Y, yes.

---

**TABLE 25–4.** Selection of Patients for Thrombolytic Therapy

Treat those most likely to respond and benefit
    Acute myocardial infarction: Within 12 hours of onset; consider percutaneous intervention
    Stroke: Ischemic stroke within 4.5 hours of symptom onset
    Peripheral arterial obstruction
        Acute occlusions
        Distal obstruction not correctable by surgery
    Deep vein thrombosis
        Large proximal thrombi with symptoms for less than 7 days (Chap. 24)
    Pulmonary embolism
        Massive or submassive embolism, especially with hemodynamic compromise
Avoid bleeding complications
    Major contraindications
        Risk of intracranial bleeding
        Recent head trauma or central nervous system surgery
        History of stroke or subarachnoid bleed
        Intracranial metastatic disease
Risk of major bleeding
    Active gastrointestinal or genitourinary bleeding
    Major surgery or trauma within 7 days
    Dissecting aneurysm
Relative contraindications
    Remote history of gastrointestinal bleeding
    Remote history of genitourinary bleeding
    Remote history of peptic ulcer
    Other lesion with potential for bleeding
    Recent minor surgery or trauma
    Severe, uncontrolled hypertension
    Coexisting hemostatic abnormalities
    Pregnancy

recent years due to control of risk factors, but total numbers are increasing as a consequence of aging of the population. Although aspirin and anticoagulants may be useful in prevention, thrombolytic therapy is the only available intervention during the acute stage.

The appropriate use of thrombolytic therapy for stroke is based on an understanding of its pathogenesis. Ischemic stroke is most commonly caused by rupture of an atherosclerotic plaque within a large or medium-sized artery in the neck or cranium. In addition, transient ischemic attacks and strokes involving small arteries can result from embolization of platelet–fibrin thrombi that form on atherosclerotic vessels in the neck and ascending aorta, or from embolization of thrombi that form in the heart in association with atrial fibrillation, valve dysfunction, artificial valves, or endocardial thrombi. Up to 30 percent of strokes have no defined etiology.

Current approaches to thrombolytic therapy for stroke are based on imaging to define the etiology, results of clinical trials, and the experience with thrombolysis for acute myocardial infarction. Modern computed tomography (CT) imaging and magnetic resonance imaging (MRI) can identify ischemic areas and localize areas of hemorrhage quite early. Additionally, arteriography can identify obstructed vessels and follow the course of recanalization during thrombolytic therapy. Clinical studies have generally followed the successful designs used for myocardial infarction that demonstrated the critical pathologic role of the occluded vessel, the importance of early recanalization in preserving myocardium, and the impressive decrease in morbidity and mortality resulting from early reperfusion. They have also characterized the bleeding risk.

The experience with thrombolytic treatment for stroke also highlights important differences from myocardial infarction. The arterial anatomy of the brain is more complex, the time from onset of ischemia to irreversible necrosis is shorter, the risk and consequences of bleeding are greater, and there is more variability in the thrombo(embolic) occluding lesion. Further, the occlusive platelet-fibrin thrombus that precipitates a myocardial infarction is quite small, whereas the occlusive lesion causing ischemic stroke may be a large *in situ* thrombus, small platelet-fibrin embolus, or large embolus of varying age and composition originating from the left atrium. Thrombolysis has had a smaller impact for stroke than it has for myocardial infarction, based largely on these differences.

### Early Thrombolytic Studies

The current therapeutic approach began with small, open-label studies that used intravenous or intraarterial streptokinase, urokinase, and t-PA to determine dose, recanalization rate, hemorrhagic potential, and clinical predictors of response.[324-339] These studies demonstrated that recanalization could be achieved, that early treatment was essential, and that the rate of intracranial hemorrhage and hemorrhagic transformation within the ischemic area was high. Phase II studies defined the optimum dosage and time window for intravenous t-PA and served as the basis for larger phase III trials that led to the current t-PA–based approach to thrombolytic therapy for stroke (Table 25–5). At present, the only FDA-approved therapy for acute stroke is intravenous alteplase (recombinant t-PA) given within 3 hours of symptom onset.

### Tissue Plasminogen Activator Therapy

The National Institute of Neurological Disorders and Stroke (NINDS) Study was a two-part randomized, double-blind, placebo-controlled study[340] to test whether t-PA improved clinical outcome at 24 hours and

**TABLE 25–5.** Major Fibrinolytic Therapy Trials in Stroke

| Study | No. of Patients | Time | Drug | Thrombolytic Dose*† | Main Efficacy Result |
|---|---|---|---|---|---|
| NINDS | 624 | ≤3 h | t-PA, IV | 0.9 mg/kg | Reduced disability at 3 months |
| ECASS I | 620 | ≤6 h | t-PA, IV | 1.1 mg/kg | No significant difference |
| ECASS II | 800 | ≤6 h | t-PA, IV | 0.9 mg/kg | No significant difference |
| ECASS III | 821 | 3–4.5 h | t-PA, IV | 0.9 mg/kg | Improved outcome at 3 months |
| ATLANTIS | 613 | ≤6 h‡ | t-PA, IV | 0.9 mg/kg | No significant difference |
| SITS-ISTR# | 11,865 vs. 664 | ≤3 vs. 3–4.5 h | t-PA, IV | 0.9 mg/kg | No significant difference |
| ASK | 340 | ≤4 h | SK, IV | 1.5 million units | Increased morbidity and mortality |
| MAST-I | 622 | ≤6 h | SK, IV¶ | 1.5 million units | Increased mortality |
| MAST-II | 310 | ≤6 h | SK, IV§ | 1.5 million units | Increased mortality |
| PROACT II | 180 | ≤6 h | pro-UK,‖ IA | 9 mg | Improved 3-month outcome |
| MELT | 114 | ≤6 h | u-PA, IA | Variable< | No significant difference in favorable outcome; significant difference in excellent functional outcome |

ASK, Australian Streptokinase; ATLANTIS, Alteplase Thrombolysis for Acute Noninterventional Therapy in Ischemic Stroke; ECASS, European Cooperative Acute Stroke Study; IA, intraarterial; MAST, Multicentre Acute Stroke Trial; MELT, The Middle Cerebral Artery Embolism Local Fibrinolytic Intervention Trial; NINDS, National Institute of Neurological Disorders and Stroke; Pro-UK, pro-urokinase; PROACT II, Prolyse in Acute Cerebral Thromboembolism II; SITS-ISTR, Safe Implementation of Treatments in Stroke—International Stroke Thrombolysis Registry; SK, streptokinase; t-PA, tissue-type plasminogen activator; u-PA, urokinase-type plasminogen activator.

*All placebo controlled.

†All given over 1 h except PROACT II, which was 2 h.

‡547/613 within 3–5 h.

#Observational study without placebo arm.

¶2 × 2 factorial design with acetylsalicylic acid (ASA) 300 mg/d.

§Acetylsalicylic acid (ASA) 100 mg/d.

‖Pro-UK and placebo group also received heparin.

<Mean doses of u-PA in patients with good and poor outcome were 555,000 IU and 789,000 IU.

3 months. All patients were treated within 3 hours of symptom onset with a total dose of 0.9 mg/kg of t-PA. The combined results showed a 30 percent improvement in clinical outcomes at 3 months and the benefit persisted at 12 months, despite a 10-fold increase in early symptomatic intracranial hemorrhage. At 3 months, there was no difference in mortality between the groups. This study formed the basis of the approval by the FDA of intravenous t-PA for stroke in 1996.

Early randomized trials of IV t-PA did not show clear benefit for patients treated beyond 3 hours after stroke onset. In the European Cooperative Acute Stroke Study (ECASS), subjects with moderate to severe symptoms were randomized to placebo or t-PA within 6 hours of symptom onset[341]; results showed no significant difference in either the primary end point of functional status at 90 days or in 30-day mortality. In the ECASS II, in which patients were randomized and stratified for presentation up to 3 hours after symptom onset or between 3 and 6 hours, there was no significant benefit of thrombolytic therapy using the primary end point of functional capacity of 90 days.[342] The Alteplase Thrombolysis for Acute Noninterventional Therapy in Ischemic Stroke (ATLANTIS) Study evaluated the safety of recombinant t-PA (rt-PA) in a double-blind, placebo-controlled study with administration of drug between 3 and 5 hours after symptom onset,[343] and the primary end point of excellent neurologic recovery was observed in 32 percent of placebo and 34 percent of rt-PA–treated patients. Early symptomatic intracranial hemorrhage occurred in 1.1 percent of control and 7.0 percent of rt-PA–treated patients. There was a nonsignificant trend toward increased mortality with rt-PA treatment at 90 days (6.9 percent vs. 11.0 percent, p = 0.09). A meta-analysis pooling data from NINDS, ATLANTIS, and ECASS II patients who received either alteplase or placebo within 6 hours showed that the odds of a favorable 3-month outcome decreased as the interval from stroke onset to the start of alteplase treatment increased. Furthermore, the study alluded to the potential benefit of extending the treatment window to 4.5 hours with favorable but decreasing odds ratio for alteplase treatment beyond 3 hours.[344]

The benefit of IV t-PA for treatment beyond the 3-hour window was established by the ECASS III trial.[345] This study showed that IV t-PA treatment initiated at 3 to 4.5 hours after ischemic stroke onset led to a modest improvement in the 3-month outcome. More patients had a favorable outcome with t-PA than with placebo (52.4 percent vs. 45.2 percent; odds ratio 1.34; 95 percent confidence interval [CI] 1.02 to 1.76). While the incidence of intracranial hemorrhage was higher with t-PA treatment (2.4 percent vs. 0.2 percent; p = 0.008), there was no difference in mortality between the two groups.

The effect of alteplase given beyond 3 hours after stroke on infarct growth and reperfusion was studied in the Echoplanar Imaging Thrombolytic Evaluation Trial (EPITHET) trial.[346] Alteplase was shown to be significantly associated with increased reperfusion in patients who had mismatch at baseline (p = 0.001), better neurologic outcome (p <0.0001), and better functional outcome (p = 0.010). The observational Safe Implementation of Treatment in Stroke International Stroke Thrombolysis Register (SITS-ISTR) study further supported the safety of administering IV t-PA between 3 and 4.5 hours after acute ischemic stroke.[347,348] Compared to patients treated within less than 3 hours (n = 11,865), those treated at 3 to 4.5 hours (n = 664) had similar rates of independence, symptomatic intracranial hemorrhage, and mortality. An updated pooled analysis of ECASS, ATLANTIS, NINDS, and EPITHET trials continues to demonstrate that patients with ischemic stroke, selected by clinical symptoms and CT, benefit from intravenous alteplase when treated no later than 4.5 hours.[349]

### Streptokinase Therapy

Streptokinase has been evaluated in three large stroke trials. The Australian Streptokinase (ASK) study showed an increase in death rate at 90 days in streptokinase-treated patients, and the study was prematurely

terminated.[350] The Multicentre Acute Stroke Trial–Italy (MAST-I) study examined benefits and risks of streptokinase treatment with or without aspirin in patients with acute ischemic stroke who presented within 6 hours of symptom onset.[351] An interim analysis resulted in early termination because streptokinase treatment was associated with a 2.7-fold increase in fatality at 10 days among patients receiving both streptokinase and aspirin. In the Multicenter Acute Stroke Trial–Europe (MAST-E) study, the mortality rate at 10 days was higher in patients who received streptokinase (34.0 percent) compared with placebo (18.2 percent, p <0.02) primarily because of hemorrhagic transformation of infarcts.[352]

### Tenecteplase Therapy

Tenecteplase is a genetically modified and genetically engineered recombinant t-PA; it has a higher fibrin specificity and greater resistance to inactivation by its endogenous inhibitor (PAI-1) compared to native t-PA. In a phase IIB study, there were no significant differences in intracranial bleeding or other serious adverse events in patients receiving alteplase versus tenecteplase.[353] However, the two tenecteplase groups had greater reperfusion (p = 0.004) and clinical improvement (p <0.001) at 24 hours compared with the alteplase group. The study outcome supports ongoing phase II–III trials of tenecteplase versus alteplase in the time window that is currently approved for stroke thrombolysis (ClinicalTrials.gov identifiers: NCT01472926 and NCT01949948).

### Intraarterial Thrombolysis

Intraarterial administration allows delivery of a high concentration of a Plg activator in proximity to the thrombus, more accurate anatomic diagnosis, the ability to observe the course of recanalization, and lower total doses of drug that might reduce intracranial hemorrhage. On the other hand, this approach requires specialized facilities and experienced personnel to perform arteriography and selective catheterization, which may delay treatment. Several small open-label trials observed a high rate of recanalization and apparent clinical benefit with intraarterial therapy using urokinase, streptokinase, or t-PA, but hemorrhagic transformation was a frequent problem.[327,331,334,337,354-360]

The Prolyse in Acute Cerebral Thromboembolism (PROACT) and PROACT II trials evaluated recombinant human prourokinase by catheter-directed intraarterial administration.[361,362] In the PROACT trial, a significantly higher recanalization rate was observed with prourokinase treatment with no increase in intracranial hemorrhage. This led to the larger PROACT II trial, which revealed a significantly higher recanalization rate with prourokinase (66 percent vs. 18 percent, p <0.001) and superior functional improvement at 90 days.[363,364] Symptomatic intracranial hemorrhage occurred in 10 percent of patients treated with prourokinase and 2 percent of controls. Although promising, these results did not lead to FDA approval of intraarterial prourokinase for treatment of stroke.

A third study, the Middle Cerebral Artery Embolism Local Fibrinolytic Intervention Trial (MELT), was underpowered because of premature study closure.[365] A favorable, but not statistically significant, outcome at 90 days was more likely with intraarterial urokinase compared with placebo. The proportion of patients with an excellent functional outcome was significantly better in the intraarterial urokinase group (42 percent vs. 23 percent, p = 0.045). Intracerebral hemorrhage within 24 hours of treatment occurred in 9 percent and 2 percent of patients, respectively ( p = 0.206). This study suggested that intraarterial fibrinolysis has the potential to increase the likelihood of excellent functional outcome in appropriate clinical settings.

Overall, these studies show that treatment of acute stroke with thrombolytic therapy can lead to recanalization of the occluded artery and improvement in clinical outcomes. The need for early treatment, which improves outcome, is currently the single largest limitation to greater application of thrombolytic therapy for stroke, and less than

5 percent of stroke patients currently receive t-PA treatment, indicating the need for focused community educational efforts.[366-368] Randomized studies with rt-PA have shown that intravenous thrombolytic therapy can be safely extended to 4.5 hours after symptom onset in selected patients, whereas streptokinase was associated with an unacceptably high rate of intracranial hemorrhage.[344,345,347] In addition, intracranial hemorrhage can be reduced by identifying patients at greatest risk using MRI diffusion–perfusion mismatch to identify reversible ischemia.[346,369-371] The combination of potent antiplatelet therapy using a glycoprotein IIb/IIIa antagonist with a lower dose of a thrombolytic agent may improve results.[372-377]

In summary, current recommendations limit thrombolytic therapy for stroke to patients presenting within 3 hours of symptom onset.[378-380] The approved therapy is with 0.9 mg/kg (maximum: 90 mg) of t-PA administered intravenously with 10 percent as an initial bolus and the remainder infused over 60 minutes. The best results are obtained in patients who meet strict eligibility requirements (Table 25-6). Patients should be closely monitored for bleeding complications, especially intracranial hemorrhage, and careful attention should be paid to blood pressure and other comorbidities.

## PERIPHERAL VASCULAR DISEASE

Acute peripheral arterial occlusion presents with the sudden onset of new, severe leg symptoms or acute worsening of chronic ischemia, and often involves embolic or thrombotic occlusion of leg arteries. The goals of treatment are to preserve limb function through restoration of flow.

**TABLE 25–6.** Guidelines for Tissue-Type Plasminogen Activator Therapy in Stroke

**Eligibility**

Time from symptom onset to therapy ≤3 hours

Results from European Cooperative Acute Stroke Study (ECASS) III trial suggest treatment within 4.5 hours of onset is beneficial

**Exclusions**

Prior intracranial hemorrhage

Major surgery within 14 days

Gastrointestinal or urinary tract bleeding with 21 days

Arterial puncture in noncompressible site

Recent lumbar puncture

Intracranial surgery, serious head trauma, or prior stroke within 3 months

Minor neurologic deficit

Seizure at time of stroke onset

Clinical findings of subarachnoid hemorrhage

Active bleeding

Persistent systolic blood pressure (BP) >185 and/or diastolic BP >110 or requiring aggressive treatment

Arteriovenous malformation or aneurysm

Evidence of hemorrhage on computed tomography scan

Platelets <100,000/μL

International normalized ratio >1.5 on warfarin

Elevated partial thromboplastin time on heparin

Blood glucose <40 or >400 mg/dL

ECASS III additionally excluded patients >80 years old, patients with a combination of previous stroke and diabetes mellitus, and patients with an National Institutes of Health Stroke Scale score of >25.

Anticoagulation is useful to prevent thrombus extension, while thrombolytic therapy or surgery can restore perfusion.

Early approaches to acute peripheral arterial occlusion involved streptokinase. Several small studies demonstrated reperfusion in approximately 40 percent of patients, with greatest success when occlusions were recent; bleeding complications occurred in up to one-third of subjects.[381] Following the report in 1974 by Dotter[382] of successful thrombolysis in peripheral arterial occlusion using locally administered thrombolysis, practice moved progressively to the nearly exclusive use of local intraarterially administered treatment. Advantages include delivery of a high concentration of drug directly to the site of thrombosis, the ability to follow the course of treatment using the treatment catheter, and identification of local vascular lesions requiring endovascular or surgical treatment after recanalization.

Treatment involves arterial access from a remote site followed by fluoroscopic guidance of the catheter to administer drug directly into the thrombus. Therapy is delivered by continuous infusion over hours to days and requires close monitoring and a large dose of thrombolytic agent. Successful reperfusion occurs in approximately three-quarters of cases.[383] Ouriel and colleagues[384] reported that thrombolytic therapy resulted in a 70 percent recanalization rate and a frequency of limb salvage that mirrored that of operative intervention. There was, however, a survival advantage in patients receiving primary thrombolytic therapy resulting primarily from a decrease in the occurrence of in-hospital complications. The Surgery versus Thrombolysis for Ischemia of the Lower Extremity (STILE) trial, which compared the optimal surgical procedure to catheter-directed thrombolysis with either t-PA or urokinase, was terminated prematurely because of ongoing or recurrent ischemia at 30 days in surgically treated patients.[385] More than half of patients receiving thrombolysis had a decrease in the magnitude of the surgical procedure eventually required, with significant reductions in the 1-year rate of major amputation. In addition, there was no difference in outcome with t-PA versus urokinase.

The Thrombolysis or Peripheral Arterial Surgery (TOPAS) I study compared recombinant urokinase or surgery for initial therapy of acute lower-extremity ischemia of less than 14 days in duration.[386] The 1-year mortality and amputation-free survival were similar in the urokinase and surgery groups. There was a significant reduction in the frequency and magnitude of surgical interventions eventually required in patients randomized to initial thrombolysis. The larger TOPAS II study showed recanalization in 80 percent of patients who received urokinase.[387] Amputation-free survival at 1 year was not significantly different between the surgical and thrombolysis groups, 70 percent and 65 percent, respectively. Major hemorrhagic complications were significantly more frequent with urokinase (13 percent) compared to surgery (6 percent; p = 0.005).

In other studies, reteplase appears to be as equally effective as t-PA or urokinase with comparable recanalization rates and clinical outcomes and bleeding complications.[388,389] Prourokinase also gave similar overall results to urokinase in a phase II study.[390] In an open-label trial, staphylokinase, a highly fibrin-specific Plg activator, resulted in revascularization in 83 percent of subjects with occluded arteries.[391] Occasional allergic reactions occurred, and severe bleeding complications were comparable to those with other agents. The addition of abciximab, a glycoprotein IIb/IIIa inhibitor, to urokinase resulted in more rapid clot like lysis in a randomized study,[392] and good results were also reported with reteplase and abciximab.[393] Intraoperative thrombolysis during thromboembolectomy has been used successfully to improve clearance of distal thromboemboli with or without adjunctive mechanical thrombectomy.[394-398]

Thrombolysis should be viewed as one part of a combined, comprehensive management approach to peripheral arterial occlusion.

Key points include early, accurate angiographic diagnosis, appropriate intrathrombic catheter positioning, and, in some cases, definitive endovascular or surgical procedures.[399-402] Evidence favors mechanical thromboembolectomy as adjunctive therapy for acute limb ischemia resulting from peripheral arterial occlusion.[403]

## OTHER INDICATIONS

Thrombolytic therapy has been useful in treating acute venous and arterial occlusions in a wide variety of sites. Reports document successful treatment of intraabdominal thrombosis including Budd-Chiari syndrome,[404] portal vein thrombosis,[405-407] and mesenteric vein thrombosis.[407-409] Thrombolytic agents are frequently used to open thrombosed central venous catheters,[410-413] as well as access devices for hemodialysis.[414-418]

## MANAGEMENT OF BLEEDING COMPLICATIONS

Bleeding complications are more frequent with fibrinolytic than with anticoagulant therapy and require rapid diagnosis and management. The most serious complication, intracranial hemorrhage, occurs in approximately 1 percent of patients and is associated with a high mortality and serious disability in survivors. Risk factors for intracranial hemorrhage, including prior stroke, serious head trauma, intracranial surgery, tumor or vascular disease such as aneurysms or arteriovenous malformation, and uncontrolled hypertension, are strong contraindications to fibrinolytic therapy.[419] Bleeding is most common at sites of invasive vascular procedures or preexisting gastrointestinal or genitourinary lesions and should not interrupt therapy if it can be managed with local pressure or other simple measures.

Treatment of bleeding involves local measures as well as correction of the systemic hypocoagulable state resulting from proteolysis of plasma proteins and platelets (Table 25-7).[420] The fibrinolytic agent should be discontinued, and most will be cleared rapidly because of the short half-life. For serious bleeding, an antifibrinolytic agent such as ε-aminocaproic acid can be administered but will be effective only if the fibrinolytic agent remains in the blood. Replacement of fibrinogen and other hemostatic proteins can be accomplished with cryoprecipitate and fresh frozen plasma, respectively; treatment should be monitored with repeated coagulation tests. Administration of platelet concentrates may also be useful because fibrinolytic therapy results in platelet dysfunction

### TABLE 25-7. Treatment of Fibrinolytic Bleeding

If intracranial bleeding is suspected, obtain imaging, consult neurosurgery, and correct hemostasis as below.

For major bleeding:

Send diagnostic test: activated partial thromboplastin time (aPTT), platelet count, and fibrinogen.

Attend to local hemostatic problems. Apply pressure if bleeding related to arterial puncture. Proceed with general supportive measures, including intravenous fluid hydration and transfusion of packed red cells if indicated. Proceed with diagnostic evaluation for gastrointestinal or genitourinary tract bleeding.

Correct abnormal hemostasis:

Prevent further fibrinolysis: stop fibrinolytic therapy; consider ε-aminocaproic acid or tranexamic acid.

Replacement therapy to repair hemostasis defect induced by fibrinolytic therapy: give cryoprecipitate 5–10 U and 2 U fresh-frozen plasma; consider platelet transfusion.

Correct other hemostatic defects: stop anticoagulant and anti-platelet agents; consider protamine to reverse heparin.

### TABLE 25-8. Principal Uses of Antifibrinolytic Agents

| Condition | Comment |
|---|---|
| **Systemic Fibrinolysis** | |
| $a_2$-Plasmin inhibitor or plasminogen activating inhibitor (PAI)-1 deficiency | Rare inherited disorders |
| Acute promyelocytic leukemia | Must distinguish fibrinolysis from disseminated intravascular coagulation (DIC) |
| Cirrhosis and liver transplantation | Occasional cases of cirrhosis; common in anhepatic phase of liver transplantation |
| Malignancy | Occasional cases of prostate and other carcinomas |
| DIC | Must be used with caution; thrombosis can result |
| Cardiopulmonary bypass | Decreases blood loss and transfusion needs |
| Fibrinolytic therapy | Can be used in treating bleeding complications |
| **Localized Fibrinolysis** | |
| Hemophilia and von Willebrand disease | Decreases bleeding after dental extractions and possibly other procedures |
| Prostatectomy | Can decrease postoperative bleeding |
| Kasabach-Merritt syndrome | May shrink hemangioma |
| Menorrhagia | Often decreases bleeding |

from proteolysis of surface proteins. Heparin can be reversed by administration of protamine sulfate, and 1-deamino-8-D-arginine vasopressin (DDAVP) may have some value in reversing platelet dysfunction.

## ANTIFIBRINOLYTIC THERAPY

Pharmacologic agents can be used to inhibit fibrinolytic bleeding, but care must be exercised given the risk of thrombosis (Table 25-8). For example, in patients with consumption coagulopathies, there may be excessive activation of both the coagulation and fibrinolytic systems, resulting in clinical manifestations of both bleeding and thrombosis. In this situation, inhibiting fibrinolysis to treat bleeding can precipitate or worsen thrombosis.

## ANTIFIBRINOLYTIC AGENTS

Both ε-aminocaproic acid and tranexamic acid are synthetic lysine analogues. These agents inhibit fibrinolysis by competitively blocking binding of Plg to lysine residues on fibrin.[421-424] Both can be administered orally or intravenously, have rapid absorption after oral administration, and are excreted primarily through the kidneys. Only ε-aminocaproic acid is approved for use in the United States, with the exception that tranexamic acid can be used for treatment of menorrhagia. Pharmacologically, tranexamic acid is approximately 10-fold more potent than ε-aminocaproic acid because of its higher binding affinity. Both drugs have a short half-life of 2 to 4 hours and must, therefore, be administered frequently. ε-Aminocaproic acid can be administered intravenously with a loading dose of approximately 100 mg/kg over 30 to 60 minutes followed by a continuous infusion of up to 1 g/h, or the dose can be divided for intermittent administration. For oral treatment, the same loading dose can be administered followed by a maximum dose of 24 g/d in divided doses given every 1 to 6 hours as indicated. The use of tranexamic acid follows similar principles. The intravenous dose is 10 mg/kg followed by 10 mg/kg every 2 to 6 hours as needed. It can also be administered orally in a dose of 25 mg/kg given three or four times daily. Both $\varepsilon$-aminocaproic acid and tranexamic acid are generally well tolerated, but patients must be observed for possible thrombotic complications. Additionally, thrombotic ureteral obstruction can occur in patients with upper urinary tract bleeding, and such patients should be treated only after careful consideration. The risks of ureteral obstruction can be decreased by insuring high urine flow. Thrombotic complications can occur in patients with hypercoagulability, and thrombotic events can be precipitated or worsened in patients with disseminated intravascular coagulation (DIC). Myonecrosis is a rare complication. Minor complications, including rash, abdominal discomfort, nausea, and vomiting, are reported.

Aprotinin is a naturally occurring, broad-spectrum, proteinase inhibitor derived from bovine lung.[425–427] It has both antiinflammatory and antifibrinolytic properties. Until recently, aprotinin was used in the United States for reducing perioperative blood loss and blood transfusions in patients undergoing cardiopulmonary bypass. However, its use is associated with an increased risk of postoperative renal dysfunction, cardiac and cerebral events,[428,429] and increased short- and long-term mortality compared to patients who received $\varepsilon$-aminocaproic acid, tranexamic acid, or placebo. In a retrospective analysis of electronic records from 33,517 aprotinin recipients and 44,682 $\varepsilon$-aminocaproic acid recipients, the unadjusted risk of death within the first 7 days after coronary artery bypass graft was 4.5 percent for aprotinin recipients compared to 2.5 percent for $\varepsilon$-aminocaproic acid recipients. The relative risk of death was significantly increased in the aprotinin group (relative risk 1.64; 95% CI 1.50 to 1.78).[430] Another retrospective study found that use of aprotinin was associated with both a significantly increased mortality risk at 1 year and a larger risk-adjusted increase in serum creatinine (p <0.001).[431] The prospective Blood Conservation Using Antifibrinolytics in a Randomized Controlled Trial (BART) study, which was designed to randomize a total of 3000 patients to aprotinin, aminocaproic acid, or tranexamic acid to further assess the safety of aprotinin, was terminated early because of a significantly higher death rate from any cause at 30 days in the aprotinin recipients.[432] Based on these studies, aprotinin was removed from the U.S. market in May 2008, and its access is limited to investigational use.

Excessive systemic fibrinolytic activation can lead to bleeding and may result in a shortened euglobulin clot lysis time, decreased Plg, decreased $\alpha_2$-plasmin inhibitor, increased plasmin–antiplasmin complexes, decreased fibrinogen, and increased fibrinogen degradation products. Screening tests, including the PT and aPTT, may be prolonged. It may be difficult to distinguish between abnormal hemostasis caused by DIC versus systemic fibrinolysis. Useful features include a more prominent decrease in fibrinogen and increase in fibrinogen degradation products and relatively less thrombocytopenia and elevation of D-dimer with primary fibrinolysis. Homozygous deficiencies of either $\alpha_2$-plasmin inhibitor or of PAI-1 can cause a lifelong bleeding disorder and have been treated effectively with antifibrinolytic agents.[297,433–436]

APL is often associated with a severe bleeding disorder that may have elements of both DIC and systemic fibrinolysis in addition to thrombocytopenia. Administration of $\varepsilon$-aminocaproic acid to inhibit fibrinolysis can be useful, but it must be given with care to avoid thrombosis.[437–440] In severe liver disease, fibrinolysis caused by reduced inhibitor synthesis can contribute to bleeding and may occasionally be the primary abnormality.[441–443] During orthotopic liver transplantation, accelerated fibrinolysis often contributes to bleeding, particularly during the anhepatic phase. Treatment with antifibrinolytic agents can improve bleeding complications and decrease blood loss.[444–447]

Primary fibrinolysis with bleeding may rarely occur with some malignant tumors, including prostatic carcinoma,[444–453] and also with heat stroke.[454] Fibrinolytic activation routinely occurs as a compensatory mechanism in consumption coagulopathy. If fibrinolytic activation is prominent in DIC and other measures do not control bleeding, use of antifibrinolytic therapy can be helpful but must be used with caution to avoid exacerbation of underlying thrombotic events.

The contact system is activated during cardiopulmonary bypass, resulting in alterations in the coagulation, fibrinolytic, and complement systems,[455,456] and both postoperative bleeding and the need for large transfusion volumes can be a major problems. Several trials of antifibrinolytic therapy have established that total blood loss and transfusion requirements can be reduced, with aminocaproic acid and tranexamic acid often used for this purpose.[450,451,457–460] Antifibrinolytic therapy can also be useful in treating bleeding associated with some snakebites and following administration of fibrinolytic therapy.

In hemophilia or von Willebrand disease, bleeding associated with a local lesion such as dental extraction may also respond to antifibrinolytic therapy. Both the oral and urinary mucosas are rich in fibrinolytic activity, and inhibition of normal fibrinolysis can prevent local bleeding, such as after prostatectomy.[461–463] Similarly, endometrial fibrinolysis contributes to menstrual bleeding, and antifibrinolytic therapy can be useful in treating menorrhagia.[464,465] Antifibrinolytic therapy may also be useful in rare cases of Kasabach-Merritt syndrome in which a giant hemangioma is associated with consumption coagulopathy.[466,467] Antifibrinolytic therapy has been used in treating gastrointestinal or genitourinary bleeding in patients with severe thrombocytopenia, ulcerative colitis, hereditary hemorrhagic telangiectasia, traumatic hyphema, following tonsillectomy, and with subarachnoid hemorrhage. However, caution is advised in the latter condition, as rebleeding may be decreased with antifibrinolytic therapy, but vasospasm and distal ischemia may worsen.[467]

# REFERENCES

1. Hajjar KA: The molecular basis of fibrinolysis, in *Nathan and Oski's Hematology of Infancy and Childhood*, 7th ed, edited by Orkin SH, Nathan DG, Ginsburg D, Look AT, Fisher DE, Lux SE, pp 1–15. Elsevier, Philadelphia, 2014.
2. Hajjar KA: Cellular receptors in the regulation of plasmin generation. *Thromb Haemost* 74:294–301, 1995.
3. Plow EF, Doeuvre L, Das R: So many plasminogen receptors: Why? *J Biomed Biotechnol* 2012:1–6, 2012.
4. Raum D, Marcus D, Alper CA, et al: Synthesis of human plasminogen by the liver. *Science* 208:1036–1037, 1980.
5. Bohmfalk J, Fuller G: Plasminogen is synthesized by primary cultures of rat hepatocytes. *Science* 209:408–410, 1980.
6. Castellino FJ: Biochemistry of human plasminogen. *Semin Thromb Hemost* 10:18–23, 1984.
7. Collen D, Tytgat G, Claeys H, et al: Metabolism of plasminogen in healthy subjects: Effect of tranexamic acid. *J Clin Invest* 51:1310–1318, 1972.
8. Forsgren M, Raden B, Israelsson M, et al: Molecular cloning and characterization of a full-length cDNA clone for human plasminogen. *FEBS Lett* 213:254–260, 1987.
9. Miles LA, Dahlberg CM, Plow EF: The cell-binding domains of plasminogen and their function in plasma. *J Biol Chem* 263:11928–11934, 1988.
10. Markus G, De Pasquale JL, Wissler FC: Quantitative determination of the binding of epsilon-aminocaproic acid to native plasminogen. *J Biol Chem* 253:727–732, 1978.
11. Markus G, Priore RL, Wissler FC: The binding of tranexamic acid to native (glu) and modified (lys) human plasminogen and its effect on conformation. *J Biol Chem* 254:1211–1216, 1979.
12. Hajjar KA, Harpel PC, Jaffe EA, Nachman RL: Binding of plasminogen to cultured human endothelial cells. *J Biol Chem* 261:11656–11662, 1986.
13. Miles LA, Plow EF: Cellular regulation of fibrinolysis. *Thromb Haemost* 66:32–36, 1991.
14. Rakoczi I, Wiman B, Collen D: On the biologic significance of the specific interaction between fibrin, plasminogen, and antiplasmin. *Biochim Biophys Acta* 540:295–300, 1978.
15. Hayes ML, Castellino FJ: Carbohydrate of the human plasminogen variants. I. Carbohydrate composition, glycopeptide isolation, and characterization. *J Biol Chem* 254:8768–8771, 1979.

16. Hayes ML, Castellino FJ: Carbohydrate composition of the human plasminogen variants. II. Structure of the asparagine-linked oligosaccharide unit. *J Biol Chem* 254:8772–8776, 1979.

17. Hayes ML, Castellino FJ: Carbohydrate of the human plasminogen variants. III. Structure of the O-glycosidically-linked oligosaccharide unit. *J Biol Chem* 254:8777–8780, 1979.

18. Saksela O: Plasminogen activation and regulation of proteolysis. *Biochim Biophys Acta* 823:35–65, 1985.

19. Wallen P, Wiman B: Characterization of human plasminogen. I. On the relationship between different molecular forms of plasminogen demonstrated in plasma and found in purified preparations. *Biochim Biophys Acta* 221:20–30, 1970.

20. Wallen P, Wiman B: Characterization of human plasminogen. II. Separation and partial characterization of different molecular forms of human plasminogen. *Biochim Biophys Acta* 157:122–134, 1972.

21. Holvoet P, Lijnen HR, Collen D: A monoclonal antibody specific for lys-plasminogen. *J Biol Chem* 260:12106–12111, 1985.

22. Hoylaerts M, Rijken DC, Lijnen HR, Collen D: Kinetics of the activation of plasminogen by human tissue plasminogen activator: Role of fibrin. *J Biol Chem* 257:2912–2929, 1982.

23. Hajjar KA, Nachman RL: Endothelial cell-mediated conversion of glu-plasminogen to lys-plasminogen: Further evidence for assembly of the fibrinolytic system on the endothelial cell surface. *J Clin Invest* 82:1769–1778, 1988.

24. Silverstein RL, Friedlander RJ, Nicholas RL, Nachman RL: Binding of lys-plasminogen to monocytes and macrophages. *J Clin Invest* 82:1948–1955, 1988.

25. Murray JC, Buetow KH, Donovan M, et al: Linkage disequilibrium of plasminogen polymorphisms and assignment of the gene to human chromosome 6q26–6q27. *Am J Hum Genet* 40:338–350, 1987.

26. Petersen TE, Martzen MR, Ichinose A, Davie EW: Characterization of the gene for human plasminogen, a key proenzyme in the fibrinolytic system. *J Biol Chem* 265:6104–6111, 1990.

27. Jenkins GR, Seiffert D, Parmer RJ, Miles LA: Regulation of plasminogen gene expression by interleukin-6. *Blood* 89:2394–2403, 1997.

28. McLean JW, Tomlinson JE, Kuang WJ, et al: cDNA sequence of human apolipoprotein(a) is homologous to plasminogen. *Nature* 330:132–137, 1987.

29. Nakamura T, Nishizawa T, Hagiya M, et al: Molecular cloning and expression of human hepatocyte growth factor. *Nature* 342:440–443, 1989.

30. Weissbach L, Treadwell BV: A plasminogen-related gene is expressed in cancer cells. *Biochem Biophys Res Commun* 186:1108–1114, 1992.

31. Yoshimura T, Yuhki N, Wang MH, et al: Cloning, sequencing, and expression of human macrophage stimulating protein (MSP, MST 1) confirms MSP as a member of the family of kringle proteins and locates the MSP gene on chromosome 3. *J Biol Chem* 268:15461–15468, 1993.

32. Byrne CD, Schwartz K, Meer K, et al: The human apolipoprotein(a)/plasminogen gene cluster contains a novel homologue transcribed in liver. *Arterioscler Thromb* 14:534–541, 1994.

33. Ichinose A: Multiple members of the plasminogen-apolipoprotein(a) gene family associated with thrombosis. *Biochemistry* 31:3113–3118, 1992.

34. Shanmukhappa K, Matte U, Degen JL, Bezerra JA: Plasmin-mediated proteolysis is required for hepatocyte growth factor activation during liver repair. *J Biol Chem* 284:12917–12923, 2009.

35. Bugge TH, Flick MJ, Daugherty CC, Degen JL: Plasminogen deficiency causes severe thrombosis but is compatible with development and reproduction. *Genes Dev* 9:794–807, 1995.

36. Ploplis VA, Carmeliet P, Vazirzadeh S, et al: Effects of disruption of the plasminogen gene on thrombosis, growth, and health in mice. *Circulation* 92:2585–2593, 1995.

37. Drew AF, Kaufman AH, Kombrinck KW, et al: Ligneous conjunctivitis in plasminogen-deficient mice. *Blood* 91:1616–1624, 1998.

38. Pennica D, Holmes WE, Kohr WJ, et al: Cloning and expression of human tissue-type plasminogen activator cDNA in E. coli. *Nature* 301:214–221, 1983.

39. Tate KM, Higgins DL, Holmes WE, et al: Functional role of proteolytic cleavage at arginine-275 of human tissue plasminogen activator as assessed by site-directed mutagenesis. *Biochemistry* 26:338–343, 1987.

40. Pohl G, Kenne L, Nilsson B, Einarsson M: Isolation and characterization of three different carbohydrate chains from melanoma tissue plasminogen activator. *Eur J Biochem* 170:69–75, 1987.

41. Spellman MW, Basa LJ, Leonard CK, Chakel JA: Carbohydrate structures of tissue plasminogen activator expressed in Chinese hamster ovary cells. *J Biol Chem* 264:14100–14111, 1989.

42. Harris RJ, Leonard CK, Guzzetta AW: Tissue plasminogen activator has an O-linked fucose attached to threonine-61 in the epidermal growth factor domain. *Biochemistry* 30:2311–2314, 1991.

43. Ny T, Elgh F, Lund B: Structure of the human tissue-type plasminogen activator gene: Correlation of intron and exon structures to functional and structural domains. *Proc Natl Acad Sci U S A* 81:5355–5359, 1984.

44. Browne MJ, Tyrrell AWR, Chapman CG, et al: Isolation of a human tissue-type plasminogen activator genomic clone and its expression in mouse L cells. *Gene* 33:279–284, 1985.

45. Degen SJF, Rajput B, Reich E: The human tissue plasminogen activator gene. *J Biol Chem* 261:6872–6885, 1986.

46. Van Zonnefeld AJ, Veerman H, Pannekoek H: Autonomous functions of structural domains on human tissue-type plasminogen activator. *Proc Natl Acad Sci U S A* 83:4670–4674, 1986.

47. Feng P, Ohlsson M, Ny T: The structure of the TATA-less rat tissue-type plasminogen activator gene. *J Biol Chem* 265:2022–2027, 1990.

48. Kooistra T, Bosma PJ, Toet K, et al: Role of protein kinase C and cyclic adenosine monophosphate in the regulation of tissue-type plasminogen activator, plasminogen activator inhibitor-1, and platelet-derived growth factor mRNA levels in human endothelial cells. Possible involvement of proto-oncogenes c-jun and c-fos. *Arterioscler Thromb* 11:1042–1052, 1991.

49. Medcalf RL, Ruegg M, Schleuning WD: A DNA motif related to the cAMP-responsive element and an exon-located activator protein-2 binding site in the human tissue-type plasminogen activator gene promoter cooperate in basal expression and convey activation by phorbol ester and cAMP. *J Biol Chem* 265:14618–14626, 1990.

50. Kooistra T, Van den Berg J, Tons A, et al: Butyrate stimulates tissue type plasminogen activator synthesis in cultured human endothelial cells. *Biochem J* 247:605–612, 1987.

51. Diamond SL, Eskin SG, McIntire LV: Fluid flow stimulates tissue plasminogen activator secretion by cultured human endothelial cells. *Science* 243:1483–1485, 1989.

52. Hanss M, Collen D: Secretion of tissue-type plasminogen activator and plasminogen activator inhibitor by cultured human endothelial cells: Modulation by thrombin, endotoxin, and histamine. *J Lab Clin Med* 109:97–104, 1987.

53. Thompson EA, Nelles L, Collen D: Effect of retinoic acid on the synthesis of tissue-type plasminogen activator and plasminogen activator inhibitor 1 in human endothelial cells. *Eur J Biochem* 201:627–632, 1991.

54. Kooistra T, Opdenberg JP, Toet K, et al: Stimulation of tissue-type plasminogen activator synthesis by retinoids in cultured human endothelial cells and rat tissue *in vivo*. *Thromb Haemost* 65:565–572, 1991.

55. Medcalf RL, Van den Berg E, Schleuning WD: Glucocorticoid-modulated gene expression of tissue- and urinary-type plasminogen activator and plasminogen activator inhibitor-1 and 2. *J Cell Biol* 106:971–978, 1988.

56. Santell L, Levin EG: Cyclic AMP potentiates phorbol ester stimulation of tissue plasminogen activator release and inhibits secretion of plasminogen activator inhibitor-1 from human endothelial cells. *J Biol Chem* 263:16802–16808, 1988.

57. Levin EG, del Zoppo GJ: Localization of tissue plasminogen activator in the endothelium of a limited number of vessels. *Am J Pathol* 144:855–861, 1994.

58. Levin EG, Santell L, Osborn KG: The expression of endothelial tissue plasminogen activator in vivo: A function defined by vessel size and anatomic location. *J Cell Sci* 110:139–148, 1997.

59. Levin EG, Osborn KG, Schleuning WD: Vessel-specific gene expression in the lung: Tissue plasminogen activator is limited to bronchial arteries and pulmonary vessels of discrete size. *Chest* 114:68S, 1998.

60. Diamond SL, Sharefkin JB, Dieffenbach C, et al: Tissue plasminogen activator messenger RNA levels increase in cultured human endothelial cells exposed to laminar shear stress. *J Cell Physiol* 143:364–371, 1990.

61. O'Rourke J, Jiang X, Hao Z, et al: Distribution of sympathetic tissue plasminogen activator (tPA) to a distant microvasculature. *J Neurosci* 79:727–733, 2005.

62. Dichek D, Quertermous T: Thrombin regulation of mRNA levels of tissue plasminogen activator inhibitor-1 in cultured human umbilical vein endothelial cells. *Blood* 74:222–228, 1989.

63. Levin EG, Marotti KR, Santell L: Protein kinase C and the stimulation of tissue plasminogen activator release from human endothelial cells. *J Biol Chem* 264:16030–16036, 1989.

64. Kasai S, Arimura H, Nishida M, Suyama T: Primary structure of single-chain pro-urokinase. *J Biol Chem* 260:12382–12389, 1985.

65. Gunzler WA, Steffens GJ, Otting F, et al: Structural relationship between high and low molecular mass urokinase. *Hoppe Seylers Z Physiol Chem* 363:133–141, 1982.

66. Riccio A, Grimaldi G, Verde P, Sebastio G, Boast S, Blasi F: The human urokinase-plasminogen activator gene and its promoter. *Nucleic Acids Res* 13:2759–2771, 1985.

67. Holmes WE, Pennica D, Blaber M, et al: Cloning and expression of the gene for pro-urokinase in *Escherichia coli*. *Nat Biotechnol* 3:923, 1985.

68. Schmitt M, Wilhelm O, Janicke F, et al: Urokinase-type plasminogen activator (uPA) and its receptor (CD87): A new target in tumor invasion and metastasis. *J Obstet Gynaecol* 21:151–165, 1995.

69. Van Hinsbergh VW, Kooistra T, Van den Berg EA, et al: Tumor necrosis factor increases the production of plasminogen activator inhibitor in human endothelial cells *in vitro* and in rats *in vivo*. *Blood* 72:1467–1473, 1988.

70. Medina R, Socher SH, Han JH, Friedman PA: Interleukin-1, endotoxin, or tumor necrosis factor/cachectin enhance the level of plasminogen activator inhibitor messenger RNA in bovine aortic endothelial cells. *Thromb Res* 54:41–52, 1989.

71. Gerwin BI, Keski-Oja J, Seddon M, et al: TGF beta 1 modulation of urokinase and PAI-1 expression in human bronchial epithelial cells. *Am J Pathol* 259:262–269, 1990.

72. Stump DC, Lijnen HR, Collen D: Purification and characterization of a novel low molecular weight form of single-chain urokinase-type plasminogen activator. *J Biol Chem* 261:17120–17126, 1986.

73. Steffens GJ, Gunzler WA, Olting F, et al: The complete amino acid sequence of low molecular mass urokinase from human urine. *Hoppe Seylers Z Physiol Chem* 363:1043–1058, 1982.

74. Lijnen HR, Zamarron C, Blaber M, et al: Activation of plasminogen by prourokinase: I. Mechanism. *J Biol Chem* 261:1253–1258, 1986.

75. Gurewich V, Pannell R, Louie S, et al: Effective and fibrin-specific clot lysis by a zymogen precursor form of urokinase (pro-urokinase). A study in vitro and in two animal species. *J Clin Invest* 73:1731–1739, 1984.

76. Colman RW: Activation of plasminogen by human plasma kallikrein. *Biochem Biophys Res Commun* 35:273–279, 1968.

77. Mandle RJ, Kaplan AP: Hageman factor-dependent fibrinolysis: Generation of fibrinolytic activity by the interaction of human activated factor XI and plasminogen. *Blood* 54:850–862, 1979.
78. Goldsmith GH, Saito H, Ratnoff OD: The activation of plasminogen by Hageman factor (factor XII) and Hageman factor fragments. *J Clin Invest* 62:54–60, 1978.
79. Ouimet H, Loscalzo J, Schafer AI: Fibrinolysis, in *Thrombosis and Hemorrhage*, vol 1, edited by Loscalzo J and Schafer AI, p 127. Blackwell Scientific, Boston, 1994.
80. Hiraoka N, Allen E, Apel IJ, et al: Matrix metalloproteinases regulate neovascularization by acting as pericellular fibrinolysins. *Cell* 95:365–377, 1998.
81. Hrafnkelsdottir T, Ottosson P, Gudnason T, et al: Impaired endothelial release of tissue-type plasminogen activator in patients with chronic kidney disease and hypertension. *Hypertension* 44:300–304, 2004.
82. Patrassi GM, Sartori MT, Viero ML, et al: Venous thrombosis and tissue plasminogen activator release deficiency: A family study. *Blood Coagul Fibrinolysis* 2:231–235, 1991.
83. Sjogren LS, Doroudi R, Gan L, et al: Elevated intraluminal pressure inhibits vascular tissue plasminogen activator secretion and downregulates its gene expression. *Hypertension* 35:1002–1008, 2000.
84. Carmeliet P, Schoonjans L, Kieckens L, et al: Physiological consequences of loss of plasminogen activator gene function in mice. *Nature* 368:419–424, 1994.
85. Rau JC, Beaulieu LM, Huntington JA, Church FC: Serpins in thrombosis, hemostasis and fibrinolysis. *J Thromb Haemost* 5:102–115, 2007.
86. Aoki N: The past, present and future of plasmin inhibitor. *Thromb Res* 116:455–464, 2005.
87. Holmes WE, Nelles L, Lijnen HR: Primary structure of human alpha2-antiplasmin, a serine protease inhibitor (serpin). *J Biol Chem* 262:1659–1664, 1987.
88. Hirosawa S, Nakamura Y, Miura O, et al: Organization of the human alpha2-antiplasmin inhibitor gene. *Proc Natl Acad Sci U S A* 85:6836–6840, 1988.
89. Plow EF, Collen D: The presence and release of alpha-2-antiplasmin from human platelets. *Blood* 58:1069–1074, 1981.
90. Lijnen HR, Okada K, Matsuo O, et al: Alpha2-Antiplasmin gene deficiency in mice is associated with enhanced fibrinolytic potential without overt bleeding. *Blood* 93: 2274–2281, 1999.
91. Aoki N, Moroi M, Tachiya K: Effects of alpha-2-plasmin inhibitor on fibrin clot lysis. Its comparison with alpha-2-macroglobulin. *Thromb Haemost* 39:22–31, 1978.
92. Huisman LG, Van Griensven JM, Kluft C: On the role of C1-inhibitor as inhibitor of tissue-type plasminogen activator in human plasma. *Thromb Haemost* 73:466–471, 1995.
93. Scott RW, Bergman BL, Bajpai A, et al: Protease nexin: Properties and a modified purification procedure. *J Biol Chem* 260:7029–7034, 1985.
94. Cunningham DD, Van Nostrand WE, Farrell DH, Campbell CH: Interactions of serine proteases with cultured fibroblasts. *J Cell Biochem* 32:281–291, 1986.
95. Sprengers ED, Kluft D: Plasminogen activator inhibitors. *Blood* 69:381–387, 1987.
96. Ny T, Sawdey M, Lawrence D, et al: Cloning and sequence of a cDNA coding for the human beta-migrating endothelial-cell-type plasminogen activator inhibitor. *Proc Natl Acad Sci U S A* 83:6776–6780, 1986.
97. Kruithof EK: Plasminogen activator inhibitor type 1: Biochemical, biological, and clinical aspects. *Fibrinolysis* 2:59–70, 1988.
98. Samad F, Yamamoto K, Loskutoff DJ: Distribution and regulation of plasminogen activator inhibitor-1 in murine adipose tissue *in vivo*. *J Clin Invest* 97:37–46, 1996.
99. Sawdey M, Podor TJ, Loskutoff DJ: Regulation of type-1 plasminogen activator inhibitor gene expression in cultured bovine aortic endothelial cells. *J Biol Chem* 264:10396–10401, 1989.
100. Van den Berg EA, Sprengers ED, Jaye M, et al: Regulation of plasminogen activator inhibitor-1 mRNA in human endothelial cells. *Thromb Haemost* 60:63–67, 1988.
101. Van Hinsbergh VW, Van den Berg EA, Fiers W, Dooijewaard G: Tumor necrosis factor induces the production of urokinase-type plasminogen activator by human endothelial cells. *Blood* 75:1991–1998, 1990.
102. Loskutoff DJ, Linders M, Keijer J, et al: Structure of the human plasminogen activator inhibitor-1 gene: Non-random distribution of introns. *Biochemistry* 26:3763–3768, 1987.
103. Mottonen J, Strand A, Symersky J, et al: Structural basis of latency in plasminogen activator inhibitor-1. *Nature* 355:270–273, 1992.
104. Declerck PJ, De Mol M, Alessi MC, et al: Purification and characterization of a plasminogen activator inhibitor-1 binding protein from human plasma. Identification as multimeric form of S protein (vitronectin). *J Biol Chem* 263:15454–15461, 1988.
105. Dupont DM, Madsen JB, Kristensen T, et al: Biochemical properties of plasminogen activator inhibitor-1. *Front Biosci* 14:1337–1361, 2009.
106. Kruithof EK: Regulation of plasminogen activator inhibitor type 1 gene expression by inflammatory mediators and statins. *Thromb Haemost* 100:969–975, 2008.
107. Nagamine Y: Transcriptional regulation of the plasminogen activator inhibitor type 1—With an emphasis on negative regulation. *Thromb Haemost* 100:1007–1013, 2008.
108. Bosma PJ, Van den Berg EA, Kooistra T, et al: Human plasminogen activator inhibitor-1 gene: Promoter and structural nucleotide sequences. *J Biol Chem* 263:9129–9141, 1988.
109. Van Zonnefeld AJ, Curriden SA, Loskutoff DJ: Type 1 plasminogen activator inhibitor gene: Functional analysis and glucocorticoid regulation of its promoter. *Proc Natl Acad Sci U S A* 85:5525–5529, 1988.
110. Westerhausen DR, Hopkins WE, Billadello JJ: Multiple transforming growth factor beta-inducible elements regulate expression of the plasminogen activator inhibitor type-1 gene in HepG2 cells. *J Biol Chem* 266:1092–1100, 1991.
111. Keeton MR, Curriden SA, Van Zonneveld AJ, Loskutoff DJ: Identification of regulatory sequences in the type 1 plasminogen activator inhibitor gene responsive to transforming growth factor. *J Biol Chem* 266:23048–23052, 1991.
112. Van Hinsbergh VW, Bauer KA, Kooistra T, et al: Progress of fibrinolysis during tumor necrosis factor infusions in humans. Concomitant increase in tissue-type plasminogen activator, plasminogen activator inhibitor type-1, and fibrin(ogen) degradation products. *Blood* 76:2284–2289, 1990.
113. Schleef RR, Bevilacqua MP, Sawdey M, et al: Cytokine activation of vascular endothelium: Effects on tissue-type plasminogen activator and type 1 plasminogen activator inhibitor. *J Biol Chem* 263:5797–5803, 1988.
114. Craik CS, Rutter WJ, Fletternick R: Splice junctions: Association with variation in protein structure. *Science* 220:1125–1129, 1983.
115. Stiko-Rahm A, Wiman B, Hamsten A, Nilsson J: Secretion of plasminogen activator inhibitor-1 from cultured human umbilical vein endothelial cells is induced by very low density lipoprotein. *Arteriosclerosis* 10:1067–1073, 1990.
116. Etingin OR, Hajjar DP, Hajjar KA, et al: Lipoprotein(a) regulates plasminogen activator inhibitor-1 expression in endothelial cells. *J Biol Chem* 266:2459–2465, 1990.
117. Vaughan DE, Lazos SA, Tong K: Angiotensin II regulates the expression of plasminogen activator inhibitor-1 in cultured endothelial cells. A potential link between the renin-angiotensin system and thrombosis. *J Clin Invest* 95:995–1001, 1995.
118. Gelehrter TD, Scyncer-Laszuk R: Thrombin induction of plasminogen activator-inhibitor synthesis in vitro. *J Clin Invest* 77:165–169, 1986.
119. Van Hinsbergh VW, Sprengers ED, Kooistra T: Effect of thrombin on the production of plasminogen activators and PA inhibitor-1 by human foreskin microvascular endothelial cells. *Thromb Haemost* 57:148–153, 1987.
120. Scarpati EM, Sadler JE: Regulation of endothelial cell coagulant properties. Modulation of tissue factor, plasminogen activator inhibitors, and thrombomodulin by phorbol 12-myristate 13-acetate and tumor necrosis factor. *J Biol Chem* 264:20705–20713, 1989.
121. Konkle BA, Kollros PR, Kelly MD: Heparin-binding growth factor-1 modulation of plasminogen activator inhibitor-1 expression. *J Biol Chem* 265:21867–21873, 1990.
122. Erickson LA, Fici GJ, Lund JE, et al: Development of venous occlusions in transgenic mice for the plasminogen activator inhibitor-1 gene. *Nature* 346:74–76, 1990.
123. Carmeliet P, Kieckens L, Schoonjans L, et al: Plasminogen activator inhibitor-1 gene-deficient mice: I. Generation by homologous recombination and characterization. *J Clin Invest* 92:2746–2755, 1993.
124. Carmeliet P, Stassen JM, Schoonjans L, et al: Plasminogen activator inhibitor-1 gene-deficient mice. II. Effects on hemostasis, thrombosis, and thrombolysis. *J Clin Invest* 92:2756–2760, 1993.
125. Fay WP, Shapiro AD, Shih JL, et al: Complete deficiency of plasminogen activator inhibitor type 1 due to a frame-shift mutation. *N Engl J Med* 327:1729–1733, 1992.
126. Ye RD, Wun TC, Sadler JE: CDNA cloning and expression in Escherichia coli of a plasminogen activator inhibitor from human placenta. *J Biol Chem* 262:3718–3725, 1987.
127. Ye RD, Aherns SM, Le Beau MM, et al: Structure of the gene for human plasminogen activator inhibitor-2. The nearest mammalian homologue of chicken ovalbumin. *J Biol Chem* 264:5495–5502, 1989.
128. Ogbourne SM, Antalis TM: Characterization of PAUSE-1, a powerful silencer in the human plasminogen activator inhibitor type 2 gene promoter. *Nucleic Acids Res* 29:3919–3927, 2001.
129. Antalis TM, Clok MA, Barnes T, et al: Cloning and expression of a cDNA coding for a human monocyte-derived plasminogen activator inhibitor. *Proc Natl Acad Sci U S A* 85:985–989, 1988.
130. Schleuning WD, Medcalf RL, Hession C, et al: Plasminogen activator inhibitor 2: Regulation of gene transcription during phorbol ester-mediated differentiation of U-937 human histiocytic lymphoma cells. *Mol Cell Biol* 7:4564–4567, 1987.
131. Chapman HA, Stone OL: A fibrinolytic inhibitor of human alveolar macrophages. Induction with endotoxin. *Am Rev Respir Dis* 132:569–575, 1985.
132. Nesheim M, Wang W, Boffa M, et al: Thrombin, thrombomodulin and TAFI in the molecular link between coagulation and fibrinolysis. *Thromb Haemost* 78:386–391, 1997.
133. Mosnier LO, Bouma BN: Regulation of fibrinolysis by thrombin activatable fibrinolysis inhibitor, an unstable carboxypeptidase B that unites the pathways of coagulation and fibrinolysis. *Arterioscler Thromb Vasc Biol* 26:2445–2453, 2006.
134. Bajzar L, Manuel R, Nesheim M: Purification and characterization of TAFI, a thrombin activatable fibrinolysis inhibitor. *J Biol Chem* 270:14477–14484, 1995.
135. Eaton DL, Malloy BE, Tsai SP, et al: Isolation, molecular cloning, and partial characterization of a novel carboxypeptidase B from plasma. *J Biol Chem* 269:21833–21834, 1991.
136. Wang W, Hendriks DF, Scharpe SS: Carboxypeptidase U, a plasma carboxypeptidase with high affinity for plasminogen. *J Biol Chem* 269:15937–15944, 1994.
137. Bajzar L, Nesheim ME, Tracy PB: The profibrinolytic effect of activated protein C in clots formed from plasma is TAFI-dependent. *Blood* 88:2093–2100, 1996.
138. Bajzar L, Morser J, Nesheim M: TAFI, or plasma procarboxypeptidase B, couples the coagulation and fibrinolytic cascades through the thrombin-thrombomodulin complex. *J Biol Chem* 271:16603–16608, 1996.
139. Minnema MC, Friederich PW, Levi M, et al: Enhancement of rabbit jugular vein thrombolysis by neutralization of factor XI: *In vivo* evidence for a role of factor XI as an anti-fibrinolytic factor. *J Clin Invest* 101:10–14, 1998.
140. Nagashima M, Yin ZF, Zhao L, et al: Thrombin-activatable fibrinolysis inhibitor (TAFI) deficiency is compatible with murine life. *J Clin Invest* 109(101):110, 2002.
141. Wang X, Smith PL, Hsu MY, et al: Deficiency in thrombin-activatable fibrinolysis inhibitor (TAFI) protected mice from ferric chloride-induced vena cava thrombosis. *J Thromb Thrombolysis* 23:41–49, 2007.
142. Mao SS, Holahan MA, Bailey C, et al: Demonstration of enhanced endogenous fibrinolysis in thrombin activatable fibrinolysis inhibitor-deficient mice. *Blood Coagul Fibrinolysis* 16:407–415, 2005.

143. Redlitz A, Tan AK, Eaton D, Plow EF: Plasma carboxypeptidases as regulators of the plasminogen system. *J Clin Invest* 96:2534–2538, 1995.

144. Miles LA, Dahlberg CM, Plescia J, et al: Role of cell surface lysines in plasminogen binding to cells: Identification of alpha-enolase as a candidate plasminogen receptor. *Biochemistry* 30:1682–1691, 1991.

145. Miles LA, Ginsberg MA, White JG, Plow EF: Plasminogen interacts with platelets through two distinct mechanisms. *J Clin Invest* 77:2001–2009, 1986.

146. Kanalas JJ, Makker SP: Identification of the rat Heymann nephritis autoantigen (GP330) as a receptor site for plasminogen. *J Biol Chem* 266:10825–10829, 1991.

147. Barnathan ES, Kuo A, Van der Keyl H, et al: Tissue-type plasminogen activator binding to human endothelial cells: Evidence for two distinct binding sites. *J Biol Chem* 263:7792–7799, 1988.

148. Hajjar KA: The endothelial cell tissue plasminogen activator receptor: Specific interaction with plasminogen. *J Biol Chem* 266:21962–21970, 1991.

149. Hajjar KA, Hamel NM: Identification and characterization of human endothelial cell membrane binding sites for tissue plasminogen activator and urokinase. *J Biol Chem* 265:2908–2916, 1990.

150. Das R, Burke T, Plow EF: Histone H2B as a functionally important plasminogen receptor on macrophages. *Blood* 110:3763–3772, 2007.

151. Lighvani S, Baik N, Diggs JE, et al: Regulation of macrophage migration by a novel plasminogen receptor Plg-R$_{KT}$. *Blood* 118:5622–5630, 2011.

152. D'Alessio S, Blasi F: The urokinase receptor as an entertainer of signal transduction. *Front Biosci* 14:4575–4587, 2009.

153. Montuori N, Ragno P: Multiple activities of a multifaceted receptor: Roles of cleaved and soluble uPAR. *Front Biosci* 14:2492–2503, 2009.

154. Roldan AL, Cubellis MV, Masucci MT, et al: Cloning and expression of the receptor for human urokinase plasminogen activator, a central molecule in cell surface, plasmin-dependent proteolysis. *EMBO J* 9:467–474, 1990.

155. Casey JR, Petranka JG, Kottra J, et al: The structure of the urokinase-type plasminogen activator receptor gene. *Blood* 84:1151–1156, 1994.

156. Behrendt N, Ronne E, Ploug M, et al: The human receptor for urokinase plasminogen receptor. *J Biol Chem* 265:6453–6460, 1990.

157. Ploug M, Ronne E, Behrendt N, et al: Cellular receptor for urokinase plasminogen activator. Carboxyl-terminal processing and membrane anchoring by glycosylphosphatidylinositol. *J Biol Chem* 266:1926–1933, 1991.

158. Cubellis MV, Andreasson P, Ragno P, et al: Accessibility of receptor-bound urokinase to type-1 plasminogen activator inhibitor. *Proc Natl Acad Sci U S A* 86:4828–4832, 1989.

159. Ellis V, Wun TC, Behrendt N, et al: Inhibition of receptor-bound urokinase by plasminogen activator inhibitor. *J Biol Chem* 265:9904–9908, 1990.

160. Cubellis MV, Wun TC, Blasi F: Receptor-mediated internalization and degradation of urokinase is caused by its specific inhibitor PAI-1. *EMBO J* 9:1079–1085, 1990.

161. Ellis V, Behrendt N, Dano K: Plasminogen activation by receptor-bound urokinase. *J Biol Chem* 266:12752–12758, 1991.

162. Kugler MC, Wei Y, Chapman HA: Urokinase receptor and integrin interactions. *Curr Pharm Des* 9:1565–1574, 2003.

163. Bugge TH, Suh TT, Flick MJ, et al: The receptor for urokinase-type plasminogen activator is not essential for mouse development or fertility. *J Biol Chem* 270:16886–16894, 1995.

164. Dewerchin M, Van Nuffelen A, Wallays G, et al: Generation and characterization of urokinase receptor-deficient mice. *J Clin Invest* 97:870–878, 1996.

165. Waltz DA, Chapman HA: Reversible cellular adhesion to vitronectin linked to urokinase receptor occupancy. *J Biol Chem* 269:14746–14750, 1994.

166. Wei Y, Waltz DA, Rao N, et al: Identification of the urokinase receptor as an adhesion receptor for vitronectin. *J Biol Chem* 269:32380–32388, 1994.

167. Wei Y, Lukashev M, Simon DI, et al: Regulation of integrin function by the urokinase receptor. *Science* 273:1551–1555, 1996.

168. Xue W, Kindzelskii AL, Todd RF, Petty HR: Physical association of complement receptor type 3 and urokinase-type plasminogen activator in neutrophil membranes. *J Immunol* 152:4630–4640, 1994.

169. Stahl A, Mueller BM: The urokinase-type plasminogen activator receptor, a GPI-linked protein, is localized in caveolae. *J Cell Biol* 129:335–344, 1995.

170. Anderson RG: Caveolae: Where incoming and outgoing messengers meet. *Proc Natl Acad Sci U S A* 90:10909–10913, 1993.

171. Okamoto T, Schlegel A, Scherer PE, Lisanti MP: Caveolins, a family of scaffolding proteins for organizing "preassembled signaling complexes" at the plasma membrane. *J Biol Chem* 273:5419–5422, 1998.

172. Gerke V, Creutz CE, Moss SE: Annexins: Linking Ca++ signalling to membrane dynamics. *Nat Rev Mol Cell Biol* 6(6):449–461, 2005.

173. Flood EC, Hajjar KA: The annexin A2 system and vascular homeostasis. *Vascul Pharmacol* 54:59–67, 2011.

174. Luo M, Hajjar KA: Annexin A2 system in human biology: Cell surface and beyond. *Semin Thromb Hemost* 39(4):338–346, 2013.

175. Chung CY, Erickson HP: Cell surface annexin II is a high affinity receptor for the alternatively spliced segment of tenascin-C. *J Cell Biol* 126:539–548, 1994.

176. Wright JF, Kurosky A, Wasi S: An endothelial cell-surface form of annexin II binds human cytomegalovirus. *Biochem Biophys Res Commun* 198:983–989, 1994.

177. Kassam G, Choi KS, Ghuman J, et al: The role of annexin II tetramer in the activation of plasminogen. *J Biol Chem* 273:4790–4799, 1998.

178. Siever DA, Erickson HP: Extracellular annexin II. *Int J Biochem Cell Biol* 29:1219–1223, 1997.

179. Falcone DJ, Borth W, Faisal Khan KM, Hajjar KA: Plasminogen-mediated matrix invasion and degradation by macrophages is dependent on surface expression of annexin II. *Blood* 97:777–784, 2001.

180. Brownstein C, Deora AB, Jacovina AT, et al: Annexin II mediates plasminogen-dependent matrix invasion by human monocytes: Enhanced expression by macrophages. *Blood* 103:317–324, 2004.

181. Menell JS, Cesarman GM, Jacovina AT, et al: Annexin II and bleeding in acute promyelocytic leukemia. *N Engl J Med* 340:994–1004, 1999.

182. Lee TH, Rhim T, Kim SS: Prothrombin kringle 2 domain has a growth inhibitory activity against basic fibroblast growth factor-stimulated capillary endothelial cells. *J Biol Chem* 273:28805–28812, 1998.

183. Tressler RJ, Updyke TV, Yeatman TJ, Nicolson GL: Extracellular annexin is associated with divalent cation-dependent tumor cell adhesion of metastatic RAW 117 large-cell lymphoma cells. *J Cell Biochem* 53:265–276, 1993.

184. Yeatman TJ, Updyke TV, Kaetzel MA, et al: Expression of annexins on the surfaces of non-metastatic human and rodent tumor cells. *Clin Exp Metastasis* 11:37–44, 1993.

185. Tressler RJ, Nicolson GL: Butanol-extractable and detergent-solubilized cell surface components from murine large cell lymphoma cells associated with adhesion to organ microvessel endothelial cells. *J Cell Biochem* 48:162–171, 1992.

186. Swairjo MA, Seaton BA: Annexin structure and membrane interactions: A molecular perspective. *Annu Rev Biophys Biomol Struct* 23:193–213, 1994.

187. Spano F, Raugei G, Palla E, et al: Characterization of the human lipocortin-2-encoding multigene family: Its structure suggests the existence of a short amino acid unit undergoing duplication. *Gene* 95:243–251, 1990.

188. Cesarman GM, Guevara CA, Hajjar KA: An endothelial cell receptor for plasminogen/tissue plasminogen activator: II. Annexin II-mediated enhancement of t-PA-dependent plasminogen activation. *J Biol Chem* 269:21198–21203, 1994.

189. Deora AB, Kreitzer G, Jacovina AT, Hajjar KA: An annexin 2 phosphorylation switch mediates its p11-dependent translocation to the cell surface. *J Biol Chem* 279:43411–43418, 2004.

190. Hajjar KA, Guevara CA, Lev E, et al: Interaction of the fibrinolytic receptor, annexin II, with the endothelial cell surface: Essential role of endonexin repeat 2. *J Biol Chem* 271:21652–21659, 1996.

191. He K, Deora AB, Xiong H, et al: Endothelial cell annexin A2 regulates polyubiquitination and degradation of its binding partner, S100A10/p11. *J Biol Chem* 283:19192–19200, 2008.

192. Hajjar KA, Gavish D, Breslow J, Nachman RL: Lipoprotein(a) modulation of endothelial cell surface fibrinolysis and its potential role in atherosclerosis. *Nature* 339:303–305, 1989.

193. Hajjar KA, Mauri L, Jacovina AT, et al: Tissue plasminogen activator binding to the annexin II tail domain: Direct modulation by homocysteine. *J Biol Chem* 273:9987–9993, 1998.

194. Kraus JP: Molecular basis of phenotype expression in homocystinuria. *J Inherit Metab Dis* 17:383–390, 1994.

195. Boushey CJ, Beresford SA, Omenn GS, Motulsky AG: A quantitative assessment of plasma homocysteine as a risk factor for vascular disease. *JAMA* 274:1049–1057, 1995.

196. Refsum H, Ueland PM, Nygard O, Vollset SE: Homocysteine and cardiovascular disease. *Annu Rev Med* 49:31–62, 1998.

197. Hajjar KA: Homocysteine-induced modulation of tissue plasminogen activator binding to its endothelial cell membrane receptor. *J Clin Invest* 91:2873–2879, 1993.

198. Jacovina AT, Deora AB, Ling Q, et al: Homocysteine inhibits neoangiogenesis in mice through blockade of annexin A2-dependent fibrinolysis. *J Clin Invest* 119:3384–3394, 2009.

199. Surette AP, Madureira PA, Phipps KD, et al: Regulation of fibrinolysis by S100A10 *in vivo*. *Blood* 118:3172–3181, 2011.

200. O'Connell PA, Surette AP, Liwski RS, et al: S100A10 regulates plasminogen-dependent macrophage invasion. *Blood* 116:1136–1146, 2010.

201. O'Connell PA, Madureira PA, Berman JN, et al: Regulation of S100A10 by the PML-RARalpha oncoprotein. *Blood* 117:4095–4105, 2011.

202. Ishii H, Yoshida M, Hiraoka M, et al: Recombinant annexin II modulates impaired fibrinolytic activity *in vitro* and in rat carotid artery. *Circ Res* 89:1240–1245, 2001.

203. Cesarman-Maus G, Cantu-Brito C, Barinagarrementeria F, et al: Autoantibodies against the fibrinolytic receptor, annexin A2, in cerebral venous thrombosis. *Stroke* 42:501–503, 2011.

204. Cesarman-Maus G, Rios-Luna NP, Deora AB, et al: Autoantibodies against the fibrinolytic receptor, annexin 2, in antiphospholipid syndrome. *Blood* 107:4375–4382, 2006.

205. Ling Q, Jacovina AT, Deora AB, et al: Annexin II is a key regulator of fibrin homeostasis and neoangiogenesis. *J Clin Invest* 113:38–48, 2004.

206. Bu G, Warshawsky I, Schwartz AL: Cellular receptors for the plasminogen activators. *Blood* 83:3427–3436, 1994.

207. Lillis AP, Van Duyn LB, Murphy-Ullrich J, Strickland DK: LDL receptor-related protein 1: Unique tissue-specific functions revealed by selective gene knockout studies. *Physiol Rev* 88:887–918, 2008.

208. Herz J, Goldstein JL, Strickland DK, et al: 39 kDa protein modulates binding of ligands to low density lipoprotein receptor-related protein/alpha-2-macroglobulin receptor. *J Biol Chem* 266:21232–21238, 1991.

209. Herz J, Clouthier DE, Hammer RE: LDL receptor-related protein internalizes and degrades uPA-PAI-1 complexes and is essential for embryo implantation. *Cell* 71:411–421, 1992.

210. Herz J, Clouthier DE, Hammer RE: Correction: LDL receptor-related protein internalizes and degrades uPA-PAI-1 complexes and is essential for embryo implantation. *Cell* 73:428, 1993.

211. Otter M, Barrett-Bergshoeff MM, Rijken DC: Binding of tissue type plasminogen activator by the mannose receptor. *J Biol Chem* 266:13931–13935, 1991.

212. Hajjar KA, Reynolds CM: Alpha-fucose-mediated binding and degradation of tissue plasminogen activator by HepG2 cells. *J Clin Invest* 93:703–710, 1994.

213. Narita M, Bu G, Herz J, Schwartz AL: Two receptor systems are involved in the plasma clearance of tissue-type plasminogen activator (t-PA) *in vivo*. *J Clin Invest* 96:1164–1168, 1995.

214. Bailey K, Bettelheim FR, Lorand L, Middlebrook WR: Action of thrombin in the clotting of fibrinogen. *Nature* 167:233–234, 1951.

215. Doolittle RF, Stamatoyannopoulos G, Nienhuis AW, et al: The molecular biology of fibrin, in *The Molecular Basis of Blood Diseases*, vol 2, edited by Stamatoyannopoulos G, pp 701–723. WB Saunders, Philadelphia, 1994.

216. Marder VJ, Budzinski AZ: Data for defining fibrinogen and its plasmic degradation products. *Thromb Diath Haemorrh* 33:199–207, 1975.

217. Furlan M, Kemp G, Beck EA: Plasmic degradation of fibrinogen. *Biochim Biophys Acta* 400:95–111, 1975.

218. Gaffney PJ, Dobos P: A structural aspect of human fibrinogen suggested by its plasmin degradation. *FEBS Lett* 15:13–16, 1971.

219. Latallo ZS, Flether AP, Alkjaersig N, Sherry S: Inhibition of fibrin polymerization by fibrinogen proteolysis products. *Am J Physiol* 202:681–686, 1962.

220. Pizzo SV, Schwartz ML, Hill RL, McKee PA: The effect of plasmin on the subunit structure of human fibrin. *J Biol Chem* 248:4574–4583, 1973.

221. Culasso DE, Donati MB, DeGaetano G, et al: Inhibition of human platelet aggregation by plasmin digests of human and bovine preparations: Role of contaminating factor VIII-related material. *Blood* 44:169–175, 1974.

222. Buluk K, Malofiejew M: The pharmacologic properties of fibrinogen degradation products. *Br J Pharmacol* 35(1):79–89, 1969.

223. Richardson DL, Pepper DS, Kay AB: Chemotaxis for human monocytes by fibrinogen degradation products. *Br J Haematol* 32(4):507–513, 1976.

224. Girmann G, Pees H, Schwarze G, Scheulen PG: Immunosuppression by micromolecular fibrin-fibrinogen degradation products in cancer. *Nature* 259:399–391, 1976.

225. Wiman B, Collen D: On the kinetics of the reaction between human antiplasmin and plasmin. *Eur J Biochem* 84:573–578, 1978.

226. Van Zonnefeld AJ, Veerman H, Pannekoek H: On the interaction of the finger and the kringle-2 domain of tissue-type plasminogen activator with fibrin: Inhibition of kringle-1 binding to fibrin by epsilon-aminocaproic acid. *J Biol Chem* 261:14214–14218, 1986.

227. Camiolo SM, Thorsen S, Astrup T: Fibrinogenolysis and fibrinolysis with tissue plasminogen activator, urokinase, streptokinase-activated human globulin and plasmin. *Proc Soc Exp Biol Med* 138:277–280, 1971.

228. Pannell R, Black J, Gurewich V: Complementary modes of action of tissue-type plasminogen activator and pro-urokinase by which their synergistic effect on clot lysis may be explained. *J Clin Invest* 81:853–859, 1988.

229. Bell W: Fibrinolytic therapy: Indications and management, in *Hematology: Basic Principles and Practice*, vol 2, edited by Hoffman R, Benz EJ, Shattil SJ, Furie B, Cohen HJ, Silberstein LE, pp 1814–1829. Churchill Livingstone, New York, 1995.

230. Coligan JE, Slayter HS: Structure of thrombospondin. *J Biol Chem* 259:3944–3948, 1984.

231. Ott U, Odermatt E, Engel J, et al: Protease resistance and conformation of laminin. *Eur J Biochem* 123:63–72, 1982.

232. Aplin JD, Hughes RC: Complex carbohydrates of the extracellular matrix structures, interactions, and biologic roles. *Biochim Biophys Acta* 694:375–418, 1982.

233. Marder VJ, Sherry S: Thrombolytic therapy: Current status. *N Engl J Med* 318:1512–1520, 1988.

234. Unkeless JC, Gordon S, Reich E: Secretion of plasminogen activator by stimulated macrophages. *J Exp Med* 139:834–850, 1974.

235. Ossowski L, Reich E: Antibodies to plasminogen activator inhibit human tumor metastasis. *Cell* 35:611–619, 1983.

236. Strickland S, Reich E, Sherman MI: Plasminogen activator in early embryogenesis: Enzyme production by trophoblast and parietal endoderm. *Cell* 9:231–240, 1976.

237. Strickland SE, Beers WH: Studies on the role of plasminogen activator in ovulation. *J Biol Chem* 254:5694–5702, 1976.

238. Moonen G, Grau-Wagemans MP, Selak I: Plasminogen activator-plasmin system and neuronal migration. *Nature* 298:753–755, 1982.

239. Pittman RN, Ivins JK, Buettner HM: Neuronal plasminogen activators: Cell surface binding sites and involvement in neurite outgrowth. *J Neurosci* 9:4269–4286, 1989.

240. Virji MA, Vassalli JD, Estensen D, Reich E: Plasminogen activator of islets of Langerhans: Modulation by glucose and correlation with insulin production. *Proc Natl Acad Sci U S A* 77:875–879, 1980.

241. Russell J, Schneider AB, Katzhendler J, et al: Modification of human placental lactogen with plasmin. *J Biol Chem* 254:2296–2302, 1979.

242. Loskutoff DJ, Quigley JP: PAI-1, fibrosis, and the elusive provisional fibrin matrix. *J Clin Invest* 106:1441–1443, 2000.

243. Romer J, Bugge TH, Pyke C, et al: Impaired wound healing in mice with a disrupted plasminogen gene. *Nat Med* 2:287–292, 1996.

244. Bugge TH, Kombrinck KW, Flick MJ, et al: Loss of fibrinogen rescues mice from the pleiotropic effects of plasminogen deficiency. *Cell* 87:709–719, 1996.

245. Ploplis VA, French EL, Carmeliet P, et al: Plasminogen deficiency differentially affects recruitment of inflammatory cell populations in mice. *Blood* 91:2005–2009, 1998.

246. Carmeliet P, Moons L, Ploplis VA, et al: Impaired arterial neointima formation in mice with disruption of the plasminogen gene. *J Clin Invest* 99:200–208, 1997.

247. Coleman JL, Gebbia JA, Piesman J, et al: Plasminogen is required for efficient dissemination of *B. burgdorferi* in ticks and for enhancement of spirochetemia in mice. *Cell* 89:1111–1119, 1997.

248. Chen ZL, Strickland SE: Neuronal death in the hippocampus is promoted by plasmin-catalyzed degradation of laminin. *Cell* 91:917–925, 1997.

249. Chapman HA: Disorders of lung matrix remodeling. *J Clin Invest* 113:148–157, 2004.

250. Hattori N, Degen JL, Sisson TH, et al: Bleomycin-induced pulmonary fibrosis in fibrinogen-null mice. *J Clin Invest* 106:1341–1350, 2000.

251. Eitzman DT, McCoy RD, Zheng X, et al: Bleomycin-induced pulmonary fibrosis in transgenic mice that either lack or overexpress the murine plasminogen activator inhibitor-1 gene. *J Clin Invest* 97:232–237, 1996.

252. Olman MA, Mackman N, Gladson CL, et al: Changes in procoagulant and fibrinolytic gene expression during bleomycin-induced lung injury in the mouse. *J Clin Invest* 96:1621–1630, 1995.

253. Fujimoto H, Gabazza EC, Taguchi O, et al: Thrombin-activatable fibrinolysis inhibitor deficiency attenuates bleomycin-induced lung fibrosis. *Am J Pathol* 168:1086–1096, 2006.

254. Sisson TH, Hanson KE, Subbotina N, et al: Inducible lung-specific urokinase expression reduces fibrosis and mortality after lung injury in mice. *Am J Physiol Lung Cell Mol Physiol* 283:L1023–L1032, 2002.

255. Krishnan S, Deora AB, Annes JP, et al: Annexin II-mediated plasmin generation activates TGF-beta3 during epithelial-mesenchymal transformation in the developing avian heart. *Dev Biol* 265:140–154, 2004.

256. Sporn MB, Roberts AB, Wakefield LM, Assoian RK: Transforming growth factor-beta: Biological function and chemical structure. *Science* 233:532–534, 1986.

257. Lyons RM, Gentry LE, Purchio AF, Moses HL: Mechanism of activation of latent recombinant transforming growth factor beta1 by plasmin. *J Cell Biol* 110:1361–1367, 1990.

258. Konstantinides S, Schafer K, Loskutoff DJ: Do PAI-1 and vitronectin promote or inhibit neointima formation? *Arterioscler Thromb Vasc Biol* 22:1943–1945, 2002.

259. Ross R: Atherosclerosis: An inflammatory disease. *N Engl J Med* 340:115–126, 1999.

260. Konstantinides S, Schafer K, Thinnes T, Loskutoff DJ: Plasminogen activator inhibitor-1 and its cofactor vitronectin stabilize arterial thrombi following vascular injury in mice. *Circulation* 103:576–583, 2001.

261. Peng L, Bhatia N, Parker AC, et al: Endogenous vitronectin and plasminogen activator inhibitor-1 promote neointima formation in murine carotid arteries. *Arterioscler Thromb Vasc Biol* 22:934–939, 2002.

262. Engelse MA, Hanemaaijer R, Koolwijk P, Van Hinsbergh VW: The fibrinolytic system and matrix metalloproteinases in angiogenesis and tumor progression. *Semin Thromb Hemost* 30:71–82, 2004.

263. Hajjar KA, Deora AB: New concepts in fibrinolysis and angiogenesis. *Curr Atheroscler Rep* 2:417–421, 2000.

264. Bajou K, Noel A, Gerard RD, et al: Absence of host plasminogen activator inhibitor 1 prevents cancer cell invasion and vascularization. *Nat Med* 4:923–928, 1998.

265. Rakic JM, Lambert V, Munaut C, et al: Mice without uPA, tPA, or plasminogen genes are resistant to experimental choroidal neovascularization. *Invest Ophthalmol Vis Sci* 44:1732–1739, 2003.

266. Lambert V, Munaut C, Noel A, et al: Influence of plasminogen activator inhibitor type 1 on choroidal neovascularization. *FASEB J* 15:1021–1027, 2001.

267. Bajou K, Peng H, Laug WE, et al: Plasminogen activator inhibitor-1 protects endothelial cells from FasL-mediated apoptosis. *Cancer Cell* 14:324–334, 2008.

268. Vogten JM, Reijerkerk A, Meijers JC, et al: The role of the fibrinolytic system in corneal angiogenesis. *Angiogenesis* 6:311–316, 2003.

269. Drinane M, Mollmark J, Zagorchev L, et al: The antiangiogenic activity of rPAI-1 23 inhibits vasa vasorum and growth of atherosclerotic plaque. *Circ Res* 104:337–345, 2009.

270. Huang B, Deora AB, He K, et al: Hypoxia-inducible factor-1 drives annexin A2 system-mediated perivascular fibrin clearance in oxygen-induced retinopathy in mice. *Blood* 118:2918–2929, 2011.

271. Aoki N, Moroi M, Sakata Y, et al: Abnormal plasminogen: A hereditary molecular abnormality found in a patient with recurrent thrombosis. *J Clin Invest* 61:1186–1195, 1978.

272. Schuster V, Hugle B, Tefs K: Plasminogen deficiency. *J Thromb Haemost* 5:2315–2322, 2007.

273. Demarmels Biasiutti F, Sulzer I, Stucki B, et al: Is plasminogen deficiency a thrombotic risk factor? A study on 23 thrombophilic patients and their family members. *Thromb Haemost* 80:167–170, 1998.

274. Sartori MT, Patrassi GM, Theodoridis P, et al: Heterozygous type I plasminogen deficiency is associated with an increased risk for thrombosis: A statistical analysis of 20 kindreds. *Blood Coagul Fibrinolysis* 5:889–893, 1994.

275. Shigekiyo T, Uno Y, Tomonari A, et al: Type I congenital plasminogen deficiency is not a risk factor for thrombosis. *Thromb Haemost* 67:189–192, 1992.

276. Tait RC, Walker ID, Conkie JA, et al: Isolated familial plasminogen deficiency may not be a risk factor for thrombosis. *Thromb Haemost* 76:1004–1008, 1996.

277. Azuma H, Mima N, Shirakawa M, et al: Molecular pathogenesis of type I congenital plasminogen deficiency: Expression of recombinant human mutant plasminogens in mammalian cells. *Blood* 89:183–190, 1997.

278. Ichinose A, Espling ES, Takamatsu J, et al: Two types of abnormal genes for plasminogen in families with a predisposition for thrombosis. *Proc Natl Acad Sci U S A* 88:115–119, 1991.

279. Schott D, Dempfle CE, Beck P, et al: Therapy with a purified plasminogen concentrate in an infant with ligneous conjunctivitis and homozygous plasminogen deficiency. *N Engl J Med* 339:1679–1686, 1998.

280. Robbins KC: Dysplasminogenemia. *Prog Cardiovasc Dis* 34:295–308, 1992.

281. Tsutsumi S, Saito T, Sakata T, et al: Genetic diagnosis of dysplasminogenemia: Detection of an Ala601-Thr mutation in 118 out of 125 families and identification of a new Asp676-Asn mutation. *Thromb Haemost* 76:135–138, 1996.

282. Lijnen HR, Collen D: Congenital and acquired deficiencies of components of the fibrinolytic system and their relationship to bleeding or thrombosis. *Fibrinolysis* 3: 67–77, 1989.

283. Rakoczi I, Chamone D, Collen D, Verstraete M: Prediction of postoperative leg vein thrombosis in gynaecological patients. *Lancet* 1:509–510, 1978.

284. Nilsson IM, Ljungner H, Tengborn L: Two different mechanisms in patients with venous thrombosis and defective fibrinolysis: Low concentrations of plasminogen activator or increased concentration of plasminogen activator inhibitor. *Br Med J* 290:1453–1456, 1985.

285. Meltzer ME, Doggen CJ, De Groot PG, et al: The impact of the fibrinolytic system on the risk of venous and arterial thrombosis. *Semin Thromb Hemost* 35:469–477, 2009.

286. Meltzer ME, Doggen CJ, De Groot PG, et al: Reduced plasma fibrinolytic capacity as a potential risk factor for a first myocardial infarction in young men. *Br J Haematol* 145:121–127, 2009.

287. Hamsten A, Wiman B, De Faire U, Blomback M: Increased plasma levels of a rapid inhibitor of tissue plasminogen activator in young survivors of myocardial infarction. *N Engl J Med* 313:1557–1563, 1985.

288. Paramo JA, Alfaro MJ, Rocha E: Postoperative changes in the plasmatic levels of tissue-type plasminogen activator and its fast-acting inhibitor: Relationship to deep vein thrombosis and influence of prophylaxis. *Thromb Haemost* 54:713–716, 1985.

289. Juhan-Vague I, Roul C, Alessi MC, et al: Increased plasminogen activator inhibitor activity in non-insulin dependent diabetic patients: Relationship with plasma insulin. *Thromb Haemost* 61:370–373, 1989.

290. Francis CW: Plasminogen activator inhibitor-1 levels and polymorphisms: Association with venous thromboembolism. *Arch Pathol Lab Med* 126:1401–1404, 2002.

291. Tsantes AE, Nikolopoulos GK, Bagos PG, et al: The effect of the plasminogen activator inhibitor-1 4G/5G polymorphism on the thrombotic risk. *Thromb Res* 122:736–742, 2008.

292. Juhan-Vague I, Alessi MC, Joly P, et al: Plasma plasminogen activator inhibitor-1 in angina pectoris: Influence of plasma insulin and acute-phase response. *Arteriosclerosis* 9:362–367, 1989.

293. Stump DC, Taylor FB, Nesheim ME, et al: Pathologic fibrinolysis as a cause of clinical bleeding. *Semin Thromb Hemost* 16:260–273, 1990.

294. Saito H: Alpha-2-plasmin inhibitor and its deficiency states. *J Lab Clin Med* 112:671–678, 1988.

295. Gresele P, Binetti BM, Branca G, et al: TAFI deficiency in liver cirrhosis: Relation to plasma fibrinolysis and survival. *Thromb Res* 121:763–768, 2008.

296. Stein E, McMahon B, Kwaan H, et al: The coagulopathy of acute promyelocytic leukaemia revisited. *Best Pract Res Clin Haematol* 22:152–163, 2009.

297. Fay WP, Shapiro AD, Shih JL, et al: Brief report: Complete deficiency of plasminogen-activator inhibitor type 1 due to a frame-shift mutation. *N Engl J Med* 327:1729–1733, 1992.

298. Suarez CR, Walenga J, Mangogna LC, Fareed J: Neonatal and maternal fibrinolysis: Activation at time of birth. *Am J Hematol* 19:365–372, 1985.

299. Albisetti M: The fibrinolytic system in children. *Semin Thromb Hemost* 29(4):339–348, 2003.

300. Summaria L: Comparison of human normal, full-term, fetal and adult plasminogen by physical and clinical analyses. *Haemostasis* 19:266–273, 1989.

301. Edelberg JM, Enghild JJ, Pizzo SV, Gonzales-Gronow M: Neonatal plasminogen displays altered cell surface binding and activation kinetics: Correlation with increased glycosylation of the protein. *J Clin Invest* 86:107–112, 1990.

302. Andrew M, Brooker L, Leaker M, et al: Fibrin clot lysis by thrombolytic agents is impaired in newborns due to a low plasminogen concentration. *Thromb Haemost* 68:325–330, 1992.

303. Corrigan JJ, Sleeth JJ, Jeter MA, Lox CD: Newborn's fibrinolytic mechanism: Components and plasmin generation. *Am J Hematol* 32:273–278, 1989.

304. Corrigan JJ, Jeter MA: Histidine-rich glycoprotein and plasminogen plasma levels in term and preterm newborns. *Am J Dis Child* 144:825–828, 1990.

305. Parmar N, Albisetti M, Berry LR, Chan AK: The fibrinolytic system in newborns and children. *Clin Lab* 52:115–124, 2006.

306. Corrigan JJ, Jeter MA: Tissue-type plasminogen activator, plasminogen activator inhibitor, and histidine-rich glycoprotein in stressed human newborns. *Pediatrics* 89:43–46, 1992.

307. Brus F, Van Oeveren W, Okkern A, Oetomo SB: Activation of the plasma clotting, fibrinolytic, and kinin-kallikrein system in preterm infants with severe idiopathic respiratory distress syndrome. *Pediatr Res* 36:647–653, 1994.

308. Cederholm-Williams SA, Spencer JA, Wilkerson AR: Plasma levels of selected haemostatic factors in newborn babies. *Thromb Res* 23:555–558, 1981.

309. Andrew M, Paes B, Milner R, et al: Development of the human coagulation system in the full-term infant. *Blood* 70:165–172, 1987.

310. Andrew M, Massicotte-Nolan PM, Karpatkin M: Plasma protease inhibitors in premature infants: Influence of gestational age, postnatal age, and health status. *Proc Soc Exp Biol Med* 173:495–500, 1983.

311. Corrigan JJ: Thrombosis and thromboembolism, in *Hemorrhagic and Thrombotic Disease in Childhood and Adolescence*, pp 147–176. Churchill Livingstone, New York, 1985.

312. Bonnar J, Daly L, Sheppard BL: Changes in the fibrinolytic system during pregnancy. *Semin Thromb Hemost* 16:221–229, 1990.

313. Brenner B: Haemostatic changes in pregnancy. *Thromb Res* 114:409–414, 2004.

314. Bremme KA: Haemostatic changes in pregnancy. *Best Pract Res Clin Haematol* 16:153–168, 2003.

315. Hellgren M: Hemostasis during pregnancy and puerperium. *Haemostasis* 26:244–247, 1996.

316. Schjetlein R, Haugen G, Wisloff F: Markers of intravascular coagulation and fibrinolysis in preeclampsia: Association with intrauterine growth retardation. *Acta Obstet Gynecol Scand* 76:541–546, 1997.

317. SantAna Dusse LM, Cooper AJ, Lwaleed BA: Thrombin activatable fibrinolysis inhibitor (TAFI): A role in pre-eclampsia? *Clin Chim Acta* 378:1–6, 2007.

318. Hajjar KA, Francis CW: Fibrinolysis and thrombolysis, *Williams Hematology*, 7th ed, edited by K Kaushansky, MA Lichtman, E Beutler, TJ Kipps, U Seligsohn, JT Prchal, pp 2089–2115. McGraw-Hill, New York, 2006.

319. Sherry S, Fletcher AP, Alkjaersig N: Fibrinolysis and fibrinolytic activity in man. *Physiol Rev* 39:343–382, 1959.

320. Adelman B, Michelson AD, Loscalzo J, et al: Plasmin effect on platelet glycoprotein Ib-von Willebrand factor interactions. *Blood* 65:32–40, 1985.

321. Loscalzo J, Vaughan DE: Tissue plasminogen activator promotes platelet disaggregation in plasma. *J Clin Invest* 79:1749–1755, 1987.

322. Rudd MA, George D, Amarante P, et al: Temporal effects of thrombolytic agents on platelet function in vivo and their modulation by prostaglandins. *Circ Res* 67:1175–1181, 1990.

323. Go AS, Mozaffarian D, Roger VL, et al: Executive summary: Heart disease and stroke statistics—2014 update: A report from the American Heart Association. *Circulation* 129:399–410, 2014.

324. Abe T, Kazama M, Naito I, et al: Clinical evaluation for efficacy of tissue culture urokinase (TCUK) on cerebral thrombosis by means of multicenter double blind study. *Blood Vessels* 12:321–341, 1981.

325. Abe T, Kazama M, Naito I, et al: Clinical effect of urokinase (60,000 units/day) on cerebral infarction comparative study by means of multiple center double blind test. *Blood Vessels* 12:342–358, 1981.

326. Atarashi J, Otomo E, Araki G, et al: Clinical utility of urokinase in the treatment of acute stage of cerebral thrombosis: Multi-center double-blind study in comparison with placebo. *Clin Eval* 13:659–709, 1985.

327. del Zoppo GJ, Ferbert A, Otis S, et al: Local intra-arterial fibrinolytic therapy in acute carotid territory stroke. A pilot study. *Stroke* 19:307–313, 1988.

328. Fletcher AP, Alkjaersig N, Lewis M, et al: A pilot study of urokinase therapy in cerebral infarction. *Stroke* 7:135–142, 1976.

329. Hacke W, Zeumer H, Ferbert A, et al: Intra-arterial thrombolytic therapy improves outcome in patients with acute vertebrobasilar occlusive disease. *Stroke* 19:1216–1222, 1988.

330. Hanaway J, Torack R, Fletcher AP, Landau WM: Intracranial bleeding associated with urokinase therapy for acute ischemic hemispheral stroke. *Stroke* 7:143–146, 1976.

331. Matsumoto K, Satoh K: *Topical Intraarterial Urokinase Infusion for Acute Stroke.* Springer-Verlag, Heidelberg, 1991.

332. Meyer JS, Gilroy J, Barnhart MI, Johnson JF: Therapeutic thrombolysis in cerebral thromboembolism. Double-blind evaluation of intravenous plasmin therapy in carotid and middle cerebral arterial occlusion. *Neurology* 13:927–937, 1963.

333. Meyer JS, Gilroy J, Barnhart MI, Johnson JF: Anticoagulants plus streptokinase therapy in progressive stroke. *JAMA* 189:373, 1964.

334. Mori E, Tabuchi M, Yoshida T, Yamadori A: Intracarotid urokinase with thromboembolic occlusion of the middle cerebral artery. *Stroke* 19:802–812, 1988.

335. Mori E: *Fibrinolytic Recanalization Therapy in Acute Cerebrovascular Thromboembolism.* Springer-Verlag, Heidelberg, 1991.

336. Otomo E, Araki G, Itoh E, et al: Clinical efficacy of urokinase in the treatment of cerebral thrombosis. *Clin Eval* 13:711–751, 1985.

337. Theron J, Courtheoux P, Casasco A, et al: Local intraarterial fibrinolysis in the carotid territory. *AJNR Am J Neuroradiol* 10:753–765, 1989.

338. Zeumer H, Freitag HJ, Grzyska U, Neunzig HP: Local intra-arterial fibrinolysis in acute vertebrobasilar occlusion. Technical developments and recent results. *Neuroradiology* 31(4):336–340, 1989.

339. Zeumer H, Freitag HJ, Zanella F, et al: Local intra-arterial fibrinolytic therapy in patients with stroke: Urokinase versus recombinant tissue plasminogen activator (r-TPA). *Neuroradiology* 35:159–162, 1993.

340. Tissue plasminogen activator for acute ischemic stroke. The National Institute of Neurological Disorders and Stroke rt-PA Stroke Study Group. *N Engl J Med* 333:1581–1587, 1995.

341. Hacke W, Kaste M, Fieschi C, et al: Intravenous thrombolysis with recombinant tissue plasminogen activator for acute hemispheric stroke. The European Cooperative Acute Stroke Study (ECASS). *JAMA* 274(13):1017–1025, 1995.

342. Hacke W, Kaste M, Fieschi C, et al: Randomised double-blind placebo-controlled trial of thrombolytic therapy with intravenous alteplase in acute ischaemic stroke (ECASS II). Second European-Australasian Acute Stroke Study Investigators. *Lancet* 352:1245–1251, 1998.

343. Clark WM, Wissman S, Albers GW, et al: Recombinant tissue-type plasminogen activator (Alteplase) for ischemic stroke 3 to 5 hours after symptom onset. The ATLANTIS Study: A randomized controlled trial. Alteplase Thrombolysis for Acute Noninterventional Therapy in Ischemic Stroke. *JAMA* 282:2019–2026, 1999.

344. Hacke W, Donnan G, Fieschi C, et al: Association of outcome with early stroke treatment: Pooled analysis of ATLANTIS, ECASS, and NINDS rt-PA stroke trials. *Lancet* 363:768–774, 2004.

345. Hacke W, Kaste M, Bluhmki E, et al: Thrombolysis with alteplase 3 to 4.5 hours after acute ischemic stroke. *N Engl J Med* 359:1317–1329, 2008.

346. Davis SM, Donnan GA, Parsons MW, et al: Effects of alteplase beyond 3 h after stroke in the Echoplanar Imaging Thrombolytic Evaluation Trial (EPITHET): A placebo-controlled randomised trial. *Lancet Neurol* 7:299–309, 2008.

347. Wahlgren N, Ahmed N, Davalos A, et al: Thrombolysis with alteplase 3–4.5 h after acute ischaemic stroke (SITS-ISTR): An observational study. *Lancet* 372:1303–1309, 2008.

348. Ahmed N, Wahlgren N, Grond M, et al: Implementation and outcome of thrombolysis with alteplase 3–4.5 h after an acute stroke: An updated analysis from SITS-ISTR. *Lancet Neurol* 9:866–874, 2010.

349. Lees KR, Bluhmki E, von Kummer R, et al: Time to treatment with intravenous alteplase and outcome in stroke: An updated pooled analysis of ECASS, ATLANTIS, NINDS, and EPITHET trials. *Lancet* 375:1695–1703, 2010.

350. Donnan GA, Davis SM, Chambers BR, et al: Streptokinase for acute ischemic stroke with relationship to time of administration: Australian Streptokinase (ASK) Trial Study Group. *JAMA* 276(12):961–966, 1996.

351. Randomised controlled trial of streptokinase, aspirin, and combination of both in treatment of acute ischaemic stroke. Multicentre Acute Stroke Trial–Italy (MAST-I) Group. *Lancet* 346:1509–1514, 1995.

352. Thrombolytic therapy with streptokinase in acute ischemic stroke. The Multicenter Acute Stroke Trial—Europe Study Group. *N Engl J Med* 335:145–150, 1996.

353. Parsons M, Spratt N, Bivard A, et al: A randomized trial of tenecteplase versus alteplase for acute ischemic stroke. *N Engl J Med* 366:1099–1107, 2012.

354. Barnwell SL, Clark WM, Nguyen TT, et al: Safety and efficacy of delayed intraarterial urokinase therapy with mechanical clot disruption for thromboembolic stroke. *AJNR Am J Neuroradiol* 15:1817–1822, 1994.

355. Barr JD, Mathis JM, Wildenhain SL, et al: Acute stroke intervention with intraarterial urokinase infusion. *J Vasc Interv Radiol* 5(5):705–713, 1994.

356. Casto L, Caverni L, Camerlingo M, et al: Intra-arterial thrombolysis in acute ischaemic stroke: Experience with a superselective catheter embedded in the clot. *J Neurol Neurosurg Psychiatry* 60:667–670, 1996.

357. Jansen O, von Kummer R, Forsting M, et al: Thrombolytic therapy in acute occlusion of the intracranial internal carotid artery bifurcation. *AJNR Am J Neuroradiol* 16:1977–1986, 1995.

358. Nesbit GM, Clark WM, O'Neill OR, Barnwell SL: Intracranial intraarterial thrombolysis facilitated by microcatheter navigation through an occluded cervical internal carotid artery. *J Neurosurg* 84:387–392, 1996.

359. Tarr R, Taylor CL, Selman WR, et al: Good clinical outcome in a patient with a large CT scan hypodensity treated with intra-arterial urokinase after an embolic stroke. *Neurology* 47:1076–1078, 1996.

360. Janjua N, Brisman JL: Endovascular treatment of acute ischaemic stroke. *Lancet Neurol* 6:1086–1093, 2007.

361. Liu M, Wardlaw J: Thrombolysis (different doses, routes of administration and agents) for acute ischaemic stroke. *Cochrane Database Syst Rev* 2:CD000514, 2000.

362. Wardlaw JM, Del Zoppo G, Yamaguchi T, Berge E: Thrombolysis for acute ischaemic stroke. *Cochrane Database Syst Rev* 3:CD000213, 2003.

363. del Zoppo GJ, Higashida RT, Furlan AJ, et al: PROACT: A phase II randomized trial of recombinant pro-urokinase by direct arterial delivery in acute middle cerebral artery stroke. PROACT Investigators. Prolyse in Acute Cerebral Thromboembolism. *Stroke* 29:4–11, 1998.

364. Furlan A, Higashida R, Wechsler L, et al: Intra-arterial prourokinase for acute ischemic stroke. The PROACT II study: A randomized controlled trial. Prolyse in Acute Cerebral Thromboembolism. *JAMA* 282:2003–2011, 1999

365. Ogawa A, Mori E, Minematsu K, et al: Randomized trial of intraarterial infusion of urokinase within 6 hours of middle cerebral artery stroke: The middle cerebral artery embolism local fibrinolytic intervention trial (MELT) Japan. *Stroke* 38:2633–2639, 2007.

366. Broderick JP: William M. Feinberg Lecture: Stroke therapy in the year 2025: Burden, breakthroughs, and barriers to progress. *Stroke* 35:205–211, 2004.

367. Kleindorfer D, Khoury J, Alwell K, et al: Eligibility for rt-PA in acute ischemic stroke: A population-based study. *Stroke* 34:281, 2003.

368. Kothari RU, Pancioli A, Liu T, Brott T, Broderick J: Cincinnati Prehospital Stroke Scale: Reproducibility and validity. *Ann Emerg Med* 33:373–378, 1999.

369. Albers GW, Thijs VN, Wechsler L, et al: Magnetic resonance imaging profiles predict clinical responses to early reperfusion: The diffusion and perfusion imaging evaluation for understanding stroke evolution (DEFUSE) study. *Ann Neurol* 60:508–517, 2006.

370. Furlan AJ, Eyding D, Albers GW, et al: Dose Escalation of Desmoteplase for Acute Ischemic Stroke (DEDAS): Evidence of safety and efficacy 3 to 9 hours after stroke onset. *Stroke* 37:1227–1231, 2006.

371. Hacke W, Albers G, Al-Rawi Y, et al: The Desmoteplase on Acute Ischemic Stroke Trial (DIAS): A phase II MRI-based 9-hour window acute stroke thrombolysis trial with intravenous desmoteplase. *Stroke* 36:66–73, 2005.

372. Abciximab in Ischemic Stroke Investigators: Abciximab in acute ischemic stroke: A randomized, double-blind, placebo-controlled, dose-escalation study. *Stroke* 31(3):601–609, 2000.

373. Qureshi AI, Suri MF, Khan J, et al: Abciximab as an adjunct to high-risk carotid or vertebrobasilar angioplasty: Preliminary experience. *Neurosurgery* 46:1316–1324, 2000.

374. Qureshi AI, Ali Z, Suri MF, et al: Intra-arterial third-generation recombinant tissue plasminogen activator (reteplase) for acute ischemic stroke. *Neurosurgery* 49:41–48, 2001.

375. Seitz RJ, Hamzavi M, Junghans U, et al: Thrombolysis with recombinant tissue plasminogen activator and tirofiban in stroke: Preliminary observations. *Stroke* 34:1932–1935, 2003.

376. Seitz RJ, Meisel S, Moll M, et al: The effect of combined thrombolysis with rtPA and tirofiban on ischemic brain lesions. *Neurology* 62:2110–2112, 2004.

377. Straub S, Junghans U, Jocanovic V, et al: Systemic thrombolysis with recombinant tissue plasminogen activator and tirofiban in acute middle cerebral artery occlusion. *Stroke* 35:705–709, 2004.

378. Adams HP Jr, Adams RJ, Brott T, et al: Guidelines for the early management of patients with ischemic stroke: A scientific statement from the Stroke Council of the American Stroke Association. *Stroke* 34:1056–1083, 2003.

379. Broderick JP, Hacke W: Treatment of acute ischemic stroke: Part I: Recanalization strategies. *Circulation* 106:1563–1569, 2002.

380. Kaste M, Thomassen L, Grond M, et al: Thrombolysis for acute ischemic stroke: A consensus statement of the 3rd Karolinska Stroke Update, October 30–31, 2000. *Stroke* 32:2717–2718, 2001.

381. Brogden RN, Speight TM, Avery GS: Streptokinase: A review of its clinical pharmacology, mechanism of action and therapeutic uses. *Drugs* 5:357–445, 1973.

382. Dotter CT, Rosch J, Seaman AJ: Selective clot lysis with low-dose streptokinase. *Radiology* 111:31–37, 1974.

383. Ouriel K: Current status of thrombolysis for peripheral arterial occlusive disease. *Ann Vasc Surg* 16:797–804, 2002.

384. Ouriel K, Shortell CK, DeWeese JA, et al: A comparison of thrombolytic therapy with operative revascularization in the initial treatment of acute peripheral arterial ischemia. *J Vasc Surg* 19:1021–1030, 1994.

385. Results of a prospective randomized trial evaluating surgery versus thrombolysis for ischemia of the lower extremity. The STILE trial. *Ann Surg* 220:251–266, 1994.

386. Ouriel K, Veith FJ, Sasahara AA: Thrombolysis or peripheral arterial surgery: Phase I results. TOPAS Investigators. *J Vasc Surg* 23:64–73, 1996.

387. Ouriel K, Veith FJ, Sasahara AA: A comparison of recombinant urokinase with vascular surgery as initial treatment for acute arterial occlusion of the legs. Thrombolysis or Peripheral Arterial Surgery (TOPAS) Investigators. *N Engl J Med* 338:1105–1111, 1998.

388. Castaneda F, Swischuk JL, Li R, et al: Declining-dose study of reteplase treatment for lower extremity arterial occlusions. *J Vasc Interv Radiol* 13:1093–1098, 2002.

389. Ouriel K, Katzen B, Mewissen M, et al: Reteplase in the treatment of peripheral arterial and venous occlusions: A pilot study. *J Vasc Interv Radiol* 11:849–854, 2000.

390. Ouriel K, Kandarpa K, Schuerr DM, et al: Prourokinase versus urokinase for recanalization of peripheral occlusions, safety and efficacy: The PURPOSE trial. *J Vasc Interv Radiol* 10:1083–1091, 1999.

391. Heymans S, Vanderschueren S, Verhaeghe R, et al: Outcome and one year follow-up of intra-arterial staphylokinase in 191 patients with peripheral arterial occlusion. *Thromb Haemost* 83:666–671, 2000.

392. Duda SH, Tepe G, Luz O, et al: Peripheral artery occlusion: Treatment with abciximab plus urokinase versus with urokinase alone—A randomized pilot trial (the PROMPT Study). Platelet Receptor Antibodies in Order to Manage Peripheral Artery Thrombosis. *Radiology* 221:689–696, 2001.

393. Drescher P, McGuckin J, Rilling WS, Crain MR: Catheter-directed thrombolytic therapy in peripheral artery occlusions: Combining reteplase and abciximab. *AJR Am J Roentgenol* 180:1385–1391, 2003.

394. Cohen LH, Kaplan M, Bernhard VM: Intraoperative streptokinase. An adjunct to mechanical thrombectomy in the management of acute ischemia. *Arch Surg* 121:708–715, 1986.

395. Comerota AJ, White JV, Grosh JD: Intraoperative intra-arterial thrombolytic therapy for salvage of limbs in patients with distal arterial thrombosis. *Surg Gynecol Obstet* 169:283–289, 1989.

396. Parent FN, Bernhard VM, Pabst TS, et al: Fibrinolytic treatment of residual thrombus after catheter embolectomy for severe lower limb ischemia. *J Vasc Surg* 9:153–160, 1989.

397. Quinones-Baldrich WJ, Zierler RE, Hiatt JC: Intraoperative fibrinolytic therapy: An adjunct to catheter thromboembolectomy. *J Vasc Surg* 2:319–326, 1985.

398. Vedantham S, Vesely TM, Parti N, et al: Lower extremity venous thrombolysis with adjunctive mechanical thrombectomy. *J Vasc Interv Radiol* 13:1001–1008, 2002.

399. Berridge DC, Kessel D, Robertson I: Surgery versus thrombolysis for acute limb ischaemia: Initial management. *Cochrane Database Syst Rev* 3:CD002784, 2002.

400. Kessel D, Berridge D, Robertson I: Infusion techniques for peripheral arterial thrombolysis. *Cochrane Database Syst Rev* 1:CD000985, 2004.

401. Thrombolysis in the management of lower limb peripheral arterial occlusion—A consensus document. Working Party on Thrombolysis in the Management of Limb Ischemia. *Am J Cardiol* 81:207–218, 1998.

402. Hirsch AT, Haskal ZJ, Hertzer NR, et al: ACC/AHA 2005 practice guidelines for the management of patients with peripheral arterial disease (lower extremity, renal, mesenteric, and abdominal aortic): A collaborative report. *Circulation* 113:e463–e654, 2006.

403. Alonso-Coello P, Bellmunt S, McGorrian C, et al: Antithrombotic therapy in peripheral artery disease: Antithrombotic Therapy and Prevention of Thrombosis, 9th ed: American College of Chest Physicians Evidence-Based Clinical Practice Guidelines. *Chest* 141:e669S–e690S, 2012.

404. Menon KV, Shah V, Kamath PS: The Budd-Chiari syndrome. *N Engl J Med* 350(6):578–585, 2004.

405. Aytekin C, Boyvat F, Kurt A, et al: Catheter-directed thrombolysis with transjugular access in portal vein thrombosis secondary to pancreatitis. *Eur J Radiol* 39:80–82, 2001.

406. Ciccarelli O, Goffette P, Laterre PF, et al: Transjugular intrahepatic portosystemic shunt approach and local thrombolysis for treatment of early posttransplant portal vein thrombosis. *Transplantation* 72:159–161, 2001.

407. Tateishi A, Mitsui H, Oki T, et al: Extensive mesenteric vein and portal vein thrombosis successfully treated by thrombolysis and anticoagulation. *J Gastroenterol Hepatol* 16:1429–1433, 2001.

408. Calin GA, Calin S, Ionescu R, et al: Successful local fibrinolytic treatment and balloon angioplasty in superior mesenteric arterial embolism: A case report and literature review. *Hepatogastroenterology* 50:732–734, 2003.

409. Savassi-Rocha PR, Veloso LF: Treatment of superior mesenteric artery embolism with a fibrinolytic agent: Case report and literature review. *Hepatogastroenterology* 49:1307–1310, 2002.

410. Haire WD, Atkinson JB, Stephens LC, Kotulak GD: Urokinase versus recombinant tissue plasminogen activator in thrombosed central venous catheters: A double-blinded, randomized trial. *Thromb Haemost* 72:543–547, 1994.

411. Semba CP, Deitcher SR, Li X, et al: Treatment of occluded central venous catheters with alteplase: Results in 1,064 patients. *J Vasc Interv Radiol* 13:1199–1205, 2002.

412. Shen V, Li X, Murdock M, et al: Recombinant tissue plasminogen activator (alteplase) for restoration of function to occluded central venous catheters in pediatric patients. *J Pediatr Hematol Oncol* 25:38–45, 2003.

413. Timoney JP, Malkin MG, Leone DM, et al: Safe and cost effective use of alteplase for the clearance of occluded central venous access devices. *J Clin Oncol* 20:1918–1922, 2002.

414. Cooper SG: Original report. Pulse-spray thrombolysis of thrombosed hemodialysis grafts with tissue plasminogen activator. *AJR Am J Roentgenol* 180:1063–1066, 2003.

415. Cynamon J, Pierpont CE: Thrombolysis for the treatment of thrombosed hemodialysis access grafts. *Rev Cardiovasc Med* 3(Suppl 2):84–91, 2002.

416. Daeihagh P, Jordan J, Chen J, Rocco M: Efficacy of tissue plasminogen activator administration on patency of hemodialysis access catheters. *Am J Kidney Dis* 36:75–79, 2000.

417. Hilleman DE, Dunlay RW, Packard KA: Reteplase for dysfunctional hemodialysis catheter clearance. *Pharmacotherapy* 23:137–141, 2003.

418. Shrivastava D, Lundin AP, Dosunmu B, et al: Salvage of clotted jugular vein hemodialysis catheters. *Nephron* 68:77–79, 1994.

419. Sobel BE: Intracranial bleeding, fibrinolysis, and anticoagulation. Causal connections and clinical implications. *Circulation* 90:2147–2152, 1994.

420. Sane DC, Califf RM, Topol EJ, et al: Bleeding during thrombolytic therapy for acute myocardial infarction: Mechanisms and management. *Ann Intern Med* 111:1010–1022, 1989.

421. Alkjaersig N, Fletcher AP, Sherry S: Xi-aminocaproic acid: An inhibitor of plasminogen activation. *J Biol Chem* 234:832–837, 1959.

422. Andersson L, Nilsson IM, Nilehn JE, et al: Experimental and clinical studies on AMCA, the antifibrinolytically active isomer of p-aminomethyl cyclohexane carboxylic acid. *Scand J Haematol* 2:230–247, 1965.

423. Brockway WJ, Castellino FJ: The mechanism of the inhibition of plasmin by xi-aminocaproic acid. *J Biol Chem* :246:4641–4647, 1971.

424. McNicol GP, Fletcher AP, Alkjaersig N, et al: The absorption, distribution and excretion of xi-aminocaproic acid following oral or intravenous administration to man. *J Lab Clin Med* 59:15, 1962.

425. Huber R, Kukla D, Ruhlmann A, Steigemann W: Pancreatic trypsin inhibitor (Kunitz). I. Structure and function. *Cold Spring Harb Symp Quant Biol* 36:141–148, 1972.

426. Ruhlmann A, Kukla D, Schwager P, et al: Structure of the complex formed by bovine trypsin and bovine pancreatic trypsin inhibitor. Crystal structure determination and stereochemistry of the contact region. *J Mol Biol* 77:417–436, 1973.

427. Wiman B: On the reaction of plasmin or plasmin-streptokinase complex with aprotinin or alpha 2-antiplasmin. *Thromb Res* 17:143–152, 1980.

428. Mangano DT, Tudor IC, Dietzel C: The risk associated with aprotinin in cardiac surgery. *N Engl J Med* 354:353–365, 2006.

429. Mouton R, Finch D, Davis I, Zacharowski K: Effect of aprotinin on renal dysfunction. *Lancet* 372:1543–1544, 2008.

430. Schneeweiss S, Seeger JD, Landon J, Walker AM: Aprotinin during coronary-artery bypass grafting and risk of death. *N Engl J Med* 358:771–783, 2008.

431. Shaw AD, Stafford-Smith M, White WD, et al: The effect of aprotinin on outcome after coronary-artery bypass grafting. *N Engl J Med* 358:784–793, 2008.

432. Fergusson DA, Hebert PC, Mazer CD, et al: A comparison of aprotinin and lysine analogues in high-risk cardiac surgery. *N Engl J Med* 358:2319–2331, 2008.

433. Aoki N, Moro M, Matsuda M, Tachiya K: The behavior of alpha-2 plasmin inhibitor in fibrinolytic states. *J Clin Invest* 60:361–369, 1977.

434. Aoki N, Sakata Y, Matsuda M, Tateno K: Fibrinolytic states in a patient with congenital deficiency of alpha 1-plasmin inhibitor. *Blood* 55:483–488, 1980.

435. Dieval J, Nguyen G, Gross S, et al: A lifelong bleeding disorder associated with a deficiency of plasminogen activator inhibitor type 1. *Blood* 77(3):528–532, 1991.

436. Lee MH, Vosburgh E, Anderson K, McDonagh J: Deficiency of plasma plasminogen activator inhibitor 1 results in hyperfibrinolytic bleeding. *Blood* 81:2357–2362, 1993.

437. Avvisati G, Ten Cate JW, Sturke A, et al: Acquired alpha-2-antiplasmin deficiency in acute promyelocytic leukemia. *Br J Haematol* 70:43–48, 1988.

438. Avvisati G, Ten Cate JW, Buller HR, Mandelli F: Tranexamic acid for control of haemorrhage in acute promyelocytic leukemia. *Lancet* 2:122–124, 1989.

439. Rodeghiero F, Avvisati G, Castaman G, et al: Early deaths and anti-hemorrhagic treatments in acute promyelocytic leukemia. A GIMEMA retrospective study in 268 consecutive patients. *Blood* 75:2112–2117, 1990.

440. Schwartz BS, Williams EC, Conlan MG, Mosher DF: Epsilon-aminocaproic acid in the treatment of patients with acute promyelocytic leukemia and acquired alpha-2-plasmin inhibitor deficiency. *Ann Intern Med* 105:873–877, 1986.

441. Booth NA, Anderson JA, Bennett B: Plasminogen activators in alcoholic cirrhosis: Demonstration of increased tissue type and urokinase type activator. *J Clin Pathol* 37:772–777, 1984.

442. Hayashi T, Kamogawa A, Ro S, et al: Plasma from patients with cirrhosis increases tissue plasminogen activator release from vascular endothelial cells *in vitro. Liver* 18:186–190, 1998.

443. Violi F, Basili V, Ferro D: Association between high values of D-dimer and tissue-plasminogen activator activity and first gastrointestinal bleeding in cirrhotic patients. *Thromb Haemost* 76:177, 1996.

444. Boylan JF, Klinck JR, Sandler AN, et al: Tranexamic acid reduces blood loss, transfusion requirements, and coagulation factor use in primary orthotopic liver transplantation. *Anesthesiology* 85:1043–1048, 1996.

445. Kaspar M, Ramsay MA, Nguyen AT, et al: Continuous small-dose tranexamic acid reduces fibrinolysis but not transfusion requirements during orthotopic liver transplantation. *Anesth Analg* 85:281–285, 1997.

446. Segal HC, Hunt BJ, Cottam S, et al: Fibrinolytic activity during orthotopic liver transplantation with and without aprotinin. *Transplantation* 58:1356–1360, 1994.

447. Soilleux H, Gillon MC, Mirand A, et al: Comparative effects of small and large aprotinin doses on bleeding during orthotopic liver transplantation. *Anesth Analg* 80:349–352, 1995.

448. Al-Mondhiry H, Manni A, Owen J, Gordon R: Hemostatic effects of hormonal stimulation in patients with metastatic prostate cancer. *Am J Hematol* 28:141–145, 1988.

449. Bennett B, Croll AM, Robbie LA, Herriot R: Tumour cell u-PA as a cause of fibrinolytic bleeding in metastatic disease. *Br J Haematol* 99:570–574, 1997.

450. Mannucci PM, Cugno M, Bottasso B, et al: Changes in fibrinolysis in patients with localized tumors. *Eur J Cancer* 26:83–87, 1990.

451. Meijer K, Smid WM, Geerards S, van der Meer J: Hyperfibrinogenolysis in disseminated adenocarcinoma. *Blood Coagul Fibrinolysis* 9:279–283, 1998.

452. Webber MM, Waghray A: Urokinase-mediated extracellular matrix degradation by human prostatic carcinoma cells and its inhibition by retinoic acid. *Clin Cancer Res* 1:755–761, 1995.

453. Zacharski LR, Memoli VA, Ornstein DL, et al: Tumor cell procoagulant and urokinase expression in carcinoma of the ovary. *J Natl Cancer Inst* 85:1225–1230, 1993.

454. Bouchama A, Bridey F, Hammami MM, et al: Activation of coagulation and fibrinolysis in heatstroke. *Thromb Haemost* 76:909–915, 1996.

455. Harker LA: Bleeding after cardiopulmonary bypass. *N Engl J Med* 314:1446–1448, 1986.

456. Williams GD, Bratton SL, Nielsen NJ, Ramamoorthy C: Fibrinolysis in pediatric patients undergoing cardiopulmonary bypass. *J Cardiothorac Vasc Anesth* 12:633–638, 1998.

457. Horrow JC, Hlavacek J, Strong MD, et al: Prophylactic tranexamic acid decreases bleeding after cardiac operations. *J Thorac Cardiovasc Surg* 99:70–74, 1990.

458. Horrow JC, Van Riper DF, Strong MD, et al: Hemostatic effects of tranexamic acid and desmopressin during cardiac surgery. *Circulation* 84:2063–2070, 1991.

459. Munoz JJ, Birkmeyer NJ, Birkmeyer JD, et al: Is epsilon-aminocaproic acid as effective as aprotinin in reducing bleeding with cardiac surgery? A meta-analysis. *Circulation* 99:81–89, 1999.

460. Soslau G, Horrow J, Brodsky I: Effect of tranexamic acid on platelet ADP during extracorporeal circulation. *Am J Hematol* 38:113–119, 1991.

461. Blomback M, Johansson G, Johnson H, et al: Surgery in patients with von Willebrand's disease. *Br J Surg* 76:398–400, 1989.

462. Hedlund PO: Antifibrinolytic therapy with Cyklokapron in connection with prostatectomy. A double blind study. *Scand J Urol Nephrol* 3:177–182, 1969.

463. Sindet-Pedersen S, Stenbjerg S: Effect of local antifibrinolytic treatment with tranexamic acid in hemophiliacs undergoing oral surgery. *J Oral Maxillofac Surg* 44:703–707, 1986.

464. Callender ST, Warner GT, Cope E: Treatment of menorrhagia with tranexamic acid. A double-blind trial. *Br Med J* 4:214–216, 1970.

465. Ong YL, Hull DR, Mayne EE: Menorrhagia in von Willebrand disease successfully treated with single daily dose tranexamic acid. *Haemophilia* 4:63–65, 1998.

466. Ortel TL, Onorato JJ, Bedrosian CL, Kaufman RE: Antifibrinolytic therapy in the management of the Kasabach Merritt syndrome. *Am J Hematol* 29:44–48, 1988.

467. Stahl RL, Henderson JM, Hooks MA, et al: Therapy of the Kasabach-Merritt syndrome with cryoprecipitate plus intra-arterial thrombin and aminocaproic acid. *Am J Hematol* 36:272–274, 1991.

# INDEX

Page numbers in **bold** indicate a major discussion of the topic. Page numbers followed by *f* and *t* indicate the location of figures and tables, respectively.